Edited by

RAFAEL ANDRADE, M.D., F.A.A.D., F.A.C.P.

Professor and Chairman, Department of Dermatology, LaSalle Medical School,
La Salle University of Mexico; Consultant in Dermatology, and Chief, Section
of Dermatopathology, Departments of Dermatology and Pathology, General
Hospital of Mexico City. Formerly Associate Professor of Dermatology,
New York University School of Medicine, and Director, Laboratory of Skin Pathology,
Skin and Cancer Unit, New York University Medical Center.

STEPHEN L. GUMPORT, M.D., F.A.C.S.

Professor of Clinical Surgery, New York University School of Medicine; Co-Director
of the Tumor Service, Department of Surgery, New York University Medical Center;
Visiting Surgeon, Bellevue Hospital; Consultant, Manhattan Veterans Administration
Hospital; Attending Surgeon, University Hospital, New York.

GEORGE L. POPKIN, M.D.

Professor of Clinical Dermatology, New York University School of Medicine;
Attending in Dermatology, University Hospital, New York.

THOMAS D. REES, M.D., F.A.C.S.

Clinical Associate Professor of Surgery (Plastic Surgery), Institute of
Reconstructive Plastic Surgery, New York University School of Medicine;
Attending Surgeon, University Hospital and Doctors Hospital; Visiting
Surgeon, Bellevue Hospital; Consultant, U.S. Naval Hospital, St. Albans;
Surgeon Director, Manhattan Eye, Ear and Throat Hospital, New York.

Volume One

CANCER
of the
SKIN

Biology-Diagnosis-Management

1976

W. B. SAUNDERS COMPANY

Philadelphia • London • Toronto

W. B. Saunders Company: West Washington Square
Philadelphia, PA   19105

1 St. Anne's Road
Eastbourne, East Sussex BN21 3UN, England

833 Oxford Street
Toronto, Ontario M8Z 5T9, Canada

Library of Congress Cataloging in Publication Data

Main entry under title:

Cancer of the skin.

Includes index.

CONTENTS: v. 1. Biology-diagnosis-management.

1. Skin—Cancer.   I. Andrade, Rafael. [DNLM: 1. Skin
   neoplasms. WR500 C215]

RC280.S5C36   616.9′94′77   73–91274

ISBN 0–7216–1245–8 (v. 1)

Cancer of the Skin

ISBN Vol 1: 0-7216-1245-8
ISBN Vol 2: 0-7216-1246-6

Print No.:   9   8   7   6   5   4   3   2   1

Contributors

A. BERNARD ACKERMAN, M.D.

Associate Professor of Dermatology and Pathology, New York University School of Medicine, New York.

ROY E. ALBERT, M.D.

Professor of Environmental Medicine, New York University School of Medicine; Associate Attending Physician, Department of Medicine, New York University Medical Center, New York.

JORGE ALBORES-SAAVEDRA, M.D.

Professor of Pathology and Chairman of the Pathology Unit, National University of Mexico School of Medicine at the General Hospital of Mexico City.

DAVID E. ANDERSON, Ph.D.

Professor of Biology, Section of Medical Genetics, The University of Texas System Cancer Center, M.D. Anderson Hospital and Tumor Institute, Houston.

RAFAEL ANDRADE, M.D.

Professor and Chairman, Department of Dermatology, LaSalle Medical School, LaSalle University of Mexico; Consultant in Dermatology, and Chief, Section of Dermatopathology, Departments of Dermatology and Pathology, General Hospital of Mexico City.

A. BASTOS ARAÚJO, M.D.

Assistant Professor of Dermatology, University Hospital, Coimbra, Portugal.

ROBERT AUERBACH, M.D.

Assistant Professor of Dermatology, New York University School of Medicine; Attending Physician, University Hospital and Bellevue Hospital, New York.

A. POIARES BAPTISTA, M.D.

Professor of Dermatology, University Hospital, Coimbra, Portugal.

ROBERT S. BART, M.D.

Associate Professor of Dermatology, New York University School of Medicine and Post-Graduate Medical School; Associate Attending Dermatologist, University Hospital; Assistant Visiting Dermatologist, Bellevue Hospital, New York.

ROBERT W. BEASLEY, M.D.

Professor of Surgery (Plastic Surgery), New York University School of Medicine, New York.

E. MARK BECKMAN, M.D.

Associate Professor of Obstetrics and Gynecology, New York University School of Medicine; Assistant Attending Physician, University Hospital; Associate Attending Physician, Bellevue Hospital, New York.

BRADLEY BIGELOW, M.D.

Associate Professor of Pathology, New York University School of Medicine; Associate Attending Pathologist, Bellevue Hospital; Associate Attending Pathologist, University Hospital, New York.

SAMUEL M. BLUEFARB, M.D.

Professor and Chairman, Department of Dermatology, Northwestern University Medical School; Senior Attending Physician, Northwestern Memorial Hospital, Chicago.

EARLE W. BRAUER, M.D.

Associate Professor of Clinical Dermatology, New York University School of Medicine; Associate Attending Dermatologist, University Hospital, New York.

MARTIN H. BROWNSTEIN, M.D.

Clinical Associate Professor of Dermatology and Clinical Assistant Professor of Pathology, New York Medical College–Metropolitan Hospital Center, New York.

WILLIAM A. CARO, M.D.

Clinical Associate Professor, Northwestern University Medical School; Associate Attending Physician, Northwestern University Hospital, Chicago.

PHILLIP R. CASSON, M.D.

Associate Professor of Surgery (Plastic Surgery), New York University School of Medicine; Associate Attending Surgeon, University Hospital, and Manhattan Eye, Ear, and Throat Hospital, New York.

JEAN CIVATTE, M.D.

Professor of Dermatology, University of Paris; Saint-Louis Hospital, Paris, France.

RICHARD J. COBURN, D.M.D., M.D.

Clinical Associate in Surgery, Mount Sinai School of Medicine; Attending Surgeon, Doctors Hospital; Assistant Surgeon, Columbus Hospital, New York.

JOHN MARQUIS CONVERSE, M.D.

Lawrence D. Bell Professor of Plastic Surgery, New York University School of Medicine; Director, Institute of Reconstructive Plastic Surgery, New York University Medical Center; Director, Plastic Surgery Service, Bellevue Hospital; Chairman, Department of Plastic Surgery, Manhattan Eye, Ear, and Throat Hospital; Director, Plastic Surgery Service, New York Veterans Administration Hospital, New York.

RODY P. COX, M.D.

Professor of Medicine and Pharmacology, New York University Medical Center; Director, Division of Human Genetics, and Attending Physician, Bellevue Hospital and University Hospital, New York.

HELEN OLLENDORFF CURTH, M.D.

Assistant Clinical Professor of Dermatology (retired), College of Physicians and Surgeons; Lecturer in Dermatology and Attending Dermatologist, Presbyterian Hospital, New York.

JOHN F. DALY, M.D.

Professor and Chairman, Department of Otolaryngology, New York University School of Medicine; Director of Otolaryngology, New York University Medical Center, New York.

CHARLES P. DeFEO, Jr., M.D.

Associate Clinical Professor of Dermatology, New York University School of Medicine.

BERNARD DUPERRAT, M.D.

Professor of Dermatology, Saint-Louis Hospital, Paris, France.

GABRIELLE NOURY-DUPERRAT, M.D.

Associate Pathologist, Saint-Louis Hospital, Paris, France.

ANTHONY T. FARINA, M.D.

Assistant Professor of Radiology, New York University School of Medicine; Attending Radiotherapist, Bellevue Hospital, New York.

ALAN H. FRIEDMAN, M.D.

Associate Professor of Ophthalmology and Associate Professor of Pathology, Albert Einstein College of Medicine; Associate Attending Ophthalmologist and Associate Attending Pathologist, Montefiore Hospital and Medical Center; Director of Ophthalmic Pathology, Albert Einstein College of Medicine/Montefiore Hospital, New York.

ALVIN E. FRIEDMAN-KIEN, M.D.

Associate Professor of Dermatology and Microbiology, New York University Medical Center; Attending Physician, University Hospital and Bellevue Hospital; Chief of Dermatology, Goldwater Memorial Hospital, New York.

PAULINO L. GETZROW, M.D.

Assistant Clinical Professor of Medicine (Dermatology Section), and of Pathology, Albert Einstein College of Medicine of Yeshiva University, New York.

ARTHUR H. GLADSTEIN, M.D.

Professor of Clinical Dermatology, New York University School of Medicine; Attending Dermatologist, Bellevue Hospital, New York.

LEON GOLDMAN, M.D.

Professor and Chairman, Department of Dermatology, and Director, Laser Laboratory, University of Cincinnati Medical Center; Director of Dermatology, Cincinnati General Children's Hospital, Cincinnati.

FREDERICK M. GOLOMB, M.D.

Associate Professor of Clinical Surgery, New York University School of Medicine.

DOUGLAS GORDON, M.B., B.S.

Professor and Head, Department of Social and Preventive Medicine, University of Queensland; Deputy-Chairman, Royal Brisbane Hospital, Brisbane, Australia.

HANS GÖTZ, M.D.

Professor of Dermatology and Director of the Dermatologische Klinik und Poliklinik der Universität Essen, Germany.

W. ROBSON N. GRIER, M.D.

Associate Professor of Clinical Surgery, New York University School of Medicine; Attending Surgeon, University Hospital; Visiting Surgeon, Bellevue Hospital; Director of Surgery, Goldwater Memorial Hospital, New York.

STEPHEN L. GUMPORT, M.D., F.A.C.S.

Professor of Clinical Surgery, New York University School of Medicine; Co-Director of the Tumor Service, Department of Surgery, New York University Medical Center.

MATTHEW N. HARRIS, M.D.

Professor of Clinical Surgery, New York University School of Medicine; Attending Surgeon, University Hospital; Visiting Surgeon, Bellevue Hospital; Attending Surgeon, Manhattan Veterans Administration Hospital, New York.

PAUL HENKIND, M.D., Ph.D.

Professor and Chairman, Department of Ophthalmology, Albert Einstein College of Medicine/Montefiore Hospital and Medical Center; Attending Ophthalmologist, Montefiore Hospital and Medical Center; Attending Ophthalmologist, Bronx Municipal Hospital Center, New York.

OTTO P. HORNSTEIN, M.D.

Professor, University of Erlangen, Nürnberg; Department of Dermatology, University Hospital, Erlangen, Germany.

ROBERT S. HOTCHKISS, M.D.

Professor Emeritus of Urology, New York University School of Medicine; Attending Urologist, University Hospital and Bellevue Hospital, New York.

J. B. HOWELL, M.D.

Clinical Professor of Dermatology, University of Texas Health Science Center at Dallas, Southwestern Medical School; Attending Dermatologist, Baylor University Hospital and Parkland Memorial Hospital, Dallas.

YASUMASA ISHIBASHI, M.D.

Associate Professor of Dermatology, University of Tokyo, Japan.

ARLETTE JACOB, M.D.

Centre de Recherches sur la Cellule Normale et Cancéreuse du Centre National de la Recherche Scientifique, Paris, France.

LAWRENCE M. JOSEPH, M.D.

Dermatology Attending Staff, Baylor College of Medicine; Acting Staff, Pasadena Bayshore Hospital, Pasadena, and Clear Lake Hospital, Webster, Texas.

†ISAAC KATZENELLENBOGEN, M.D.

Professor and Chairman, Department of Dermatology, Tel-Aviv University Medical School; Head, Department of Dermatology, Beilinson Medical Center, Petah-Tiqvah, Israel.

HOWARD J. KESSELER, M.D.

Associate Professor of Clinical Surgery, New York University School of Medicine; Attending Surgeon, University Hospital; Attending Surgeon, Lenox Hill Hospital, New York.

---

†Deceased.

A. KINT, M.D.

Professor of Dermatology, State University of Ghent; Clinic for Dermatology, Akademisch Ziekenhuis, Ghent, Belgium.

EDMUND KLEIN, M.D.

Chief, Department of Dermatology, Roswell Park Memorial Institute; Research Professor of Dermatology, State University of New York at Buffalo, School of Medicine, Buffalo.

GEORG KLINGMÜLLER, M.D.

University of Bonn; Skin Hospital, Bonn-Venusberg, Germany.

JOHN M. KNOX, M.D.

Professor and Chairman, Department of Dermatology and Syphilology, Baylor College of Medicine; Chief of Dermatology, Ben Taub General Hospital and Texas Children's Hospital, Houston, Texas.

ALFRED W. KOPF, M:D.

Professor of Dermatology, New York University School of Medicine; Attending Dermatologist, University Hospital; Attending Dermatologist and Syphilologist, Bellevue Hospital; Head of Oncology Section, Skin and Cancer Unit, New York University Medical Center, New York.

LEOPOLD G. KOSS, M.D.

Professor and Chairman, Department of Pathology, Albert Einstein College of Medicine/Montefiore Hospital and Medical Center; Chairman, Department of Pathology, Montefiore Hospital and Medical Center, New York.

ADOLF KÚTA, M.D.

Associate Professor, Hautklinik der Städtischen, Kliniken Darmstadt, Darmstadt-Eberstadt, Germany.

ERICH LANDES, M.D.

Professor der Joh. Wolfgang-Goethe-Universität, Frankfurt; Direktor der Hautklinik der Städtischen, Kliniken Darmstadt, Darmstadt-Eberstadt, Germany.

RAFFAELE LATTES, M.D.

Professor of Surgical Pathology, Columbia University College of Physicians and Surgeons; Director of Surgical Pathology Division, New York Presbyterian Hospital, New York.

ELIANE LE BRETON, M.D.

Professor and Honorary Director of the Centre de Recherches sur la Cellule Normale et Cancéreuse du Centre National de la Recherche Scientifique, Paris, France.

DONALD D. LEONARD, M.D.

Visiting Lecturer in Pathology and Assistant Clinical Professor of Dermatology, University of North Carolina, Chapel Hill; Pathologist, Moses H. Cone Memorial Hospital, Greensboro, North Carolina.

HERBERT Z. LUND, M.D.

Visiting Professor of Pathology and Clinical Professor of Dermatology, University of North Carolina, Chapel Hill; Pathologist, Moses H. Cone Memorial Hospital, Greensboro, North Carolina.

JOSEPH G. McCARTHY, M.D.

Assistant Professor of Surgery (Plastic Surgery), New York University School of Medicine; Attending Physician in Plastic Surgery, University Hospital, Bellevue Hospital, Veterans Administration Hospital, and Manhattan Eye, Ear, and Throat Hospital, New York.

JOSÉ M. MASCARÓ, M.D.

Professor and Chairman of Department of Dermatology, University of Valencia, Spain.

AMIR H. MEHREGAN, M.D.

Clinical Professor of Dermatology, Wayne State University School of Medicine; Senior Associate Staff, Detroit General Hospital, Detroit.

NICOLAS MELCZER, M.D., D.Sci.

Professor and Director, Department of Dermatology and Venereology, University Pécs, Hungary.

LEONARD P. MERKOW, M.D., Ph.D.

Head, Division of Experimental Pathology and Electron Microscopy, William H. Singer Research Institute; Senior Attending Pathologist, Allegheny General Hospital, Pittsburgh.

BURKHARD METZ, M.D.

Hautklinik der Stätischen Kliniken Darmstadt, Darmstadt-Eberstadt, Germany.

GEORGE E. MOORE, M.D., Ph.D.

Professor of Surgery, University of Colorado Medical Center; Director of Surgical Oncology, Department of Surgery, Denver General Hospital, Denver.

ARCELIA MORA-TISCAREÑO, M.D.

Assistant Pathologist, Pathology Unit, National University of Mexico School of Medicine at the General Hospital of Mexico City.

JOSEPH NEWALL, M.D.

Professor of Radiology, New York University School of Medicine; Attending Radiotherapist, University Hospital and Bellevue Hospital, New York.

HERBERT E. NIEBURGS, M.D.

Associate Professor of Pathology, Mount Sinai School of Medicine; Director of Laboratory of Cell Pathology, Mount Sinai Hospital, New York.

H. OBERSTE-LEHN, M.D.

Professor and Director, Hautklinik, Städtische Ferdinand-Sauerbruch-Krankenanstalten, Wuppertal-Elberfeld, Germany.

RUBEN OROPEZA, M.D.

Assistant Professor of Surgery, New York University School of Medicine; Attending General Surgeon, New York Infirmary; Attending Surgeon and Chairman of Tumor Service, Cabrini Health Center; Attending Surgeon, Doctors Hospital, New York.

LILLY PFLEGER, M.D.

Associate Professor, University Clinic of Skin Diseases (I), Vienna, Austria.

HERMANN PINKUS, M.D.

Professor of Dermatology, Wayne State University School of Medicine; Senior Attending Dermatologist, Detroit General Hospital, Detroit.

JOAQUÍN PIÑOL AGUADÉ, M.D., Ph.D.

Professor and Head, Professional School of Dermatology and Venereology, Faculty of Medicine, University of Barcelona; Head, Department of Dermatology and Venereology, Hospital Clínico y Provincial, Barcelona, Spain.

GEORGE L. POPKIN, M.D.

Professor of Clinical Dermatology, New York University School of Medicine; Attending Dermatologist, University Hospital, New York.

SIRIA POUCELL, M.D.

Assistant Pathologist, Pathology Unit, National University of Mexico School of Medicine at the General Hospital of Mexico City.

FELIX T. RAPAPORT, M.D.

Professor of Surgery, New York University School of Medicine; Visiting Surgeon, Bellevue Hospital; Attending Surgeon, University Hospital, New York.

THOMAS D. REES, M.D.

Clinical Associate Professor of Surgery (Plastic Surgery), Institute of Reconstructive Plastic Surgery, New York University School of Medicine; Attending Surgeon, University Hospital and Doctors Hospital.

BRUNO von B. RISTOW

Chief, Plastic and Reconstructive Surgery, Presbyterian Hospital–Pacific Medical Center; Attending Surgeon, Childrens Hospital, San Francisco.

GUY F. ROBBINS, M.D.

Associate Clinical Professor of Surgery, Cornell University Medical School; Attending Surgeon, Breast Service, Memorial Hospital for Cancer and Allied Diseases, New York.

PERRY ROBINS, M.D.

Associate Professor of Clinical Dermatology, New York University School of Medicine; Attending Physician at University Hospital, Bellevue Hospital, and Manhattan Veterans Administration Hospital, New York.

HECTOR A. RODRÍGUEZ-MARTINEZ, M.D.

Professor of Pathology and Chief, Surgical Pathology Department, Pathology Unit, National University of Mexico School of Medicine at the General Hospital of Mexico City.

HAROLD H. SAGE, M.D.

Associate Professor of Surgery, New York University School of Medicine; Attending Surgeon, Bellevue Hospital, New York.

HERNANDO SALAZAR, M.D., M.P.H.

Associate Professor of Pathology, University of Pittsburgh; Pathologist, Magee-Women's Hospital, Pittsburgh.

MIRIAM SANDBANK, M.D.

Senior Lecturer in Dermatology, Tel-Aviv University Medical School; Deputy Chief, Department of Dermatology, Beilinson Medical Center, Petah-Tiqvah, Israel.

KENNETH V. SANDERSON, M.B.

Senior Lecturer in Dermatology, St. George's Hospital Medical School; Physician to the Skin Department, St. George's Hospital, London.

CHARLES F. SCHETLIN, M.D.

Assistant Professor of Clinical Surgery, New York University School of Medicine; Attending Surgeon, St. Luke's Hospital, New York.

MARGARETE SCHLÜTER, D.M.D.

Formerly Department of Dermatology, University of Cologne, Germany. Presently in private dental practice.

†RUDOLF SCHULZE, M.D.

Professor of Dermatology, University of Hamburg, Germany.

LEWIS SHAPIRO, M.D.

Clinical Professor of Dermatology and Pathology, College of Physicians and Surgeons, Columbia University, New York.

†HAROLD SILVERSTONE, M.A., Ph.D.

Reader in Medical Statistics, Department of Social and Preventive Medicine, University of Queensland, Brisbane, Australia.

LAWRENCE M. SOLOMON, M.D.

Professor and Head, Department of Dermatology, University of Illinois; Chief, Dermatology Service, University of Illinois Hospital, Chicago.

GERD KLAUS STEIGLEDER, M.D.

Professor and Chairman, Department of Dermatology, University of Cologne, Germany.

MARION B. SULZBERGER, M.D.

Clinical Professor of Dermatology (Emeritus), University of California, San Francisco; Professor Emeritus of Dermatology, New York University School of Medicine, New York.

JOSEF TAPPEINER, M.D.

Professor of Dermatology, University of Vienna; Head, Department of Dermatology (I), Vienna, Austria.

ALEXANDER C. TEMPLETON, M.D.

Pathology Department, St. Vincent Hospital, Worcester, Massachusetts.

DOUGLAS TORRE, M.D.

Clinical Professor of Dermatology, Cornell University Medical College; Attending Physician, The New York Hospital; Attending Dermatologist, Memorial Hospital, New York.

GEORGE TSOÏTIS, M.D.

Lecturer in Dermatology, University of Thessaloniki; Lecturer in Dermatological Histopathology, University of Paris, Saint-Louis Hospital, Paris, France; Director, Laboratory of Dermatological Histopathology, Venereal and Skin Disease Hospital at Thessaloniki, Greece.

CHRISTOPHER VIRTUE, M.D.

Instructor in Dermatology, University of Illinois; Resident, University of Illinois Hospital, Chicago.

---

†Deceased.

KLAUS WOLFF, M.D.

Professor of Dermatology, University of Vienna; Head, Division of Experimental Dermatology, Department of Dermatology (I), Vienna, Austria.

JANE C. WRIGHT, M.D.

Professor of Surgery, New York Medical College; Attending Physician, Flower and Fifth Avenue Hospitals, Metropolitan Hospital Center, and Westchester County Medical Center Hospital, New York.

Foreword

This book is a natural outgrowth of a cooperative effort begun many years ago at the New York University Medical Center, when different specialists with a common interest in cancer of the skin began working together on the challenging problems presented by this spectrum of disorders. The group includes dermatologists, pathologists, surgeons, radiotherapists, and plastic surgeons. Regular meetings are held to discuss cases of mutual interest, and many research projects have evolved from this collective consideration of difficult therapeutic problems. Hence, this book is a tribute to the expanding enthusiasm generated by an interdisciplinary group working together on shared projects.

The book is more than a collection and distillation of the very considerable experience gained by this group over the past two decades or more, however. Significant contributions to present knowledge of the biology of the skin and the pathology of its malignant disorders have been made elsewhere in the world, often where occupational or environmental factors are very different from those in North America. The discussions of pathogenesis and clinical course of the many individual diseases have thus deliberately been made extensive, with a firm effort to enlist as contributors the world's outstanding authorities on their respective subjects. The results of their investigations are now made widely available to the general reader for the first time.

Bringing together in a single work the diverse experience and knowledge of so many specialists is a remarkable achievement in itself. But those who use this book to help them provide more intelligent, more rational care for patients afflicted with these, the most common of all cancers, will be making their own real contribution to medical progress. For any volume such as this can only be a symbol of the state of the science. Readers will agree that progress to date in this complex field has been steady and promising, and the present work is a milestone along the path.

Frank C. Spencer, M.D.

Preface

Modern management of the complicated entity known as cancer is best accomplished by a multidisciplinary approach. For over 25 years such an approach has been the basis of the Oncology Conference conducted by the Skin and Cancer Unit of the New York University Medical Center. These conferences have provided a lucid interchange of ideas among specialists, including dermatologists, pathologists, radiologists, and surgeons, and others interested in cancer of the skin. Representatives of these disciplines share their knowledge and provide stimulating exchanges. All too often specialists are trained along rigid lines and are inclined to believe that the particular modality of treatment offered by their specialty is always the treatment of choice. The give and take provided by an open conference quickly dispels such insular thinking.

The idea for *Cancer of the Skin* was born and carried to fruition through the stimulus of this coordinated interdisciplinary effort. The editors have long been associated with this Oncology Conference and are grateful to their colleagues, who have provided so many enlightening and stimulating discussions through the years.

Early in the planning of this book, it became apparent that the knowledge of experts on the subject of cancer of the skin throughout the world must be sought to provide an up-to-date and meaningful presentation. To the many contributors to this book we owe our deep appreciation and thanks for their untiring efforts. It is our hope that their work will provide a useful reference for those interested in this fascinating subject.

Before embarking on the details of the material in the following chapters, it is important to recognize that an overall philosophy of treatment of cancer of the skin, just as with treatment of cancer elsewhere in the human organism, should be formulated and constantly kept in mind by those who undertake the therapy of these lesions.

RAFAEL ANDRADE
STEPHEN L. GUMPORT
GEORGE L. POPKIN
THOMAS D. REES

Contents

37

38

39

40

41

42

43

44

45

46

47

Introduction

By far the most common form of cancer in man is cancer of the skin. According to recently published statistics from the American Cancer Society, the number of new cases of skin cancer reported annually in the United States population varies between 300,000 and 600,000. In agreement with this are the statistics from the Third National Cancer Survey which indicate an incidence of about 300,000 new cases of cancer of the skin per year, as well as the statistics of the National Center for Health Statistics which indicate a prevalence of about 536,000 malignant skin tumors in the United States. Our experience, based on over 200,000 computerized diagnoses, at the Skin and Cancer Unit of the Department of Dermatology of New York University is that more than 2 per cent of these are skin cancers.

These statistics, however, do not provide a true picture of the extent of skin cancer, since basal cell cancer, the most common form seen on the skin, preferentially affects certain age and ethnic groups. Furthermore, there is a much higher occurrence of basal cell cancer in geographic regions where the population is subjected to particularly intensive and extensive exposure to sunlight.

A much more accurate view of the importance of the problem emerges when essentially precancerous skin lesions—actinic keratoses, in particular—are taken into consideration. This prevalence figure, according to the National Center for Health Statistics, is over 4 million.

The authors, in presenting their multidisciplinary approaches to diagnosis, treatment, and follow-up, have made significant contributions toward recognizing the problem. These are physicians who not only are expert in their own medical and surgical specialties but also have participated for many years in a combined weekly tumor conference serving patients at the Skin and Cancer Unit and as a result have amassed the kind of enormous experience necessary to produce a unique volume such as this.

RUDOLF L. BAER, M.D.

Part

I

General Topics

1

An Approach to Cancer Therapy

Observations on the Treatment of Skin Cancer

Marion B. Sulzberger, M.D.

Skin cancers serve as excellent examples of how studies of skin lesions lead to medical knowledge and techniques which are quite generally useful and, conversely, how diagnostic and therapeutic procedures derived from many disciplines are required for the management of skin lesions.

To illustrate these points I shall draw upon my knowledge of the history, the people, and the workings of the institution with which I was associated for the major part of my medical life.

The New York Skin and Cancer Hospital was established in 1882. It was, therefore, one of the first multidisciplinary hospitals in the United States — and perhaps in the world — devoted to the study, prevention, and treatment of cancer.

The rather unusual emphasis upon skin tumors, in a hospital devoted to the management of all cancer, could not fail to produce great benefits, perhaps unexpected by the founders. For skin cancers are so numerous, so accessible, and so varied (ranging from basal cell epithelioma, which is usually almost entirely benign, to that often most malignant of all human tumors, the malignant melanoma)

that their study has yielded valuable information about almost every type of cancer. Moreover, the approaches required for the optimal management of skin tumors are so diverse (ranging from minor, major, and plastic surgery to radiation therapy, immunotherapy, chemotherapy, and cryosurgery) that many different skills and disciplines must be brought to focus in order to achieve the greatest success.

In addition, many skin diseases are the outer signs of inner tumors; and still other skin lesions (the precanceroses) are the earliest forewarnings of malignancy to follow.

It is also noteworthy that the first known causes of cancer (arsenic, tars, tobacco, radiation and thermal burns, sunlight, and virus) were discovered because they produced visible tumors of the skin or of the accessible mucous membranes. Consequent to these dermatologic observations of clinical cancers of known cause, the first experimentally induced cancers were produced in the skins of laboratory animals by deliberate exposure to chemical, physical, and infective carcinogens. This provided the tools and opportunities for modern laboratory research into carcinogenesis

3

and cancer therapy in general. Observations of the responses of both clinical and experimental skin tumors have led to new and more effective forms of treatment of all cancers; for example, through radiation, immunotherapy, cryo- and chemo-surgery.

I have mentioned but a few of the ways in which the combined endeavors to treat skin and general cancer in one institution inevitably improve the understanding and management of skin cancers and of cancers elsewhere. For in such an institution every up-to-date preventive, diagnostic, and therapeutic approach known to medicine and surgery must be available; and a smooth collaboration between dermatologists, surgeons, radiologists, pathologists, and other specialists becomes imperative.

This kind of smooth collaboration was guaranteed by the composition and quality of the staff of the New York Skin and Cancer Unit, from its beginning through today. Its earlier staffs included dermatologists such as Bulkley, George Henry Fox, Pollitzer, MacKee, Wise, and Rosen; surgeons such as Willy Meyer, Torek, and Herbert Willy Meyer; physicians and pediatricians such as Janeway and Abraham Jacobi; and radiation experts such as MacKee, Cipollaro, and Bucky. These are but a few of the stars in its galaxy. Unfor-

tunately, I have had to omit the names of many dozens of its illustrious physicians of the past and, of course, have made no mention of any of its outstanding specialists of the present.

In the 1880's the many-pronged, simultaneous attack upon cancer was a pioneering approach. But it has now been adopted by practically every modern institution. The present Charles C. Harris Skin and Cancer Unit of New York University Medical Center, directed by Dr. Rudolf L. Baer, is a fine example of this. Its oncology section, established in my time under the direction of Dr. Alfred W. Kopf, is dedicated to the principle of eclecticism — the continued study and selection of better methods for cancer diagnosis and therapy, drawn from every source through the close collaboration of specialists in many fields.

The selected methods which have resulted from this kind of collaboration, not only in their own but also in sister institutions, are set forth in useful, practical terms in this textbook edited by four outstanding members of the staff of the New York University Medical Center's Skin and Cancer Unit: its dermatologist and pathologist; its general and tumor surgeon; its dermatologist and dermatologic surgeon; and its plastic and reconstructive surgeon.

General Principles for the Treatment of Cancer
of the Skin

Stephen L. Gumport, M.D., and Matthew N. Harris, M.D.

There are several general principles to be followed in the treatment of cancer of the skin which must be understood in order to obtain optimal results. Essentially, the principles involved center around just six words — early diagnosis, adequate treatment, careful follow-up. As with all rules these may have to be broken at times, but the physician should know he is doing so and it should be done only for good reasons.

Early diagnosis requires the physician to be constantly alert as to whether even the

most innocuous-appearing lesion could conceivably represent a malignancy. It is easy to recognize an advanced and fungating lesion, but early unpigmented subungual melanoma or early dermatofibrosarcoma protuberans, for example, requires acumen and experience on the part of the observer for the correct diagnosis to be made. It is therefore wise to keep in mind that any cutaneous lesion or nodule that increases in size, bleeds, ulcerates, becomes infected, or changes in color may possibly represent a neoplasm.

Adequate and representative biopsies should be obtained of all suspicious lesions. Even the direction in which the biopsy incision is placed is important. The placement of this incision in an ill-considered direction may make the definitive surgical procedure much more difficult. A detailed chapter on biopsy (Chap. 66) is included in this book.

The clinician and the pathologist should have a very close working relationship so that the clinical information can be shared, and the microscopic slides reviewed together. If the diagnosis is difficult, these slides should be circulated to other pathologists for consultation, and possibly even another biopsy should be performed.

The physician should keep in mind that no potentially disfiguring or disabling procedure should ever be performed without a confirmed tissue diagnosis of malignant disease. It is far better to do too small a procedure for a patient with cancer than too large a procedure for one in whom the process is later diagnosed as benign.

Once the diagnosis of malignancy has been confirmed, the appropriate definitive treatment should be promptly undertaken. Consideration should be given to the particular modality apt to produce the best result for the patient with this particular tumor. Should it be surgery, radiation therapy, chemotherapy, or chemosurgery? Among the factors to be considered in the selection of the treatment are the age and physical condition of the patient, the microscopic appearance of the tumor being treated, the location of the tumor, the presence of nearby important or vital structures, the availability of therapeutic modalities, and the skill and experience of the physicians who will be administering treatment. There are also other factors. It must be kept in mind that radiation therapy when given to very young people may produce serious secondary effects years later. Also, there is a potential hazard in moving large flaps of skin and subcutaneous tissue over surgical defects, since these flaps may conceal recurrences for an unduly long period of time.

It is extremely helpful to have a "tumor board" that meets regularly and frequently to discuss difficult problems and to make suitable recommendations. This board should be composed of the most experienced dermatologists, surgeons, plastic surgeons, radiotherapists, chemotherapists, rehabilitation physicians, and pathologists. At times, members of other specialties may be included.

No discussion of the planned treatment is ever complete without consideration of the disability and deformity which the method may produce and recommendations regarding the best way of overcoming these problems. Reconstruction and rehabilitation are essential to the treatment of patients with cancer.

Once the appropriate therapy has been decided upon, it should be thoroughly discussed with the patient and his family. Their questions in regard to the diagnosis and prognosis should be answered as fully as possible. Their apprehension should be appreciated and every effort made to convey to them the physician's understanding of their feeling and the fact that he is deeply concerned and interested in both the patient and the disease process. A realistic approach is necessary, but this does not preclude an optimistic attitude. Hope should never be taken away. Happily, we have not always been right in our more unfavorable predictions as to the future.

Once the treatment has been selected it should be skillfully and thoroughly performed. Every effort should be made to eliminate the neoplasm with the first procedure. Recurrences are much harder to deal with and reduce chances for success.

After treatment has been completed and the patient rehabilitated, he should be carefully followed over a lifetime, if possible. This lengthy follow-up is desirable not only to make certain there is no reappearance of the original tumor, but also to make sure no other malignancy develops. Patients who have had one major malignancy have an increased incidence of second major malignancies. One should keep in mind that while careful follow-up is important, it should be done in a considerate manner so as not to alarm an already apprehensive patient or to make him unduly dependent on the examiner.

When all is said and done, the qualities expected from a physician treating patients with cancer are exactly the same as those expected from a physician treating any patient with a serious and life-threatening disease. These are good judgment, great interest in the patient and the disease process, willingness to seek experienced help, careful planning of treatment and subsequent care, and, above all, compassion.

Organization and Function of an Oncology Service for Skin Tumors

Alfred W. Kopf, M.D.

The principal objectives of an Oncology Service for Skin Tumors are to accumulate a large amount of factual data about neoplasms of the skin; to improve the care of patients with skin tumors; to further training of physicians on both undergraduate and postgraduate levels in the field of cutaneous oncology; and to develop a basis for scientific investigations in neoplasia. To meet these objectives requires a considerable amount of careful planning. In this chapter an outline of the organization and function of an Oncology Service for Skin Tumors is presented.

AN ONCOLOGY SERVICE

Recording System. A properly designed patient record is essential to gathering meaningful data concerning tumors of the skin. The format in current use in the Oncology Section of the Skin and Cancer Unit of the New York University Medical Center allows for rapid retrieval of data. The pertinent information concerning the patient and the presenting tumor(s) is recorded on a specially prepared oncology chart (Fig. 1–1). This chart has been devised in such a manner that the data can be readily abstracted for coding purposes. This information can be fed onto International Business Machine (IBM) punch cards for tabulation and statistical study (Fig. 1–2). The precise site of each skin tumor recorded is indicated on anatomical charts (Fig. 1–3). The perimeter of each lesion is outlined with a glass marking pencil on a sheet of clear plastic held over the tumor. This outline is then transferred onto millimeter-square, ruled graph paper (Fig. 1–4). In this manner, over 8000 skin neoplasms have been recorded in the Oncology Section of the Skin and Cancer Unit since 1955. Within minutes, information concerning any of the recorded and punched data can be retrieved automatically. A number of clinical investigations have been published by our group based on this recording system (Baer and Kopf, 1963, 1965; Brodkin, Kopf, and Andrade, 1969; Gellin, Kopf, and Garfinkel, 1965; Kopf, 1960; Kopf and Andrade, 1966; Lightstone, Kopf, and Garfinkel, 1965; Silberberg, Kopf, and Baer, 1962; Sulzberger, Witten, and Kopf, 1957).

Following the initial work-up of the patient, the lesion in point is photographed and the patient is then referred to the appropriate section of the Skin and Cancer Unit (Surgery, Radiation Therapy, Cryosurgery, Chemotherapy, or Chemosurgery) or to another department (Surgery, Radiation Therapy, or Plastic and Reconstructive Surgery) for biopsy and treatment. After completion of therapy, the patient is followed at intervals (average: first year, every three months; second year, every four months; third year, every six months; fourth and more years, every 12 to 24 months) in the Oncology Section in order to assess the result of the particular treatment rendered. In this way, a single group of physicians can judge the ultimate adequacy of various modalities of therapy.

Tumor Conference. Difficult diagnostic and therapeutic problems are seen weekly by the members of the Combined Skin Tumor Conference. This conference
(Text continued on page 14.)

NEW YORK UNIVERSITY MEDICAL CENTER

UNIVERSITY HOSPITAL
SKIN AND CANCER UNIT

Patient No.

ONCOLOGY SECTION

1-6

---

7   Service: I   II   III   IV   V   Photography No.: _____

Date: _____ Clinic Biopsy No.: _____

Clinic No.: _____

Hospital No.: _____ Hospital Biopsy No.: _____

Name: _____
            Last   First   Middle

Address: _____

            _____ Phone _____

Occupation: _____

Other Means of Contact: _____

            _____ Phone _____

Age: _____

8   Color:
            (1) _____ White
            (2) _____ Negro
            (3) _____ Yellow
            (4) _____ Other

- -

Clinical Diagnosis: (1) _____

                       (2) _____

                       (3) _____

Pathological Diagnosis:
                       (1) _____

                       (2) _____

                       (3) _____

Figure 1-1   Face sheet of Oncology Section chart. The numbers appearing in the boxes on the left refer to the IBM punch card columns. The numbers in parentheses refer to the specific punch made in a column. For example, if the patient is Negro, a number 2 is punched in column 8. The total record has 10 pages and utilizes 63 columns on the punch card (see Fig. 1-2).

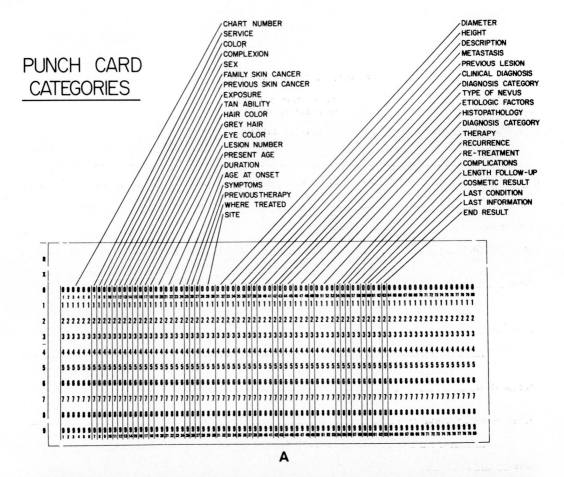

A

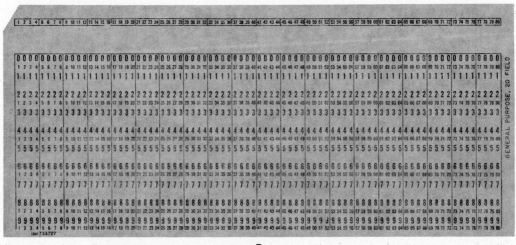

B

Figure 1–2   The punch card. *A*, The various categories of information which are coded are indicated. *B*, Sample unused IBM punch card.

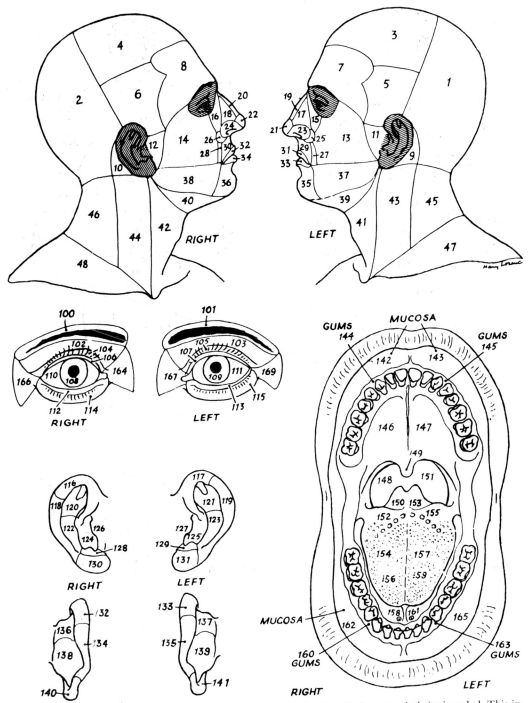

NEW YORK UNIVERSITY MEDICAL CENTER
University Hospital - Skin and Cancer Unit
ONCOLOGY SECTION

Figure 1–3 A set of anatomical charts used in the Oncology Section. Each anatomical site is coded. This information is entered onto the abstract form (Fig. 1–5) and, from this, punched into columns 28, 29, and 30 of the punch card. Thus, if one is interested in reviewing all tumors seen in the left little fingernail bed one merely sets the sorter for 335 on columns 28, 29, and 30.

(Illustration continued on following pages.)

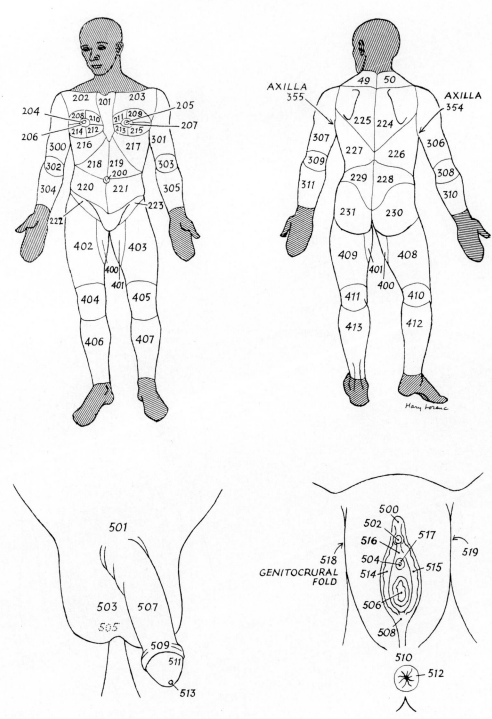

Figure 1–3 *Continued.*

(*Illustration continued on opposite page.*)

NEW YORK UNIVERSITY-BELLEVUE MEDICAL CENTER
University Hospital – Skin and Cancer Unit
ONCOLOGY SECTION

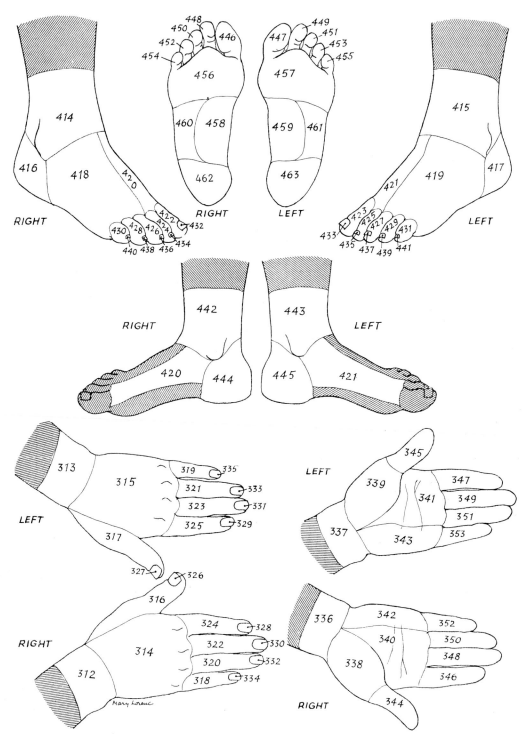

Figure 1–3   *Continued.*

ONCOLOGY SECTION

Midline

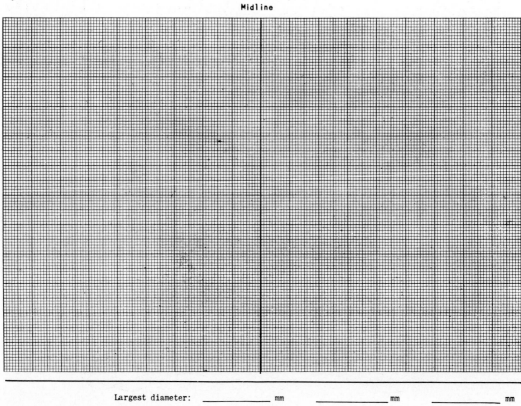

Largest diameter: _____ mm   _____ mm   _____ mm

Height: _____ mm   _____ mm   _____ mm

DESCRIPTION:

ADDITIONAL HISTORY:

Signature: _____

Figure 1–4 Sample of millimeter-ruled paper on which the precise size of the perimeter of the lesion is drawn, as explained in the text.

ONCOLOGY SECTION
DECODING FORM

Patient No.   1-6 ☐☐☐☐☐☐   Puerto Rican   No ☐   Yes ☐

ITEM	COL.			ITEM	COL.		
Service	7			Where treated Prev.	27		
Color	8			Anat. Chart No.	28-30		
Complexion	9			Largest Diam in mm.	31-32		
Sex	10			Height in mm.	33-34		
Fam Hist. Skin Ca.	11			Descrip. of Lesion(1)	35		
Past Hist. Skin Ca.	12			Descrip. of Lesion(2)	36		
Activities Outdoors	13			Met. before visit	37		
Ability to tan	14			How lesion arose	38		
Orig. Color Hair	15			Clinical Diag.	39-41		
Is Hair Graying	16			Malig. or Benign	42		
Color Patient's Eyes	17			Cellular Nevus	43		
No. this lesion	18			Poss. etiol. factors	44		
Pres. Age Patient	19-20			Nature etiol. factors	45		
Dur. Pres. Lesion	21-22			Histopath. Diag.	46-48		
Age Pat. Les. Onset	23-24			Malig. or Benign	49		
Subjective Symptoms	25			Therapy given	50-51		
Previous Therapy	26			Schedule of Therapy	52		

FOLLOW-UP INFORMATION

Was Ther. Comp.	RE-curr?	Ther. to Recur	Com-plica-tions	Time Elapsed		Cosm. Effect	Cond.	Time Last Info.		End Res.
53	54	55	56	57	58	59	60	61	62	63

Figure 1-5   Form used to abstract data from oncology chart. This form is used by the operator to key-punch the IBM cards.

brings together experts from the various branches of medicine including chemosurgery, dermatology, dermatopathology, radiation therapy, reconstructive surgery, and tumor surgery. Often guests from other departments (e.g., ophthalmology, otolaryngology, and neurology) participate. The regular members as well as the guests give their opinions and recommendations about how patients with complex skin tumor problems may be managed best. This mode of consultation is particularly fruitful in improving the care of patients with the more serious skin cancers and those cancers presenting special problems in diagnosis or therapy. The assemblage of an interested group of specialists also serves as a peer review group which enhances the quality of patient care (Sandler, 1970). By means of the Combined Skin Tumor Conference, approximately 350 patients are seen in the Skin and Cancer Unit in this type of special consultation yearly.

Each patient sent to the tumor conference has a special form filled out by the referring source. A typed summary of the opinions and recommendations of the members of the tumor conference, which is dictated during the conference, is sent to the referring physician.

Staff.   It is essential that a dermatologist with a dedicated interest in cutaneous oncology be in charge of such a section. The work must be meticulously accurate and, therefore, requires that a proper amount of time be made available for this purpose. Depending on the patient load, other staff physicians and residents can aid in working-up new patients and in conducting follow-up examinations. All records should be typed. This requires a secretary, preferably one who can take dictation. As the patient load increases, a follow-up secretary may be needed. The data processing can be handled by any computer center, private or university based, at relatively low cost, or, as in our set-up, by a key punch operator who has other administrative functions in the Oncology Section. The abstract form prepared for the keypunch operator is shown in Figure 1–5.

Teaching Opportunities. An Oncology Service dealing with cutaneous neoplasms can serve as an excellent focus for undergraduate, postgraduate, and continuing medical education. Teaching by the faculty is facilitated in the Oncology Section of the Skin and Cancer Unit by the fact that clinical photographs and histologic sections are stored right in the Oncology Section and are freely available for educational purposes. The Combined Skin Tumor Conference is especially of great teaching value since all present, including students and faculty, are exposed to multidisciplinary approaches to given diagnostic and therapeutic problems.

Research Activities. The concentration of patients with skin tumor problems in our Section has great advantages for an organized approach to clinical and basic research. An Oncology Service can provide biologic materials (tumor tissue, blood samples, and so forth) from such patients. The areas of need for research are more clearly identified as those where present approaches generally fail to achieve cures for cutaneous neoplasms. This type of "targeted" research is important if we are to eventually improve the outlook for those lesions which currently present unresolved therapeutic challenges.

Summary   There are many advantages to the establishment of an Oncology Service for Skin Tumors in the departments of dermatology in medical centers. Such a service provides an ideal setting for improved patient care, for the accumulation of factual data about cutaneous neoplasms, for teaching on both undergraduate and postgraduate levels, and for clinical as well as basic research on cutaneous neoplasms. Such a service can serve as the focal point for the organization of a Combined Skin Tumor Conference where the members, representing the various medical specialties concerned with skin cancer, can take the needed multidisciplinary approach to the diagnosis and management of the more difficult cutaneous neoplasms.

REFERENCES

Baer, R. L., and Kopf, A. W.: Keratoacanthoma, leading article, 1962–1963 series. Year Book of Dermatology. Chicago, Year Book Medical Publishers, 1963, pp. 7–41.

Baer, R. L., and Kopf, A. W.: Complications of therapy of basal-cell epitheliomas (based on 1,000 histologically verified cases), 1964–1965 series. Year

Book of Dermatology. Chicago, Year Book Medical Publishers, 1965, pp. 7–26.

Brodkin, R. H., Kopf, A. W., and Andrade, R.: Basal-cell epithelioma and elastosis: a comparison of distribution. *In* Urbach, F. (ed.): Biologic Effects of Ultraviolet Radiation, Oxford, Pergamon Press Ltd., 1969, pp. 581–618.

Gellin, G. A., Kopf, A. W., and Garfinkel, L.: Basal-cell epithelioma: a controlled study of associated factors. Arch. Dermatol., 91:38, 1965.

Kopf, A. W.: Skin cancer therapy: some dermatological surgical aspects. Minn. Med., 43:156, 1960.

Kopf, A. W., and Andrade, R.: Benign juvenile melanoma, leading article, 1965–1966 series. Year Book of Dermatology, Chicago, Year Book Medical Publishers, 1966, pp. 7–52.

Lightstone, A. C., Kopf, A. W., and Garfinkel, L.: Diagnostic accuracy—a new approach to its evaluation. Arch. Dermatol., 91:497, 1965.

Sandler, H. C.: A retrospective study of a head and neck cancer control program. Cancer 25:1153, 1970.

Silberberg, I., Kopf, A. W., and Baer, R. L.: Recurrent keratoacanthoma of the lip. Arch. Dermatol., 86:44, 1962.

Sulzberger, M. B., Witten, V. H., and Kopf, A. W.: Diagnosis and treatment of skin cancer of the face. Symposium on Cancer of the Head and Neck, Annual Scientific Session, American Cancer Society, October 28–29, 1957, New York City (pp. 193–201 in the Proceedings published by the American Cancer Society).

2

Anatomy and Embryology of the Skin

Hermann Pinkus, M.D.

The skin is not only a protective envelope, it also has vital metabolic functions related to body homeostasis. In addition, it possesses many morphologic characteristics of great esthetic significance to the individual and therefore to the skin cancer therapist. The physician dealing with skin cancer also must be thoroughly familiar with cutaneous tissue structure which determines the nature and spread of tumors and the therapeutic approaches.

In all these structural and functional respects, the concept "skin" is an abstraction. In reality, there is scalp, facial skin, skin of the trunk, extremities, palms, soles, and many other regions which show gross or microscopic differences, based on developmental tendencies. The dermatologist, surgeon, and radiologist dealing with skin cancer must be familiar with all of these regions in order to choose treatment wisely. An example of an undesirable therapeutic result is the transplantation of abdominal skin to cover a defect of the palm in a young patient. Not only is the grafted skin deficient in structural toughness, but also it may bulge with fat tissue when the bearer later develops embonpoint.

The following discussion will present the development and structure of skin in relation to function, and will emphasize points important in the diagnosis and treatment of skin cancer. Comprehensive accounts of this field are available in the 3rd edition of Montagna's well-known monograph (Montagna and Parakkal, 1974) and in the supplement to Jadassohn's *Handbuch* (1963, 1964, 1968), which contains several chapters in English. References to detailed accounts of individual features will be given in the appropriate places. Recent American publications have been given preference for easy access.

EMBRYOLOGY

The skin develops through the interaction of ectodermal and mesodermal components. Ectodermal differentiation is presented in diagrammatic fashion in Figure 2–1 (Pinkus and Mehregan, 1969). The mesodermal portions are derived in part from the somites, and in part from nonsegmental mesenchyma. Nervous supply is later added on a segmental basis from the spinal and sympathetic ganglia, with the exception of the head region, which is

16

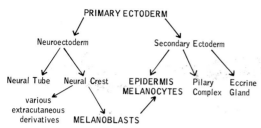

Figure 2-1 Ectodermal derivatives. (*From* Pinkus and Mehregan: A Guide to Dermatohistopathology, 1969. Courtesy of Appleton-Century-Crofts, Publishing Division of Prentice-Hall, Inc., Englewood Cliff, N.J.)

supplied by cranial nerves. For a comprehensive discussion see Pinkus and Tanay (1968). Electron microscopic data on many features were reported by Hashimoto (1965, 1970).

Ectoderm

Along the dorsal midline of the embryo, the single cuboidal layer of the primary ectoderm thickens and folds in (Fig. 2–2) to form the neural system, from which the skin is supplied with sensory and autonomic nerves. Cells along the elevated rim of the neural groove (the neural crest) contribute to many tissues and organs of the body. Some neural crest cells develop into melanoblasts, which migrate widely and eventually become located in the skin as

well as in some other tissues. That part of the ectoderm which remains after the separation of the neuroectoderm may be called the secondary ectoderm. It differentiates (Fig. 2–1) into the epidermis and its adnexa, and also forms conjunctiva and the lining of the external auditory meatus, the lining of a large part of the nasal cavity, and the lining of the mouth. Ectoderm is continuous with entodermal epithelium in the pharynx and at the anus, and with urogenital epithelium at the urethral opening.

In discussing the development of epidermis and adnexa, one has to keep in mind the important role of the mesoderm. While epithelial morphology is more impressive, it is induced and supported by mesodermal influences.

Epidermis. Through mitotic division exceeding that needed to keep pace with body growth, the epidermis becomes two layered and later multilayered (Fig. 2–3). The original two layers are known as basal layer and periderm (the name epitrichium for the latter is obsolete). While in young embryos mitosis may occur in both layers, it soon becomes restricted to the basal layer, which throughout life is the germinal layer of the epidermis. The periderm has metabolic functions. Its surface is beset with microvilli during the tenth to the sixteenth weeks, an indication that it serves as the place of exchange between body and amniotic fluid (Hoyes 1968) be-

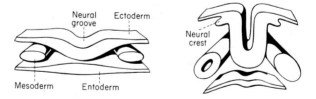

Figure 2-2 Development of the neural crest and its derivatives. (Adapted from Hamilton et al., 1952; and Zimmermann and Becker, 1959.)

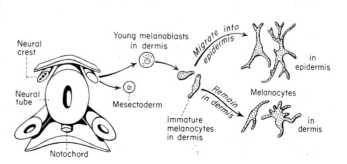

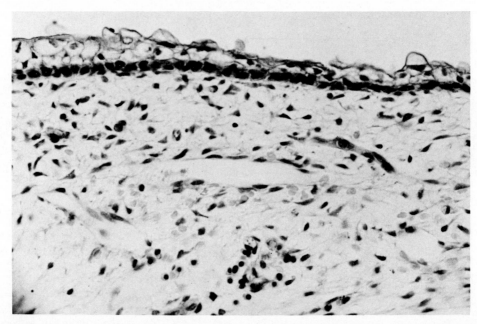

Figure 2–3 Fetal human skin. The epidermis consists of a basal layer and a periderm layer, between which an intermediary layer begins to form. The dermis contains mesenchymal cells embedded in ground substance with few fibrils. Some early capillary vessels are lined by endothelial cells. *H & E,* ×*360.*

fore specialized excretory organs develop. All layers of the early epidermis contain much glycogen. Later this substance disappears from the basal cells but persists in the developing multiple layers of prickle cells and in the periderm. After the sixteenth week, the periderm is shed and replaced by keratinizing cells from the germinal layer. It should be noted here that the old hypothesis that certain forms of ichthyosis (collodion baby) represent persistent periderm is utterly without foundation (Lentz and Altman, 1968; Schnyder, 1970). From about the sixth fetal month on, the epidermis resembles that of postnatal life. It shows regional differences quite early.

Pilar Apparatus. Beginning in the third fetal month, focal crowding of basal cells takes place at regular intervals (Pinkus, 1958a). These very first anlagen of the hair follicles (pregerm) are due to locally increased mitotic activity which a little later leads to downward bulging of the columnar basal cells. There is no invagination of the epidermis. Almost simultaneously, mesenchymal cells accumulate around the basal buds to make the *hair germ* (Fig. 2–4). Thus, the development of

the pilosebaceous apparatus shows evidence of epithelial-mesenchymal interaction (Fleischmajer and Billingham, 1968) from the very beginning. Numerous experiments in animals indicate (Kollar, 1970) that the mesoderm actually has the leading, determining role, which it retains all through life in controlling the hair cycle. The term "primary epithelial germ," which disregards mesodermal-epithelial interaction, should be discarded in favor of the older name hair germ (Stöhr, 1904) or, if one wants to be highly accurate, pilosebaceous germ. Each of these units arises through an act of embryonic differentiation (see Chap. 17) and, once formed, acts as a separate small organ.

Hair germs develop at relatively even intervals, and as the first ones are pulled apart by growth of body and skin, additional anlagen are formed. Furthermore, secondary germs develop laterally to the primary ones, forming the characteristic three-hair group. Occasionally two or more tertiary hairs are added to make five-hair or seven-hair groups. Rarely, only a single secondary hair will develop posterior to the primary follicle. With few exceptions, hair neogenesis is completed by

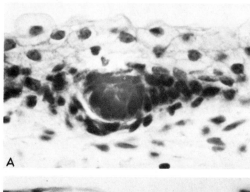

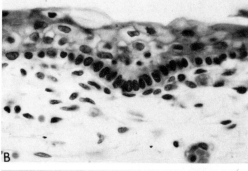

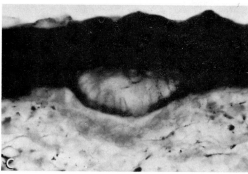

Figure 2–4 Hair germs. *A*, Sagittal section, anterior end to left. *H & E*, ×400. *B*, Frontal section. *H & E*, ×400. *C*, Frontal section. *Periodic acid-Schiff and light green*, ×400.

Note that the hair germs develop from the basal layer and that there is no invagination of the upper layers. Mesodermal nuclei have accumulated around the epithelial bud. In *C* the epidermis is full of glycogen, while the hair germ contains only traces. The dark line between epithelial and mesenchymal portions of the germ is the earliest formation of a PAS-positive (and diastase-resistant) basement membrane. (*From* Pinkus: Embryology of the hair. *In* Montagna and Ellis (Eds.): The Biology of Hair Growth. New York, Academic Press, Inc., 1958).

the seventh fetal month (Muller, 1971). From then on, differential growth of body areas leads to variable dilution of the number of pilary apparatuses per unit area of skin surface.

The use of the terms lateral and posterior (Pinkus, 1927) indicates that the hair germ has bilateral symmetry from the beginning. It grows in a slanting fashion down into and through the developing dermis until its end comes to rest in the subcutaneous fat tissue (Fig. 2–5). This is true for all hairs of the first fetal generation, while in adult life only strong hairs reach the panniculus. The slant of the follicles determines the later direction of the hairs, the hair streams and whorls. That portion of the skin which is shaded by the protruding hair shaft is said to be posterior to the pilosebaceous complex. The degree of slanting varies, the strong, straight follicles of Orientals being implanted more steeply. In fetuses destined to have curly or spiraling hair, the follicle curves as it grows down (Fig. 2–6), and the bulb may become situated perpendicularly below the point of origin (Fig. 2–17).

As the hair germ lengthens, its lower end becomes bulbous because the epithelium grows around the knob of mesodermal cells and becomes a bell-shaped structure, the hair matrix (Fig. 2–5), the hollow of which is occupied by metachromatic connective tissue, the dermal papilla. Simultaneously, two or three buds develop at the posterior (lower) circumference of the follicle. The lowest one is known as the bulge and marks the site at which the arrector pili muscle later will insert and to which the dying hair in catagen will rise. Above the bulge, a similar roundish bud develops into the sebaceous gland. The third and highest bud (Fig. 2–7) furnishes the apocrine gland, which in man develops only in relatively small areas of the body surface. Development of the arrector pili muscle completes the pilary complex. The muscle forms in a metachromatic zone of mesoderm behind the follicle and grows upward toward the epidermis and downward toward the bulge region of the hair root.

At the same time that the pilosebaceous anlage grows down into the dermis, it also grows upward through the epidermis to the surface (Pinkus, 1958a). The cells of the intraepidermal portion soon begin to form keratohyalin and keratin, and thus produce a central lumen, the hair canal (Fig. 2–8). The hair canal, into which the

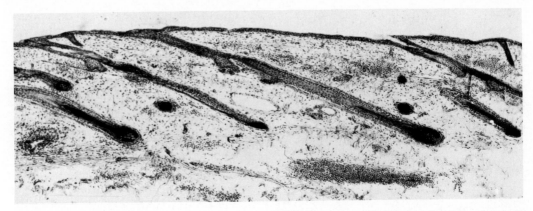

Figure 2–5 Fetal skin with straight slanting hair follicles which have attained their full length, their bulbs being in the subcutaneous fat tissue. The two thinner epithelial formations near the right and left borders of the picture are eccrine germs. Note the two buds at the lower surface of the follicles (bulge and sebaceous gland) and the thin streaks of arrector muscle. *H & E, ×30.*

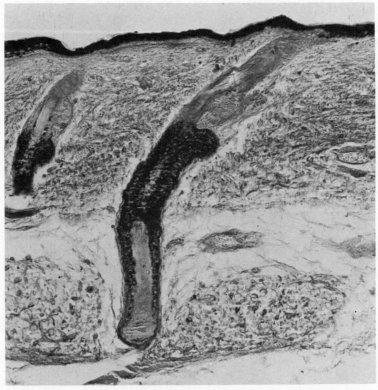

Figure 2–6 Fetal skin with curved hair follicle. The dark material represents glycogen in this PAS-stained section. Note the difference between the glycogen-rich bulge and the glycogen-free sebaceous gland, the cells of which appear vacuolated. Note also the rich vascularization of the two fetal fat organs to the right and left of the follicle. ×60. (*From* Pinkus: Embryology of the hair. *In* Montagna and Ellis (Eds.): The Biology of Hair Growth. New York, Academic Press, Inc., 1958.)

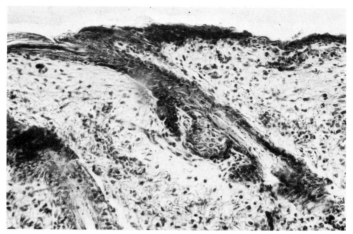

Figure 2-7 Fetal scalp. The hair follicle has an apocrine gland rudiment sprouting from the follicular wall above the sebaceous gland. The hair follicle opens at the surface by means of the cornified hair canal. *H & E, ×80. (From* Pinkus: Embryology of the hair. *In* Montagna and Ellis (Eds.): The Biology of Hair Growth. New York, Academic Press, Inc., 1958.)

hair later enters from below, is a long oblique structure, a fetal differentiation (Hashimoto, 1970b), most of which dissapears before birth. The persistent lower end becomes the infundibulum, recently named the acrotrichium (Duperrat and Mascaro, 1963).

Eccrine Apparatus. The eccrine glands, the true sweat glands of man, develop independently of hair follicles (Ellis, 1968), although some spatial relationship has been suggested. Their first anlage is a tiny bud of basal cells which elongates into a solid cord (Fig. 2-9) and grows almost vertically down through the dermis until it reaches the subcutaneous fat tissue, where it coils up. The mesodermal component of the eccrine germ, while present, is less conspicuous. Eccrine glands begin to form on the palms in the third fetal month, on the soles some weeks later, and on the general body surface in the fifth month. New buds arise between the earlier ones as these become separated by a critical distance during body growth. A full complement is reached in the seventh month. The eccrine germ also extends upward through the epidermis in a spiral fashion and forms the acrosyringium (Pinkus et al., 1956) or intraepidermal eccrine sweat duct unit. The great biologic significance of acrosyringium and acrotrichium will be discussed later in this chapter under the heading Interactions Between Dermis, Epidermis, and Adnexa, but one peculiar feature of its embryologic formation must be mentioned

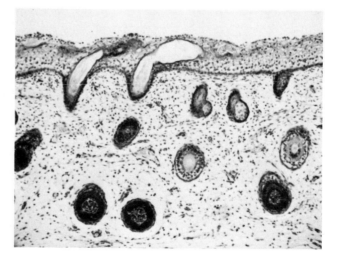

Figure 2-8 Fetal eyebrow. A dozen hair follicles are cut obliquely at different levels. Two of them exhibit curved hair canals extending through the epidermis to the surface. Their lumina are filled with keratin, although the epidermis still exhibits periderm and no stratum corneum. *H & E, ×60.*

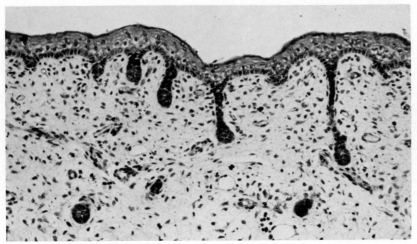

Figure 2–9   Fetal palm. Eccrine germs of different length extend down from the epidermis at fairly even intervals. They have a knobby lower end and show alignment of mesenchymal cells to form the mesodermal portion of the eccrine apparatus. *H & E, ×90.*

here because it has achieved relevance in the diagnosis of sweat gland tumors. While the intradermal duct acquires a lumen through cleft formation between cells, the lumen of the acrosyringium is formed by the confluence of intracellular vacuoles, which finally unite by breaking through the cell walls of neighboring cells. This peculiar process was investigated by Hashimoto et al. (1965) and is similar in eccrine and apocrine glands (Hashimoto, 1970a).

Nail.   Even though the earliest anlage of the nail may be at the border of ventral and dorsal skin of the digit (Alkiewicz, 1951), the developing nail field (Zaias,

1963) is on the dorsal surface, and its distal end marks the boundary against the ventral (later ridged) skin. The nail field is an almost rectangular area of thickened epithelium from which a solid bar grows at a slant down into the dermis (Fig. 2–10) toward the distal interphalangeal joint. Thus the proximal nail fold is formed. The epithelial bar keratinizes in its center to form the early nail plate and thereby is split into a lower portion which becomes the true nail matrix and an upper portion from which the eponychium is formed (Fig. 2–11). The nail plate slides distally over the nail bed and reaches the free

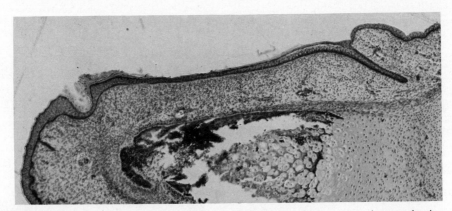

Figure 2–10   Distal phalanx of fetal thumb. The future nail matrix is seen in cross-section as a slanting plate of cells growing in the direction of the interphalangeal joint. The nail field is covered with epidermoid epithelium and has an elevated distal wall covered with thick horny material. This is the site of the future distal matrix. To the left of it is the sweat gland–bearing skin of the thumb tip, separated from the distal matrix by a deep groove. *H & E, ×30.*

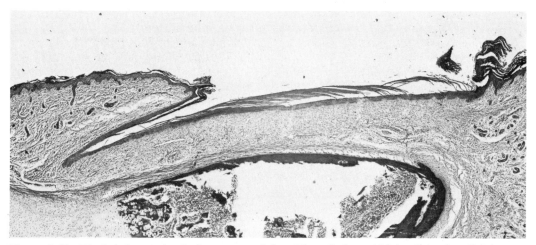

Figure 2–11 Distal phalanx and nail of a premature infant. The nail plate, which is split into lamellae through technical artifact, has not quite reached the distal matrix at the right end of the picture. The roof of the proximal nail fold forms the cuticle. Although the lamellation of the nail plate is artificial, it indicates the oblique positioning of the isochronous material in the nail (see Fig. 2–21). *H & E*, ×*15.*

margin at fetal maturity. Details of nail structure will be discussed in the macroscopic and microscopic portions of this chapter (p. 78).

Mesoderm and Ectodermal-Mesodermal Interaction

In the early embryo, the developing epithelium of the skin is supported by undifferentiated mesenchyma. Fusiform and stellate cells (Fig. 2–3) are embedded in ground substance rich in mucinous substances and glycogen (Pinkus and Tanay, 1968). Collagen fibers form from the second month on and later organize into bundles. PAS-positive basement membranes appear first (Fig. 2–4C) around early hair germs, and later between epidermis and dermis. Elastic fibers develop relatively late, from the fifth fetal month on (Varadi, 1970) and continue to increase after birth. Blood vessels form by local differentiation, or from sprouts of the segmental arteries (Töndury, 1964). The subpapillary plexus and the papillary capillaries are not fully developed until several months after birth (Perera et al., 1970, Syme and Riley, 1970). At certain periods the skin is a blood-forming organ and gives rise to both red cells (Popoff and Popoff, 1958) and lymphocytes. These potentialities may be revived later in life

under pathologic circumstances. Details of mesodermal organization will be discussed later, along with the description of adult skin.

It is, however, necessary to discuss here the field of ectodermal-mesodermal interaction in cutaneous development, a field long known to experimental embryologists but relatively recently called to the attention of pathologists and dermatologists (Pinkus, 1953) and developed with significant results in the last decade (Fleischmajer and Billingham, 1968). It has been established that differentiation and maturation of epidermis and cutaneous adnexa are not only induced by mesodermal factors, but need their continuous support. Epidermis transplanted onto the chorioallantoic membrane of chick embryos survives in organized form only if it is in contact with its own mesoderm, although the latter need not be viable (Briggaman and Wheeler, 1971). Embryonic development of either feathers or scales in chick skin is determined by specific mesoderm, and the same is true for differentiation of hairs in mice (Hardy, 1951; Kollar, 1970). Later in life, the dermal papilla seems to be the leading partner in the events of the hair cycle, and destruction of only the papilla by means of the galvanic current (electrolysis) eliminates hair growth permanently. On the other hand, an anagen hair may be plucked and most of the matrix and the root sheaths destroyed, and yet the hair root will soon reconstitute itself and give rise to a new hair. Other details will be discussed on pages 65 to 72.

Another recently established fact is that basement membrane material (Hay, 1964; Pierce, 1965) and even collagen (Pruniéras et al., 1969) are formed by epithelial cells interacting with mesoderm. The basement membrane (for definition, see p. 63) is not a barrier but a product of biologic interaction, exchange, and organization. Basement membranes are absent in early fetal life before cells are capable of interaction, and in carcinogenesis after they have lost that ability.

Neuroectoderm

Neuroectodermal derivatives enter the skin in the form of sensory nerves, autonomic nerves, and pigment-forming cells. Only the face receives motor innervation to the striated muscles (Fig. 2–49), which are found there in the deep portions of the skin.

Nerves. Voluntary and autonomic nerves have segmental distribution according to their derivation from spinal or cranial ganglia and from the sympathetic chain. The term dermatome, originally referring to embryonic metameric organization, is now being used in clinical practice to refer to those parts of the skin which are supplied by sensory nerves from one segmental root or one cranial nerve. Nerve endings may be free or organized into special structures, which will be described on page 80. Autonomic innervation of glands and smooth muscle is entirely sympathetic, but may be cholinergic or adrenergic.

Pigment Cells. The neuroectodermal derivation of melanocytes has been so thoroughly established by experimental means in many lower and higher vertebrates that it must be accepted also for the human species in spite of absence of experimental proof (Starck, 1964; Montagna and Hu, 1967). Actually, the careful observations of Zimmermann (1948), Zimmermann and Becker (1959), and later workers (Pinkus and Tanay, 1968) give suggestive evidence of migration of melan-

oblasts into the skin from underlying tissues in human fetuses.

Some of these cells (Fig. 2–2) remain in the dermis where they become the substrate of Mongolian spots, blue nevi (Jadassohn-Tièche), and brown-blue nevi (Ota and Ito), and probably also of the periocular umbra. Most melanoblasts reach the epithelial structures and settle eventually in the basal layer of epidermis and hair matrix. They mature into melanocytes which contain tyrosinase and are the only cells in the skin capable of producing melanin. Either melanoblasts or embryologically deviated nevoblasts (Mishima, 1967) give rise to nevus cell nevi of junction, compound, and intradermal types and to malignant melanomas. Melanocytes are involved in the formation of freckles (ephelides), lentigines of the simplex and senilis type, nevus spilus, cafe au lait spots, and any other type of pigmentary disorder.

The dendritic cell of Langerhans is mentioned here because it was believed to be related to melanocytes. This belief has been thoroughly shaken by investigations which have shown that Langerhans cells develop in embryonic mouse epidermis transplanted into the spleen of adult mice (Breathnach et al., 1968) from limb buds before these are invaded by neuroectodermal elements. Langerhans cells therefore are not of neuroectodermal origin. Their actual derivation, whether mesodermal or ectodermal, awaits clarification. Cells resembling them form the substrate of the granulomas of histiocytosis X (Gianotti and Caputo, 1969).

GROSS ANATOMY

The attention which primitive as well as civilized people pay to the appearance and artificial modification of their skin, and the tremendous growth of the cosmetic industry in recent years testify to the psychologic (esthetic) importance of gross characteristics of the skin. The factor of a cosmetically acceptable result must be taken into account whenever possible in the treatment of skin cancer, and the details of gross anatomy of the skin must therefore be well known to the cancer therapist.

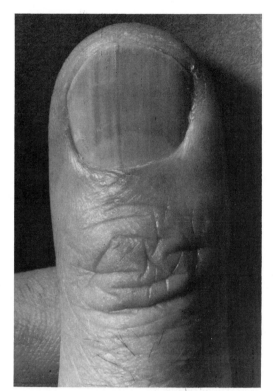

Figure 2-12 Thumb and part of the volar ridged skin of forefinger. Note the change from the hairy skin on the dorsum of the basal phalanx, to the coarsely wrinkled glabrous skin of the joint area, to the smooth periungual skin, and to the nail and its proximal, lateral, and distal folds. There are at least five quite different types of skin in close proximity. The nail shows a large lunula and early senile longitudinal ridges.

Moreover, knowledge of normal surface characteristics, which can be recognized with the naked eye or a magnifying glass, is very helpful in the clinical diagnosis of certain skin tumors which influence these characteristics.

The skin of one person differs from that of another in many respects. Sex, age, racial and other genetic factors, environmental exposure, and topographical differences (Figs. 2-12 and 2-42) interact to produce a great variety of skins. The following discussion will deal with surface characteristics, physical dimensions, and topographical and individual differences. It is based on the published work of many authors, and especially on the respective chapters of F. Pinkus (1927) and H. Pinkus (1964) in Jadassohn's *Handbuch.* The latter

should be consulted if no other source is given.

Surface Characteristics

Visual examination of the skin takes into account reflection of light, which is modified by unevenness of the surface and various pigments, and the products of the cutaneous adnexa in the form of hairs, nails, and glandular secretions.

Elevations and Furrows. Normal skin is perfectly smooth and shiny only in very limited areas, mainly around the proximal part of the nails. (Figs. 2-12 and 2-20). Everywhere else, it appears dull due to the presence of fine wrinkles and coarser folds. The latter are either flexure creases or are caused by attachment of the skin to deeper structures. They generally increase with age and are important to the surgeon,

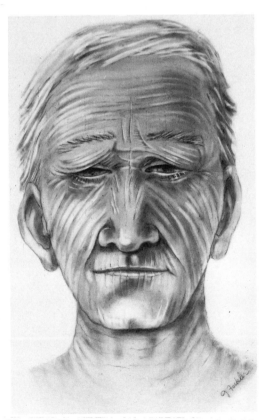

Figure 2-13 Exaggerated illustration of facial wrinkle lines for guidance in making surgical incisions.

especially when they are located on the face (Fig. 2–13) where they should guide the direction of his incision. Linear scars following wrinkle lines are much less conspicuous than scars which deviate from them or cross them. On other parts of the body, Langer lines (pp. 46, 47) are more important.

The very fine wrinkles are a great factor in the reflection of light. They disappear in severely atrophic skin, which then looks unnaturally shiny. They divide the skin surface into irregular polygonal or triangular facets which have a characteristic arrangement in various regions of the body (Chinn and Dobson, 1964; Tring and Murgatroyd, 1974), although relatively little is known concerning their exact distribution (F. Pinkus, 1927; Dillon, 1963) and possible inheritance. They influence

the matching of transplanted skin with its new surroundings.

More exact data are known about these fine furrows in those areas where they form regular patterns: the friction surfaces (Fig. 2–12) of digits, palms, and soles. The science of "ridged skin" (dermatoglyphics—Cummins and Midlo, 1943) has associated with it a great array of data (for short reviews see Stough and Seely, 1969; and Verbov, 1970) which, however, is of less importance to the cancerologist than to the geneticist (Holt, 1968), criminologist, and anthropologist. The pattern of ridged skin remains constant throughout life and is influenced by relatively few diseases (Pinkus and Plotnick, 1958) because deep dermal changes are required to destroy it. Disturbances related to cancer are atrophy in chronic x-ray skin, develop-

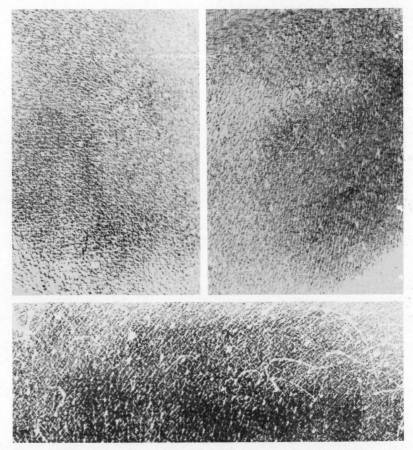

Figure 2–14   Dermatograms produced by pressing the inked skin of the forearm against smooth paper. The pattern of fine wrinkles is interrupted by the roundish pores of hair follicles and streaks produced by some hairs. The fine details (minutiae) of such patterns can be used for individual identification.

ment of arsenical and x-ray keratoses, and peculiar pits pathognomonic of the nevoid basal cell carcinoma syndrome (Howell and Mehregan, 1970). Dobson's (1965) claim that small palmar keratoses are more commonly found in patients with internal cancer awaits confirmation.

The pattern of fine wrinkles may be studied in dermatograms (Bettman, 1927) obtained by inking the skin and pressing it on smooth paper (Fig. 2–14). A variety of other methods have been developed (see Pinkus, 1964; Sivadjan, 1970), many of which use replica techniques (Wolf and Hanušová, 1970; Tring and Murgatroyd, 1974).

Horny Layer and Pores. The stratum corneum consisting of more or less coherent keratinized epidermal cells ordinarily is supple and follows all elevations and depressions of the underlying tissues. Although probably one layer of horny cells is exfoliated each day, this process involves single cells or small groups and is imperceptible except on the scalp where a small amount of dandruff is normally retained on the hairy skin. If, however, the horny layer is dehydrated, the edges of small areas curl up and later deep cracks may develop. Other types of scaliness indicate a variety of skin diseases. Ichthyosis and other processes accompanied by a thickened horny layer make the skin less supple.

Roughness of the skin surface can be measured photometrically by applying a dye solution (methylene blue) or suspension (hostapermblue) which is retained in superficial cracks (Tronnier and Eisbacher, 1970). Many methods have been developed to document the surface of normal and abnormal skin permanently by making replicas from molds. Dental mass, plaster of paris, and special compounds may be used (see Cseplála and Marton, 1967). More recently, the method of scanning electron microscopy has begun to add to our knowledge (Orfanos et al., 1969).

Various other methods are available to test the physiologic functions of the skin surface. Extraction and analysis of lipids (Nicolaides, 1961; Reinertson and Wheatley, 1959; Pochi and Strauss, 1964), histochemical tests for esterases (Steigleder and Schultis, 1957), and histochemical and biochemical analysis of water-extractable substances have been used on normal and pathologic skin. Kleine-Natrop (1967) recently combined wetting ability using methylene blue solution, spreading ability of sebum, and tests for neutralization of alkali and acid in order to obtain a fairly comprehensive picture of surface activity of the epidermis.

Another feature of considerable significance are the pores of the skin which indicate the opening of pilosebaceous complexes and eccrine glands. The latter are so tiny that they are not usually seen except when a drop of sweat exudes. They can be recognized on the ridges of digits and palms with a magnifying glass. Sweat pores can be stained specifically on the living skin surface by electrophoresis of acid or basic dyes, or by *o*-phthalaldehyde (Ohman and Shelley, 1969), which combines with minimal amounts of ammonia in the duct. Activity of eccrine glands can be demonstrated by Minor's starch-iodine method and its modifications, or by application of plastic films. The latest method described is that of Sarkany and Gaylarde (1969), who let a silicone film form on the skin and then expose it to silver nitrate, which blackens the spots where eccrine glands have been active. The test has the advantages that it is convenient, produces permanent records, and can be repeatedly used on the same area of skin. Pilosebaceous pores are easily visible on the face even if no hair protrudes from them. There are small pores (vellus follicles) and larger ones (sebaceous follicles); the latter are particularly prominent on the nose and central parts of the face. Individual differences are marked, and large-pored skin, a complaint of many young girls, is an innate characteristic that can be hidden but not changed. Pore patterns can be made visible on the skin, or preferably on tissue paper impressions lifted from it, by exposure to osmic acid, which blackens the lipids.

Pigments. The word pigment is used here in the wide sense of coloring matter. Normally this includes melanin, hemoglobin, sebum, elastic fiber pigment, and some less well understood colored substances. It is also important to point out that the colorless keratohyalin granules act as a diffusing screen, and so does the white collagen of the dermis. Foreign material, introduced into the skin accidentally or as a tattoo, must be considered, and in some diseases there are abnormal metabolic substances (as in hemosiderosis, calcinosis, ochronosis, and xanthoma).

The tinge of normal skin is determined mainly by melanin and hemoglobin and is influenced by the diffusing effect of keratohyalin and collagen. Melanin may be present in the basal layer or in all strata of the epidermis as well as in the dermis at varying depth. The color produced by it ranges from blackish-brown to light brown, yellow, and blue, depending on the amount and the distance from the surface. The color of hemoglobin differs in its oxidized and reduced forms, but it is further influenced by keratohyalin in the epi-

dermis and by the turbid whiteness of the dermis.

The diffusing influence of the keratohyalin layer can be demonstrated neatly by holding a pencil lead below a partly frosted glass slide (Fig. 2–15). When the lead touches the glass, it looks black under the frosted part as well as under the clear portion. If it is removed a little way, the contours become indistinct and the color gray (Jesionek, 1916). Similarly, the color of hemoglobin in the dermal capillaries is modified. The vermilion of the lips derives much of its vivid color from an absence of keratohyalin, while the pale color of the lips of older people is in part due to the development of a granular layer in actinic cheilitis. The vivid red of most inflamma-

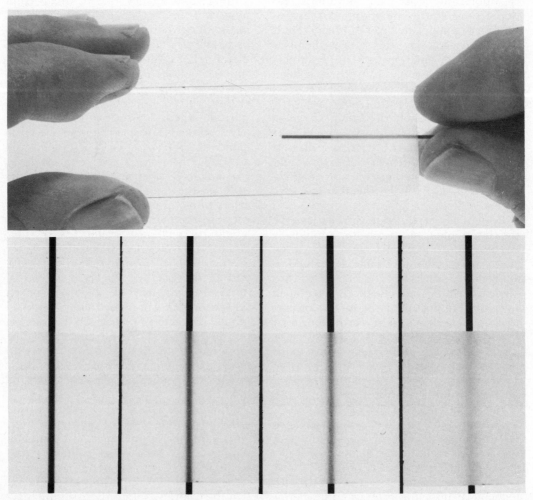

Figure 2–15 Effect of a ground-glass surface on the visualization of a pencil lead held at various distances below the glass slide. This illustrates the diffusing effect of the keratohyalin layer.

tory dermatoses is due in part to absence of the granular layer, while lichen planus, having a thick keratohyalin layer, is apt to have a violaceous hue. Keratohyalin also is responsible for the white color of leukoplakia of the mucous membranes.

The vivid red color of skin lesions can be due to blood in dilated inflamed vessels, to noninflammatory telangiectasia, to extravasated blood in fresh purpura, or to red dyes in tattoos, usually cinnabar. Application of a glass slide under pressure (diascopy) permits differentiation of inflammatory redness from purpura, but trapped red cells in ectatic capillaries may not disappear unless they are displaced by seesaw or rotating movements of the slide.

Yellow color is produced by sebum in sebaceous glands; by massed elastic fibers in pseudoxanthoma elasticum and actinic elastosis; by lipids in xanthoma, necrobiosis lipoidica, and follicular retention cysts; by leukocytes in pustules; and by caseation necrosis in lupus miliaris disseminatus. Carotinemia may produce an orange-yellow discoloration, especially on the palms of young children and in some food faddists, and there is of course the bile pigment of icteric skin.

Blue color may be due to deep-seated melanin in Mongolian spots and blue nevi, to carbon in tattoos and occupational abrasions in miners, and to pencil lead or other black substances in scars from accidental injuries. The principal factor modifying brown and black to blue is the dermal collagen (Findlay, 1970). Silver in very fine distribution produces a gray or bluish-gray diffuse discoloration in argyria. Hemoglobin looks blue not only in veins, but also outside the vascular system in bruises. The rainbow colors of the decomposition products of blood are well known, and the final long-lasting product, hemosiderin, is the substrate of shades varying from yellow to rusty brown and brownish-black.

Other substances known as melanoids may cause the horny layer to assume yellowish, dirty brown, gray, and almost black hues, especially in thick deposits.

Measurement and Recording of Skin Color. The skin presents many hues under normal conditions, and even more in disease. Their objective description has been a troublesome problem and has not been fully resolved. The most common but scientifically least satisfactory method has been to use comparison with the colors of the spectrum or with familiar objects. Expressions such as rose pink, salmon, boiled ham color, and violet are examples and mean different things to different observers, especially when the object of comparison becomes obsolete (e.g., heliotrop) or varies in color in different parts of the world (e.g., apple jelly, which is made from green apples in Europe and from red apples in the United States). Attempts to describe skin color by comparison with standardized colors in tables have been made but have not met universal acceptance (Pinkus, 1964).

Modern methods use either three-color schemes or photometric measurements. Two relatively modern ways of utilizing color blending are the color top and the Lovibond tintometer. Both use, in addition to three pure colors, a correction for saturation of color. The color top (Todd et al., 1928) consists of a disk with variable sections of black and of the three principal colors red, blue, and yellow. If the disk is rotated quickly on its axis, the eye perceives the mixture of the four sections and the observer can match this impression to the color of the skin by varying the size of the sections. In the tintometer (Plotnick, 1966), tinted glass filters are superimposed on one another and are compared to skin color in a gun-like instrument, the viewing part of which is held close to the skin. Both methods are open to subjective error and require considerable experience. Photometric methods are objective, but require rather cumbersome instrumentation. The Hardy recording spectrophotometer and similar instruments have been used widely. Recently, monochromators have become available. In choosing the proper type of instrument, one has to decide whether actual color differences have to be identified, or whether one can be content to measure lightness and darkness. In the first case one may have to go as far as Barnicot (1958), who measured reflection at nine different wavelengths. In the latter case, one may use a fairly simple device constructed by Lasker (1954) for field work, which employs only one wavelength (420 mμ). The two main factors in skin coloration are hemoglobin and melanin, and as the latter has no characteristic spectral peak but absorbs increasingly from the red to the violet end of the spectrum, it just modifies the saturation of the blood color in combination with the white reflection (albedo) induced by keratohyalin. Sheard and Brunsting (1929) therefore recommended measurements at 580 to 590 mμ.

Finally, a word should be said about the photographic recording of skin, skin lesions, and skin color. In order to obtain comparable pictures, especially for the evaluation of progression or regression of lesions and of therapeutic results, conditions must be strictly standardized for any one office or hospital. Reflecting background, intensity of light source, distance between camera and patient, and positioning of the patient must be kept constant. For black and white photography, the incident angle of light must be controlled in order to produce similar shadows. In color photography, the same emulsion must be employed for a sequence of pictures.

Hairs. Hair follicles are distributed over most of the skin surface although in uneven number. The hairs they produce, however, vary so widely in caliber and length that large areas are commonly described as glabrous (hairless), a term which in the strict sense applies only to palms and soles and a few adjoining areas. With the exceptions of eyelashes and eyebrows, hairs of the first fetal generation are alike all over the body and are called lanugo. The second generation, which forms either in the older fetus or after birth, is differentiated into long scalp hair and vellus hair of the rest of the skin surface. Persistence of long lanuginous hair all over the body is a rare dominant characteristic (hypertrichosis lanuginosa universalis; for a recent review see Felgenhauer, 1969). Acquired hypertrichosis of this type usually is a dermadrome of internal malignancy (Fretzin, 1967; Herzberg et al., 1969; Chadfield and Khan, 1970).

Later in life, especially in the male, further differentiation takes place. The formation of axillary and pubic hair depends on the presence of sex hormones, but is fairly even in boys and girls. In men, larger or smaller parts of the body and extremi-

ties develop terminal hair, which is considerably thicker than vellus and reaches a length of 1 to 3 cm. In addition, sexually mature men grow beards and still later in life develop strong hairs in nose and ears. There is no doubt that the differentiation of these specialized hairs takes place under the stimulus of sex hormones, but once formed they continue to grow even after castration. If women develop stronger hairs in areas of the male pattern, this is known as hirsutism.

SCALP. The delineation of scalp hair in children and women usually is very sharp, although less distinct on the nape of the neck than around the ears and the face. Diameter of scalp hair varies from about 40 μ to 150 μ, the most common measurements being 60 to 100 μ (F. Pinkus, 1927). The thickness increases gradually during childhood. Hairs below 65 μ in thickness rarely contain medulla; most of those above 100 μ do. Scalp hairs grow for several years. The average increment is 0.3 to 0.5 mm a day or 11 to 18 cm a year. Since untrimmed hair of young Caucasian men grows to below the shoulders, and that of women commonly reaches the hips and may reach the knees or even the feet, continuous growth for five years and more is not exceptional. Maximal length of hair evidently is a genetically determined characteristic and varies greatly in different races.

The shape of hairs also varies on a genetic basis from straight to wavy, curly, and spiraled. It is associated with variations in the shape of the cross-section of the hair. Straight hair usually has a round contour, while that of curly hairs is oval or kidney shaped. Both properties are determined by the shape of the hair follicle and hair matrix. The follicles of straight and wavy hairs are straight and extend down on a slant corresponding to their fetal development. Even very thick hair that seems to emerge vertically is implanted at an angle (Fig. 2–16). The hair root of strongly curled (Negroid) hair, on the other hand, is curved and may describe a semicircle (Fig. 2–17). The hair matrix may be perpendicularly below the surface opening or may be deflected in an unforeseeable direction. In these hairs there is a more or less sharp kink between the matrix and the

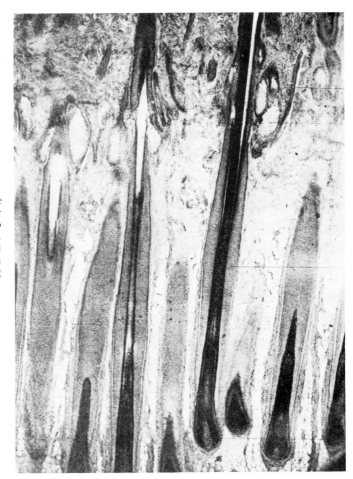

Figure 2–16 Vertical section of the scalp of a Chinese. The straight hair roots slant slightly and extend deep into the subcutaneous fat tissue. *(From* Fritsch: Das Haupthaar und seine Bildungstätte bei den Rassen des Menschen. Berlin, Georg Reimer, 1912.)

keratogenous zone (Fig. 2–17*A*) and the follicle has an asymmetric cross-section.

Knowledge of these differences is important in the cosmetic transplantation of hair. In the usual method of taking small specimens from the occipital region, the direction of the skin punch must be slanted in straight-haired people to follow the direction of the hair root (Orentreich, 1970). In persons with curved follicles, larger punch specimens are recommended, and the percentage of undamaged hair roots per specimen may be smaller. Furthermore, hairs must be implanted on a bald scalp so that they are inclined toward the forehead following the natural direction on the frontal scalp of most persons. Similar attention must be paid to the slant of the hair when flaps of scalp are used to reconstruct eyebrows or bearded upper lip.

The number of scalp hairs per square centimeter has been counted by various authors, and figures between 128 and 626 have been published (Pinkus, 1964). Values between 300 and 500 are most common. Hairs usually stand in groups of two to eight, three and five hairs to the group being most common. In some individuals the follicles merge below the surface (compound follicles (Fig. 2–18) and several hairs protrude from one opening. These persons are said to be particularly susceptible to folliculitis (Loewenthal, 1947; Oberste-Lehn, 1957).

Changes in the area covered with scalp hair are well known. Most boys develop a glabrous temporal triangle at puberty, while women develop it only in the menopause. Only too many men find that the balding process continues toward the vertex, or that a bald spot starts at the vertex,

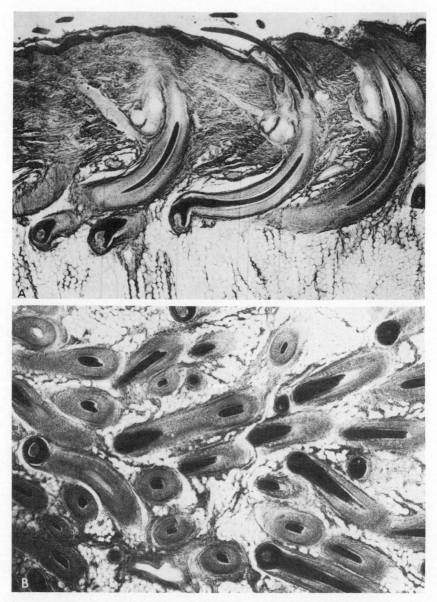

Figure 2–17   *A*, Vertical and, *B*, horizontal sections of scalp of a Hottentot. The hair follicles producing the tightly curled hair of this tribe are semicircular with a nearly right angle between the matrix and the keratogenous zone. The deep ends of the follicles deviate in different directions and the follicles do not extend as deep as those in Figure 2–16. *(From* Fritsch: Das Haupthaar und seine Bildungstätte bei den Rassen des Menschen. Berlin, Georg Reimer, 1912.)

enlarges, and possibly meets the temporal zones. In this process of patterned baldness, no hair follicles are destroyed. Instead, every matrix produces progressively thinner and shorter hair with each new generation; turnover time is accelerated, until eventually only extremely fine and short vellus is produced.

The status of hair growth on a scalp can be estimated and used for diagnostic and prognostic purposes in cases of increased falling hair (telogen effluvium) (Kligman, 1961a) by the use of one of two methods. The older one (F. Pinkus, 1928) is based on counts and measurements of the hairs lost. Hair loss of up to 100 hairs a day from

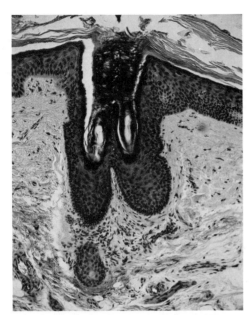

Figure 2–18 Merging infundibula of two hair roots, forming a compound follicle. *H & E, ×90.*

a full scalp is within the range of normal. The percentage of short hairs (hairs up to 12 cm. long and having a natural tip representing hairs of less than one year's life span) should not exceed 20 percent. If more hairs are lost but the percentage is normal, one deals with an effluvium due to sudden causes such as febrile disease, surgical shock, or childbirth. These cases have a good prognosis. The hair will regrow after two to three months. A higher percentage of short hairs signifies intrinsic weakening of hair growth and shortening of the cycle. These cases have a poor prognosis and will probably result in pattern baldness.

The newer method, elaborated by Van Scott et al. (1957), Kligman (1961a), and others, uses 50 to 100 hairs pulled from the scalp by a quick forceful pull. Hair roots are examined and divided into resting (telogen) and growing (anagen) hairs. A normal scalp should not contain more than 20 percent of hairs in telogen, and a higher percentage signifies telogen effluvium regardless of cause. Extremely high values speak for loss from sudden extraneous causes. The two methods nicely complement each other and may be combined with microscopic examination of the shafts

of growing hairs for evidence of the Pohl-Pincus mark. This mark (Fig. 2–19) consists of slight constriction of the shaft and interruption of the medulla, if the medulla is present. It is therefore best to examine strong hairs, preferably white ones, which show the medulla well. Pohl-Pincus mark corresponds to the Beau line on the nail and indicates severe but temporary impairment of health. Distance from the hair bulb can be used to estimate the time that has elapsed since the illness (Pinkus and Mehregan, 1969).

The basic color of hair is determined by the number and density of pigment granules contributed to the keratinizing cells by melanocytes in the hair matrix. The surface appearance is influenced by several other factors. Loss of integrity of the cuticula or foreign material deposited on the hair makes it appear dull. Twists in the shaft (pili torti) and gas bubbles in the cortex (pili annulati) produce uneven reflection of light. Gas in the medulla of senile or albino hairs and reflection at interfaces within the hair (Orfanos et al., 1970) make the colorless fiber appear white in reflected light. The natural color of hair varies on a genetic basis from black to brown and blond. Red tinges are produced by a different pigment, the nature of which is not completely agreed upon, (Flesch, 1968). Red is inherited as a separate factor. It may be the only color in a person's hair or may be added to varying amounts of the brown coloration. Even black hair may have a hidden component of genetic red which is revealed in the red-headed child of two dark-haired parents.

With advancing age—in some persons as early as the third decade and in the majority after the fiftieth year—individual hairs lose their color. The process is sudden (Herzberg and Gusek, 1970) and in most cases complete, and usually is tied to the hair cycle: a dark hair falls out and is replaced by a white hair through loss of the matrix melanocytes in catagen. The increasing admixture of white hairs makes a person's head increasingly gray, but there are few if any "gray hairs." Instances of sudden "turning white" have recently been explained as diffuse alopecia areata (Helm and Milgrom, 1970; Aram, 1970).

FACE. The number of hair follicles,

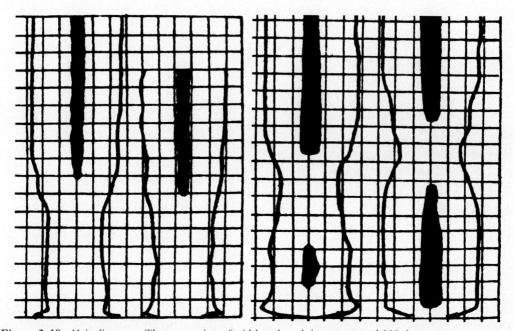

Figure 2–19   Hair diagrams. The proportion of width to length is exaggerated 100 times.

    The two hairs on the left were plucked from the scalp of a 21 year old man eight days after defervescence of severe erythema multiforme. The bottom part of the hairs shows decreased diameter and loss of medulla.

    The two hairs on the right were taken a week later and show beginning restitution of diameter of the shaft and medulla. The constricted portion would have become visible later as Pohl-Pincus mark. (*From* Pinkus, F.: **Die** Einwirkung von Krankheiten auf das Kopfhaar des Menschen. Ed. 2. Berlin, S. Karger, 1928.)

given variously as from 400 to over 1000 per square centimeter but most commonly as 500 to 800, is higher on the face than on any other part of the body, but the number of visible hairs may be very small. There are basically three different types of follicles, tiny ones producing vellus, large ones producing beard hairs, and a third type called sebaceous follicles (Fig. 2–48), in which the hair root appears as an appendage to the very large, and often multiple, sebaceous gland. Inasmuch as no new follicles are formed after birth, it is assumed that vellus follicles enlarge and begin to produce beard hairs (Fig. 2–49) under the influence of sex hormones. This phenomenon is among the most puzzling of the many mysteries of hair growth. There is no doubt that beard hairs develop only under the influence of testicular hormones in males, but once a man has a beard, castration does not make it disappear. In the female, development of a beard is associated with various forms of hormonal dysfunction, but often regresses if virilizing tumors are removed. The tendency to be-

come a beard follicle seems to be innate in certain hair roots: not a few adolescents start growing beard hairs inbetween scalp hairs in a limited area anterior to the ear, a phenomenon easily visible if scalp hair is dark and straight and beard hair is red and curly.

    Beard hairs often have the thickest shafts and may have round, oval, angular, or fluted cross-sections. Multiple hairs (pili multigemini) (Pinkus, 1951a) are found exclusively in the beard. The histologic reasons are discussed in the legend of Figure 2–53. The beard may differ from head hair in color, commonly being more red, and it may be multi-colored and have white portions already early in life. It may turn universally gray and white earlier or later than the capillitium. These matters, as well as the extent and density of the beard, are genetically determined.

    The face presents other specialized forms of hair. The two most important ones are eyelashes and eyebrows. Both are distinct already in fetal life, being the earliest sites of hair formation anywhere on the body. They resemble in this respect vibrissae and tactile hairs on the face of mammals.

As Montagna (1970a) has shown recently, the eyebrows (supercilia), although they are not sinus hairs, have certain characteristics in adult life that suggest a relation to animal tactile hairs. The individual eyebrow hair has a limited length which it achieves in a few weeks of growth. The root then goes into a prolonged resting state lasting several months. This must be kept in mind when eyebrows are shaved preoperatively. They may not grow back for quite some time.

Eyelashes (cilia) are longest in children, often 10 to 11 mm.; a length above 12 mm. is extremely rare (Pinkus, 1964). Their length is reduced with age, approximately a millimeter per decade. They often are not longer than 3 to 4 mm. in elderly people, even in the absence of disease.

Still other facial hairs are the vibrissae in the nose and the terminal hairs on the ears. While the former are present in both sexes, they are much stronger in men and are apt to grow more profusely with age. Hairs around the tragus of the ear are an almost exclusively male characteristic. They usually are not very noticeable before the age of 40, and grow stronger from then on. Terminal hair on the helix is very rare in men of European stock but are fairly common in certain parts of India where it is considered a sign of virility. These hairs begin to grow in the third decade of life and the trait is said to be carried on the Y chromosome (Dronamraju, 1960).

SEXUAL HAIR. It has already been said that growth of a beard and patterned loss of scalp hair are triggered by male hormones. Boys castrated before puberty do not get bald even if they come from balding families and do not grow beards. Both events can be induced by giving testosterone later in life (Porter and Lobitz, 1970).

In addition to beard hairs, those of the axillae (hirci) and the genital region (pubes) are induced by sex hormones, but equally so in boys and girls. The words puberty and pubescence indicate growth of the pubic hair, which usually is restricted to the triangular escutcheon in women, while it extends toward the umbilicus in men and may merge diffusely with terminal hair on the abdomen and chest.

HAIR OF THE GENERAL BODY SURFACE. After it has lost the fetal lanugo, the child's body may have very little visible hair or may be covered with more or less prominent fuzz, which usually is colorless but which may be pigmented. This intermediate hair generally persists in women but gradually transforms into terminal hair on parts of the body surface of many men. Women may grow terminal hair on legs and forearms. In men, terminal hair is the rule on all extremities and is variably developed on the trunk. At least some strong hairs grow around and between the mamillae and may cover chest, abdomen, and back. Great racial and genetic differences exist.

A peculiar feature is the loss of terminal hair on the lower legs of men, especially on the lateral surface. This almost universal phenomenon has been "discovered" and related to various disease states a number of times, but has no pathologic significance. On the other hand, loss of hair on the dorsal surface of the big toe is a sign of longstanding ischemia, and hairs may grow again when the circulation improves (Naide, 1953).

Nails. Nails grow continuously throughout life at the rate of about 0.1 mm. a day. The rate becomes somewhat slower with advancing age, but the actual amount of nail substance formed does not necessarily decrease because the nail plate often grows thicker. Nails have surface characteristics which change with age. Children often have oblique ridges which converge toward the center at the distal end. These disappear in early adult life. Much later, longitudinal ridges (Fig. 2–20) appear and increase in old age. They may be smooth or interrupted (moniliform) and are due to intrinsic curling of layers in the nail plate. They may lead to splitting at the free edge of the nail.

The nail plate (Fig. 2–12) is semitranslucent, and its color is strongly influenced by the color of the nail bed; it is pink in Caucasians and more or less brown in Negroes. That the nail appears white at the free edge is due mainly to the air space below it, and any dirt or other foreign sub-

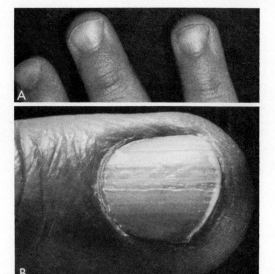

Figure 2–20   *A*, Lateral portions of middle and ring fingernails of a 2 year old child show oblique striations which converge distally toward the center where they meet longitudinal striations.

B, Ring fingernail of a 65 year old man exhibiting three types of senile ridging. There are several thin elevated longitudinal lines. Near the center of the nail there is a slightly sinuous groove which threatens to lead to splitting of the free end of the nail. Just to the left is a moniliform arrangement of alternating thicker and thinner portions of nail.

stance below the nail influences its color. Similarly, the lunula, representing the distal part of the matrix, looks whitish owing to factors of reflectance which are not fully understood. White spots in the nail plate (leukonychia) are caused by slight trauma to the nail at the site of its formation and are due to persistent nuclei and to air bubbles in the plate. Dark longitudinal streaks are very rare in Caucasians and arouse suspicion of a junction nevus or melanoma in the matrix. They are common in Negroes and other pigmented ethnic groups and simply reflect local activity of melanocytes in the matrix. Livid nails are found in cyanosis, and azure lunulae in Wilson's disease. The so-called yellow line which parallels the free border of the nail will be discussed later in this chapter under Microscopic Anatomy.

The form and shape of nails vary widely. Most commonly, fingernails are longer than wide, slightly convex along their long axis, and more convex along their transverse diameter. Flat or concave (coilony-

chia) nails are found in certain pathologic conditions (e.g., anemia), but may be a family trait. "Coffin lid" nails with an almost flat center and sloping sides usually are strong, healthy nails which run in families. Toenails, with the exception of the first ray, are broader than long. Size and shape of nails can be expressed in onychodiagrams (Pfister and Weirich, 1956).

The slow growth of nails makes them a repository of pathologic changes which were active as long as six months earlier. A hematoma produced by trauma to the matrix will move forward with the nail and disappear after five to six months. Transverse lines and depressions may be due to trauma or inflammation of the matrix region, but are usually the result of sudden systemic disease if they occur on several nails at the same time. These transverse grooves (Beau lines) (Fig. 2–21) are analogous to the Pohl-Pincus mark of the hair. Tiny pits are a diagnostic sign in psoriasis, and irregular depressions usually result from acute dermatitis. Severe injury of the nail matrix leads to permanent deformity of the nail, while trauma to the nail bed rarely affects the nail. Therefore, it is safe to take biopsies of the nail bed, but biopsy of the matrix should be done only if strictly necessary and then by a clean incision along the growth axis of the nail. Even then, it may lead to a longitudinal ridge or groove. Transplantation of nails has been achieved by excising and grafting the nail matrix. If a U-shaped portion of the matrix is left behind, it will restore a nail on the donor digit (Sheehan, 1929).

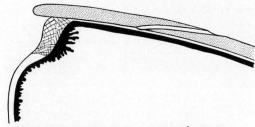

DISTAL END OF HUMAN NAIL WITH BEAU'S GROOVE

Figure 2–21   Diagram of the histomechanics of Beau groove. During an acute illness, an isochronous lamella of nail was poorly formed and has now moved forward. Its outer surface is eroded and becomes visible as a transverse depression.

Dimensions and Physical Properties

Dimensions. Skin surface is very large in comparison to thickness. The area for an average man usually is given as 1.8 m.², but thickness is only 0.3 to 8 mm. Inasmuch as direct measurements on the living are difficult or impossible, various formulas have been developed to determine skin surface area (*S*) from height (*H*) and weight (*W*). One of these, proposed by Schmitz (1954) as particularly accurate is

$$S = 0.8 \left[\frac{0.01\ W}{H} + 2 \times (0.01\ WH)^{0.5} \right]$$

A simple formula by the same author is

$$S = \frac{W}{6 \times 10} + \frac{6H}{10} - c$$

where $c = 0.1175$ for adults, and $c = 0.0893$ for children above three years.

Sendroy and Cecchini (1954) devised diagrams for the same purpose (Fig. 2-22). The surface area of individual body parts, highly important in burn cases and for transplantation surgery, usually is expressed by the rule of nine (Table 2-1). More accurate data, published by Skerlj

TABLE 2-1 BODY SURFACE: RULE OF NINE	
Head and neck	9%
Trunk, front	18%
Trunk, back	18%
Right upper extremity	9%
Left upper extremity	9%
Right lower extremity	18%
Left lower extremity	18%
Genitals	1%
Total	100%

(1957), are summarized in Table 2-2. The mean surface area of the hands was determined by Kirk (1966) as 503– 547 cm² in several groups of men, and as 414– 436 cm² in women.

Thickness of the skin has been measured by several authors in the living body as well as in cadavers. Some pertinent data are listed in Table 2-3. Thickness of the panniculus varies much more widely in different areas than does thickness of the skin proper. The propensity of certain regions to develop a thick adipose layer must be kept in mind in full-thickness transplants because the graft follows the rules of the donor site and may thicken more or less than the host site in later life. While adipose tissue, with the exception of the abdomen, develops fairly evenly in men, women have many predisposed sites, only some of which may become fat in any one individual (Fig. 2-23).

Weight and Specific Gravity. Published values for the weight of the average skin vary from 10 kg. to 3.5 kg., because some authors included more or less panniculus in their definitions of the integument. If we follow Leider's (1949) proposal to include that part of the subcutaneous tissue that envelops hair roots and sweat coils, we may use 4 kg., or 1/16 (6 percent) of the weight as a fair estimate for a 65 kg body. Specific gravity of whole skin is 1.10, that of nail is 1.30, and that of hair is 1.31 (Leider and Buncke, 1954).

Elasticity and other Physical Properties. The normal skin is elastic in the sense that it can be deformed by either compression or stretching and will return to its original condition when the force is released. On the living body, compression by a known weight is most easily measured. The response to stretching can be mea-

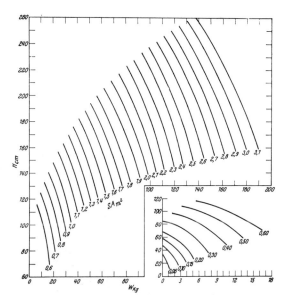

Figure 2-22 Diagrams for the determination of skin surface area (SA) from height and weight for adults and children. *(From Sendroy and Cecchini: J. Appl. Physiol., 7:1, 1954.)*

TABLE 2–2 RELATIVE SURFACE AREAS OF BODY REGIONS EXPRESSED AS A PERCENTAGE OF TOTAL BODY SURFACE[*]

Region	6–10 Years M	6–10 Years F	11–15 Years M	11–15 Years F	16–20 Years M	16–20 Years F	21–55 Years M	21–55 Years F
Head and neck	12.5	12.0	10.5	10.0	9.0	10.0	9.0	10.0
Trunk	26.5	25.5	26.0	25.5	26.0	25.5	26.5	26.0
Both upper arms	9.5	9.5	10.0	9.5	10.0	9.5	11.0	9.5
Both forearms and hands	13.0	13.0	13.0	13.0	14.5	13.0	14.5	13.0
Both thighs	20.0	20.0	20.5	22.0	20.5	22.0	20.0	21.5
Both lower legs and feet	18.5	20.0	20.0	20.0	20.0	20.0	19.0	20.0
Total	100.0	100.0	100.0	100.0	100.0	100.0	100.0	100.0

[*]Adapted from Skerlj, 1957.

TABLE 2–3 THICKNESS OF TOTAL SKIN, DERMIS, AND EPIDERMIS IN VARIOUS REGIONS[*]

Region	Entire Skin (μ)	Dermis (μ)	Epidermis (μ)
Scalp	—	722–1352	45– 90
Face	750–2950	1411–2271	52
Forehead	940–1702	—	74– 94
Cheek	—	611	52– 117
Eyelid	330– 700	625	54
Tip of nose	—	—	85– 101
Upper lip	—	—	66– 91
Retroauricular	558– 686	—	53– 91
Chin	—	—	65– 93
Neck	762–1850	—	45– 103
Axilla	—	466–1296	39– 123
Upper arm, extensor	—	—	78– 129
Upper arm, flexor	—	—	80– 166
Upper arm, medial	635–1300	496–1275	30– 137
Upper arm, lateral	762–2600	464–1843	23– 94
Forearm, extensor	—	—	74– 142
Forearm, flexor	—	—	68– 120
Forearm, medial	559–1400	551–1248	29– 85
Forearm, lateral	800	681–1234	37– 88
Hand, dorsal	850	—	157– 246
Finger, volar	—	894–1326	330– 539
Palm	—	—	205– 334
Chest	762–1350	536–1960	25– 77
Abdomen	762–2050	301–1933	23– 125
Pubes	—	826–1107	37– 55
Back	1524–2600	527–2492	22– 116
Buttocks	3100	—	77– 119
Scrotum	—	—	64– 137
Thigh, extensor	889–1850	—	78– 122
Thigh, flexor	1016–1900	863–1314	33– 114
Thigh, medial	737–2250	510–1369	18– 114
Thigh, lateral	940–1850	561–1802	27– 112
Lower leg, extensor	—	647–1118	53– 161
Lower leg, flexor	1500	506–1565	24– 175
Lower leg, medial	—	505–1634	23– 113
Lower leg, lateral	—	440–1573	42– 80
Foot, dorsal	—	—	150– 243
Toe, tip	—	—	454– 698
Sole	—	867–1805	529–1377

[*]Adapted from Pinkus (1964) with additional data from Odagiri (1969).

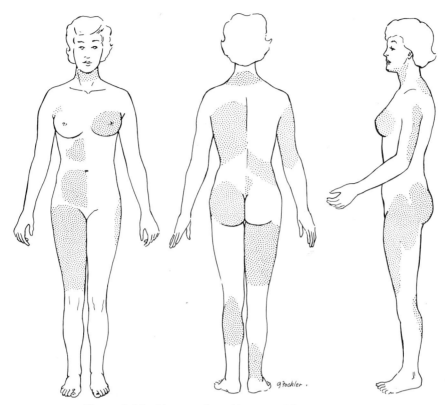

Figure 2–23 Diagram of specific areas of female obesity.

sured on strips of excised skin (Jansen and Rottier, 1957). Available methods and their advantages and disadvantages were reviewed by Keller (1963a). The fine structural basis for the skin's mechanical properties is discussed on page 65.

When pressure is applied to a circumscribed area of normal skin and is quickly released, the deformity will disappear immediately, and we measure purely physical phenomena. If pressure is maintained for several minutes, part of the deformation will be restored more slowly because physiologic factors such as displacement of tissue fluid and blood enter the picture. These phenomena are accentuated in edematous skin and under other pathologic conditions. Similarly, quick and slow stretching of the skin will give different results, because the weave of the collagen bundles can be altered with time. Under pathologic conditons, when skin is stretched very gradually by underlying adiposity or slow-growing tumors, still

other factors, either atrophy or reactive growth, complicate the picture. It has been shown clearly that the so-called stretch marks (striae distensae) are caused mainly by hormonal influences, e.g., in pregnancy, in Cushing's syndrome, and in stressful situations, which weaken the elastic fibers; the direction of the stria is determined by the direction of the stretching force (Pinkus et al., 1966). Any portion of the skin is more easily stretched in one direction than in others. This is due to the preferential arrangement of collagen bundles and elastic fibers in the reticular dermis and is expressed in the Langer lines of cleavage.

Other physical properties of skin are its electrical resistance and its barrier function with respect to absorption of water-soluble and lipid-soluble substances. These, however, need not be discussed here. Recent reviews are those of Keller (1963b) and Malkinson and Rothman (1963).

Topographical Differences

There are more profound differences between scalp and palm than the obvious presence or absence of hair. Differences between other parts of the skin (Fig. 2–42) may be more subtle but are very real and have to be known to physicians dealing with skin cancer in diagnosis as well as in therapy. Some data have already been given. Additional features are the following:

Hair. Topographical differences of size and shape of hair have already been discussed. Another regional characteristic of hair is its slant (Fig. 2–24), which produces hair streams, whorls, and crosses. The head of most individuals carries one whorl; 6 to 10 percent of people have two. Clockwise rotation is four times as common as is counterclockwise rotation, and the vertex is more often on the right side than on the left. Frontal scalp hair is directed toward the forehead, and this direction usually continues down to the eyebrows (44 percent in Caucasians). If, however, forehead hair is slanted upward (Fig. 2–25), the so-called cowlick results (28 percent). In another 28 percent of persons hairs grow downward on one side of the forehead, upward on the other. The inheritance of these features was investigated by Kiil (1948). More or less constant whorls and crosses are found on the trunk and extremities and are listed as follows according to Ludwig (1921): 9 points of divergence – 1 vertex, 2 eye centers, 4 ear centers, and 2 trunk centers; 12 points of convergence – 2 ear whorls, 1 umbilical whorl, 1 penis whorl, 1 scrotal whorl, 1 rump whorl, 2 elbow whorls, 2 hand convergences, and 2 foot convergences; 19 crosses – 1 frontal, 1 nasal, 4 anal, 2 preauricular, 1 cervical, 1 thoracic, 1 abdominal, 1 penile, 1 coccygeal, 2 scapular, 2 ulnar, and 2 patellar.

Although hair follicles are formed at fairly even intervals all over the body surface in the fetus, they are later thinned out by the uneven growth of the body regions. Thus, in the adult, according to Szabo (1958), the numbers of pilar apparatuses per unit area on head, trunk, arm, and leg have a relation of 58:16:15:11. Absolute figures were collected mainly by Japanese authors (Pinkus, 1964). A few are listed in Table 2–4. These differences explain in part the poorer healing tendency of denuded areas on the lower extremities, inasmuch as hair roots contribute greatly to the reepithelialization of wounds. Cosmetic planing of skin has better results on the face because the number of follicles (and sweat ducts) is so large that complete loss of the epidermis is restored within a few days before the dermis has occasion to form appreciable amounts of granulation tissue. Since hair follicles are also a source for repigmentation of the epidermis, their relative number influences the chances for return of normal skin color in large superficial burns, in donor sites of split skin grafts, and in vitiligo.

Sebaceous Glands. Sebaceous glands are rarely obvious on gross inspection except in a few regions. These include the shaft of the penis, the scrotum, the labia minora, the mouth, and the neck and supraclavicular region, especially in women where sebaceous glands may be seen as rows of tiny papules. The glands are usually associated with hair follicles and therefore are absent on palms,

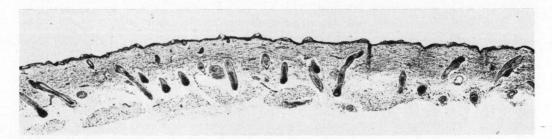

Figure 2–24 Fetal skin of trunk in the area of hair divergence. The reversal of follicle slant is clearly seen. *H & E*, ×9. (*From* Pinkus: Embryology of hair. *In* Montagna and Ellis (Eds.): The Biology of Hair Growth. New York, Academic Press, Inc., 1958.)

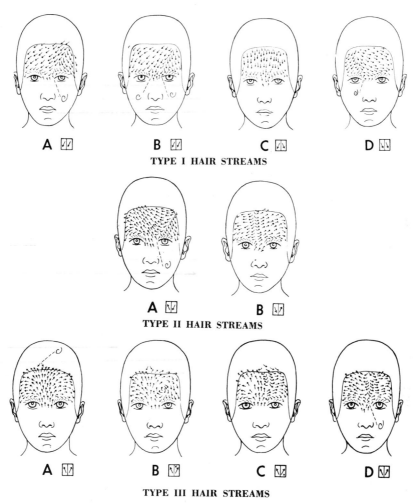

A ⊡ B ⊡ C ⊡ D ⊡

TYPE I HAIR STREAMS

A ⊡ B ⊡

TYPE II HAIR STREAMS

A ⊡ B ⊡ C ⊡ D ⊡

TYPE III HAIR STREAMS

Figure 2–25 Diagrams of the direction of frontal hair. Persons of type III have the so-called cowlick if the streams of forehead and scalp meet above the frontal scalp hair line. (Reprinted with permission from the *Journal of Heredity* 39:206–216, 1948. Copyright 1948, by the American Genetic Association.)

soles, and the adjacent portions of truly glabrous skin. They do, however, occur by themselves on the lips, the oral mucosa (Fordyce bodies), the labia minora, and the inner aspect of the labia majora. They have been found a few times on the tongue (Guiducci and Hyman, 1962). With these exceptions, the number of sebaceous glands should be proportional to the number of hair follicles. However, while pilosebaceous units usually have only one gland, they may have several, and this is particularly true for those regions where individual glands are large. The amount of sebaceous epithelium therefore shows tremendous topical differences, being largest on the central parts of the

face and smallest on the dorsum of hands and feet. Actual size of individual sebaceous glands varies from 0.0005 mm.³ to more than 1 mm³. On the nose and adjoining parts of the face they may occupy almost 30 percent of the volume of the skin (Figs. 2–48 and 2–49).

Apocrine Glands. The distribution of apocrine glands is much more restricted in man than in other mammals, but they reach appreciable size (Fig. 2–42C) in those regions where they are concentrated (Fig. 2–26). The armpit contains a solid aggregate of apocrine glands that has been called an axillary organ (Montagna, 1959), and glands are diffusely present in the genitoanal region. From there, they ex-

TABLE 2–4   NUMBER OF HAIR GROUPS PER CM² °

Region	Adults	Children
Forehead	320–846	541–1061
Vertex	236–504	270– 775
Occiput	289–626	–
Cheek	880	–
Neck	86	–
Chest	45– 87	50– 402
Abdomen	36– 65	12– 196
Back	54–108	87– 461
Buttocks	78–115	55– 488
Upper arm	37–119	54– 392
Forearm	39–104	66– 418
Thigh	42– 97	55– 447
Lower leg	38– 79	42– 281

*Adapted from Pinkus (1964).

tend in decreasing number to the lower abdomen and are potentially present in the apocrine triangle formed by the two axillae and the pubic region. Some may be found more laterally, but the back of the trunk and the distal parts of the extremities may be considered as regions free of apocrine glands. Most people, on the other hand, have some apocrine glands on the neck, face, and scalp, and specialized apocrine glands are present regularly on the eyelids (glands of Moll) and in the ear canals (ceruminous glands).

Apocrine secretion usually is turbid or milky but may be yellow, red, green, or bluish-black (chromhidrosis). The amount of fluid produced by apocrine glands is small and gradually fills the wide lumina until it is excreted by myoepithelial contraction. Containing protein and other organic substances, it becomes odorous through bacterial action. On the other hand, the profuse sweat arising in the axillae is the product of eccrine glands.

Eccrine Glands. Eccrine glands are the true sweat glands of man. In most other mammals they are restricted to the foot pads; only the great apes show a wider distribution. In the human skin, eccrine glands are present everywhere except in the ear canal, the glans penis, and the

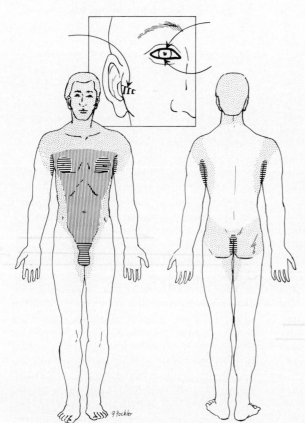

Figure 2–26 Diagram of apocrine gland distribution. Horizontal bars indicate areas of apocrine gland concentration. Vertical bars indicate the "apocrine triangle," in which accessory mammae also are found most frequently. Dots indicate areas in which a few apocrine glands normally occur. The eyelids and the external ear canal regularly have apocrine glands.

TABLE 2–5 NUMBER OF SWEAT DUCTS PER CM² *

Region	Adults	Children
Forehead	212–424	399–1083
Scalp	115–369	453–1056
Cheek	55–320	260– 870
Neck	124–169	333–1193
Chest	121–175	271–1018
Abdomen	93–220	245– 816
Back	75–388	381–1370
Buttocks	153–533	446–1812
Upper arm	110–335	433–1989
Forearm	123–280	502–2113
Hand, dorsal	287–350	837–1950
Palm	630	910–2890
Thigh	120–489	435–2113
Lower leg	145–273	534–2321
Foot, dorsal	250	690–4140
Sole	620	1000–4140

*Adapted from Pinkus (1964).

labia. Size and number vary somewhat (Table 2–5) and reach a maximum on palms and soles. Face and scalp also are richly endowed. On the trunk they are more prominent near the midline of the body; on the extremities they increase distally. Mucous and semimucous membranes have no eccrine glands.

Mucinous Glands. Mucin-producing cells are present in conjunctival epithelium and in organized glands in the nasal and oral mucosa. The latter also contains serous glands (minor salivary glands).

Horny Layer. The thickness and consistency of the protective outer coat of the skin varies considerably from place to place (Fig. 2–42), but exact data are difficult to come by. Simple inspection of vertical sections shows that the stratum corneum is thin on the scalp and face, and thicker on the trunk and extremities. It not only increases in thickness toward the hands and feet, but also appears more compact. The horny layer of the palms and, even more so, of the soles is 10 to 20 times as thick as that of the general body surface and usually exceeds the thickness of the living portion of the epidermis. A method for counting keratinized cells was first developed by Pinkus and his associates (Hunter et al., 1956), who reported values between 500,000 and 1,200,000 per cm.² on the shoulder and the flexor surface of the forearm. More recent work with other

methods was done by McGinley et al. (1969), who were interested in counting only the desquamating dehiscent portion of the horny layer. They found a mean of 82,000 cells per cm.² on the forehead, 187,000 on the arm, 218,000 on the abdomen, and 319,000 on the heel. Pinkus (1951b) estimated the number of horny layers on the forearm as 20 to 30 on the basis of tape-stripping experiments. Goldschmidt and Kligman (1963) described a method to count horny layers in tissue sections. Other details are discussed later in this chapter.

Pigmentation and Other Color Differences. Major topographical differences of pigmentation are due to differences in sun exposure, not only in Caucasian skin but also in the more deeply pigmented races. In addition, there are zones of inherited pigmentary tendency, which are influenced by hormonal action. These are mainly the mamilla and its areola, the midabdominal linea nigra, and the genital skin. Garn et al. (1965) reported that reflectance of the female areola (measured at 480 mμ) is reduced from about 15 percent to about 8 percent in pregnancy, and that a relative decrease of 20 percent is a rather reliable indication of pregnancy. Lines of pigment demarcation have been described mainly in Japan, but are perhaps even more common among not too darkly skinned Negroes. The most common one (Fig. 2–27) extends along the lateral surface of the arm, the dorsal skin being darker than the ventral skin. Similar lines occur on the thighs and chest (Fig. 2–28).

Other color differences are due to increased vascularity, red cheeks being the outstanding example. The red color of the lip vermilion is partly due to rich vascularity, partly to absence of the diffusing keratohyalin layer of the epithelium. When the latter becomes more epidermis-like in older age, and especially under actinic influence, the lips become pale.

Matching of skin coloration is one of the most difficult tasks in skin transplantation, and all factors must be taken into consideration. In addition, there is the danger that a matching flap may later change color owing to increase or decrease of vascularity.

root system. One therefore speaks of "systemized" nevus, and so forth.

There are indeed several "linear" systematizations in the skin. Hair streams, which are the expression of fetal growth directions, were mentioned previously. General distribution of blood vessels is influenced by the segmental arteries springing from the fetal aorta. The course of peripheral nerves constitutes another systematized pattern. Two additional systems of lines, commonly known as Langer lines (cleavage lines) and Voigt lines, warrant discussion.

Langer lines, named after a nineteenth century surgeon, remain of great importance to surgeons since these lines determine the best position of incisions. They were originally determined by piercing the skin of a cadaver with a sharp round instrument. On withdrawal, the round puncture will be seen to look like a slit. By making additional punctures at the ends

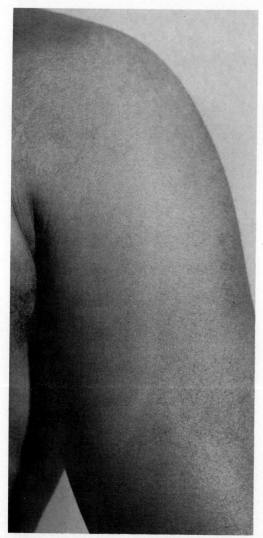

Figure 2–27 Pigment demarcation line on left upper arm of an American Negro (Courtesy Dr. Robert Heidelberg.)

Systematizations. Some skin diseases follow linear patterns which have a degree of similarity in different patients. The best known linear dermatosis is zoster, and there is no doubt that the eruption is related to the nervous system and follows the distribution of sensory nerve roots. In other cases, such as lichen striatus, incontinentia pigmenti, linear Darier disease, and linear nevi, the factors determining localization are less clear. One suspects, however, that innate differences in the skin are responsible and are caused by the distribution of systems other than the nerve

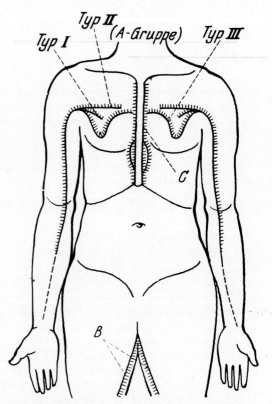

Figure 2–28 Diagram of pigment demarcation lines in Japanese. (*From* Miura: Tohoku J. Exp. Med., 54:135, 1951.)

of the slit, one can develop a system of lines which mark the prevalent direction of collagen bundles and elastic fibers. Surgical incisions made along cleavage lines will transect a minimal number of fibers and will heal with less disfigurement than incisions deviating from the lines. Diagrams like those shown in Figs. 2–29 and 2–30 can be prepared because the lines have a similar course in most adults. They change, however, during fetal development and have modified direction in the newborn and in early childhood. Langer lines can be determined on the living patient by stretching or lifting the skin. It stretches more easily perpendicular to the lines than parallel to them. On the face, wrinkle lines (Fig. 2–13) usually take the place of Langer lines in guiding the surgeon's knife for best cosmetic results.

Voigt lines are boundary lines between areas of distribution of segmental nerves (Figs. 2–29 and 2–30). They seem to represent loci of biologic fragility in the skin and correspond most closely to the distribution of many linear "systematized" dermatoses, including the pigment demarcation lines mentioned on page 44.

Differences of Age, Sex, and Race

The skin of the child undergoes gradual changes (Kantner, 1968) which concern its thickness, hairiness, and texture. The first two factors are readily discernible and measurable; the third is more difficult. Changes in texture are at least in part due to subtle changes in the solubility of the fibrous proteins of the dermis, the increasing thickness of collagen bundles, the changing ratio of elastic and collagen fibers, the rearrangement of fat tissue, and other even less well defined factors (Cerimele and Serri, 1969). It may sound surprising, but it is undoubtedly true that sebaceous glands are practically nonfunctional in prepuberal skin after the newborn period. Apocrine glands also either are not fully developed or are non functional.

Later, many of the changes generally attributed to age are really due to reaction of the skin to external influences (see Chap.

17). The covered skin of the body changes relatively little with age except when it becomes truly senile and atrophic. Progressive rise of the module of elasticity with age was demonstrated with a suction cup method by Grahame and Holt (1969), but the module was low in the "transparent skin" of senile individuals.

Hormonal influences on the skin, especially the differential action of male and female sex hormones, are well known. Effects on hair growth are particularly obvious and are mainly responsible for the "feminine" or "masculine" appearance of an individual's skin. Texture, however, also is important, and the peculiarly soft and smooth skin of some men having hepatic cirrhosis probably is due to excess of female steroid hormones.

Genetic differences (Becker, 1968) range from very striking ones between the major races to subtle characteristics inherited in families. Pigmentation of the epidermis and the shape, color, and distribution of hair are the most obvious ones, but many other features of the skin are also inherited. Characteristics of dermatoglyphics are a favorite subject of geneticists (Holt, 1968) and anthropologists. A conspicuous racial character is the blue sacral spot of newborn children (Pinkus, 1964; Uribe, 1970), which was called the Mongolian Spot because it is found in almost all babies of the Oriental race. Further investigation, however, has shown that it is an almost universal feature of mankind to have functional dermal melanocytes in the lower dorsal region at birth. The color does not usually show in fair-skinned children but is found in 3 to 15 percent of children in Southern Europe. The blue tinge may be overshadowed in dark Negroes by epidermal pigment but is present in more than 80 percent of infants and may be so extensive that almost the entire back is involved. Another area of inherited dermal pigmentation which is of considerable cosmetic significance is the periocular umbra (Goodman and Belcher, 1969), which may persist even in cases of universal vitiligo (personal observation).

There is little doubt about the racial prevalence of a tendency to form keloids, but I know of no systematic study. Among surgeons, this observation has led to a

(*Text continued on page 48.*)

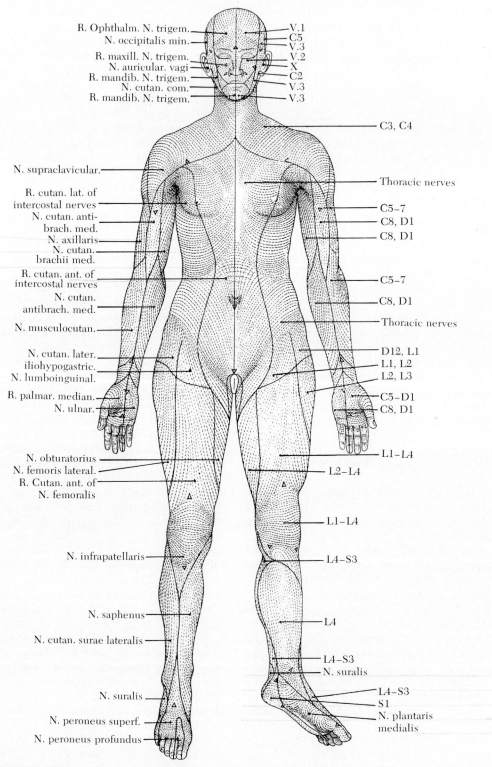

R. Ophthalm. N. trigem. — V.1
N. occipitalis min. — C5
— V.3
R. maxill. N. trigem. — V.2
N. auricular. vagi — X
R. mandib. N. trigem. — C2
N. cutan. com. — V.3
R. mandib. N. trigem. — V.3

— C3, C4

N. supraclavicular. — Thoracic nerves

R. cutan. lat. of intercostal nerves — C5–7
N. cutan. anti-brach. med. — C8, D1
N. axillaris — C8, D1
N. cutan. brachii med.
R. cutan. ant. of intercostal nerves — C5–7
N. cutan. antibrach. med. — C8, D1
N. musculocutan. — Thoracic nerves

N. cutan. later. iliohypogastric. — D12, L1
N. lumboinguinal. — L1, L2
— L2, L3
R. palmar. median. — C5–D1
N. ulnar. — C8, D1

— L1–L4

N. obturatorius — L2–L4
N. femoris lateral.
R. Cutan. ant. of N. femoralis

— L1–L4

N. infrapatellaris — L4–S3

N. saphenus — L4

N. cutan. surae lateralis — L4–S3
— N. suralis

— L4–S3
— S1
N. suralis — N. plantaris medialis
N. peroneus superf.
N. peroneus profundus

Figure 2–29 Diagram of Langer cleavage lines, peripheral sensory nerves, and dorsal nerve roots on anterior body surface.

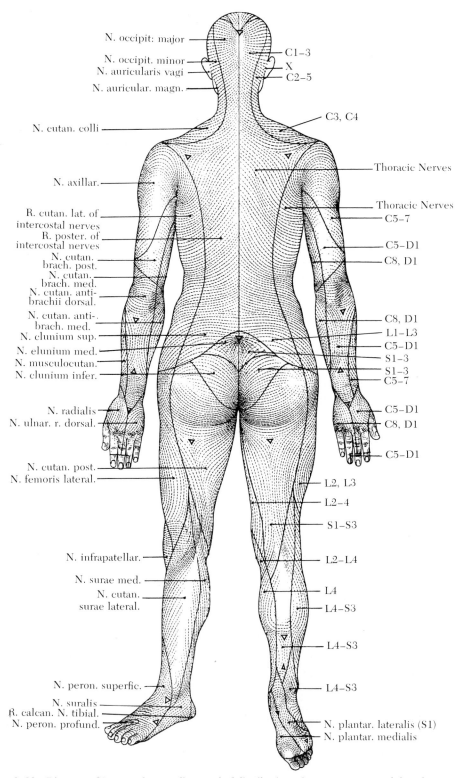

N. occipit: major

N. occipit. minor
N. auricularis vagi
N. auricular. magn.

N. cutan. colli

N. axillar.

R. cutan. lat. of
intercostal nerves
R. poster. of
intercostal nerves
N. cutan.
brach. post.
N. cutan.
brach. med.
N. cutan. anti-
brachii dorsal.
N. cutan. anti-
brach. med.
N. clunium sup.
N. elunium med.
N. musculocutan.
N. clunium infer.

N. radialis
N. ulnar. r. dorsal.

N. cutan. post.
N. femoris lateral.

N. infrapatellar.

N. surae med.
N. cutan.
surae lateral.

N. peron. superfic.

N. suralis
R. calcan. N. tibial.
N. peron. profund.

C1–3
X
C2–5

C3, C4

Thoracic Nerves

Thoracic Nerves
C5–7

C5–D1
C8, D1

C8, D1
L1–L3
C5–D1
S1–3
S1–3
C5–7

C5–D1
C8, D1

C5–D1

L2, L3

L2–4

S1–S3

L2–L4

L4

L4–S3

L4–S3

L4–S3

N. plantar. lateralis (S1)
N. plantar. medialis

Figure 2–30 Diagram of Langer cleavage lines and of distribution of sensory nerves and dorsal root segments on posterior body surface.

hypothesis of general "fibroplastic" tendency in Negroes.

Peculiar racial differences in apocrine glands will be mentioned later in this chapter.

Specialized Regions

Some relatively small areas of the body surface are distinct from their surroundings in specific ways, which include embryologic development, macroscopic features, and histologic details, usually in adaptation to specific functions. Although some of their features have been mentioned on preceding pages and others will be discussed in the microscopic portion of this chapter, it seems best to consider these regions as individual units. They comprise the eyelids, eyebrows, nose, external ear, lips, axillae, areola and nipple, umbilicus, anal and genital parts, and distal portions of the extremities.

Facial Features. Facial skin (Figs. 2–48 and 2–49) is more highly specialized than other regions partly because it is closely associated with underlying bones, cartilage, and striated muscle, and partly because it surrounds and molds the openings of eyes, ears, nose, and mouth. In addition, it presents esthetically significant differences of hairiness.

Eyelids. The eyelids develop as folds of the orbital skin and grow from above and below over that part of the skin which is destined to become cornea and conjunctiva. Between the fourth and sixth fetal months, the lids are joined by an epithelial bridge (Fig. 2–31). During this time the lashes develop near the outer rim and the meibomian glands develop near the inner rim. The lids separate again before birth. Nevus cells developing in the epidermis while the lids are joined give rise to a split nevus, one-half of which is in the upper lid, the other half in the lower lid (Harrison and Okun, 1960).

The lids enclose the elastic cartilaginous plates called tarsi, which harbor the meibomian glands, and the musculus orbicularis oculi. They are lined by the mucin-producing stratified epithelium of the conjunctiva on the inside and by thin epidermis on the outside. Eyelashes (cilia) protrude from the external rim and usually form a row of parallel, slightly curved fibers, but occasionally they grow in irregular bushy fashion (Pinkus, 1964). Details of the special-

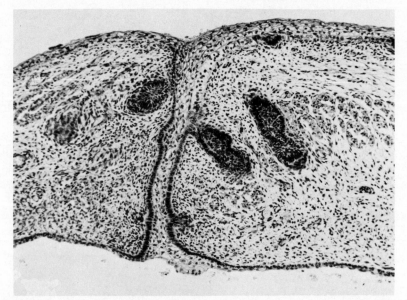

Figure 2–31   Fetal lids during the period of epithelial junction. Upper lid on right shows the development of two eyelash follicles and the bud of a meibomian gland near the bulbar surface. Another eyelash follicle is visible in the lower lid.

ized histology of the lids were recently investigated by Montagna and Ford (1969). The skin, epidermis as well as dermis, is probably the thinnest of the entire body. It gradually merges into the similarly thin orbital skin, which in turn is fairly suddenly replaced by much thicker integument at the rim of the orbit. The orbital skin, especially that below the eyes, often contains dermal melanocytes of varying degrees of activity. These produce the periocular umbra, especially in brunet Caucasians. In addition, differences of filling of blood vessels and accumulation of tissue fluid can cause rapidly changing bagginess of the orbital skin in conditions as varied as tiredness, postalcoholic hangover, and renal failure. Thickening of the lower orbital skin also is characteristic of atopic children (Morgan line).

EYEBROWS. The upper rim of the orbit carries hairy skin with many specialized features. Human eyebrow hairs (supercilia, ophrya) grow in a place characterized by sensory vibrissae in many animals. While man has no true vibrissae (although intranasal hairs go by that name), eyebrow follicles are richly vascularized and innervated (Montagna, 1970a). The hairs have arrector muscles. Eccrine glands, on the other hand, are sparse or absent, a feature that one may link with the function of the eyebrows to keep forehead sweat from flowing toward the eyes. The area occupied by eyebrows, and the profusion and length of the eyebrows vary considerably, and these features have always been of considerable esthetic significance. Whether they are too weak or too strong, they are often tampered with by both sexes. Complete surgical obliteration of eyebrows is a cosmetic defect that should be avoided and may have to be corrected by transplantation of scalp. One should also keep in mind that shaved eyebrows may not regrow for many months. Loss of the lateral portion is seen in thyroid deficiency and leprosy, but is not diagnostic of these diseases. Spotty loss of eyebrows and eyelashes used to be a diagnostic sign of secondary syphilis. In porphyria cutanea tarda, the region between lateral eyebrows and temporal scalp may become so hypertrichotic that both seem to merge. Merging of the eyebrows medially across the glabella is a genetically determined feature (synophrys).

NOSE. The skin of the nose adheres tightly to underlying bone and cartilage and allows little leeway for closure of excisional wounds. It is full of large sebaceous glands, which may occupy considerably more than 50 percent of its volume. Therefore, electrosurgical destruction of actinic keratoses or small skin cancers may leave cosmetically undesirable deep depressions because destroyed sebaceous glands are rarely regenerated. On the other hand, nasal skin usually carries no visible hairs, except in some men in old age. The pores of the pilosebaceous canals vary greatly in size on an inherited basis, and generally tend to become more prominent with age. Large-pored skin of the nose and adjoining central parts of the face is cosmetically undesirable to many women, but no effective remedy is available except heavy make-up. Progressive enlargement of sebaceous glands with age, especially in association with rosacea, leads to bulbous thickening of the nose and to rhinophyma. A rare congenital malformation is a median fistula from which hairs may protrude or which may give rise to abscesses (Johnson, 1969). They may extend quite deep because they are usually connected with dermoid cysts located below the nasal bones (Brownstein et al., 1974).

The nasal cavity is lined with hair-bearing skin for some distance. The size of the nasal vibrissae increases with age and is much more pronounced in men. Inept cosmetic removal of the hairs often leads to acute or chronic inflammation, but one should not forget that benign and malignant skin tumors may develop in the vestibulum nasi.

EXTERNAL EAR. The external ear canal including the eardrum is lined by highly specialized skin and is surrounded by the concha with its intricately folded elastic cartilage and integument. The skin of the ear canal (Perry, 1957) possesses pilosebaceous units and specialized apocrine (ceruminous) glands but no eccrine glands in its bony portion. The stratum corneum formed by the epidermal covering of the eardrum moves outward from the center, perhaps by a mechanism based on the progressive increase of cellular diameter as the cells are transformed from basal cells into horny cells. This movement assures a degree of self-cleaning under normal circumstances.

The skin of the concha adheres tightly to the concave side of the cartilage, while the external side has a fair amount of mobility due to the presence of fat tissue. Both sides carry numerous small pilosebaceous and eccrine apparatuses, and surgical defects not involving the perichondrium will heal by granulation fairly readily if they cannot be sutured. In excisional surgery, one should avoid stretching the skin too tightly over the cartilage and, rather, should excise a corresponding portion of the cartilage. It is, however, surprising how difficult it is to persuade patients to undergo a mutilation of the ear, and cosmetically acceptable results should be strived for without sacrificing thoroughness in cancer surgery.

A not too infrequent minor malformation are sinuses or appendages in front of the external ear (Pinkus, 1964). These are often associated with deeply situated fragments of ear cartilage. Protruding appendages of this type sometimes are called supernumerary auricles and may be mis-

taken for moles or neoplasms. Fistulas may be the site of chronic infection. In a personally observed case, basal cell epithelioma had developed in the wall of the sinus in a 24 year old man.

LIPS.   The lips are highly motile muscular folds covered by hair-bearing skin on the outside and by gland-bearing mucosa with stratified epithelium on the buccal side. In between there is a zone called the vermilion, which is covered by stratified keratinizing epithelium and which may bear free sebaceous glands, but which has no hairs or other glands. The relative absence of keratohyalin over a richly vascularized membrana propria explains the characteristic redness of youthful lips. Later in life, under actinic exposure, the granular layer thickens and produces pale lips. Actinic elastosis adds a yellow tinge. The border between vermilion and skin is absolutely sharp, and must be lined up carefully in suturing surgical defects. On the other hand, large portions of the lower lip can be excised with surprisingly little cosmetic defect, either by vermilionectomy or by wedge or block excision of as much as 40 percent of the lip.

Peculiar developmental defects of the lips are fistulas, which may occur near the midline or near the corners of the mouth and are often symmetrical (Pinkus, 1964,

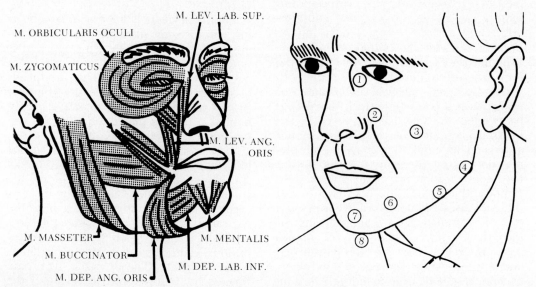

Figure 2–32   Distribution of facial muscles and sites of dental fistulas according to Vriezen. (*From* Ned. Tijdschr. Geneeskd., 112:65, 1968.)

McConnel et al., 1970). Acquired inflammatory sinuses in the lip region usually are of dental abscess origin and may occur in surprising locations (Fig. 2–32) (Vriezen, 1968).

Special Areas of the Trunk. Specialized skin is found in the axillae, the nipple region, the umbilicus, and the genitoanal area.

AXILLA. The armpit has a fairly sharply defined oval area bearing strong hairs (hirci). Its size is proportionately similar in men and women (Gloor-Rutishauser, 1953) and is associated with large apocrine glands (Fig. 2–42C) forming a veritable "organ" (Montagna, 1959). The hairs develop in puberty but may rarely be absent on a hereditary basis. They may get weaker but they do not disappear in old age. Apocrine glands also usually do not mature until puberty and persist in old age to varying degree. Eccrine glands are well developed and are the producers of profuse axillary sweat, while apocrine glands contribute only small quantities of a turbid, milky, or colored fluid, which is easily dissociated (Shelley et al., 1953) into smelly compounds by bacterial growth. Axillary hyperhidrosis can be ameliorated surgically by excising a relatively small central area with a fusiform incision (Hurley and Shelley, 1963), while excision of the axillary organ for bromhidrosis requires removal of the entire hair-bearing area (Takami, 1960).

NIPPLE AND AREOLA. Embryonic development of the skin region related to the mamma is similar in both sexes and forms the knob-like central nipple (mamilla) and a surrounding halo which contains many smooth muscles but barely any glands or hairs except a peripheral ring of specialized apocrine glands, which are the basis of the Montgomery tubercles (Montagna, 1970b). The epidermis of nipple and areola usually is more deeply pigmented than the surrounding skin, but may be prominently pink in light-skinned individuals.

The man's nipple and areola resemble those of the child, except that the mamilla becomes somewhat larger and erectile. The average diameter of the areola increases from 13.1 ± 0.7 mm. in 9 and 10 year old boys to 21.5 ± 1.2 mm. in 17 to 20 year old young men (Garn, 1952).

The diameter of the areola in females increases from 11.9 ± 0.7 mm. at 9 and 10 years to 33.1 ± 2.2 mm. in sexually mature girls (Garn, 1952). The erectile mamilla assumes cylindrical shape in normal development but may become long and pendulous in older women, or it may not protrude at all or may be inverted. Final growth often is not achieved until pregnancy, when even inverted nipples may take on a functional shape (Hytten and Baird, 1958). Based on the regular presence of hair germs in fetal development, occasional hairs may grow from the center of the female mamilla as well as from Montgomery tubercles. Free sebaceous glands and apocrine sweat glands are more commonly associated with the lactiferous ducts.

Supernumerary nipples occur in men and women. Their expression may vary from a single hair or a tiny pigmented spot to full development of a functioning mamma and all its cutaneous accessory structures. F. Pinkus (1927) reported an 8.24 percent incidence in men and a 7.1 percent incidence in nonpregnant women. More recent statistics also show that hyperthelia is slightly more common in men (1.9 to 4.3 percent) than in women (1.2 to 3.6 percent) and occurs more often on the left side of the body. Hirasawa (1932) reported the very high incidence of 15.0 percent in Japanese lactating mothers. The number in any one individual may vary from one to four. Mammary tissue is more frequently associated above than below the breast. Accessory nipples and mammae usually are located along the fetal mammary line from the axilla to the labia majora but have been reported in such unusual sites as the nape of the neck, the nasofrontal region, the flexor surface of the wrist, and the posterior deltoid region.

UMBILICUS. The navel may vary from the usual wrinkled pit to a protruding nodule. It should be remembered that some patients consider removal or obliteration of the umbilicus as mutilation. The skin of the umbilicus itself is usually free of cutaneous adnexa, but may contain remnants of the structures which are related to it in fetal life: the urachus and Meckel's diverticulum of the gut. It can also become the seat of Paget's disease derived from these

epithelial sources, or of metastatic adenocarcinoma extending along the ligamen-
tum teres. Occasionally, pigmented
cellular nevi develop in the navel.

ANOGENITAL REGION. Perianal skin is
separated from rectal mucosa by a ring of
anal mucosa which is derived from the
cloacal membrane. Details of this region
can be left to proctologic treatises. Similarly, the anatomy of the female genitalia is
detailed in many gynecologic books, for instance, the volume by Gardner and Kaufman (1969).

The skin of the male parts is generally
thin and stretchable. That of the scrotum
owes its rugosity to a layer of smooth muscle, the tunica dartos, and bears some pilosebaceous complexes. These also are
found to some extent on the proximal part
of the shaft of the penis, while the distal
part has only a few free sebaceous glands.
The skin of the glans usually is completely
free of adnexa except for the frequent formation of paraurethral sinuses lateral to
the frenulum. The "glands" bearing Tyson's name (Hyman and Brownstein,
1969) are simply papillary protrusions
(Fig. 2–33*A*), which may be so numerous
and large (Winer and Winer, 1955) that
they give rise to "hirsuties penis" (Fig. 2–
33*B*). From the frenulum, a pigmented

line or ridge, the raphe, extends along the
ventral surface of the penis and the midline of the scrotum to the ventral rim of
the anus. The raphe may be the seat of
epithelium-lined sinuses.

The epidermis of male and female genitalia usually is not only more pigmented
than the surrounding skin but also contains an unusually high number of melanocytes per square centimeter. The epidermis of the scrotum is much more
permeable to many chemicals than the rest
of the skin surface, a fact that must be
taken into account in surgical practice.

The skin surrounding the genitalia
bears many strong hairs (pubes) which are
under the control of sex hormones. In addition, the perigenital and perianal skin
contains variable numbers of apocrine
glands. While these, according to Kling-
man and Shehadeh (1964), do not produce
a smelly secretion, they may become the
seat of chronic purulent infection (hidradenitis suppurativa), often in combination
with similar involvement of axillary glands.
The great chronicity of this process may
lead to establishment of deep epithelialized sinuses and even cutaneoanal fistulas,
and may be the occasional source of squamous cell carcinoma.

Well known to surgeons is the pilonidal

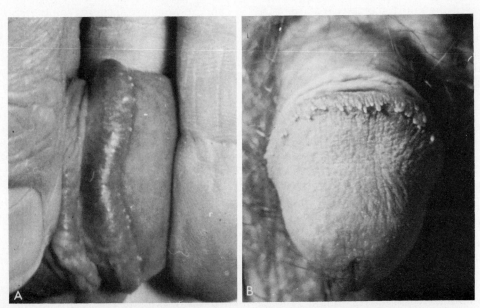

Figure 2–33 *A,* Tyson "glands" of corona glandis penis. *B,* Papillomatosis ("hirsuties") penis. (Courtesy Dr.
Louis Winer.)

sinus which develops in the anal cleft on a congenital basis, presumably through the deposition of extraneous hair and foreign body inflammation complicated by infection.

Distal Portions of the Extremities. Hands and feet have highly specialized ridged skin on their volar surfaces (Fig. 2–42*B*) and peculiar hairless skin (Fig. 2–12) on the knuckles and around the nails. Dermatoglyphic characteristics of the volar skin and their significance in genetics and other areas have been mentioned previously. The pattern of palmar flexor creases has attracted the attention of soothsayers more than that of the medical profession. The presence of a single four-finger line (monkey line, simian crease), however, has assumed significance in the diagnosis of Down's syndrome, and other variations may have significance in other congenital disease states (Alter, 1970).

Pale color of the creases is a bedside sign of severe anemia.

It is important to keep in mind that horny layer and epidermis are much thicker on the palmar and plantar surfaces, and that the texture of the underlying dermis is much more rigid than in any other area. Beneath the skin are fat pads traversed by tough connective septa (retinacula), which bind the dermis to the fascia and influence the spread of infections. Acrosclerosis causes the pads on the distal phalanges to become atrophic. The number and size of eccrine glands are exceptional, while elements of the pilar apparatus are absent. Eccrine coils form a layer in the deeper portion of the volar dermis. Their ducts open at regular intervals on top of the epidermal ridges. Their activity is regulated more by emotional stimuli than by heat, although their innervation is of a cholinergic nature similar to that of

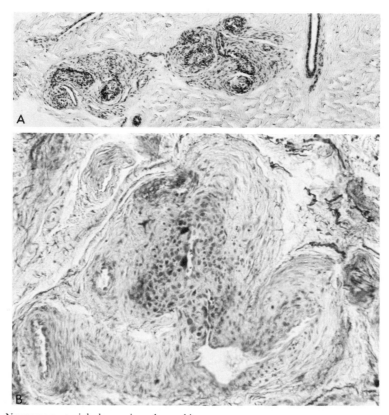

Figure 2–34 Neuromyoarterial glomus in palmar skin.
A, Low power view of twin arteriovenous anastomoses. A sweat duct is at the right. *H & E, ×30.*
B, Sucquet-Hoyer canal surrounded by glomus cells. A few hyperchromatic nuclei are not infrequently found. *H & E, ×180.*

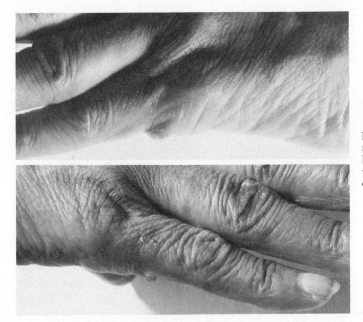

Figure 2–35 Rudimentary super-numerary digits on the right and left hands of an American Negro woman. The location near the base of the fifth digit is characteristic.

other eccrine glands. The usefulness of our hands is in part due to the highly developed sense of touch which is subserved by special end organs, the Meissner corpuscles. These are not only situated directly below the epidermis, but their arrangement in the slant of the friction ridges insures maximal directional perception of stimuli (Cauna, 1956b).

The acral parts of our extremities also are more involved in heat regulation and emotional sweating than are other portions of skin. Special arteriovenous shunts in the reticular dermis can divert blood from the superficial layers. These shunts (Fig. 2–34) are known as the neuromyoarterial glomus of Masson. They consist of coiled thick-walled vessels (Sucquet-Hoyer canal) containing peculiar contractile elements, the so-called glomus cells, which are also the characteristic feature of glomus tumors (glomangiomas). These vessels, which connect arteries and veins, normally are contracted but may relax and permit blood to be shunted through them. Large nerve trunks are part of the glomus. Supernumerary digits are occasionally found, especially in the rudimentary form (Fig. 2–35) of small nodules situated at the lateral surface of the fifth metacarpal or basal phalanx.

MICROSCOPIC ANATOMY

Histologic examination of abnormal skin frequently is necessary for exact diagnosis of inflammatory as well as neoplastic conditions. A basic prerequisite for meaningful interpretation of histopathologic changes is intimate knowledge of normal histology. The better anatomist becomes the superior pathologist especially if morphologic knowledge is laced with the ability to interpret the picture of tissue sections in terms of skin biology.

We shall first discuss the epidermis, next the dermis (cutis or corium), and then the cutaneous adnexa, which are composed of ectodermal epithelium and mesodermal stroma. Finally, neuroectodermal derivatives will be described.

Epidermis

When the vernix caseosa, consisting of exfoliated keratinized cells, shed lanugo, and sebum, has been wiped off, the epidermis of the newborn is essentially mature. Throughout life, epidermis (Fig. 2–36) consists of one basal layer; several layers of prickle cells (stratum spinosum), the uppermost of which contain kerato-

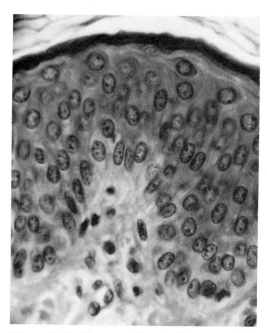

Figure 2-36　Human epidermis. Two rete ridges separated by dermal papilla. Suprapapillary plate has approximately six rows of prickle cells between the columnar basal cells and the stratum granulosum. *H & E*, ×600.

hyalin granules (stratum granulosum); and many layers of keratinized cells (stratum corneum).

All these cells represent successive life phases of the single species "epidermal cell," now usually called the keratinocyte. Mature keratinized cells flake off from the surface and are replenished by slow transport of cells upward from the basal layer, which is the principal seat of mitotic division in normal skin (Pinkus, 1970). The normal life span of a keratinocyte is approximately one month. One horny layer probably is shed each day. In hyperplastic (acanthotic) epidermis with more rapid turnover (e.g., psoriasis), basal and several suprabasal layers may constitute the stratum germinativum, and epidermal turnover may be much accelerated. The life span of a keratinocyte may be reduced to three to four days. The physiologic term germinal layer should be carefully distinguished from the anatomic term basal layer, which refers to those cells in immediate contact with mesoderm. All other cells of similar morphology are best re-

ferred to as "basaloid" cells. Because terminology is complex in the field of skin histology and has been confused by imprecise usage, the terms used in this chapter and their exact definitions are listed in Table 2-6. Proper usage is not pedantry but an expression of clear understanding of the facts and a prerequisite of proper interpretation of pathologic events.

Keratinocytes, like all cells, consist of nucleus, cell body, and cell membrane (Odland and Reed, 1967; Brody, 1968). The following special features identify them.

Nucleus.　The nucleus is relatively small and dark-staining in basal and basaloid cells, and is larger and vesicular with one or more angular nucleoli in the prickle cells. It shrinks, becomes pyknotic, and eventually disappears in keratohyalin cells and the lower stratum corneum, whether this is organized into a stratum lucidum or not. Chromatin content of all normal nuclei is in diploid range (Kint, 1963), meaning that basal cells reach tetraploid values in the S phase preceding a mitotic division, which reduces DNA again to the diploid amount (Fig. 2-37).

Cell Body.　The cell body (Fig. 2-38) contains within the cytoplasm the usual organelles, such as endoplasmic reticulum, ribosomes, Golgi apparatus, centriole, and mitochondria, but it also contains characteristic structures known as tonofilaments, keratohyalin granules, lamellar bodies (Odland bodies, membrane-coating granules, or keratinosomes), and in many cases melanin granules.

Owing mainly to the presence of tonofilaments, keratinocytes stain with hematoxylin and basic dyes more heavily than do many other cells. Tonofilaments aggregate into bundles in the stratum spinosum and are then demonstrable by light microscopic methods as tonofibrils. They usually respect a narrow perinuclear zone (Fig. 2-40) rich in endoplasmic reticulum and mitochondria (endoplasm), but mitochondria (Fig. 2-39) become sparse as the cells move upward.

Keratohyalin granules, which are both hematoxylinophilic and osmiophilic, make their appearance in the uppermost layer or layers of the stratum spinosum. They

TABLE 2–6   DEFINITIONS AND RECOMMENDED TERMS FOR THE
EPITHELIAL COMPONENTS OF THE SKIN

Ectodermal Epithelium	Epidermis
Definition Epithelial cells and tissues derived from the ectoderm (outer germ layer) of the embryo, including epidermis, epithelium of certain mucosal surfaces, and the glandular adnexa and hair follicles derived from these surface epithelia.	*Definition* Stratified squamous epithelium covering the skin surface and keratinizing normally with the formation of keratohyalin. Note: Epidermis (and epidermal) is not synonymous with ectoderm (and ectodermal). It consists of epidermal cells (epidermal keratinocytes).
Recommended Terms 1. EPIDERMIS and EPIDERMAL CELL are the terms that describe the surface epithelium of the skin. 2. MUCOSAL EPITHELIUM is used to refer to the surface epithelium of the oral cavity and other mucous membranes. 3. ADNEXAL EPITHELIUM (follicular, sebaceous, eccrine, apocrine, salivary) denotes the epithelial parts of hair follicles and glandular adnexa. 4. ECTODERMAL EPITHELIUM should be used when all or several of the above are meant. 5. ECTODERMAL MODULATED CELL is the term for the quasiembryonic cell in wound healing or other emergency situations. 6. STRATIFIED refers to any multilayered epithelium. 7. SQUAMOUS denotes any multilayered epithelium in which the cells flatten toward the surface (and usually keratinize). 8. EPIDERMOID is the term for any epithelium resembling the epidermis, especially if it keratinizes in the epidermal manner with keratohyalin formation.	*Recommended Terms* 1. KERATINOCYTE is the generic term for all cells capable of keratinization. There are epidermal, mucosal, and adnexal keratinocytes. 2. BASAL CELL is the anatomical term for any cell of a multilayered epithelium which is in contact with the dermis. There are epidermal, mucosal, and adnexal basal cells. 3. MATRIX CELL is a biologic term for the immature cells of an epithelial structure, which divide to produce the maturing (differentiating) cells. They may or may not be basal cells. 4. BASALOID CELL should be used for cells having morphologic resemblance to basal cells, but not bordering on connective tissue. In histopathology this is the recommended term for immature cells of benign tumors and so-called basal cell cancers. 5. PRICKLE CELL (malpighian cell), although a misnomer, is generally used for maturing cells before they become visibly keratinized. 6. GRANULAR CELL (keratohyalin cell) denotes cells containing hematoxylinophilic granules as evidence of beginning keratinization (no relation to the tumor cells of granular cell myoblastoma). 7. HORNY CELL (keratinized cell, corneocyte) refers to the non-nucleated cells composing the stratum corneum. 8. NONKERATINOCYTES is a generic term for cells in the epidermis, which do not keratinize. It refers to melanocytes, Langerhans cells and indeterminate dendritic cells living as symbionts in the epidermis.

are seen as angular bodies under the light microscope, and as very irregular masses (Fig. 2–39) on electron microscopic examination. The long-debated nature of the keratohyaline granules has been clarified as a proteinaceous material (Voorhees et al., 1968) synthetized in the upper layers (histidine-rich protein); this material is essential for normal keratinization because it fills the interfilamentous spaces and compacts the cell contents into the electron microscopic keratin pattern.

Lamellar bodies, described by Selby (1957) and Odland (1960), have been the subject of many investigations and much speculation. They have a single membrane (Fig. 2–39) and contain packets of lamellae. Many also contain acid phosphatase, and they are now usually considered to be a special type of lysosome. They empty onto the cell surface in the keratogenous zone, and their contents become part of the intercellular substances of the horny layer. Melanin granules are acquired by transfer from melanocytes.

Cell Membrane and Intercellular Space. The cell membrane is highly organized through the presence of innumerable desmosomes. While these organelles (Fig. 2–39) are not specific for keratinocytes or even for ectodermal cells or epithelial cells in general (they are found

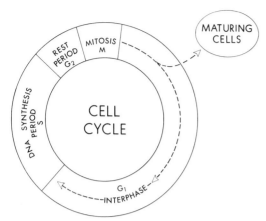

Figure 2–37 Diagram of mitotic cell cycle.

also on fibroblasts, heart muscle cells, and so forth), they are developed to an extraordinary degree. Through their close structural association with the cytoplasmic tonofilaments, they give keratinocytes in the prickle cell phase their distinctive appearance.

In well-fixed electron microscopic prep-

arations, the three-layered cell membranes run parallel to each other, separated by a narrow intercellular space. They often form an interlocking zigzag pattern. At the site of a desmosome, the electron-dense outer and inner leaflets of the opposite membranes are thickened, and the intercellular cleft is filled with material organized into a central dense layer between two less-dense layers. We thus see five electron-dense lines separated by four lighter lines. In three-dimensional view, the desmosome is a roundish nine-layered plate, and to this is added within each cell an "attachment plaque" to which tonofilaments are anchored (tonofilament-desmosome complex) and which in cross-section appears as a less well defined electron-dense line (Fig. 2–39).

In routine light microscopic sections the desmosome appears as the bridge nodule of Bizzozero. In routine processing, cells shrink away from each other, the intercellular space widens, but the cell membranes remain glued together at the site of desmosomes. Thus the electron microscopic

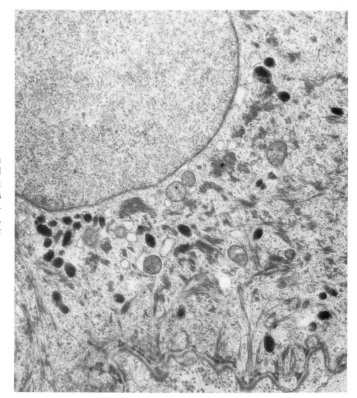

Figure 2–38 Electron micrograph of part of a basal cell. The basal lamina and superficial dermis are at lower border of picture. The nucleus is at the upper left. Cytoplasm contains tonofilaments, mitochondria, melanin granules, and endoplasmic reticulum. ×12,000.

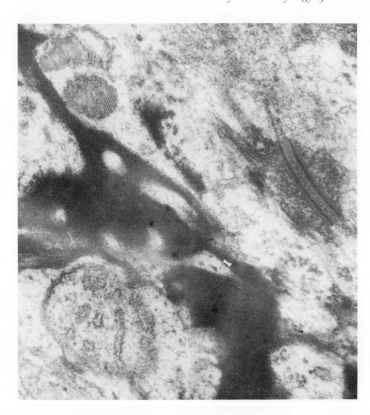

Figure 2–39 Electron micrograph of part of two keratohyalin cells. A desmosome is at the right; a mitochondrion is at the lower left; two lamellated bodies (keratinosomes) are at the upper left. Masses of keratohyalin are in the center. ×48,000.

undulation of the cell surfaces is converted into abrupt protrusions of membrane-covered cytoplasm which we call intercellular bridges. In transverse or oblique section, the bridges resemble the spines or prickles on the surface of a sea urchin and have given the entire cell layer its name. It is, however, a misnomer because there are no free spines. In reality, the light microscopic preparation (Fig. 2–40) shows cytoplasmic bridges spanning the shortest distance between two cells as straight cords and bearing the bridge nodule or desmosome near the center. The terms prickle cell, spinous layer, and stratum spinosum, and their derived application in pathology (acanthosis, prickle cell carcinoma), are so ingrained that we continue using them, but their basic inappropriateness must be kept in mind.

The cell membrane and the desmosomes of basal cells are in all respects similar to those of prickle cells where they are in contact with other epidermal cells, although there are relatively few desmosomes between the lateral surfaces of basal cells, and tonofilament-desmosome com-

plexes are less well organized. At their lower surface, the basal cells possess cytoplasmic prolongations known as pedicles, which interlock with mesodermal structures. Details will be discussed later.

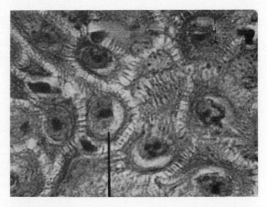

Figure 2–40 Photomicrograph of prickle cells in edematous epidermis. Cellular bridges are stretched across the slightly widened intercellular spaces. The line points to the widened perinuclear space (endoplasm). Bridge nodules (desmosomes) are clearly visible. The small dark bodies in intercellular spaces are parts of nuclei of polymorphonuclear leukocytes. *H & E*, ×1200.

Until recently little was known about permanency or fragility of desmosomal connection, although one had to assume that they can be dissolved and reconstructed in order to permit movement of keratinocytes as well as that of migrating leukocytes between them. Examination of keratin-stripped skin (Mishima and Pinkus, 1968) has shown that during the period of active regeneration following this procedure cells break their connections within a few hours and make new connections later. The desmosomes do not split but instead retract to one side of the widened intercellular space, while a break develops in the opposite cell membrane. The break is quickly repaired and the cells form numerous microvilli. The process is different from the events in bullous dermatoses such as pemphigus.

At the level of transition from stratum granulosum to corneum, the cell membrane thickens. Latest information shows that this is due to apposition of electron-dense material from the inside. Desmosomes persist in the horny layer and a considerable amount of intercellular material accumulates. Much of this appears to be mucopolysaccharide in nature and related to similar material (glycocalyx) already present in the stratum spinosum (Wolff and Schreiner, 1970). Eventually, though, connections break, and single intact cells are exfoliated from the surface. In light microscopic preparations, the characteristic basket weave appearance of the horny layer is due to the fact that only cell membranes stain and the cell bodies appear as spaces. If the horny layer looks dense in some regions, mainly on the distal end of the extremities, this is due to the compacting of very flat cells.

Special mention must be made of the stratum lucidum, which is seen as a bright-staining, structureless line in vertical sections of the thick epidermis of the extremities. Electron microscopic studies show no such distinct transition zone, and the light microscopic appearance probably is due to transient physicochemical conditions which obliterate differences of refractivity.

Histochemistry and Radioautography. Much has been learned about life processes in the epidermis by means of histochemical and radioautographic studies.

Relatively simple methods, applicable to routine paraffin sections, demonstrate polysaccharides. It was mentioned previously that all layers of early fetal epidermis contain much glycogen and that this substance is later restricted to prickle cells and periderm. Normal adult epidermis contains little or no stainable glycogen, but the stratum spinosum of acanthotic epidermis does. The basal layer, on the other hand, contains glycogen only under exceptional circumstances and for a few hours at a time (stripping effect, ultraviolet radiation, and other trauma (Lobitz et al., 1962). Intercellular spaces contain acid mucopolysaccharides. The organized basement membrane is strongly PAS positive. A variety of enzymes have been demonstrated in the human epidermis. These are catalogued in Table 2–7.

Biologic synthesis (Bernstein et al., 1970) has been studied by radioautography using labeled amino acids and thymidine. Many of these investigations used animal skin, but there is enough evidence from human material to consider the results applicable to man (Rothberg et al., 1961). Injected amino acids are quickly absorbed into the epidermis through the basement membrane and incorporated into proteins (Fukuyama and Epstein, 1968). This hap-

TABLE 2–7   ENZYMES OF THE EPIDERMIS[*]

Name	Localization
Cytochrome oxidase	Living epidermal layers
Monoamine oxidase	Strongest in basal layer
Succinic dehydrogenase	Strongest in basal layer
NADH- and NADPH-tetrazolium reductases	Noncornified epidermis
Coenzyme-linked dehydrogenases	Noncornified epidermis
Phosphorylase and branching enzyme	Basal and spinous layers
Esterases	Variable, including living and nonliving strata and skin surface
Acid phosphatase	All layers; strongest in the transitional zone
Alkaline phosphatase	Negative; or positive in stratum intermedium
Adenosine triphosphatase	Cell membranes, especially Langerhans cells
Nucleases	Zones of nuclear breakdown
Beta-glucuronidase	Whole epidermis
Carbonic anhydrase	Strongest in basal layer
Ubiquinone	Stratum basale, spinosum, intermedium

[*]Listed mainly according to Brody (1968).

pens in all living layers, but in differential fashion. Histidine, for instance, is incorporated more in the higher layers where the formation of histidine-rich protein parallels the morphologic appearance of keratohyalin. ³H-Thymidine is incorporated into nuclei during the S phase preceding mitotic division (Fig. 2–37) or during repair after exposure to ultraviolet light (Cleaver, 1970). In normal epidermis, thymidine is accepted mainly by basal cells. The labeled products of mitotic division of these cells gradually move outward and permit us to follow the path and life span of keratinocytes. Studies of this type have confirmed the earlier suggestion (Hunter et al., 1956) that the normal life span of an epidermal cell is approximately four weeks. Under pathologic circumstances, however, the life span may be reduced to three to four days, as in active psoriasis (Weinstein and Frost, 1968). If the epidermis is deprived of its horny layer by tape stripping, a burst of mitosis that has its peak after 48 hours is capable of doubling the number of cells within 24 hours (Pinkus, 1952).

Epidermal Architecture and Biology. The epidermis consists of living building blocks without intercellular fibrous substance. Its components, the keratinocytes, are held tightly together by desmosomes, but can move against each other and generally follow a vertical path from the basal layer outward (Pinkus, 1970). Basal cells (Fig. 2–41) are small in diameter (6 to 10 μ) and either cuboidal or columnar in shape. When they ascend into the prickle cell layer they become more bulky, are at first polyhedral, and later are broad and flattened. Nuclei of basal cells are ovoid,

with their long axis vertical to the basement membrane. Nuclei of prickle cells are more spherical, those of granular cells are flat resembling the yolk in a fried egg. Keratinized cells that have lost their nuclei are still flatter, with diameters ranging from 30 to 45 μ (Hunter et al., 1956; Plewig and Marples, 1970) and surface areas from 746–1222 μ^2. Due to the differences in size and shape between basal cells and horny cells, a much smaller number of cells cover the same area on the skin surface than at the basement membrane (Fig. 2–41). The proportion of number of basal cells to number of keratinized cells is further increased by the fact that the dermoepidermal junction usually is not flat, but its area is greatly enlarged by the presence of papillae and rete ridges. Thus a relatively low mitotic rate in the basal layer suffices to cover the loss of keratinized cells (Fular, 1953). Mitotic rates have been determined in the range of 1:1000 to 1:10,000. The rate of renewal of one horny layer has been estimated as 20 to 47 hours (Baker and Blair, 1968) the time increasing with age. The normal life span of one epidermal cell is approximately one month, the transit time through the horny layer may vary from 13 days in young people to 17 to 36 days in elderly people.

Dermis

The derma, cutis, or corium (Montagna et al., 1970; Schmidt, 1968), in American usage referred to as dermis, constitutes the major portion of skin volume and has

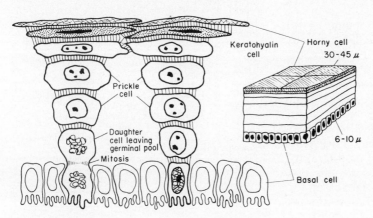

Figure 2–41 Diagram of epidermal biology and relative size and number of cells in the basal and horny layers. (Modified from Pinkus, 1964.)

mechanical functions in addition to intricate biologic ones. Its ability to serve as a supple and tough protective envelope for the body is based on a mixture of two fibrous proteins, collagen and elastin, arranged in the form of fibers, ribbons, and bundles in a mucinous ground substance. A rich sensory nerve supply makes the dermis a highly effective warning system for environmental influences transmitting the qualities of cold, warmth, touch, pain, and tickle or itch. A blood supply far in excess of nutritional needs subserves thermal homeostasis and is supplemented by the ability of eccrine glands to produce large quantities of hypotonic sweat. In addition, the dermis serves as a vast storehouse for water, salt, glucose, fat, and other substances, and is involved in many allergic and immunologic reactions. Last but not least, it maintains and regulates the integrity and function of epidermis and ectodermal adnexa, which matured under its inductive influence in fetal life.

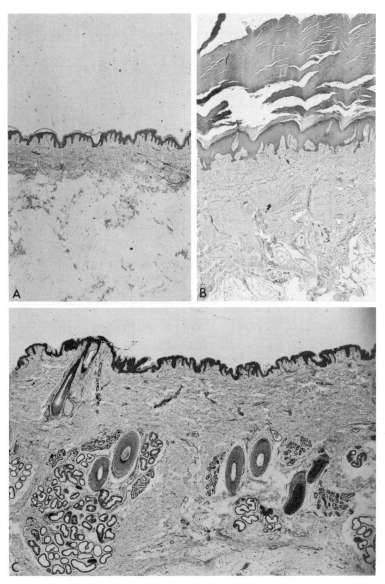

Figure 2–42 Three regions of skin at identical magnification. *A,* Abdomen. *B,* Sole. *C,* Axilla exhibiting small and large hair follicles, sebaceous glands, and eccrine and apocrine glands. *H & E, ×14.*

The dermis (Fig. 2–42) has three major portions: the pars papillaris, consisting of papillae and a subpapillary layer; the pars reticularis, in which pilosebaceous and eccrine apparatuses are embedded; and, by the definition given on page 65, a certain amount of fat tissue. Inclusion of fat tissue, which really is part of the subcutis or hypoderm, is advisable because of two facts: Not only is the border between fibrous corium and subcutis never sharp (fat lobes often protrude upward (Fig. 2–50) around hair roots and eccrine glands, and fibrous tissue extends down in the form of retinacula) but also the roots of strong hairs (Figs. 2–16 and 2–17) and the coils of many eccrine glands are truly embedded in the hypoderm.

Pars Papillaris. Subpapillary Layer and Papillae. The uppermost dermal layer (papillary dermis or pars papillaris) forms a biologic unit with the epidermis. Both react together under many normal and abnormal circumstances. Many inflammatory processes are restricted to the epidermis and the papillary dermis, and the same holds true for precancerous lesions, carcinoma in situ, and superficial basal cell epithelioma. The pars papillaris consists of fibers and thin bundles of collagen and of thin elastic fibers in special arrangement. It contains the subpapillary plexus of arterioles and venules from which capillary loops enter the papillae. A similar lymphatic plexus also is present, as are terminal ramifications of sensory nerves. The blood supply far exceeds the nutritional needs of the epidermis and serves a thermoregulatory function. Blood flow can be completely diverted from the papillary layer by deeper arteriovenous anastomoses.

Collagen fibers are bathed in relatively abundant ground substance, which consists mainly of a dilute gel of hyaluronic acid. Collagen and reticulum fibrils envelop vessels (Berger and Berger, 1970) and nerves as a three-dimensional felt. It

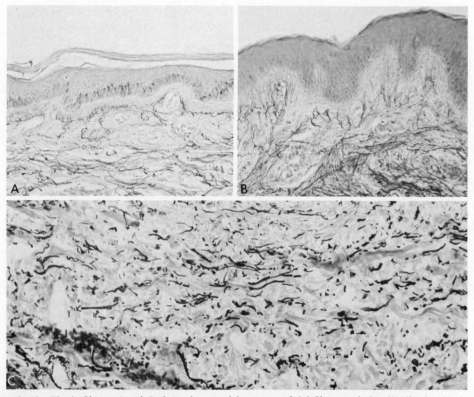

Figure 2–43 Elastic fibers. *A* and *B* show short and long superficial fibers and the distribution in the pars papillaris. *C* shows the thick fibers of the pars reticularis, which are cut into shorter or longer pieces by the microtome knife. *Acid orcein and Giemsa*, ×*90*.

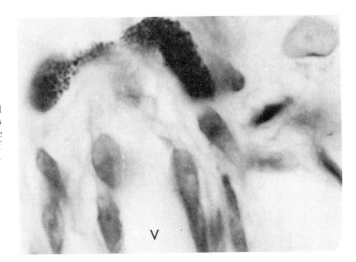

Figure 2–44 A small blood vessel (*V*) lined by endothelial cells. There is a mast cell at the upper left of the picture. The other nuclei are those of perivascular fibrocytes and histiocytes. *Acid orcein and Giemsa,* ×*1000.*

is, however, the elastic fibers which give the pars papillaris its special signature. The elastic fibers of the subpapillary layer (Fig. 2–43) form a three-dimensional loose net around the vascular plexus and may form a distinct basket around lymph vessels, especially on the lower extremities. At a variable distance below the epidermis, very thin fibers form a coherent felt from which free ending fibrils rise toward the epidermis like shoots of shrubbery. They end just below the basement membrane, but their mucosaccharide sheath enters into the junctional zone (Cooper, 1969). Knowledge of this generally neglected feature of dermal structure provides valuable information in many pathologic situations (Pinkus, 1960 and 1970; Pinkus and Mehregan, 1969).

The pars papillaris (papillary dermis) is relatively rich in fixed tissue type cells, some of which are fibrocytes, others histiocytes, and still others cells of the perivascular coat. Few of the small vessels have smooth muscle coats when viewed with ordinary stains. Mast cells are present normally in small numbers (Fig. 2–44).

DERMOEPIDERMAL JUNCTION. Dermis and epidermis adhere tightly under most circumstances. Their union is assured by a series of structural mechanisms ranging from almost macroscopic to submicroscopic. In many areas, the normal epidermis carries on its lower surface a system of interconnecting ridges. The depressions between them (Fig. 2–45) are filled with finger-like dermal projections, the blood-bearing papillae. This arrangement is easily demonstrated by separating epidermis from dermis by means of dilute acetic acid or other fluids. Inspection of the lower surface of the epidermal sheet at low magnification shows clearly that rete "pegs" do not exist as is illustrated in the diagram.

Higher magnification is needed to recognize the pedicles of the basal cells which fit into the felt of collagenous and elastic fibers. Silver staining reveals a dense array of reticulin fibrils at the junction. The PAS and similar procedures show a fairly broad homogeneous band (Winter and Levan, 1970). One might compare the arrangement (Fig. 2–46) with the pile of a rug impregnated with mucilage into which the fibers of a broom (the epidermal pedicles) are pressed from above. Finally, at the electron microscopic level, one recognizes that the lower membrane of the basal cells is accompanied in all its flexions by an electron-dense line called the basal lamina (adepidermal membrane), from which it is separated by an electron-lucent space about 300 Å wide (Fig. 3–38). The cell membrane possesses half-desmosomes, from which very thin fibrils cross to the basal lamina which itself is secured to the dermis below by anchoring fibrils (Fig. 2–46). Thus, a most intimate cohesion is assured.

Recent studies have shown that the basal lamina (Hay, 1964; Briggaman et al., 1970) and the light microscopic PAS-posi-

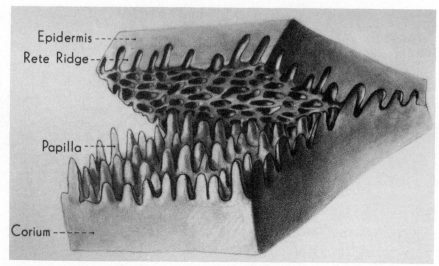

Figure 2–45   Diagram of dermoepidermal interface as it might appear when the tissues are pulled apart after treatment with acetic acid or other macerating fluids. (*From* Pinkus and Mehregan: A Guide to Dermatohisto-pathology, 1969. Courtesy of Appleton-Century-Crofts, Publishing Division of Prentice-Hall, Inc., Englewood Cliffs, N.J.)

tive membrane are, at least in part, products of the epidermal cells, formed under the influence of mesoderm. Furthermore, the basement membrane is not a barrier to biochemical exchange, although perhaps a regulator. Most soluble substances injected into the dermis (amino acids, dyes) cross the junction within seconds or minutes. Even ferritin particles go through. Within the epidermis, the intercellular spaces appear to be open channels, blocked only at the keratogenous level (Pinkus, 1970).

Pars Reticularis.   The major portion of the dermis below the pars papillaris consists of interconnecting bundles of collagen fibers and a three-dimensional network of thick elastic fibers (Fig. 2–43*C*) with mucinous ground substance in the interfascicular compartment (pars reticularis or reticular dermis). This portion (see Table 2–3) varies in thickness from 0.3 to 8 mm. in man, constitutes the leather of tanned animal hides, and has mainly a mechanical function. Its structure may be compared

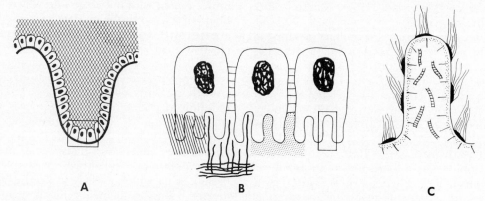

Figure 2–46   Diagram of dermoepidermal junction at different levels of magnification.

A, A rete ridge with basal cells is shown.

B, Three basal cells with their pedicles are shown. On the left are the silver-stainable reticulum fibers; in the middle are the elastic fibers; and on the right are the PAS-positive mucopolysaccharides.

C, Parts of two pedicles with basal lamina, hemidesmosomes, and tonofilaments are shown. Anchoring fibrils extend from the basal lamina toward collagen fibrils in the dermis.

with the construction of an elastic garment in which nonstretchable fibers are woven into a stretchable fabric containing rubber threads which cause the garment to return to the original size and shape when stretch is released. The garment develops bulges when the rubber threads are weakened or broken. Similarly, nonstretchable collagen fibers are arranged in wavy bundles which are interconnected, but permit considerable stretch. The three-dimensional network of stretchable elastic fibers serves the role of the rubber threads in the garment. Whenever they have disappeared through injury or disease, the skin is apt to bulge unless it has been made inelastic by fibrosis. Examples are flabby surgical scars, striae distensae, and macular atrophy. Directional arrangement of collagen bundles as the basis of Langer's lines was discussed previously.

The reticular dermis contains almost no reticulin fibers except around vessels, hair follicles, and sweat glands. The proportion of elastic fibers and collagen fibers varies topographically and with age. There are no good quantitative data, but it has been my impression that elastic fibers are prominent in childhood, are outgrown by collagen and reach a low point in early adulthood, and become relatively plentiful in senile skin. This statement does not take into consideration the elastotic changes seen in exposed skin with advancing age (see p. 45). There are probably great individual variations. Elastic fibers are easily destroyed by inflammatory and granulomatous processes. When disease processes or surgical incisions heal, new fibers form fairly readily in young persons, but poorly in older individuals. This influences the conditions of scars and striae.

The reticular dermis contains relatively few blood vessels (Moretti, 1968) connecting the subpapillary and deep cutaneous plexus, the latter situated at the border of the hypoderm. Blood vessels are more numerous around pilosebaceous and eccrine apparatuses. Nerves usually follow the vessels. The neuromyoarterial glomus was discussed previously. The pars reticularis also is relatively acellular when compared to either the pars papillaris or the subcutis. It is for these reasons that wounds and incisions penetrating into the subcutaneous fat tissue heal better by either primary or secondary intention, fibrocytes, and vascular supply coming mainly from the hypoderm. Another reason to extend biopsies and excisional defects into the hypoderm is found in the much greater ease with which such wounds are sutured when no tough connective tissue resists approximation of the edges.

Hypoderm. The subcutaneous tissue (Schmidt, 1968) consists of fat lobes (Fig. 2–49) separated from each other and held in position by narrow or broad connective tissue septa in which the major vessels are located. The fat lobules are richly vascularized by terminal vessels (Smahel and Charvát, 1964) and constitute, according to their fetal development, individual small organs with a much more active metabolism than they are usually given credit for. Small lobes often are associated with relatively superficial sweat coils located within the dermis. Scalp hair roots (Fig. 2–16) and other strong hairs extend into the fat tissue, a feature to be kept in mind in the transplantation of hair.

Cutaneous Adnexa

Developmental stages of the three adnexal structures are completed before birth. Later in life two of them, the eccrine apparatus and the nail, have relatively constant microscopic features. The third one, the pilar apparatus, is at the same time the most variable and the most complicated one, consisting of hair root, sebaceous gland, apocrine gland, and arrector muscle.

Pilar Apparatus. The relative size and development of the components of the pilary complex (Fig. 2–47) may vary greatly, and any one or several may be entirely absent. Apocrine glands are connected with only a minority of pilosebaceous follicles in human skin. Many vellus hairs have no arrector muscle. The hair root, usually the most conspicuous portion of the complex, is a mere appendage in the large sebaceous follicles of the face (Fig. 2–48) and is absent in the free sebaceous glands of semimucous and mucous membranes and the female nipple. Sebaceous glands can undergo temporary atrophy

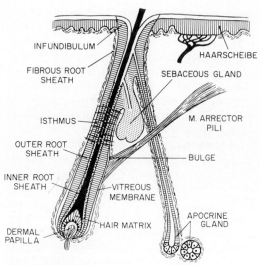

Figure 2-47 Diagram of the pilary complex. The Haarscheibe and the isthmus are supplied with sensory nerve fibers. (*From* Pinkus, H.: Static and dynamic histology and histochemistry of hair growth. *In* Baccaredda-Boy, A., et al. (Eds.): Biopathology of Pattern Alopecia. Basel, S. Karger, 1968.)

and may be regenerated from elements in the outer root sheath. Thus their absence on any one follicle does not necessarily imply agenesis.

HAIR AND HAIR FOLLICLE. While the hair shaft protrudes naked from the skin, its root below the surface is surrounded by the hair follicle which carries the hair matrix at its lower bulbous end.

Morphology. The hair follicle (Fig. 2-47) usually is divided for descriptive purposes into an upper permanent portion and a lower expendable one. It seems preferable, however, to recognize a middle portion extending from below the opening of the sebaceous duct to the insertion of the arrector muscle at the bulge which marks the site to which the club hair ascends in telogen (Pinkus, 1968).

The opening of the follicle onto the skin surface is roundish and filled with loose keratin, in the center of which the hair shaft may be present. The opening is surrounded by stratified epithelium (Figs. 2-18 and 2-48) keratinizing in an epidermis-like manner and lining a funnel-shaped lumen (infundibulum) at the lower end of which one or several sebaceous ducts open (Fig 2-49). The infundibulum therefore is actually the pilosebaceous canal and includes the lower portion of the fetal hair canal, which in fetal life grows from the hair germ in the basal layer of the epi-

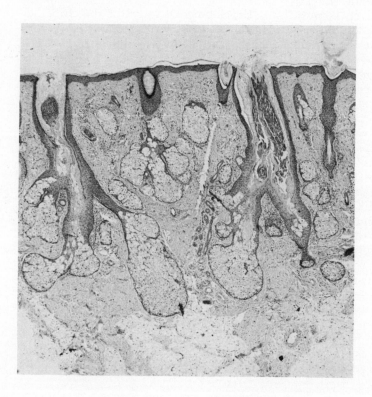

Figure 2-48 Skin of forehead with three sebaceous follicles. Vellus hair follicles are at the right. The sebaceous follicles contain plugs, which correspond to small blackheads. *H & E,* ×60.

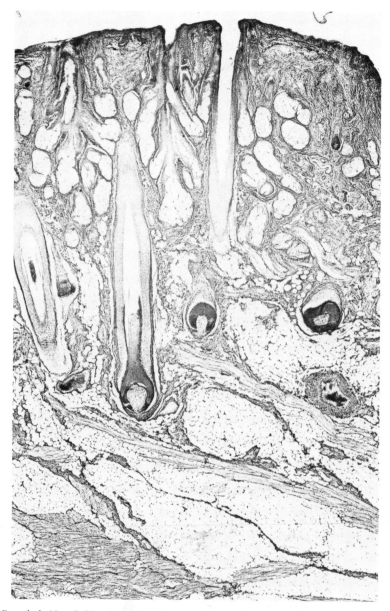

Figure 2–49 Bearded skin of chin. Beard follicles extend into subcutaneous fat tissue, which contains strands of striated muscle. There are sebaceous follicles between the beard hairs. A small vellus follicle is at the right. *van Gieson,* ×*30.*

dermis obliquely upward to the surface. Therefore, and this is highly important in epidermal carcinogenesis, the infundibulum is not an invagination of the epidermis and is not lined by epidermis, but consists of adnexal keratinocytes maturing in an epidermoid manner. In this respect, it is more similar to the sebaceous duct than to the outer root sheath (trichilemma) below the infundibulum. Ducts of free sebaceous glands on the oral mucosa have identical structure, although neither epidermis nor hair root is available as sources of keratohyalin-forming epithelium.

While the infundibulum contains loose keratin mixed with sebum, is open to the outside world, and often is colonized by cocci and yeasts (Fig. 2–48), there is no

open lumen in the follicle below the sebaceous duct level (Fig. 2–50) . Outer root
sheath, inner root sheath, and hair are
tightly apposed in the next stretch, the
isthmus of the hair follicle (Fig. 2–51). If
the keratinized inner root sheath begins to
disintegrate some distance below the sebaceous duct, then the outer root sheath
produces trichilemmal keratin (Fig. 2–50),

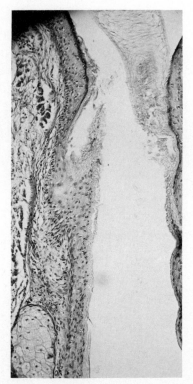

Figure 2–51 Isthmus portion of a scalp hair follicle. The hair shaft is absent. The opening of the
sebaceous duct on the left side marks the border between the epidermoid infundibulum and the trichilemma, which forms a thick keratin layer without
keratohyalin. The upper end of the keratinized internal root sheath is seen at the lower rim of the picture.
H & E, ×200.

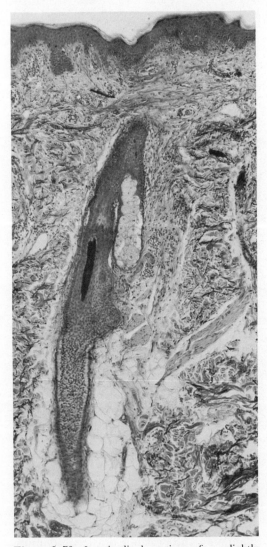

Figure 2–50 Longitudinal section of a slightly
curved terminal hair follicle of male dorsal skin. The
dark material in the center of the follicle is the
tangentially cut inner root sheath. The sebaceous
gland, bulge, and arrector muscle are shown. The
lower follicle segment is embedded in fat tissue, thus
exhibiting the fibrous root sheath on the outside of
the tall, light-staining basal cells of the trichilemma.
Acid orcein and Giemsa, ×180.

which is formed without a keratohyalin
layer and consists of bulky non-nucleated
cells with PAS-positive intercellular substance. The isthmus (Fig. 2–47) is surrounded by a stromal sheath of collagenous and elastic fibers and is supplied
with an intricate basket of sensory fibers
(Roman et al., 1969), which represents a
mechanoreceptor end organ, responding
to minor movements of the free hair (Orfanos, 1967).

Below the isthmus, the trichilemma
thickens, especially on that side of the
follicle that forms an open angle with the
epidermis (Fig. 2–50). This is the remnant
of the bulge which was so prominent in
fetal skin. In the adult, the bulge often is
rather inconspicuous, but it may produce
branching epithelial proliferations (Madsen, 1964) mimicking trichoepithelioma,
or it may form an epithelial tendon for the

arrector muscle which inserts here by means of a network of elastic fibers. The bulge marks the upper limit to which the club hair ascends in the resting phase (telogen) and the lower limit of elastic fibers coating the follicle.

Below this level, the follicle waxes and wanes with each hair cycle. During the active growth phase (anagen), the hair root (Fig. 2–52) consists of the central hair shaft surrounded by the concentric tubes of epithelial inner, epithelial outer, and fibrous root sheaths. The latter consists of fibrocytes forming circular and longitudinal strands of collagen and is richly vascularized. It is separated from the epithelial parts by a hyaline basement membrane, the vitreous (glassy) membrane, on which the high columnar basal

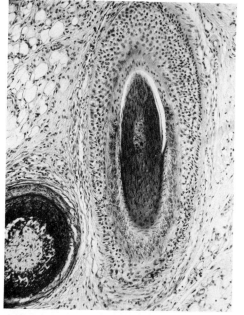

Figure 2–52 Oblique section of the keratogenous zone and transverse section of the bulb of scalp hairs. The oblique section shows the epithelial outer root sheath (trichilemma) surrounded by the vascularized fibrous root sheath. The hair shaft consists of medulla, cortex, and cuticle, of which only the cuticle is fully keratinized (light portion). Huxley layer of the inner root sheath is in transition from the trichohyalin stage at the lower circumference to the keratinizing stage with pyknotic nuclei at the upper pole. The cross-section of the bulb shows the dermal papilla in the center surrounded by the epithelial matrix and the outer and fibrous root sheath. Dendritic melanocytes are mixed with the basal layer of the matrix. *H & E, ×360.*

cells of the trichilemma (epithelial outer root sheath) rest. These cells contain much glycogen and therefore look light in routinely stained sections. They produce just enough mitoses to assure a slow movement of the inner layers of stratified epithelium obliquely upward to keep pace with the movement of hair and inner root sheath.

At its deep end, the follicle widens into the bulb. This is the site of hair formation (Figs. 2–49 and 2–53) and consists of the central ovoid dermal papilla surrounded by the bell-shaped hair matrix. On longitudinal section the matrix resembles pincers which almost touch at the bottom. Only a narrow stem bearing blood capillaries connects the mucopolysaccharide-rich dermal papilla with the fibrous root sheath covering the outer surface of the bulb. The epithelial matrix consists of a mass of immature small cells, which are among the most actively proliferating body tissues, undergoing mitosis more than once a day. By not completely understood mechanisms (Pinkus, 1968), the matrix cells undergo differentiation in six distinct fashions. Those close to the bottom of the papilla, next to the ring where matrix joins the trichilemma, produce a single circumferential layer of quickly keratinizing flat elongated cells called the Henle layer. The next several rows of matrix cells produce the multilayered Huxley layer, which keratinizes somewhat more slowly. Next follow two rows of cells which make two interlocking cuticles, the cuticle of the inner root sheath and the cuticle of the hair. The major portion of the matrix above these rows produces hair cortex, and in large hair roots, the cells capping the papilla produce medulla. Still another feature of the bulb is the presence of dendritic melanocytes (Fig. 2–52) in the upper half of the matrix. These contribute melanin granules to the keratinizing cells of the cortex and medulla. They disappear at the time when a pigmented hair turns irrevocably white.

The keratinizing hair and inner root sheath, their cuticles tightly interlocked, are pushed upward through the stationary tube of trichilemma and fibrous root sheath at the rate of 0.3 to 0.5 mm. a day. The trichilemma produces just enough new cells to let its inner surface keep pace

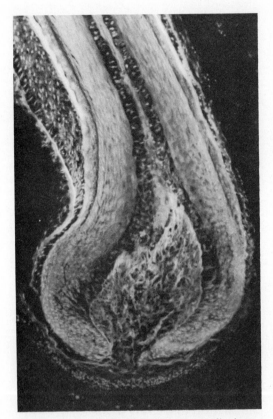

Figure 2–53 Thioflavin-stained longitudinal section of the lower portion of a beard hair photographed with ultraviolet illumination. The dermal papilla is continuous with the fibrous root sheath through a narrow neck between the pincer-like matrix. The hair, consisting of medulla (dark with light nuclei), cortex (gray), and cuticle (striated), is surrounded by cuticle, Huxley layer, and Henle layer of the inner root sheath. Henle layer is keratinized in the upper half of the picture (broad, light streak). The trichilemma is much thicker on the concave side of the follicle. Note that the dermal papilla has two tips, above which the medulla is formed, while an abnormal central column of cortex arises from the depression between the two tips. This slight abnormality is found once in a while in beard hairs and produces a double medulla. It indicates that the type of keratinization of hair matrix cells is determined by their distance from the base of the papilla (see Pinkus, 1968). ×500.

with the moving contents. This completes the description of the hair root during the anagen phase of the hair cycle.

Hair Cycle. Hairs grow for a few weeks or up to several years according to their length (Saitoh et al., 1970). Eventually, due to causes lodged in the individual follicle, the dermal papilla loses its rich store of sulfated mucopolysaccharides, its capillaries collapse, and it becomes almost completely atrophic. The hair matrix also undergoes atrophy and ceases to produce hair and inner root sheath. This involutionary stage is called catagen (Fig. 2–54). During catagen, the lower follicle shortens and is absorbed, the lower end of the hair coming to rest at the level of the bulge, where it is embedded in a trichilemmal sac. The cells of the trichilemma keratinize around the pilar stub (Fig. 2–55), adding their specific keratin material to it. They produce a club-shaped thickening and firmly anchor the dead hair (club hair), which remains in this condition (telogen) for from eight weeks to five months or longer.

If one plucks a telogen hair or collects one that has fallen out, one sees and feels the tiny hard knob at the end of the club hair. This is in contrast to the appearance of a plucked anagen hair. If a hair is pulled in anagen, one usually pulls out hair shaft, inner root sheath, the major part of the matrix, and sometimes even portions of the outer root sheath. Macroscopically, the plucked hair has a soft lower portion surrounded by a transparent, viscous coat. If the hair is pigmented, a dark, soft knob is seen at the lowest point. Catagen hairs, which are rarely seen because this phase of the cycle is short, have no viscous coat but instead a soft end without definite club. In very rare cases, an anagen hair may be plucked complete with all sheaths, matrix, and papilla intact (Ludwig, 1967). Pathologic hair shapes need not be considered here.

We do not know the causes initiating spontaneous catagen, the forces acting during the disintegration of the lower follicle, and even the exact histomechanisms by which it is accomplished. We know that one can induce catagen by stopping mitosis by means of x-ray or cytotoxic drugs, but a normal club is not formed under these circumstances and the hairs fall out within two to three weeks. Systemic stress, such as high fever or major surgery, often induces many scalp hairs to enter catagen and telogen. These hairs become typical club hairs and will not be lost until 80 to 90 days later, when a new hair cycle dislodges them.

The foreshortening of the lower follicle has been attributed to cell death, but there

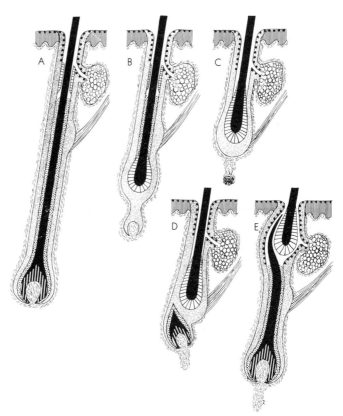

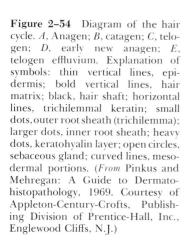

Figure 2–54 Diagram of the hair cycle. *A*, Anagen; *B*, catagen; *C*, telogen; *D*, early new anagen; *E*, telogen effluvium. Explanation of symbols: thin vertical lines, epidermis; bold vertical lines, hair matrix; black, hair shaft; horizontal lines, trichilemmal keratin; small dots, outer root sheath (trichilemma); larger dots, inner root sheath; heavy dots, keratohyalin layer; open circles, sebaceous gland; curved lines, mesodermal portions. (*From* Pinkus and Mehregan: A Guide to Dermatohistopathology, 1969. Courtesy of Appleton-Century-Crofts, Publishing Division of Prentice-Hall, Inc., Englewood Cliffs, N.J.)

is little histologic evidence of cell degeneration. It seems likely that the anagen hair matrix is kept in place through the turgor of the large number of newly formed hair cells which are confined in a cul-de-sac. While they are forced upward through the follicular tube, they exert an equal force downward on the matrix. Once mitotic activity ceases, the hydrostatic forces of the surrounding connective tis-

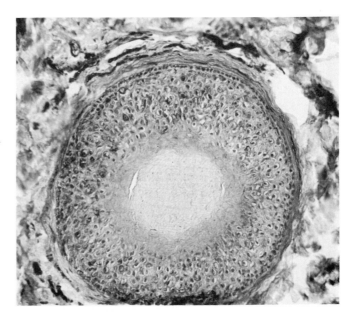

Figure 2–55 Cross-section of catagen follicle showing the lower end of the hair shaft surrounded by trichilemmal keratin, producing the "club" of the telogen hair. *PAS-van Gieson, ×600.*

sue gain the upper hand. The hair shaft escapes upward, similar to a stick in the center of a bag of beans that is being kneaded. Cells of the outer root sheath decrease in volume through loss of glycogen and conversion into the dense material of the keratinized club. It is, however, questionable whether these two factors are sufficient to explain all the shrinkage. Actual cell death must still be invoked to explain the phenomena observed.

For reasons that are just as unknown as those inducing catagen, the dermal papilla, a mere knob of fibrocyte-like cells during telogen, reorganizes and induces a new hair germ at the lowest pole of the trichilemmal sac. A sequence of events, very similar to those of fetal life, leads to formation of a new hair root which pushes downward into the collapsed remnants of the fibrous root sheath and eventually pushes the tip of the new hair upward and past the old club hair, loosening the latter and causing it to fall out. Telogen hair loss, therefore, in most cases indicates regrowth of a new hair, which may be similar, or stronger, or weaker than the old one, depending on circumstances.

Hair Neogenesis. For all practical purposes, new formation of hair roots ceases in man before birth. Increased hairiness later in life, for instance the growth of the male beard or excessive hair in women, is due to the conversion of small follicles into large ones. Experimental results suggest that neogenesis of hairs may take place in rodents, and hopeful voices have called attention to the massive new formation of hairs in the velvet covering the new antlers of deer. In this case, however, complete new skin is produced in great quantity, and nothing comparable takes place in human life. It is probable that accessory hair roots are formed very occasionally in human skin, but most of those encountered in biopsy material are rudimentary and often grow in an abnormal direction. Other instances of rudimentary root formation are seen in benign tumors such as trichofolliculomas (Kligman and Pinkus, 1960; Pinkus and Sutton, 1965) and histiocytomas. The suggestion (Kligman and Strauss, 1956) that new hair roots form in abraded facial skin is not entirely convincing. For other details, see Muller's (1971) review. The possibility of producing new hairs in man must remain a dream for the present.

Sebaceous Gland. It was mentioned previously that the sebaceous gland forms as a knobby bud from the lower (or posterior) wall of the fetal hair germ above the bulge. The bud grows into a more or less spherical mass, the central cells of which acquire lipid and eventually degenerate. They accumulate in a lumen-like space which opens into the follicular canal. During childhood, sebaceous glands remain small and seem to be inactive. Puberty produces variable growth. One or more sebaceous glands may open into a follicle; the largest usually occupies the original position at the posterior surface. The gland (Fig. 2–56) consists of a secretory portion and a duct. The secretory portion is lobated and has no definitive shape, because lobules collapse and new lobules form continuously. They consist of a flat layer of basal cells in which mitotic activity takes place. Inward, the cells become bulky through accumulation of lipid droplets. Small amounts of glycogen also are found in human glands. The lipid droplets are

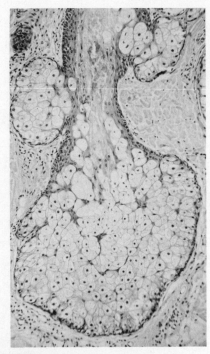

Figure 2–56 Sebaceous gland. *H & E, ×180.*

coarse, and in paraffin sections the nucleus is seen in the center of a network of vacuolated cytoplasm. Toward the center of the lobe, the nuclei become pyknotic and the cells disintegrate to form an amorphous mass which enters the short sebaceous duct. Turnover studies using tritiated thymidine (Grana and Bosco, 1969) have shown that DNA of basal cells remains labeled for from four to seven days. Label can be demonstrated in the central mass of sebum for as long as four weeks. The duct consists of stratified epithelium, often showing some evidence of epidermoid keratinization, and traverses the trichilemma in an oblique course. Its lower wall (Fig. 2–51) is seen in favorable sections as a spur of stratified epithelium, the ductal surface of which contains keratohyalin granules, while the surface facing the follicular lumen exhibits trichilemmal keratinization without keratohyalin. The sebaceous and the follicular lumina merge to form the pilosebaceous canal which opens onto the skin surface through the epidermoid (but not epidermal) infundibulum.

APOCRINE GLAND. The least constant component of the human pilar apparatus is the apocrine gland. Only a small percentage of fetal hair follicles develop a third bud (Fig. 2–7) above the bulge and the sebaceous gland, and even that remains rudimentary except in some regions of the body (see p. 42). While apocrine glands in the axilla may be fully formed at birth, they usually reach a functional stage only at puberty, and at that time apocrine components may also mature in pathologic formations, such as organoid nevi (Pinkus, 1954).

The fully developed apocrine gland (Montagna, 1959) consists of a relatively short and inconspicuous duct and a coiled tubular secretory portion (Fig. 2–42C). The duct usually traverses the wall of the follicular infundibulum (Fig. 2–58A) but may open on the skin surface close to the follicle. It extends fairly straight down and is lined with two layers of cuboidal cells similar to the eccrine duct. The secretory tubule, on the other hand, has a much wider lumen (Fig. 2–57) than its eccrine counterpart, and it may have blind sacculations. It is lined by two layers of cells, the outer one being a flat myoepithelial layer, which is much better developed than in the eccrine gland; and the inner one being a lining of secretory cells which vary from flat to cuboidal to high columnar, depending on the secretory phase. Segments of different configuration are found in the

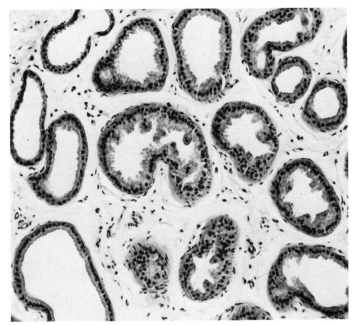

Figure 2–57 Axillary apocrine gland. Secretory cells vary from cuboidal to high columnar and are surrounded by a flat layer of myoepithelial cells. *H & E, ×180.*

same gland. The secretory cells have a basal nucleus and contain a variety of granules in their central portion, which may protrude into the lumen in the shape of a cap. The old view, however, that the cells decapitate themselves in the process of secretion (apocrine secretion) has been proved erroneous by electron microscopy. The cell surface carries numerous microvilli, and the granules are secreted through these. The granules give a variety of staining reactions. Some are of lipid nature, others contain molecular iron, still others are PAS-positive or are naturally pigmented. The pigment generally has a yellow or pale brown tinge, but may be very dark or green or blue. It, then, is the basis of colored sweat (chromhidrosis) which may be excreted in some individuals

not only from the axillae but also from the face or other potentially gland-bearing area. For a tabulation of histochemical enzyme activities in apocrine and eccrine glands, see page 77. Figure 2–58 illustrates the presence of phosphorylase activity in the apocrine duct and its almost complete absence in apocrine secretory epithelium, in contrast to strong activity throughout the eccrine apparatus.

The epithelial portion is surrounded by baskets of elastic and reticulum fibers, which are less well developed than in eccrine glands. The coils usually reside in the subcutaneous tissue between fat lobules. They are innervated by adrenergic fibers. The secretion contains corpuscular elements and may be turbid, milky white, or colored. It accumulates in the wide lumina,

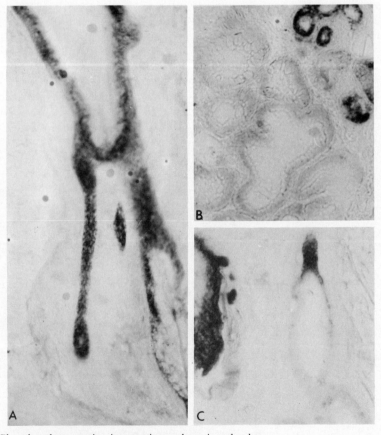

Figure 2–58 Phosphorylase reaction in apocrine and eccrine glands.

A, There is strong enzyme activity in the apocrine duct entering the similarly positive hair follicle. A sebaceous gland is at lower right.

B, There is reactivity of the eccrine coil (upper right) and nonreactivity of the apocrine secretory epithelium.

C, There is abrupt loss of reactivity at the transition from apocrine duct to secretory portion. *Phosphorylase reaction, ×180.* (Courtesy Dr. Melita Svob.)

from which it is excreted onto the skin surface by myoepithelial contraction under adrenergic stimulation. Containing protein and lipids, apocrine sweat is a breeding ground for bacteria and thus becomes the principal source of axillary odor (Shelley et al., 1953).

Peculiar genetically controlled differences exist between the major human races. Most individuals of Oriental stock have differently constructed apocrine glands in the axilla as well as in the ear canal. The ceruminous glands of the auditory meatus secrete a crumbly whitish material in contrast to the soft yellow-brown ear wax of Caucasians and Negroes. The axillary glands of Orientals do not give rise to odors (Adachi, 1937; Pinkus, 1964). Cholinergic innervation of axillary apocrine glands is found in Negroes (Montagna, 1962).

Development and function of apocrine glands depend to a large extent on hormonal regulation. They often remain rudimentary until puberty and undergo some degree of involution in senescence. Well-developed axillary glands, however, persist in women into old age (Montagna, 1959). It has been said and denied that axillary glands have a growth phase during pregnancy. It is sure, in any case, that pathologic conditions, such as Fox-Fordyce disease and hidradenitis suppurativa, show amelioration in pregnancy (Cornbleet, 1952).

Eccrine Apparatus. The eccrine apparatus (Figs. 2–42 and 2–59) consists of a single tube which may be divided into two major portions (Ellis, 1968). These are the secretory (glandular) and the excretory (ductal) portions. The latter is conveniently subdivided into the coiled intradermal part, the "straight" intradermal part, and the intraepidermal part (acrosyr-

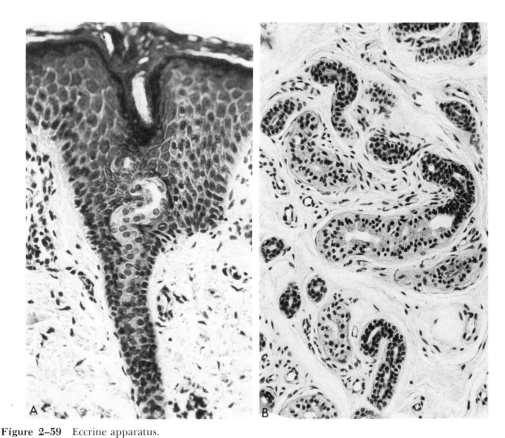

Figure 2–59   Eccrine apparatus.
A, Acrosyringium within the epidermis.
B, Part of the coil of a palmar sweat gland. Note "ampulla" at the sudden transition from ductal to secretory epithelium. *H & E, ×360.*

ingium). All subdivisions are lined by a two-layered epithelium, a general characteristic of sweat and salivary glands, which is often preserved in their tumors.

The acrosyringium (Fig. 2–59*A*) follows a spiraling course through the living and keratinized layers of the epidermis. It is formed by two or more layers of cells which surround a star-shaped lumen lined by a PAS-positive cuticle. The cells produce keratohyalin granules and begin to keratinize at a lower level than the epidermis itself. They are gradually carried to the outside with the slow outward movement of the epidermal keratinocytes, with which they are tightly connected by desmosomes. The acrosyringium is maintained by mitotic divisions taking place in the subepidermal portion of the duct. It appears to have a fixed length (eccrine epidermal sweat duct unit): it is almost straight under acanthotic conditions, but forms a steep spiral in normal epidermis and a tight coil in epidermal atrophy.

Below the epidermis the duct follows a course that has been described as a three-dimensional meander (Wells and Landing, 1968) but which is relatively straight. Its direction may be vertical to the skin surface or it may deviate considerably. One can never be sure in single paraffin sections which coil belongs to which sweat pore. The duct is lined by two layers of cuboidal epithelium surrounded by a tenuous mesodermal sheath. The outer (basal) epithelial layer contains infrequent mitoses, especially in a zone a short distance below the epidermis. Removal of the horny layer by stripping induces numerous mitoses in this area (Pinkus and Mehregan, 1969), which evidently is a matrix zone for the acrosyringium. The ductal cells usually contain much glycogen and are rich in mitochondria and other organelles related to their function of reabsorbing salt from the sweat. A PAS-positive, diastase-resistant cuticle covers the luminal surface.

Deep in the dermis or in the subcutaneous tissue the duct changes direction and forms part of the eccrine coil without changing its cytologic characteristics. About halfway into the coil, however, the ductal epithelium suddenly gives way to the secretory type. The border is quite sharp and usually at a slant. The lumen at this point is slightly widened to form what has been called the eccrine ampulla (Loewenthal, 1961).

The glandular portion has an inner layer of secretory cells and an outer layer represented by a basket of myoepithelial cells, which are less numerous than in the apocrine gland. The epithelium rests on a PAS-positive basement membrane around which is spun a basket of regularly arranged elastic and reticulum fibrils. The secretory cells are divided into light and dark cells according to the depth of staining of their cytoplasm. The light cells are concerned mainly with the secretion of sweat, while the dark cells probably form mucoid substances, including the characteristic diastase-resistant and PAS-positive cuticle of the eccrine duct. In some individuals, all cells have a foamy structure, but there is no obvious relation to function. Both light and dark cells rest on the basket of myoepithelial cells and the basement membrane. The light cells, however, are broader at the base, and the dark cells are broader at the luminal surface. Thus, a false impression of a two-layered secretory epithelium may be produced. The true outer layer is the network of myoepithelial cells. The light cells contain no light microscopic granules and resemble the cells of serous glands. The dark staining of the other cell type is due to larger amounts of basophilic RNA. They contain granules which are stainable by PAS and alcian blue, and are basophilic and metachromatic. The Ziehl-Neelsen reaction for acid-fast substances also demonstrates large granules.

Enzyme histochemistry has demonstrated a characteristic set of activities in the eccrine apparatus which is more or less faithfully maintained in tumors related to eccrine glands. Table 2–8, modified from one published by Hashimoto and Lever (1968), shows that there are differences and overlaps in the "enzyme signature" of eccrine and apocrine glands.

Relatively little is known about regenerative processes in the eccrine apparatus. Mitoses are seen rarely in normal glands and ducts; they are increased in the subepidermal zone when the acrosyringium must be replaced after stripping. Removal of epidermis and upper duct leads to prolifer-

TABLE 2–8   ENZYMES OF ECCRINE AND APOCRINE APPARATUSES*

Localization	Amylophosphorylase and Branching Enzyme		Succinic and Malic Dehydrogenases		Leucine Aminopeptidase		Acid Phosphatase		Alkaline Phosphatase		Beta-Glucuronidase		Indoxyl Esterase		Acetyl-cholinesterase	
	E†	A†	E	A	E	A	E	A	E	A	E	A	E	A	E	A
Intraepithelial duct	++++	+++	?	?	?	?	?	?	?	?	?	?	?	?	?	?
Intradermal duct	++++	+++	+++	−	+++	+	++	+++	−	−	−	+	+	−	−	−
Secretory portion	++++ + to −	+	+++	+	+++	++	++	++++	++++	++++ in myoepithelial cells	−	++++	+	++	+++	++ to − in peripheral nerve fibers

*Modified from Hashimoto and Lever (1968) with additional, unpublished data.
†E = eccrine apparatus.
 A = apocrine apparatus.

ation of the stump (Lobitz et al., 1954), which regénerates the acrosyringium and then contributes to the epidermization of the wound surface. Division of the duct below the epidermis by cutting leads to abnormal regenerative processes from the deep portion. An acrosyringium-like structure with spiraling lumen may be formed, or milium-like keratinizing cysts may result. Destruction of the coil seems to cause degeneration of the upper portion of the duct (author's unpublished results). All these data suggest but do not prove that there is a slow movement of cells from the bottom upward, comparable perhaps to the gradual migration of cells from intestinal crypts to the villi of the gut.

Specialized Glands. Several body regions possess special glands. These include the ceruminous glands of the auditory meatus, the meibomian and Moll glands of the eyelids, and the Montgomery glands of the areola. The ceruminous glands are modified apocrine glands which produce a semisolid product, the ear wax. Their histologic structure is not too much different from other apocrine glands. Similarly, the glands of Moll are fairly typical apocrine glands associated with the eyelashes. They sometimes give rise to simple cysts characteristically located along the lid margins. Meibomian glands, on the other hand, are related to sebaceous glands and

consist of multiple lobules opening into a long central duct. The glands in Montgomery tubercles of the areola, while sharing many features of apocrine sweat glands, have a peculiar embryologic history, which relates them to the mamma but also sets them apart as truly specialized glands of the integument. They have an alveolar structure (Pinkus and Tanay, 1968). The so-called Tyson glands of the corona penis have been recognized as nothing but small papillary excrescences of the skin (Fig. 2–33).

Nail. The adult nail (Achten, 1968; Lewis, 1954) grows from the proximal matrix which forms the floor of the proximal nail fold (Fig. 2–60). Stratified epithelium keratinizes without keratohyalin to form the strongly interconnected horny cells in which keratin fibrils are arranged vertical to the growth axis. The nail plate grows forward out of the cul-de-sac in which it is formed because each individual cell gains in longitudinal diameter as it flattens (Kligman, 1961a). A thin dorsal portion seems to be added to the plate from cells in the most proximal portion of the roof of the nail fold. More distal cells of the roof form the eponychium or cuticle, which adheres to the dorsal nail surface. When the nail plate reaches the distal end of the lunula, it comes into contact with the nail bed and glides over it with the apposition

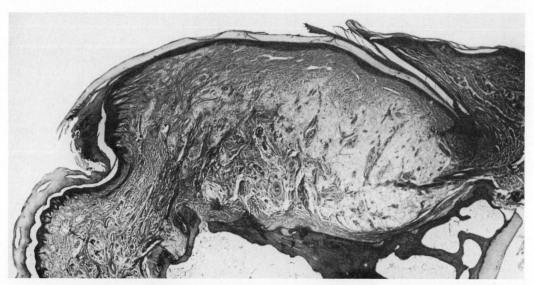

Figure 2–60   Distal phalanx of adult toe. Compare with Figures 2–10 and 2–11. *H & E*, ×8.

of a minimal amount of keratinizing cells formed by the bed. When the nail approaches the free end of the digit, it meets the distal matrix,* a narrow band of epithelium which adds specialized keratin to the lower surface of the nail in the region of the macroscopic "yellow line." This material (horn of the sole) fastens the nail much more tightly at the distal edge, as the surgeon can feel when he starts to evulse a nail by pushing the blade of a hemostat under it. Once the instrument breaks through this adhesive band, it slides easily between nail and nail bed. The horn of the sole is homologous to the mass of horn composing the horse's hoof and takes its name from that comparison. It becomes hyperplastic in pachyonychia congenita (Achten and Wanet-Rouard, 1970). Still further distalward, the epidermis forms loose masses of keratin which easily mix with dirt and are removed cosmetically.

The nail bed consists of stratified epidermis resting on long ridges of dermis with closely arrayed papillae. The lower surface of the epithelium resembles corrugated board. Between the main area of the nail bed and the distal yellow line, one can macroscopically define a band that blanches easily from pressure from below. In this area, the dermal papillae begin to slant forward and become very long. The capillaries in them are easily emptied by pressure, and in very thin nails they can be seen as longitudinal loops. Bleeding from these capillaries produces the so-called splinter hemorrhages under the nail.

Electron microscopic and x-ray diffraction studies have done much to clarify the intimate structure and the remarkable physical properties of the nail plate (Baden, 1970; Forslind, 1970).

Interactions Between Dermis, Epidermis, and Adnexa

In order to understand normal, regenerative, and neoplastic life processes in the

skin, it is necessary to be aware of interactions between epithelium and mesoderm, and also between the specialized components of the epithelial system. Interest in these matters has increased greatly over the years. A recent conference on epithelial-mesenchymal interaction (Fleischmajer and Billingham, 1969) has produced a good review. Not only does the epithelium of epidermis and adnexa differentiate and mature under the inductive influence of mesoderm, but it also seems to need constant association and support to maintain its integrity. This has been shown in a variety of transplantation and explantation experiments. The morphologic expression of this interaction is the formation of basement membranes which develop in the fetus first at the sites of hair germs and persist through life unless malignant neoplasia deprives the epithelial cells of the ability to interact properly.

Less frequently emphasized, but of considerable significance in wound healing, in restitution after inflammatory disturbances, and in the early stages of neoplasia, is the fact that the pluripotential epithelia of the adnexa live in symbiotic relationship with the epidermal keratinocytes (Pinkus, 1958b). The fetal adnexal apparatuses grow from the basal layer upward through the epidermis to the surface and in later life form intraepidermal biologic units, the acrotrichium and the acrosyringium (Fig. 2–61). Whenever epidermis is lost in blistering or necrotizing disease, in burns, or in donor sites of skin grafts, the stumps of the adnexal units first regenerate themselves, then become modulated to form new epidermis. If the epidermis becomes neoplastic in actinic skin or in Bowen dermatosis, the normal balance between epidermal keratinocytes and adnexal keratinocytes is disturbed. The two types of epithelium do not recognize each other any more as "self," and grow competitively past each other, the healthy adnexal keratinocytes spreading on the surface and the neoplastic epidermal keratinocytes extending along the dermal junction. These matters are discussed in more detail in Chapter 17. Symbiotic relationships of the keratinocytes of epidermis and hair root to the Langerhans cells and neuroectodermal melanocytes will be discussed later.

---

*The distal matrix is being referred to as hyponychium in American literature, following the example of *Lewis* (1954). Hyponychium was and is being used in European literature to refer to the nail bed. The term hyponychium is avoided in this chapter in order to prevent confusion.

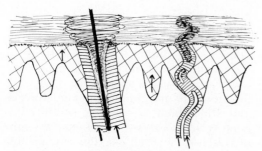

Figure 2–61 Diagram illustrating the symbiosis of epidermal, follicular, and eccrine keratinocytes.

Still more subtle organizational relationships in the skin are suggested by spatial distribution of hairs, sweat glands, and their associated nerves and vessels. These were alluded to by F. Pinkus (1927) under the designation hair field, and were later elaborated upon by Horstmann (1957) in his concept of repetitive motifs in the arrangement of eccrine glands around hair groups. A thoughtful article by Straile (1971) suggests that epithelial and dermal structures are organized in repeating vertical units, each containing a highly systematized population of nerves and nerve endings, blood vessels and blood vessel endings, hair follicle groups, and glands.

Neuroectoderm

Nerves and Nerve Endings. When axons of sensory and sympathetic ganglion cells and their sheathing Schwann cells have reached their final distribution in the skin, they innervate epithelial structures and blood vessels as free endings or form specifically organized nerve end organs. Myelinated sensory nerves (Winkelmann, 1960) approach and possibly enter the epidermis and certain portions of the hair follicle, while glands, hair muscle, and blood vessels receive autonomic innervation (Montagna, 1962; Hagen, 1968). The effects of surgical interruption of the respective connections are well known. Restitution of sensory function often is achieved after nerves are severed in or near the skin, or in transplanted skin, because new axons grow along the old channels.

Specifically structured nerve end organs

are of four types: (1) capsulated organs of the Vater-Pacinian type, (2) coiled organs of the Meissner type, (3) perifollicular nerve networks, and (4) Haarscheiben (hair disks) possessing Merkel cells. Some other forms described by earlier anatomists are variants of these four main types or examples of morphologic misinterpretation (Winkelmann, 1960). The Vater-Pacinian corpuscle usually is situated in subcutaneous tissue, is so large it can be seen with the naked eye, and is a fluid-filled ovoid mass with multiple connective tissue lamellae forming a capsule around the central axon. The Meissner corpuscle (Cauna, 1956a and 1956b) is always situated in a cutaneous papilla close to the lower surface of the epidermis. It is a tiny egg-shaped structure consisting of stacked Schwann cells on which multiple endings of a sensory axon are distributed. It, or its variants (Fig. 2–62), are found only in the hairless skin of volar surfaces and mucocu-

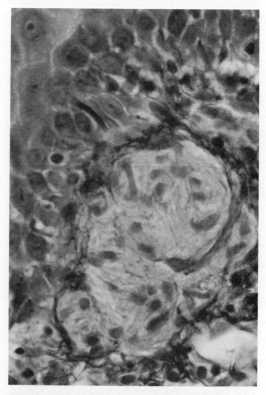

Figure 2–62 Sensory nerve corpuscle from glans penis, the mucocutaneous end organ of Winkelmann (1960). It resembles a deformed Meissner corpuscle. *Acid orcein and Giemsa, ×800.*

taneous junctions. Meissner corpuscles subserve the sensation of touch.

In the hairy skin, the function of acute touch perception is in part fulfilled by nerve baskets surrounding the isthmus of the hair root and activated by slight movement of the long lever of the hair. The haarscheibe, described under this name almost 70 years ago, had its unique function as a slow-reacting touch perceptor clarified only in recent years (Straile, 1971). It is always found close to a hair and consists of a disk-like array of Merkel cells in the epidermal basal layer to which a thick myelinated nerve fiber extends hederiform endings. Merkel cells, which appear as clear roundish elements under the microscope, are modified epidermal keratinocytes possessing special submicroscopic granules (Smith, 1970).

Dendritic Cells. Under the noncommittal name dendritic cells, we unite melanocytes and Langerhans cells. While the melanocytes are of neuroectodermal origin, the cells of Langerhans probably are not. They may be either of ectodermal or mesodermal origin, but additional information is needed to settle this issue.

MELANOCYTES. Melanocytes occur in adult skin in three principal locations: in the epidermis, in the hair matrix, and in the dermis (Montagna and Hu, 1967). They are commonly found in some benign epithelial tumors, such as seborrheic verruca and trichoepithelioma, and in basal cell epithelioma; but they are rare in truly malignant lesions, such as squamous cell carcinoma, and in the precursor lesion, actinic keratosis. Malformed derivatives of fetal melanoblasts, and possibly also of adult melanocytes, are known as nevus cells and form brown moles. The cells of malignant melanoma may be derived either from nevus cells or from melanocytes (Mishima, 1967).

Epidermal melanocytes (Fig. 2–63) are intercalated between basal cells and are seen by light microscopy either as the clear cells of Masson or as dendritic elements full of tiny, evenly sized brown granules. They often sit between the lower portions of two basal cells or may hang down from the epidermis like spiders. In the examina-

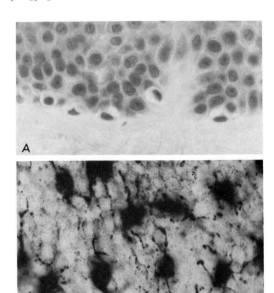

Figure 2–63 Melanocytes.

A, Masson clear cells in a vertical section of nonpigmented skin. *H & E,* ×*360.*

B, A photograph of a dopa-treated sheet of isolated epidermis showing the dendritic shape of junctional melanocytes. ×*400.*

tion of dopa-treated epidermal sheets separated from the dermis by trypsin or sodium bromide solutions, they are seen as dendritic cells (Fig. 2–63*B*), very much resembling the shape of astrocytes of the brain. They are histochemically identifiable by the dopa reaction because they contain an enzyme, now generally accepted as being tyrosinase, which also acts on dioxyphenylalanine (dopa) to produce black, insoluble melanin. This reaction demonstrates even unmelanized melanocytes, except for those in albinos. Counts have shown that very light as well as very dark skins contain similar numbers of melanocytes per square millimeter of skin surface (Staricco and Pinkus, 1957). On the other hand, considerable topographic differences exist, ranging from about 600 on the abdomen to 2000 on the face and genitalia (Szabo, 1959). A convenient mean value to remember is 1000 melanocytes per square millimeter. In vertical sections, about one cell in every 10 basal cells is normal (Cochran, 1970). The color difference between light and dark skin is a purely physiologic one, depending on the level of melanin-forming activity of the melanocytes.

Similarly, differences in hair color are attributable to varying levels of activity of the melanocytes of the hair matrix. Albino hairs also contain melanocytes, while senile white hairs have lost their complement of these cells.

Dermal melanocytes, which form a widespread system in the skin of many mammals and other vertebrates, are rudimentary in man and are usually restricted to the area of the sacral or dorsal blue spot of newborn babies and to the periocular umbra.

The individual melanocyte consists of a nucleus, which appears shrunken under the light microscope and irregularly lobular under the electron microscope; and cytoplasm, which usually is drawn out into two or more processes called dendrites. The cell does not possess tonofibrils or desmosomes but does contain many mitochondria and other organelles. The cell membrane is backed by an electron-dense plate at the surface which faces the dermis (Tarnowski, 1970). A constant feature is the presence of melanosomes, which are visible under the light microscope only when they are melanized (melanin granules).

Electron microscopic and histochemical studies have shown that melanosomes arise as vesicles in the region of the Golgi apparatus and develop a fibrillar proteinaceous skeleton, on which the precursors of melanin are formed from tyrosine under the action of tyrosinase. Melanin is deposited as a polymerized insoluble end product and eventually obscures all structural details of the melanosome. Melanin is argentaffin and precipitates silver out of solutions of its salts. Melanosomes in the unmelanized state, either when they are young or if they are incapable of melanin production in albinos, are not argentaffin but argyrophilic (Mishima, 1960b). That means they can be demonstrated by Fontana-Masson's ammoniacal silver nitrate method (Mishima's premelanin reaction). Furthermore, the protein base of the me-

lanin granule binds methylene blue (and other basic dyes), thereby converting the brown tinge of melanin into greenish-black and differentiating it from hemosiderin and other pigments.

Normal human melanin granules are elongated ovoid bodies and have been compared to lemons and American footballs. They are easily transferred into other cells through phagocytosis of parts of the dendrites containing them. Under physiologic conditions, the keratinocytes of the epidermis (Fig. 2–38) and the hair matrix acquire a smaller or larger number of melanin granules by this process and carry them to the surface. Epidermal cells of Caucasians and Orientals have been shown to segregate the granules into lysosomes and to fragment and disintegrate them, while the keratinocytes of Negroes (Szabo et al., 1969) and Australian aborigines (Mitchell, 1968) retain the granules intact in their cytoplasm. These physiologic differences probably accentuate the macroscopically visible color differences.

The enzyme tyrosinase is inhibited in Caucasian epidermal melanocytes and is demonstrable only by dopa. It becomes activated by ultraviolet or ionizing radiation and can then be shown also by incubation with tyrosine. Even in Negro skin, sunlight and x-rays will produce a marked activation of tyrosinase, as is evidenced by the color difference between exposed and nonexposed skin of relatively light brown individuals and the considerable darkening effect of even small doses of x-ray therapy. The enzyme appears to be more strongly inhibited, but not absent, in albino skin. The inhibiting factors in albinos seem to be present in the dermis, inasmuch as separated epidermal sheets and the matrix of plucked growing hairs give a positive dopa reaction.

Keratinocytes and melanocytes live in symbiotic relationship (Pinkus et al., 1959), and it seems that each melanocyte has its territory and supplies melanin granules to a more or less fixed number of keratinocytes in an epidermal melanin unit (Fitzpatrick and Breathnach, 1963; Frenk and Schellhorn, 1969). The symbiosis is disturbed under three circumstances. If keratinocyte metabolism is deranged either in inflammatory disease or in neoplasia, the

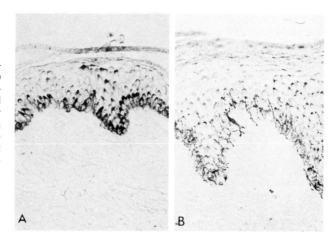

Figure 2-64 Fontana-Masson silver reaction in normal (*A*) and inflamed (*B*) portion of the epidermis in a case of pityriasis rosea in Negro skin. The normal basal layer contains distinct supranuclear caps of melanin, which are also present in many prickle cells. Melanocytes are inconspicuous. The edematous and acanthotic epidermis shows large dendritic melanocytes, but less pigment in keratinocytes. ×180.

cells temporarily or permanently stop phagocytosing melanin granules. The melanocytes, if active, then become engorged with granules which fill their dendrites to the extreme. Inflamed Negro skin thus is apt to acquire a darker hue by a physical phenomenon similar to the darkening of the skin of frogs when their dendritic melanophores expand. Under the microscope and in vertical section (Fig. 2–64) such

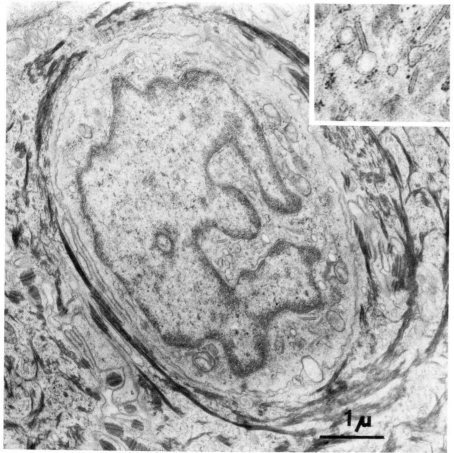

Figure 2-65 Electron micrograph of epidermal Langerhans cell. ×17,400. Insert shows the characteristic racket-shaped granules. ×45,600.

epidermis may appear lighter because the concentrated deep pigmentation of the basal layer disappears and melanin is distributed over a larger surface. In diseases such as lupus erythematosus or lichen planus, in which there is severe disturbance of basal cells, melanocytes discharge their granules into dermal macrophages, where it is stored for prolonged times. In neoplasia, e.g., in actinic keratoses or Bowen's disease, the melanocytes quickly die out in most cases.

If melanocytes become neoplastic, they are apt to loose their territorial behavior and to crowd together. This is seen in all nevus cell lesions, whether benign or malignant, and also in lentigo maligna (Dubreuilh's precancerous melanosis), where large dendritic melanocytes honeycomb the basal layer in a diagnostic pattern (Mishima, 1960a).

Finally, in wound healing, regeneration of the epidermis far outstrips the ability of the melanocytes to multiply. While some melanocytes usually are carried along with the epithelium advancing from the rim of the wound or from follicular stumps, the new epidermis is free of visible pigmentation; this is most evident in Negro skin. Weeks later, pigment spreads from the wound periphery and from follicular pores (Staricco, 1963). Similarly, pigmentation advances in healing areas of vitiligo. It has been shown that this process can be initiated by transplanting individual hair roots into vitiliginous areas (Nosaki and Yokota, 1968).

LANGERHANS CELLS. Dendritic cells, first demonstrated by Langerhans by means of gold chloride, are present in the higher epidermal layers. Electron microscopy (Fig. 2–65) has shown that they contain highly characteristic cytoplasmic bodies called Langerhans cell granules, although they usually have an elongated shape. Very similar granules have been identified in the specific cells of histiocytosis X (Gianotti and Caputo, 1969). More work is needed to establish the histogenesis and function of these dendritic cells, but their existence as a separate morphologic element in the epidermis is established beyond doubt. They play a peculiar role in vitiligo, where melanocytes become inactive, and are first replaced by dendritic cells without any granules, and later by Langerhans cells (Zelickson and Mottaz, 1968; Mishima et al., 1969).

REFERENCES

Achten, G.: Normale Histologie und Histochemie des Nagels. *In* Jadassohn's Handbuch der Haut- und Geschlechtskrankheiten. Ergänzungswerk, Vol. I. 1:339, Berlin, Springer-Verlag, 1968.

Achten, G., and Wanet-Rouard, J.: Pachonychia, Br. J. Dermatol., 83:56, 1970.

Adachi, B.: Das Ohrenschmalz als Rassenmerkmal und der Rassengeruch ("Achselgeruch") nebst dem Rassenuntersshied der Schweissdrüse. Z. Rassenkunde, 6:273, 1937.

Alkiewicz, J.: On the original location of the germ of human nails. Bull. Soc. Amic. Sci. Poznan., Ser., C2:56, 1951.

Alter, M.: Variations in palmar creases. Am. J. Dis. Child., 120:424, 1970.

Aram, H.: Scalp hair. Arch. Dermatol., 102:562, 1970.

Baden, H. P.: The physical properties of nail. J. Invest. Dermatol. 55:115, 1970.

Baker, H., and Blair, C. P.: Cell replacement in the human stratum corneum in old age. Br. J. Dermatol., 80:367, 1968.

Barnicot, N. A.: Reflectometry of the skin in Southern Nigerians and in some Mulattoes. Hum. Biol., 30:150, 1958.

Becker, P. E.: Humangenetik. Ein Kurzes Handbuch in fünf Bänden. Stuttgart, Georg Thieme, 1968.

Berger, H., and Berger, C.: Elektronenmikroskopische Befunde zur Verankerung kleiner Hautgefässe im Bindegewebe. Arch. Klin. Exp. Dermatol., 236:207, 1970.

Bernstein, I. A., Chakrabarti, S. G., Kumaroo, K. K., and Sibrack, L. A.: Synthesis of protein in the mammalian epidermis. J. Invest. Dermatol., 55:291, 1970.

Bettmann, S.: Über Dermatogramme und ihre Verwertung. Arch. Dermatol. Syph. (Berlin), 153:637, 1927.

Breathnach, A. S., Silvers, W. S., Smith, J., and Heyner, S.: Langerhans cells in mouse skin experimentally deprived of its neural crest component. J. Invest. Dermatol., 50:147, 1968.

Briggaman, R. A., Dalldorf, F. G., and Wheeler, C. E., Jr.: Basal lamina formation in adult human skin. J. Invest. Dermatol., 54:346, 1970.

Briggaman, R. A., and Wheeler, C. E., Jr.: Epidermal-dermal interactions in adult human skin. II. The nature of the dermal influence. J. Invest. Dermatol., 56:18, 1971.

Brody, I.: The epidermis. *In* Jadassohn's Handbuch der Haut- und Geschlechtskrankheiten. Ergänzungswerk Vol. I, 1:1, Berlin, Springer-Verlag, 1968.

Brownstein, M. H., Shapiro, L., and Slevin, R.: Fistula of the dorsum of the nose. Arch. Dermatol., 109:227, 1974.

Cauna, N.: Structure and origin of the capsule of Meissner's corpuscle. Anat. Rec., 124:77, 1956a.

Cauna, N.: Nerve supply and nerve endings in Meissner's corpuscles. Am. J. Anat., 99:315, 1956b.

Cerimele, D., and Serri, F.: Le vieulissement physiologique et pathologique de la peau; revue des données histologiques et biochimiques. Arch. Belg. Dermatol. Syphiligr., 25:1, 1969.

Chadfield, H. W., and Khan, A. U.: Acquired hypertrichosis lanuginosa. Trans. St. Johns Hosp. Dermatol. Soc., 56:30, 1970.

Chinn, H. D., and Dobson, R. L.: The topographic anatomy of human skin. Arch. Dermatol., 89:267, 1964.

Cleaver, J. E.: DNA damage and repair in light sensitive human skin disease. J. Invest. Dermatol., 54:181, 1970.

Cochran, A. J.: The incidence of melanocytes in normal human skin. J. Invest. Dermatol., 55:65, 1970.

Cooper, J. H.: Histochemical observations on elastic sheath–elastofibril system of dermis. J. Invest. Dermatol., 52:169, 1969.

Cornbleet, T.: Pregnancy and apocrine gland diseases: hidradenitis, Fox-Fordyce disease. Arch. Dermatol., 65:12, 1952.

Cseplala, G., and Marton, T.: New method for documentation of healthy or diseased skin surface. Arch. Klin. Exp. Dermatol., 228:414, 1967.

Cummins, H., and Midlo, C.: Finger Prints, Palms, and Soles. An Introduction to Dermatoglyphics. Philadelphia, Blakiston Company, 1943.

Dillon, D. J.: The identification of impressions of nonfriction–ridge-bearing skin. J. Forensic Sci., 8:576, 1963.

Dobson, R. L., Young, M. R., and Pinto, J. S.: Palmar keratoses and cancer. Arch. Dermatol., 92:553, 1965.

Dronamraju, K. R.: Hypertrichosis of the pinna of the human ear; y-linked pedigrees. J. Genet. 57:230, 1960.

Duperrat, B., and Mascaro, J. M.: Une tumeur bénigne développée aux dépens de l'acrotrichium ou partie intraépidermique du follicule pilaire: porome folliculaire (acanthome folliculaire intraépidermique; acrotrichoma. Dermatologica, 126:291, 1963.

Ellis, R. A.: Eccrine sweat glands: electron microscopy, cytochemistry and anatomy. *In* Jadassohn's Handbuch der Haut- und Geschlechtskrankheiten. Ergänzungswerk, Vol. I. 1:224, Berlin, Springer-Verlag, 1968.

Felgenhauer, W.-R.: Hypertrichosis lanuginosa universalis. J. Genet. Hum., 17:1, 1969.

Findlay, G. H.: Blue skin. Br. J. Dermatol., 83:127, 1970.

Fitzpatrick, T. B., and Breathnach, A. S.: Das epidermale Melanin-Einheit-System. Derm. Med. Wochenschr., 147:481, 1963.

Fleischmajer, R., and Billingham, R. E.: Epithelial-Mesenchymal Interactions. Baltimore, The Williams & Wilkins Co., 1968.

Flesch, P.: The epidermal iron pigments of red species. J. Invest. Dermatol., 51:337, 1968.

Forslind, B.: Biophysical studies of the normal nail. Acta Derm. Venereol., 50:161, 1970.

Frenk, E., and Schellhorn, J. P.: Zur Morphologie der epidermalen Melanineinheit. Dermatologica, 139:271, 1969.

Fretzin, D. H.: Malignant down. Arch. Dermatol., 95:294, 1967.

Fritsch, G.: Das Haupthaar und seine Bildungstätte bei den Rassen des Menschen. Berlin, Georg Reimer, 1912.

Fukuyama, K., and Epstein, W. L.: Synthesis of RNA and protein during epidermal cell differentiation in man. Arch. Dermatol., 98:75, 1968.

Fular, W.: Der Zellersatz in der menschlichen Epidermis.Gegenbauers Morphol. Jahr., 96:1, 1953.

Gardner, H. L., and Kaufman, R. H.: Benign Diseases of the Vulva and Vagina. St. Louis, The C. V. Mosby Co., 1969.

Garn, S. M.: Changes in areolar size during the steroid growth phase. Child Develop., 23:55, 1952.

Garn, S. M., Selby, S., and Crawford, N. R.: Skin reflectance during pregnancy. J. Obstet., 72:974, 1956.

Gianotti, F., and Caputo, R.: Skin ultrastructure in Hand-Schüller-Christian disease. Arch. Dermatol., 100:342, 1969.

Gillespie, J. A., and Kane, S. P.: Evaluation of a simple surgical treatment of axillary hyperhidrosis. Br. J. Dermatol., 83:684, 1970.

Gloor, M., and Friederich, H. C.: Experimental investigations on secretion of sebum from autografts in man. Hautarzt, 21:219, 1970.

Gloor-Rutishauser, N.: Zur makroskopischen Anatomie der apokrinen Achseldrüsen. Acta Anat., 19:197, 1953.

Goldschmidt, H., and Kligman, A. M.: Quantitative estimation of keratin production by the epidermis. Arch. Dermatol., 88:709, 1963.

Goodman, R. M., and Belcher, R. W.: Periorbital hyperpigmentation. Arch. Dermatol., 100:169, 1969.

Grahame, R., and Holt, P. J. L.: Influence of aging on in vivo elasticity of human skin. Gerontologia, 15:121, 1969.

Grana, A., and Bosco, M.: Il turnover delle ghiandole sebacee umane. Ann. ital. di Dermatologia clin. e sperimentale. 23:279, 1969.

Guiducci, A. A., and Hyman, A. B.: Ectopic sebaceous glands: a review of the literature regarding their occurrence, histology and embryonic relationships. Dermatologica, 125:44, 1962.

Hagen, E.: Zur Innervation des Haut. In Jadassohn's Handbuch der Haut- und Geschlechtskrankheiten. Ergänzungswerk, Vol. I. 1:377, Berlin, Springer-Verlag, 1968.

Hamilton, W. J., Boyd, J. D., and Mossman, H. W.: Human Embryology. Ed. 2. Cambridge, Heffer, 1952.

Hardy, M. H.: The development of pelage hairs and vibrissae from skin in tissue culture. Ann. N. Y. Acad. Sci., 53:546, 1951.

Harrison, R., and Okun, M.: Divided nevus. Arch. Dermatol, 82:235, 1960.

Hashimoto, K.: The ultrastructure of the skin of human embryos. VII. Formation of the apocrine gland. Acta Dermatol. Venereol., 50:241, 1970a.

Hashimoto, K.: The ultrastructure of the skin of human embryos. IX. Formation of the hair cone and intraepidermal hair canal. Arch. Klin. Exp. Derm., 238:333, 1970b.

Hashimoto, K., Gross, B. G., and Lever, W. F.: The ultrastructure of the skin of human embryos. I. The intraepidermal eccrine sweat duct. J. Invest. Dermatol., 45:139, 1965.

Hashimoto, K., and Lever, W. F.: Appendage

Tumors of the Skin. Springfield, Illinois, Charles C Thomas, Publisher, 1968.

Hay, E. D.: Secretion of a connective tissue protein by developing epidermis. *In* Montagna, W., and Lobitz, W. C., Jr.: The Epidermis. New York, Academic Press, Inc., 1964.

Helm, F., and Milgrom, H.: Can scalp hair suddenly turn white? A case of canities subita. Arch. Dermatol, 102:102, 1970.

Herzberg, J., and Gusek, W.: Das Ergrauen des Kopfhaares; eine histo- und fermentchemische sowie elektronenmikroskopische Studie. Arch. Klin. Exp. Dermatol., 236:368, 1970.

Herzberg, J. J., Potjan, K., and Gebauer, D.: Hypertrichose lanugineuse acquise. Un nouveau syndrome paranéoplasique cutané. Ann. Dermatol. Syphiligr., 96:129, 1969.

Hirasawa, M. Über akzessorische Brüste. Zbl. Gynakol., 56:585, 1932.

Holt, S. B.: The Genetics of Dermal Ridges. Springfield, Illinois, Charles C Thomas, Publisher, 1968.

Horstmann, E.: Die Haut. *In* Mollendorf-Bergmann (Eds.): Handbuch der mikroskopischen Anatomie des Menschen. Berlin, Springer-Verlag, 1957.

Howell, J. B., and Mehregan, A. H.: Pursuit of the pits in the nevoid basal cell carcinoma syndrome. Arch. Dermatol., 102:586, 1970.

Hoyes, A. D.: Electron microscopy of surface layer (Periderm) of human fetal skin. J. Anat. 103:321, 1968.

Hunter, R., Steele, C. H., and Pinkus, H.: Examination of the epidermis by the strip method. III. The number of keratin cells in the human epidermis. J. Invest. Dermatol., 27:31, 1956.

Hurley, H. J., and Shelley, W. B.: Simple surgical approach to management of axillary hyperhidrosis. J.A.M.A., 186:109, 1963.

Hyman, A. B., and Brownstein, M. H.: Tyson's "glands"; ectopic sebaceous glands and papillomatosis penis. Arch. Dermatol., 99:31, 1969.

Hytten, F. E., and Baird, D.: The development of the nipple in pregnancy. Lancet, I:1201, 1958.

Jadassohn, J.: Normale und Pathologische Physiologie. *In* Jadassohn's Handbuch der Haut- und Geschlechtskrankheiten. Ergänzungswerk, Vol. I. 3, Berlin, Springer-Verlag, 1963.

Jadassohn, J.: Normale und Pathologische Anatomie 2. *In* Jadassohn's Handbuch der Haut- und Geschlechtskrankheiten. Ergänzungswerk, Vol. I. 2, Berlin, Springer-Verlag, 1964.

Jadassohn, J.: Normale und Pathologische Anatomie 1. *In* Jadassohn's Handbuch der Haut- und Geschlechtskrankheiten. Ergänzungswerk, Vol. I. 1, Berlin, Springer-Verlag, 1968.

Jansen, L. H., and Rottier, P. B.: Elasticity of human skin related to age. Dermatologica, 115:106, 1957.

Jesionek, A.: Biologie der gesunden und kranken Haut. Leipzig, F. C. W. Vogel, 1916.

Johnson, M. L.: Median nasal dermoid fistula. Trans. St. John Dermatol. Soc., 55:241, 1969.

Kantner, M.: Entwicklungsmorphologie der Haut im Kindesalter. *In* Opitz, H., and Schmid, F. (Eds.): Handbuch der Kinderheilkunde. Berlin, Springer-Verlag, 1968.

Keller, P.: Mechanische Eigenschaften der Haut. *In* Jadassohn's Handbuch der Haut- und Geschlechtskrankheiten. Ergänzungswerk, Vol. I. 3:1, Berlin, Springer-Verlag, 1963a.

Keller, P.: Elektrophysiologie der Haut. *In* Jadassohn's Handbuch der Haut- und Geschlechtskrankheiten. Ergänzungswerk, Vol. I. 3:36, Berlin, Springer-Verlag, 1963b.

Kiil, V.: Inheritance of frontal hair directions in man. J. Hered., 39:206, 1948.

Kint, H.: Histophotometric investigation of the nuclear DNA-content in normal epidermis, seborrheic keratosis, keratosis senilis, squamous cell carcinoma and basal cell carcinoma. J. Invest. Dermatol., 40:95, 1963.

Kirk, J. E.: Hand washing. Quantitative studies on skin lipid removal by soaps and detergents based on 1500 experiments. Acta Dermatol. Venereol., 46:1, 1966.

Kleine-Natrop, H. E.: Die Grenzflächenaktivität der gesunden Epidermis und gleichsinnige Ergebnisse bekannter Oberflächen-Funktionsprüfungon. Jap. J. Derm., Ser. B., 77:7, 1967.

Kligman, A. M.: Pathologic dynamics of human hair loss. I. Telogen effluvium. Arch. Dermatol., 83:175, 1961a.

Kligman, A. M.: Why do nails grow out instead of up? Arch. Dermatol., 84:181, 1961b.

Kligman, A. M., and Pinkus, H.: The histogenesis of nevoid tumors of the skin: The folliculoma, a hair follicle tumor. Arch. Dermatol., 81:922, 1960.

Kligman, A. M., and Shehadeh, N.: Pubic apocrine glands and odor. Arch. Dermatol., 89:461, 1964.

Kligman, A. M., and Strauss, J. S.: The formation of vellous hair follicles from human adult epidermis. J. Invest. Dermatol., 27:19, 1956.

Kollar, E. J.: The induction of hair follicles by embryonic dermal papillae. J. Invest. Dermatol., 55:374, 1970.

Lasker, G. W.: Photoelectric measurement of skin color in a Mexican mestizo population. Am. J. Phys. Anthropol., 12:115, 1954.

Leider, M.: On the weight of the skin. J. Invest. Dermatol., 12:187, 1949.

Leider, M., and Buncke, M. C.: Physical dimensions of the skin. Determination of the specific gravity of skin, hair and nail. Arch. Dermatol., 69:563, 1954.

Lentz, C. L., and Altman, J.: Lamellar ichthyosis: the natural clinical course of collodion baby. Arch. Dermatol., 97:3, 1968.

Lewis, B.: Microscopic studies of fetal and mature nail and surrounding soft tissue. Arch. Dermatol., 70:732, 1954.

Lobitz, W. C., Jr., Brophy, D., Larner, A. E., and Daniels, F.: Glycogen response in human epidermal basal cell. Arch. Dermatol., 86:207, 1962.

Lobitz, W. C., Jr., Holyoke, J. B., and Montagna, W.: Responses of the human eccrine sweat duct to controlled injury. J. Invest. Dermatol., 23:329, 1954.

Loewenthal, L. J. A.: "Compound" and grouped hairs of the human scalp; their possible connection with follicular infections. J. Invest. Dermatol., 8:263, 1947.

Loewenthal, L. J. A.: The eccrine ampulla: morphology and function. J. Invest. Dermatol., 36:171, 1961.

Ludwig, E.: Morphologie und Morphogenese des Haarstrichs. Z. Anat. Entwicklungsgesch., 62:59, 1921.

Ludwig, E.: Removal of intact hair papilla and connective tissue sheath by plucking anagen hairs. J. Invest. Dermatol., 48:595, 1967.

Madsen, A.: Studies on the "bulge" (Wulst) in superficial basal cell epithelioma. Arch. Dermatol., 89:698, 1964.

Malkinson, F. D., and Rothman, S.: Percutaneous absorption. *In* Jadassohn's Handbuch der Haut- und Geschlechtskrankheiten. Ergänzungswerk, I. 3:90, Berlin, Springer-Verlag, 1963.

McConnel, F. M. S., Zellweger, H., and Lawrence, R. A.: Labial pits: cleft lip and/or palate syndrome. Arch. Otolaryngol., 91:407, 1970.

McGinley, K. J., Marples, R. R., and Plewig, G.: A method for visualizing and quantitating the desquamating portion of the human stratum corneum. J. Invest. Dermatol., 53:107, 1969.

Mishima, Y.: Melanosis circumscripta precancerosa (Dubreuilh), a non-nevoid premelanoma distinct from junction nevus. J. Invest. Dermatol., 34:361, 1960a.

Mishima, Y.: New technic for comprehensive demonstration of melanin, premelanin, and tyrosinase sites. Combined dopa-premelanin reaction. J. Invest. Dermatol., 34:355, 1960b.

Mishima, Y.: Cellular and subcellular activities in the ontogeny of nevocytic and melanocytic melanomas. *In* Montagna, W., and Hu, F. (Eds.): The Pigmentary System. New York, Pergamon Press, 1967.

Mishima, Y., Kawasaki, H., and Pinkus, H.: Dendritic cell dynamics in progressive depigmentations. Presented at the 7th International Pigment Conference, Seattle, Washington, September, 1969.

Mishima, Y., and Pinkus, H.: Electron microscopy of keratin stripped human epidermis. J. Invest. Dermatol., 50:89, 1968.

Mitchell, R. E.: The skin of the Australian aborigine; a light and electron microscopical study. Australas. J. Dermatol., 9:314, 1968.

Miura, O.: On the demarcation lines of pigmentation observed among the Japanese. Tohoku J. Exp. Med., 54:135, 1951.

Montagna, W.: Histology and citochemistry of human skin. XIX. The development and fate of the axillary organ. J. Invest. Dermatol., 33:151, 1959.

Montagna, W.: Histology and cytochemistry of human skin. XXXIV. The eyebrows. Arch. Dermatol., 101:257, 1970a.

Montagna, W.: Histology and cytochemistry of human skin. XXV. The nipple and areola. Br. J. Dermatol., 83 (Jubilee Issue):2, 1970b.

Montagna, W., Bentley, J. P., and Dobson, R. L. (Eds.): The Dermis. Advances in Biology of Skin. New York, Appleton-Century-Crofts, 1970.

Montagna, W., and Ford, D. M.: Histology and cytochemistry of human skin. XXIII. The eyelid. Arch. Dermatol., 100:328, 1969.

Montagna, W., and Hu, F. (Eds.): The Pigmentary System. Advances in Biology of Skin. New York, Pergamon Press, 1967.

Montagna, W., and Parakkal, P. F. (Eds.): The Structure and Function of Skin. Ed. 3. New York, Academic Press, 1974.

Moretti, G.: The blood vessels of the skin. *In* Jadassohn's Handbuch der Haut- und Geschlechtskrankheiten. Ergänzungswerk, I. 1:471, Berlin, Springer-Verlag, 1968.

Muller, S. A.: Hair neogenesis. J. Invest. Dermatol., 56:1, 1971.

Naide, M.: Relation of growth of hair on digits to severity of ischemia. N. Engl. J. Med., 248:179, 1953.

Naruse, N., and Fujita, T.: Changes in the physical properties of human hair with age. J. Am. Geriatr. Soc., 19:308, 1971.

Nicolaides, N.: Gas chromatographic analysis of the waxes of human scalp skin surface fat. J. Invest. Dermatol., 37:507, 1961.

Nosaki, T., and Yokota, N.: Spot skin grafting and hair follicle transplantation in vitiligo vulgaris: Mechanism of pigment spread induced by these methods. Jap. J. Dermatol., Ser. B., 78:450, 1968.

Oberste-Lehn, H.: Die Bedeutung der Bündelhaare im menschlichen Haarkleid fur die chronischen Follikulitiden. Arch. Klin. Exp. Dermatol., 206:506, 1957.

Odagiri, H.: The histological studies on the epidermis, especially on its regional differences. Jap. J. Dermatol., Series B, 79:62, 1969.

Odland, G. F.: A submicroscopic granular component in human epidermis. J. Invest. Dermatol., 34:11, 1960.

Odland, G. F., and Reed, T. H.: Epidermis. *In* Zelickson, A. S.: Ultrastructure of Normal and Abnormal Skin. Philadelphia, Lea & Febiger, 1967.

Ohman, S., and Shelley, W. B.: o-Phthalaldehyde staining of coiled and uncoiled intraepidermal sweat ducts. J. Invest. Dermatol., 53:29, 1969.

Orentreich, N.: Hair transplants. *In* Maddin, S. (Ed.): Current Dermatologic Management. St. Louis, The C. V. Mosby Co., 1970.

Orfanos, C.: Elektronenmikroskopischer Nachweis epithelio-neuraler Verbindungen (Mechano-Receptoren) am Haarfollikelepithel des Menschen. Arch. Klin. Exp. Dermatol., 228:421, 1967.

Orfanos, C., Christenhasz, R., and Mahrle, G.: Die normale und psoriatische Hautoberfläche; vergleichende Beobachtungen mit dem Raster-Elektronenmikroskop. Arch. Klin. Exp. Dermatol., 235:284, 1969.

Orfanos, C., Ruska, H., and Mahrle, G.: Das weisse Haar alternder Menschen. IV. Uber die Feinstruktur der Haare. Arch. Klin. Exp. Dermatol., 236:395, 1970.

Perera, P., Kurban, A. K., and Ryan, T. J.: The development of the cutaneous microvascular system in the newborn. Br. J. Dermatol., Suppl. No. 5, 82:86, 1970.

Perry, E. T.: The Human Ear Canal. Springfield, Illinois, Charles C Thomas, Publisher, 1957.

Pfister, R., and Weirich, E.: Wachstum u. Gestaltung der Nägel I. u. II. Hautarzt, 7:98, 1956.

Pierce, G. B., Jr.: Basement membranes. VI. Synthesis by epithelial tumors of the mouse. Cancer Res., 25:636, 1965.

Pinkus, F.: Die Normale Anatomie der Haut. *In* Jadassohn, J. (Ed.): Handbuch der Haut- und Geschlechtskrankheiten. Vol. I. 1:1, Berlin, Springer-Verlag, 1927.

Pinkus, F.: Die Einwirkung von Krankheiten auf das Kopfhaar des Menschen. Ed. 2. Berlin, S. Karger, 1928.

Pinkus, H.: Multiple hairs (Flemming-Giovannini). J. Invest. Dermatol., 17:291, 1951a.

Pinkus, H.: Examination of the epidermis by the strip method. I. Observations on the thickness of the horny layer and on mitotic acticity after stripping. J. Invest. Dermatol., 16:383, 1951b.

Pinkus, H.: Examination of the epidermis by the strip method. II. Biometric data on regeneration of the human epidermis. J. Invest. Dermatol., 19:431, 1952.

Pinkus, H.: Premalignant fibroepithelial tumors of skin. Arch. Dermatol., 67:598, 1953.

Pinkus, H.: Life history of nevus syringadenomatous papilliferus. Arch. Dermatol., 69:305, 1954.

Pinkus, H.: Embryology of hair. *In* Montagna, W., and Ellis, R. A. (Eds.): The Biology of Hair Growth. New York, Academic Press, Inc., 1958a.

Pinkus, H.: The concept of symbiosis applied to normal and abnormal growth in the human epidermis. Dermatologica, 117:369, 1958b.

Pinkus, H.: Four-dimensional histopathology. Arch. Dermatol., 82:681, 1960.

Pinkus, H.: Die Makroskopische Anatomie der Haut. *In* Jadassohn's Handbuch der Haut- und Geschlechtskrankheiten. Ergänzungswerk, Vol. I. 2:1, Berlin, Springer-Verlag, 1964.

Pinkus, H.: Static and dynamic histology and histochemistry of hair growth. *In* Baccaredda-Boy, A., et al. (Eds.): Biopathology of Pattern Alopecia. Basel, S. Karger, 1968.

Pinkus, H.: The direction of growth in human epidermis. Br. J. Dermatol., 83:556, 1970.

Pinkus, H., Keech, M. K., and Mehregan, A. H.: Histopathology of striae distensae. J. Invest. Dermatol., 46:283, 1966.

Pinkus, H., and Mehregan, A. H.: A Guide to Dermatohistopathology. New York, Appleton-Century-Crofts, 1969.

Pinkus, H., and Plotnick, H.: Destruction of fingerprint pattern by superficial late syphiloderm. Arch. Dermatol., 78:744, 1958.

Pinkus, H., Rogin, J. R., and Goldman, P.: Eccrine poroma; tumors exhibiting features of the epidermal sweat duct unit. Arch. Dermatol., 74:511, 1956.

Pinkus, H., Staricco, R. J., Kropp, P. J., and Fan, J.: The symbiosis of melanocytes and human epidermis under normal and abnormal conditions. *In* Gordon, M. (Eds.): Pigment Cell Biology. New York, Academic Press, Inc., 1959.

Pinkus, H., and Sutton, R. L., Jr.: Tricholfolliculoma. Arch. Dermatol., 91:46, 1965.

Pinkus, H., and Tanay, A.: Embryologie der Haut. In Jadassohn's Handbuch der Haut- und Geschlechtskrankheiten. Ergänzungswerk, Vol. I. 1:624, Berlin, Springer-Verlag, 1968.

Plewig, G., and Marples, R. R.: Regional differences of cell sizes in the human stratum corneum, Part 1. J. Invest. Dermatol., 54:13, 1970.

Plotnick, H.: Use of a portable colorimeter in dermatology. Cutis, 2:578, 1966.

Pochi, P. E., and Strauss, J. S.: Sebum production, casual sebum levels, titratable acidity of sebum, and urinary fractional 17-ketosteroid excretion in males with acne. J. Invest. Dermatol., 43:383, 1964.

Popoff, H., and Popoff, N.: L'hémopoièse cutanée au cours de la vie intra-uterine. Ann. Dermatol. Syphiligr., 85:157, 1958.

Porter, P. S., and Lobitz, W. C., Jr.: Human hair: a genetic marker. Br. J. Dermatol., 83:225, 1970.

Pruniéras, M., Frey, J., Gazzolo, L., and Delescluse, C.: Synthèse de collagène par les cellules de l'épiderme. Bull. Soc. Fr. Dermatol. Syphiligr., 76:20, 1969.

Reinertson, R. P., and Wheatley, V. R.: Studies on the chemical composition of human epidermal lipids. J. Invest. Dermatol., 32:49, 1959.

Roman, N. A., Ford, B. A., and Montagna, W.: The demonstration of cutaneous nerves. J. Invest. Dermatol., 53:328, 1969.

Rothberg, S., Crounse, R. C., and Lee, J. L.: Glycine-C^{14} incorporation into the proteins of normal stratum corneum and the abnormal stratum corneum of psoriasis. J. Invest. Dermatol., 37:497, 1961.

Saitoh, M., Uzuka, M., and Sakamoto, M.: Human hair cycle. J. Invest. Dermatol., 54:65, 1970.

Sarkany, I., and Gaylarde, P.: A method for demonstration of sweat gland activity. Br. J. Dermatol., 80:601, 1969.

Schmidt, W.: Die normale Histologie von Corium und Subcutis. *In* Jadassohn's Handbuch der Haut- und Geschlechtskrankheiten. Ergänzungswerk, Vol. I. 1:430, Berlin, Springer-Verlag, 1968.

Schmitz, K. L: Die Berechnung der Körperoberfläche. Z. Biol., 106:325, 1954.

Schnyder, U. W.: Inherited ichthyoses. Arch. Dermatol., 102:240, 1970.

Selby, C. C.: An electron microscopic study of thin sections of human skin. II. Superficial cell layers of footpad epidermis. J. Invest. Dermatol., 29:131, 1957.

Sendroy, J., Jr., and Cecchini, L. P.: Determination of human body surface area from height and weight. J. Appl. Physiol., 7:1, 1954.

Sheard, C., and Brunsting, L. A.: The color of the skin as analyzed by spectrophotometric methods. I. Apparatus and procedures. J. Clin. Invest., 7:559, 1929.

Sheehan, J. E.: Replacement of thumb nail. J.A.M.A., 92:1253, 1929.

Shelley, W. B., Hurley, H. J., Jr., and Nichols, A. C.: Axillary odor. Arch. Dermatol., 68:430, 1953.

Sivadjan, J.: Application de l'hydrophotographie aux études dermatoglyphiques. Dermatologica, 140:93, 1970.

Skerlj, B.: Age changes in absolute and relative surface areas of the human body. Br. J. Plast. Surg., 10:146, 1957.

Smahel, J., and Charvát, A.: Fatty tissue in plastic surgery. Acta Chir. Plast., 6:223, 1964.

Smith, K. R., Jr.: The ultrastructure of the human Haarscheibe. J. Invest. Dermatol., 54:150, 1970.

Späth, U., und Steigleder, G. K.: Zahl der Mastzellen (MZ) bei Alopecia areata. Z. Haut. Geschlechtskr., 45:435, 1970.

Starck, D.: Herkunft und Entwicklung der Pigmentzellen. Jadassohn's Handbuch der Haut- und Geschlechtskrankheiten. Ergänzungswerk, Vol. I. 2:139, Berlin, Springer-Verlag, 1968.

Staricco, R. G.: Amelanotic melanocytes in the outer sheath of the human hair follicle and their role in the repigmentation of regenerated epidermis. Ann. N. Y. Acad. Sci., 100:239, 1963.

Staricco, R. G., and Pinkus, H.: Quantitative and qualitative data on the pigment cells of adult human epidermis. J. Invest. Dermatol., 28:33, 1957.

Steigleder, G. K., und Schultis, K.: Zur Histochemie der Esterasen der Haut. Arch. Klin. Exp. Dermatol., 205:196, 1957.

Stöhr, P.: Entwicklungsgeschichte des menschlichen Wollhaares. Anat. Hefte, Abt. 1, 23:1, 1904.

Stough, T. R., and Seely, J. R.: Dermatoglyphics in medicine. Clin. Pediatr., 8:32, 1969.

Straile, W. E.: Vertical cutaneous organization. J. Theor. Biol., 24:203, 1971.

Straile, W. E.: Dermal-epidermal interaction in sensory hair follicles. *In* Montagna, W., and Dobson, R. L. (Eds.): Hair Growth. New York, Pergamon Press, 1968.

Syme, J., and Riley, I. D.: Nail-fold capillary loop development in the infant of low birth weight. Br. J. Dermatol., 83:591, 1970.

Szabo, G.: The regional frequency and distribution of hair follicles in human skin. *In* Montagna, W., and Ellis, R. A. (Eds.): The Biology of Hair Growth. New York, Academic Press, Inc., 1958.

Szabo, G.: Quantitative histological investigations on the melanocytic system of the human epidermis. *In* Gordon, M. (Ed.): Pigment Cell Biology. New York, Academic Press, Inc., 1959.

Szabo, G., Getald, A. B., Pathak, M. A., and Fitzpatrick, T. B.: Racial differences in fate of melanosomes in human epidermis. Nature, 222:1081, 1969.

Takami, Y.: A study on axillary odor. Jap. J. Dermatol., 70:242, 1960.

Tarnowski, W. M.: Ultrastructure of the epidermal melanocyte dense plate. J. Invest. Dermatol., 55:265, 1970.

Todd, T. W., Blackwood, B., and Beecher, H.: Skin pigmentation: the color top method of recording. Am. J. Phys. Anthropol., 11:197, 1928.

Töndury, G.: Embryologie u. Hauttopographie. Arch. Klin. Exp. Dermatol., 219:12, 1964.

Tring, D. C., and Murgatroyd, L. B.: Surface microtopography of normal human skin. Arch. Dermatol., 109:223, 1974.

Tronnier, H., and Eisbacher, I.: Über eine neue Methode zur Messung der Rauhigkeit der Haut. Berufsdermatosen, 18:89, 1970.

Uribe, G. A.: La mancha mongolica. Int. J. Dermatol., 9:180, 1970.

Van Scott, E. J., Reinertson, R. P., and Steinmuller, R.: The growing hair roots of the human scalp and morphologic changes therein following amethapterin therapy. J. Invest. Dermatol., 29:197, 1957.

Varadi, D. P.: Elastin in embryonic skin and aorta. J. Invest. Dermatol. (Abst.), 54:351, 1970.

Verbov, J.: Clinical significance and genetics of epidermal ridges—a review of dermatoglyphics. J. Invest. Dermatol., 54:261, 1970.

Voorhees, J. J., Chakrabarti, S. G., and Bernstein, I. A.: The metabolism of "histidine-rich" protein in normal and psoriatic keratinization. J. Invest. Dermatol., 51:344, 1968.

Vriezen, C.: Cutaneous fistulas of dental origin. Ned. Tijdschr. Geneeskd., 112:65, 1968.

Weinstein, G. D., and Frost, P.: Abnormal cell proliferation in psoriasis. J. Invest. Dermatol., 50:254, 1968.

Wells, T. R., and Landing, B. H.: The helical course of the human eccrine sweat duct. J. Invest. Dermatol., 51:177, 1968.

Winer, J. H., and Winer, L. H.: Hirsutoid papillomas of coronal margin of glans penis. J. Urol., 74:375, 1955.

Winkelmann, R. K.: Nerve Endings in Normal and Pathologic Skin. Springfield, Illinois, Charles C Thomas, Publisher, 1960.

Winter, V., and Levan, N. E.: Basement membrane of normal skin. (A study using the fluorescent periodic acid-acriflavine method). Arch. Dermatol., 102:418, 1970.

Wolf, J., and Hanušova, S.: Influence of the age of skin relief in man. Folia Morphol., 18:262, 1970.

Wolff, K., and Schreiner, E.: Zur ultrastrukturellen Histochemie des Intercellularraumes der Epidermis. Arch. Klin. Exp. Dermatol., 237:290, 1970.

Zaias, N.: Embryology of the human nail. Arch. Dermatol., 87:37, 1963.

Zelickson, A. S., and Mottaz, J. H.: Epidermal dendritic cells. A quantitative study. Arch. Dermatol., 98:652, 1968.

Zimmermann, A. A.: The development of epidermal pigmentation in the Negro fetus. Anat. Rec., 100:96, 1948.

Zimmermann, A. A., and Becker, S. W., Jr.: Melanoblasts and melanocytes in fetal Negro skin. Illinois Monogr. Med. Sci., 6:1, 1959.

3

*Transplantation Biology**

Felix T. Rapaport, M.D., and John Marquis Converse, M.D.

The replacement of diseased or worn organs with normal tissues has been one of mankind's fondest dreams since the beginning of recorded history. The mythologic chimera, the data inscribed in Egyptian papyri, numerous allusions to transplantation in Medieval times, and the depiction of an actual limb transplantation in a classical painting of the Renaissance are particularly striking illustrations of this ever-recurring dream (Converse and Casson, 1968). In more modern times, transplantation has gained increasing recognition as an extremely useful model for the study of a wide variety of biologic problems. These include the actual transplantation of a variety of organs, with the associated problems of organ procurement, preservation, and perfusion. Of equal importance is the massive research effort centered on the problem that normal mammalian hosts confronted with tissues obtained from another donor, i.e., allografts, will respond to this intrusion by triggering mechanisms which are normally designed to protect them from invasive microorganisms and rapidly mutating cells (Lawrence, 1959b).

This brief review will be concerned with the allograft rejection reaction and its biologic implications. Autografts, i.e., tissues transplanted from one site to another on the same host, and tissues exchanged between identical twins, neither of which evokes a rejection reaction, will not be discussed. There will also be no attempt to delve into the very extensive literature on nonvital allografts (or homostatic allografts), such as frozen skin or bone, which do not usually evoke a rejection response, but instead act as biologic dressings or as scaffolding for the subsequent ingrowth of host tissues or cells (Woodruff, 1960). Rather, an attempt will be made to place into the overall perspective of modern medicine a number of significant stages in transplantation which have directly led to a broadening of our understanding of immunologic reactions and to significant improvements in current methods of management of end-stage disease of vital organs. It must be noted in this regard that the actual transplantation of such organs constitutes only one of the facets of the dramatic impact of this field upon the sum total of mammalian biology. The exponential growth of modern immunology and

*Work by the authors has been supported by a grant from the John A. Hartford Foundation, Inc.

especially our increased understanding of cellular response mechanisms are a striking example of the contribution of transplantation to science. Much of the information gathered during studies of allograft reactivity may also in the not too distant future became focused upon one of the main health problems threatening human survival—cancer. As was originally suggested by Thomas (1959) and Burnet (1965), it is not unlikely that the primordial mechanisms triggered by allogenic tissues may have been originally intended by nature to protect the host from newly proliferating neoplastic cells. The apparent inability of cancer patients to mount vigorous cellular immune responses (Solowey and Rapaport, 1965) may thus be a reflection of an alteration in immunologic reactivity which makes possible the development of malignant disease and its unchecked growth.

GENERAL CONSIDERATIONS IN TRANSPLANTATION IMMUNOLOGY

The tempo and intensity of the allograft rejection response have long been known to be directly related to the degree of antigenic or genetic disparity between donor and recipient. As a consequence, a considerable portion of transplantation research has been concerned with the immunogenetics of transplantation, leading to the development of a whole new field of endeavor, histocompatibility testing or "tissue typing." As early as 1903, Jensen observed that mice of different "races" differed in their susceptibility to spontaneous tumors, and suggested the presence of a state of active immunity in the resistant animals. The careful studies of Loeb and of Tyzzer during this same period provided suggestive evidence of the genetic background for host resistance or susceptibility to such transplantable tumors (Billingham and Silvers, 1971). The classic studies of Little in 1914 then provided evidence that host susceptibility to transplantable tumors was determined by a large number of inherited factors, each determined by an independent gene (Little, 1956). Finally, Little's distinguished successor at the Jackson Laboratory, George D. Snell, and the late Peter Gorer of Guy's Hospital in London, through a series of brilliant experiments provided the basis for modern immunogenetics of histocompatibility (Gorer, 1937; Snell, 1956). Their studies culminated in the demonstration of a serologically detectable, multiallelic major system of histocompatibility in the murine species, termed H-2. Largely based upon this experimental model, similar major histocompatibility systems have now been defined in every species studied thus far, including HL-A in man (Dausset and Rapaport, 1966b; Rapaport and Dausset, 1968 and 1969), AgB or RtH_1 in the rat (Palm, 1971; Stark et al., 1971), GPL-A in the guinea pig (DeWeck et al., 1971), SL-A in the pig (Vaiman, 1970), DL-A in the dog (Rapaport et al., 1970; Dausset et al., 1971), ChL-A in the chimpanzee (Balner et al., 1971), and RhL-A in the rhesus monkey (Balner et al., 1971a).

A significant portion of the early studies of histocompatibility has been based upon the tumor allograft model; evidence that mammalian host responses to normal tissues generally paralleled earlier findings with tumors then led to the adoption of the skin allograft as the classic experimental model for immunologic studies of transplantation responses (Rapaport and Converse, 1968). Indeed, the fact that skin contains most if not all transplantation antigens present in other tissues, the readily accessibility of this tissue, and the ease of observation of the experimental results make this tissue a particularly useful instrument for transplantation studies, particularly in human subjects.

Schöene (1908) and Lexer (1911) were the first to suggest that allografts of skin are rejected through a process which Schöene termed "transplantations—immunität." These studies were continued by Loeb, who concluded in 1930 that the biologic uniqueness of the individual provided an unbreachable barrier to successful allotransplantation. It remained, however, for the classic studies of Medawar (1944 and 1945) and, in particular, of Gibson and Medawar (1942) to provide definitive evidence in man that skin allografts were rejected as a consequence of the acquisition by the recipient of an active state of immunity specifically directed against the donor's tissues.

THE SKIN ALLOGRAFT REACTION IN MAN

The responses of normal human donors to skin allografts may be of particular interest to the readers of this volume. For this reason, an attempt will be made to outline the experimental parameters and methods which have led to the modern definition of the range of human responsiveness to skin allografts. The experimental model for these studies was standardized by the authors in 1956. Briefly, it consists of incision (under local infiltration anesthesia) of donor sites on the anterior surfaces of the forearms of the recipients with a circular Castroviejo trephine, yielding defects measuring 11 mm. in diameter. Full-thickness skin grafts are excised, and the superficial portion of the host's dermis is left intact, as a graft-recipient bed. Full-thickness skin specimens obtained from another subject are then placed upon the prepared graft beds, and the grafts are approximated to the surrounding host skin by interrupted 5–0 nylon sutures. A pressure dressing is applied, and the grafts are examined daily after the first postoperative day.

In order to provide more precise criteria for the diagnosis of allograft rejection, the surface of the grafts is examined with a Bausch and Lomb stereomicroscope, with visualization of the small superficial vessels of the graft and of blood flow through these vessels. Through the combined use of gross and microscopic techniques of graft examination, a set of specific criteria was developed for the determination of graft rejection. These criteria, which were an essential prerequisite for further studies of the host's immunologic responses to skin allografts, included (1) erythema and edema surrounding the skin graft, (2) dark red or cyanotic color of the graft, (3) edema, (4) cessation of blood flow in all superficial graft vessels, and (5) appearance of small punctate thrombi and/or hemorrhages throughout the graft surface. Subsequent escharification and sloughing of

the graft confirmed the diagnosis of rejection.

The vascular changes observed in the skin transplants were of particular interest. During the first 48 hours after operation, skin allografts and autografts did not differ significantly. There were multiple dilated capillaries filled with blood on the graft surface, with little if any blood circulation. Blood flow usually developed by the third or fourth postoperative days, then increased in extent during the fifth and sixth days. At that time, dilated vessels seen earlier were replaced by small calibered vessels exhibiting rapid blood flow. This vascular pattern became predominant in the autografts, whose surface resembled normal skin within two to three weeks after transplantation. In contrast, this phase of normalization gradually ceased in the allografts, and was followed by a renewed dilation of the superficial vessels, with an eventual cessation of blood flow by the eighth or ninth day after transplantation. The dilated vessels developed multiple punctate thrombi and hemorrhages during the next 24 to 48 hours, and the graft became progressively opacified, with eventual escharification and sloughing of the graft (Converse and Rapaport, 1956).

Upon rejection of the first skin graft obtained from a donor, the recipient acquires a state of generalized hypersensitivity to additional grafts from that particular donor (Rapaport and Converse, 1957 and 1958). The type of response elicited by these second set skin grafts depends upon the waiting period between first-set rejection and the second challenge. If the second-set graft is given within one to seven days after rejection, a white graft reaction develops, characterized by dead white pallor of the graft and a complete absence of vascularization. When the latent period between first and second-set grafts is extended beyond one week, the grafts undergo a second-set or accelerated rejection reaction. In this case, the events of allograft rejection described with first-set grafts are telescoped into a shorter, four to five day period, with full escharification by the seventh or eighth postoperative day. Extension of the latent period beyond 80 days permits the host to revert to a first-set state of reactivity (Rapaport and Converse, 1957 and 1958).

Accelerated skin graft rejection reactions (four to five days) are usually associated with the flare up of erythema and edema, and with occasional intradermal hemorrhage and necrosis at the formerly quiescent site of rejection of the first-set graft, which was from the same donor. This response, termed the recall flare, is individual-specific, and may constitute an expression of the retention at the first-set graft site of some of the donor's histocompatibility antigens (Rapaport and Converse, 1958). In this regard, the recall flare resembles similar responses observed at tuberculin skin test sites in negative human reactors given a transfer of delayed hypersensitivity with leukocyte extracts obtained from tuberculin-sensitive donors (Lawrence, 1957). This observation provided one of the early links between mechanisms of skin allograft rejection and the delayed or cellular type of hypersensitivity response in man (Lawrence, 1959a).

GENETIC DETERMINANTS OF HUMAN HISTOCOMPATIBILITY

Two principal but by no means exclusive histocompatibility systems are currently known in man—the ABO erythrocyte antigen groups and the HL-A system of leukocyte antigens. The ability of A_1,B and AB erythrocytes in O recipients to induce sensitivity to skin allografts obtained from other donors of the corresponding erythrocyte group has provided definitive evidence that the A_1 and B antigens act as potent and group-specific transplantation antigens in man (Dausset and Rapaport, 1966a; Rapaport and Dausset, 1967). This interpretation is further supported by the ability of cell-free soluble A and B substances isolated from heterologous sources to induce the same results in O recipients (Rapaport et al., 1968b). Although it is not certain that the kind of immunologic response evoked in sensitized recipients by erythrocyte antigens is the same as that produced by histocompatibility antigens

isolated from nucleated cells, the evidence clearly points to the predominant role played by ABO incompatibility in experimental as well as clinical (Starzl et al., 1964; Wilson and Kirkpatrick, 1964) transplantation.

The possibility that a major system of histocompatibility similar to the murine H-2 system might exist in man received its first support in the observation that unrelated members of the random human population share greater or lesser numbers of transplantation antigens (Rapaport et al., 1960 and 1962b). In these studies, it was observed that the more recipients included in a panel of subjects tested with skin allografts obtained from the same donor, the greater the chances of locating individuals who were *more* as well as *less* compatible with this particular donor. In addition, when recipients immunized with a first-set skin graft from a given donor were challenged simultaneously with one or more skin grafts obtained from other donors, some of the latter grafts were rejected in an accelerated manner, suggesting cross-sensitization by the skin allograft obtained from the first donor. Similar cross-reactions were observed after sensitization with transplantation antigens obtained from blood leukocytes (Friedman et al., 1961; Rapaport et al., 1962a, 1964, and 1965). In order to test the possibility that such cross-sensitizations were the result of a sharing of transplantation antigens between the donor of the sensitizing grafts and some of the donors of the subsequent first-set grafts, skin grafts were then exchanged between those donors who appeared to share antigens on the basis of such cross-reactions, as well as between donors in whom this did not occur. Grafts exchanged between putatively antigen-sharing subjects regularly survived for significantly longer periods of time than did grafts exchanged between those donors who were negative in this regard (Rapaport et al., 1962b). These studies were subsequently extended to a "third man test" of histocompatibility by Küss and Legrain (1961), by Mathé (1962), and by Wilson et al., (1963).

Interest in leukocytes for studies of human histocompatibility was initially stimulated by the report of Medawar (1946)

that the intradermal injection of leukocytes from a given rabbit donor sensitized
other rabbits to skin allografts obtained
from that particular donor. This observation, which established the sharing of histocompatibility antigens by leukocytes and
skin, was extended to man soon thereafter
(Friedman, 1961; Rapaport et al., 1962a,
1964, and 1965), and set the stage for a
series of intensive serologic studies of
antigens located on the surface of human
leukocytes. Historically, this endeavor
began with the observation that the serum
of polytransfused patients contains leu-
koagglutinating antibodies (independent
of erythrocyte group antibodies) which
have the capability to react with leukocytes
of some but not all donors tested (Dausset
and Nenna, 1952; Miescher and Fauconnet, 1954). The first leukocyte group, Mac,
was characterized by Dausset in 1958.
Since then, largely as the result of an international effort sponsored by the National
Institute of Allergy and Infectious Diseases (Transplantation and Immunology
Collaborative Branch), a series of remarkable advances by a number of distinguished laboratories has resulted in the
isolation of most of the components of the
human analogue of H-2—the HL-A system. Payne and Bodmer defined a system
of three alleles, termed L-A1,2, and 3; van
Rood and van Leeuwen introduced computer methods of analysis for studies of
sera obtained from multiparous women
and developed a biallelic system which
they termed 4a4b; and Dausset and his associates postulated in 1965 that all of these
leukocyte surface antigens were part of a
single complex histocompatibility system
for which the term Hu-1 was proposed
(Dausset and Rapaport, 1968a). Further
studies by these and other investigators,
including Amos, Kissmeyer-Nielsen, Terasaki, Ceppellini, van Rood, and their associates, have since provided definitive evidence for this hypothesis. It is then
generally accepted today that this system,
now known as HL-A, is an immunogenetic
system of enormous complexity. whose
products are governed by at least two discrete loci or regions on the same autosomal
chromosome. The first locus determines
antigens HL-A1,2,3,9,10,11,28, W29, 30,
31, and 32 as alternative alleles, and the

second locus determines antigens HL-
A5,7,8,12,13,14,27, W5, FJH, BB, JA,
LND, AA, HL-A17, W16, W18, W21, and
TT in similar fashion (Dausset et al.,
1970).

An impressive array of data points to the
implication of the HL-A system in human
histocompatibility responses. The survival
of skin allografts in HL-A identical and
haploidentical individuals (Dausset and
Rapaport, 1969), and the results of living-
related donors (Rapaport et al., 1967;
Dausset and Hors, 1971) and cadaver
donors (Payne et al., 1971) reflect the potential role of HL-A compatibility in transplantation. It is equally clear, however,
that HL-A is only *one* of the determinants
of allograft survival, and that there is a
great need for additional guidelines for
the selection of optimally compatible
donor-recipient pairs for transplantation
(Dausset and Rapaport, 1971). One of the
direct consequences of this consideration
has been an intensive search for alternative
techniques designed to identify histocompatible individuals. These include in vivo
tests, performed with skin allografts or
lymphocytes obtained from prospective
organ donors and recipients, and an in
vitro test, the mixed lymphocyte culture
test, which has recently acquired great importance in genetic studies of histocompatibility determinants.

The three main currently known in vivo
tests include the third man test, the normal
lymphocyte transfer test, and the irradiated hamster test of Ramseier and
Streilein. As noted earlier, the *third man test*
is based upon sensitization of an unrelated
person (i.e., a third man) with a skin allograft obtained from the future transplant
recipient. Two weeks later, skin grafts
from each prospective organ donor and a
second-set graft from the patient are
placed on the third man. That donor
whose first-set skin graft behaves most like
the second-set graft from the patient is
considered to share the greatest number of
histocompatibility antigens with that particular patient. This test only detects
similarities between donors and recipients,
but does not provide a satisfactory measure of the actual antigenic differences
which may also exist between these two individuals. This serious disadvantage, and

the time element required before the results can be interpreted, significantly hinder the clinical application of this test (Nelson and Russell, 1968).

In the *normal lymphocyte transfer test*, blood lymphocytes obtained from the patient (test cells) and from two healthy unrelated donors (control cells) are given intradermally to a number of prospective organ donors. The size and intensity of the cutaneous reactions are assessed two days later, and the compatible donor is the individual in whom the intradermal reaction to the patient's lymphocytes was the smallest. Although this test can eliminate grossly incompatible donors, it has, however, not been able to select consistently the best donor, even in panels of living-related donor candidates (Billingham and Silvers, 1971).

The *irradiated hamster test* resembles the normal lymphocyte transfer test in that it depends upon the reactivity of donor and recipient lymphocytes against each other in a supralethally irradiated hamster. Lymphocyte suspensions from the patient and from a number of prospective donors, and mixed suspensions of lymphocytes from the patient and each donor are injected intradermally into an irradiated hamster. The most compatible donor is the individual whose lymphocytes caused the smallest skin reaction in the hamster, upon mixing with the recipient's cells. This model has been studied extensively as a test of histocompatibility in rats and mice, and to a lesser extent in man. While it was of usefulness in detecting gross incompatibilities, it has not been successful in differentiating between donors bearing lesser degrees of histoincompatibility with the recipient (Nelson and Russell, 1968).

The mixed leucocyte culture (MLC) test, developed by Bain and Lowenstein (1964) and by Bach and Hirschhorn (1964), is based upon the in vitro assessment of the immunologic competence of human peripheral blood lymphocytes. It has gained increasing acceptance as a sensitive model for studies of the recognition phase of the allograft response. The MLC test originates from the observation that leukocytes exposed to HL-A incompatible antigens present in leukocytes obtained from another donor became stimulated, and transform into blast cells which have the capacity to take up tritiated thymidine and undergo division. The one-way MLC test of Bach and Voynow (1966), where the cells obtained from one of the two donors are rendered nonreactive (i.e., are present only as *antigens*) by exposure to mitomycin-C, is generally accepted today as the standard method for these studies.

The close correlation originally observed between genotypically HL-A identical individuals and MLC nonreactivity (Amos and Bach, 1968) has provided the chief evidence supporting the existence of the HL-A locus in man. More recently, however, Bach and Segall (1972), Eijsvoogel and his associates (1972), and Sasportes et al., (1972) have reported convincing data supporting the possibility that MLC reactivity may actually be controlled by a separate genetic system which appears to be closely linked to, but not identical with, the HL-A region. The MLC "region" has been tentatively localized to the right side of the second HL-A locus on the basis of recombinations within family studies. Preliminary evidence suggests that this newly identified genetic determinant may also be of great importance in conditioning human allograft responses. The situation is not clear at this time, however, and it is not unlikely that continuing studies will result in the identification of many other probably multigenic determinants of human histocompatibility.

TRANSPLANTATION ANTIGENS

Transplantation antigens are genetically determined molecular structures, present on the surface and within mammalian cells, which are capable of provoking sensitization to tissue allografts when administered to genetically disparate recipients of the same species. Much of the early work on transplantation antigens was done with whole tissues, using skin as the prototype. The observation by Medawar (1946) that blood leukocytes were as effective as skin allografts in the induction of donor-specific accelerated skin graft rejection in rabbits then suggested a readily available source of materials for the isolation and study of transplantation antigens in different animal species. This finding was extended to man by Friedman and his associates (1961) and by Rapaport et al. (1962a, 1964, 1965), and resulted in the isolation of cell-free cytoplasmic components of human blood leukocytes (mitochondria, microsomes, and cell membrane fragments) which retained the capacity to induce strong individual-specific skin allograft sensitivity in this species (Rapaport et al. 1965). Further attempts to isolate transplantation antigens from these particulate components were not successful, however. Although some of the solubilized extracts retained serologic activity in vitro, they generally lost their biologic activity after a variety of solubilization procedures. Recent studies by Nathenson and Davies (1966) and by Kahan and Reisfeld (1969) may, however, hold promising leads for further progress in this vitally important field. The latter studies in particular hold considerable promise. On the basis of ultrasound disruption and extraction of water-soluble cell components, these authors appear to have isolated a protein which retains serologic specificity and biologic activity in lower mammals, and considerable interest is currently focused upon extension of this approach to the human species. This possibility has evident potential from the clinical standpoint, since it appears clear that the eventual solution of the transplantation problem will depend upon the availability of a variety of soluble transplantation antigen extracts for the induction of specific graft unresponsiveness in the recipient.

HL-A serologic studies have contributed significantly to our understanding of some of the properties of transplantation antigens. An extreme degree of polymorphism has been an almost constant feature of the main histocompatibility systems studied thus far in different species. One consequence of this polymorphism in man, for example, has been the multitude of cross-reactions which have been observed between different HL-A antigens. Such cross-reactions have recently been shown to extend to the isoantigens of other species, as reported for rabbits and mice by Abeyounis and Milgram (1969), for rats and mice by Sachs et al. (1971), and for primates and man by van Rood et al. (1972). A growing body of evidence also points to the presence, in dogs, rabbits, guinea pigs, rats, and mice, of histocompatibility antigens which cross-react with Group A streptococcal membrane antigens (Billingham et al., 1954; Rapaport and Chase, 1964 and 1965; Chase et al., 1965; Rapaport et al., 1966, 1968c, and 1971b; Rapaport, 1967, 1968, and 1970; Rapaport and Markowitz, 1969). These data also appear to suggest that each of these species, in turn, share histocompatibility antigens with each other, and that a significant portion of these determinants, which have thus far been considered to be species-restricted, may actually be highly ubiquitous throughout nature. As a consequence, there may exist throughout different living cells a wide ranging and occasionally completely unexpected spectrum of cross-reacting determinants capable of affecting allograft responsiveness in a given species. Moreover, the intensity of host responses to allografts or even xenografts may be conditioned by the degree to which this particular host's surface cellular components cross-react with the antigenic structures to which he has been exposed. In this regard, the specific transplantation antigen configuration present on the cell surface may be an important basic factor in the antigenic recognition process.

IMMUNOLOGIC EFFECTOR MECHANISMS IN ALLOGRAFT REJECTION

As in many other areas in transplantation, the skin allograft has provided the principal model for studies of the mediation of allograft sensitivity. Billingham et al. (1954), Brent et al. (1962), and Lawrence et al. (1960) have described in detail the overwhelming body of evidence incriminating cellular immunologic mechanisms in the rejection of first-set allografts composed of solid tissues. The classic experiments of Gowans and his associates (1962, 1965, and 1965) have demonstrated that the small lymphocyte is the key participant in the in vivo process of the host's recognition of foreign transplantation antigens, and in the initiation of the changes which eventually result in destruction of the allograft. The reader is referred to the extensive reviews by Billingham and Silvers (1963), Brent and Medawar (1967), and Gowans (1965) for a more detailed discussion of these important data.

In man, Lawrence and his associates (1960) demonstrated that leukocyte extracts prepared from specifically sensitized donors have the capacity to transfer individual-specific allograft sensitivity to normal recipients both by local infiltration of target skin grafts with this transfer factor, and by systemic sensitization, where transfer factor is injected at a site distant from the test skin grafts. Although the situation is not as clear experimentally for other organs, Strober and Gowan (1965) have demonstrated that lymphocytes isolated from the thoracic duct of sensitized donors can mediate kidney allograft rejection in rats. It would thus appear that in the majority of, if not all, instances the first-set rejection of allografts of normal tissues in nonsensitized recipients is mediated through the same type of cellular effector mechanisms.

The preponderant role of cellular immune mechanisms in first-set allograft rejection under well-defined clinical or experimental conditions does not, however, rule out an involvement of humoral antibodies in this process. The white graft rejection reaction accorded skin allografts after passive transfers of sensitivity with heterologous antisera (Chutna, 1961; Rapaport et al., 1969), or in human O recipients given erythrocyte-group–incompatible grafts after sensitization with the appropriate A or B antigen, constitutes an important example of antibody mediated allograft rejection responses. The latter situation has also been observed in hyperacute renal allograft rejection in man (Starzl et al., 1964; Wilson and Kirkpatrick, 1964), and the evidence indicates that the presence of preformed HL-A antibodies (i.e., transplantation antibodies) in the host may result in similar rejection responses (Kissmeyer-Nielsen et al., 1966; Terasaki et al., 1968). It is quite possible, therefore, that the degree to which cellular and humoral mechanisms intervene in the mediation of allograft rejection may be significantly conditioned by the host's previous exposure to antigens present in that particular graft.

IMMUNOLOGIC TOLERANCE AND ENHANCEMENT

The classic studies of Billingham et al. (1956a) in London provided definitive evidence that in utero exposure of prospective recipients to immunologically competent cells from a given mouse strain before the development of immunologic competence results in a specific state of allograft unresponsiveness when these recipients are tested later with a skin allograft from the same donor strain. For this purpose, 15 to 16 day old CBA mouse embryos were injected with a suspension of viable adult cells obtained from A strain mice. Eight weeks after birth, the recipients and a series of controls were tested with A strain skin grafts, and with grafts obtained from an unrelated AU strain. Mice injected in utero with spleen cell suspensions (but not with testis or kidney cells) either accepted A grafts permanently, or accorded such grafts a prolonged survival time, while AU grafts were rejected in first-set fashion. These studies heralded a new era in immunobiology, and the theoretical implications of the concept of immunologic tolerance are still a subject of intensive investigation today. One point of particular importance has been the establishment of the concept that the duration of the induced tolerance is conditioned by the degree to which the inoculated cells succeed in migrating, proliferating, and becoming permanently established in the host's immunologic response centers.

In recent years, it has been observed that immunologic tolerance can also be induced in adult animals, and that the neonate or the in utero phase is not an essential prerequisite for the induction of tolerance, particularly across weak histocompatibility barriers. An alternative technique for the induction of tolerance in adult animals has been the use of immunosuppressive adjuncts, such as irradiation, antimetabolites, or antilymphocyte serum. Of considerable theoretical and possible practical importance to transplantation is the suggestion of Main and Prehn (1955) that bone marrow transplantation may have the capacity to induce a state of long-term unresponsiveness to other tissues obtained from the same donor. This thesis has been confirmed for kidney and skin allografts in the canine species (Rapaport et al., 1971a, 1972a, 1972b, 1973).

Immunologic enhancement was originally observed by Flexner and Jobling (1907), who reported that the rate of growth of a transplanted rat sarcoma was increased by pretreatment of the recipients with an emulsion of heat-killed tumor cells. This phenomenon, which has since been studied extensively by Casey (1932), Snell (1952), and Kaliss (1958,), essentially consists of the enhancement of survival of an allograft (usually a tumor allograft) by treatment of the recipient with a nonliving preparation of the future donor's tissue antigens. The ability of serum obtained from such enhanced animals to transfer passively this state of enhancement to normal recipients has been a particularly important characteristic of the phenomenon. Although the overwhelming majority of successful enhancement experiments has been performed with tumor transplants, Snell (1957), Batchelor (1963), and others have suggested that a similar mechanism may be invoked in conditioning host responses to normal tissues. Billingham et al. (1956b) have, for example, observed relative prolongations in skin graft survival after pretreatment of mice with lyophilized donor strain-specific tissue antigens; Nelson (1961) has reported similar results in guinea pigs; and Heslop (1966) has observed prolongations in skin graft survival after treatment of rats with formalin-treated donor-specific spleen cell suspensions. In man, Rapaport et al. (1968a) have observed that freezing and storage of cytoplasmic extracts of human leukocytes abrogate their capacity to sensitize recipients to donor-specific skin allografts; rather, subjects pretreated with such altered antigen(s) (1) have accorded prolongations in survival time to donor-specific grafts and (2) have developed antidonor lymphocytotoxic serum antibodies.

A discussion of this important segment of transplantation biology would not be complete without noting the recent data which support the possibility that the dividing lines between tolerance and enhancement may eventually become quite tenuous (Levey, 1972). Tolerance and enhancement share the common property of depending upon the continued presence of antigenic stimulation for their persistence. The work of the Hellströms and their associates (Hellström and Hellström, 1970; Quadracci et al., 1970; Hellström et al., 1970) has demonstrated the presence, in tolerant as well as in enhanced animals, of immunologically competent cells which are prevented from attacking their tissue targets by specific serologic factors (immunoglobulins) loosely complexed with antigen(s) present in the host's circulation. The two "different" immunologic mechanisms, originally termed tolerance and enhancement, may therefore actually represent the end-product of the greater or lesser influence of a number of variables, including antigen dosage, route of administration, age of the recipient, state of immunologic reactivity, method used for the detection of allograft reactivity, and the relative role of different cells and antibodies at various stages during and after sensitization.

CONCLUSIONS

A complete review of transplantation biology is clearly beyond the scope of this manuscript. Instead, an attempt has been made to highlight some of the salient features which may eventually have a significant impact on medicine.

The exponential growth of transplantation as a scientific discipline is well exemplified by the steady increase in the size of the published proceedings of the international transplantation conferences held at two-year intervals since 1954. The reader is referred to the References (Rogers, 1955, 1958, and 1962; Converse, 1957 and 1960; Converse et al., 1964; Rapaport, 1966; Dausset et al., 1968; Transplant. Proc., 1969 and 1971) for a more complete overview of this fascinating field. The impact that transplantation has had upon the practice of medicine is reflected by the fact that over 12,000 kidney, 200 heart, 200 liver, 370 bone marrow, 40 lung, and 35 pancreas and intestine transplants have been performed in man thus far, and the old dream of organ replacement may thus not be too far from its final fruition.

In addition, however, transplantation biology has been of inestimable service in furthering our understanding of developmental phenomena, and in broadening the horizons of modern immunology far beyond the fondest dreams of the earlier classical serologists. This progress, in turn, may be of great significance to clinical medicine. Indeed, it is by providing a unique experimental setting for the study of mechanisms of human disease that transplantation biology may eventually make its greatest and most significant contributions. In this respect, transplantation biology is a rather unique discipline, which has provided a common forum and shared goals for representatives drawn from a multitude of different specialties. It is this special flavor and effervescence that has made transplantation biology a particularly rich and exciting field of endeavor.

REFERENCES

Abeyounis, C. J., and Milgram, F.: Tissue isoantigens shared by rabbits and mice. Transplant Proc., 1:556, 1969.

Amos, D. B., and Bach, F. H.: Phenotypic expressions of the major histocompatibility locus in man (HL-A): Leukocyte antigens and mixed leukocyte culture reactivity. J. Exp. Med., 128:623, 1968.

Bach, F., and Hirschhorn, K.: Lymphocyte interaction: a potential histocompatibility test in vitro. Science, 143:815, 1964.

Bach, F., and Segall, M.: The genetics of the mixed leucocyte culture response. A re-examination. Transplant Proc., 4:205, 1972.

Bach, F., and Voynow, N. K.: One-way stimulation in mixed leucocyte culture. Science, 153:545, 1966.

Bain, B., and Lowenstein, L.: Genetic studies on the mixed leucocyte reaction. Science, 145:1315, 1964.

Balner, H., Gabb, B. W., Dersjant, H., van Vreeswijk, W., and van Rood, J. J.: The major histocompatibility locus of Rhesus monkeys (RhL-A). Nature, 230:177, 1971a.

Balner, H., van Vreeswijk, W., van Leeuwen, A., and van Rood, J. J.: Identification of chimpanzee leukocyte antigens (ChL-A) and their relation to HL-A. Transplantation, 11:309, 1971b.

Batchelor, J. R.: The mechanism and significance of immunological enhancement. Guy's Hosp. Rep., 112:345, 1963.

Billingham, R., and Silvers, W.: Sensitivity to normal tissues and cells. Ann. Rev. Microbiol., 17:531, 1963.

Billingham, R., and Silvers, W.: The Immunobiology of Transplantation. Englewood Cliffs, New Jersey, Prentice-Hall, Inc., 1971, p. 25.

Billingham, R., Brent, L., and Medawar, P. B.: Quantitative studies on tissue transplantation immunity. II. The origin, strength and duration of actively and passively acquired immunity. Proc. R. Soc. (B), 143:58, 1954.

Billingham, R., Brent, L., and Medawar, P. B.: Quantitative studies on tissue transplantation immunity. III. Actively acquired tolerance. Philos. Trans. R. Soc. Lond., 239:357, 1956a.

Billingham, R., Brent, L., and Medawar, P. B.: "Enhancement" in normal homografts, with a note on its possible mechanism. Transplant. Bull., 3:84, 1956b.

Brent, L., and Medawar, P. B.: Cellular immunity and the homograft reaction. Br. Med. Bull., 23:55, 1967.

Brent, L., Brown, J., and Medawar, P. B.: Quantitative studies on tissue transplantation immunity. VI. Hypersensitivity reactions associated with rejection of homografts. Proc. R. Soc. (B), 156:187, 1962.

Burnet, S.: Somatic mutation and chronic disease. Br. Med. J., 1:338, 1965.

Casey, A. E.: Experimental enhancement of malignancy in the Brown-Pearce rabbit tumor. Proc. Soc. Exp. Biol. Med., 29:819, 1932.

Chase, R. M., Jr., and Rapaport, F. T.: The bacterial induction of homograft sensitivity. 1. Effects of sensitization with Group A Streptococci. J. Exp. Med., 122:721, 1965.

Chutna, J.: White graft reaction and passive transfer of immunity in inbred strains of mice. Plast. Reconstr. Surg., 28:121, 1961.

Colombani, J., and Dausset, J.: L'Histocompatibilité Humaine. Path. Biol., 17:281, 1969.

Converse, J. M., (Ed.): Second tissue homotransplantation conference. Ann. N. Y. Acad. Sci., 64:735, 1957.

Converse, J. M. (Ed.): Fourth tissue homotransplantation conference. Ann. N. Y. Acad. Sci., 87:1–607, 1960.

Converse, J. M., and Casson, P. R.: The historical background of transplantation. In Rapaport, F. T.: and Dausset, J. (Eds.): Human Transplantation. New York, Grune & Stratton, Inc., 1968, p. 3.

Converse, J. M., and Rapaport, F. T.: The vascularization of skin autografts and homografts. An experimental study in man. Ann. Surg., 143:306, 1956.

Converse, J. M., Rogers, B. O., Rapaport, F. T. (Eds.): Sixth International Transplantation Conference. Ann. N.Y. Acad. Sci., 120:1–806, 1964.

Dausset, J., and Hors, J.: Analysis of 221 renal transplants. In: Rapaport, F. T., and Dausset, J. (Eds.): Tissue Typing Today. New York, Grune & Stratton, Inc., 1971, p. 26.

Dausset, J., and Nenna, A.: Présence d'une leucoagglutinine dans le sérum d'un cas d'agranulocytose chronique. C.R. Soc. Biol., 146:1539, 1952.

Dausset, J., and Rapaport, F. T.: Role of ABO erythrocyte groups in human histocompatibility reactions. Nature, 209:209, 1966a.

Dausset, J., and Rapaport, F. T.: The role of blood group antigens in human histocompatibility. Ann. N.Y. Acad. Sci., 129:408, 1966b.

Dausset, J., and Rapaport, F. T.: Blood group determinants of human histocompatibility. In: Rapaport,

F. T., and Dausset, J. (Eds.): Human Transplantation. New York, Grune & Stratton, Inc., 1968a, p. 383.

Dausset, J., and Rapaport, F. T.: The Hu-1 system of human histocompatibility. *In* Rapaport, F. T., and Dausset, J. (Eds.): Human Transplantation. New York, Grune & Stratton, Inc., 1968b, p. 369.

Dausset, J., and Rapaport, F. T.: Histocompatibility studies in haploidentical genetic combinations. Transplant. Proc., 1:649, 1969.

Dausset, J., and Rapaport, F. T.: Current problems in analysis of results of renal transplantation in man. Transplant Proc., 3:979, 1971.

Dausset, J., Colombani, J., Legrand, L., Feingold, N., and Rapaport, F. T.: Genetic and biological aspects of the HL-A system of human histocompatibility. Blood, 35:591, 1970.

Dausset, J., Hamburger, J., and Mathé, G.: Advance in Transplantation — Proceedings of the First International Congress of the Transplantation Society. Munksgaard, Copenhagen, 1968.

Dausset, J., Rapaport, F. T., Cannon, F. D., and Ferrebee, J. W.: Histocompatibility studies in a closely bred colony of dogs. III. Genetic definition of the DL-A system of canine histocompatibility, with particular reference to the comparative immunogenicity of the major transplantable organs. J. Exp. Med., 134:1222, 1971.

DeWeck, A. L., Polak, L., Sato, W., and Frey, J. R.: Determination of histocompatibility antigens by leucocyte typing in outbred guinea pigs and effect of matching on skin graft survival. Transplant. Proc., 3:192, 1971.

Eijsvoogel, V. P., Koning, L., Groot-Kooy, L., Huismans, L., van Rood, J. J., and Schellekens, P.Th.A.: Mixed lymphocyte culture and HL-A. Transplant. Proc., 4:199; 1972.

Flexner, S., and Jobling, J. W.: On the promoting influence of heated tumor emulsions on tumor growth. Proc. Soc. Exp. Biol. Med., 4:156, 1907.

Friedman, E. A., Retan, J. W., Marshall, D. C., Henry, L., and Merrill, J. P.: Accelerated skin graft rejection in humans pre-immunized with homologous leucocytes. J. Clin. Invest., 40:2162, 1961.

Gibson, T., and Medawar, P. B.: The fate of skin homografts in man. J. Anat., 77:299, 1942.

Gorer, P. A.: The genetic and antigenic basis of tumor transplantation. J. Path. Bact., 44:691, 1937.

Gowans, J. L.: The role of lymphocytes in the destruction of homografts. Br. Med. Bull., 21:106, 1965.

Gowans, J. L., and McGregor, D. D.: The immunological activities of lymphocytes. Progr. Allergy, 9:1, 1965.

Gowans, J. L., McGregor, D. D., Cowen, D. M., and Ford, C. E.: Initiation of immune responses by small lymphocytes. Nature, 196:651, 1962.

Hellström, I., Hellström, K. E., Storb, R., and Thomas, E. D.: Colony inhibition of fibroblasts from chimeric dogs mediated by the dogs' own lymphocytes and specifically abrogated by their serum. Proc. Natl. Acad. Sci. U.S.A., 66:65, 1970.

Hellström, K. E., and Hellström, I.: Immunological enhancement as studied by cell culture techniques. Ann. Rev. Microbiol., 24:373, 1970.

Heslop, B. F.: Immunological enhancement of skin allografts in rats following pretreatment of the re-cipients with nonviable allogeneic cells. Transplantation, 4:37, 1966.

Kahan, B. D., and Reisfeld, R. A.: Transplantation antigens. Solubilized antigens provide chemical markers of biologic individuality. Science, 164:514, 1969.

Kaliss, N.: Immunological enhancement of tumor homografts in mice. Cancer Res., 18:992, 1958.

Kissmeyer-Nielsen, F., Olsen, S., Petersen, V. P., and Fjeldborg, O.: Hyperacute rejection of kidney allografts, associated with pre-existing humoral antibodies against donor cells. Lancet, 2:662, 1966.

Küss, R., and Legrain, M.: Homologous transplantation of the human kidney. Trans. Am. Soc. Artif. Organs., 7:116, 1961.

Lawrence, H. S.: Similarities between homograft rejection and tuberculin type allergy: a review of recent experimental findings. Ann. N.Y. Acad. Sci., 64:826, 1957.

Lawrence, H. S.: Delayed hypersensitivity and the behavior of the cellular transfer system in animal and man. *In* Shaffer, J. H., et al. (Eds.): Mechanisms of Hypersensitivity., Boston, Little, Brown & Co., 1959a, p. 453.

Lawrence, H. S.: Homograft sensitivity. An expression of the immunological origins and consequences of individuality. Physiol. Rev., 39:811, 1959b.

Lawrence, H. S., Rapaport, F. T., Converse, J. M., and Tillett, W. S. Transfer of delayed hypersensitivity to skin homografts with leukocyte extracts in man. J. Exp. Med., 39:185, 1960.

Lexer, E.: Ueber freie transplantationen. Arch. Klin. Chir., 95:827, 1911.

Little, C. C.: The genetics of tumor transplantation. *In* Snell, G. D. (Ed.): Biology of the Laboratory Mouse. New York, Dover Publications, Inc., 1956, p. 279.

Loeb, L.: The biological basis of individuality. Physiol. Rev., 10:547, 1930.

Main, J. M., and Prehn, R. T.: Successful skin homografts after the administration of high dosage x-radiation and homologous bone marrow. J. Natl. Cancer Inst., 15:1023, 1955.

Mathé, G.: *In* Proceedings, Fifth International Tissue Homotransplantation Conference. N.Y. Acad. Sci., 99:262, 1962.

Miescher, P., and Fauconnet, M.: Nise en évidence de différents groupes leucocytaires chez l'homme. J. Suisse Méd., 84:597, 1954.

Medawar, P. B.: Behavior and fate of skin autografts and skin homografts in rabbits. J. Anat., 78:176, 1944.

Medawar, P. B.: A second study of the behavior and fate of skin homografts in rabbits. J. Anat., 79:157, 1945.

Medawar, P. B.: Immunity to homologous grafted skin. II. The relationship between the antigens of blood and skin. Br. J. Exp. Pathol., 27:15, 1946.

Nathenson, S. G., and Davis, D. A. L.: Transplantation antigens: Studies of the mouse model system, solubilization and partial purification of H-2 isoantigens. Ann. N.Y. Acad. Sci., 129:6, 1966.

Nelson, D. S.: Immunological enhancement of skin homografts in guinea pigs. Br. J. Exp. Pathol., 43:2, 1961.

Nelson, D. S., and Russell, P. S.: In vivo histocompatibility testing. *In* Rapaport, F. T., and Dausset, J. (Eds): Human Transplantation. New York, Grune and Stratton, Inc., 1968, p. 394.

Palm, J.: Classification of inbred rat strains for AgB histocompatibility antigens. Transplant. Proc., 3: 169, 1971.

Payne, R., Perkins, H. A., Kountz, S. L., and Belzer, F. O.: Unrelated kidney transplants and matching for HL-A antigens. *In* Rapaport, F. T., and Dausset, J.: Tissue Typing Today. New York, Grune and Stratton, Inc., 1971, p. 58.

Quadracci, L. J., Hellström, I. E. Striker, G. E., Marchioro, T. L., and Hellström, K. E.: Immune mechanisms in human recipients of renal allografts. Cell. Immunol., 1:561, 1970.

Rapaport, F. T. (Ed.): Seventh International Transplantation Conference. Ann N.Y. Acad. Sci., 129:1–884, 1966.

Rapaport, F. T.: Heterologous cross-reactions in mammalian transplantation. *In* Trentin, J. (Ed.): Cross-Reacting Antigens and Neo-Antigens. Baltimore, The Williams & Wilkins Co., 1967, p. 15.

Rapaport, F. T.: Heterologous antigens and antibodies in transplantation. *In* Rapaport, F. T., and Dausset, J. (Eds.): Human Transplantation. New York, Grune & Stratton, Inc., 1968, p. 39.

Rapaport, F. T.: Role of streptococcal and other heterologous antigens in transplantation. Transplant. Proc., 2:447, 1970.

Rapaport, F. T., and Chase, R. M., Jr.: Homograft sensitivity induction by Group A streptococci. Science, 145:407, 1964.

Rapaport, F. T., and Chase, R. M., Jr.: The bacterial induction of homograft sensitivity. II. Effects of sensitization with staphylococci and other microorganisms. J. Exp. Med., 122:733, 1965.

Rapaport, F. T., and Converse, J. M.: Observations on immunological manifestations of the homograft rejection phenomenon in man: the recall flare. Ann. N.Y. Acad. Sci., 64:836, 1957.

Rapaport, F. T., and Converse, J. M.: The immune response to multiple-set skin homografts. An experimental study in man. Ann. Surg., 147:273, 1958.

Rapaport, F. T., and Converse, J. M.: Skin transplantation. *In* Rapaport, F. T., and Dausset, J. (Eds.): Human Transplantation. New York, Grune & Stratton, Inc., 1968, p. 304.

Rapaport, F. T., and Dausset, J.: Erythrocyte antigens as determinants of human histocompatibility. Surg. Forum, 18:225, 1967.

Rapaport, F. T., and Dausset, J.: The HL-A system as a determinant of human histocompatibility. *In* Rose, N. R., and Milgrom (Eds.): International Convocation on Immunology, Buffalo, New York. Basal, S. Karger, 1968.

Rapaport, F. T., and Dausset, J.: Immunological principles of donor selection for human cardiac transplantation. Prog. Cardiovasc. Dis., 12:119, 1969.

Rapaport, F. T., and Markowitz, A. S.: Streptococcal antigens and antibodies in transplantation. Transplant. Proc., 1:638, 1969.

Rapaport, F. T., Cannon, F. D., Blumenstock, D. A., Watanabe, K., and Ferrebee, J. W.: Long-term survival of bone marrow and kidney allografts in irradiated DL-A identical dogs. Transplant. Proc., 3:1337, 1971a.

Rapaport, F. T., Cannon, F. D., Blumenstock, D. A., Watanabe, K., and Ferrebee, J. W.: Induction of unresponsiveness to canine renal allografts by total body irradiation and bone marrow transplantation. Nature [New Biol.], 235:190, 1972a.

Rapaport, F. T., Chase, R. M., Jr., Markowitz, A. S., McCluskey, R. T., Shimada, T., and Watanabe, K.: Cross-reactions in mammalian transplantation—with particular reference to streptococcal antigens and antibodies. Transplant. Proc., 3:89, 1971b.

Rapaport, F. T., Chase, R. M., Jr., and Solowey, A. C.: Transplantation antigen activity of bacterial cells in different animal species and intracellular localization. Ann. N.Y. Acad. Sci., 129:102, 1966.

Rapaport, F. T., Dausset, J., Converse, J. M., and Lawrence, H. S.: Biological and ultrastructural studies of leucocyte fractions as transplantation antigens in man. Transplantation 3:490, 1965.

Rapaport, F. T., Dausset, J., Hamburger, J., Hume, D. M., Kano, K., Williams, G. M., and Milgrom, F. Serologic factors in human transplantation. Ann. Surg., 166:596, 1967.

Rapaport, F. T., Dausset, J., Lawrence, H. S., and Converse, J. M.: Enhancement of skin allograft survival in man. Surgery, 64:25, 1968a.

Rapaport, F. T., Dausset, J., Legrand, L., Barge, A., Lawrence, H. S., and Converse, J. M.: Erythrocytes in human transplantation: effects of pretreatment with ABO group-specific antigens. J. Clin. Invest., 47:2206, 1968b.

Rapaport, F. T., Hanoaka, T., Shimada, T., Cannon, F. D., and Ferrebee, J. W.: Histocompatibility studies in a closely bred colony of dogs. I. Influence of leucocyte group antigens upon renal allograft survival in the unmodified host. J. Exp. Med., 131:881, 1970.

Rapaport, F. T., Kano, K., and Milgrom, F. Heterophile antibodies in human transplantation. J. Clin. Invest., 47:633, 1968c.

Rapaport, F. T., Lawrence, H. S., Converse, J. M., and Mulholland, J. H.: Leucocyte fractions as transplantation antigens in man. Surg. Forum, 14:146, 1964.

Rapaport, F. T., Lawrence, H. S., Thomas, L., and Converse, J. M.: Biological properties of leukocyte fractions in the induction and detection of skin homograft sensitivity in man. Fed. Proc., 21:40, 1962a.

Rapaport, F. T., Lawrence, H. W., Thomas, L., Converse, J. M., Tillett, W. S., and Mulholland, J. H. Cross-reactions to skin homografts in man. J. Clin. Invest., 41:2166, 1962b.

Rapaport, F. T., Markowitz, A. S., and McCluskey, R. T.: The bacterial induction of homograft sensitivity. III. Effects of Group A streptococcal membrane antisera. J. Exp. Med., 129:623, 1969.

Rapaport, F. T., Thomas, L., Converse, J. M., and Lawrence, H. S.: The specificity of skin homograft rejection in man. Ann. N.Y. Acad. Sci., 87:217, 1960.

Rapaport, F. T., Watanabe, K., Matsuyama, M., Cannon, F. D., Mollen, N., Blumenstock, D., and Ferrebee, J. W.: Immunologically specific allogeneic unresponsiveness in DL-A identical radiation chimerae—a follow-up report. Transplant. Proc., 4:537, 1972.

Rapaport, F. T., Watanabe, K., Matsuyama, M., Cannon, F. D., Mollen, N., Blumenstock, D. A., and Ferrebee, J. W.: The induction of immunological tolerance to allogeneic tissues in the canine species. Ann. Surg., 176:529, 1972b.

Rogers, B. O. (Ed.): The Relation of immunology to tissue homotransplantation. Ann. N.Y. Acad. Sci., 59:277, 1955.

Rogers, B. O. (Ed.): Third tissue homotransplantation conference. Ann. N.Y. Acad. Sci., 73:539, 1958.

Rogers, B. O. (Ed.): Fifth tissue homotransplantation conference. Ann. N.Y. Acad. Sci., 99:335, 1962.

Sachs, D. H., Winn, H. J., and Russell, P. S.: Histocompatibility relationships between species. Transplant. Proc., 3:210, 1971.

Sasportes, M., Lebrun, A., Dausset, J., and Rapaport, F. T.: Studies of skin allograft survival and mixed lymphocyte culture reaction on HL-A-genotyped families. Transplant. Proc., 4:209, 1972.

Schöene, G. E.: Vergleichende untersuchungen uber die transplan. von Geschwulsten und von normalen Geweben. Bruns. Beitr. Klin. Chir., 61:1, 1908.

Snell, G. D.: Enhancement and inhibition of the growth of tumor homotransplants by pretreatment of the hosts with various preparations of normal and tumor tissue. J. Natl. Cancer Inst., 13:719, 1952.

Snell, G. D.: Biology of the Laboratory Mouse. New York, Dover Publications, Inc., N.Y., 1956.

Snell, G. D.: The homograft reaction. Ann. Rev. Microbiol., 11:445, 1957.

Solowey, A. C., and Rapaport, F. T.: Immunologic responses in cancer patients. Surg. Gynecol. Obstet., 121:756, 1965.

Stark, O., Kren, V., and Gunther, E.: RtH-1 antigens in 39 rat strains and six congenic lines. Transplant. Proc., 3:165, 1971.

Starzl, T. E., Marchioro, T. L., Holmes, J. H., and Waddell, W. R.: The incidence, cause and significance of immediate and delayed oliguria or anuria after human renal transplantation. Surg. Gynecol. Obstet., 118:819, 1964.

Strober, S., and Gowans, J. L.: The role of lymphocytes in the sensitization of rats to renal homografts. J. Exp. Med., 122:347, 1965.

Terasaki, P. I., Thrasher, D. L., and Hauber, T. H. Serotyping for homotransplantation. XII. Immediate kidney transplant rejection and associated preformed antibodies. Advance in Transplantation— Proceedings of the First International Congress of the Transplantation Society. Munksgaard, Copenhagen, 1968, p. 225.

Thomas, L.: *In* Lawrence, H. S. (Ed.): Cellular and Humoral Aspects of the Hypersensitivity States. New York, Hoeber, 1959, p. 530.

Transplant. Proc., 1:1–682, 1969.

Transplant. Proc., 3:1–978, 1971.

Vaiman, M., Renard, C., Lafage, P., Ameteau, J., and Nizza, P.: Evidence for a histocompatibility system in swine (SL-A). Transplantation, 10:155, 1970.

van Rood, J. J., van Leeuwen, A., and Balner, H.: HL-A and ChL-A: Similarities and differences. Transplant. Proc., 4:55, 1972.

Wilson, R. E., Henry, L., and Merrill, J. P.: A model system for determining histocompatibility in man. J. Clin. Invest., 42:1497, 1963.

Wilson, W. E. C., and Kirkpatrick, C. H.: Immunologic aspects of renal homotransplantation. *In* Starzl, T. E. (Ed.): Experience in Renal Transplantation. New York, Grune & Stratton, Inc., 1964, p. 239.

Woodruff, M. F. A.: The Transplantation of Tissues and Organs. Springfield, Illinois, Charles C Thomas, Publisher, 1960.

4

Cutaneous Wound Healing

Joseph G. McCarthy, M.D., and John Marquis Converse, M.D.

While the successful eradication of the neoplasm remains the primary goal of the physician treating a skin tumor, he must also concern himself with the secure closure and ultimate cosmetic appearance of the resulting cutaneous defect. The latter considerations depend on an understanding of the biology of wound healing and repair.

Skin is a complex organ capable of performing many essential functions. As it possesses no regenerative ability, it relies on the phenomenon of wound healing to restore any disruption of physical continuity. Healing is the process by which closure of a skin defect is achieved through the ingrowth and deposition of viable cells. Wound healing cannot be accelerated in any clinically significant way. Consequently, the surgeon must be prepared to promote favorable wound conditions so that the basic healing process is neither hindered nor retarded.

BASIC MECHANISMS OF WOUND HEALING

To understand wound healing, it is best to consider individually those basic mecha-

nisms which are present in all healing wounds: epithelialization, contraction, connective tissue reaction, and, finally, maturation or remodeling of the wound scar.

Epithelialization. Epithelization occurs in all types of wounds and is the primary mechanism in dermal wounds (abrasions, first- and second-degree burns, and donor areas for split-thickness skin grafts). Epithelial reaction is rapid and has first priority. The rate of growth and repair of injured epithelium differs for each source (Gillman and Ordman, 1965). It is most rapid in the epidermis, and is followed by the hair follicles and sebaceous glands; the injured sweat ducts are the slowest source.

In any wound the earliest concentration of epithelial mitotic activity is seen in the basophilic-staining areas of the epidermis. The highest mitotic activity is just adjacent to the edge of the wound (Bullough and Laurance, 1960). There is no such epidermal reaction when the dermis is damaged from below and the epidermis is left intact. Mitotic activity reaches a peak in 48 to 72 hours following injury. The marginal basal epithelial cells lose their attachment to the dermis and, following mitosis and enlargement, migrate upward to the prickle cell layer. This is histologically demonstrated by flattening of the rete pegs.

Precise histologic studies of cleanly incised wounds (Ordman and Gillman, 1966) have shown that the two advancing epithelial sheets invade the incision line and upper layers of the paraincisional dermis. The ability of the epithelial sheets to shear through the wound tissue is attributed to a collagenolytic system present in epithelial tissue (Grillo and Gross, 1964). In some wounds the two advancing epithelial margins can unite within 24 to 48 hours (e.g., eyelid wounds) and cover the dermis. The epithelial cells may use strands of fibrin that bridge the wound as a substrate for their migration (Ross and Odland, 1969). The thin epithelial layer then thickens and epithelial growth extends deeper into the dermis in the form of epithelial spurs. By the seventh to eighth day, the surface scar epithelium is fully healed and remodeling of both the surface epithelium and epithelial spurs begins.

In wounds where the defect is so large that coverage cannot be achieved by epithelialization alone, the end result of the repeated, and often unsuccessful, attempts to resurface in this way can lead to epidermoid cancer. Peacock (1969) has pointed out that wounds resulting from radiant energy develop carcinoma in a time sequence directly related to the wavelength of the radiant energy. Gamma or x-ray wounds can develop carcinoma within months, while injuries caused by thermal burns (radiation almost in the visible spectrum) require 20 years or more for the appearance of invasive carcinoma. Similarly, carcinoma in chronic sinus tracts will require even longer periods of time to develop than these radiant energy induced lesions.

Uncontrolled epithelialization can also be demonstrated in the epithelialized tracts and cysts caused by suture material and the driving needle. In comparison with the intraepithelial and intradermal injury produced by the suture, the healing of the incision itself is a relatively insignificant event (Gillman and Ordman, 1965).

Contraction. In large cutaneous defects which cannot be resurfaced by epithe-lialization alone or which have not been covered by skin grafts, contraction is the most important aspect of wound healing. When the adjacent tissue has only minimal underlying attachments (e.g., cheeks, eyelids, neck), contraction closes the wound at the expense of disfiguring and disabling contractures. Conversely, in areas in which the tissues are firmly attached (e.g., hand, pretibial region, scalp), contraction is limited. As epithelialization cannot take over the entire task of resurfacing the wound, an indolent ulcer is the usual sequel unless skin grafting provides a new epithelial cover.

Contraction is essentially a cellular process, and since it occurs in scorbutic animals it must be independent of protein synthesis. The rate of contraction is not determined by the size of the defect. Contraction proceeds at a uniform rate of 0.6 to 0.75 mm. per day. In the first five to seven days after injury, there is little change in the size or shape of the wound. However, following this "lag phase," movement of the skin edges proceeds rapidly (Peacock and van Winkle, 1970).

Currently there are two theories concerning the source and mechanism of the contracting cellular forces:

1. The "picture frame theory" (Watts et al., 1958) places the wound margins as the location of the contraction forces. Excision of the central granulation tissue from a contracting open wound failed to interfere with the rate and extension of contraction. Excision of the wound edges and separation of the advancing skin margins, however, inhibited contraction.

2. The "pull theory" attributes skin movement to contraction of fibroblasts within the granulation tissue, with consequent pulling on the margin of the wound. A recent electron miscroscopic study (Majno et al., 1971) showed that the fibroblasts in the granulation tissue developed morphologic characteristics intermediate between those of typical fibroblasts and those of smooth muscle cells. Strips of granulation tissue, when treated with substances that induce contraction of smooth muscle, will likewise contract in vitro. The data support the view that fibroblasts can differentiate into a cell type structurally and functionally similar to smooth muscle,

and that this cell, the "myofibroblast," plays an important role in wound contraction.

Connective Tissue Reaction. Since collagen is the principal component of connective tissue, an understanding of the biology of this unique macromolecule is essential. Ultrastructural and biophysical studies have demonstrated that collagen is a rod-like molecule 3000Å in length and 14 Å in width with a molecular weight of 240,000. The collagen molecule consists of three polypeptide chains of equal length and each chain contains approximately 1000 amino acids. This unit molecule, tropocollagen, consists of two such identical chains (α_1) and a third chain with a slightly different composition (α_2). The α chains are left-handed helices and the three helices are then twisted into a right-handed "superhelix" (Peacock and van Winkle, 1970). The molecules aggregate in a three-dimensional array, overlapping each other by 25 percent of their length. The quarter-staggering accounts for the 640 Å periodicity seen in electron miscroscopic studies.

The role of the accompanying ground substance (mucopolysaccharides, protein polysaccharides, glycoprotein, ions, and bound water) is as yet ill defined. It may, however, be responsible for the orientation of the collagen fibril during aggregation and growth (Peacock and van Winkle, 1970).

As mentioned earlier, epithelial activity commences immediately after the injury, but cellular reaction deep to the epithelium cannot be demonstrated until the third to fifth day (Gillman and Ordman, 1965). This initial lag period prior to fibroplasia represents the phase of inflammatory cell influx, during which wound toilet is accomplished. Consequently, any wound strength present at this stage must be accounted for simply by epithelial apposition or fibrin plug.

About the fourth day, newly formed fibroblasts, identifiable by their large amounts of rough endoplasmic reticulum (Ross, 1968), develop in the subcutaneous fat and papillary layer of the dermis and migrate diffusely into the wound space. The papillary layer of the dermis is quite reactive and is the source of the newly formed cellular repair tissue, and the re-

ticular layer plays a more passive role (Ordman and Gillman, 1966). Fibroblast formation is most vigorous in the loose perivascular areolar connective tissue and has caused speculation that the first fibroblasts may have a hematogenous origin (Gillman and Ordman, 1965). However, experiments (Grillo, 1963) employing x-irradiation of epithelial wounds both 20 minutes and 28 hours after wounding caused a greater than 50 percent decrease in subsequent fibroblast and capillary endothelial cell proliferation. It was therefore concluded that since the depressive action of irradiation antedated the vascular influx of cellular elements into the wound, fibroblasts arose predominantly from proliferation of locally resident connective tissue cells.

By the fifth day, collagen fibers can be seen as fine reticulin fibers, and there is an accompanying rapid increase in wound tensile strength. The collagen concentration (hydroxyproline) of the wound then rapidly expands until the fifteenth day, when it ceases (Adamsons et al., 1964).

The intraincisional collagen fibers are initially vertical in orientation, but gradually become oblique and more abundant. They run across the incision, achieving a weave with the undamaged dermal collagen bundles on either side of the wound.

Maturation or Remodeling of the Wound Scar. Clinicians have long observed that a scar remains in a dynamic state for some time after the period of peak collagen formation. A scar can become hypertrophic and, indeed, keloidal, months after surgery. Conversely, the scar may whiten and become depressed in cross-section. The classic scorbutic wounds were actually late dehiscences of previously healed wounds.

A working concept for the production and maturation of collagen can be outlined as follows: proline $\longrightarrow$ hydroxyproline $\longrightarrow$ saline extractable collagen $\longrightarrow$ acid extractable collagen $\longrightarrow$ mature insoluble collagen. The rate of new collagen deposition can be determined in this way by measuring hydroxyproline levels (Peacock, 1961). While the amount of soluble collagen in uninjured skin continues to decrease with aging, scar tissue has a high proportion of soluble collagen for months after injury (Banfield and Brindley, 1959). Similarly, the collagen concentration (hydroxyproline) bears little relationship to the tensile strength of the wound (Adamsons et al., 1964). The rate of gain of wound tensile strength can be correlated with the synthesis of collagen only up to 45 days after injury (Peacock, 1966). Despite this relatively stable level of collagen, cutaneous scars will exhibit rapid increases in breaking and tensile strength for months thereafter. Without a measurable increase in the concentration of the collagen molecules, a basic reorganization and remodeling of the molecule by the insertion of cross-links must account for this increase in scar tensile strength. With time, as fibrils mature, weak hydrogen bonds and intermolecular forces are replaced by covalent bonds, the strongest union between atoms (Jackson and Bentley, 1960). Such covalent unions between polypeptides can lead to unlimited intramolecular and intermolecular cross-bonding with a stronger and more efficient collagen weave.

The sophisticated experiments of Grillo and Gross (1964) have demonstrated a collagenolytic system (collagenase) present in wound and injured epidermis and injured mesenchymal tissue. Such activity was absent in normal mesenchymal tissue. The wound margins were particularly rich in collagenase.

Using the above information, Peacock has proposed an "equilibrium theory" (Riley and Peacock, 1967). A healed wound can be regarded as a source of connective tissue, either in or out of balance, in terms of the rate of collagen synthesis and aggregation, and the rate of collagen degradation (collagenase system). Such a hypothesis could explain the late development of a scorbutic dehiscence (degradation without synthesis) and late keloid formation (synthesis without collagenolysis). The recent clinical successes with the use of triamcinolone for the treatment of keloids may be attributed to the enhancement of the collagenase system (Peacock et al., 1970).

Another promising area of investigation in the remodeling of scar tissue is the experimental work with induced lathyrism (Peacock, 1966). Lathyrism is a disease seen in animals who have eaten the common ground pea or flowering sweet pea of the genus *Lathyrus*. It results in a generalized loss of connective tissue tensile strength, which can be manifest as dissecting aneurysms, scoliosis, and abdominal hernias. The sequelae vary with the species affected. The active agent is beta-aminoproprionitride (BAPN), which interferes with aldehyde formation and subsequent covalent cross-linkage. The drug has recently been employed to prevent the development of harmful scar tissue between repaired flexor tendons and adjacent soft tissue, and to protect immobilized small joints of the fingers from developing periarticular scar tissue. It has also been shown that BAPN significantly reduces the degree of pulmonary fibrosis in rats subjected to intratracheal instillation of quartz crystals (Levine and Bye, 1964).

THE HEALING OF DIFFERENT TYPES OF WOUNDS

Healing of Clean, Incised Sutured Wounds (Primary Intention). The basic biologic phenomena involved in the repair of this most optimal wound healing situation have been discussed above. The careful histologic, multilevel studies of Gillman can be simply outlined (Gillman and Ordman, 1965).

DAY 1. Initially there is shedding of blood, fibrin, and lymph into the wound. Polymorphonuclear leukocytes rapidly spread throughout the length and depth of the incision. The epidermis thickens at the cut edges and the epithelial sheets advance by cleaving between the surface and intraincisional clot.

DAY 2. The second day is characterized by phagocytosis of polymorphonuclear leukocytes and erythrocytes by mononuclear cells. Epithelial spurs are noted in the upper part of the incision along with hyperplasia of the epithelium of the periincisional zone. The wound is now covered by epithelium. There is also a round cell reaction in the papillary layer of the dermis.

DAY 3. Round cells, which had been present in the dermal papillary layer, stream into the incisional area; the reticular layer remains inert.

DAY 4.   The fibroblasts make their first appearance and are oriented vertically to the surface. Frequent mitoses are noted within the intraincisional new connective tissue and the abutting zone of loose areolar connective tissue.

DAYS 5 TO 12.   Collagen fibrils are seen. With passage of time there is rearrangement of new collagen across the incision, with interdigitation and union of the new collagen with the original transected dermal collagen bundles. A keratin layer develops in the new incisional epithelium and the scab becomes loose.

DAYS 13 TO 24.   There is remodeling of the epithelium invading the dermis, and the collagen bundles become more dense. Fine, delicate elastic fibrils make their first appearance.

DAYS 25 AND ONWARD.   Scar epithelium becomes apparent, and the collagen bundles rearrange in a more compact form. With time, the scar shows less cellularity and vascularity.

Healing of Wounds with Loss of Substance (Secondary Intention).   When there is substantial full-thickness loss of skin, the initial event remains an outpouring of lymph, blood, and serum into the defect. As in wounds which heal by primary intention, there is mitotic activity in the basal layer of the marginal epithelium. If the defect is small in size, epithelialization can keep pace with the formation of granulation tissue (blood vessels, connective tissue, and cellular infiltrate). In wounds of larger size, the phenomenon of contraction is responsible for reducing the area to be epithelialized. As discussed earlier, the process is dependent on the mobility of adjacent tissue. Unsightly contractures and functional defects can be the end products of contraction.

When a large wound has been allowed to heal solely by contraction and epithelialization, the wound is covered by a thin layer of flattened epithelial cells with a thick, heavily desquamative layer of corneum. The convoluting rete pegs are conspicuously absent. Such epithelial surfaces, as seen in the extensively burned patient, are extremely vulnerable to minor trauma, bleed easily, and separate at the dermoepi-

dermal junction. The dryness of the skin is attributed to the absence of normal accessory skin structures, e.g., hair follicles, sebaceous glands, and sweat glands.

Healing of Partial-Thickness Wounds. Partial-thickness wounds include those in which the whole epidermis but only part of the dermis has been lost. Abrasions, split-thickness skin graft donor sites, and partial-thickness burns are common examples.

With an intact dermis, fibroplasia and the development of granulation tissue play a lesser role; epithelialization is the dominant process. The wound edges, the hair follicles, and the sebaceous and sweat glands, in that order, are the sources of epithelial regeneration. When skin grafts are cut from the deeper portions of the dermis, where hair follicles are fewer, the sweat ducts can supply epithelium. The regenerating epithelial sheets spread across the reticular layer of the dermis deep to the clot, and initially there is no accompanying connective tissue regrowth.

The rapidity of healing of partial thickness wounds is dependent on multiple factors (Converse and Robb-Smith, 1944). With thin grafts, the donor site can heal within 6 to 10 days. Conversely, when the graft is taken toward the base of the dermis, where lobules of fat begin to appear in the donor site, healing can require 21 to 58 days. The thickness of the skin in the donor site also plays a role. An abdominal donor site with its thicker dermis will heal in an average of 12 days, while a thigh donor site requires an average of 16 days. If the region of the donor site is loosely bound to the underlying structures, then contraction will hasten wound healing. Finally, local wound sepsis, particularly with *Pseudomonas*, can cause necrosis of the residual dermis and retard healing by creating a wound of thicker loss.

FACTORS INFLUENCING WOUND HEALING

Although many factors are generally cited as influencing wound healing, only a few have been substantiated by critical analysis. Moreover, local factors, such as wound sepsis or hematoma formation, play a statistically more significant role in interfering with wound healing.

Steroids. The presumed depressive effect of cortisone on wounds is felt to be due to the retardation of the production of all mesenchymal cellular elements without which the healing sequence cannot proceed. While chronic steroid administration has been shown to decrease the breaking strength and tensile strength in healing wounds, short-term use of steroids has little clinical effect on wound healing (McNamara et al., 1969).

Local use of vitamin A in experimental studies can be helpful in overcoming the depressing effect of cortisone (Hunt et al., 1969). Similarly, anabolic steroids such as testosterone can restore normal healing in the face of concurrent administration of cortisone (Ehrlich and Hunt, 1969). Both testosterone and vitamin A are believed to labilize the lysosomal membrane; cortisone stabilizes the membrane.

Protein Depletion. Prolonged protein depletion has an adverse effect upon wound healing in experimental animals. The decrease in tensile strength is associated with a decrease in the number of fibroblasts and the amount of collagen in the wound (Ross, 1968). However, the addition of a single amino acid, methionine, restores the pattern of hexosamine and hydroxyproline concentrations toward normal (Dunphy et al., 1956). Serum protein levels correlate poorly with the undernourished state of a patient with poor wound healing. Careful protein estimation of rectus sheath, peritoneum, and muscle in normal patients, debilitated patients, and those with recent wound disruptions demonstrates a marked difference in protein content between the different groups.

Vitamin C. Scurvy came to the attention of physicians in the eighteenth century by reports of late wound dehiscences in sailors subsisting on a diet lacking fresh fruits and vegetables. The basic defect of repair in scurvy is a deficiency of collagen synthesis. Ultrastructure studies have shown subcellular alterations within the scorbutic fibroblast. In addition, the concentration of hexosamines in scorbutic wounds is less than in a normal wound (Dunphy et al., 1956). The ground substance alteration probably results from a

defect in the sulfation of mucopolysaccharides. Hyaluronic acid accumulates and chondroitin sulfate formation lags (Ross, 1968). Vitamin C deficiency is improbable in healthy, well-nourished individuals, but elderly, debilitated patients may have borderline scurvy which can be aggravated by prolonged illness and acute trauma. Under such conditions, this group of patients may benefit from the use of ascorbic acid.

Anemia. Retrospective clinical studies have always emphasized the frequent association of anemia in patients with wound dehiscences. Local wound oxygen-tension studies (Hunt and Zederfelt, 1969) have demonstrated that with impairment of local circulation by injury, transport of nutritional substances across the wound is retarded. In addition, oxygen requirements of the injured tissue is elevated. Uncorrected hypovolemia will result in an additional drop in local wound oxygen. Consequently, the role of anemia may in reality only be a reflection of a decreased blood volume.

TECHNICAL CONSIDERATIONS

The physician can employ his knowledge of wound healing to promote this process in the most expedient and least conspicuous manner. Some regions of the body, endowed with an especially rich blood supply, like the head and neck, will demonstrate rapid healing. Incisions can be planned for hidden areas of the body. Hair-bearing skin, the oral cavity, skin lines of tension such as wrinkle lines and lines of dependency offer such opportunity. Simple pinching of the skin is helpful in determining the axis of the natural wrinkle lines.

The classic Halstedian technique of gentle handling of tissues and avoidance of bundle tissue ligation results in improved wound statistics. Careful hemostasis should be practiced to avoid the formation of hematomas. The latter impede wound healing because they retard the ingrowth of proliferating mesenchymal cells and small blood vessels. Hematomas, in providing an ideal culture medium, are a common cause of wound sepsis. Infection will delay healing and damage delicate regenerating tissue. In partial-thickness wounds, sepsis can convert the wound to a full-thickness defect.

The spectrum of suture material reactivity ranges from stainless steel to catgut in terms of degree of reactivity. Wounds with monofilament suture demonstrate a lower incidence of suture abscess, because the interstices of braided material are more susceptible to infestation by microorganisms. The tension with which the sutures are tied is the greatest cause of skin suture marks. Sutures tied too tightly, the hallmark of the beginning surgeon, will necrose the intervening tissue. The resulting fibrous tissue replacement is called a "stitch mark." Within reasonable limits, the size of suture or the size of needle plays only a minor role (Crikelair, 1958). To avoid stitch marks, epidermal sutures can be removed early and the wound reinforced with tape. Because of the long period of cutaneous scar remodeling, a buried intradermal nylon suture should be employed to prevent scar widening. This suture can be left in place for several weeks without fear of tissue reaction. Buried sutures, provided the material is fine and nonreactive, should be used to promote coaptation of the tissue. The smallest possible number of skin sutures should be used to close the wound, and they should be of the everting type. Epithelialization suture tracts can be avoided by early suture removal; and if tracts develop, they are best handled by marsupialization (Converse, 1966).

Hypertrophic scars and keloids have always presented a dilemma in treatment. While histologic differentiation between these two types of abnormal wound responses remains controversial, a hypertrophic wound tends to maintain its original configuration, while a keloid extends beyond the original confines of the wound. Reports of success with triamcinolone injection are encouraging (Griffith et al., 1970). The drug can be employed in three ways: Keloids in less conspicuous areas of the body are best handled by multiple intralesional injections without any surgery. Other keloids, especially those in the facial region, can be treated by excision and injection of the dermis at the time of surgery. Finally, the steroid injections can be withheld until at least three weeks following excision. Peacock has proposed that steroids may act by promoting collagenolytic activity (Peacock et al., 1970).

REFERENCES

Adamsons, R. L., Musco, F., and Enquist, I. E.: The relationship of collagen content to wound strength in normal and scorbutic animals. Surg. Gynec. Obstet., 119:323, 1964.

Banfield, W. B., and Brindley, D. C.: Acetic acid-soluble collagen in human scars. Surg. Gynec. Obstet., 109:367, 1959.

Bullough, W. S., and Laurance, E. B.: Control of epidermal mitotic activity in the mouse. Proc. R. Soc. Lond., B151:517, 1960.

Converse, J. M.: Treatment of epithelized suture tracts of the eyelid by marsupialization. Plast. Reconstr. Surg., 38:576, 1966.

Converse, J. M., and Robb-Smith, A. H. T.: The healing of surface cutaneous wounds: its analogy with the healing of superficial burns. Ann. Surg., 120:873, 1944.

Crikelair, G. F.: Skin suture marks. Am. J. Surg., 96:631, 1958.

Dunphy, J. E., Udupua, K. N., and Edwards, L. C.: Wound healing. A new perspective with particular reference to ascorbic acid deficiency. Ann. Surg., 144:304, 1956.

Ehrlich, H. P., and Hunt, T. K.: The effects of cortisone anabolic steroids in the tensile strength of healing wounds. Ann. Surg., 170:203, 1969.

Gillman, T., and Ordman, L. J.: Tissue Reactions during Healing of Cutaneous Wounds, in Structure and Function of Connective and Skeletal Tissue. London, Butterworths, 1965.

Griffith, B. H., Monroe, C. W., and McKinney, P.: A follow-up study of the treatment of keloids with triamcinolone acetonide. Plast Reconstr. Surg., 46:145, 1970.

Grillo, H. C.: Origin of fibroblasts in wound healing: An antoradiographic study of inhibition of cellular proliferation by local X-irradiation. Ann. Surg., 157:453, 1963.

Grillo, H. C., and Gross, J.: Collagenolytic activity and epithelial-mesenchymal interaction in healing mammalian wounds. J. Cell. Biol., 23:39A, 1964.

Hunt, T. K., and Zederfelt, B.: Nutritional and environmental aspects of wound healing. *In* Dunphy, J. E., and van Winkle, W. (eds.): Repair and Regeneration, New York, McGraw-Hill Book Company, 1969.

Hunt, T. K., Ehrlich, H. P., Garcia, J. A., and Dunphy, J. E.: Effect of vitamin A on reversing the inhibitory effect of cortisone on healing of open wounds in animals and man. Ann. Surg., 170:633, 1969.

Jackson, D. S., and Bentley, J. P.: On the significance of the extractable collagens. J. Biophys. Biochem. Cytol., 7:37, 1960.

Kazanjian, V. H., and Converse, J. M.: The Surgical Treatment of Facial Injuries. Ed. 3. Baltimore, The Williams & Wilkins Co., 1972.

Levine, C. I., and Bye, I.: The effect of B-aminoproprionitrite in silicatic fibrosis in rats. Fed. Proc., 23:236, 1964.

Majno, G., Gabbiani, G., Hirschel, B. J., Ryan, G. B., and Stratkov, P. R.: Contraction of granulation tissue in vitro: similarity to smooth muscle. Science, 173:548, 1971.

McNamara, J. J., Lamborn, P. J., Mills, D., and Aaby, G. V.: Effect of short-term pharmacologic doses of adrenocortical therapy on wound healing. Ann. Surg., 170:199, 1969.

Ordman, L. J., and Gillman, T.: Studies on the healing of cutaneous wounds. I. The healing of incisions through the skin of pigs. Arch. Surg., 93:857, 1966.

Peacock, E. E.: The effects of acid extract of collagen, cold neutral solutions of collagen and reconstituted collagen fibrils in wound healing and protein-depleted rats. Surg. Gynec. Obstet., 113:329, 1961.

Peacock, E. E.: Inter- and intramolecular bonding in collagen of healing wounds by insertion of methylene and amide cross-links into scar tissue. Ann. Surg., 163:1, 1966.

Peacock, E. E.: Wound healing and wound care. *In* Schwarz, S. I. (Ed.): Principles of Surgery. New York, McGraw-Hill Book Company, 1969.

Peacock, E. E., and van Winkle, W.: Surgery and Biology of Wound Repair. W. B. Saunders Company, 1970.

Peacock, E. E., Madden, J. W., and Trier, W. C.: Biologic basis for the treatment of keloids and hypertrophic scars. South. Med. J., 63:755, 1970.

Riley, W. B., and Peacock, E. E.: Identification, distribution and significance of a collagenolytic enzyme in human tissue. Proc. Soc. Exp. Biol. Med., 124:207, 1967.

Ross, R.: The fibroblast and wound repair. Biol. Rev., 43:51, 1968.

Ross, R., and Odland, G.: Fine structure observations of human skin wounds and fibrogenesis. In Dunphy, J. E., and van Winkle, W. (Eds.): Repair and Regeneration, New York, McGraw-Hill Book Company, 1969.

Watts, G. T., Grillo, H. C., and Gross, J.: Studies in wound healing. II. The role of granulation tissue in contraction. Ann. Surg., 148:153, 1958.

5

Skin Carcinogenesis

Roy E. Albert, M. D.

The purpose of this chapter is to present an overview of the current status of skin carcinogenesis research involving the major classes of carcinogens: (1) ionizing radiation, (2) ultraviolet radiation, (3) chemical carcinogens, and (4) viruses.

IONIZING RADIATION

Upton (1967) has summarized the early history of radiation carcinogenesis. The ability of ionizing radiation to cause skin cancer was first noted in man at the turn of the century. Experimental production of sarcomas in animals by means of high doses of x-radiation was made in 1910, and carcinoma of the skin was experimentally produced in 1918. Little progress was made in the experimental study of the carcinogenic action of penetrating radiation on the skin until the use of electron beams and β-rays made it possible to limit the action of irradiation to the skin of small laboratory animals without causing injury to deep-seated organs.

The use of radiation for the experimental induction of skin tumors has certain advantages over that of the chemical carcinogens. Various spatial and temporal distributions of dosage can de defined precisely. The effect of irradiation on target cells is direct, and there is no ambiguity about penetration into target cells or about the extent of biochemical transformation to the active form of the carcinogen. With externally applied radiation, there is no persisting exposure such as occurs when chemicals are applied to the skin.

Physical Aspects. The ionizing radiations include electromagnetic radiations (x-rays and γ-rays), and particulate radiations (electrons, protons, neutrons, α-particles, and heavy nuclei). Both types of radiations cause their biologic effects primarily by ionizing important cell constituents; however, electromagnetic and particulate radiations differ quantitatively because of differences in penetrating power and in the microscopic pattern in which they deposit their energy within cells. As ionizing radiations of any type penetrate matter, they tend to lose energy by interacting with atoms and molecules in their path, exciting or ionizing them in the process.

The distance an impinging particle may penetrate into an absorbing material varies directly as a function of the energy of the radiation, and inversely as a function of its charge and the density of the absorber.

Particulate radiations, such as α-particles and protons, produce dense linear tracks of ionization, whereas electrons and the

111

electromagnetic radiations, x-rays and γ-rays, produce a much more scattered pattern of ionization. The more specific characteristics of penetration and rate of energy deposition, or linear energy transfer (LET) will be described later in the appropriate section.

Most methods used to detect and measure ionizing radiation depend on the collection of ions formed through the interaction of the radiation with a gas or solid in a detecting device. Other approaches include the use of photographic techniques and scintillation counters.

Dosimetry involves the measurement of the amount and distribution of the absorbed energy within the absorbing mass. The unit of absorbed dose is the rad, which is the deposition of 100 ergs per gram of tissue. The roentgen, or R, is that quantity of x- or γ-radiation which produces one electrostatic unit of charge in one ml. of air at standard temperature and pressure.

Sources generally used for skin irradiations emit "soft" radiations which do not penetrate much beyond the skin in order to avoid the complicating effects of radiation damage to deeper structures. Devices for this purpose include low voltage x-ray machines, and various types of accelerators (van de Graaff generators, cyclotrons, and linear accelerators) which are used to produce beams of electrons, protons, α-particles, and occasionally larger atomic nuclei. Isotope sources for skin irradiations contain a pure or almost pure β-emitting isotope (e.g., ^{90}Sr, ^{32}P, ^{91}Y, ^{208}Tl) distributed in a plastic sheet, deposited on the surface of filter paper, or bonded to a metallic foil.

Subcellular, Cellular, and Tissue Effects. Radiation produces damage by ionization and excitation. The primary targets are cellular macromolecules. Disruption of macromolecules is produced by direct interaction, and also indirectly through formation of highly reactive free radical water products. DNA strand breakage is readily demonstrable by ultracentrifugation methods, and chromosome breaks and aberrations are a consequence of DNA damage. Reproductive cell death is a characteristic effect in which death is delayed until attempted division.

In the last decade major advances have been made in the quantitative characterization of cell damage (see Elkind, 1967, for a comprehensive review). Cells grown in culture can be dispersed by trypsinization into a suspension of single cells. When inoculated into a flat culture dish, single cells attach to the glass floor of the dish and proliferate to form individual colonies in about two weeks. Exposure of the inoculated cells to graded doses of radiation causes a reduction in colony formation. The extent of reduction in colony formation provides a quantitative means of measuring cell lethality in terms of reproductive capability. Serial measurements of the number of cells in each colony provide additional information about effects of radiation on reproduction. There are also techniques for obtaining suspensions of cells which are in the same stage of the cell cycle. Such synchronized cell cultures provide information about the susceptibility of cells to injury at different stages of the cell cycle. Fractionated radiation exposures provide information on the rates of recovery from lethal damage.

High LET radiation causes an exponential decrease in colony survival with increasing dose characteristic of a one hit process. Low LET radiation shows an initial shoulder in the survival curve followed by an exponential decrease. Split doses of low LET radiation show very rapid and complete recovery similar to the tumorigenic response. Intracellular recovery does not occur with high LET radiation, but comparable tumorigenic studies have not yet been done.

Irradiation is always followed by a period of division delay. The duration of this period is dose dependent. After division delay, both killed and surviving cells divide with approximately the same doubling time. Ultimately, nonsurviving cells are able to carry out a limited number of divisions, i.e., one to five depending on the dose. Cells which lose the ability to divide commonly enlarge to a giant size before disintegrating.

The age of a cell is counted from the time the division of its parent is complete. The generation time of culture cells commonly ranges from about 10 to 20 hours. The M stage is the stage of mitotic cell division. G_1 is the period following the completion of the M stage. The G_1 stage is then followed by the S stage, in which DNA is replicated. The S stage is followed by the G_2 stage, and precedes the M stage of mitosis and cytokinesis (cell cleavage).

The sensitivity of the cell to radiation increases progressively with cell age reaching a maximum in G_2. Hence, it is characteristic of an irradiated cell population to have substantial numbers of cells held up in the G_2 period. These cells enter mitosis after the end of the delay period, producing a transient rebound in the number of mitotic cells. The relation of cell age to induction of chromosomal damage is analogous: i.e., there is an increased tendency to damage during the S period, reaching a maximum in the G_2 period.

DNA strand breakage can be shown by ultracentrifugation studies to be linearly dependent on dose, with a very rapid rate of restitution of the broken DNA strands (Lett et al., 1967). Although it is tempting to postulate this mechanism as the basis for chromosomal damage and cell lethality, it cannot be the only mechanism since the cell cycle stage has no effect on strand breakage (Lett and Sun, 1970).

Skin irradiation involves epidermal cell loss and repopulation (Fig. 5–1). Epidermal repopulation may overshoot to the level of hyperplasia, which subsides over a period of weeks.

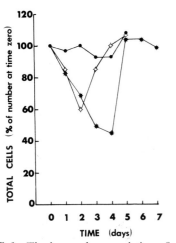

Figure 5–1 The loss and repopulation of rat epidermal cells following exposure to 10 kilovolt peak x-rays. •—• = controls; ⋄—⋄ = 1000 R; ✦—✦ = 2500 R. (*From* Burns: Radiat. Res., 43:219, 1970.)

The penetration of ionizing radiation is known to be an important factor in the production of acute radiation injury in the skin. Witten et al. (1953) demonstrated that α-radiation from a sealed ^{224}Ra (thorium X) source, applied directly to the surface of human skin, was much less effective in producing erythema than was the β-radiation from ^{224}Ra which had been introduced into the skin by iontophoresis. Moritz and Henriques (1952) reported that for equal surface doses, the soft β-rays of ^{35}S caused much less acute injury to porcine skin than did the more deeply penetrating β-rays of ^{90}Sr and ^{91}Y. Irradiations of the skin which penetrate deeper than the hair follicle can produce follicle atrophy (Fig. 5–2). The mechanism of this effect is unknown; its quantitative dose-effect aspects have an important bearing on tumorigenesis and are discussed later. High doses of deeply penetrating radiation produce ulceration which develops in one to two weeks and eventually results in a contracted scar.

Transformation of short-term cultured hamster embryo cells by ionizing radiation has been reported. Transformation is evident by the outgrowth of cell clones with altered morphology and excessive growth due to reduced contact inhibition. Inoculation of transformed cells into an antigenically compatible host results in the formation of connective tissue tumors. As the dose of x-rays is increased, the percentage of transformation increases to a plateau of about 1 percent between 100 and 300 rads; a further increase in dose results in an appreciable decrease in the proportion of cells transformed (Borek, 1973).

Temporal Aspects of Tumor Formation and Dose-Response Relationships. A striking feature of radiation tumorigenesis is that a single radiation exposure produces tumors, after a latent period, at an appreciable rate for the rest of the animal's life. This is illustrated by the response of the rat skin to single ^{91}Y β-ray exposures (Albert et al., 1961). Male rats were given single exposures on a 35 cm.^{2} skin area, with doses at the skin surface ranging from 230 rads to 10,000 rads at an average age of 21 weeks; dose rates were on the order of 20 rads per minute. Multiple tumor formation on individual rats was very com-

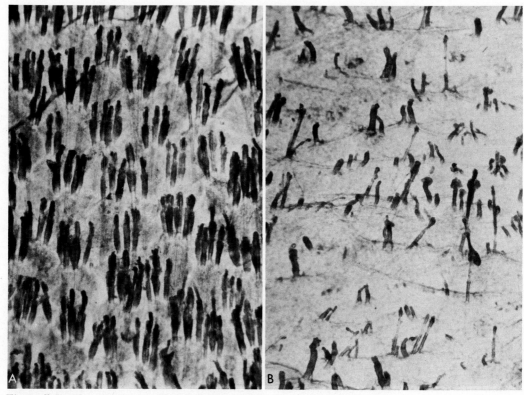

Figure 5–2 The appearance of hair follicles on whole-skin mount preparations.
A, Unirradiated sample. *B,* Severe follicle loss and atrophy from a single nonulcerating electron irradiation after 72 weeks. (*From* Albert et al.: Radiat. Res., 30:515, 1967a.)

mon, the maximum number being 16. Tumors developed independently, since the frequency distribution of the number of tumors which developed on individual rats followed a Poisson distribution. Most of the tumors were adnexal (Albert et al., 1969). The tumor formation sites were located only within the irradiated skin area, even where shrinkage of the irradiated skin occurred owing to high β-ray doses.

The time characteristics of tumor formation are shown in Figure 5–3 in terms of the number of tumors per rat. Tumor formation started between 8 and 20 weeks at doses equal to or greater than 4000 rads. At lower doses, the onset occurred somewhat later, between 28 and 44 weeks. The onset of tumor formation was relatively independent of dose in the dosage range of 230 to 2000 rads. The epidermoid carcinomas produced by severely ulcerogenic doses (above 5000 rads) were the earliest tumors to develop. An increasing age-

specific incidence of skin tumors after single exposures was observed by Jones et al. (1968) following single whole-body x-ray and neutron exposure in rats.

The dose-tumor incidence curves for tumors of all types are presented in Figure 5–4 at various times after irradiation. It will be seen that tumors appeared earliest at the higher doses. At 72 weeks the tumor incidence was comparatively low up to doses of about 2000 rads; with increasing doses, the incidence rose very rapidly, passing through a maximum at about 4000 rads, and then dropped rapidly. The decreased tumor formation at the high ulcerogeneic doses was limited to adnexal tumors. At doses which produced the maximum yield of tumor induction, there was a heavy predominance of adnexal tumors. The maximal yield of tumors was produced in the marginally ulcerogenic dose range.

The dose-tumor incidence curves are in good agreement with those obtained by

Raper et al. (1951) who used whole-skin β-irradiation by placing rats in a box lined with ^{32}P impregnated walls. It appears quite certain that the dependence of tumor incidence on dose is highly nonlinear over the range of 230 to 10,000 rads. These dose-response relationships, therefore, cannot be explained solely on the assumption that tumors are caused by somatic mutations.

The effect of age on tumor response has not been studied carefully; however, there is no difference in response between rats irradiated at the ages of 20 weeks and 40 weeks. There does not appear to be a significant difference in response among Sprague-Dawley, Holtzmann, and Wistar rats.

The Effect of Penetration of Ionizing Radiation. Glucksmann (1963) reported that 0.3 Mev electrons did not produce skin tumors in the mouse, in contrast to 0.7 Mev electrons. Lamerton (1963) also re-

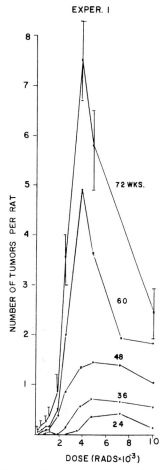

Figure 5–4 Incidence of epithelial skin tumors of all types according to the dose of yttrium-91 β-radiation (single exposures) for various times after exposure. Bar lines indicate standard errors. (*From* Albert et al.: Radiat. Res., 15:410, 1961.)

ported the lack of tumor production in the mouse skin by external α-radiation.

From studies with rats, there is now strong evidence that the surface epidermis and the upper 100 to 150 microns, the hair follicle, are completely unresponsive to the tumorigenic effect of ionizing radiation. Rats were irradiated with 5 Mev protons from a van de Graaff generator at doses ranging from 300 to 9500 rads (Albert et al., 1967a). No tumors occurred during a postirradiation period of 44 weeks. The only evidence of skin damage was the loss of the brown scale normally present on male albino rats. The same observation was made with an α-beam that penetrated the skin to a depth of 0.12 mm. (Heimbach et al., 1969). Here again, no tumors were

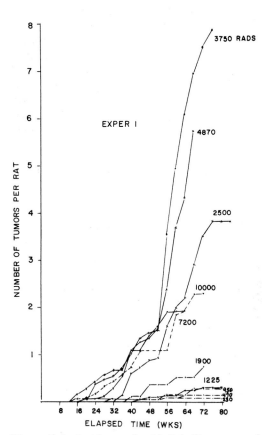

Figure 5–3 Incidence of epithelial skin tumors of all types according to time after single exposure to yttrium-91 beta radiation at the indicated doses.

produced in a 72 week postirradiation period with doses of 1230 and 2460 rads.

In view of the evident importance of penetration depth of ionizing radiation on the production of skin tumors, the tumor incidence and skin damage from graded doses and depths of penetration was studied in detail (Albert et al., 1967a). An electron beam from a 1.0 Mev electron van de Graaff accelerator was used with three different penetration depths. Figure 5–5 shows the depth-dose curves for the three maximum electron penetrations of 0.36 mm., 0.75 mm., and 1.40 mm. used in this experiment. The rats were rotated through the beam in small wooden boxes with a 3 by 8 cm. area of dorsal skin exposed to the electrons. Tumor formation had the same temporal characteristics described above for β-radiation for all three penetration depths. The same kinds of tumors were produced regardless of penetration, most of them being adnexal.

The surface dose-tumor incidence curves for the postirradiation time of 80 weeks are plotted in Figure 5–6 for the three electron penetration depths. To produce an equal tumor incidence, the shallower penetration required surface doses seven to eight times as great as those for the deeper penetration. The response of the 0.75 mm. penetration was intermediate between the 0.36 mm. and 1.40 mm. responses.

There is only one level in the skin where the tumor response is independent of the

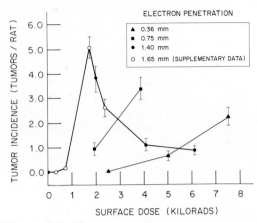

Figure 5–6 The tumor incidence with respect to surface dose at 80 weeks for three penetration depths of electrons. The shallower penetrations require higher surface doses for equal tumor incidence. (*From* Albert et al.: Radiat. Res., 30:515, 1967a.)

depth-dose characteristics of the electron radiation beam. The disparity between these curves disappears when the tumor incidence is related to the dose at a skin depth of 0.3 mm. (Fig. 5–7).

The hair follicles in the telogen (resting) stage of hair growth are about 0.5 mm. long and lie at an angle of about 30 to 45 degrees with respect to the skin surface. A depth of 0.3 mm. is, therefore, close to the bottom of the resting follicles. The existence of a critical depth near the bottom of the resting hair follicles indicates that the tumor yield is independent of the dose to the surface epithelium and more superficial parts of the hair follicle. One possible explanation for this finding is that the epithelial tumors arise from cells that were near the bottom of the follicles at the time of irradiation.

Irradiation of the rat skin with growing hair follicles indicates that the critical depth remains about 0.3 mm. in spite of the marked elongation of the hair follicles (Burns et al., 1973b).

The Effect of Linear Energy Transfer (LET). Particulate forms of radiation such as α-particles, protons, and neutrons produce densely ionized tracks in tissue in contrast to the more diffusely distributed ionization pattern from x-rays and electrons. Hence, for equal amounts of absorbed energy per gram of tissue, the energy deposition is much more concentrated with high LET radiations.

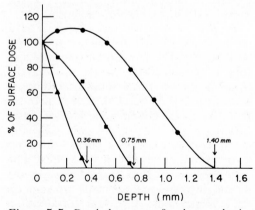

Figure 5–5 Depth-dose curves for electrons having maximum penetrations of 0.36 mm., 0.75 mm., and 1.40 mm. (*From* Albert et al.: Radiat. Res., 30:515, 1967a.)

The relative biologic effectiveness (RBE) of high LET radiations is 3 to 10 times greater than that for low LET radiations for many biologic responses. Furthermore, the dose-response pattern can be quite different. The dose-survival curve for cultured cells with high LET radiation is exponential without any threshold, whereas for low LET radiations there is a large shoulder region in which increasing doses produce little effect. Dose fractionation studies have shown that this difference is related to the substantial reversibility of injury caused by low LET radiations, and the lack of recovery from injury produced by high LET radiation. Presumably this difference is due to the very severe molecular damage produced by the densely ionized tracks of high LET particles.

In addition to its theoretical importance, the RBE of high LET radiations is of considerable practical concern in the protection of radiation workers. The skin tumor RBE for α-particles was found to be three times greater than that for electrons in cases where the depth-dose curve of the two forms was matched by use of a spinning filter wheel in the α-beam (Burns et al., 1968). As shown in Figure 5–8, the shapes of the dose-response curves for electron and α-particle radiations were not significantly different. An RBE of 3 for high LET radiations is consistent with the

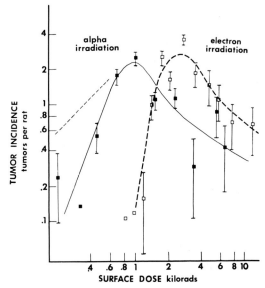

Figure 5–8 Tumor incidence at 76 weeks after irradiation, versus surface dose for α-particle and electron irradiation. The depth-dose characteristics of the α-particle and electron radiations were similar, having a maximum penetration of one millimeter in skin. The dose-incidence curves have the same shape but are displaced by a dose factor of 2.9. (*From* Burns et al.: Radiat. Res., 36(2):225, 1968.

observations of Jones et al. (1968) and of Hulse (1969).

Nonuniform Surface Patterns of Irradiation. Nonuniform surface applications of radiation are known to have marked effects on the injury response of the skin. The use of a sieve irradiation pattern to minimize skin damage is standard practice in radiation therapy. The effect of the size and proximity of irradiated areas on the injury response in the skin has been studied by Jolles (1950).

The effect of sieve pattern irradiation on the tumorigenic response of the rat skin has been studied in some detail because it involves an important theoretical question: is the tumor response only a function of the number of cells that are irradiated, or are there tissue factors that play an important role in tumor response? The question was first investigated by Passonneau et al. (1952). They showed that when the skin was exposed to the same ^{90}Sr activity, which was either distributed uniformly in a plane source or concentrated in a few beads, the tumor response from the few concentrated sources was not as great as that from the

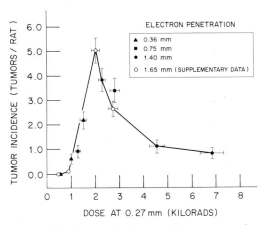

Figure 5–7 Tumor incidence with respect to the dose at a skin depth of 0.27 mm. at 80 weeks for three penetration depths of electrons. This is the only skin depth at which the dose-tumor incidence curves are congruent. (*From* Albert et al.: Radiat. Res., 30:515, 1967a.)

uniform source. This did not answer the question because the focal irradiation doses were much larger and could have been much higher than the range for optimal tumorigenesis.

The issue was further studied by use of sieve pattern radiation (Albert et al., 1967b). The first experiment with electron radiation showed a marked reduction in tumor yield for sieve pattern radiation normalized to the same amount of skin irradiated in the uniform surface pattern (Fig. 5–9). The same result was obtained (Albert and Burns, 1973b) with soft x-irradiation, where, unlike electron irradiation, there was negligible side scattering of radiation within the skin into the shielded areas (Fig. 5–10). Hence, it appears established that sieve pattern exposure to low LET radiation affords a marked protective effect against tumor formation. On the other hand, no such protective effect was observed in another experiment in which the sieve irradiation was done with protons having a high LET radiation (Burns et al., 1972). As indicated previously, it is well established that intracellular recovery from the lethal effects of ionizing radiation is an important characteristic of low LET radiation in contrast to high LET radiation. It would appear that the tumorigenic injury from high LET radiation is nonreparable, and there is consequently no protective effect obtained from the sieve pattern irradiation.

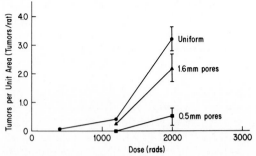

Figure 5–10 Dose-tumor incidence curves at 72 weeks after a single exposure to 25 kilovolt peak x-rays with uniform and sieve patterns. A marked protective effect of sieve irradiation is seen where the pore size is 0.5 mm. in diameter. (*From* Albert and Burns: Proc. Radiat. Res. Soc., Abstract Cd-2, 1973b.)

The Association of Follicle Atrophy and Skin Tumors. In rats irradiated when the hair follicles are in the resting stage, optimal skin tumor formation with single irradiation exposures occurs at doses which are just below the level required to produce ulceration. These doses produce permanent and partial epilation. There is a quantitative association between the numbers of tumors and atrophic follicles—about one tumor per 2000 to 4000 atrophic follicles (Fig. 5–11)—regardless of the penetration depth or the LET characteristics of the irradiations (Albert et al., 1967a, 1972). The same critical skin depth of about 0.3 mm. holds for the production of atrophic follicles as well as for tumors. These findings suggest that the atrophic follicles are a necessary precursor lesion for adnexal tumor formation. However, shallow irradiation of the rat skin when the follicles were in the growing stage shows that adnexal tumors develop without follicle atrophy. The critical depth for follicle atrophy in the growing hair moves down to about 0.8 mm., whereas the critical depth for tumor formation remains at about 0.3 mm. There is evidently a spatial dissociation of the critical depths for tumorigenesis and follicle damage (Burns et al., 1973b).

The character of the follicle injury response is part of the marked difference in tumor response of rats and mice to ionizing radiation (Albert et al., 1972). Relatively few skin tumors can be produced in the mouse, and of the epithelial tumors that do occur, most are epidermoid car-

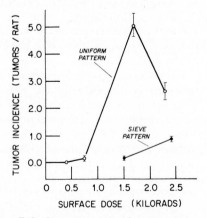

Figure 5–9 Dose-tumor incidence curves at 80 weeks after single exposures to electrons with either a uniform or a sieve pattern of surface irradiation. There is a marked protective effect of sieve pattern irradiation, particularly at 1700 rads. (*From* Albert et al.: Radiat. Res., 30:525, 1967b.)

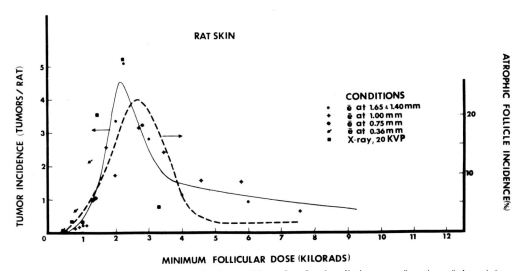

Figure 5–11 The dose-response curves in the rat 80 weeks after irradiation, as a function of the minimum follicular dose for incidence of epithelial skin tumors (solid line), and as a function of the percent atrophic follicles per control (broken line); ē indicates electron irradiation. These curves show similar dose-response relationships for the incidence of skin tumors and atrophic follicles. (*From* Albert et al.: J. Natl. Cancer Inst., 49:1131, 1972.)

cinomas rather than adnexal tumors. The dose-response curve for skin tumor induction following graded doses of electron radiations for mice with resting hair is shown in Fig. 5–12. The peak epithelial tumor response is more than an order of magnitude lower than that for rats. In terms of follicle loss, the mouse is twice as sensitive as the rat: the dose for 50 percent follicle loss is 3000 rads in rats and 1500 rads in mice. Follicle atrophy is not an important intermediate stage of injury in mice; follicles tend to be either totally destroyed or completely normal. Relative to follicle damage, the amount of dermal injury is less severe in mice.

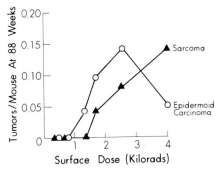

Figure 5–12 The surface dose versus incidence of sarcomas and epidermoid carcinomas in mouse skin 88 weeks after irradiation with electrons having a maximum penetration of 0.4 mm. (*From* Albert et al.: J. Natl. Cancer Inst., 49:1131, 1972.)

This results in large areas of irradiated mouse epidermis completely denuded of follicles; whereas in the rat, comparable levels of complete follicle destruction are associated with very severe ulceration and marked shrinkage of the residual scar. The lack of adnexal tumor formation in the mouse may be due to a high susceptibility to lethal damage of the follicles, which precludes a significant amount of neoplastic cell transformation.

Effect of Dose Fractionation. The effect of dose fractionation on tumor formation has an important bearing on the issue of recovery from tumorigenic radiation injury. Observations by Raper et al. (1951) showed that the cumulative dose from daily β-ray exposures in rats was much greater than that from a single exposure for an equivalent skin tumor response. Similar findings were obtained for x-rays by Zackheim (1964). There is a striking lack of accumulation of tumorigenic radiation injury in the rat skin, as shown by split-dose experiments (Burns et al., 1973a). A single subtumorigenic electron exposure of 750 rads during the resting stage of hair growth in rats has virtually no effect on the tumor response of the same animals reirradiated 31 days later, when their skin was again in the resting stage of hair growth (Fig. 5–13). The almost complete recovery from the effects of the initial

Skin Carcinogenesis

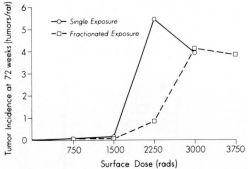

Figure 5–13 The single-exposure dose-incidence curve shows the tumor response 72 weeks after a single electron irradiation at the indicated doses. The fractionated dose-incidence curve represents animals that received the identical treatment as the single-exposure animals, except that they had been irradiated 31 days earlier with 750 rads. The two curves would be congruent if the fractionated dose-incidence curve were replotted with the initial 750 rads subtracted from the total dose. The lack of effect of the initial 750 rads means that tumorigenic recovery was almost complete. (*From* Burns et al.: Radiat. Res., 53:235, 1973a.)

750 rads could have been due to intracellular repair processes or to proliferative recovery where the damaged cells were replaced. The fact that essentially the same results were obtained when the interval between doses was 24 hours (Fig. 5–14) suggests that intracellular recovery was the dominant process, since 24 hours is insufficient time for proliferative repair (Albert and Burns, 1973a).

ULTRAVIOLET (UV) RADIATION

The etiologic role of sunlight in human skin cancer was suggested around the turn of the century and has been amply sub-

stantiated since then. The occurrence of skin cancer is correlated to UV exposure, since the incidence tends to be high in sunny regions, in outdoor workers, and in people with light complexions, and in the most exposed skin areas of the body (Epstein, 1970). The induction of skin cancer in experimental animals has been extensively studied with UV alone and to some extent in combination with chemical carcinogens. DNA repair processes, first detected with UV radiation, have been of particular importance in opening a new area of carcinogenesis research.

Physical Aspects. The photochemical effects of UV are due to electron excitation in the absorbing atoms and molecules, which induces damaging chemical reactions. UV is a weakly penetrating radiation, but unlike ionizing radiation the depth-dose characteristics in skin are difficult to measure. UV absorption is determined by the chemical composition of the different layers of skin, and much scattering occurs by refraction and reflection. Transmission through the epidermis is generally low but varies markedly according to wavelength and to thickness (Blum, 1959). The effective wavelength range for biochemical damage is 230 to 320 μm. DNA strongly absorbs UV at 280 μm.

DNA Damage and Repair. Chemical changes induced in DNA by radiation constitute important sites of damage which may be responsible for cell death and neoplastic transformation. The damaging action of UV arises chiefly from the formation of two unwanted chemical bonds, called dimers, between adjacent thymine bases on one DNA strand. The presence of excessive numbers of dimers blocks DNA

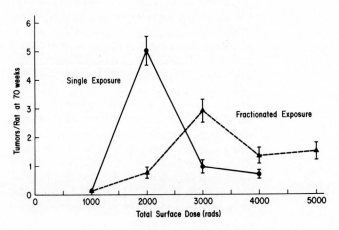

Figure 5–14 Dose-response relationships for singly and doubly electron-exposed rats. This experiment is the same as that shown in Figure 5–13, except that the doubly exposed rats received 1000 rads 24 hours before the second exposure. (*From* Albert and Burns: Proc. Am. Assoc. Cancer Res., 14:86, 1973a.)

replication. In 1949, Kelner discovered a repair process called photoreactivation. The number of soil organisms that survived large doses of ultraviolet radiation could be increased by a factor of several hundred thousand if the irradiated bacteria were subsequently exposed to an intense source of ultraviolet light. Photoreactivation is a form of DNA repair which occurs in lower phylogenic orders (bacteria and molds, up through marsupials) by which a light-activated (300 to 500 μm.) enzymatic reaction splits thymine dimers in situ (Hanawalt and Haynes, 1967).

Another DNA repair mechanism which is not dependent on light has been demonstrated in bacteria and human fibroblasts. In this process, segments of DNA strands containing thymine dimers are excised and replaced. This is done in a cut and patch operation by enzymes which sever the DNA strand at either side of the site of thymine dimer formation; the excised strand segment is resynthesized using the opposite normal DNA strand as a template, and the ends are rejoined to re-form the continuous DNA molecule.

There are several methods for detecting this form of unscheduled DNA synthesis. One method uses radioactive bromodeoxyuridine (BUdR), a metabolic analogue of thymidine which becomes incorporated into DNA (Cleaver, 1969). Incorporation of radioactive BUdR during DNA synthesis associated with cell replication produces abnormally heavy strands which can be detected by cesium chloride density gradient centrifugation. With unscheduled DNA synthesis due to DNA repair, small patches of DNA incorporate radioactive BUdR in insufficient quantities to make the strands heavy. Hence, the demonstration of normal density DNA containing radioactive BUdR is evidence of repair synthesis. Another method involves the use of radioautography to detect a generalized low level of [3]HTdR tritiated thymidine uptake into the DNA of cell nuclei. The DNA synthesis associated with cell replication is either represented as very heavily [3]HTdR-labeled cell nuclei, or it is selectively blocked by the use of hydroxyurea, which has little effect on DNA repair synthesis (Stich et al., 1973). Unscheduled DNA synthesis has been observed in the connective tissue of the upper dermis within minutes after exposure to UV radiation (Epstein et al., 1969).

Excision repair ends in about six hours, but it is incomplete with about half the dimers remaining. Rodent cells do not show this early form of excision repair, but they do show repair that occurs during replication (Rauth, 1967). Newly synthesized DNA strands formed against the complementary dimer-containing strand have blank segments corresponding to the dimers. These are subsequently removed either by excision repair or by a process analogous to recombination, where segments of preformed DNA are inserted into the gaps (Witkin, 1969).

The skin fibroblasts from patients with xeroderma pigmentosum (XP) show a pronounced increase in susceptibility to the lethal effects of UV (Cleaver, 1968). XP cells have an abnormally low ability to carry out excision repair of the thymine dimers. This deficiency is due to a defect in the enzymes which carries out the first step in excision repair—that of cutting the DNA strand (Setlow et al., 1969). The high susceptibility of XP patients to UV-induced skin cancer is strong evidence that DNA damage underlies both the lethal and the carcinogenic responses to UV.

Cellular Effects. The lethal effect of UV on cultured cells, measured in terms of colony-forming ability, differs from that described previously for ionizing radiation in that the shape of the survival is sigmoid instead of having an initial shoulder followed by an exponentially decreasing slope (Lee and Puck, 1960). These differences in the shape of the survival curve indicate a fundamental difference in mechanism of action; the response to UV radiation clearly does not fit the concept of one or more targets in the cells which determine lethality.

The effect of UV radiation on the progression of cells through the mitotic cycle appears mainly to be a slowing in their movement through the S phase due to a reduced rate of DNA synthesis (Djordjevic and Tolmach, 1967). The formation of thymine dimers in DNA is the most probable explanation for the slow rate of DNA synthesis. The depression of DNA synthesis is much greater with UV than with ionizing radiation at comparable levels of cell lethality.

The cellular effects of both ultraviolet and ionizing radiation are strongly affected by the stage in the cycle in which the cells are exposed. With UV, the sensitivity to damage is greatest in the G_1 stage and progressively decreases with cell age (Djordjevic and Tolmach, 1967). X-radiation has the opposite effect as described previously, since the sensitivity rises to a peak in G_2. The decreasing sensitivity to UV with increased cell age is consistent with the concept that the damage is proportional to the amount of dimers in the DNA which is yet to be replicated. This is the case in terms of lethality, lengthened generation time, and depressed DNA synthesis. However, for reasons unknown, chromosomal damage peaks with UV in the S period (Humphrey et al., 1963).

When cells are irradiated in G_1 with UV at a dose which has low survival (e.g., 5 percent) in terms of colony formation, almost all of the nonsurviving cells die before or as they enter mitosis. The cells destined to survive G_1 irradiation take about six times longer than normal to complete the cycle, but thereafter behave normally. Cells irradiated in the late S or early G_2 stage are about eight times more resistant than those irradiated in G_1 — the survivors complete the cell cycle without delay but are very slow in the next generation; thereafter, they return to normal (Thompson and Humphrey, 1970).

This response pattern with UV differs from ionizing radiation in the following features: Both radiations lengthen the irradiated cell cycle, but the effect is greater with UV. The slowing with UV radiation occurs in S, while the delay from ionizing radiation occurs in G_2. With UV radiation almost all cell death occurs in the irradiated generation, whereas with ionizing radiation both survivors and nonsurvivors divide and the nonsurvivors degenerate after as many as a half dozen cycles (Thompson and Suit, 1969); hence, there is a much more delayed cell death with ionizing radiation. Chromosomal damage with UV is largely of the chromatid variety, which is single stranded in character and occurs only during the DNA replication period when the complementary strands are separated in the process of replication (Humphrey et al., 1963). Ionizing radiation causes greater energy deposition: it produces chromosomal aberrations (double-strand damage) when the cells are irradiated in G_1, and it produces chromatid damage in the S period and later; the dominant form of DNA damage with ionizing radiation is strand breakage which is quickly repaired (Lett and Sun, 1970). The repair of UV thymine dimer formation and other damage is much slower: recovery of UV-exposed cells in terms of colony-forming ability as measured by split-dose experiments with Chinese hamster cells requires about 30 hours for completion (Todd et al., 1969). Recovery measured in a similar way with split-dose experiments using ionizing radiation requires only a few hours for completion (Elkind and Whitmore, 1967). Both forms of radiation have the common property of a large proportion of cell deaths associated with mitotic abnormalities. With both forms of irradiation, factors which modify lethality have a parallel effect on skin tumor induction.

Tissue Reactions to UV. Early inhibition of DNA synthesis and cell mitosis in the UV-exposed epidermis is also characteristic of chemical carcinogens (Iversen and Evensen, 1962). Similar effects are seen with ionizing radiation. Suppression of DNA synthesis and mitotic inhibition in the skin of hairless mice and in human skin has also been observed with single UV exposures (Epstein et al., 1969). These effects with doses of 4.5×10^6 ergs per cm.[2] develop in one to two hours and persist for several hours. There is a rebound acceleration of DNA synthesis and mitosis associated with the development of hyperplasia, which reaches a peak by about two weeks and disappears by four weeks. The hyperplastic stimulus spreads beyond the immediately irradiated area (Blum, 1959).

With continuing UV exposures there are increasing mitotic and [3]HTdR labeling indices as the epidermis progresses from normal through the hyperplastic state to a premalignant or early malignant state (Epstein, 1970). There is also a reduction in the duration of the DNA synthetic period (S), and in the interval between the S period and mitosis (the G_2 period). In addition, this is a marked acceleration in the epidermal transit time. There is no evidence of delayed maturation, but rather there is an accelerated cell formation, maturation, and turnover.

The hyperplastic epidermal response is associated with striking changes in the basement membrane, which becomes thick and ropelike, then becomes frayed, and finally disappears with the development of frank malignancy. The degeneration of the basement membrane with sustained UV exposure is associated with the appearance of pleomorphic basal cells in which mitotic abnormalities are frequent (Epstein, 1970). A similar pattern has been shown for chemically induced tumors (Dobson, 1963).

The role of dermal damage in epidermal tumor formation has been reviewed by Epstein (1970). Degeneration of the dermal connective tissue, called actinic elastosis, characteristically occurs in heavily exposed humans but does not appear to be essential to the development of epidermal malignancies. There is some evidence that dermal damage results from radiation injury of the dermal fibroblasts. A series of connective tissue changes has been correlated with epidermal tumor formation. This series includes collagen and elastic tissue dissolution, increased amounts of acid mucopolysaccharides, and increased numbers of mast cells and abnormal dermal vasculature.

Carcinogenic Action. The effective wavelengths for both the inflammatory and carcinogenic effects of UV radiation range from 230 to 320 μm.; the most potent range is 280 to 320 μm. (Blum, 1943; Kelner and Taft, 1956). Longer wavelengths can also be phototoxic and carcinogenic when administered concomitantly with a photosensitizer. The effective UV dose to the skin is reduced by the presence of hair, melanin, and a thick stratum corneum; the latter is suggested as the basis for the resistance of the hairless rat (Hueper, 1941).

The tumorigenic response of the skin of the ear of the albino mouse has been studied extensively. However, unlike the case in humans, most of the UV tumors are sarcomas (Grady, 1941; Grady et al., 1943). A greater proportion of carcinomas are pro-

duced in this system with shorter UV wavelengths of 254 μm. (Blum and Lippincott, 1942; Kelner and Taft, 1956). Hairless mice develop carcinoma almost exclusively in response to UV radiation (Winkelmann, 1960), and melanomas have been produced in pigmented hairless mice (Epstein et al., 1967).

Classic studies in the quantitative tumorigenic response to UV at relatively high dose rates have been carried out by Blum (1959). These studies were done by rotating male strain A mice under an intermediate pressure mercury arc lamp (wavelengths shorter than 313 μm.) with three exposure schedules: once per week, five times per week, and seven times per week. Single doses ranged from 0.32 to 8.6×10^7 ergs/cm.^{2} Tumor appearance was scored at a size of approximately 60 mm.^{3} At each dose schedule, the cumulative incidence had a log probability distribution (Fig. 5–15), indicating that the dose schedule simply shifted the time scale of tumor development (Fig. 5–16).

No effects of dose rate were observed above 0.35×10^4 ergs/cm.^{2} Below this level a very pronounced delay in tumor formation was obtained for the same dose. Discontinuation of the exposure before the onset of tumor formation (which occurred with continuous exposure) also markedly delayed the appearance of tumors (Fig. 5–17). For each of the three dosage schedules, there is a log-linear decrease in the median time of tumor formation with increasing dose, to a minimum level which remains unchanged with further increases in dose. Blum developed a model which explains these results on the basis that each UV dose not only produces new clones of transformed cells but, more importantly, also accelerates the growth rate of those already formed.

Blum found that tumors could not be produced unless the exposures were extended over a longer period than $2\frac{1}{2}$ months. However, short periods of exposure do have an effect because application of the promoting agent croton oil after a single UV exposure of 1.3×10^7 ergs/cm.^{2} does result in tumor formation (Epstein and Roth, 1968).

Subtumorigenic doses of UV radiation administered after a single application of

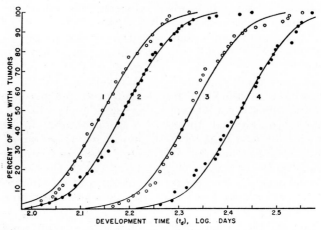

Figure 5-15   The incidence of chronic ultraviolet-induced skin tumors in albino mice showing a temporal displacement with progressively lower doses (curves 1, 2, and 3) and dose rates (curve 4). The data for the curves are the following:

Curve Number	Number of Mice	Single Dose, D (ergs cm.$^{-2}$ $\times$ 10^7)	Interval Between Doses, i (days)	Dose Rate (ergs cm.$^{-2}$ sec.$^{-1}$)
1	47	2.0	1.0	4.3
2	98	2.6	1.4	4.3
3	41	1.8	1.4	3.3
4	44	1.8	1.4	0.18

(*From* Blum: Carcinogenesis by Ultraviolet Light. Princeton University Press, 1959.)

7,12-dimethylbenz(*a*)anthracene (DMBA) will produce a substantial increase in the yield of malignancies but not of papillomas, in contrast to the action of a promoting agent (Epstein and Epstein, 1962). A single dose of DMBA before a carcinogenic UV exposure will accelerate the

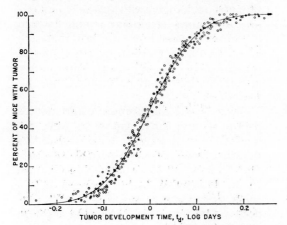

Figure 5-16   Same data as given in Figure 5-15 but normalized to the same median tumor development time (zero log days). (*From* Blum: Carcinogenesis by Ultraviolet Light. Princeton University Press, 1959.)

development of malignancies. These summation effects are similar to those obtained with chemical carcinogens (Saffiotti and Shubik, 1956; Poel, 1963) and support the concept that promotion by a potent carcinogen results in the progressive formation of malignancies (Shubik, 1950).

In vitro cell transformation by UV radiation has not been reported. However, there is ample evidence that UV radiation of cultured cells that have been exposed to chemical carcinogens or viruses increases the yield of transformed cells.

CHEMICAL CARCINOGENESIS

The history of chemical carcinogenesis has been summarized by Clayson (1962). That chemical agents applied to the skin could cause cancer in man was recognized by Pott in 1775, when he ascribed the high incidence of scrotal cancer in chimney sweeps to soot and chronic irritation. About 100 years later the common occurrence of skin cancers in workers exposed

PERCENT OF MICE WITH TUMOR
100
80
60
40
20
0
END OF
EXPOSURES
CD
CE
CF
CH
CD
1.9
2.0
2.1
2.2
2.3
2.4
2.5
DEVELOPMENT TIME, t_d, LOG DAYS.

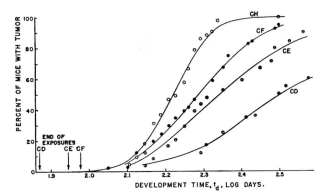

Figure 5–17 These data show the marked delay in tumor formation when chronic exposure is terminated before the onset of tumor formation. The ultraviolet dosing schedule is the same for each of the four treatment groups, but except for group CH the exposures were stopped at the indicated times. (*From* Blum: J. Natl. Cancer Inst., 11:463, 1950.)

to paraffin, pitch, and shale oil tar was discovered. In 1918 Yamagiwa and Ichikawa were able to produce skin cancer on the ears of rabbits by the prolonged application of gas works tar.

Classes of Chemical Carcinogens. The identification of the active carcinogen in pitch was made by Kennaway and his associates in the early 1930's. The success in this landmark series of investigations was based on the inspired guess that the carcinogens in pitch were responsible for its fluorescence. Without this approach, it would have been a hopeless task to do animal tests on the many fractions of such a complex material as pitch. By comparing the fluorescence of various fractions of pitch with that of known organic compounds, a series of polycyclic aromatic compounds were found which proved to be carcinogenic. There followed an intensive period of activity to determine the relationship of polycyclic aromatic structure to carcinogenic activity. The hope that the specificity of carcinogenic polycyclic structure would be a simple key to understanding the cellular biochemical changes associated with carcinogenesis proved illusory with the discovery of a whole series of organic compounds of unrelated structure that also have carcinogenic activity. These are shown in Figures 5–18 and 5–19. The primary classes of carcinogens are the polycyclic aromatic hydrocarbons, the aromatic azo dyes, the alkylating agents, and the nitrosamines, and also a variety of natural products including the aflatoxins, pyrrolizidine alkaloids, and cycasin. A number of inorganic metals, such as beryllium, cadmium, zinc, lead, chromium, nickel, and arsenic are also carcinogens.

Metabolism of Chemical Carcinogens. Miller (1970) has reviewed the intense effort in the last decade to deduce the

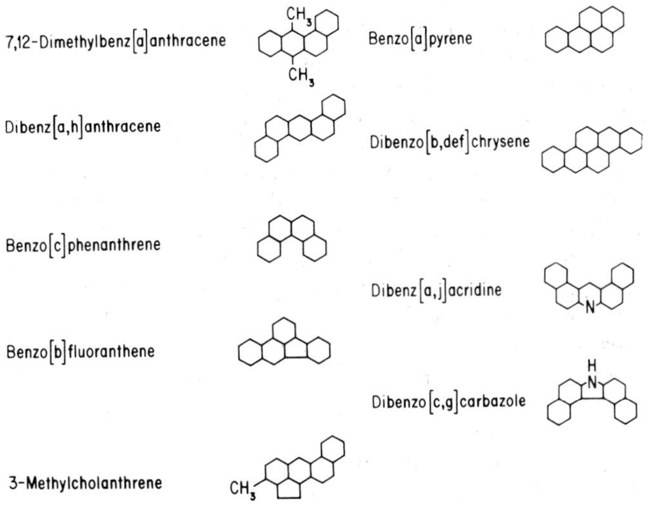

7,12-Dimethylbenz[a]anthracene
CH_3
CH_3
Benzo[a]pyrene
Dibenz[a,h]anthracene
Dibenzo[b,def]chrysene
Benzo[c]phenanthrene
Dibenz[a,j]acridine
N
Benzo[b]fluoranthene
Dibenzo[c,g]carbazole
H
N
3-Methylcholanthrene
CH_3

Figure 5–18 Representative polycyclic aromatic hydrocarbon carcinogens.

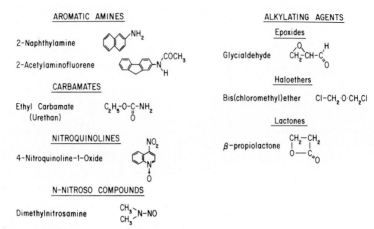

Figure 5–19 Representative chemical carcinogens of different structural classes.

metabolism of these various classes of carcinogens, particularly the biochemical transformations that convert the carcinogen to its active form. All of the organic carcinogens, except the alkylating agents, require biochemical transformation to an active form. The alkylating agents are essentially in their final reactive form as administered, and take part in substitution reactions in which a relatively positive, or electrophilic, atom in the alkylating agent combines with a relatively negative, or nucleophilic, atom of the molecule in the cell.

Biochemical Interactions. The essential feature of the biochemical interaction of carcinogens in cells is the covalent bonding of carcinogen residues with cellular macromolecules: RNA, DNA, and protein. The essential feature of the biochemical activation of carcinogens is their conversion to a reactive electrophilic form in which they behave as alkylating agents. For example, the nitrosamines become methyl donors which attach to the N-7 position of guanine bases in DNA. The aromatic amines become N-hydroxylated and esterified to the active form and interact with the C-8 position of guanine in DNA. The biochemical mode of activation of the polycyclic hydrocarbons is not yet clear. Although epoxide derivatives of polycyclics have been implicated as metabolic derivatives, they are not found in exposed skin (Brookes and Baird, 1973), and it is possible that the reactive form is a hydroperoxide or a free radical.

The enzyme system called benzopyrene or aryl hydrocarbon hydroxylase, primarily responsible for the metabolism of polycyclic hydrocarbons, is located in the cell microsomes of most tissues including skin (Gelboin, 1967). The enzyme is inducible by polycyclic hydrocarbons and other agents such as drugs and pesticides. It is probably responsible for the metabolic activation to the active form of the carcinogen, but the enzyme is also responsible for metabolic degradation to a variety of phenols, dihydrodiols, quinones, and other water-soluble conjugated products (National Academy of Sciences, 1972). The inhibition of aryl hydrocarbon hydroxylase by benzoflavone markedly reduces mouse skin tumorigenesis caused by repeated treatment with 7,12-dimethylbenz (*a*) anthracene (Gelboin, 1970; Wattenberg and Leong, 1970). There is substantial evidence that chemical carcinogens in the activated form characteristically interact with DNA to produce mutations (Miller and Miller, 1971) and initiate DNA repair (Lieberman, 1972).

Cell and Tissue Effects. The cell population kinetic responses of the epidermis with single and repeated doses of polycyclic carcinogens such as 3-methylcholanthrene have been summarized by Iverson (1964). A single carcinogen application causes a prompt suppression of DNA synthesis and mitotic block when applied to the mouse epidermis. The period of increased cell loss during the first three days is followed by a regenerative hyperplasia with increased rate of cell production. Repeated carcinogen applications are associated with a sustained

irritant such as turpentine or wounding of the skin. He interprets promotion as a conversion of the dormant initiated cell into a neoplastically transformed cell; tumor development can then be hastened by nonspecific proliferative stimuli.

The dose-response relationships for the promoting agent phorbol ester are unusual in that the total yield of tumors depends on total dose, but the time of tumor occurrence is constant regardless of the dose (van Duuren, 1973). It appears that the initiator produces potential tumor sites; the number of these sites that develop into tumors depends on the total dose of phorbol ester. However, the dose rate of a promoter is also important, since there is an optimal regimen of exposing the skin two to three times a week, higher or lower dose rates for the same total amount of promoter are considerably less efficient (Boutwell, 1964). This dose rate effect suggests that the action of promoting agents is reversible.

There are a number of factors which modify the initiation-promotion process. The induction of hyperplasia by an irritant before the application of the initiating agent will increase the yield of tumors subsequent to the application of a promoting agent (Pound, 1968). Other agents, such as nitrogen mustard and actinomycin, block the initiating action of carcinogens, but the mechanism for this effect is unknown (Berenblum, 1969). There are also agents which will reduce the effectiveness of tumor promotion. This includes a number of antiproteolytic compounds (Klassen et al., 1972), cyclic AMP (adenosine monophosphate) (Belman and Troll, 1973), and cortisone (Belman and Troll, 1972). Some of these agents depress the inflammatory response, and others depress proliferation caused by promoters.

The initiation-promotion process is applicable to the mouse skin only in the epidermis; it has not been demonstrated to hold true for dermal tumor production. There is only limited evidence that initiation-promotion applies to other experimental systems. Cigarette smoke carcinogenesis may be predominantly a promotion effect both in the human lung and in the mouse skin as a test system.

Some agents have been shown to be pure initiators (van Duuren et al., 1970). The existence of such materials makes the problem of the control of environmental cancer hazards considerably more difficult, because it expands the range of possible agents that need to be controlled.

Major advances have been made relatively recently in the development of tissue culture systems for studying neoplastic cell transformation (DiPaolo et al., 1971). The metabolic activation of chemical carcinogens is a prerequisite for an effect. The dose-response relationships are linear, in terms of the yield of transformed clones with respect to the carcinogen concentration in the culture media. The initially transformed cells are not very neoplastic, since large numbers are required to produce tumors in antigenically compatible hosts. The malignancy of these transformed cells increases with serial passage in culture or animals.

Chemically and radiation-induced neoplasms differ from viral tumors in their antigenic character. Tumors produced by a given type of virus have common antigenic properties. Individual tumors produced by chemicals and ionizing radiation are all different with respect to the kind and degree of antigenicity.

Dermal Sarcoma Induction by Plastic Films. Many plastics induce malignant tumors when implanted subcutaneously in the form of a sheet in rats, mice, or hamsters, but their mode of action is still disputed. Work in this area stemmed from the original observation by Oppenheimer that cellophane films wrapped around the kidney to produce hypertension caused sarcomas, with a latent period of about one year (see review by Clayson, 1962). The most compelling argument that tumors are caused by the plastic film acting as a physical barrier is that the carcinogenic activity of several plastics is lost or greatly reduced if the same amount of the material is implanted in the animal as a powder. The carcinogenic effect may be chemical in some cases where sarcomas are produced by the plastic in shredded form (Carter and Roe, 1969).

The plastic film provokes a granulation tissue reaction. The encapsulated pocket thickens for about five to six months, when fibrotic and capillary activity diminish and the pocket becomes practically in-active. Brand and Buon (1968) have shown by use of animals with chromosomal markers that during this period the transformed cells are attached to the film in a nonproliferative state; the film can be removed with the attached cells and transferred to an immunologically compatible host where these cells proliferate to form tumors. The mechanism of transformation of the cells attached to the film is unknown, but it is of interest that the transformation occurs in a nondividing cell population throughout the premalignant phase.

VIRAL CARCINOGENESIS

Early in this century it was discovered that infectious agents could produce tumors. In 1907 Smith and Townsend isolated the bacterium which causes the crown gall tumor in plants. In 1908 Ellerman and Bang found that cell-free filtrates could transmit chicken leukemia. In 1910 Rous discovered that fowl sarcoma could also be transmitted by cell-free agents. In 1932 Shope found that skin fibromas in wild cotton-tailed rabbits could be transmitted by the cell-free extracts. A year later Shope discovered another mammalian tumor of viral origin which causes benign epidermal papillomas in the rabbit (Shope, 1933). In 1936 the Bittner milk factor, a mouse mammary tumor virus, was recognized; this tumor virus was found to be one of several factors in the causation of mammary tumors, including hormonal stimulation and genetic susceptibility. The virus is primarily responsible for causing hyperplastic nodules; these conditional adenomas provide the bed for carcinoma formation under hormonal stimulation.

In 1951 Gross found that cell-free extracts of leukemic tumors from AK mice caused leukemia in C_3H mice inoculated soon after birth, i. e., prior to the development of immunologic competence. It was soon found that these extracts contained both a leukemia virus as well as a polyoma virus which caused a wide variety of solid tumors, including those of hair follicles (Gross, 1953; Stewart, 1953). In 1961 Eddy et al. found that the simian-40 virus

(SV_{40}) was tumorigenic when inoculated into newborn rodents. More recently a number of commonly found human adenoviruses can also cause tumors in certain newborn rodents.

Classification of Oncogenic Viruses. Oncogenic viruses are classified into two broad categories according to the type of nucleic acid—DNA or RNA—they contain. The DNA viruses are responsible for naturally occurring benign tumors, e.g., papillomas in man and rabbits. The RNA viruses are responsible for the naturally occurring leukemia-sarcoma complexes of chickens and mice and the hormone-dependent mammary carcinoma of mice. Both kinds of virus can produce malignant transformation in cell cultures. Papillomas produced by the Shope virus experimentally in domestic rabbits, as well as those occurring naturally in wild cotton-tailed rabbits, can become malignant. However, the viral genome disappears in the carcinomas and there is no evidence that the carcinogenic transformation of papillomas is due to the virus (Syverton, 1952). None of the oncogenic RNA viruses is cytopathic in tissue culture, and none of the many cytopathic RNA viruses is oncogenic (Sabin, 1968).

Transformation by Viruses. In vitro transformation by viruses involves the following characteristics: increased growth rate and shortened doubling times of the cultured cells, an unlimited lifetime in culture and the formation of permanent cell lines, the lack of contact inhibition with the production of multilayer clones, chromosomal abnormalities of increased incidence and types, and production of tumors on transplantation to an immunologically compatible host (Habel, 1968).

The nature of interaction with cells is different for DNA and RNA viruses. With RNA virus, cell transformation can occur either with or without active production of virus. With DNA virus, cells that are infected and actively produce virus particles die in the process, whereas those cells that are infected and transformed do not produce virus particles.

There is substantial evidence that the transforming effect of viruses on cultured cells is direct. This is indicated by the promptness with which transformation takes place and by the linear dose-response characteristics, suggesting a single hit phenomenon (Stoker and Macpherson, 1961). The nucleic acid of core DNA viruses can produce transformation, although at a reduced efficiency (Crawford et al., 1964).

The reason why some viruses are oncogenic and others are not is unknown. The mere presence of virus in cells is an insufficient condition for oncogenicity, since nononcogenic viruses can be carried by cells. However, the interaction of oncogenic viruses with transformed cells is not a transient hit and run affair. RNA viruses continue to be produced by transformed multiplying cells. There is strong evidence that the DNA viral genome is integrated in transformed cells even though the virus is not produced. In the case of the rabbit papilloma, infectious DNA is extractable (Ito and Evans, 1961), and there are viral structural antigens present in the transformed cells (Huebner et al., 1964). Only 20 to 50 percent of the DNA viral genome is necessary for transformation (Benjamin, 1965). RNA viruses are also integrated into the genome, since they carry a reverse transcriptase enzyme into the host cell; this enzyme is responsible for the production of complementary DNA, which is then integrated in the host cell genome.

There are a number of cell factors that determine transformation. Cells must have proper receptor sites that permit viral attachment, penetration, and uncoating, so that the viral genetic core can interact. There is some evidence that viral integration and, thus, cell transformation may depend on homogeneous base sequences in the DNA of viral and host cells (Axlerod, 1964). Biologic and morphologic transformation with either DNA or RNA virus requires at least one cell division after integration (Todaro et al., 1966). With polyoma virus and x-irradiation–induced transformation in cultured cells, cell division must occur within three to five days after exposure in order to obtain transformation (Sachs, 1965). Chromosomal damage by x-radiation, UV radiation, aging, or chemical treatment increases the efficiency of viral transformation. SV_{40} transformation is 10 times more efficient in cultured cells from patients with the Fanconi syndrome, an autosomal recessive disease associated with a high incidence of chromosomal breaks and neoplasms (Todaro et al., 1966).

There is evidence that integration of viral DNA is responsible for derepression of cell division, which in turn prevents virus maturation. In the case of the Shope papilloma virus, production occurs only in the nonproliferating keratinizing cells that are released from the basal layer of the skin (Noyes and Mellors, 1957). The importance of the persisting viral genome in the transformed cell is indicated by the fact that it determines the surface antigens and the morphology of the transformed cells. Cells doubly transformed by a second DNA virus infection have increased oncogenicity (Todaro et al., 1965). Cell hybrids between DNA transformed cells and normal mouse cells retain their neoplastic transformation (Defendi et al., 1967). This indicates that transformation is not due to the loss of genetic material in the original transformed cells, but instead represents an added genetic factor. The finding that a single cell can be transformed by two different DNA tumor viruses and thereby acquire heightened growth potential suggests that there are different sites of action on cell control mechanisms (Habel, 1968).

Interaction of Viruses and Chemical Carcinogens. Studies on skin tumor induction caused by the interaction of viruses and chemical carcinogens have been summarized by Roe (1968). Treatment of the skin with coal tar of 3-methylcholanthrene (MC) before or after the application of Shope papilloma virus increases the number and the malignancy of tumors. Systemic administration of polycyclic hydrocarbons, cortisone, or 6-mercaptopurine enhances the skin tumorigenic induction by the Shope papilloma virus, probably by means of immune suppression. The skin tumor response to carcinogenic polycyclic aromatic hydrocarbons is strongly enhanced by inoculation of newborn mice with polyoma virus or West Nile virus (an RNA arbor virus) during the treatment period. The basis for these interactions is unknown.

SUMMARY

The efficiency of carcinogenic action is clearly affected by factors which determine the extent to which a given carcinogen actually reaches cells in an active form, and by factors which determine the susceptibility of the cell to transformation. Susceptibility must encompass a variety of factors determining the extent of initial injury and the effectiveness of repair.

At present, it is not clear whether there is a common pathway for cellular neoplastic transformation, although this has been suggested in terms of the activation of a latent viral oncogen (Huebner and Todaro, 1969). It is also not clear whether the inheritable abnormalities transmitted to successive generations of proliferating cancer cells are caused by genetic damage or by abnormal differentiation involving the deranged expression of the normal genome.

Neoplastic transformation at the cellular level is not a simple all or none phenomenon. Transformed cells show differences in the extent to which they acquire the several independent properties of neoplasia: unrestrained proliferation, invasiveness, and antigenicity. Neoplasia is also not an immutable property which is transmitted equally to all the progeny of a transformed cell. The clonal outgrowth of single cultured cells shows a spectrum of neoplastic and non-neoplastic properties among progeny, which has been related to chromosomal balance (Hitotsumachi, 1972). Single cells isolated from malignant teratomas also produce clones of cells, some neoplastic and others undergoing normal differentiation. The neoplastic character of a tumor, therefore, appears to depend on the average behavior of its component cells.

It is possible that the carcinogenic process will prove to be similar to the process for the evolution of species, in that random genetic damage of somatic cells produced by carcinogens is combined with selection pressures to breed out a race of cells having growth advantages over their normal counterparts. It would be expected that the process would be generally slow, progressive in character, and wasteful of cells due to lethal injury; cell lethality, however, could undoubtedly facilitate the selection process, especially in tissues, such as the dermis, which normally have a low proliferative rate.

Pitot and Heidelberger (1963) have formulated an epigenetic scheme for neoplasia based on abnormal differentiation. Braun (1969) has also elaborated this alternative, based on plant tumorigenesis experiments. These studies show that plant tumors can arise from an epigenetic differentiation abnormality which is characterized by the production of large amounts of growth hormone by the tumor cells. These anaplastic tumors, after years of propagation in tissue culture, can permanently revert to normal plant tissue when grown under certain conditions.

It is evident that in spite of tremendous research efforts and impressive advances, some very basic questions about cancer are still unanswered: What makes cells neoplastic? How do they acquire defective control of proliferation? How do they develop invasive metastatic properties? How do carcinogens produce these neoplastic cellular disturbances, and what makes for wide differences in susceptibility? Such knowledge would greatly facilitate the identification and control of environmental carcinogens and, perhaps, provide a more rational basis for cancer therapy.

REFERENCES

IONIZING RADIATION

Albert, R. E., and Burns, F. J.: The effect of dose fractionation on the recovery of radiation-induced oncogenesis in rat skin. Proc. Am. Assoc. Cancer Res., 14:86, 1973a.

Albert, R. E., and Burns, F. J.: The sieve effect for tumor induction with low voltage x-rays in rat skin. Proc. Radiat. Res. Soc., Abstract Cd-2, p. 24, 1973b.

Albert, R. E., Burns, F. J., and Bennett, P.: Radiation-induced hair-follicle damage and tumor formation in mouse and rat skin. J. Natl. Cancer Inst., 49:1131, 1972.

Albert, R. E., Burns, F. J., and Heimbach, R. D.: The effect of penetration depth of electron radiation of skin tumor formation in the rat. Radiat. Res., 30:515, 1967a.

Albert, R. E., Burns, F. J., and Heimbach, R. D.: Skin damage and tumor formation from grid and sieve patterns of electron and beta radiation in the rat. Radiat. Res., 30:525, 1967b.

Albert, R. E., Newman, W., and Altshuler, B.: The dose-response relationships of beta-ray-induced skin tumors in the rat. Radiat. Res., 15:410, 1961.

Albert, R. E., Phillips, M. E., Bennett, P., Burns, F. J., and Heimbach, R. D.: The morphology and growth characteristics of radiation-induced epithelial skin tumors in the rat. Cancer Res., 29:658, 1969.

Borek, C.: In-vitro cell transformation by x-rays. Proc. Radiat. Res. Soc., Abstract Cd-1, p. 24, 1973.

Burns, F. J.: The loss of basal cells in the rat epidermis following irradiation. Radiat. Res., 43:219, 1970.

Burns, F. J., Albert, R. E., and Heimbach, R. D.: The RBE for skin tumors and hair follicle damage in the rat following irradiation with alpha particles and electrons. Radiat. Res., 36:225, 1968.

Burns, F. J., Albert, R. E., Bennett, P., and Sinclair, I. P.: Tumor incidence in rat skin after proton irradiation in a sieve pattern. Radiat. Res., 50:181, 1972.

Burns, F. J., Albert, R. E., Sinclair, I. P., and Bennett, P.: The effect of fractionation on tumor induction and hair follicle damage in rat skin. Radiat. Res., 53:235, 1973a.

Burns, F. J., Sinclair, I. P., and Albert, R. E.: The oncogenic response of anagen phase rat skin to electron radiation of various penetrations. Proc. Am. Assoc. Cancer Res., 14:88, 1973b.

Elkind, M. M., and Whitmore, G. F.: The Radiobiology of Cultured Mammalian Cells. New York, Gordon and Breach, Science Publishers, Inc., 1967.

Glucksmann, A.: *In* Harris, R. J. C. (Ed.): Cellular Basis and Aetiology of Late Somatic Effects of Ionizing Radiation. London, Academic Press, 1963, pp. 121–128.

Glucksmann, A., Lamerton, L. F., and Mayneord, W. V.: Carcinogenic effects of radiation. *In* Raven, R. W. (Ed.): Cancer. London, Butterworths, 1957, Vol. 1, p. 497.

Heimbach, R. D., Burns, F. J., and Albert, R. E.: An evaluation by alpha-particle Bragg peak radiation of the critical depth in the rat skin for tumor induction. Radiat. Res., 39:332, 1969.

Hulse, E. V.: Osteosarcomas, fibrosarcomas and basal-cell carcinomas in rabbits after irradiation with gamma-rays or fission neutrons: an interim report on incidence, site of tumours and RBE. Int. J. Radiat. Biol., 16:27, 1969.

Jolles, B.: The reciprocal vicinity effect of irradiated tissues on a "diffusible substance" in irradiated tissues. Br. J. Radiol., 23:18, 1950.

Jones, D. C., Castanera, T. J., Kimeldorf, D. J., and Rosen, V. J.: Radiation induction of skin neoplasms in the male rat. J. Invest. Dermatol., 50:27, 1968.

Lamerton, L. F.: *In* Harris, R. J. C. (Ed.): Cellular Basis and Aetiology of Late Somatic Effects of Ionizing Radiation. New York, Academic Press, 1963, p. 129.

Lamerton, L. F.: Radiation carcinogenesis. Br. Med. Bull., 20:134, 1964.

Lett, J. T., and Sun, C.: The production of strand breaks in mammalian DNA by x-rays: at different stages in the cell cycle. Radiat. Res., 44:771, 1970.

Lett, J. T., Caldwell, I., Dean, C. J., and Alexander, P.: Rejoining of x-ray induced breaks in the DNA of leukaemia cells. Nature, 214:790, 1967.

Moritiz, A. R., and Henriques, F. W.: Effect of beta rays on the skin as a function of the energy, intensity and duration of radiation. II. Animal experiments. Lab. Invest., 1:167, 1952.

Passonneau, J. V., Hamilton, K., and Brues, A. M.: Carcinogenic effects of diffuse and point source beta radiation on rat skin. Final summary document No. ANL-4932, p. 31, 1952.

Raper, J. R., Henshaw, P. S., and Snider, R. S.: Delayed effects of single exposures to external beta rays. *In* Zirkle, R. E. (Ed.): Biological Effects of External Beta Radiation, National Nuclear Energy Series IV-22E. New York, McGraw-Hill, 1951, Chap. 13, p. 206.

Upton, A. C.: Radiation carcinogenesis. *In* Busch, H. (Ed.): Methods in Cancer Research. New York, Academic Press, 1967, Vol. III.

Witten, V., Braver, E. W., Holmstrom, V., and Loevinger, R.: Studies of thorium X applied to human skin. III. The relative effects of alpha and beta-gamma radiation in the production of erythema. J. Invest. Dermatol., 21:249, 1953.

Zackheim, H. S., Krobock, E., and Langs, L.: Cutaneous neoplasms in the rat produced by Grenz ray and 80 KV x-ray. J. Invest. Dermatol., 43:519, 1964.

ULTRAVIOLET RADIATION

Blum, H. F.: Wavelength dependence of tumor induction by ultraviolet radiation. J. Natl. Cancer Inst., 3:533, 1943.

Blum, H. F.: Carcinogenesis by Ultraviolet Light. Princeton, New Jersey, Princeton University Press, 1959.

Blum, H. F., and Lippincott, S. W.: Carcinogenic effectiveness of ultraviolet radiation of wavelength 2537A. J. Natl. Cancer Inst., 3:211, 1942.

Cleaver, J. E.: Defective repair replication of DNA in xeroderma pigmentosum. Nature, 218:652, 1968.

Cleaver, J. E.: Repair replication of mammalian cell DNA: effects of compounds that inhibit DNA synthesis or dark repair. Radiat. Res., 37:334, 1969.

Djordjevic, B., and Tolmach, L. J.: Responses of synchronous populations of HeLa cells to ultraviolet irradiation at selected stages of the generation cycle. Radiat. Res., 32:327, 1967.

Dobson, R. L.: Anthramine carcinogenesis in the skin of rats. I. The epidermis. J. Natl. Cancer Inst., 31:841, 1963.

Epstein, J. H.: Ultraviolet carcinogenesis. *In* Giese, A. C. (Ed.): Photophysiology. Current Topics in Photobiology and Photochemistry. New York, Academic Press, 1970, Vol. V, pp. 235–273.

Epstein, J. H., and Epstein, W. L.: Cocarcinogenic effect of ultra-violet light on DMBA tumor initiation in albino mice. J. Invest. Dermatol., 39:455, 1962.

Epstein, J. H., and Roth, H. L.: Experimental ultraviolet light carcinogenesis: A study of croton oil promoting effects. J. Invest. Dermatol., 50:387, 1968.

Epstein, J. H., Epstein, W. L., and Nakai, T.: Production of melanomas from DMBA-induced "blue nevi" in hairless mice with ultraviolet light. J. Natl. Cancer Inst., 38:19, 1967.

Epstein, W. L., Fukuyama, K., and Epstein, J. H.: Early effects of ultraviolet light on DNA synthesis in human skin in vivo. Arch. Dermatol., 100:84, 1969.

Grady, H. G., Blum, H. F., and Kirby-Smith, J. S.: Pathology of tumors of the external ear in mice induced by ultraviolet radiation. J. Natl. Cancer Inst., 2:269, 1941.

Grady, H. G., Blum, H. F., and Kirby-Smith, J. S.: Types of tumor induced by ultraviolet radiation and factors influencing their relative incidence. J. Natl. Cancer Inst., 3:371, 1943.

Hanawalt, P. C., and Haynes, R. H.: The repair of DNA. Sci. Am., 216:36, 1967.

Hueper, W. C.: Cutaneous neoplastic responses elicted by ultraviolet rays in hairless rats and in their haired litter mates. Cancer Res., 1:402, 1941.

Humphrey, R. M., Dewey, W. C., and Cork, A.: Relative ultraviolet sensitivity of different phases in the cell cycle of Chinese hamster cells grown *in vitro.* Radiat. Res., 19:247, 1963.

Iversen, O. H., and Evensen, A.: Experimental Skin Carcinogenesis in Mice. Oslo, Norway, Norwegian University Press, 1962.

Kelner, A.: Effect of visible light on the recovery of streptomyces griseus conidia from ultraviolet injury. Proc. Nat. Acad. Sci., 35:73, 1949.

Kelner, A., and Taft, E. B.: Influence of photoreactivating light on type and frequency of tumors induced by ultraviolet radiation. Cancer Res., 16:860, 1956.

Lee, H. H., and Puck, T. T.: The action of ultraviolet radiation on mammalian cells as studied by single-cell techniques. Radiat. Res., 12:340, 1960.

Poel, W. E.: Skin as a test site for the bioassay of carcinogens and carcinogen precursors. Natl. Cancer Inst. Monogr. 10:611, 1963.

Rauth, A. M.: Evidence for dark-reactivation of ultraviolet light damage in mouse L cells. Radiat. Res., 31:121, 1967.

Saffiotti, U., and Shubik, P.: Effects of low concentrations of carcinogen in epidermal carcinogenesis. Comparison with promoting agents. J. Natl. Cancer Inst., 16:961, 1956.

Setlow, R. B., Regan, J. D., German, J., and Carrier, W. L.: Evidence that xeroderma pigmentosum cells do not perform the first step in the repair of ultraviolet damage to their DNA. Proc. Natl. Acad. Sci., U.S.A., 64:1035, 1969.

Shubik, P.: Growth potentialities of induced skin tumors in mice; effects of different methods of chemical carcinogenesis. Cancer Res., 10:713, 1950.

Stich, H. F., San, R. H. C., and Kawazoe, Y.: Increased sensitivity of xeroderma pigmentosum cells to some chemical carcinogens and mutagens. Mutat. Res., 17:127, 1973.

Thompson, L. H., and Humphrey, R. M.: Proliferation kinetics of mouse L-P59 cells irradiated with ultraviolet light: a time-lapse photographic study. Radiat. Res., 41:183, 1970.

Thompson, L. H., and Suit, H. D.: Proliferation kinetics of x-irradiated mouse L cells studied with time-lapse photography. II. Int. J. Radiat. Biol., 15:347, 1969.

Todd, P., Coohill, T. P., Hellewell, A. B., and Mahoney, J. A.: Post-irradiation properties of cultured Chinese hamster cells exposed to ultraviolet light. Radiat. Res., 38:321, 1969.

Winkelmann, R. K., Baldes, E. J., and Zollman, P. E.: Squamous cell tumors induced in hairless mice with ultraviolet light. J. Invest. Dermatol., 34:131, 1960.

Witkin, E. M.: Ultraviolet-induced mutation and DNA repair. *In* Roman, H. L., et al. (Eds.): Annual Review of Genetics. Palo Alto, California, Annual Reviews, Inc., 1969, Vol. 3, pp. 525–552.

CHEMICAL CARCINOGENESIS

Albert, R. E., and Altshuler, B.: Considerations relating to the formulation of limits for unavoidable population exposures to environmental carcinogens. *In* Ballou, J. E., et al. (Eds.): Radionuclide Carcinogenesis. AEC Symposium Series, CONF-720505. Springfield, Virginia, NTIS, 1973.

Belman, S., and Troll, W.: The inhibition of croton oil-promoted mouse skin tumorigenesis by steroid hormones. Cancer Res., 32:450, 1972.

Belman, S., and Troll, W.: The effect of 12-0-tetradecanoylphorbol-13-acetate on cyclic AMP levels in mouse skin. Proc. Am. Assoc. Cancer Res., 14:21, 1973.

Berenblum, I.: The two-stage mechanism of carcinogenesis as an anlytical tool. *In* Emmelot, P., and Muhlbock, O. (Eds.): Cellular Control Mechanisms and Cancer. Amsterdam, Elsevier Publishing Company, 1964.

Berenblum, I.: A re-evaluation of the concept of cocarcinogenesis. Progr. Exp. Tumor Res., 11:21, 1969.

Berenblum, I., Haran-Ghera, N., and Trainin, N.: An experimental analysis of the "hair cycle effect" in mouse skin carcinogenesis. Br. J. Cancer, 12:402, 1958.

Boutwell, R. K.: Some biological aspects of skin carcinogenesis. Progr. Exp. Tumor Res., 4:207, 1964.

Brand, K. G., and Buoen, L. C.: Polymer tumorigenesis: multiple preneoplastic clones in priority order with clonal inhibition. Proc. Soc. Exp. Biol. Med., 128:1154, 1968.

Brookes, P., and Baird, W. M.: The role of the K-region epoxide of 7-methylbenz(a)anthracene in the in-vivo binding of parent hydrocarbon. Proc. Am. Assoc. Cancer Res., 14:30, 1973.

Carter, R. L., and Roe, F. J. C.: Induction of sarcomas in rats by solid and fragmented polyethylene: experimental observations and clinical implications. Br. J. Cancer, 23:401, 1969.

Clayson, D. B.: Chemical Carcinogenesis. Boston, Little, Brown and Company, 1962.

DiPaolo, J. A., Nelson, R. L., and Donovan, P. J.: Morphological, oncogenic, and karyological characteristics of Syrian hamster embryo cells transformed in vitro by carcinogenic polycyclic hydrocarbons. Cancer Res., 31:1118, 1971.

Frei, J. V., and Stephens, P.: The correlation of promotion of tumour growth and of induction of hyperplasia in epidermal two-stage carcinogenesis. Br. J. Cancer, 22:83, 1968.

Gelboin, H. V.: Carcinogens, enzyme induction, and gene action. *In* Haddow, A., and Weinhouse, S.: Advances in Cancer Research. New York, Academic Press, Vol. 10, 1967.

Gelboin, H. V., Wiebel, F., and Diamond, L.: Dimethylbenzanthracene tumorigenesis and aryl hydrocarbon hydroxylase in mouse skin: inhibition by 7,8-benzoflavone. Science, 170:169, 1970.

Giovanella, B. C., Liegel, J., and Heidelberger, C.: The refractoriness of the skin of hairless mice to chemical carcinogenesis. Cancer Res., 30:2590, 1970.

Howell, J. S.: Skin tumors in the rat produced by 9,10-dimethyl-1,2-benzanthracene and methylcholanthrene. Br. J. Cancer, 16:101, 1962.

Iversen, O. H.: Discussion on cell destruction and population dynamics in experimental skin carcinogenesis in mice. Progr. Exp. Tumor Res., 4:169, 1964.

Klassen, A., Altshuler, B., and Troll, W.: Inhibition of initiation and complete carcinogenesis in mouse skin by tosyl phenylalanine chloromethyl ketone. Proc. Am. Assoc. Cancer Res., 13:75, 1972.

Lee, P. N., and O'Neill, J. A.: The effect both of time and dose applied on tumor incidence rate in benzopyrene skin painting experiments. Br. J. Cancer, 25:759, 1971.

Lieberman, M. W., and Forbes, P. D.: Demonstration of DNA repair in normal and neoplastic tissues after treatment with proximate chemical carcinogens and ultraviolet radiation. Nature [New Biol.], 241:199, 1973.

Marchant, J., and Orr, J. W.: Further attempts to analyze the roles of epidermis and deeper tissues in experimental chemical carcinogenesis by transplantation and other methods. Br. J. Cancer, 7:329, 1953.

Miller, E. C., and Miller, J. A.: The mutagenicity of chemical carcinogens: correlations, problems, and interpretations. *In* Hollaender, A. (Ed.): Chemical Mutagens. Plenum Press, New York, 1971, Vol. I, pp. 83–119.

Miller, J. A.: Carcinogenesis by Chemicals: An Overview — G. H. A. Clowes Memorial Lecture. Cancer Res., 30:559, 1970.

National Academy of Sciences: Particulate Polycyclic Organic Matter; Biologic Effects of Atmospheric Pollutants. Washington, D.C., National Academy of Sciences, 1972.

Poel, W. E.: Effect of carcinogenic dosage and duration of exposure on skin-tumor induction in mice. J. Natl. Cancer Inst., 22:19, 1959.

Pound, A. W.: Carcinogenesis and cell proliferation. N.Z. Med. J., 67:88, 1968.

Raick, A. N., Thumm, K., and Chivers, B. R.: Early effects of 12-0-tetradecanoyl-phorbol-13-acetate on the incorporation of tritiated precursor into DNA and the thickness of the interfollicular epidermis, and their relation to tumor promotion in mouse skin. Cancer Res., 32:1562, 1972.

Rous, P., and Kroo, J. G.: Conditional neoplasms and subthreshold neoplastic states. J. Exp. Med., 73: 365, 1941.

Sivak, A., and van Duuren, B. L.: A cell culture system for the assessment of tumor promoting activity. J. Natl. Cancer Inst., 44:1091, 1970a.

Sivak, A., and van Duuren, B. L.: RNA synthesis induction in cell culture by a tumor promoter. Cancer Res., 30:1203, 1970b.

Steinmuller, D.: A reinvestigation of epidermal transplantation during chemical carcinogenesis. Cancer Res., 31:2080, 1971.

Tarim, D.: Further electron microscopic studies of the mechanism of carcinogenesis: the specificity of the changes in carcinogen-treated mouse skin. Int. J. Cancer, 3:734, 1968.

Turusov, V., Day, N., Andrianov, L., and Jain, D.: Influence of dose on skin tumors induced in mice by single application of 7,12-dimethylbenz-(a)anthracene. J. Natl. Cancer Inst., 47:105, 1971.

van Duuren, B. L.: Tumor promoting agents in two-stage carcinogenesis. Progr. Exp. Tumor Res., 11:31, 1969.

van Duuren, B. L.: Unpublished data. 1973.

van Duuren, B. L., Sivak, A., Goldschmidt, B. M., Katz, C., and Melchionne, S.: Initiating activity of aromatic hydrocarbons in two-stage carcinogenesis. J. Natl. Cancer Inst., 44:1167, 1970.

Wattenberg, L. W., and Leong, J. L.: Inhibition of the carcinogenic action of benzo(a)pyrene by flavones. Cancer Res., 30:1922, 1970.

VIRAL CARCINOGENESIS

Axelrod, D., Habel, K., and Bolton, E. T.: Polyoma virus genetic material in a virus-free polyoma-induced tumor. Science, 146:1466, 1964.

Benjamin, T. L.: Relative target sizes for the inactivation of the transforming and reproductive abilities of polyoma virus. Proc. Natl. Acad. Sci., U.S.A., 54:121, 1965.

Crawford, L., Dulbecco, R., Fried, M., Montagnier, L., and Stoker, M.: Cell transformation by different forms of polyoma virus DNA. Proc. Natl. Acad. Sci., U.S.A., 52:148, 1964.

Defendi, V., Ephrussi, B., Koprowski, H., and Yoshida, M. C.: Properties of hybrids between polyoma-transformed and normal mouse cells. Proc. Natl. Acad. Sci., U.S.A., 57:299, 1967.

Eddy, B. E., Borman, G. S., Berkeley, W. H., and Young, R. D.: Tumors induced in hamsters by injection of rhesus monkey kidney cell extracts. Proc. Soc. Exp. Biol. Med., 107:191, 1961.

Gross, L.: A filterable agent, recovered from Ak leukemic extracts, causing salivary gland carcinomas in C3H mice. Proc. Soc. Exp. Biol. Med., 83:414, 1953.

Habel, K.: The biology of viral carcinogenesis. Cancer Res., 28:1825, 1968.

Huebner, R. J., Pereira, H. G., Allison, A. C.,

Hollinshead, A. C., and Turner, H. C.: Production of type-specific C antigen in virus-free hamster tumor cells induced by adenovirus type 12. Proc. Natl. Acad. Sci., U.S.A., 51:432, 1964.

Ito, Y., and Evans, C. A.: Induction of tumors in domestic rabbits with nucleic acid preparations from partially purified Shope papilloma virus and from extracts of the papillomas of domestic and cottontail rabbits. J. Exp. Med., 114:485, 1961.

Noyes, W. F., and Mellors, R. C.: Fluorescent antibody detection of the antigens of the Shope papilloma virus in papillomas of the wild and domestic rabbit. J. Exp. Med., 106:555, 1957.

Roe, F. J. C.: The induction of cancer by combinations of viruses and other agents. Int. Rev. Exp. Pathol., 6:181, 1968.

Sabin, A. B.: Viral carcinogenesis: phenomena of special significance in the search for a viral etiology in human cancers. Cancer Res., 28:1849, 1968.

Sachs, L.: An analysis of the mechanism of carcinogenesis by polyoma virus, hydrocarbons, and x-irradiation. *In* Moleculare Biologie des Maligner Wachstums. New York, Springer-Verlag, New York, Inc., 1965.

Shope, R. E.: Infectious papillomatosis of rabbits, with a note on the histopathology. J. Exp. Med., 58:607, 1933.

Stewart, S. E.: Leukemia in mice produced by a filterable agent present in AKR leukemic tissues with notes on a sarcoma produced by the same agent. Anat. Rec., 117:532, 1953.

Stoker, M., and Macpherson, I.: Studies on transformation of hamster cells by polyoma virus in vitro. Virology, 14:359, 1961.

Syverton, J. T.: The pathogenesis of the rabbit papilloma-to-carcinoma sequence. Ann. N.Y. Acad. Sci., 54:1126, 1952.

Todaro, G. J., and Green, H.: Cell growth and the initiation of transformation by SV40. Proc. Natl. Acad. Sci., U.S.A., 55:302, 1966.

Todaro, G. J., Green, H., and Swift, M. R.: Susceptibility of human diploid fibroblast strains to transformation by SV40 virus. Science, 153:1253, 1966.

Todaro, G. J., Habel, K., and Green, H.: Antigenic and cultural properties of cells doubly transformed by polyoma virus and SV40. Virology, 27:179, 1965.

SUMMARY

Braun, A. C.: The Cancer Problem: A Critical Analysis and Modern Synthesis. New York, Columbia University Press, 1969.

Hitotsumachi, S., Rabinowitz, Z., and Sachs, L.: Chromosomal control of chemical carcinogenesis. Int. J. Cancer, 9:305, 1972.

Huebner, R. J., and Todaro, G. J.: Oncogenes of RNA tumor viruses as determinants of cancer. Proc. Nat. Acad. Sci., U.S.A., 64:1087, 1969.

Pitot, H. C., and Heidelberger, C.: Metabolic regulatory circuits and carcinogenesis. Cancer Res., 23:1694, 1963.

6

Genetics and Cancer

Rody P. Cox, M.D.

The genetic basis of cutaneous cancer is but one facet of a broad biologic problem: the genetics of neoplasia. A review of the various theories, the evidence supporting and contradicting each of these theories, and the innumerable speculations on the genetic basis or genetic contributions to the genesis of tumors would be diffuse, confusing, and probably misleading. Many of these theories are based on tenuous evidence and show little appreciation of the complexity of neoplasia and little understanding of the nature of genetic systems and inheritance.

This presentation will discuss the difficulties in assessing the genetic components in the etiology of cancer as well as describe several instances in which the genetic contributions are well defined. Rather than cataloguing clinical evidence for a genetic basis for certain skin cancers, a discussion of genetic principles and mechanisms as they relate to the initiation and propagation of tumors in a broad biologic context will be presented. Specific examples of skin tumors illustrating these mechanisms will be used when evidence suggests they are appropriate.

The genetic concept for the origin of cancer is an old one.

As early as the seventeenth century physicians speculated about hereditary factors

in malignancy. Bashford (1908) appreciated the interplay of environmental, cultural, and genetic factors in the etiology of carcinoma. Boveri (1914) noted the presence of atypical cell division in embryonic tissue and reasoned that these aberrant mitoses might under certain conditions lead to alterations in chromosome number. This genetic imbalance might produce aberrations in cell growth and lead to cancer. Although Boveri's suggestions were largely ignored for many years, they have recently attracted a good deal of attention and experimental support (see p. 148). For many years scientists have also recognized that some mutagens are also carcinogens, and they have speculated on somatic cell mutations as a causation of cancer (see p. 152). The concept of somatic mutation as a cause of tumors illustrates one of the complexities of the cancer problem, for one must consider not only the genetic constitution of the host and his germinal inheritance but also the interaction of this genetic constitution with a somatic cell containing one or more mutations. The recent elucidation of cellular control mechanisms and epigenesis as related to embryonic development and differentiation has stimulated speculation about an epigenetic basis of certain tumors and their clinical manifestations (see p. 154).

137

PITFALLS IN ASSESSING THE GENETIC COMPONENTS IN NEOPLASIA

Cancer cannot be considered a single or unit disease to the same degree that we regard tuberculosis as a unit disease. Tuberculosis may affect a variety of tissues and produce a multiplicity of symptoms and signs. However, etiologic, pathologic, and epidemiologic similarities exist between patients with pulmonary, renal, or osseous tuberculomas. On the other hand, a squamous cell carcinoma of the skin bears little relationship to a squamous cell carcinoma of the uterine cervix. Therefore, in assessing the role of genetic factors in the etiology of neoplasia, we may have to consider the location and type of tumor rather than pooling data on different neoplasms. A second difficulty is that errors in the diagnosis of malignant disease are not infrequent, although they are much less common in skin neoplasia than in tumors involving inaccessible sites.

Most malignant tumors occur late in life. This complicates genetic studies, and they are made even more difficult by the variable time of onset of cancer. P. A. Gorer (1953) has pointed out that these difficulties are substantial even under experimental conditions where genetic and nongenetic factors are controlled as much as possible; in assessing clinical material, they are formidable. For instance, in one family when three of four brothers developed a squamous cell carcinoma of the skin, one developed it at 45 years of age, the second at 70, and the third at 84. The fourth brother died of myocardial infarction at the age of 50. With this evidence it is not possible to decide whether genetic or environmental factors are primary. For example, the importance of sunlight in the genesis of squamous cell carcinoma is well recognized. If the three brothers with this tumor were farmers exposed to ultraviolet radiation for many years, the significance of a genetic contribution might be less than if they were clerical workers. When such family pedigrees are analyzed for inheritance of tumor susceptibility, with few exceptions tumors are not found. (Certain of these exceptions will be discussed later. For example, see Fanconi anemia, p. 148.)

There are a number of factors besides genetic ones that tend to concentrate neoplasms in certain families. Families share the same environment and have similar dietary habits. Often sibs follow the same occupation and generally belong to the same social class. In particular, they often share infective agents, and recent evidence suggests that certain human neoplasms may have a viral etiology.

An example of the complexity of analyzing genetic factors in susceptibility to neoplasms is provided by studies on mammary cancer in mice. Inbred strains of mice show marked differences in the incidence of mammary cancer: some strains have a high incidence and others develop the disease rarely. Initially these differences were attributed solely to genetic factors. However, it soon became apparent that mendelian genetic factors (i.e., chromosomal inheritance) could not explain completely the occurrence of the disease (Bittner, 1958). When inbred cancer-prone strains were crossed with inbred strains having a low incidence of cancer, the occurrence of mammary tumor in the F_1 generation depended in large part on which strain provided the mother (Fig. 6–1). By using high incidence and low incidence strains of mice for nursing newborn of various genotypes, it was shown that the maternal influence on the development of mammary cancer was transmitted through the milk. This infectious agent has many properties of a virus and is known as MTA (mammary tumor agent).

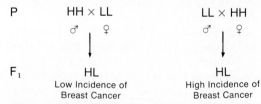

Figure 6–1 *HH*, parent derived from a strain of mice with a high incidence of mammary carcinoma. *LL*, parent derived from a strain of mice with a low incidence of mammary carcinoma. Reciprocal crosses show the difference in the incidence of mammary cancer in the F_1 generation (HL), depending on which strain nurses the progeny. This maternal effect is due to a mammary tumor virus transmitted through the milk. The genotype of the mouse contributes to susceptibility to the mammary tumor virus, but the relationship is complex (see text).

The genotype of the mouse in part does determine susceptibility to this agent, but the interaction is complex. For example, in some strains of mice it was found that the genetic influence on mammary cancer was mediated through alterations in the hormonal environment (Little, 1934). Certain strains of mice have shorter breeding periods than others, and therefore the mammary glands are subjected to reduced hormonal stimulation, which leads to a reduced incidence of cancer. Administration of hormone to these strains of mice increases the incidence of tumors. Genetic analysis indicates that a number of different genetic loci contribute to cancer susceptibility. The complex interaction of genetic constitution, a tumor virus, and hormonal milieu is further complicated when one compares the incidence of mammary tumors in identical strains studied in different laboratories (Bittner, 1958). Not only did the incidence of tumors vary, but even more impressive were the ages of onset of the neoplasm, which differed markedly from one laboratory to another. Apparently unidentified environmental factors influence the development and time of onset of mammary tumors.

The relevance of the study of mammary cancer in mice to the study of cancer proneness in man is readily apparent. In mice one deals with a nearly ideal experimental population which includes highly inbred strains that are genetically homogeneous, controlled matings, and a relatively standard environment. In human populations genetic variability is the rule; matings, although not completely random, are highly unstructured; the number of progeny is small; the generation time is long; and the environment is variable and includes toxins, carcinogens, and, in the female, hormones for contraceptive purposes. The difficulty in sorting out and assigning an etiologic role to each factor in human populations is extremely difficult. Nevertheless, important contributions have been made, and even more impressive accomplishments appear certain. Studies in man (Dmochowski et al., 1969) indicated that in human breast cancer, B- and C-type particles which resemble a virus are present. The analogy between breast cancer in mice and man may be much closer than we had imagined a few years ago.

STUDIES ON CANCER FAMILIES

The earliest contribution to the genetics of cancer were individual pedigrees showing a high incidence of tumors. Such studies may be misleading, since they may represent rare events that occur by chance. Warthin (1913) identified families showing a susceptibility to cancer involving a number of anatomic sites. He was among the first to emphasize the importance of histologic diagnosis in all malignancy involving families. Much of the earlier data relies on mortality statistics which are primarily clinical and consequently subject to error. A follow-up of certain of Warthin's families has been published by Lynch (1967). One of these, family G, shows an extremely high frequency of carcinoma, particularly adenocarcinoma, of many different sites.

Waaler (1931) made a thorough investigation of cancer-prone families in Norway. He compared the incidence of cancer in relatives of cancer patients, using their spouses as controls, and he also separated his groups according to the site of malignancy. His data tend to show a slight genetic susceptibility to certain carcinomas, for example, carcinomas of the esophagus, abdominal viscera, prostate gland, breast, uterus, and ovary. Cancer of the skin and lips did not show such genetic susceptibility. An objection to Waaler's data is the heterogeneity in ascertainment, since the diagnostic skills of large numbers of clinicians (over 100 physicians) used in this investigation must be variable and the reliability of data on death certificates is also in question. In recent years a number of investigators have published studies of families with a high incidence of cancer involving either a single organ or multiple anatomic sites. In general, these studies display a high standard of clinical and pathologic skill, although the statistical aspects are subject to the difficulties described above (see monograph by Lynch, 1967).

STUDIES ON TWINS

Studies on twins are a valuable method for assessing the relative importance of heredity and environment where family studies fail to show simple mendelian inheritance. One of the earliest and most extensive investigations was published by Macklin (1940), in which she combined her own series of twins with published cases. Her finding of an excess of concordance of neoplasia in monozygotic twins when compared to dizygotic twins must be evaluated with caution, since she pooled selected and unselected cases. There is a tendency to publish concordant twin pairs, which seriously biases data. Moreover, her study included exostoses, cysts, and polyps as tumors, which adds to the heterogeneity of her clinical material. It is difficult to obtain unbiased data. Surveys of twin pairs in large populations is a time-consuming and formidable venture but is probably the ideal method. A second technique is to determine all cancer patients in a large population and ascertain if they are members of a twin pair. Each set of twins is classified as monozygotic or dizygotic; however, the criteria for this classification is rarely complete. If malignant disease is concentrated in certain families, an excess of concordance with both monozygotic and dizygotic twins should be observed. If this susceptibility has a genetic component, the excess should be greater for the monozygotic pairs. Harvald and Hauge (1963) have investigated nearly 7000 sets of twins from the Danish twin registry and found the incidence of cancer in twins to be no greater than the expected rates. Concordance for monozygotic twins was not statistically different than that for dizygotic twins. Nevertheless, from these data one cannot conclude that the genetic constitution is unimportant in the genesis of neoplasia. Twin studies suffer from some of the difficulties in assessing the genetic component in neoplasia described previously. For example, aging is important in the onset of neoplasia, and certain twin pairs studied may be too young or may be lost to follow-up studies. Also, after one twin has developed neoplasia, one cannot conclude that the co-twin will remain free of the disease unless the study continues for a number of years. All of these factors re-emphasize the difficulties in human population studies of malignancy. Gorer (1953), in an excellent and balanced presentation of this subject,

has set forth preliminary evidence that in unselected monozygotic twins concordance for cancer in the same organ is high when compared to dizygotic pairs, although the time of onset varies markedly. Clearly, nongenetic factors play a role in determining the time at which a malignancy develops in man, as they certainly do in mice. Heredity and environment are not mutually exclusive factors in determining the etiology of cancer, and twin studies emphasize the difficulties in assigning responsibility to either of these agents.

CANCER SUSCEPTIBILITY DUE TO SINGLE GENES

A few cancers in man have a clear-cut and indisputable genetic basis which segregate as simple mendelian characters (i.e., showing dominant, recessive, or sex-linked inheritance). Several of them have major dermatologic associations and will be discussed in detail later. A listing of these disorders and their mode of inheritance is shown in Table 6–1. Sporadic cases of most of these disorders probably occur and may confuse studies on the mode of inheritance. Phenocopies, that is, abnormalities produced by developmental or environmental factors, which mimic certain genetic disorders may also complicate interpretation. It should be clearly understood that the assigning of a mendelian inheritance to a certain tumor does not explain the etiology of the disease. Frequently complex interactions between the genetic constitution and environmental factors are required before neoplasia is expressed (see p. 00).

Table 6–2 lists certain cancers of the skin in which genetic factors have been proposed to play a role in the etiology. However, the mode of inheritance in these families is not clear cut and the data are consistent with a common environmental agent within a family which may trigger the neoplasm. The difficulty in ascribing familial diseases to genetic factors or to a common environmental agent — for example, a virus — has been discussed previously.

Genetics is a rapidly developing subject which only recently has received attention

TABLE 6–1   CANCER SUSCEPTIBILITY SHOWING MENDELIAN INHERITANCE

Disorder	Mode of Inheritance	Tumor	References
Xeroderma pigmentation	autosomal recessive	epitheliomas	Siemens and Kohn (1925) Cockayne (1933) El-Hefnawi et al. (1965)
Multiple nevoid basal cell carcinoma syndrome	autosomal dominant	basal cell carcinoma	Straith (1939) Gorlin and Goltz (1960)
Neurofibromatosis	autosomal dominant	neurofibromas sarcomas gliomas meningiomas pheochromocytoma	Gates (1946)
Fanconi anemia	autosomal recessive	leukemia multisite cancers	Swift and Hirschhorn (1966)
Bloom syndrome	autosomal recessive	leukemia multisite cancers	Sawitsky et al. (1966)
Familial polyposis	autosomal dominant	adenocarcinoma of colon	Dukes (1952)
Retinoblastoma	autosomal dominant	retinoblastoma	Griffith and Sorsby (1944)
Gardner syndrome	autosomal dominant	adenocarcinoma of colon epidermal cysts osteoma fibromas	Gardner and Richards (1953)
Polyendocrine adeno-matosis	autosomal dominant	multiple endocrine tumors	Werner (1954)
Multiple exostosis	autosomal dominant	exostosis	Solomon (1963)
Tylosis and esophageal cancer	autosomal dominant	esophageal carcinoma	Howel-Evans et al. (1958)
Thyroid carcinoma with amyloidosis	(?) autosomal dominant	medullary thyroid car-cinoma	Williams et al. (1966)
Werner syndrome	autosomal recessive	sarcomas meningiomas	Epstein et al. (1966)
Ataxia-telangiectasia	autosomal recessive	lymphoreticular malignancy	Peterson et al. (1964)
Chédiak-Higashi syn-drome	autosomal recessive	(?) lymphoma	Page et al. (1962)

in the medical curriculum. A review section on inheritance and gene action seems appropriate. For a more detailed discussion of the interrelationships of genetics and molecular biology, see the review by King and Cox (1967).

Definitions. At this point, it is appropriate to review some of the terms that will be frequently mentioned in this chapter:

1. *Gene*—an independently segregating unit of heredity which controls or contributes to the development of a character.

2. *Alleles*—alternate forms of a gene which may occupy a given locus (or place) on a chromosome. The alleles control alternate expressions of a character (e.g., tall or short).

3. *Diploid*—In man and higher forms each chromosome is paired. One is inherited from the father and the other

TABLE 6–2   CANCER OF THE SKIN TO WHICH GENETIC FACTORS MAY CONTRIBUTE

Disorder	Mode of Inheritance	Tumor	References
Kaposi sarcoma	(?) Dominant with incomplete penetrance	sarcoma	Oettle (1962)
Generalized kerato-acanthoma	(?) autosomal dominant	keratoacanthoma (?) squamous cell car-noma	Butterworth and Strean (1962)
Malignant melanoma	(?) autosomal dominant with incomplete penetrance	malignant melanoma	Lynch (1967)

from the mother. Therefore, there are two representatives of each gene at two homologous loci, one on the maternal chromosome and the other on the paternal chromosome.

4. *Homozygous*—when alleles (genes at homologous loci on both chromosomes) are alike (both normal or both mutant).

5. *Heterozygous*—when alleles (genes at homologous loci on both chromosomes) are unlike (one normal and the other mutant).

6. *Genotype*—the sum of an individual's genetic constitution, or the genetic potential; the genetic information coded in the DNA of a person.

7. *Phenotype*—the appearance of an individual with respect to a particular character (or characters). The phenotype is the result of interaction of the genome and the environment.

8. *Dominant*—trait expressed whenever the corresponding allele is present.

9. *Recessive*—trait expressed only in individuals homozygous for the allele (double dose).

10. *Codominant*—traits expressed by both alleles when persent in the heterozygote; for example, blood groups A and B are both expressed in the heterozygote AB.

11. *Penetrance*—the proportion of individuals in a population who carry a particular gene *and* evidence it phenotypically. For example, a trait that depends upon a simple dominant gene may "skip" a generation and be transmitted by an individual who carries it but shows no manifestation of that gene; in this case it is nonpenetrant. Penetrance is usually expressed as a percentage of those individuals with a gene who manifest it phenotypically.

12. *Expressivity*—variations in the degree to which a gene expresses itself in an individual. Some individuals may have a full-blown clinical picture, while others may show only a slight manifestation (*forme fruste*).

13. *Polygenic systems*—traits or characters determined by several different genetic loci. A trait is quantitative, varying along a graded continuum rather than falling into clear-cut categories. For example, pigmentation, height, weight, and blood pressure are determined by many different loci,

probably with multiple alleles at each locus.

14. *Modifiers*—alleles at different loci which modify the expression of a trait.

15. *Epistasis*—"to stand upon," used in the situation where an allele at one locus acts to suppress the expression of an allele at another.

16. *Sex-linked*—genes occurring on a sex chromosome, usually restricted to the X-chromosome.

17 *Autosome*—any chromosome except the sex chromosome.

Patterns of Inheritance. The classical geneticists knew little of the nature of gene action. They made deductions from observations on the pattern of transmission of characters from parent to offspring. It became apparent very early that what was inherited was not a character but a potentiality to produce one under proper conditions. Molecular biology is giving us greater and greater insight into the complex succession of events between gene and character, but certain of the classical terms for the types of transmission of phenotypic expression are still of value, particularly as applied to pedigrees of individuals. Classification of human phenotypes according to patterns of inheritance may be of great value in predicting the probability of occurrence of a phenotype among the offspring of a given mating and in framing hypotheses and designing experiments concerning the biochemical mechanism producing the trait.

DOMINANT INHERITANCE. In human genetics a phenotype is said to be dominant when a single mutant gene on one of the chromosome pairs is sufficient to cause the clinical effect. Thus, the heterozygote shows the abnormality. Homozygotes for dominant genes are very rare in human genetics and they are often lethal. Figure 6–2 shows the inheritance of an autosomal dominant disorder. The segregation of a chromosome carrying the mutant gene leads, on the average, to one-half of the children being affected. Figure 6–3 shows a pedigree of a family with brachydactyly, a minor trait showing dominant inheritance. The affected individual in the second generation probably is the result of a mutation in the gonad of one parent, since there was no previous history of the abnor-

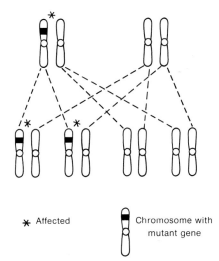

* Affected   Chromosome with mutant gene

Figure 6–2 Transmission of autosomal dominant disease.

mality in the family. Thereafter a *vertical pattern* of inheritance is observed, with affected members in each generation passing the mutant gene to, on the average, 50 percent of their progeny. Autosomal dominant traits are transmitted equally to males and females. The number of generations through which a mutant gene persists depends upon the number of children born to affected individuals. If the gene is very deleterious and affected subjects do not reproduce, then the occurrence of the disease will be equal to the mutation rate for that locus. If, as in the pedigree shown,

there is little selection against affected individuals ("fitness" is near normal), then the disease will be passed on to about one-half of their progeny.

An important consideration in genetics is the modification of gene expression by environmental or genetic interactions (for a more detailed discussion see p. 154). The *expression* of a genetic disease in an individual may be so mild as to be barely detectable, or it may be full blown with severe clinical manifestations. Variations in *expressivity* of mutant genes in different persons are the result of interactions between a gene determining a potential character and other genes which modify or modulate its expression. The environment, including that in utero, also may modify or alter the genetic potential. The final phenotype depends on these complex interactions.

Occasionally in pedigrees in which a dominant mutant gene is segregating, a person who appears completely normal has an affected child. In this case the parent is obviously carrying the mutation but shows no manifestation of the gene. In this case the mutation is nonpenetrant. *Penetrance* is a population concept, and is defined as the proportion of individuals with a particular mutant gene who show manifestations of the mutation. Obviously, pedigrees in which penetrance is low complicate the interpretation of modes of inheritance.

Figure 6–3 Pedigree showing autosomal dominant inheritance.

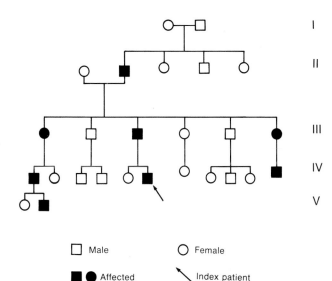

□ Male   ○ Female

■ ● Affected   ↖ Index patient

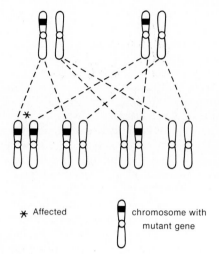

* Affected

chromosome with mutant gene

Figure 6–4 Transmission of an autosomal recessive disease.

RECESSIVE INHERITANCE. A characteristic is recessive when it appears only in individuals homozygous for the allele. Often the heterozygous carriers of such an allele cannot be diagnosed, and in pedigrees the characteristic will appear frequently among the offspring of parents, neither of whom show it, since they are both heterozygous. Figure 6–4 shows a diagram of an autosomal recessive disease. Each parent transmits a chromosome carrying the mutant gene to one-half of his progeny. The probability of a child getting a mutant gene from each parent is 25 percent. On the average, half of the children will be carriers. The ratio of affected to clinical normal then will be 1 to 3. Figure 6–5 shows a typical pedigree of albinism showing a recessive inheritance. This mode of transmission in pedigrees is often called *horizontal*, since sibs of the index patient are frequently affected and it is unusual for other members of the family to show the trait. Figure 6–5 also shows consanguinity—marriage between first cousins (III generation)—which is commonly present in pedigrees showing rare recessive mutant alleles. If a recessive gene is rare, related persons have an increased probability of each having a mutant allele derived from a common ancestor. Consanguinity is less often seen in pedigrees showing recessive inheritace of relatively common genes, for example, cystic fibrosis. The probability of two unrelated heterozygotes marrying is relatively high in this disorder.

SEX-LINKED INHERITANCE. Genes located on the X-chromosome show a peculiar pattern of transmission, since carrier females pass their X-chromosomes to their sons. The males are *hemizygous*, that is, they have only one X-chromosome which they receive from their mother. Therefore, males having an X-chromosome with a recessive mutant allele express the trait. This leads to the oblique pattern of inheritance seen in Figure 6–6. There is a one-in-two risk of disease in the sons of women heterozygous for a sex-linked recessive mutation. Half of the daughters will also receive the mutant chromosome and be heterozygous carriers like their mother (Fig. 6–6). The result of this inheritance is that mutant sex-linked genes most often manifest themselves in males who inherit

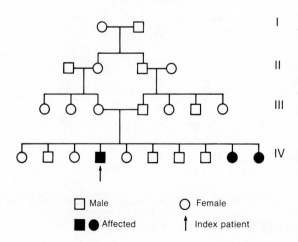

I

II

III

IV

Figure 6–5 Pedigree showing autosomal recessive inheritance.

☐ Male   ○ Female

■● Affected   ↑ Index patient

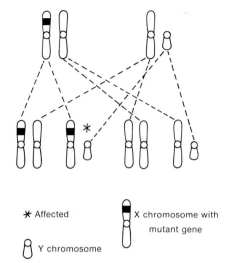

Figure 6–6 Transmission of a sex-linked recessive disease.

every somatic cell of the female zygote at an early time in embryonic development (Lyon, 1962). The inactivation of an X-chromosome in female cells may not be complete, since certain X-linked loci show a heterozygous expression; for example, the Xg blood group locus shows a heterozygous expression in red cells (Fialkow, 1970; Fialkow et al., 1970b; Lawler and Sanger, 1970). Moreover, Merey (1970) has recently shown that as much as 30 percent of the inactivated X-chromosome replicates early in DNA synthesis and therefore may contain genetically active euchromatin. Those loci that are inactivated during embryonic development are apparently permanently inactive in every cell line. However, there is more to the metabolic differences between the sexes than merely the random inactivation of one X-chromosome. A human zygote with a single X and no Y is a sterile female with somatic aberrations (Turner syndrome). In mice, the same karyotype is a fertile female. We have much more to learn about the control of differentiation of sex and about differences in metabolic controls.

POLYGENIC INHERITANCE.   The majority of observable traits in most organisms do not manifest themselves as sharply defined pairs of alternate phenotypes, nor do they show a simple mendelian pattern of inheritance. Such human traits as skin pigmentation, height, blood pressure, and resistance to certain diseases differ along graded continua, not by clear-cut categories. These quantitative traits undoubtedly result from complex interactions between the many different alleles of a polygenic system and environmental influences all acting

them from their mothers. Thus, a sex-linked mutation commonly descends from grandfather to grandson through a female heterozygous carrier. As shown in Figure 6–7, this pattern of inheritance is relatively easy to identify in any reasonably extensive pedigree.

In species such as man where the female is the homogametic sex — her X-chromosomes are paired — one would expect her to have twice the gene activity of the male for those genes found on the X-chromosome. However, this is not the case. Normal human females and males have similar levels of glucose-6-phosphate dehydrogenase and antihemophilic globulin. Both these proteins are under the control of X-linked genes. This dosage compensation appears to be result of a random inactivation of one of the X-chromosomes in

Figure 6–7 Pedigree showing sex-linked recessive inheritance.

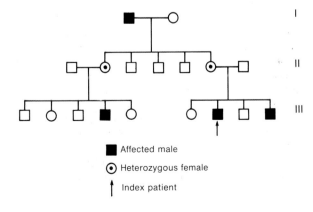

throughout ontogeny. Sometimes the extremes of these continua are produced by the coincidence in an individual of many genes, of small individual effect, all acting in one direction. In others the same phenotype may result from the effect of one or a pair of alleles at a single locus. For example, a very short person may have a single gene for dwarfism or a genotype in which many genes reducing stature happen to have segregated together. In pedigree studies, traits attributable to single genes are more likely to be distinctively recognizable than those due to polygenic systems. Polygenic inheritance is more likely to produce a smoothly graded series. One must be wary of analyzing this complex pattern by setting an arbitrary cut-off point for a quantitative trait and then partitioning the progeny in proportions consistent with a preconceived genetic ratio.

GENE INTERACTION. Cells and organisms are complex systems with delicately interrelated controls, and it is obvious that genes must interact to produce a viable functioning organism. Mendel's most important contribution was his demonstration that genetic units were particulate and unchanging. However, his experiments also showed that in producing a phenotype the two alleles of a pair did not produce independent effects. This is the basis of classical dominance and recessiveness. Interactions between genes at different loci were discovered early in the development of genetics. A number of terms have been coined to describe and classify these interactions, and many of them are still in use.

The term epistasis is used to describe the situation where a dominant allele at one locus acts to suppress the expression of the dominant allele at another. Epistasis is often used, in a more general sense, to describe any case in which alleles at different loci interact to modify the phenotype. For example, the mutant Bombay blood group type is epistatic to the ABO locus, since the normal allele at the Bombay locus is responsible for the synthesis of the blood group precursor upon which the enzymes determined by the ABO alleles act.

Modifiers are genes which reduce or enhance the expression of other genes. An extreme form of a modifier is a suppressor gene, which restores the wild type phenotype in a genotype which would otherwise have been mutant. The phenomenon of penetrance may in some cases be due to suppressors, but no clear-cut examples are known in human populations. Other kinds of modifiers have easily measurable effects, but many are less precise and often have variable effects. Modifiers sometimes have cumulative effects, but more often than not this cumulation is not strictly additive. A polygenic system, in a sense, consists of a series of modifiers each segregating independently and each of small individual effect. Such modifiers sometimes can be demonstrated in animal populations by a program of selection for an increase in the expression of a given trait, or by showing the differences in the degree of expression of a given gene when it is transferred by crossing from the genetic background of one strain into that of another.

Obviously two concepts previously introduced, penetrance and expressivity, are in part based upon modifiers. Expressivity refers to the degree to which a characteristic is observable in a single individual. On the other hand, penetrance is a yes-or-no determination on whether an individual who carries a given gene has any observable manifestations of the phenotype. For a population, penetrance is measured by the number of individuals who carry the gene and who express it phenotypically. This must not be confused with the frequency of a gene in the population.

Environmental factors influence both penetrance and expressivity. The contribution of environmental and genetic factors in determining penetrance and expressivity can be estimated by statistical methods in experimental animals, although there are often serious complications. In human family studies these measurements are even more formidable. Generally, when an animal geneticist uses genes as markers, he selects those which have a high probability of penetrance and a relatively uniform degree of expression. Variable expressivity and low penetrance are often more serious problems for the human geneticist, for he must deduce the relative genetic and environmental contributions to the phenotype from what is often incomplete and unsatisfactory information. He cannot select his strains and arrange his crosses. Often the critical cross is unavailable.

All these terms for different types of gene interaction in diploid organisms are descriptive rather than analytical. They were coined during that period of genetics when the organism was a kind of black box. One used a gene as input and obtained a phenotype as output. With the development of molecular and biochemical genetics, the understanding of gene action has increased. The old terms are often applied to later observations, and there have been numerous shifts in their meaning and some confusion in their application. As our knowledge of molecular biology increases, a more detailed understanding of gene interactions will be apparent, and the old terms and concepts may become obsolete unless they are precisely redefined.

RACIAL AND GEOGRAPHIC FACTORS IN CANCER

The incidence of specific neoplasms varies in different populations. However, careful analysis is needed to decide how many of these differences are genetically determined and how any are due to environment. Thus, in skin cancer the incidence of squamous cell carcinoma depends on the degree of pigmentation which is genetically determined and the intensity of ultraviolet light. The almost total absence of cancer of the penis in the Jewish population might be interpreted as having a genetic basis, but it has been shown to depend on very early circumcision (Kennaway, 1957). Similarly, the very high incidence of liver cancer among Bantu Africans, Chinese, and Javanese appears to have a predominantly dietary rather than genetic basis (Bonne, 1935). Gastric cancer is common in Japan but rare in China. Eskimos are said to have cancer only rarely, but how often does an Eskimo have adequate medical diagnosis and how often does he survive to an age when cancer is common? For further discussion of other examples, see the monograph edited by Shivas (1967).

Study of geographic and racial pathology is important in detecting environmental differences which may contribute to neoplasia; it is much less useful in detecting a genetic predisposition. For example, nasopharyngeal carcinoma is a rare neoplasm in most countries of the world. However, it is one of the leading cancer problems of the Far East. In Singapore, Chinese have a very high incidence of this tumor, while Chinese in the United States have a very low rate. This suggests an environmental factor, and recent evidence implicates infection with Epstein-Barr (EB) virus as the etiologic agent (Old et al., 1966).

The above caveats do not exclude genetic differences between populations as contributing to cancer susceptibility, but they indicate the difficulties in separating complex genetic, cultural, and environmental interactions. An appreciation of the genetics of population structure and evolution are beyond the scope of this review. For further discussion see James C. King's book Biology of Race (1971), a preceptive and accurate presentation of this subject.

ASSOCIATIONS BETWEEN GENETIC POLYMORPHISM AND CANCER

The existence in a population of more than one allele at a locus leads to the appearance of several genotypes. If the frequency of various alleles is high, then the population may be divided into several classes on the basis of genetic heterogeneity for this trait. For example, populations differ in the frequency of the ABO blood group antigens. Most populations consist of four classes: A, B, AB, and O. Maintenance of this polymorphism in a population has been attributed to selective processes which tend to maintain the gene frequencies. Associations between certain diseases and a particular polymorphic genotype has been found, although the pathogenetic basis of this association and the role of the disease as a selective factor are very much in doubt. Aird and coworkers (1953) demonstrated an association between gastric carcinoma and blood group A (also see Vogel, 1970). Blood group A was later associated with pernicious anemia and atrophic gastritis (Clarke, 1959; Roberts, 1959). More recently, blood group A is claimed to be associated with neoplastic diseases of the ovary (Osborne and De George, 1963) and with multiple primary malignancies including those of the skin (Fadhi and Dominguez, 1963). On the other hand xeroderma pigmentosum shows a statistical correlation with blood group O (El-Hefnawi et al., 1965).

The significance of the statistical association between blood group antigens and certain cancers is not known. The data are extensive enough and from sufficiently different geographical areas to probably exclude the possibility that patients belong to a subpopulation in which both the specific blood group allele and the disease happen to be more frequent than in the control group (but see Wiener, 1970). Moreover, the relative incidence of the disease among patients and their healthy sibs differs according to blood group frequencies in the same general way it does among patients and unrelated controls (Stern, 1960). Nevertheless, the incidence of the disease depends on complex interactions, and only a few individuals contract the disease. The strength of the association is relatively limited, and the full implications of the observed associations remain to be realized.

CHROMOSOMAL ABNORMALITIES ASSOCIATED WITH NEOPLASIA

The association of chromosomal abnormalities with malignant neoplasms has been recognized for many years (Boveri, 1914). Whether these abnormalities are a cause or an effect of the tumor is still a subject for controversy. Recently evidence has accumulated that several diseases, for example, Bloom syndrome and Fanconi anemia, which are under simple genetic control, are accompanied by a high frequency of chromosomal rearrangements in somatic cells and a striking increase in the prevalence of malignancy. German et al. (1965) reported that Bloom syndrome was accompanied by chromosome aberrations in somatic cells, and similar observations

were made in Fanconi anemia by Schroeder, Anschütz, and Knopp (1964). The association of these diseases with malignancy has been stressed by Swift and Hirschhorn (1966) and by Sawitsky et al. (1966). The relationship between chromosomal aberrations and the onset of malignancy has been the subject of considerable investigation, and the mechanism is still in doubt. The chromosomal changes are essentially structural and result from chromosome breakage (Fig. 6–8). They consist of chromatid gaps, isochromatid breaks, fragments, minute chromosomes, dicentric chromosomes, and quadrilateral formation, which is the result of chromatid breaks in two chromosomes followed by fusion of the broken arms and chromatid exchanges. The basic event is an interruption of the continuity of the chromosome. This may be barely apparent as a gap in a single chromatid, or so large that the continuity of the chromatid is broken (Fig. 6–8A). The broken ends are sticky, and this accounts for the chromosome exchanges and dicentric chromosomes (Fig. 6–8D) which are frequently observed. If damage to a chromatid occurs after replication (S phase of the cell cycle), only one chromatid of the pair will show the discontinuity—a chromatid gap or break. If damage to a chromatid occurs prior to replication of the chromosome, both the old and newly synthesized chromatids will show the defect—isochromatid breaks. Some breaks lead to the formation of fragments which remain free or translocate onto other broken chromosomes. Dicentric and ring chromosomes represent bizarre translocation figures in which more than one chromatid break is required. Many of these aberrations are not compatible with an equal partitioning of genetic material during mitosis and are probably lethal to the cells that contain them. Other abnormalities may favor unregulated cell growth.

The cause of the chromosomal breaks in these two diseases is not known. It might be an effect of the mutation per se (Bloom et al., 1966) or it may be the result of a metabolic abnormality that impedes repair of chromosome breakages due to irradiation, virus infection, or other environmental agents. Allison and Paton (1965) have postulated that activation of lysosomal en-

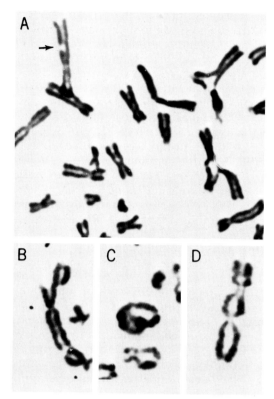

Figure 6–8 Cytogenetic abnormalities in Fanconi anemia.

A, Chromatid gap (*arrow*) and two translocation figures, lymphocytes, Case 2.

B, Chromatid break, bone marrow, Case 1.

C, Ring chromosome and fragment, fibroblasts, Case 1.

D, Dicentric chromosome, fibroblasts, Case 1.

(*From* Swift and Hirschhorn: Ann. Intern. Med., 65:500, 1966.)

1966). This important study showed that cell strains derived from normal individuals have a low frequency of transformation, <0.05 percent. Cell strains from patients with Fanconi anemia show a 0.05 to 0.75 percent incidence (Fig. 6–9). A finding of great importance is that heterozygous carriers of Fanconi anemia who show *no* chromosomal abnormalities also have an increased susceptibility (0.2 to 0.3 percent) to transformation by oncogenic viruses and possibly an increased incidence of neoplasms (Garriga and Crosby, 1959; Swift, 1971). This implies that chromosomal breakage and reorganization is not the only factor that enhances susceptibility to viral transformation. While certain heterozygous carriers of the Fanconi mutation have chromosomes that appear to be cytologically normal, their susceptibility to virus transformation in vitro and perhaps to neoplasia in vivo raises the possibility that certain cancer-prone individuals might be detected by using Todaro's quantitative test. The exciting possibility exists that heterozygous carriers of these genes which may confer increased cancer susceptibility may account for a significant proportion of apparently normal persons who develop cancer. For example, Fanconi anemia (homozygote) is very rare, one in 1,400,000 persons is affected. However, carriers of the gene (heterozygotes) occur with an incidence of 1 in 600, as predicted by the Hardy-Weinberg equation. The he-

zymes may release DNAase, which produces chromosomal damage.

Chromosome breaks are also known to be associated with increased susceptibility of cells to infection by oncogenic viruses (Pollock and Todaro, 1968). A quantitative test using human diploid skin fibroblast cultures has been devised to test "susceptibility" to transformation by oncogenic viruses. In this test fibroblast cultures are established from skin biopsies. Exponentially growing cultures are inoculated with a standard titer of oncogenic virus, for example, simian-40 virus (SV_{40}), and the number of transformed cells are identified by a dense, disordered, heaping up of the cells unlike the ordered monolayer of normal cells (Todaro et al.,

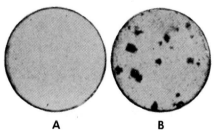

Figure 6–9 Culture of human diploid cell strain HG (normal) fixed and stained 17 days after inoculation of 5×10^4 cells. *A,* Control. *B,* Culture which had been infected with $10^{9.0}$ TCID/ml. of SV_{40} one day prior to plating. Photograph shows transformed colonies as dense areas of disordered cell growth on a background of normal cells. (*From* Todaro et al.: Science, 153:1253, 1966. Copyright 1966 by the American Association for the Advancement of Science.)

terozygotes appear normal without anemia, excess pigmentation, skeletal deformation, or tendency to chromosome
breakage. The clinically normal heterozygotes for rare autosomal recessive syndromes associated with predisposition to
cancer constitute a relatively large group
which may contribute significantly to the
incidence of neoplasia (Swift, 1971). Heterozygotes for other mutant genes which
confer an increased susceptibility to
tumors may account for many so-called
spontaneous cancers.

One type of cancer, chronic myelogenous leukemia, almost invariably is associated with a specific chromosomal defect—the Philadelphia chromosome Ph[1]
(Nowell and Hungerford, 1960). This abnormal chromosome is probably produced
by a partial deletion or translocation of the
long arm of a G group chromosome, number 22 (Fig. 6–10), and probably represents an acquired chromosomal aberration
(Nowell and Hungerford, 1964). It has
been suggested that genetic loci controlling
leukocyte maturation may be located on
the deleted chromosome and thereby account for the increase in granulocyte survival and immaturity associated with this
disease.

Chronic lymphatic leukemia in a family

in Australia was associated in two siblings
with a deletion of the short arms of group
G chromosome, which has been named the
Christ Church chromosome, Ch[1]. Several
unaffected relatives also showed the chromosomal abnormality (Gunz et al., 1962).
Table 6–3 presents certain diseases in
which chromosomal aberrations and malignancies are associated.

While a specific chromosome defect
(Ph[1]) is nearly present in chronic myelogenous leukemia, chromosome analysis
of solid tumors, including cancer of the
skin, fails to show chromosome aberrations
specific for each kind of tumor. However,
nearly every solid tumor seems to have a
chromosome complement characteristic of
the particular lesion in an individual.
Thus, the karyotypic findings differ not
only between different kinds of tumor but
also between individuals with identical
tumors. The uniqueness of chromosome
aberrations in each individual tumor may
be fortuitous and coincidental, reflecting a
selection of a particular stem cell line, or it
may be that a particular chromosome complement has a selective advantage in a particular patient because of his unique genetic composition. For a more detailed
review of chromosome studies in solid
tumors, see Makino et al. (1964).

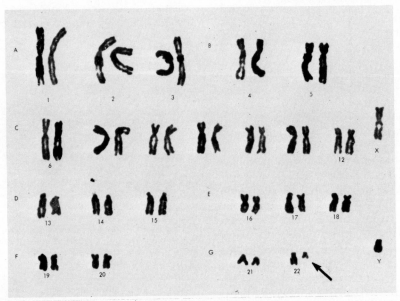

Figure 6–10 Karyotype of granulocyte from a patient with chronic myelogenous leukemia showing the
Philadelphia chromosome Ph[1] (arrow). (Courtesy of Dr. S. R. Wolman.)

TABLE 6–3   CHROMOSOMAL ABNORMALITIES ASSOCIATED WITH NEOPLASIA

Disorder	Mode of Inheritance	Chromosomal Aberration	Tumor	References
Fanconi anemia	autosomal recessive	multiple chromosome breaks and rearrangements	carcinomas leukemia	Swift (1971)
Bloom syndrome	autosomal recessive	multiple chromosome breaks and rearrangements	acute leukemia	Sawitsky et al. (1966)
Ataxia-telangiectasia	autosomal recessive	(?) chromosome breaks	lymphoreticular malignancy	Peterson et al. (1914)
Chronic myelogenous leukemia	— acquired	deletion G group (Ph¹)	leukemia	Nowell and Hungerford (1964)
Chronic lymphatic leukemia	familial chromosome aberration	deletion or translocation G group (Ch¹)	leukemia	Gunz et al. (1962)

HERITABLE DISORDERS OF METABOLISM WHICH PREDISPOSE TO SKIN CANCER

Although the metabolism of tumors differs from that of normal cells of the same tissue the significance of these changes in the genesis of cancer is not known (Warburg, 1956). When the metabolism of neoplastic cells from a tissue is compared to undifferentiated or embryonic cells from the same source rather than to normal cells, the metabolic activities of the neoplastic and immature cells are very similar (Silber and Bertino, 1972).

Recently, the probable basis of skin cancer in a rare inherited autosomal recessive disorder, xeroderma pigmentosum, has been elucidated. This disease is characterized by a peculiar sensitivity to ultraviolet radiation which results in multiple cutaneous malignancies within the first year of life. The basic defect in this disease appears to be a deficiency of the enzyme which repairs DNA by excision of segments of DNA damaged by ultraviolet light. Ultraviolet radiation induces mutations and damages cells by a photochemical change in the nucleic acid of exposed cells (Witkin, 1966). The first photochemical lesion found in DNA of ultraviolet irradiated bacteria was the thymine dimer, which is formed by the linking of adjacent thymine bases in the same strand of DNA. Normally the purine and pyrimidine bases in a single strand of DNA are connected via the sugar phosphate groups, not directly to each other. Less frequently, other

pyrimidine dimers, for example, cytosine-cytosine and cytosine-thymine, are also formed. Dimers apparently block DNA replication and are responsible for the lethal and mutational effects of ultraviolet radiation (Witkin, 1966). Pyrimidine dimers can be repaired in bacteria and in mammalian cells by excision of short segments of single-strand DNA that includes the dimers (Regan et al., 1968). The gap left by excision is then repaired enzymatically (Epstein et al., 1970). Patients with xeroderma pigmentosum are either unable to excise the damaged DNA or are unable to repair the defect (Epstein et al., 1970). The increased incidence of skin cancer in these patients after exposure to the sun is apparently due to the mutational effects of unrepaired pyrimidine dimers. However, a direct relation between a lack of DNA repair and cancer formation remains to be determined.

Table 6–4 shows several inborn errors of metabolism in which the skin cancer is especially prevalent. Oculocutaneous albinism is a rare recessive disease characterized by decrease or absence of melanin in the skin, hair, and eyes. The marked susceptibility of albinos to skin cancer with metastasis and death was described in 1699 by Wafer. Albinism is in fact a heterogenous group of diseases affecting the skin and eyes to a varying degree. Complete albinism or oculocutaneous albinism occurs between 1 in 5000 and 1 in 25,000 births and involves the melanocytes of both the skin and eyes, producing the characteristic milk-white color and the lack of eye pigment with photophobia and nys-

TABLE 6–4 HERITABLE DISORDERS OF METABOLISM WHICH
PREDISPOSE TO SKIN CANCER

Disorder	Mode of Inheritance	Mechanism	References
Xeroderma pigmentosum	autosomal recessive	defective DNA repair following UV irradiation	Epstein et al. (1970)
Albinism	autosomal recessive	absent pigmentation predisposes skin to UV damage	Keeler (1963)
Phenylketonuria	autosomal recessive	decreased pigmentation due to phenylalanine hydroxylase deficiency predisposes skin to UV damage	

tagmus. Other varieties of albinism involve only the eyes (ocular albinism) or only the skin (cutaneous albinism). Cutaneous albinism shows an autosomal dominant inheritance, and the loss of pigment is often patterned. Ocular albinism has a sex-linked inheritance.

The basic defect in these diseases is a failure of melanin to form within the melanocytes which are normally present in albinos. The enzymatic lesion(s) responsible for the defect in melanin synthesis in the various types of albinism is not known. Subnormal melanogenesis observed in human albinos could result from (1) unavailability in melanocytes of tyrosine, the substrate which is polymerized to form melanin; (2) specific melanogenic inhibitors; and (3) decreased activity of tyrosinase, the enzyme required to convert tyrosine to dihydroxyphenylalanine (Fitzpatrick and Quevedo, 1966). Evidence suggests that one or more of these various mechanisms may be operative in albinism.

Melanin acts as a protective barrier against the sun, and it has been known for many years that fair-complexioned whites are much more susceptible to skin cancer than are dark-skinned races. Pigmentation is a genetic trait determined by a polygenic system. Single gene defects such as albinism or phenylketonuria can greatly modify melanin synthesis and enhance neoplasia. However, the carcinogenic agent is exposure to sun, and the degree of pigmentation is merely a predisposing factor. The interplay of genetics and environment in the causation of skin cancer is a striking example of the complex interactions which plague research on the genetics of neoplasia.

SOMATIC CELL MUTATIONS AND THE GENESIS OF CANCER

Heritable mutations involve germ cells and are the basis of classic genetic analysis, since they are the prime source of variation in all living things. Mutations may also occur in somatic cells, and although not transmitted to future generations they may have dramatic effects on the function and regulation of cellular activities. Mutation is probably a chemical process involving the gene (DNA). Mutations are a permanent change in the information coded in the DNA and can occur by the replacement of one base by another or by the deletion or intercalation of one or more bases. A change having arisen, the precise mechanisms of DNA replication insures its perpetuation.

An attractive hypothesis which attempts to unify various concepts of both benign and malignant tumor etiologies is the somatic cell mutation theory. Stewart (1970) and Stewart and Kneale (1970a and 1970b) have elaborated on this hypothesis and have provided evidence to support certain aspects of it. The theory attributes all tumors to a primary event involving a somatic mutation which "endows future generations of cells with more freedom of action and therefore more power over neighboring cells than normal tissue" (Stewart, 1970). Supporting evidence for this theory is provided by studies on the incidence of tumors in newborn and young children subjected to x-rays in utero during obstetric radiology. The data show an increased incidence of many tumors with, in some cases, a surprisingly short latent period, (Stewart and Kneale, 1970b). In the past, an objection to the somatic mutation theory was that the induction of cancer by x-rays did not follow a linear dose response but seemed to require a threshold of induction before tumor initiation. However, Stewart and Kneale (1970a) have presented evidence that the induction of tumors in fetuses does show a near linear dose response to x-ray. In adults, however, such a linear response between x-rays and cancer induction has not been conclusively demonstrated.

Tumorigenesis in certain cancers may be a multistep process in which the initiating event is a genetic alteration (?mutation) and a second event is required for expression of the tumor. Berenblum (1954) has made the important discovery that in some kinds of experimental chemical carcinogenesis in mouse skin, two steps—initiation and promotion—are involved. Initiation is a sudden and irreversible event akin to a somatic mutation. On the other hand, promotion is apparently a lengthy process and demands a considerable time (latency). Latency suggests a multistep process of damage to surrounding cells and inhibition or excess production of substances leading to nonlimited growth (this topic is discussed in greater detail in Chapter 5). Nevertheless, the initial event may be a genetic change in a somatic cell.

Evidence for a single cell origin of certain, but not all, tumors that is consistent with the somatic mutation hypothesis is provided by the ingenious studies of Gartler and his associates (1966). However, other tumors, including most carcinomas, seem to arise from more than one cell. The cellular origin of tumors can be investigated in neoplasms developing in patients with two or more genetically distinct cell types. One example is the mammalian female who has a cellular mosaicism because of the inactivation of one of the two X-chromosomes in each somatic cell. Inactivation apparently occurs early in embryologic development, and all descendents from a particular cell have the same X-chromosome active. For example, the locus determining glucose-6-phosphate dehydrogenase (G-6-PD) is located on the X-chromosome, and there are several alleles at this locus for electrophoretically

distinguishable types (A and B G-6-PD). Culture of skin fibroblasts from females heterozygous for the A and B gene at the X-linked G-6-PD locus show both enzyme types. However, clones originating from single cells derived from the mass culture show only one type, either A or B enzyme, never both (Davidson et al., 1963). Therefore, neoplasms arising in single cells in heterozygous females also should exhibit only one enzyme type, while those with multiple cell origins should contain both enzyme types. This technique has furnished strong evidence for a clonal origin of leiomyomas of the uterus (Linder and Gartler, 1965), chronic myelogenous leukemia (Fialkow et al., 1967), and Burkitt tumors (Fialkow et al., 1970). Multiple cell origin has been suggested for the hereditary skin disorder trichoepithelioma (Gartler et al., 1966) and in a few cases of carcinoma (Beutler et al., 1967; McGurdy, 1968). The important finding of Fialkow et al. (1970) that Burkitt tumors (an apparent multifocal tumor of presumed viral etiology) have a single type of G-6-PD raises the possibility that a single enzyme type does not necessarily mean that the original oncogenic agent affected only one cell. It is possible that initially many cells were altered but only one cell had a marked proliferative advantage and overgrew the others.

Some support for the theory of somatic mutation as the cause of cancer comes from the fact that certain carcinogenic agents react chemically with nucleic acids and are also mutagens. However, the correlation is not entirely clear, especially with respect to acidic dyes and carcinogenic hydrocarbons. For example, some acridines are mutagenic and others are carcinogenic, and there is little overlapping of these effects (Lerman, 1964; Dulbecco, 1964). The most powerful carcinogens, such as the aromatic hydrocarbons, are not mutagenic or are only weakly mutagenic. However, in the case of chemical carcinogens there is an additional difficulty in assessing their mutagenicity, since the substances are sometimes metabolized by the cell, and we don't know which metabolite is the true carcinogen. Comparison of the mechanisms of mutagenesis and carcinogenesis requires examination of the chemical alterations that these substances produce in cells. Mutagens ultimately react with DNA; however, studies on carcinogens are more controversial. In general, it has been found that most carcinogens interact with all the macromolecules of the cells. Interaction of hydrocarbons with DNA is still ambiguous (Brookes and Lawley, 1964; Heidelberger, 1964). Alkylating agents appear to be different from aromatic hydrocarbons since they react most strongly with DNA. However, they do react with other cellular components as well. The crux of the problem is to determine whether a particular chemical is both a carcinogen and a mutagen by studying it in the same host. This has yet to be done in sufficient detail to provide a firm answer. For technical reasons, mutagenesis is primarily investigated in microorganisms, molds, and *Drosophila*. Carcinogenesis is studied in mammals. These studies must now converge in an experimental system where meaningful answers can be provided. Tissue culture promises to be such a system, where in the same cell type mutagenic and carcinogenic acitivty can be investigated (Dulbecco, 1964; Chu and Malling, 1968).

At present there is no compelling reason for accepting or rejecting the somatic mutation theory for the origin of cancer. If the final conclusions are that chemical carcinogenesis does not involve alterations in DNA, we are faced with the problem of explaining the persistence of the malignant state for many cell generations. This dilemma leads us to the next and final section, that of epigenetics.

EPIGENETICS AND CANCER

Epigenetics is the branch or subdivision of genetics that analyses individual development (ontogeny) with its central problem of differentiation. It holds that the developing embryo contains more information than the zygote, since it derives information not only from the genotype but also from the embryonic environment and from interaction between tissue and organs. For example, *induction* in an embryologic sense implies the influence of one cell type on another. The responding or *induced* cell, if capable of reacting to the inductive stimulus, is *competent* and undergoes *differentiation*. Differentiation is basically a cellular alteration leading, in general, to a more specific and selective function. Within a tissue, normal differentiation is progressive and directed so that development proceeds toward the formation of an organ or functionally specialized tissues, such as muscle or skin. Cell interactions often are highly specific, and our knowledge of basic mechanism is indeed primitive.

Cancer can be regarded as a loss of special function and a return to a more autonomous or "primitive state." Genetic theory attempts to analyze this process and to understand neoplasia in terms of the complex and poorly understood laws of embryology (Willis, 1962; Ebert, 1965). As yet, the outline of the problem is hazy and ill defined; nevertheless, derangements of epigenetic mechanisms may well be the aberrations responsible for initiation and promotion of neoplasia.

One of the most obvious changes in a malignant cell is alteration of surface properties that leads to autonomous proliferation, invasion of normal tissues, and metastasis. Normal tissues placed in tissue culture show the property of contact inhibition of mitosis and locomotion, while malignant cells in culture lack these properties. Contact inhibition of mitosis, as displayed by normal cells, prevents them from dividing when they are surrounded on all sides by other cells. Contact inhibition of locomotion arrests normal cell movement when a cell touches another cell so as to prevent the cells from moving over one another and heaping up. When cells from a normal tissue of a mouse are placed in cell culture and grown for many cell generations in vitro, certain of these cells undergo an alteration called "malignant transformation," which permits them to propagate indefinitely in cell culture rather than undergo the usual senescence. These established cell lines show chromosomal aberrations and are usually aneuploid. Most of these established "normal" mouse cell lines capable of continuous propagation in culture lose contact inhibition. When these cell lines are injected into a histocompatible recipient, they produce tumors (Aaronson and Todaro, 1968). If, however, normal mouse cells are grown in culture under conditions (subculturing when population density is low) which preserve responsiveness to contact inhibition, these cell lines are unable to initiate tumors when injected into a compatible recipient (Aaronson and Todaro, 1968). These contact-inhibited established cell lines are able to be grown indefinitely in cultures and have aberrant chromosomes and aneuploidy similiar to the lines that have lost contact inhibition. This effect appears to be epigenetic, since the degree of chromosomal abnormalities is similar in contact-sensitive and contact-insensitive cell lines. The molecular basis of contact inhibition in cell culture is not known, although a serum factor seems to be involved (Todaro et al., 1965) and perhaps the saccharide constituents of mammalian cell surfaces are also important determinants (Cox and Gesner, 1965, 1967a, 1967b, 1968).

Mammalian cell surfaces contain saccharide components which are synthesized under genetic control and are able to interact with structures in the environment. Recent work suggests that cell associations in tissue culture may be mediated through interaction of surface sugars on one cell with complementary sites on another (Cox and Gesner, 1965). The effects are characterized by specificity of the cell lines affected, and by specificity of the sugars which produce the effects. For example, all cell lines studied were not affected by the same sugar. In some, such as $3T_3$ mouse embryo cells, an established cell line with a high degree of contact inhibition, L-fucose markedly altered the morphology of cells and inhibited their growth, as shown in Figures 6–11 and 6–12. $3T_3$ cells infected with an oncogenic virus (SV_{40}) lose contact inhibition, achieve a high population density, and are capable of causing tumors. L-Fucose correspondingly has much less effect on the oncogenic virus-transformed cells, as shown in Figures 6–13 and 6–14. Thus, the specific and selective effects of a sugar which is a naturally occurring component of the surface heterosaccharides of mammalian cells correlate with the degree

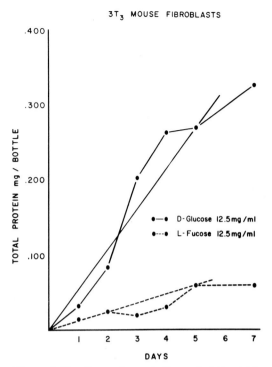

Figure 6–11 Comparison of effects of adding 12.5 mg./ml. of D-glucose or L-fucose to Waymouth's medium, on the growth of $3T_3$ mouse fibroblasts.

of contact inhibition and malignant potential exhibited. If the mechanism whereby L-fucose inhibits $3T_3$ cells is related to that which occurs in cell contact inhibition, one possible explanation for the parallelism between the phenomena might be that L-fucose produces its effects by substituting for a fucose-containing natural constituent of $3T_3$ cells. This surface component, combining with complementary structures at the surface or within susceptible cells, may induce the cells to undergo the changes characteristic of cell contract inhibition (Cox and Gesner, 1968). Such a fucose-containing constituent might occur at the surface of normal cells and act by combining with complementary sites at the surfaces of susceptible cells, or it might occur as a macromolecular constituent of normal cells which gains entrance into susceptible cells and acts intracellularly.

Other cell lines, for example, those of established monkey kidney cells BSC-1 (Fig. 6–15) and certain strains of human skin

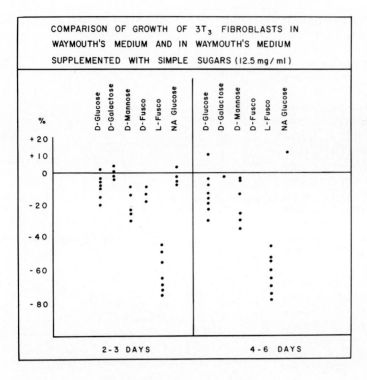

Figure 6–12 Comparison of growth of 3T$_3$ mouse fibroblasts in Waymouth's medium, and in Waymouth's medium containing 12.5 mg./ml. of various added sugars. It should be noted that Waymouth's medium contains 5 mg./ml. glucose. Each sugar to be studied was added to complete Waymouth's medium so as to provide 12.5 mg./ml. of added sugar. Each dot represents the average total cellular protein of three replicate bottles growth in a sugar when compared to the average total cellular protein of three replicate bottles growth in Waymouth's medium without added sugar (solid line). The percent reduction of growth in medium containing a sugar (ordinate) was calculated by taking the total protein in cells grown in Waymouth's medium (W), minus total protein in cells grown with added sugar (12.5 mg./ml.) (S), divided by total protein in cells grown in Waymouth's medium alone (W). Percent reduction in growth $= \dfrac{W - S}{W} \times 100$.

fibroblasts, respond dramatically to D-mannose, with alterations in cellular morphology and inhibition of cell growth. Moreover, in other cell lines, for example, the highly undifferentiated mouse L cells, none of the simple sugars which constitute the heterosaccharide components of mammalian cell surfaces affects cell morphology or growth. It is noteworthy that the high degree of structural specificity

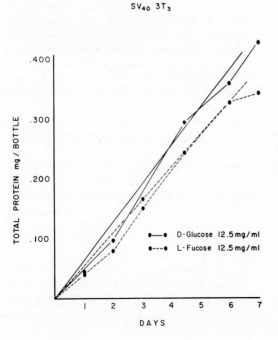

Figure 6–13 Comparison of effects of adding 12.5 mg./ml. of D-glucose or L-fucose to Waymouth's medium on the growth of 3T$_3$ mouse fibroblasts transformed by infection with oncogenic virus SV$_{40}$ (SV$_{40}$ 3T$_3$).

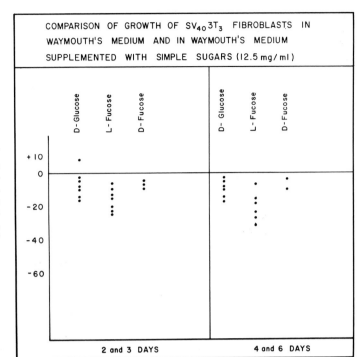

Figure 6–14 Comparison of growth of 3T₃ mouse fibroblasts transformed by infection with oncogenic virus (SV₄₀ 3T₃) in Waymouth's medium, and in Waymouth's medium containing 12.5 mg./ml. of various added sugars. See legend of Figure 6–12 for further experimental details.

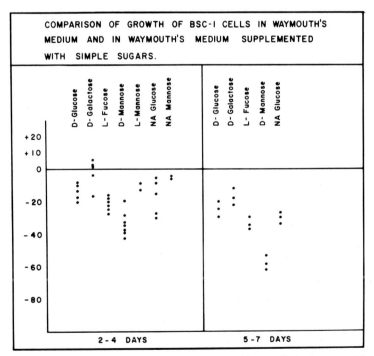

Figure 6–15 Comparison of growth of BSC-1 green monkey kidney cells in Waymouth's medium, and in Waymouth's medium containing 12.5 mg./ml. of various added sugars. See legend of Figure 6–12 for further experimental details.

required to produce these alterations is further demonstrated by the finding that stereoisomers of the effective sugars in an individual cell line had no apparent effect. The mechanism(s) of selective inhibition of cell growth by simple sugars is not known. Nevertheless, the findings demonstrate that naturally occurring saccharide constituents can profoundly alter the metabolism of selected mammalian cells, and this raises the possibility that the saccharide components of mammalian glycoproteins and cell structures might play an important role in the epigenetic regulation of cell growth and metabolism.

Further support of an epigenetic mechanism in cancer is provided by the recent experiments of Henry Harris and his coworkers (1969) on suppression of malignancy by fusing or hybridizing malignant and normal cells. These experiments show that certain nonmalignant cells contain a factor which can prevent the malignant potential from being expressed by a tumor line. Such effects are probably most compatible with regulating mechanisms associated with epigenetic controls. A possible candidate for such regulatory substances are the chalones, which inhibit cellular mitosis (Bullough and Laurence, 1968a). It has been shown that certain skin cancers (epidermal carcinoma, and melanotic and amelanotic melanomas) have reduced levels of chalones, although chalones continue to be synthesized in small amounts in these tumor cells. These cancer cells apparently retain their ability to respond to the tissue-specific epidermal chalones by a reduced mitotic rate when the chalone content of the tumors is artificially raised (Bullough and Laurence, 1968a, 1968b). Moreover, when epidermal chalones are administered to animals bearing metastatic melanomas, the tumor completely regresses (Mohr et al., 1968). These results support an epigenetic mechanism for tumor formation, since the neoplastic cells apparently retain the ability to respond in a normal fashion to a mitotic regulatory substance. It is of interest that the chalones are also synthesized by malignant cells; however, there appears to be an increased permeability of the neoplastic cell membrane to this substance, so that the concentration of chalones is reduced in tumors (Bullough and Laurence, 1968a; Rytömoa and Kiviniemi, 1968).

Epigenetic mechanisms for the origin of neoplasia predict that tumor cells are dedifferentiated, less specialized, and perhaps regressive in a functional sense. Support for this prediction is afforded by a study of protein and peptide products produced by tumor cells. Many neoplasms in humans produce hormone-like peptides—e.g., adrenocorticotropin, antidiuretic hormone, insulin, and parathormone (Hobbs and Miller, 1966). Some patients with hepatoma have a fetal α-globulin in their serum (Alpert et al., 1968). Fishman and his associates (1968) have found an unusual fetal-like alkaline phosphatase, the Regan isozyme, in the serum and tumors of some patients with disseminated carcinomas. Elson and Cox (1969) have characterized the immunologic and phenotypic characteristics of this enzyme in a human cervical carcinoma cell (HeLa) in tissue culture. They have shown that it is nearly identical to the fetal form of alkaline phosphatase found in the placentas of fetuses which are heterozygous for the F and S alleles.

The mechanism by which a neoplasm may inappropriately synthesize a biologically active protein normally produced only in certain specialized tissues (e.g., endocrine glands) or at a particular stage of development (e.g., intrauterine development) is not clear. One suggestion is that it may be due to somatic mutation or chromosomal rearrangement in malignant cells which lead to random alterations in the proteins normally produced, possibly resulting in partial duplication of the active sequences of some hormones or enzymes. This may be possible because the active site of a protein, which is responsible for its biologic effects, may represent only a small part of the molecule: for example, only 20 of the 84 amino acids in parathyroid hormone are required for biologic activity, and among these 20 some are more important than others (Potts et al., 1966). However, this probability of modifying a protein by chance to create a catalytic or endocrine activity seems remote, and this mechanism based on somatic mutation or chromosomal aberrations appears unlikely.

Another mechanism is based on the studies of Ghose et al. (1962), who have shown that some tumors can take up intact proteins from their environment. This raises the possibility that tumors may accumulate circulating hormones during their slow stages of growth and then release them in large amounts during their necrotic stage. This mechanism is also unlikely, since secretion of biologically active protein is not associated with necrotic changes in the neoplasm.

An epigenetic mechanism is the third and the most likely explanation (Gellhorn, 1963; Fishman et al., 1968; Elson and Cox, 1969). All somatic cells bear the same genetic complement in various states of repression. Derepression of a portion of the genotype in association with loss of cellular regulatory mechanism which characterizes malignant transformations might lead to the ectopic production of specialized protein by tumors.

If a unifying hypothesis for the origin of cancer is worth entertaining, it must explain certain rare but well-documented events. One of these is the spontaneous remission and/or maturation of certain malignant neoplasms, particularly in children. Metastatic nephroblastomas and neuroblastomas of childhood occasionally regress. In part, this might be due to the development of immunologic competence, which is then followed by rejection of the tumor (Burnet, 1967). In other cases it appears to be a maturation of a malignant tumor toward differentiated cell types (Willis, 1962). This maturation is reminiscent of embryologic differentiation and is again suggestive of epigenetic events.

An epigenetic mechanism as the cause of cancer has a corollary that the malignant state be reversible, and this is occasionally observed. Recent studies in cell culture further support this conclusion. Silagi and Bruce (1970) have shown that mouse melanoma cells grown in medium containing 5-bromodeoxyuridine (BUDR), an analogue of thymidine, regain contact inhibition of mitosis and locomotion and lose their tumorigenicity when injected into histocompatible hosts. The pyrimidine analogue does not affect cell growth or viability, although pigment production is greatly reduced. The effects of BUDR are reversed by growing cells in medium without the analogue. The reversible suppression of malignancy in a melanoma cell line suggests that both malignancy and differentiation may be regulated by similar mechanisms.

At the subcellular level, the two most probable theories on the origin of cancer are that (1) the fundamental event is a change in a gene or genes probably due to a chemical reaction involving DNA (somatic mutation), and (2) the decisive step occurs extragenetically (epigenetically) (Editorial, 1965). The failure to demonstrate a convincing connection between mutagenicity and carcinogenicity damages but does not exclude the somatic mutation theories, since mutagenesis is studied in unicellular organisms and carcinogenesis in mammals. Theories of epigenetic mechanisms are based in large part on the process of gene regulation in bacterial systems (Jacob and Monod, 1961) and in higher forms (Bonner et al., 1968). Gene regulation appears to be effected by small molecules which combine with repressors in microorganisms and alter the affinity of the repressor for DNA. In higher forms, regulator substances, for example, hormones, combine with receptors and the complex then alters the binding of nuclear proteins to segments of chromosomes. These regulator substances control the transcription of genes into messenger RNA. When this RNA is translated, it determines the spectrum of proteins produced and, thereby, also the biochemical function of cells. Elaborate theories which account for cancer on the basis of alterations in gene expression have been proposed (Hughes, 1965). Certain of these theories are based upon the cascade theory of multiple gene regulators (Britten and Davidson, 1969). The theories propose interlocking loops of sensors and receptors which control gene expression. However, these theories remain speculations until more is known about cell regulation and metabolic adaption in higher forms. Our ignorance of the way in which cancer arises is accurately reflected by the multitude of theories and speculations put forward in this review.

REFERENCES*

Aird, I., Bentall, H. H., and Roberts, F. J. A.: A relationship between cancer of stomach and ABO blood groups. Br. Med. J., 1:799, 1953.

Allison, A. C., and Paton, G. R.: Chromosome damage in human diploid cells following activation of lysosomal enzymes. Nature, 207:1170, 1965.

Alpert, M. E., Uriel, J., and de Nechaud, B.: Alpha fetoglobulin in the diagnosis of tumor hepatoma. N. Engl. J. Med., 278:984, 1968.

Aaronson, S. A., and Todaro, G. J.: Development of 3T3-like lines from Ba16/c mouse embryo cultures: Transformation susceptibility to SV40. J. Cell Physiol., 72:141, 1968.

Bashford, E. F.: Heredity in cancer. Lancet, II:1508, 1908.

Berenblum, I.: A speculative review: the probable nature of promoting action. Cancer Res., 14:471, 1954.

Beutler, E., Collins, Z., and Irwin, L. E.: Value of genetic variants of glucose-6-phosphate dehydrogenase in tracing the origin of malignant tumors. N. Engl. J. Med., 276:389, 1967.

Bittner, J. J.: Genetic concepts in mammary cancer in mice. Ann. N.Y. Acad. Sci., 71:943, 1958.

Bloom, G. E., Warner, S., Gerald, P. S., and Diamond, K.: Chromosome abnormalities in constitutional aplastic anemia. N. Engl. J. Med., 274:8, 1966.

Boone, C.: Cancer in Java and Sumatra. Am. J. Cancer, 25:811, 1935.

Bonner, J., Dahmus, M. E., Fambrough, D., Huang, R. C., Marushige, K., and Tuan, D. Y. H.: The biology of isolated chromatin. Science, 159:47, 1968.

Boveri, T.: The Origin of Malignant Cells. (Translation by M. Boveri.) Baltimore, The Williams & Wilkins Co., 1914.

Britten, R. J., and Davidson, E. H.: Gene regulation for higher cells: a theory. Science, 165:349, 1969.

Brookes, P., and Lawley, P. D.: Reaction of some mutagenic and carcinogenic compounds with nucleic acids. J. Cell Physiol., Suppl. 1, 64:111, 1964.

Bullough, W. S., and Laurence, E. B.: Epidermal chalone and mitotic control in the V x Z epidermal tumor. Nature, 220:134, 1968a.

Bullough, W. S., and Laurence, E. B.: Melanocyte chalone and mitotic control in melanoma. Nature, 220:137, 1968b.

Burnet, F. M.: Immunological aspects of malignant disease. Lancet, I:1171, 1967.

Butterworth, T., and Strean, L. P.: Clinical Genodermatology. Baltimore, The Williams & Wilkins Co., 1962.

Chu, E. H. Y., and Malling, H. V.: Mammalian cell genetics. II. Chemical induction of specific locus mutations in Chinese hamster cells in vitro. Proc. Nat. Acad. Sci. U.S.A., 61:1306, 1968.

Clarke, C. A.: Correlation of ABO groups with peptic ulcer, cancer and other diseases. J. Med. Educ., 34:400, 1959.

Cockayne, E. A.: Inherited Abnormalities of the Skin and Its Appendages. London, Oxford University Press, 1933.

Cox, R. P., and Gesner, B. M.: Effect of simple sugars on the morphology and growth pattern of mammalian cell cultures. Proc. Nat. Acad. Sci. U.S.A., 54:1571, 1965.

Cox, R. P., and Gesner, B. M.: Comparison of effects of simple sugars on 3T3 cells transformed by infection with oncogenic viruses. Cancer Res., 27:974, 1967a.

Cox, R. P., and Gesner, B. M.: Selective effects of L-fucose on BHK21 hamster fibroblasts and on BHK21 cells transformed by infection with polyoma virus. Exp. Cell Res., 49:682, 1967b.

Cox, R. P., and Gesner, B. M.: Studies on the effects of simple sugars on mammalian cells in culture and characterization of the inhibition of 3T3 fibroblasts by L-fucose. Cancer Res., 28:1162, 1968.

Davidson, R. G., Nitowsky, H. M., and Childs, B.: Demonstration of two populations of cells in the human female heterozygous for glucose-6-phosphate dehydrogenase variants. Proc. Nat. Acad. Sci. U.S.A., 50:481, 1963.

Dmochowski, L., Seman, G., and Gallagher, H. S.: Viruses as possible etiologic factors in human breast cancer. Cancer, 24:1241, 1969.

Dukes, C. E.: Familial intestinal polyposis. Ann. Eugen., 17:1, 1952.

Dulbecco, R.: Summary of 1964 Biology Research Conference, J. Cell. Physiol., Suppl. 1, 64:181, 1964.

Ebert, J. D.: Interacting Systems in Development. New York, Holt, Rinehart & Winston, Inc, 1965.

Editorial: Cancer theories. Lancet, I:1375, 1965.

El-Hefnawi, H., Smith, S. M., and Penrose, L. M.: Xeroderma pigmentosa—its inheritance and relationship to the ABO blood groups. Ann. Hum. Genet., 28:273, 1965.

Elson, N. A., and Cox, R. P.: Production of fetal-like alkaline phosphatase by HeLa cells. Biochem. Genet., 3:549, 1969.

Epstein, C. J., Martin, G. M., Schultz, A. L., and Motulsky, A. G.: Werner's syndrome: a review of its symptomatology, natural history, pathologic features, genetics and its relationship to the natural aging process. Medicine, 45:177, 1966.

Epstein, J. H., Fukuyama, K., Reed, W. B., and Epstein, W. L.: Defect in DNA synthesis in skin of patients with xeroderma pigmentosum demonstrated in vivo. Science, 168:1477, 1970.

Fadhi, G. G., and Dominguez, R.: ABO blood groups and multiple cancers. J.A.M.A., 185:757, 1963.

Fialkow, P. J.: X chromosome inactivation and the Xg locus. Am. J. Hum. Genet., 22:460, 1970.

Fialkow, P. J., Gartler, S. M., and Yoshida, A.: Clonal origin of chronic myelocytic leukemia in man. Proc. Nat. Acad. Sci. U.S.A., 58:1468, 1967.

Fialkow, P. J., Klein, G., Gartler, S. M., and Clifford, P.: Clonal origin for individual Burkett tumors. Lancet, I:384, 1970a.

Fialkow, P. J., Lisher, R., Giblett, E. R., and Zavola, R.: Xg locus: failure to detect inactivation in females with chronic myelocytic leukemia. Nature, 266:367, 1970b.

*Review of the literature was completed in June, 1970. For more recent references on the viral etiology of human tumors, the role of chromosome aberrations in neoplasia, and somatic mutations, see Wolman, S. R., and Horland, A. A.: Genetics of tumor cells. *In* Becker, F. F. (Ed.): Cancer: A Comprehensive Treatise. Vol. 3. New York, Plenum Press, 1975, pp. 155–198.

Fishman, W. H., Inglis, N. R., Green, S., Anstess, C. L., Ghose, N. K., Reif, A. E., Rustigian, R., Krant, M. J., and Stolback, L. L.: Immunology and biochemistry of Regan isoenzyme of alkaline phosphatase in human cancer. Nature, 219:697, 1968.

Fitzpatrick, T. B., and Quevedo, W. C.: Albinism. *In* Stanbury, J. B., Wyngaarden, J. B., and Frederickson, D. S. (Eds.): The Metabolic Basis of Inherited Disease. Ed. 2. New York, The McGraw-Hill Book Company, 1966.

Gardner, E. J., and Richards, R. C.: Multiple cutaneous and subcutaneous lesions occurring simultaneously with hereditary polyposis and osteomatosis. Am. J. Hum. Genet., 5:139, 1953.

Garriga, S., and Crosby, W. H.: The incidence of leukemia in families of patients with hypoplasia of the marrow. Blood, 14:1008, 1959.

Gartler, S. M., Ziprokowski, L., Krakowski, A., Ezra, R., Szeinberg, A., and Adams, A.: Glucose-6-phosphate dehydrogenase mosaicism as a tracer in the study of hereditary multiple trichoepithelioma. Am. J. Hum. Genet., 18:282, 1966.

Gates, R. R.: Cancer: the genetic aspects. *In* Human Genetics, 2:1170, 1946. New York, The Macmillan Company.

Gellhorn, A.: The unifying thread. Cancer Res., 23:961, 1963.

German, J., Archibald, R., and Bloom, D.: Chromosomal breakage in a rare and probably genetically determined syndrome of man. Science, 148:506, 1965.

Ghose, T., Nairn, R. C., and Fothergill, J. E.: Uptake of proteins by malignant cells. Nature, 196:1108, 1962.

Gorer, P. A.: Cancer. *In* Sorsby, A. (Ed.): Clinical Genetics. St. Louis, The C. V. Mosby Co., 1953, p. 558.

Gorlin, R. J., and Goltz, R. W.: Multiple nevoid basal cell epitheliomas, jaw cysts and bifid ribs. A syndrome. N. Engl. J. Med., 262:908, 1960.

Griffith, A. D., and Sorsby, A.: The genetics of retinoblastoma. Br. J. Ophthalmol. 28:279, 1944.

Gunz, F. W., Fitzgerald, P. N., and Adams, A.: Abnormal chromosome in chronic lymphocytic leukemia. Br. Med. J., 2:1097, 1962.

Harris, H., Miller, O. J., Klein, G., Worst, P., and Tachibana, T.: Suppression of malignancy by cell fusion. Nature, 223:363, 1969.

Harvald, B., and Hauge, M.: Heredity of cancer elucidated by a study of unselected twins. J.A.M.A., 186:749, 1963.

Heidelberger, C.: Studies on the molecular mechanism of hydrocarbon carcinogenesis. J. Cell Physiol., Suppl. 1, 64:129, 1964.

Hobbs, C. B., and Miller, A. L.: Review of endocrine syndromes associated with tumors of non-endocrine origin. J. Clin. Pathol., 19:119, 1966.

Howel-Evans, A. W., McConnel, R. B., Clarke, C. A., and Sheppard, P. M.: Carcinoma of the oesophagus with keratosis palmaris et plantaris (tylosis): a study of two families. Quart. J. Med., 22:413, 1958.

Hughes, P. E.: Chemical carcinogen and oncogenic virus: a possible interaction mechanism. Nature, 205:871, 1965.

Jacob, F., and Monod, J.: On the regulation of gene activity. Cold Spring Harbor Symp. Quant. Biol., 26:193, 1961.

Keeler, C. E.: Albinism, xeroderma pigmentosum and skin cancer. National Cancer Institute: International Conference of the Biology of Cutaneous Cancer (Monograph 10). U.S. Department of Health, Education and Welfare, 1963.

Kennaway, E. L.: Some biological aspects of Jewish ritual. Man, 57:65, 1957.

King, J. C.: Biology of Race. New York, Harcourt Brace Jovanovich, Inc., 1971.

King, J. C., and Cox, R. P.: The development of current genetic concepts. Semin. Hematol., 4:1, 1967.

Lawler, S. D., and Sanger, R.: Xg blood-groups and clonal origin theory of chronic myeloid leukemia. Lancet, I:584, 1970.

Lerman, L. S.: Acridine mutagens and DNA structure. J. Cell Physiol., Suppl. 1, 64:1, 1964.

Linder, D., and Gartler, S. M.: Distribution of glucose-6-phosphate dehydrogenase electrophoretic variants in different tissues of heterozygotes. Am. J. Hum. Genet., 17:212, 1965.

Little, C. C.: The relation of coat color to the spontaneous incidence of mammary tumors in mice. J. Exp. Med., 59:229, 1934.

Lynch, H. T.: "Cancer families.": adenocarcinomas (endometrial and colon carcinoma) and multiple primary malignant neoplasms. *In* Lynch, H. T. (Ed.): Hereditary Factors in Carcinoma—Recent Results in Cancer Research, 12:125. New York, Springer-Verlag New York, Inc., 1967.

Lyon, M. F.: Sex chromatin and gene action in the mammalian X-chromosome. Am. J. Hum. Genet., 14:135, 1962.

Macklin, M. T.: Analysis of tumors in monozygous and dizygous twins; with report of 15 unpublished cases. J. Hered., 31:277, 1940.

Makino, S., Sasaki, M. S., and Tonomura, A.: Cytological studies of tumors. XL. Chromosome studies in fifty-two human tumors. J. Nat. Cancer Inst., 32:741, 1964.

McCurdy, P. R.: Discussion: The genetics of glucose-6-phosphate dehydrogenase deficiency. *In* Beutler, E. (Ed.): Hereditary Disorders of Erythrocyte Metabolism. New York, Grune & Stratton, Inc., 1968, p. 121.

Merey, D. B.: The complete replication pattern of the allocyclic X chromosome in a normal female. Ph.D. Thesis, New York University, 1970.

Mohr, U., Althoff, J., Kinzel, V., Süss, R., and Valm, M.: Melanoma regression induced by "chalone": a new tumor inhibiting principle acting in vivo. Nature, 220:138, 1968.

Nowell, P. C., and Hungerford, D. A.: A minute chromosome in human chronic granulocytic leukemia. Science, 132:1497, 1960.

Nowell, P. C., and Hungerford, D. A.: Chromosome changes in human leukemia and a tentative assessment of their significance. Ann. N.Y. Acad. Sci., 113:654, 1964.

Oettle, A.: Geographical and racial differences in the frequency of Kaposi's sarcoma as evidence of environmental or genetic causes. Acta Un. Int. Cancer, 18:330, 1962.

Old, L. J., Boyse, E. A., and Oettgen, H. F.: Precipitating antibody in human serum to an antigen present in cultured Burketts lymphoma cells. Proc. Nat. Acad. Sci. U.S.A., 56:1699, 1966.

Osborne, R. H., and De George, F. V.: The ABO blood groups in neoplastic disease of the ovary. Am. J. Hum. Genet., 15:380, 1963.

Page, A. R., Berendes, H., Warner, J., and Good, R. A.: Chediak-Higashi syndrome. Blood, 20:330, 1962.

Peterson, R. D., Kelly, W., and Good, R. A.: Ataxia-telangiectasia. Its association with a defective thymus, immunologic deficiency disease, and malignancy. Lancet I:1189, 1964.

Pollock, R. J., and Todaro, G. J.: Radiation enhancement of SV40 transformation in 3T3 and human cells. Nature, 219:520, 1968.

Potts, J. T., Aurbach, G. D., and Sherwood, L. M.: Parathyroid hormone: chemical properties and structural requirements for biological and immunological activity. Recent Progr. Horm. Res., 22:101, 1966.

Regan, J. D., Trosko, J. E., and Carrier, W. L.: Evidence for excision of ultraviolet induced pyrimidine dimers from the DNA of human cells in vitro. Biophys. J., 8:319, 1968.

Roberts, J. A. F.: Some association between blood groups and disease. Br. Med. Bull., 15:129, 1959.

Rytömoa, T., and Kiviniemi, K.: Control of cell production in rat chloroleukemia by means of granulocytic chalone. Nature, 220:136, 1968.

Sawitsky, A., Bloom, D., and German, J.: Chromosomal breakage and acute leukemia in congenital telangiectatic erythema and stunted growth. Ann. Int. Med., 64:487, 1966.

Schroeder, T. M., Anschütz, F., and Knopp, A.: Spontane chromosomenaberrationen bei familiären Panmyelopathie. Humangenetik, 1:194, 1964.

Shivas, A. A. (Ed.): Racial and Geographical Factors in Tumor Incidence. Medical Monograph 2. Edinburgh University Press, 1967.

Siemens, W., and Kohn, E.: Z. Indukt. Abstamm-u Vereblehre, 38:1, 1925.

Silagi, S., and Bruce, S. A.: Suppression of malignancy and differentiation in melanotic melanoma cells. Proc. Nat. Acad. Sci., 66:72, 1970.

Sibler, R., and Bertino, J.: Metabolism of granulocytes. *In* Williams, W. J., et al. (Eds.): Hematology. McGraw-Hill Book Co., 1972, p. 575.

Solomon, L.: Hereditary multiple exostosis. J. Bone-Joint Surg. (Br.), 4513:292, 1963.

Stern, C.: Selection and polymorphism. *In* Human Genetics, San Francisco, W. H. Freeman & Company, 1960.

Stewart, A. M.: Gene-selection theory of cancer causation. Lancet, I:923, 1970.

Stewart, A. M., and Kneale, G. W.: Radiation dose effects in relation to obstetric X-rays and childhood cancer. Lancet, I:1185, 1970a.

Stewart, A. M., and Kneale, G. W.: Age distribution of cancer caused by obstetric X-rays and their relevance to cancer latent periods. Lancet, II:4, 1970b.

Straith, F. E.: Hereditary epidermoid cyst of the jaw. Am. J. Orthod., 25:673, 1939.

Swift, M. R.: Fanconi's anemia in the genetics of neoplasia. Nature, 230:370, 1971.

Swift, M. R., and Hirschhorn, K.: Fanconi's anemia: inherited susceptibility to chromosome breakage in various tissues. Ann. Int. Med., 65:496, 1966.

Todaro, G. J., Green, H., and Swift, M. R.: Susceptibility of human diploid fibroblast strains to transformation by SV40 virus. Science, 153:1252, 1966.

Todaro, G. J., Lazar, G. K., and Green, H.: Initiation of cell division in a contact-inhibited mammalian cell line. J. Cell Physiol., 66:325, 1965.

Vogel, F.: ABO Blood groups and disease. Am. J. Hum. Genet., 22:464, 1970.

Waaler, G. H. M.: Uber die erblichkeit des krebses. Norsk. Vidensk. Akad. Skt. Mat. Nat. Kl. No. 2, 1931.

Warburg, O.: On respiratory impairment in cancer cells. Science, 124:269, 1956.

Warthin, A. S.: Heredity with reference to carcinoma. Arch. Intern. Med., 12:546, 1913.

Werner, P.: Genetic aspects of adenomatoses of endocrine glands. Am. J. Med., 16:363, 1954.

Wiener, A. S.: Blood groups and disease. Am. J. Hum. Genet., 22:476, 1970.

Williams, E. D., Brown, C. L., and Doniach, I.: Pathological series of 67 cases of medullary carcinoma of the thyroid. J. Clin. Path., 19:103, 1966.

Willis, R. A.: The Borderland of Embryology and Pathology. Ed. 2. London, Butterworths, 1962.

Witkin, E. M.: Radiation-induced mutations and their repair. Science, 152:1345, 1966.

7

*The Biology of Cutaneous Aging**

Lawrence M. Solomon, M.D.,
and Christopher Virtue, M.D.

Time writes no wrinkle on thine azure brow,
Such as creation's dawn beheld, thou rollest now.

Lord Byron: Childe Harold

Unlike the never-changing face of the ocean in the poet's vision the skin provides man with a constant visible reminder of his aging body. Not all people, however, show the ravages of time and the elements equally, nor does the entire skin surface age uniformly. Both the epidermis and dermis undergo an aging process, but, depending on the individual's genetic background, his lifelong exposure to light, the degree of his cutaneous pigmentation, and other factors, there are marked variations in visible aging suffered by the component parts of the skin.

This chapter will briefly review some of the currently held views about the biology of aging and the effects of aging on cutaneous morphology and function.

Theories of Aging

A number of theories have been advanced to explain the morphologic and biochemical events occurring in senescence. The theories may all be partially in accord with data accumulated by a variety of experiments dealing with the subject, but all of them are, at least in part, deficient to explain other observable phenomena. For this reason the cause (if there is a single cause) of aging remains unknown; however, a very brief review of some of the major hypotheses may be of interest. There is no special significance or importance intended in the order of presentation of these theories.

Fibrosis Theory (Verzar, 1957; Gross, 1961). This theory holds that aging is the result of the deposit of excessive connective tissue, mainly collagen and amorphous ground substance. Collagen is said to have an extremely low turnover rate, so that little is absorbed; therefore, it is said to interfere with the gaseous interchanges required for cellular respiration and cellular nutrition.

---

*This chapter originally appeared in Internatl. J. Dermatol., 14:172–181, 1975.

The Effete Metabolism (Wear and Tear) Theory (Rubner, 1908). With time, certain metabolic processes wear out, and the required elements are not replaced. Some of these losses may include protein synthesis and hormones.

The Accumulation of Breakdown Products Theory (Packer et al., 1967). Tied to the previous theory, this theory states that certain breakdown products accumulate with time and injure normal cellular processes. Some of these insoluble products include lipofuscin pigments, calcium salts, proteins, and nucleic acids.

Molecular Errors Theory (Orgel, 1963). During synthesis, an occasional mistake may occur in which a wrong amino acid is substituted in a protein chain. The results may be of little importance if the error occurs at the end stage of synthesis — that is, in the protein itself. If the mistake occurs in a protein-synthesizing enzyme, however, then all the proteins produced by that enzyme will be abnormal, leading to an expotentially increasing error which may be incompatible with life.

The Increased Cross-linking Theory (Verzar, 1962; Piez, 1968). Strands of collagen and DNA become increasingly stable by chemical bonds bridging appropriately reactive molecules, thus decreasing the neoformation of young collagen and impairing cellular DNA regeneration.

The Gene Mutation Theory (Curtis and Gebhard, 1958; Curtis, 1965). Gene mutations may occur spontaneously or as a result of radiation. Mutant genes may then proliferate and carry misinformation, which eventually results in senescence.

The Chromosomal Theory (Sandberg et al., 1967; Court-Brown et al., 1966). Aside from gene mutations, abnormalities may exist in a number of aberrant chromosomal mitotic figures. These, in turn, produce abnormal cells, which increase in number with the passage of time.

The Free Radical or Auto-oxidation Theory (Harman, 1968). Polyunsaturated fatty acids in the presence of biologic metal complexes undergo oxidation-degradation to yield free hydroxyl, hydroperoxy radicals and malondialdehyde, which in turn attack cellular membranes and mitochondria, thus disrupting their integrity. This leads to cellular destruction and the formation of pigments such as lipofuscin. The free radical theory is a variant of the older theory concerning the accumulation of noxious by-products of metabolism.

The Autoimmune Theory (Walford, 1967). This theory hypothesizes that as age advances there is an increased number of mutated immunocytes whose clones will increasingly attack normal cells, since they become less capable of differentiating "self" from "nonself." Or it hypothesizes that there is a loss of histocompatibility tolerance homeostatic mechanisms, which in turn may reflect the results of a retardation in thymic function. In other words, mutated clones which would normally be eliminated become tolerated, and these clones attack normal tissue as a "graft"-versus-"host" reaction.

Programmed Death (Hayflick, 1965). It has been observed that cells kept in tissue culture undergo a finite number of divisions which end in loss of the clone. It should be pointed out that not all tissues undergo cellular division, but the experiments of Hayflick do suggest that aging may appear to be related to a programmed message within organelles of cells that have some finite number of normal replication activities built into them. If programmed death has relevance to the human life span, it does not attempt to explain the prevailing limitations on human life span, since the organism dies long before cell replication has stopped.

Noncycling Cells. A more recent theory arising from the observations of Hayflick also ties aging to cellular turnover, which in turn is related to the cell cycle. Gelfant and Graham Smith (1972) have suggested that tissue aging may be the consequence of an increasing number of cells converting from a cyclical to a noncyclical state. This cell-specific and tissue-specific phenomenon was found to be present in vivo and in vitro in those tissues capable of proliferation. After undergoing mitosis cells normally enter a G_1 phase, followed by an S phase (DNA synthesis), enter a G_2 phase, and then re-enter mitosis. Aging, it is believed by the authors, results when cells are blocked in the G_1 phase (interrupting DNA synthesis) or G_2 phase (inhibiting mitosis). It was found that release from these blocks inhibits aging. Block release may be achieved by decreasing cell density, removing some of the tissue, or administering corticosteroids.

Genetic Variability

Pedigree studies have not settled the recurring question of whether the offspring of long-lived individuals live longer. In part, the difficulties encountered in these studies lie in the inadequacy of birth documentation in parts of the world prior to 1900. Monozygotic and dizygotic twin studies have so far not given completely satisfactory answers either, though in general monozygotic twins are more concordant for longevity than dizygotic twins (Jarvik, 1971).

CUTANEOUS AGING

Several of the proposed causes of aging discussed previously may enter into the cutaneous aging process, since skin is a dynamic organ sharing the remainder of the body's common metabolic resources. Two elements play a particularly important role in the development of "old" skin: the skin's exposed position in regard to ultraviolet light, and the individual's genetic background.

Premature aging of the skin may be seen in a variety of hereditary conditions which permit study of several of its biologic characteristics. In *xeroderma pigmentosum* the skin undergoes an extremely rapid aging process, primarily epidermal in its manifestations and affecting both melanocytes and keratinocytes. The dermis is also affected, but clinically it is the epidermal changes which are most marked. Xeroderma pigmentosum is transmitted by a recessive autosomal gene and results in an enzymatic defect in DNA repair. When DNA is altered by ultravio-

let light, one enzyme (an endonuclease) is responsible for excising the affected pyrimidine base and another (a ligase) for replacing it with a normal one (Cleaver, 1970). In xeroderma pigmentosum the excising enzyme is defective, resulting in skin which is highly susceptible to ultraviolet light damage. The damaged DNA then goes on to proliferate, resulting in the very early formation of tumors such as basal cell epitheliomas, squamous cell epitheliomas, malignant melanomas, and their precursors. The skin acquires the mottled hyperpigmentation of the aged. The defect is apparently limited to ultraviolet light repair; other radiation (such as X radiation) repair is not involved. In *progeria* and *Werner's syndrome*, the skin also ages very rapidly, the predominant feature being dermal loss including the appendages, such as hair. The subjects affected by progeria at age 10 years look like little old people. This appearance of old age is supported by the histologic finding of lipofuscin in the organs and by fibroblasts incapable of existence in culture beyond two cell divisions (Goldstein, 1969; Martin et al., 1970). Other hereditary diseases may result in the *appearance* of premature aging, but the phenotypic changes do not necessarily indicate the presence of true premature aging.

The environment, including diet and light, plays an important role in premature aging. The person whose occupation requires work in the sun or the sun-worshiping fair-skinned individual risks the early appearance of an aged skin because of the noxious effects of ultraviolet light on the epidermis and dermis (see below).

Morphologic Changes in Cutaneous Aging

We are all familiar with the overt changes that occur in the skin of the aged. The exposed parts are affected most. The skin becomes "dry," wrinkled, and unevenly hyperpigmented; it acquires actinic and seborrheic keratoses, has a greater propensity to the development of neoplasia, loses its firmness, develops elastotic nodules, and changes its hair distribution and quality. These changes may be examined at a histologic level and will be reviewed in the subsequent paragraphs.

The Epidermis (Montagna, 1965; Montagna and Parakkal, 1974; Andrews, 1971). The component cells of the epidermis are keratinocytes, melanocytes, and Langerhans' cells (the function of Langerhans' cells remains elusive). The keratinocytes, as they ascend from basal layer to surface, are gradually converted to anucleic containers of the protein keratin. At the exterior of the epidermis, the keratinocytes form the stratum corneum.

With increasing age the following changes may be seen: the epidermis decreases in thickness, and the rete ridges become flatter. An increasing disparity in the size and shape of the nuclei and cells of the basal and malpighian layers develops. The cells are no longer aligned in an orderly fashion. The basement membrane becomes irregular. The staining qualities of the epidermal cells change, and glycogen appears in the upper layers of the epidermis. The thickness of the stratum corneum itself does not change in the aged, nor is there a change in the number of cells in the stratum corneum. The flattening of the epidermis may also be looked upon as the result of a decrease in the number of rete pegs, since with increasing years there is a steady decrease in dermal papillae and their corresponding rete pegs. We will not discuss here the increased incidence in the epidermis of the aged of the common benign and malignant epidermal tumors of keratinocyte and melanocyte dealt with extensively in the remainder of this text.

THE MELANOCYTIC SYSTEM (Fitzpatrick et al., 1965). The melanocyte and the keratinocytes which it supplies with melanin form a functional unit providing the skin with its basic protective response to noxious ultraviolet irradiation. As aging takes place, the number of DOPA-positive melanocytes decreases in both exposed and covered areas. In sun-exposed regions, pigmentary discontinuity in the basal layer results. The loss of functioning melanocytes is accompanied by a loss of pigmented basal cells; but melanin remains in keratinocytes that are still being fed by DOPA-positive melanocytes and in those that phagocytose cell-free melanin. These changes result in an increase of the keratinocyte/melanocyte ratio. This ratio is about 16:1. The increase in lentigos in the aged is due to *localized* abnormal proliferations of melanocytes at the dermo-epidermal junction. In spite of the overall loss of active melanocytes, the general effect of aging is spotty hyperpigmentation in the parts of the body chronically exposed to ultraviolet light. Hyperpigmentation is interspersed with areas of hypopigmentation.

Hair pigment decreasing with age results in the familiar and often unwelcome graying. Graying results from the replacement of fully pigmented hair by an increasing number of depigmented or lightly pigmented hairs. Premature graying is a dominant familial trait, but even the common graying phenomenon is determined by genetic background, age, and hair distribution on the body surface. Graying with age occurs mostly between the ages of 45 and 55 years. It starts at the temples and moves toward the scalp's vertex. The hairy areas away from the head may uncommonly participate in the graying phenomenon. Graying results from a decrease in tyrosinase-positive melanocytes in the hair bulbs of the depigmented hairs. White hair bulbs examined by electron microscopy are found to be lacking in both pigment and melanocytes.

The Cutaneous Appendages

THE HAIR. (Montagna, 1965; Giacometti, 1965). In addition to the pigmentary changes described above, the quality, quantity, and distribution of hair undergo considerable change with advancing age. The factors causing these changes are, in part, unknown. Those factors known to play a role are endocrine changes, sex of the individual, general state of health, nutrition, and the genetically controlled end-organ responsiveness to androgens and estrogens. The quality of hair undergoes a change which results in an increase in the number of vellus hairs on the scalp, a decrease in facial hair in men, and an increasing thickness of hair on the face of women. The eyebrows become thicker and longer. The number of hair follicles on the scalp decreases by about one-third, resulting in a distinctively patterned hair loss. Male pattern baldness is an expression not only of age but also of genotype and androgen activity. The hair in the aged scalp is very small compared to the sebaceous gland to which it is attached. In addition, there are visible changes in the arrectores pilorum muscle, which loses its attachment to the hair follicle. The follicle itself undergoes a relentless change in male pattern alopecia; the coarse terminal (young adult) hair is replaced by a fine vellus hair which, because of its decreased pigment and thin structure, becomes less visible. Some (but not all) of these vellus hairs may then be lost. From the cosmetic viewpoint, hair loss, although it may not be as complete as many patients believe, is as real as it seems. Hair follicles are usually clustered in groups of four or five. Aging results in vellus hair formation, first within the groups, then in entire groups, then in entire areas.

THE NAILS. The nails' rate of growth decreases with advancing age.

Sebaceous Glands (Montagna, 1965; Giacometti, 1965). These cannot be considered completely apart from the hair follicle, since the hair with its appended sebaceous gland forms a functional unit. Nor can the activity of sebaceous glands be clearly correlated with their histologic appearance, since there is little difference in the morphologic characteristics of a less active and a more active gland. According to Montagna (1965), however, "The sebaceous glands in the aged face have fewer blood vessels around them; and the gland parenchyma contains much more phosphorylase and glycogen than does that of young subjects. These features, while not all absolutely peculiar to aged skin, are more pronounced than in the skin of young subjects."

The Apocrine Glands. The apocrine glands have not been shown to undergo specific changes in old age. Some aged glands appear to have dilated segments and to become cystic, while others remain normal (Montagna and Parakkal, 1974).

Eccrine Glands. (Montagna, 1965; Oberste-Lehn, 1965). The eccrine sweat glands are activated within the first few months of life and remain active until senescence, at which time a degenerative process takes place. The coiled secretory portion of the gland undergoes a change in which its epithelium becomes irregular and the clear cells and the dark cells lining the lumen change in some of their staining properties. Rosette-shaped pigmented granules accumulate within the cellular portion of the gland, and the intercellular canaliculi become less clearly visible with argyrophilic stains. Some glands may be completely lost. In the scalp, sweat gland density does not change once adulthood has been achieved.

The Dermis. The dermis consists primarily (about 80 percent) of the fibrous protein collagen, but it also contains mucopolysaccharides, elastic tissue, water, electrolytes, fibroblasts, histiocytes, plasma cells, polymorphonuclear leukocytes, mast cells and other mononuclear cells, blood vessels, and nerves.

COLLAGEN (Andrews, 1971; Sams and Smith, 1965; Rasmussen et al., 1965; Jackson, 1965; Joseph, 1971; Elden, 1971; Pearce and Grimmer, 1972). The collagenous portion of the dermis undergoes profound change with the aging process; yet one must consider collagen in the context of the complex matrix it forms in conjunction with ground substance, water, electrolytes, and elastin. Collagen is formed by fibroblasts which extrude a precursor as a three-stranded, helical, elongated rod. These rods aggregate into fibrils and become increasingly organized into larger, thicker bundles or fibers. As age increases, less collagen is formed, and the turnover of older collagen decreases. The anatomic changes in collagen include a thickening of the collagen fibrils into bundles or fibers with decreasing interfibrillar ground substance. Fine structural changes in the fibroblast include the appearance of irregular crystal in the mitochondria and dense particles in the matrix, and the formation of vesicular changes in the endoplasmic reticulum. Functional changes in collagen also occur with the passage of time, but these are difficult to ascribe *solely* to the aging process. The reported changes (with many conflicting statements) are biochemical and physical. There is a decreased solubility of aged collagn in neutral salt, weak acids, and cold alkali; there is a decrease in collagen-bound water and an increase in collagen nitrogen. The extensibility of collagen decreases with age, possibly because the cohesion of collagen molecules increases, thus increasing its tensile properties. This observation persists in the face of the decreasing thickness of the dermis with age. The collagen molecules undergo an increase in intra- and intermolecular bonding (cross-linking), which augments their stability. The bonds formed are of the covalent type (esters). This stability also results in a small increase, with age, in the temperature at which rapid shrinkage of collagen begins (shrinkage temperature). Isometric tension produced by thermally treated collagen increases markedly with age.

ELASTIC TISSUE. Elastin is an insoluble, amorphous, extensible protein which makes up about 2 percent of the dry weight of the dermis. Its physical, chemical, tinctorial, and morphologic characteristics are quite unlike those of collagen. Morphologically, it is extremely difficult to distinguish changes in elastic tissue that occur as a result of aging from those caused by actinic damage. Some chemical changes in elastin, however, have been observed in aged dermis. There is some evidence that, like collagen, elastin undergoes an increased cross-linking process with age. Furthermore, the amino acid, lysine, contained in elastin is found to decrease with age. The reasons for this are unknown, but lysine is believed to participate in the cross-linking process. Additional chemical changes include the appearance of sugars, lipids, and polar amino acids (e.g., glutamic and aspartic acids) within the elastic tissue. Partridge (1971) believes that this last finding may be a result of free radical action. Patchy mineralization with calcium also occurs, but its cause and effect is unknown. Pearse and Grimmer (1972) found a nearly threefold relative increase in dermal elastin between the ages of 20 and 80 years.

GROUND SUBSTANCE (Samitz et al., 1965). The ground substance is a gel-like matrix of mucopolysaccharides, water, electrolytes, serum proteins, vasoactive peptides, and so forth. The major constituents of ground substance are the mucopolysaccharides, hyaluronic acid, chondroitin sulfate B (dermatan sulfate), chondroitin sulfate C, and heparin. Mucopolysaccharides function as a colloid able to hold water and to impede the flow of cells, antigens, and antibodies; they join with fibrous collagen and elastin in providing a flexible, resilient, compressible body cover as well as a source of nutrition for and interaction with the epidermis. Anyone working with aged and youthful skin experimentally must be impressed by the fibrous "toughness" of the latter and the gel-like nature of the former.

Chemical examination of the aged skin in some studies suggests a decrease in dermal water and acid mucopolysaccharides. The decrease in hyaluronic acid, occurring mostly in the period from birth to childhood, exceeds that of chondroitin sulfate. A consideration of dermal hydration has led to some interesting hypotheses regarding dermal water binding. Loosely bound water is thought to be the first lost in the process of senescent dehydration. The studies of Pearce and Grimmer (1972), in contrast to others, have found an *increase* in dermal water content with increasing age. They reasoned that increased water in ground substance may lead to erroneous conclusions about how much mucopolysaccharide is present, and in fact, they believe there is no decrease in MPS with age. They further believe that some of the dermal clearance changes might in fact be due to the physicochemical changes (gel to sol) which may result from the water increase.

The amount of water present in the dermis depends on many variables, including electrolyte balance, adrenal, pituitary, thyroid, and gonadal hormones, and neurohypophyseal activity. Water metabolism in aging skin remains an interesting and fertile area for further investigation.

NERVES (Winkelmann, 1965). The effect of aging on dermal nerves has been studied by Cauna and also by Winkelmann. Both authors found a steady decrease in the number of Meissner's corpuscles with increasing age. The form of the corpuscle changed as well, resulting in its progressive elongation, coiling, and lobulation. The nerve endings within Meissner's corpuscles were found to become coarser and irregular. Pacinian corpuscles also underwent some changes in size and form. Free nerve endings were not found to change significantly.

It should be stressed that the neural changes seen in the aging dermis do not necessarily reflect the process of aging but may represent a process of adaptation to changing needs in the internal environmental milieu.

VESSELS. The occurrence of senile purpura is common in the aged skin. This is more likely the result of changes in the vascular support tissue, collagen and ground substance, than in the vessels themselves. Cutaneous vessels may undergo a series of nonspecific changes after damage by sunlight, dermatitis, minor trauma, and so forth. Microangiopathic changes may also be seen in association with diabetes mellitus, in which the damaged vessels show thickening of the endothelial lining and a deposit of PAS-positive material between the basement membrane and the endothelial cells. These changes, though commonly found in aged skin, cannot be shown to be due to age alone, since they may also be found in young patients whose skin has undergone an inflammatory episode (Bercovici et al., 1964). Ellis (1961) found disorganization of the normal architectural arrangement of the blood vessels in the scalp of the aged; as the epidermis flattened, so did the capillary loops in the papillae.

Functional Variations in Aging Skin

Epidermal Hydration. The clinician is extremely familiar with the common complaint of "dry skin" in the elderly. The sensation of dryness is frequently the result of a mild dermatitis which leads to itchiness in dry winter conditions. Humidity in centrally heated houses may reach levels below 10 percent, and this condition is poorly tolerated by the elderly. In fact, studies of the horny layer in the aged has shown that, although there are some cytologic abnormalities in it, the stratum corneum shows no decrease in its ability to restrict water loss (Orentreich, 1971).

Epidermal Permeability. In vitro the epidermis of the aged is *more* permeable than that of the young, yet in vivo it appears to be *less* permeable. This apparent contradiction should be seen from the perspective of the reduced clearance rates of substances entering the aged dermis. The movement of foreign substances through old collagen and ground substance is decreased. As a result, substances enter senescent skin readily but have trouble being quickly removed. The retention of foreign chemicals may lead to increased reactivity to primary irritants. The dermis exposed to chronic solar radiation has a greater diffusion capacity, and thus percutaneous absorption and clearance are increased (Orentriech, 1971).

Sweating. Spontaneous sweating decreases as a function of age, and this is true of both males and females. The decrease in digital sweating observed by Silver et al. (1965) was in the range of 70 percent. The cause of reduced sweating may be in part, a reduction in the number of active glands, but the reduction in the output per gland probably also plays a role.

Pharmacologic Changes. Since aged stratum corneum is more permeable and the clearance rate from its dermis is decreased, the risk of primary irritant contact dermatitis is increased. The potential for allergic sensitization, however, does not increase. In the younger individual, a parallel situation exists in the area of chronic stasis dermatitis of the legs. The epidermis is damaged and has increased permeability, while the chronic fibrotic and vascular changes in the dermis decrease clearance from the dermis. In the latter circumstances, there is an increased potential for allergic sensitization. The difference between the incidence of allergic contact dermatitis in the two groups must therefore be a function of age rather than of change in the skin itself.

The sweating response to certain pharmacologic agents also has been shown to change with age. The sweat response to epinephrine decreases in men and women, whereas the response to methacholine chloride (Mecholyl) decreases only in men (Silver et al., 1965).

Wound Healing (Orentreich, 1971). Superficial epithelial wounds show a diminished healing rate in aging skin. The differences, though real, may not be great enough to be apparent in gross surgical repair healing time.

Sebaceous Gland Function (Pochi and Strauss, 1965). Changes in endocrine secretion with advancing age profoundly affect sebum secretion. As androgen production falls in both men and women, so does the activity of the sebaceous glands.

REFERENCES

Andrews, W.: The Anatomy of Aging in Man and Animals. New York, Grune and Stratton, 1971, p. 71.

Bercovici, E., Solomon, L. M., and Beerman, H.: Microangiopathy in diabetes mellitus and nondiabetic dermatoses. Am. J. Med. Sci., 248:54, 1964.

Christophers, E., and Kligman, A. M.: Percutaneous absorption in aged skin. *In* Montagna, W. (Ed.): Advances in Biology of Skin: Aging. Vol. 6. New York, Pergamon Press, 1965, p. 163.

Cleaver, J. E.: DNA damage and repair in light sensitive human skin disease. J Invest. Dermatol., 54:181, 1970.

Court-Brown, W. M., Buckton, K. E., Jacobs, P. A., Tough, I. M., Kuenssberg, E. V., and Knox, J. D. E.: Chromosome Studies in Adults. London, Cambridge University Press, 1966.

Curtis, H. J.: The role of somatic mutations in aging. *In* Krohn, P. L. (Ed.): Topics in the Biology of Aging. New York, Interscience, 1965, p. 63.

Curtis, H. J., and Gebhard, K. L.: Comparison of life-shortening effects of toxic and radiation stresses. Radiat. Res., 9:104, 1958.

Elden, H. R.: Biophysical properties of aging skin. *In* Montagna, W., Bentley, J. P., and Dobson, R. L. (Eds.): Advances in Biology of Skin: The Dermis. Vol. X. New York, Appleton-Century-Crofts, 1971, p. 231.

Ellis, R. A.: Vascular patterns of the skin. *In* Montagna, W., and Ellis, R. A. (Eds.): Advances in Biology of Skin: Blood Vessels and Circulation. Vol. 11. New York, Pergamon Press, 1961, p. 20.

Fitzpatrick, T. B., Szabo, G., and Mitchell, R. E.: Age changes in the human melanocyte system. *In* Montagna, W. (Ed.): Advances in Biology of Skin: Aging. Vol. 6. New York, Pergamon Press, 1965, p. 17.

Gelfant, S., and Graham Smith, J.: Aging: Noncycling cells—an exploration. Science, 178:357, 1972.

Giacometti, L.: The anatomy of the human scalp. *In* Montagna, W. (Ed.): Advances in Biology of Skin: Aging. Vol. 6. New York, Pergamon Press, 1965, p. 97.

Goldstein, S.: Lifespan of cultured cells in progeria. Lancet, 1:424, 1969.

Gross, J.: The aging of connective tissue: The extracellular components. *In* Bourne, G. H. (Ed.): Structural Aspects of Aging. New York, Hafner, 1961.

Harman, D.: Free radical theory of aging: Effect of free radical reaction inhibition on the mortality rate of male LAF₁ mice. J. Gerontol., 23;476, 1968.

Hayflick, L.: The limited in vitro lifetime of human diploid cell strains. Exp. Cell. Res., *37*:614, 1965.

Jackson, D. S.: Temporal changes in collagen—Aging or essential maturation? *In* Montagna, W. (Ed.): Advances in Biology of Skin: Aging. Vol. 6. New York, Pergamon Press, 1965, p. 219.

Jarvik, L.: Genetic aspects of aging. *In* Rossman, I. (Ed.): Clinical Geriatrics. Philadelphia, J. B. Lippincott Company, 1971, p. 85.

Joseph, N. R.: Physical chemistry of aging. *In* Blumenthal, H. T., (Ed.): Interdisciplinary Topics in Gerontology. Vol. 8. New York, S. Karger, 1971.

Martin, G. M., Sprague, C. A., and Epstein, C. S.: Replicative life span of cultivated human cells: Effects of donor's age, tissue and genotype. Lab. Invest., 23:86, 1970.

Montagna, W.: Morphology of aging skin. *In* Montagna, W. (Ed.): Advances in Biology of Skin: Aging. Vol. 6. New York, Pergamon Press, 1965, p. 2.

Montagna, W., and Parakkal, P. F.: The Structure and Function of Skin. Ed. 3. New York, Academic Press, 1974, p. 355.

Oberste-Lehn, H.: Effects of aging on the papillary body of the hair follicles and on the eccrine sweat glands. *In* Montagna, W. (Ed.): Advances in Biology of Skin: Aging. Vol. 6. New York, Pergamon Press, 1965, p. 17.

Orentreich, N.: Biological aspects of the aging skin. *In* Montagna, W., Bentley, J. P., and Dobson, R. L. (Eds.): Advances in Biology of Skin: The Dermis. Vol. X. New York, Appleton-Century-Crofts, 1971, p. 253.

Orgel, L. E.: The maintenance of the accuracy of protein synthesis and its relevance to aging. Proc. Natl. Acad. Sci. USA, 49:517, 1963.

Packer, L., Deamer, D. W., and Heath, R. L.: Regulation and deterioration of structures in membranes. *In* Strehler, B. L. (Ed.): Advances of Gerontological Research. New York, Academic Press, 1967, p. 77.

Partridge, S. M.: Biological role of cutaneous elastin. *In* Montagna, W., Bentley, J. P., and Dobson R. L., (Eds.): Advances in Biology of Skin: The Dermis. Vol. X. New York, Appleton-Century-Crofts, 1971, p. 69.

Pearce, R. H., and Grimmer, B. J.: Age and the chemical constitution of normal human dermis. J. Invest. Dermatol., 58:347, 1972.

Piez, K. A.: Crosslinking of collagen and elastin. Ann. Rev. Biochem., 37:547, 1968.

Pochi, P. E., and Strauss, J. S.: The effect of aging on the activity of the sebaceous gland in man. *In* Montagna, W. (Ed.): Advances in Biology of Skin: Aging. Vol. 6. New York, Pergamon Press, 1965, p. 121.

Rasmussen, D. M., Wakim, K. G., and Winkelmann, R. K.: Effects of aging on human dermis: Studies of thermal shrinkage and tension. *In* Montagna, W. (Ed.): Advances in Biology of Skin: Aging. Vol. 6. New York, Pergamon Press, 1965, p. 151.

Rubner, N.: Probleme des Wachstums und der lebensdauer. Mitt. Gesellch. Inn. Med. Kinderh. (Vienna), 7:58, 1908.

Samitz, J. G., Jr., Davidson, E. A., and Taylor, R. W.: Human cutaneous acid mucopolysaccharides; The effects of age and chronic sun damage. *In* Montagna, W. (Ed.): Advances in Biology of Skin: Aging. Vol. 6. New York, Pergamon Press, 1965, p. 211.

Sams, W. M., Jr., and Smith, J. F., Jr.: Alterations in human dermal fibrous connective tissue with age and chronic sun damage. *In* Montagna, W. (Ed.): Advances in Biology of Skin: Aging. Vol. 6. New York, Pergamon Press, 1965, p. 199.

Sandberg, A. A., Cohen, M. N., Renim, A. A., and Levin, M. L.: Aneuploidy and age in a population survey. Am. J. Hum. Genetc., 19:633, 1967.

Silver, A. F., Montagna, W., and Karacan, I.: The effect of age on human eccrine sweating. *In* Montagna, W. (Ed.): Advances in Biology of Skin: Aging. Vol. 6. New York, Pergamon Press, 1965, p. 129.

Verzar, F.: The aging of connective tissue. Gerontologia, 1:363, 1957.

Verzar, F.: The aging of collagen. Sci. Amer., 28:104, 1962.

Walford, R. L.: The role of autoimmune phenomena in the ageing process. Sympos. Soc. Exp. Biol., 134:22, 1967.

Winkelmann, R. K.: Nerve changes in aging skin. *In* Montagna, W. (Ed.): Advances in Biology of Skin: Aging. Vol. 6. New York, Pergamon Press, 1965, p. 51.

8

Geographic Distribution of Carcinogenic Sun Radiation

Rudolf Schulze

INTRODUCTION

The following observations deal almost exclusively with UV-B solar radiation, because solar radiation on the earth's surface does not contain UV-C, and UV-A does not cause skin cancer. The separation of the spectral distribution of ultraviolet radiation into UV-C (<280 nm.), UV-B (280 nm. to 315 nm.), and UV-A (315 nm. to 400 nm.) has proved useful and seems reasonable because UV-C and UV-B, but not UV-A, are directly harmful to DNA (the adsorption curve of DNA ends at 320 nm.). Therefore, radiation-induced skin cancer can be expected only after UV-C and UV-B radiation. The same applies to solar erythema, which is principally provoked by UV-C and UV-B, whereas direct pigmentation is due to UV-A.* Only UV-A can reverse altera-

tions of DNA caused by UV-C and UV-B (photoreactivation). Specialists in the United States avoid UV-C radiation in artificial radiation, as was done in Germany in the 1930's.

THE EARTH'S ATMOSPHERE AS A DISPERSING MEDIUM

The UV-B component of sun radiation is subject to multiple dispersion by the molecules of the earth's atmosphere (Raleigh's law), so that all the sky is filled with it. UV-B radiation of the sky at the earth's surface is usually much higher than that of direct sun radiation (Bener, 1964; Urbach, 1969). Thus living things receive UV-B radiation from the sun (= direct sun radiation) and from the sky (= sky radiation); consequently total radiation = direct solar radiation + sky radiation.

In the following, all figures refer to "total radiation" thus defined, measured with a receiving surface adjusted to the earth's surface (Larché sphere; especially reliable measurements can be found in Bener, 1964). The influence of the aerosol on the intensity of UV-B radiation is

---

*The gradation of solar erythema (increase of redness with the dosis) is steep, and that of direct pigmentation shallow. The threshold reaction with sun radiation (position of the sun 50°) is reached in 42 minutes in solar erythema, and in 17 minutes in the case of direct pigmentation. Solar erythema is removed by pressure with the glass spatula; direct pigmentation is not.

172

small; according to Hinzpeter (1955, 1956, and 1957) (high mountains equal to 100), the values are as follows:

Position of the sun:	10°	30°	60°	90°
High mountains:	100	100	100	100
Plains:	99	98	93	93
Big cities:	98	96	92	92

THE TWO WINDOWS OF THE EARTH'S ATMOSPHERE

The earth's atmosphere, which feeds and protects living things, absorbs the ionizing radiation from space (including that of the sun) almost completely, acting like a filter of 10 m. water or 90 cm. lead and like a reactor for the production of isotopes. Optical radiation can pass through the atmosphere practically unimpeded, i.e., at least part of the UV-B, the UV-A, visible light, and the IR-A passes through. High-frequency radiation also partly reaches the earth's surface in full strength.

This is what is called the two windows of the earth's atmosphere (Fig. 8–1 and 8–2). The sharp, short wave limitation of window I is caused by ozone degradation; on the other hand, the ozone absorbs all ultraviolet radiation with wavelengths of less than 290 nm. Thus the sunlight reaching the biosphere is cut off at 290 nm. This short wave limit of the sun's spectrum is designated as limit A = 290 nm. Water vapor begins to absorb noticeably at wavelength 1400 nm. and practically limits the sun's spectrum at the long wave limit, designated as limit B = 1400 nm. Between limits A and B there is the first spectral region of high optical permeability of the earth's atmosphere [window I (optical window)]. Between 8000 nm. and 13.000 nm. the absorption of infrared radiation also decreases, but not as much as in window I.

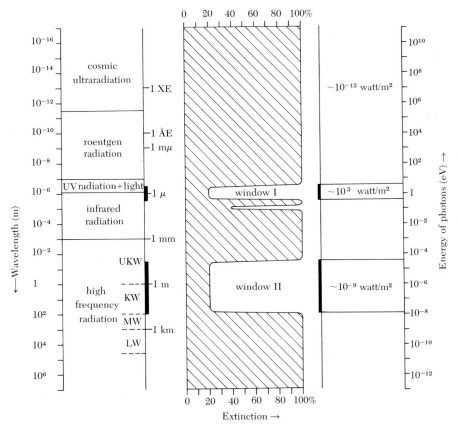

Figure 8–1 The two windows of the earth's atmosphere and the radiation intensities of the various electromagnetic radiations at the earth's surface.

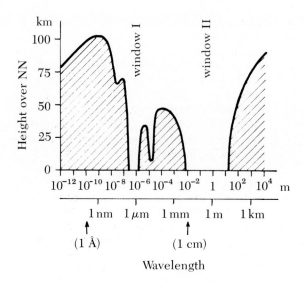

Figure 8–2 Absorption height of electromagnetic radiations coming into the earth's atmosphere. (According to Mandelstam, 1964.)

Radiation of wavelengths longer than 13.000 nm. is again totally absorbed by the molecules of the atmospheric gases. This applies to wavelengths up to about 1 cm. From wavelengths of about 100 m. on, there is absorption in the electrons of the Heaviside layers. That locates window II (radio window) between wavelengths of 1 cm. and 100 m.

Limit A (at 290 nm.) is of special interest to us here, because it seems that only those biologic molecules which could not be degraded by solar radiation with wavelengths of more than 290 nm. could have become important for the development of life on earth. This conclusion is false, however. We can see from the absorption curves of the proteins that their long wave limit is not exactly at limit A but at the slightly longer wavelength of 320 nm. This fact is borne out by the appearance of skin cancer and sunburn.

The development of organisms would have been impeded by radiation below 320 nm. (i.e., between 290 nm. and 320 nm.). This leads to the conclusion that, at the place where organisms developed, radiation on our earth should have had a short wave limit at 320 nm. This would be true in the ocean, because the upper layers of the ocean already absorb UV radiation below 320 nm.; radiation of shorter waves can no longer become effective in the deeper parts of the ocean. This makes us assume, on the basis of completely different theories (i.e., theory of evolution), that early development did take place in the ocean.

Later, when some organisms left the ocean and spread over the surface of the earth, there had to be a development of protective measures against the still existent radiation below 320 nm.; the living organism was surrounded by a radiation

TABLE 8–1 OPTICAL PERMEABILITY OF OZONE (2.5 MM.O_3) IN PERCENTAGES FOR DIFFERENT WAVELENGTHS, DEPENDING ON SUN HEIGHT, h, AND ON THE LENGTH OF THE OPTICAL PATH OF THE DIRECT SOLAR RADIATION, m, THROUGH THE OZONE

h = m =	5° 8.5	10° 5.3	15° 3.7	20° 2.9	30° 1.995	60° 1.154	90° 1.0
300 nm.	—	—	0.003	0.028	0.36	3.9	6.0%
305 nm.	—	0.031	0.35	1.20	4.7	17.2	22%
310 nm.	0.075	1.12	4.4	8.6	18.5	38	43%
315 nm.	2.8	10.8	21	30	43	61	66%
320 nm.	12.8	28	41	50	62	76	79%
325 nm.	35	52	63	70	80	87	88%
330 nm.	73	82	87	90	93	96	96%
335 nm.	84	90	93	94	96	98	98%
340 nm.	98.5	99.1	99.4	99.5	99.7	99.8	99.8%

filter which absorbed radiation below 320 nm. Examples of this are the chitin shell of flies, beetles, and worms, the fur of mammals, and the feathers of birds. Plants have a cell layer which is impermeable to UV radiation on the surface of their leaves. Man, too, developed a radiation filter in the form of the horny layer of the skin surface.

OZONE AS A RADIATION FILTER

As mentioned above, the sharp optical cut-off of solar radiation at limit Å of win-dow I is due to the special absorption properties of ozone (Table 8–1). By multiplying the numerical values of Table 8–1 with the radiation intensity of extraterrestrial solar radiation, while taking the Raleigh dispersion into consideration, we arrive at Figures 8–3 and 8–4, i.e., a statement on the displacement of the spectral distribution of total UV-B radiation in relation to ozone concentration.

Generally ozone concentration in the earth's atmosphere is taken to be 2.5 mm. This also applies to the following calcula-

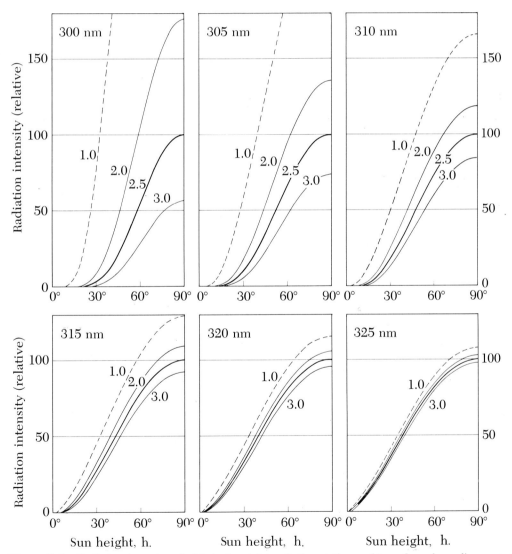

Figure 8–3. Radiation intensity of global ultraviolet radiation at the earth's surface, depending on sun height for various ozone concentrations: 1 mm.; 2 mm.; 2.5 mm.; 3 mm.; adjusted to 2.5 mm. O_3 to 100 with sun height 90°. $100 = 7.6 \times 10^{-3}$ mW./cm.^{2} at 300 nm.; $100 = 5.7 \times 10^{-2}$ (305 nm.); $100 = 1.36 \times 10^{-1}$ (310 nm.); $100 = 2.7 \times 10^{-1}$ (315 nm.); $100 = 4.1 \times 10^{-1}$ (320 nm.) and $100 = 5.5 \times 10^{-1}$ mW./cm.^{2} at 325 nm.

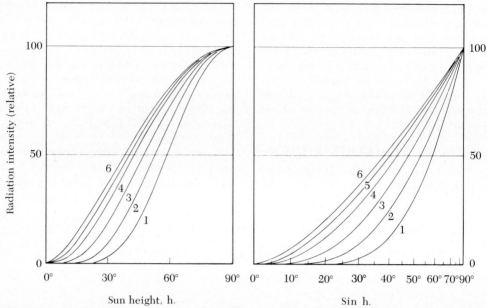

Figure 8–4 Same as Fig. 8–3, but all curves adjusted to 100 at sun height 90°; curve 1 is for 300 nm.; 2 for 305 nm.; 3 for 310 nm.; 4 for 315 nm.; 5 for 320 nm.; and 6 for 325 nm. $100 = 7.6 \times 10^{-3}$mW./cm.^{2} at 300 nm.; $100 = 5.7 \times 10^{-2}$(305 nm.); $100 = 1.36 \times 10^{-1}$(310 nm.); $100 = 2.7 \times 10^{-1}$(315 nm.); $100 = 4.1 \times 10^{-1}$(320 nm.) and $100 = 5.5 \times 10^{-1}$mW./cm.^{2} at 325 nm.

tions and measurements, which, especially in regions with a high cancer incidence (30° N–equator–30°S), lead us to expect an almost uniform ozone concentration of this magnitude throughout the year (Fig. 8–5). In the temperate zones we find a maximum in March and a minimum in October, and extreme values in the north

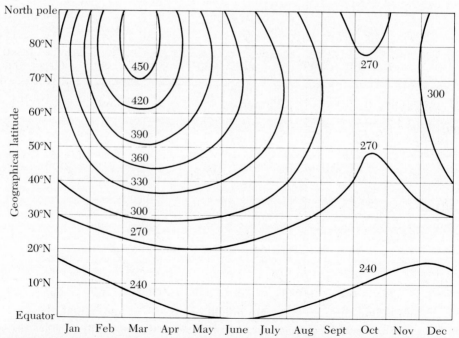

Figure 8–5 Geographic distribution of ozone concentration dependent on season. (According to Godson, 1960.)

Position of the sun:	5°	10°	30°	60°	(90°)
300 nm.	—	—	1.08 −4	3.10 −3	(8.23 −3) mW./cm.² (100 Å.)
305 nm.	2.02 −5	6.00 −5	3.12 −3	3.78 −2	(5.70 −2) mW./cm.² (100 Å.)
310 nm.	1.73 −4	5.52 −4	1.67 −2	9.90 −2	(1.39 −1) mW./cm.² (100 Å.)
315 nm.	1.17 −3	4.34 −3	6.37 −2	2.13 −1	(2.72 −1) mW./cm.² (100 Å.)
(320 nm).	4.08 −3	1.31 −2	1.09 −1	3.30 −1	(4.11 −1) mW./cm.² (100 Å.)
(325 nm).	9.63 −3	2.54 −2	1.57 −1	4.50 −1	(5.51 −1) mW./cm.² (100 Å.)

polar region. Reports on this subject have been published by Godson; Bojkov; and Kulkarni, Angaji, and Ramathan (see Technical Note No. 36 of the World Meteorological Organization, Geneva).

RADIATION INTENSITIES OF UV-B RADIATION

Radiation intensity of the extraterrestrial UV-B solar radiation above the earth's atmosphere is indicated by Thekaekara and Drummond (1971) (as the result of high-altitude flights) in mW. per cm. (100 Å.) as follows:

300 nm.	305 nm.	310 nm.
0.514	0.602	0.686

315 nm.	320 nm.	325 nm.
0.757	0.819	0.958

These numbers correspond to vertical radiation, i.e., a sun position of 90°. If we assumed that the earth had no atmosphere, we would use the cosine law for an estimate of the biologic effect of the radiation and multiply the numbers with sine h (e.g., sine 30° = 0.5; sine 10° = 0.17).

The fact is, however, that extraterrestrial solar radiation loses energy in the earth's atmosphere through dispersion and absorption, and these two processes in turn are dependent upon the position of the sun, because the length of the optical path (m) of solar radiation through the atmosphere increases with the decline of sun height. Values for the Raleigh dispersion are as follows:

Position of the sun (h)	Length of the optical path (m)
5°	10.4
10°	5.6
30°	1.995
60°	1.154
90°	1.00

Usually, the absorption of solar radiation in the ozone is described as a fictitious thickening of the ozone layer. The values for 2.5 mm. ozone are as follows:

Position of the sun	Fictious ozone layer
5°	21.2
10°	13.2
30°	5
60°	2.9
90°	2.5 nm. O^3

On this basis we can calculate the radiation intensity of UV-B radiation as it reaches the earth's surface after these processes. Our result is shown in Figure 8–3 (total radiation − horizontal receiving plane). It is thought, however, that measurements made on the earth's surface are more reliable. Such measurements have been obtained by Bener (1964) at Davos, Switzerland, at a height of 5.550 ft. (1.850 m.) for 2.5 mm. ozone. See preceding text and table at top of page 177. (The values for a sun position of 90° were extrapolated by the author according to the theory of Chandrasekhar.) Winter values are higher, because of reflection against the snow and repeated Rayleigh dispersion.

Boshoff and Kok (1969) published their

	300 nm.	305 nm.	310 nm.	315 nm.	320 nm.	325 nm.	
Very hot summer day:	0.013	0.054	0.124	0.246	0.409	0.485	mW./cm.² (100 Å.)
Average summer day:	0.011	0.044	0.102	0.202	0.336	0.398	mW./cm.² (100 Å.)

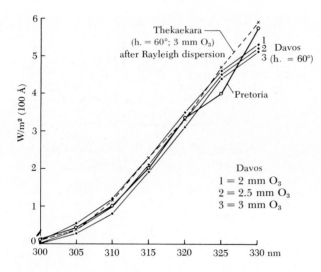

Figure 8-6 Comparison of radiation intensities of global ultraviolet radiation [measured by Bener (Davos, 1964), Boshoff and Kok (Pretoria, 1969) and calculated by Schulze], taking the spectral distribution of extraterrestrial solar radiation into consideration (Thekaekara et al., 1971).

measurements of UV radiation made in Pretoria, South Africa, without indicating ozone concentration and sun position, however.

Figure 8-6 shows the results as compared with calculated values according to Thekaekara and measured values according to Bener. We might then conclude that the values indicated by Boshoff and Kok (1969) are based on serial measurements obtained with an average of 60° sun height and 2.5 mm. ozone concentration. On the basis of this assumption, the values agree surprisingly well.

Biologic tests were carried out in man to check the influence of the mountains on the radiation intensity of the UV-B.

The threshold of the erythema provoked by UV-B was tested. The result is shown in Figure 8-7. When taking the serial measurements of other authors into consideration also, we come to the following conclusions. The intensity of UV-B radiation for the same sun height is primarily independent of geographic latitude. The lesser ozone concentration in the tropics is compensated for by the greater tropical vapor (according to Büttner, 1938). Radiation intensity is higher in the fall than in the spring (according to Götz, 1938). The vapor over big cities decreases the UV-B by approximately 10 per cent. With 1.000 m. over NN, the UV-B increases by about 15 per cent, and in the tropics

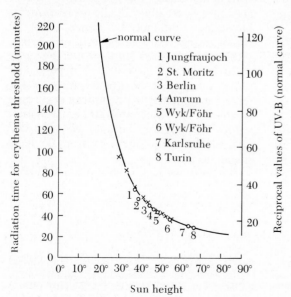

Figure 8-7 Radiation time for provocation of a first solar erythema (threshold), dependent on sun height, measured at various places and altitudes. (Drawn curve: normal UV-B curve according to Büttner, 1938.)

Height:	200	1.000	1.500	2.000	3.000
UV-B (relative):	100	118	125	130	134
%/1.000 m.:	—	22%	12%	8%	3%

by about 20 per cent to 25 per cent (according to Büttner, 1938). Sauberer (1951) found the above values for the Alps.

UV-B RADIATION IN DOSIS UNITS

Physicians and biologists need radiation doses instead of intensity in order to be able to interpret the biologic results in relation to the radiation. For this purpose we multiply the radiation intensity indicated by the physicist (energy/surface, time) with the time and obtain a dosis (energy/surface). In this way the values obtained by Bener (1964) and shown above in mW. per cm.^{2} (100 Å.) were translated into mWh. per cm.^{2} (100 Å.) in relation to a radiation time of 1 hour.

Also, the indication of a certain wavelength $\Delta\lambda$ (here $\Delta\lambda = 100$ Å.) often is a difficult concept for the physician and the biologist. This can be avoided by relating the indicated values to a definite wide spectral area, i.e., in our case, to the UV-B radiation of the sun between 300 nm. and 315 nm. With these calculations we obtain the UV-B doses in terms of mWh. per cm.^{2} for each hour of the day from sunrise to sundown. When adding up the results for the whole day, we obtain the "daily doses" of the UV-B in nature. Table 8–2 sums up the result—to the right, the yearly sums in terms of mWh. per cm.^{2} year.

By taking the yearly sum at the equator to be equal to 100, the result is as follows:

North pole:	6.7	Equator:	100
70°N	: 17.9	30°S	: 76
60°N	: 29	50°S	: 44
50°N	: 44	60°S	: 29
30°N	: 75	70°S	: 18.6

South pole: 7.0

In the course of one year, the equator zone (30°N–equator–30°S) receives the greatest portion of UV-B radiation.

The basis for these calculations is the knowledge of the sun's positions in the various geographic latitudes at the various times of the year. The sun positions were calculated for each full hour of the day for the following dates:

21.I.	8.II.	23.II.	8.III.
16.IV.	1.V.	21.V.	21.VI.
10.IX.	23.IX.	6.X.	20.X.

21.III.	4.IV.	
24.VII.	12.VIII.	28.VIII.
3.XI.	22.XI.	22.XII.

(The values can be obtained from the author.)

CARCINOGENIC SOLAR RADIATION

A calculation of the UV-B doses as indicated above gave us purely physical data, without considering the specific biologic effect of certain wavelengths. Physicians and biologists, however, require the evaluation of UV radiation according to biologic points of view. This can be achieved with the internationally approved erythema effect by multiplying, as in the usual calculation of Finsen units, the physical values in mWh. per cm.^{2} with the erythema effect. The reasoning behind this is as follows: in order to elucidate the primary erythematous process, Hamperl, Henschke, and Schulze in 1939 produced microtome sections of their own living skin. After UV-B radiation, the thymonucleic acid of the nuclei could no longer be colored. With UV-A radiation, only a darker pigmentation was found. Accordingly, the curve of the erythema effect in human skin should be similar to the curve of the absorption of thymonucleic acid. This is correct if the spectral absorption properties of the horny layer covering the living cells are taken into consideration (Fig. 8–8). The superimposition of the absorption curve of thymonucleic acid and the permeability curve of the human horny

TABLE 8-2 Geographic Distribution of Monthly and Yearly Sums of Global UV-B Radiation at the Earth's Surface on Clear Days with 2.5 mm. Ozone Concentration in MW. per CM.² Month and MW. per CM.² Year, Respectively

	Jan.	Feb.	March	April	May	June	July	Aug.	Sept.	Oct.	Nov.	Dec.	Yearly Sum
North pole	—	—	3.3 −2	1.05	4.8	8.4	7.2	3.1	3.0 −1	—	—	—	25
70°N	9.3 −2	8.4 −2	1.40	5.7	1.27+1	1.76+1	1.61+1	9.3	3.2	3.1 −1	—	—	66
60°N	1.33	9.8 −1	4.0	1.07+1	2.0 +1	2.4 +1	2.3 +1	1.57+1	6.6	2.2	2.4 −1	—	104
50°N	9.3	3.3	9.3	1.83+1	2.7 +1	3.0 +1	2.9 +1	2.3 +1	1.32+1	5.6	1.95	8.1 −1	159
30°N	1.44+1	1.39+1	2.4 +1	3.0 +1	3.5 +1	3.5 +1	3.5 +1	3.3 +1	2.6 +1	1.85+1	1.11+1	8.1	280
23.45°N	3.1 +1	1.83+1	2.7 +1	3.2 +1	3.5 +1	3.5 +1	3.6 +1	3.4 +1	2.9 +1	2.3 +1	1.53+1	1.27+1	310
Equator	3.8 +1	3.0 +1	3.5 +1	3.2 +1	3.0 +1	2.7 +1	2.8 +1	3.1 +1	3.3 +1	3.4 +1	3.1 +1	2.9 +1	370
23.45°S	3.8 +1	3.2 +1	3.0 +1	2.1 +1	1.50+1	1.14+1	1.29+1	1.51+1	2.5 +1	3.3 +1	3.6 +1	3.8 +1	310
30°S	3.8 +1	3.3 +1	2.6 +1	1.62+1	1.02+1	7.1	8.7	1.41+1	2.4 +1	3.1 +1	3.5 +1	3.9 +1	280
50°S	3.1 +1	2.1 +1	1.13+1	5.0	1.86	9.9 −1	1.34	3.1	8.1	1.77+1	2.7 +1	3.3 +1	163
60°S	2.4 +1	1.36+1	6.4	1.65 −1	3.1 −1	6.0 −2	6.2 −2	7.8 −1	3.3	1.04+1	1.98+1	2.6 +1	108
70°S	1.72+1	8.9	3.7	4.5 −1	—	—	—	9.3 −2	1.05	5.8	1.26+1	1.94+1	69
South pole	7.7	2.9	3.1 −1	—	—	—	—	—	3.0 −2	1.09	4.8	9.3	27

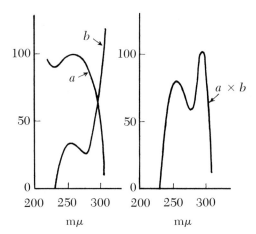

Figure 8–8 Left curves: absorption of the DNA *(a)*; optical permeability of the horny layer of human skin *(b)*. Right curve: product *(a)* × *(b)*, which is similar to the erythema effect. (According to Hamperl, Henschke, and Schulze, 1939a and 1939b.)

layer then results in a curve in which the maxima and the striking descent at 280 nm. are similar to those in the curve obtained by Hussser and Vahle.

In the 1930's the first reports on the experimental production of skin cancers in the nonhairy ear or depilated mouse and rat skin by means of radiation with high-pressure mercury lamps over many months were published (Findlay, 1930; Pustschar, and Holtz, 1930; Herlitz, Jundell, and Wahlgren, 1931; Huldschinsky, 1933; Roffo, 1933). The more often the threshold dosis for an inflammatory radiation reaction was exceeded, the earlier radiation cancer occurred (Miescher, 1939). The wavelengths $\lambda < 320$ nm. and the Hg lines 313 nm. and 302 nm. (Wetzel, 1959), 297 nm. (Friedrich, 1949), and 254 nm. (Blum and Lippincott, 1942; Kellner and Taft, 1956) were carcinogenic.

In summary, the results showed that only wave lengths of $\lambda < 320$ nm. have a carcinogenic effect, with $\lambda = 300$ nm. having a stronger effect than $\lambda = 310$ nm. and $\lambda = 254$ nm. To date, no exact curve of this effect has been established. Such a curve, however, would presumably correspond to the action curve of the inflammatory skin reaction. The most important factor for the carcinogenesis and for the inflammatory skin reaction is the alteration of the epidermal DNA.

It is noteworthy that, in the mouse, UV light does not produce a clear erythema, but predominantly an edema. The action curve of the delayed UV edema, however, corresponds (in relation to the hair growth cycle) exactly to the action curve of human erythema (Johnson, 1969).

Accordingly, it seems reasonable to evaluate the calculated UV-B doses in mWh. per cm.^{2} of the particular wavelengths in terms of their specific erythema-producing effect. For this we generally use internationally accepted values without dimension:

300 nm.: 83	305 nm.: 33	310 nm.: 11
315 nm.: 1.0	320 nm.: 0.5	325 nm.: 0.3

Up to now, two methods have been used:

1. *Radiation doses at wavelength 307.5:* When calculating the product of the spectral distribution of the global ultraviolet radiation and x erythema effect (Schulze, 1966), we obtain the "action curve of solar radiation," as shown in Figure 8–9, which shows that the radiation of wavelength 307.5 is the most effective. Table 8–3 shows the method of calculation, and at top right we find the defined product with a maximum at 307.5.

From the measurements of Bener (1964), the radiation intensities for $\lambda = 307.5$ dependent on the position of the sun were taken, and with these tables were worked out for each full hour of the day in the various geographic latitudes and for the various seasons of the year—similar to the procedure followed for UV-B radiation described above (see p. 000). By summing up these hourly sums, we could then obtain the daily, monthly, and yearly sums. The result of this lengthy calculation is shown in Table 8–4; the yearly sum for the equator was taken to be equal to 100. The data in terms of physical units are available from Figures 8–10, 8–11, and 8–12, and in the book Radiation Climate of the Earth (Schulze, 1970).

2. *Radiation doses in "biologic units":* For this section, the calculation process just described also included the radiation intensities of the following wavelengths:

300 nm.   305 nm.   310 nm.
315 nm.   320 nm.   and
325 nm.

In detail, the procedure was as follows:

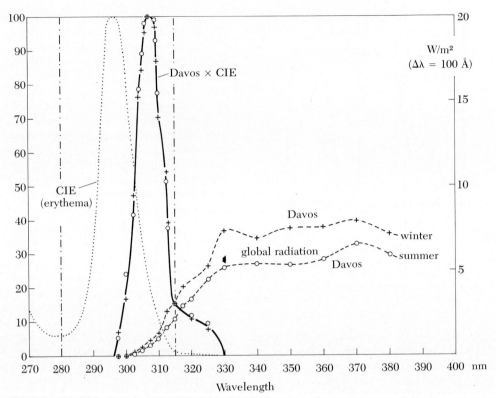

Figure 8–9   Erythema effect according to CIE (dotted line); spectral distribution of global ultraviolet radiation according to Bener (1964) (dashed line); product of both, which indicates the "action curve of solar radiation" (solid line = Davos × CIE); circles: summer data; crosses: winter data.)

(a) For the 20 days indicated on p. 179, the positions of the sun at the full hours were coordinated with radiation intensities according to Bener (1964) and the hourly sums calculated in mWh. per cm.²

(b) The daily sum was calculated for each of the wavelengths indicated.

(c) Each of these daily sums was multiplied with the erythema effect.

(d) These biologically evaluated daily

TABLE 8–3   RESULTS OF MEASUREMENTS OF GLOBAL RADIATION OVER DAVOS WITH
60° SUN HEIGHT (ACCORDING TO BENER, 1964); ERYTHEMA EFFECT (CIE);
RELATIVE BIOLOGIC EFFECT OF GLOBAL RADIATION (DAVOS × CIE)
ADJUSTED TO 100 AT 307.5 NM.

nm.	Global UV-Radiation at Davos (Bener, 1964) Summer mW./cm.² (100 A.)	Winter	Relative Erythema Effect CIE (1935)	Global Radiation Times Erythema (CIE) (307.5 nm. = 100) Summer	Winter
297.5	0.00077	0.00145	99	5.5	6.9
300	0.0041	0.00415	83	25	17
302.5	0.0110	0.0185	53	42	48
305	0.0378	0.0520	33	90	83
307.5	0.063	0.0940	22	100	100
310	0.0990	0.132	11	78	70
312.5	0.167	0.260	4.3	52	54
315	0.213	0.315	1.0	15	15
317.5	0.293	0.410	0.7	15	14
320	0.330	0.445	0.5	12	11
325	0.450	0.525	0.3	9.7	7.7

TABLE 8–4 MONTHLY SUMS OF UV RADIATION AT 307.5 NM. – RIGHT: YEARLY SUMS (YEARLY SUM AT THE EQUATOR = 100) (ACCORDING TO SCHULZE AND GRÄFE)

	Jan.	Feb.	March	April	May	June	July	Aug.	Sept.	Oct.	Nov.	Dec.	Year
North pole	–	–	–	0.11	0.5	1.4	0.7	0.14	–	–	–	–	2.8
80°N	–	–	0.018	0.5	1.4	2.1	1.8	0.7	0.11	–	–	–	6.6
70°N	–	0.02	0.18	1.4	3.0	3.9	3.5	1.8	0.5	0.09	–	–	14
60°N	0.02	0.11	0.8	3.0	5.0	6.2	5.7	3.4	1.6	0.4	0.04	–	26
50°N	0.2	0.5	2.1	5.0	7.1	8.0	7.6	5.5	3.2	1.2	0.4	0.11	41
40°N	0.7	1.8	4.2	6.7	8.5	9.2	9.0	7.3	5.0	2.3	1.0	0.5	56
30°N	2.0	3.5	5.8	8.2	9.4	9.7	9.6	8.5	6.9	4.2	2.5	1.8	72
20°N	3.9	5.5	7.6	9.0	9.6	9.7	9.6	9.2	8.1	6.2	4.4	3.5	86
10°N	6.2	7.4	8.9	9.0	9.0	8.7	8.9	9.2	8.9	7.8	6.6	5.9	96.5
Equator	8.2	8.7	9.2	8.5	8.0	7.4	7.4	8.5	8.9	8.9	8.3	8.0	100
10°S	9.6	9.4	9.2	7.4	6.4	5.5	5.8	7.3	8.3	9.2	9.4	9.5	97
20°S	10.3	9.4	8.3	5.8	4.2	3.4	3.7	5.5	7.3	9.0	9.7	10.5	87
30°S	10.5	9.0	7.1	3.7	2.3	1.6	1.7	3.5	5.6	8.1	9.6	10.6	73
40°S	9.6	7.6	5.1	2.1	0.9	0.5	0.7	1.8	3.5	6.6	8.5	10.1	57
50°S	8.2	5.9	3.2	0.9	0.2	0.12	0.2	0.7	2.0	4.8	7.1	8.7	42
60°S	6.2	3.7	1.4	0.2	0.04	–	0.02	0.12	0.7	2.7	5.6	6.7	27
70°S	3.9	2.0	0.5	0.02	–	–	–	0.09	0.2	1.2	3.0	4.4	15
80°S	2.0	0.7	0.11	–	–	–	–	–	0.018	0.4	1.2	2.3	6.8
South pole	0.7	0.18	–	–	–	–	–	–	–	0.07	0.5	1.4	2.9

sums of the various wavelengths were added to the daily sums from 300 nm. to 325 nm.

(e) These last daily sums finally yielded the monthly and yearly sums.

The data obtained in this way will be called "biologic units" and abbreviated "BU." Table 8–5 contains the final results and shows that more than 70 per cent are concentrated in the equatorial zone (30°N–equator–30°S). This becomes clear if we again take the yearly sum at the equator to be equal to 100:

North pole:	4.3	30°N	: 68	40°S	: 53
80°N	: 7.9	20°N	: 85	50°S	: 39
70°N	: 15	10°N	: 96	60°S	: 24
60°N	: 23	Equator:	100	70°S	: 15
50°N	: 38	10°S	: 96	80°S	: 8.1
40°N	: 53	20°S	: 85	South pole:	4.5
		30°S	: 69		

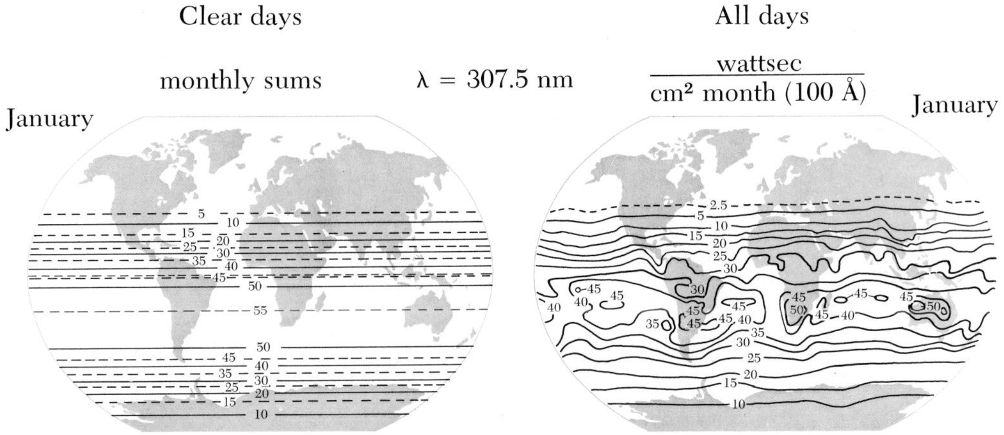

Clear days   All days

monthly sums   λ = 307.5 nm $\dfrac{\text{wattsec}}{\text{cm}^2 \text{ month (100 Å)}}$

January   January

Figure 8–10 Geographic distribution of monthly sums of global ultraviolet radiation (wavelength: 307.5 nm.) in January. Left: clear days; right: all days; in Ws./cm.² month (100 Å). Geographic distributions for the months of March, June, September, and December, can be found in Schulze, R.: Radiation Climate of the Earth. Darmstadt, Verlag Dr. Dietrich Steinkopff, 1970, p. 98.

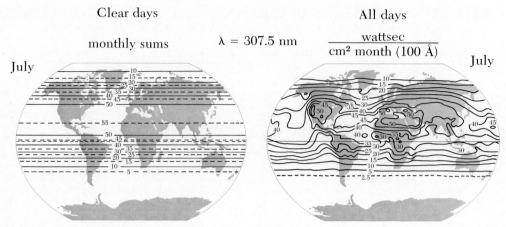

Figure 8–11 Geographic distribution of monthly sums of global ultraviolet radiation (wavelength: 307.5 nm.) in July. Left: clear days; right: all days; in Ws./cm.² month (100 Å.).

INFLUENCE OF POLLUTION CAUSED BY MAN

At the suggestion of the Massachusetts Institute of Technology, the two Royal Swedish Academies of Sciences and Engineering Sciences held a meeting on the subject "inadvertent climate modification" (Report of the Study of Man's Impact on Climate). On this occasion the question of a decrease in ozone concentration due to industrial waste gases was discussed, among others. Subsequently, the calculation of the "biologic units" (BU), as detailed on pp. 181 to 183, was modified.

With the help of computers, it was calculated for the purpose of this report by how many percentage points the number of biologic units increases if there is a decrease in ozone concentration of 25 per cent. The result is shown in Table 8–6 for four days of the year: in the equatorial zone there would be a 40 per cent increase in UV radiation, in the temperate zones the increase would be approximately 50 per cent, and in the polar regions 60 per cent (see also Table 8–7 for UV-B).

Another result of these extensive calculations can be described as follows: The percentage of the constituent part of the particularly carcinogenic 300 nm. radiation increases with decreasing ozone concentration. If the ozone concentration is decreased by 25 per cent, the percentage of the constituent part is doubled at 60°N and 60°S (March 21 and September 23) and quadrupled at 70°N and 70°S. With an ozone concentration of minus

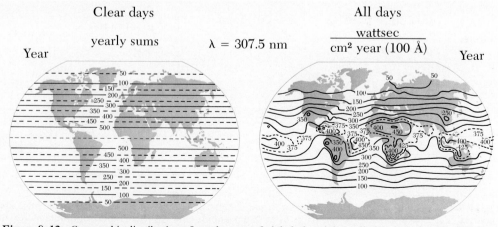

Figure 8–12 Geographic distribution of yearly sums of global ultraviolet radiation (wavelength: 307.5 nm.). Left: clear days; right: all days; in Ws./cm.² year (100 Å.).

TABLE 8–5 GEOGRAPHIC DISTRIBUTION OF GLOBAL ULTRAVIOLET RADIATION (SOLAR AND SKY RADIATION) IN BIOLOGIC UNITS (BU)

	Jan.	Feb.	March	April	May	June	July	Aug.	Sept.	Oct.	Nov.	Dec.	Yearly Sum BU
North pole	—	—	3.1 −1	9.0	4.0 +1	6.9 +1	6.2 +1	2.5 +1	3.0	—	—	—	200
80°N	—	—	2.5	2.0 +1	7.0 +1	1.20+2	1.00+2	4.6 +1	1.14+1	3.1 −1	—	—	370
70°N	—	5.6 −1	1.24+1	4.2 +1	1.33+2	1.88+2	1.74+2	8.5 +1	2.7 +1	3.1	—	—	660
60°N	6.2 −1	8.4	3.4 +1	1.04+2	2.2 +2	2.7 +2	2.6 +2	1.57+2	5.9 +1	1.70+1	2.4	—	1100
50°N	1.18+1	2.9 +1	8.9 +1	1.94+2	3.2 +2	3.6 +2	3.5 +2	2.6 +2	1.33+2	5.1 +1	1.80+1	9.3	1800
40°N	3.7 +1	7.0 +1	1.69+2	2.8 +2	3.9 +2	4.2 +2	4.1 +2	3.4 +2	2.1 +2	1.12+2	4.8 +1	2.9 +1	2500
30°N	9.0 +1	1.46+2	2.7 +2	3.5 +2	4.3 +2	4.5 +2	4.5 +2	3.6 +2	3.0 +2	2.1 +2	1.12+2	7.9 +1	3200
23.45°N	1.46+2	1.97+2	3.6 +2	4.1 +2	4.6 +2	4.9 +2	4.9 +2	4.4 +2	3.7 +2	2.7 +2	1.68+2	1.24+2	3900
20°N	1.75+2	2.3 +2	4.0 +2	4.2 +2	4.6 +2	4.5 +2	4.6 +2	4.4 +2	3.8 +2	2.9 +2	1.88+2	1.57+2	4000
10°N	2.7 +2	3.0 +2	4.2 +2	4.4 +2	4.3 +2	3.9 +2	4.1 +2	4.4 +2	4.4 +2	3.8 +2	2.8 +2	2.6 +2	4500
Equator	3.9 +2	3.8 +2	4.7 +2	4.1 +2	3.8 +2	3.3 +2	3.6 +2	4.0 +2	4.2 +2	4.3 +2	3.8 +2	3.7 +2	4700
10°S	4.6 +2	4.2 +2	4.5 +2	3.5 +2	2.7 +2	2.4 +2	2.5 +2	3.0 +2	4.0 +2	4.6 +2	4.4 +2	4.4 +2	4500
20°S	4.9 +2	4.2 +2	4.0 +2	2.7 +2	1.86+2	1.43+2	1.58+2	2.2 +2	3.3 +2	4.3 +2	4.6 +2	4.9 +2	4000
23.45°S	5.0 +2	4.1 +2	3.8 +2	2.4 +2	1.58+2	1.13+2	1.33+2	1.95+2	3.1 +2	4.2 +2	4.7 +2	5.1 +2	3900
30°S	4.7 +2	3.6 +2	3.3 +2	1.79+2	9.9 +1	6.8 +1	8.2 +1	1.46+2	2.5 +2	3.7 +2	4.4 +2	5.0 +2	3300
40°S	4.4 +2	3.0 +2	2.2 +2	9.9 +1	4.6 +1	2.7 +1	3.4 +1	6.8 +1	1.53+2	2.8 +2	3.8 +2	4.6 +2	2500
50°S	3.6 +2	2.2 +2	1.30+2	4.5 +1	1.55+1	7.5	9.9	2.7 +1	8.1 +1	1.91+2	3.1 +2	4.3 +2	1840
60°S	2.6 +2	1.37+2	5.9 +1	1.50+1	2.2	6.0 −1	9.3 −1	6.7	2.9 +1	1.02+2	2.1 +2	2.9 +2	1140
70°S	1.77+2	6.6 +1	2.2 +1	4.5	—	—	—	6.7 −1	9.0	4.7 +1	1.29+2	2.1 +2	670
80°S	1.07+2	3.6 +1	7.8	—	—	—	—	—	2.4	2.0 +1	7.4 +1	1.32+2	380
South pole	6.2 +1	1.68+1	3.1	—	—	—	—	—	—	9.3	3.9 +1	8.1 +1	210

TABLE 8-6 INCREASE AND DECREASE OF BIOLOGIC UNITS (BU) OF GLOBAL ULTRAVIOLET RADIATION IN THE CASE OF CHANGE OF OZONE CONCENTRATION BY ± 25 PER CENT, DEPENDING ON SEASON AND GEOGRAPHIC LATITUDE, IN TERMS OF 2.5 MM. O_3

	21.III. −25%	21.III. +25%	21.VI. −25%	21.VI. +25%	23.IX. −25%	23.IX. +25%	22.XII. −25%	22.XII. +25%
North pole	–	–	+60%	−31%	–	–	–	–
70°N	+59%	−32%	+49%	−29%	+59%	−32%	–	–
60°N	+53%	−31%	+46%	−28%	+53%	−31%	+65%	−32%
50°N	+51%	−30%	+44%	−27%	+51%	−30%	+59%	−31%
23.45°N	+42%	−27%	+40%	−26%	+42%	−27%	+48%	−29%
Equator	+40%	−26%	+42%	−27%	+40%	−26%	+42%	−27%
23.45°S	+42%	−27%	+48%	−29%	+42%	−27%	+40%	−26%
50°S	+51%	−30%	+59%	−31%	+51%	−30%	+44%	−27%
60°S	+53%	−31%	+65%	−32%	+53%	−31%	+46%	−28%
70°S	+59%	−32%	–	–	+59%	−32%	+49%	−29%
South pole	–	–	–	–	–	–	+60%	−31%

60 per cent, the percentage of the constituent part is increased 8 times (60°N) or 28 times (70°N). In detail, the data are as follows (see also Tables 8-8 and 8-9):

Decrease in ozone
concentration: −25%   −60%
    Equator: 1.3 ×   2.2 ×
    23.45° :   1.5 ×   2.5 ×
    50°   :   1.7 ×   4.4 ×
    60°   :   2 ×   8 ×
    70°   :   4 ×   28 ×

During these computer calculations, the question was checked out by how many percentage points the number of biologic units decreases if the ozone concentration increases by 25 per cent, i.e., from 2.5 mm. to 3.0 mm. O_3. The result is also contained in Table 8-7; it answers the question of the decrease in number of biologic units,

if theoretically we move from the equatorial zone toward the temperate zones, where the ozone concentration is higher, especially in the spring.

SUMMARY

A study of investigations of the dependence of the carcinogenic UV radiation on wavelengths showed that the action spectrum for human skin cancer more or less corresponds to the curve of the erythema-producing effect. On this basis "biologic units," in analogy to the calculation of the Finsen units, were calculated for the various geographic latitudes in relation to the seasons. The result showed that more than 70 per cent of the carcinogenic UV radiation is con-

TABLE 8-7 INCREASE AND DECREASE OF THE UV-B OF GLOBAL RADIATION IN THE CASE OF CHANGE OF OZONE CONCENTRATION BY ± 25 PER CENT, DEPENDING ON SEASON AND GEOGRAPHIC LATITUDE, IN TERMS OF 2.5 MM. O_3

	21.III. −25%	21.III. +25%	21.VI. −25%	21.VI. +25%	23.IX. −25%	23.IX. +25%	22.XII. −25%	22.XII. +25%
North pole	–	–	+441%	−26%	–	–	–	–
70°N	+51%	−32%	+29%	−22%	+51%	−32%	–	–
60°N	+37%	−24%	+28%	−20%	+27%	−24%	+112%	−51%
50°N	+32%	−22%	+26%	−19%	+32%	−22%	+54%	−35%
23.45°N	+25%	−19%	+23%	−17%	+25%	−19%	+29%	−22%
Equator	+23%	−17%	+25%	−19%	+23%	−17%	+25%	−19%
23.45°S	+25%	−19%	+29%	−22%	+25%	−19%	+23%	−17%
50°S	+32%	−22%	+54%	−35%	+32%	−22%	+26%	−19%
60°S	+37%	−24%	+112%	−51%	+37%	−24%	+28%	−20%
70°S	+51%	−32%	–	–	+51%	−32%	+29%	−22%
South pole	–	–	–	–	–	–	+41%	−26%

TABLE 8–8 PERCENTAGE PART OF RADIATION OF VARIOUS WAVELENGTHS IN THE CARCINOGENIC EFFECT IN THE CASE OF DECREASE OF OZONE CONCENTRATION BY 25 PER CENT OR 60 PER CENT, RESPECTIVELY, IN TERMS OF 2.5 MM. O_3

	Equator −25%	Equator −60%	23.45°N + S −25%	23.45°N + S −60%	50°N and 50°S −25%	50°N and 50°S −60%	60°N and 60°S −25%	60°N and 60°S −60%	70°N and 70°S −25%	70°N and 70°S −60%
300 nm.	18%	40%	15%	38%	7%	31%	3%	24%	0.5%	14%
305 nm.	37%	36%	36%	36%	31%	37%	23%	38%	11.5%	36%
310 nm.	32%	19%	35%	21%	40%	24%	43%	28%	38%	35%
315 nm.	5.5%	2.5%	6.1%	2.4%	8.9%	3.8%	12%	4.5%	15%	6.5%
320 nm.	4.3%	1.5%	4.3%	1.5%	7.0%	2.4%	10%	3.1%	16%	4.7%
325 nm.	3.2%	1.0%	3.6%	1.1%	6.1%	1.8%	9%	2.4%	19%	3.8%

TABLE 8–9 INCREASE AND DECREASE OF RADIATION INTENSITY OF GLOBAL ULTRAVIOLET RADIATION IN THE CASE OF CHANGE OF OZONE CONCENTRATION BY ± 25 PER CENT, DEPENDING ON SUN HEIGHT AND WAVELENGTH, IN TERMS OF 2.5 MM. O_3

Sun Height / Ozone Concentration	5° −25%	5° +25%	10° −25%	10° +25%	30° −25%	30° +25%	60° −25%	60° +25%	90° −25%	90° +25%
300 nm	(×121)	(×0.008)	(×20)	(×0.05)	+208%	−68%	+92%	−48%	+76%	−43%
305 nm	(×13)	(×0.075)	(×5.0)	(×0.20)	+82%	−46%	+42%	−30%	+36%	−27%
310 nm	+321%	−76%	+145%	−59%	+40%	−29%	+22%	−18%	+18%	−16%
315 nm	+104%	−51%	+56%	−36%	+18%	−15%	+10%	−9%	+9%	−8%
320 nm	+51%	−34%	+28%	−23%	+10%	−9%	+6%	−5%	+5%	−5%
325 nm	+24%	−19%	+14%	−12%	+5%	−5%	+3%	−3%	+3%	−2%

centrated in the equatorial zone (30°N–equator–30°S). Finally, it was calculated by how much UV radiation increases if, due to industrial pollution, the ozone concentration decreases by 25 per cent; the result showed that there would be a 40 per cent increase in the equatorial zone.

ACKNOWLEDGMENTS

I wish to express my sincere gratitude for their advice and generous help with the extensive calculations to Drs. Kasten and Schröder of the Meteorological Observatory of the German Meteorology Station at Hamburg, to Dr. Wiskemann, Skin Clinic of Hamburg University, and to Director Münch and Engineer Steck, both of OSRAM, Munich.

REFERENCES

Bener, P.: Tages-und Jahresgang der Spektralen Intensität der Ultravioletten Global-und Himmelsstrahlung bei wolkenfreiem Himmel in Darvos (1590 m/M). Strahlentherapir, 123:306, 1964.
Blum, H. F., and Lippincott, S. W.: Absence of hypervitaminosis in mice subjected to ultraviolet radiation. J. Nat. Cancer Inst., 3:211, 1942.
Bojkov, R.: Idojaras, 3:140, 1968.
Bojkov, R.: Idojaras, 4:233, 1968.
Boshoff, M. C., and Kok, C. S.: Plastics, Paint and Rubber, Vols. III and IV, 1969.
Büttner, K.: Physikalische Bioklimatologie. Leipzig, 1938.
Findlay, G. M.: Lancet, I:1229, 1930.
Friedrich, W.: Arch. Geschwulstforsch., 1:137, 1949.
Godson, K.: Quart. J. R. Meterol. Soc., 301, 1960.
Götz, F. W. P.: Ergeb. Kosm. Physik, 3:253, 1938.
Hamperl, H., Henschke, U., and Schulze, R.: Virchows Arch. [Pathol. Anat.], 304:19, 1939a.
Hamperl, H., Henschke, U., and Schulze, R.: Naturwissenschaften, 27:486, 1939b.
Henschke, U., and Schulze, R.: Naturwissenschaften, 26:142, 1938.
Henschke, U., and Schulze, R.: Strahlentherapie, 64:14, 1939.
Herlitz, C., Jundell, J. and Wahlgren, F.: Acta Paediatr. Scand., 10:321, 1931.
Hinzpeter, H.: Z. Meteorol., 9:308, 1955.
Hinzpeter, H.: Z. Meteorol., 10:100, 1956.
Hinzpeter, H.: Z. Meteorol., 11:1, 1957.
Huldschinsky, K.: Dtsch. Med. Wochenschr., 59:530, 1933.
Johnson, B. E.: Action spectra for acute effects of monochromatic ultraviolet light in mouse skin. In Urbach, F. (Ed.): The Biologic Effects of Ultraviolet Radiation. New York, Pergamon Press, Inc., 1969.
Kelner, A., and Taft, E. B.: Influence of photoreactivating light on type and frequency of tumors induced by ultraviolet radiation. Cancer Res., 16:860, 1956.
Larché, K.: Licht, 12:110, 1942.
Larché, K., and Schulze, R.: Z. Techn. Physik, 23:114, 1942.
Mandelstam, S. L.: Selecta, 43:1316, 1964.
Miescher, G.: Z. Krebsforsch., 49:339, 1939.
Pfleiderer, H., and Büttner, K.: Bioklim. Lehrb. Bâder- Klimakunde, 1940.
Putschar, W., and Holtz, F.: Z. Krebsforsch., 33:219, 1930.
Roffo, A. H.: Biol. Inst. Med. Estud. Cancer [Buenos Aires], 10:417, 1933.
Sauberer, F.: Arch. Met. Geophys. Bioklimat., B2, 347, 1951.
Schulze, R.: Measurement of sunlight—the ultraviolet "B" in sunlight. Conference on sunlight and skin cancer, 1964. Blum, F. and Urbach, F. (Eds.). Z. Bäder-Klimaheilkd., 13:242, 1966.
Schulze, R.: Strahlenklima der Erde. Darmstadt, Dietrich Steinkopff, 1970.
Schultze, R., and Gräfe, K.: Consideration of sky ultraviolet radiation in the measurement of solar ultraviolet radiation. In Urbach, F. (Ed.): The Biologic Effects of Ultraviolet Radiation. New York, Pergamon Press, Inc., 1969.
Thekaekara, M. P., and Drummond, A. J.: The solar constant and the spectrum measured from a research aircraft at 38,000 feet, Goddard Center, Greenbelt, Maryland, X-322-68-304, 1968. Nature Phys. Sci., 229:6, 1971.
Urbach, F.: Geographic pathology of skin cancer. In Urbach, F. (Ed.): The Biologic Effects of Ultraviolet Radiation. New York, Pergamon Press, Inc., 1969.
Urbach, F., Davies, R. E., and Forbes, P. D.: Ultraviolet radiation and skin cancer in man. In Montagna, W. (Ed.): Advances in Biology of the Skin. 75:195, 1966, New York, Pergamon Press, Inc.
Wetzel, R.: Arch. Geschwulstforsch. Press, Inc., 14:75, 120, 1959.
Winch, G. T., Boshoff, M. C., Kok, C. J., and du Toit, A. G.: J. Opt. Soc. Am., 56:456, 1966.

9

Cancer of the Skin and the Precancerous Stages in the Epidermal-Dermal Interface

H. Oberste-Lehn, M.D.

IMPORTANCE OF THE EPIDERMAL-DERMAL INTERFACE FOR THE UNDERSTANDING OF PATHOLOGIC ALTERATIONS OF THE SKIN

Through maceration of an excised piece of skin, the epidermis can be separated from the dermis and the surface of each can be represented. While the usual histologic sections permit a view of the architecture of the cell structure of the tissue, the epidermal-dermal interface gives us an idea of the dimensional structure of the epidermis, its appendages, and the corium. There is no doubt that the histologic procedure has become an indispensable tool for diagnosis and is an investigational method which has much contributed to the differentiation of morphologically similar diseases and to the understanding of the pathogenesis of the most diverse dermatoses (histochemistry). However, the view of the papillary body and the rete ridges obtained through a histologic section is not only incomplete but also in some aspects incorrect. The fault lies in the fact that the section does not give an idea of the spatial form of the changeable structures of the skin. Moreover, the shrinkage of the tissue plays a greater role in the evaluation of a section than is usually granted.

Cowdry and Nielson, for instance, determined that the shrinkage of the skin in adolescents amounts to approximately 38 to 58 percent, and in older people to about 12 to 20 percent. Since the shrinkage occurs predominantly in the corium, however, the epidermis of young people appears unproportionally thickened in the section, thus suggesting papillary bodies and rete ridges. Consequently, the richly differentiated terminology of dermatologic histology concerning the multiple alterations of the malpighian layer and the interpapillary epithelial formations in atrophy, the enlargement and deviation of the epithelium, and so forth does not always reflect the true picture. Finally, we have to take into consideration

189

that, if the sections represent certain aspects of certain structures, it is more or less due to chance. Microscopically, the stereometric representation of the epithelium is possible only through a painstaking reconstruction by means of serial sections (F. Pinkus, 1910 and 1927; Madsen, 1965; and others). Such attempts consume a great deal of effort and time, much more than the result warrants.

DEVELOPMENT OF THE TECHNIQUE FOR REPRESENTATION OF THE EPIDERMAL-DERMAL INTERFACE

The maceration technique is an adequate procedure for the production of plastic figures of the epidermis. This procedure has been known for a long time. The first systematic and extensive investigations regarding the effect of chemical agents on animal tissue were carried out by Donders (1910). Sappey (1897), Wilson (1889), Henle (1866), Kölliker (1889), Kollmann (1883), and Hebra (1880) also worked on a method for the separation of the epidermis from the dermis. For this purpose they boiled the skin or allowed it to decompose. It turned out, though, that both measures were too drastic to permit a true representation of the structure of the epidermis and the dermis.

In the course of his studies on the topographic differences in newborns, fetuses, and children, Blaschko (1887) produced preparations of the skin of decomposed fetuses, in which the epidermis can easily be separated from the dermis. In his discussion of these studies, Unna (1888) remarked that this new, practical method might be able to reveal a great number of new exact details. He felt that Blaschko (1887) had left the old method and the customary description of the papillary body according to vertical skin sections behind and embarked in a direction which must appear logical to all competent histologists.

Blaschko's (1887) systematization of topographic differences is faulty, however, because of the differences in his material and because he neglected the appendages

and their importance for the total structure of the papillary body. Consequently, his work could not be the basis for further morphologic studies. Philippson (1889), who, following Unna's suggestion, took up the maceration procedure, was likewise unable to give an exact representation of the topography of the papillary body. His representations lacked conceptual order. Nevertheless, his studies of the influence of the depressed furrows, or sulci superiores, on the structure of the basal layer are remarkable. After having tried a great number of acids, he used acetic acid for maceration. Kölliker (1889) had also been aware of this macerating agent, which he indicates had already been used before him. It appears, however, that the usefulness of acetic acid had been forgotten and was then rediscovered by Philippson (1889).

Erich Hoffmann (1939), during his nevogenetic studies, made another attempt to use the maceration procedure in order to find a solution for some problems. Together with a student of his, the zoologist Lehmensieck (1936), he used amniotic fluid as a macerating agent for the preparation of tissues. His textbook contains one figure representing the appendages of the skin. More recently Greb (1940) studied the form and structure of the papillary body with acetic acid macerations. Although he did then stress the importance of the appendages for the total structure, he did not take these results into consideration in his attempt to systematize the complicated structures of the rete ridges and the papillary body.

Until now the results obtained with the maceration technique have been unsatisfactory in giving an insight into the structures of the epidermal-dermal interface. The immediate cause of this lies in the problems encountered in tissue preparation. As mentioned above, boiling and decomposition are interventions which are too aggressive and which destroy the structure. Acetic acid maceration has the advantage of preserving the epidermal structures, but that alone does not solve the problem of making the structures visible and of preserving the preparations. It was this problem that frustrated all the investigators. Blaschko (1887) dyed the preparations while still wet with hematoxylin and studied them under a magnifying glass. Philippson (1899), on the contrary, avoided dyes; he studied the preparations against the light in order to recognize differences in structure through the shadows they cast. Greb (1940) dyed the papillae of the connective tissue with iodine. Like all other investigators before him, he worked with wet preparations. Since there existed no appropriate means of conservation, keeping and storing the preparations was impossible. This, however, is the precondition for a comparative morphologic analysis.

On the other hand, the attempts to gain definite knowledge from the maceration preparations were unsuccessful because, instead of dividing the overall structure into separate, differentiated morphologic units, the anatomoanalytic method was followed in studying only the surface view of isolated elements of the section, such as the rete ridges or the papillae. Only relatively recently has Horstmann (1952) been able to overcome both these difficulties: impregnation with turpentine made lasting preparations possible. This constituted the basis for a collection of preparations and consequently for comparative studies and photographic evaluation.

PRINCIPLES OF ORIENTATION OF THE STRUCTURES AT THE EPIDERMAL-DERMAL INTERFACE

The most important aspect of Horstmann's work, however, lies in the fact that he established *morphologically*, not through anatomic subdivisions, those forms which recur constantly in the overall orientation of the epidermal-dermal interface. These principles of orientation, which he calls motives, are dependent on the appendages of the skin. Through them it is possible to detect and define certain laws in the bewildering complexity of the epidermal-dermal structures. From then on, etiologic processes and pathologic alterations at the level of the epidermal border could be successfully studied.

In the following we shall briefly explain these principles of orientation to facilitate the understanding of the different morphologic units. The rete ridges are coordinated to the appendages of the skin and take the form of a cockade. In the immediate vicinity of the hair follicles and the sweat glands there is, in part, no structuring at all, and the borders are formed by concentrically arranged rete ridges. On the other hand, these rete ridges support epidermal structures around the appendages, which are shaped like rosettes. The arrangement of the rete ridges in relation to the sweat glands and the hair follicles is radial. This differentiation brings to mind the observations by F. Pinkus (1910 and 1927) (hair fields) and Maurer (1895) (hair regions). Both these terms meant the above structuring in relation to the appendages. These results, which are based on the studies of de Meijere (1894), were not sufficiently recognized, probably because of their phytogenous importance. The concentric, parallel, epithelial envelopes, which characterize the cockade, can involve in some cases, especially in the vellus of the ear, even the hair follicle, where they form a kind of collar (Horstmann, 1952 and 1957). Zimmermann mentioned this collar for the first time in 1935 and showed that the hair is frequently embedded in the appendages in these places. Sometimes two or three of these collars are found on top of the other. Horstmann (1952 and 1957) saw these formations as comparable to the concentric epidermal envelopes of the cockades.

Another principle of orientation is the coordination of the sweat glands to the hair follicles. These glands are arranged around the hair follicles like the numbers on a watch dial. These same form elements are found all over the skin with more or less marked variations. Their regularity and frequency induced Horstmann to consider these groups of rete ridges as special formations in the epidermis. Even in articulation folds, which interrupt the rete ridges, there are still cockades and rosettes, and those regions of the skin which do not have appendages show neither these formations nor the usual netlike epithelial ridges. Here the rete ridges are parallel and show a tendency to whorl formation. These whorls were already mentioned by Blaschko (1887). There are the most diversified transitions between the netlike arrangement of the papillae and a purely linear deposition. As demonstrated by Horstmann (1952), the ridges are more continuous in the skin of the abdomen, the back, and the chest. Other studies have shown that there is also a phylogenetic explanation for the motives (Fleischhauer, 1953b).

METHOD FOR THE PRODUCTION OF FIGURES OF THE EPIDERMAL-DERMAL INTERFACE

In general, we used 1 percent acetic acid as a macerating agent for our studies. The separation of epidermis and dermis is usually complete within two to five days. Sometimes, however, the epidermolysis is insufficient because of marked acanthosis of the epithelium with long, thin rete ridges, such as we often see in dermatologic diseases. The search for a procedure which would work better against the epidermal-dermal adhesion brought no results. Cowdry, for instance, described the epidermolysis after heating a piece of skin on a copper plate heated up to 50 or 60° C., and Medawar mentioned the epidermolysis obtained with a 0.5 percent trypsin solution, but both methods are unsatisfactory because they are too drastic. Studies of the hyaluronic acid of the hyaluronidase ferment system suggested, however, that hyaluronidase might be tried as a macerating agent, because at the same time it preserves the structures and performs an especially complete epidermolysis. Maceration with preparations of testicle hyaluronidase yielded, in effect, a complete separation of the epidermis from the corium at the basal border, even in cases of marked acanthosis of the epithelium (Oberste-Lehn, 1952b).

After about six to 12 hours the various skin specimens appear edematous, so that a stratification can clearly be recognized. The epidermis appears as a narrow, yellowish layer, followed by the paper-white edematous connective tissue and then the yellowish fragile fatty layer. In this stage the epidermis is also fragile because it is so thin, but after another 48 to 72 hours it can be separated without damage from the dermis. In addition, sodium bromide can be used for the epidermolysis (Szabo, 1954). These preparations can be dyed and used for cytologic studies, such as the distribution of the melanocytes (Szabo, 1965).

According to the procedure used by Horstmann (1952), the excised pieces of skin are usually put in 1 percent acetic acid after having been fixed and slightly extended on cork plates by means of the pricks of a hedgehog or steel needles. Hyaluronidase is used only when it is doubtful, because of the epithelial acanthosis, whether an adequate epidermolysis can be obtained with acetic acid. After two to five days, the epidermis has usually separated from the dermis, and it is carefully taken off and again fixed with hedgehog pricks or steel needles. The preparations are put into water for a short time, then processed through an ascending alcohol line and put into turpentine oil. The turpentine oil must be changed once again. American turpentine is very pure and makes the preparations appear transparent. For this reason Pinkus has recommended that beeswax be added to the turpentine. These preparations are comparable to those made with European turpentine. The preparations, which are now hard and almost white, are air-dried and finally glued to a slide with transparent glue. Then the preparations can be studied under the microscope with incident light and photographed. The comparison of the preparations is easier and clearer in photographs. Principally, it is possible to study the forces of orientation which operate at the epidermal-dermal interface from the reverse side of the separated epidermis, as well as from the surface of the papillary body superimposed on the epidermis. In the photographic reproduction, the representation of the reverse side of the epidermis is preferable, however, because the epidermis can easily be evened out in these preparations, with the rete ridges and the appendages forming a stronger contrast than the papillary body.

EXAMPLES OF THE TYPOLOGY OF PATHOLOGIC FIGURES OF THE EPIDERMAL-DERMAL INTERFACE

The decisive question is whether the many pathologic alterations recognizable in the epidermal-dermal interface are such that not only certain recurring structures can be typified, but also a relation to the known and defined morphologic efflorescences can be established. On the basis of the analysis of more than 800 different preparations, we can say that the epidermal-dermal interface does indeed permit diagnostic conclusions. Let us illustrate in a few examples the outstandingly clear and characteristic features certain dermatoses can present in the figures of the epidermal-dermal interface.

Figure 9–1 shows the usual aspect of the epidermal-dermal interface and the border of a scar. The border of the scar runs through the right upper quarter. The division of the skin into fields is as clearly visible as in the other sections of the preparation. Superimposed is a net of rete ridges. The region of the scar is characterized by the absence of the net of epithelial ridges. Coarse, parallel, and often largely continuous ridges running toward the upper right are clearly visible. The appendages are clearly outlined at the borders of the scar as well as in the normal surrounding skin. The hair follicles appear in the form of longer epithelial pads. These are loosely distributed in rows running from the upper right to the lower left. The hair line is oriented toward the upper right. Because of the magnification, the hair bulb and sebaceous gland of each hair follicle are not recognizable. Between the hair follicles we find the excretory sweat ducts, with their upper end mostly broken off. In this figure their spatial relationship to the hair follicles cannot be established.

An ordinary eczema presents a completely different epidermal-dermal interface. Figure 9–2 demonstrates the border zone, in which the differences can be shown more clearly. In the left third we see the usual net of rete ridges, the same that predominates on the dorsal aspect of the forearm. There is the beginning of a maplike demarcation of coarsening rete ridges, which becomes clearer toward the right. The hair follicles are thickened, and the rete ridges closest to

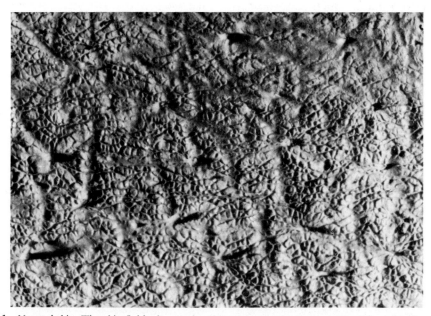

Figure 9–1   Normal skin. The skin fields show a rhombic pattern at the reverse side of the epithelium. Normal net of rete ridges. From upper right to lower left there are hair follicles in loose rows. Hair orientation is toward the upper right. Blunted ends of excretory sweat gland ducts are found between the hair follicles. At the right upper edge of the figure the epithelium shows only a few coarse rete ridges. ×20.

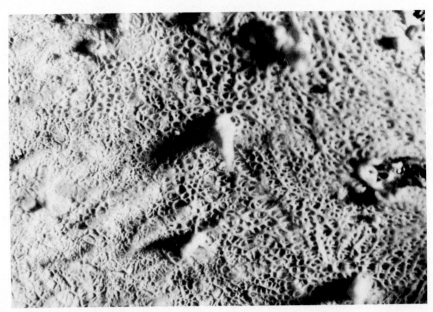

Figure 9–2   Eczema. In the left third there is a normal net of rete ridges with transition toward coarser epithelial ridges from left to right. The hair follicles also appear thickened. ×20.

them are more marked than in the other regions of the preparation. Close to the right edge of the figure there are two epithelial defects. These are artifacts due to the preparation. The eczematous aspect of the epidermis can also be recognized because of the irregular coarsening of the rete ridges, which is especially marked around the hair follicles. The hair

follicles in particular appear coarser than usual. The demarcation against the normal skin is maplike again, but clear.

Circumscribed neurodermatitis gives a different picture (Fig. 9–3). While the characteristic feature of the eczema is the varying elevation of the system of epithelial ridges, the net here presents much wider meshes. The rete ridges are thinner

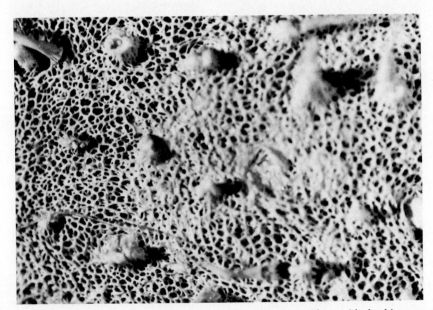

Figure 9–3   Circumscribed neurodermatitis. Wide-mesh net of rete ridges with beehive structure and thickened hair follicles. ×20.

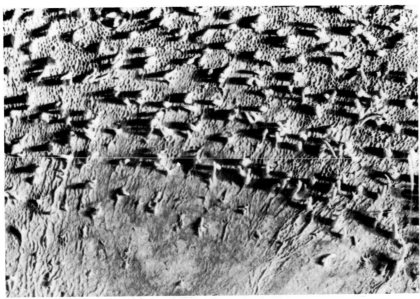

Figure 9–4 Border region of a scar. In the upper two thirds are hair groups in loose rows and isolated hair follicles. Between the hair follicles are excretory sweat gland ducts. Uniform net of rete ridges. In the lower third are some coarse epithelial ridges. No appendages. ×*18.*

and resemble a beehive rather than a sponge. The hair follicles are thickened as before and are likewise disposed in loose, parallel rows. The rete ridges arranged around them show a greater variety of forms than normal.

A new aspect again is that of the border zone of a scar in the transitional region between the eyebrow and the skin of the forehead (Fig. 9–4). The hair follicles can be seen in the lower part of the picture. They are mostly grouped; that is, next to isolated hair follicles there are also hair follicles arranged in a row. These hair follicle groups again form rows, the direction of which depends on the group ar-

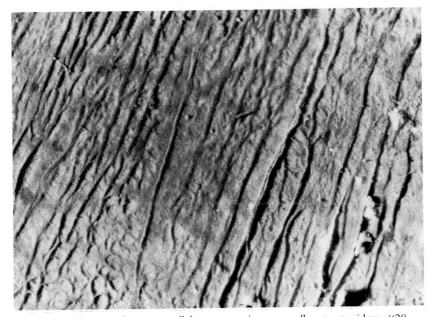

Figure 9–5 Scar. Coarse, parallel, anastomosing, or confluent rete ridges. ×*20.*

rangement. Between the hair follicle rows there are the ends of the sweat glands. The rete ridges form a net, which, with this magnification, is barely visible. Toward the lower edge of the figure the appendages become scarce and the system of epithelial ridges disappears, leaving just a few coarse, parallel ridges oriented toward a central focus situated in the upper right of the picture. The scar as such begins just above the picture and is represented in Figure 9–5. It is characterized by coarse, anastomosing, or rather confluent rete ridges, which every now and then are connected by cross-ridges. The surface relief is barely visible. The ridges are slightly darker. At the appendages, isolated excretory sweat gland ducts are recognizable, and there are no hair follicles at all. The fact that, close to the scar and in the regions devoid of appendages, the net of epithelial ridges is replaced by rests of parallel rete ridges means that the atrophied appendages of the skin have lost their organizational function for the normal structure of the basal epidermis (Horstmann, 1957; Oberste-Lehn, 1954a, 1962, 1964a, and 1964b). Such changes of the epidermal-dermal interface are irreversible. Similar forms, which vary in their particular structure, however, can be found in cir-

cumscribed scleroderma, lichen sclerosus et atrophicus, acrodermatitis atrophicans, and lichen ruber planus, but only in the zones affected by the lichenoid eruptions.

The example of the eczema and the neurodermatitis showed that the pathologic alterations of the basic structure of the epidermal-dermal interface consist only in a distortion of the normal proportions, but in the atrophic and scar-formation processes the changes in the configuration of the epithelial ridges are more thorough. The reversibility of the pathologic alterations of the epidermis depends on the conservation of the motives of Horstmann in the vicinity of the appendages (Oberste-Lehn, 1954a, 1962, 1964a, and 1964b).

An example of this is senile atrophic skin (Fig. 9–6). In these cases the net of epithelial ridges is preserved in large regions, though in a much reduced state, and it has been proved that there is neoformation of hair follicles and sweat glands (Oberste-Lehn, 1962, 1964a, and 1964b; Oberste-Lehn and Nobis, 1963). Nevertheless, in many small areas in the preparation the appendages and consequently the rete ridges are missing. These may be the pseudoscars described by Colomb et al. (1967), but investigations regarding the relation of these phenomena

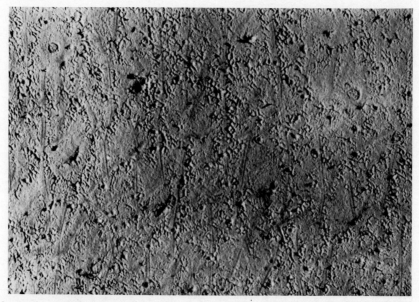

Figure 9–6   Senile atrophy. Severely reduced net of rete ridges with small hair follicles and excretory sweat gland ducts. ×*18*.

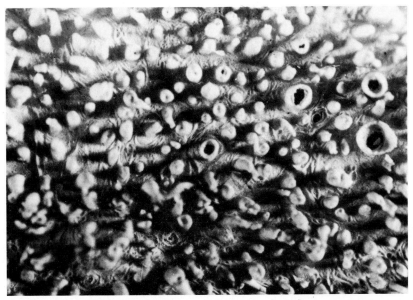

Figure 9–7 Chronic discoid lupus erythematosus. Markedly thickened hair follicles with upper end often missing. Normal excretory sweat gland ducts. Remainders of a few coarse rete ridges. ×*30.*

have not yet been concluded. Similar to these cicatricial and atrophic alterations is chronic discoid lupus erythematosus (Fig. 9–7). In this figure we are struck by the marked edema and thickening of the follicles. Their upper end has mostly been lost through maceration. This picture of the follicles corresponds to the keratotic

keratin plugs which are found in the follicles and produce the so-called tapestry-nail phenomenon. As far as we can see, the excretory sweat gland ducts are not affected. Between the hair follicles the net-like distribution of the rete ridges has been lost, and only a few coarse epithelial ridges are left, a fact that can be seen also

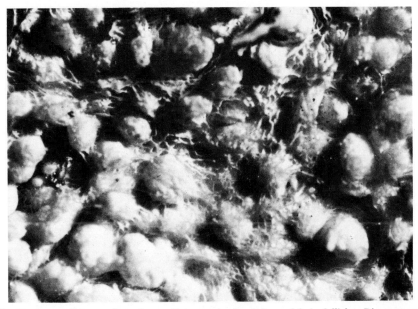

Figure 9–8 Verrucous lichen ruber planus. Dense, spheric, deformed hair follicles. Disappearance of rete ridges. ×*30.*

in histologic sections. The motives of Horstmann have disappeared. This aspect of chronic lupus erythematosus in the epidermal-dermal interface is characteristic and always recognizable. In older, almost healed foci of chronic discoid lupus erythematosus, the scarlike final stage is due to the disappearance of the ridge structures described by Horstmann and the rete ridges.

The alterations in lichen ruber planus are similar (Wilson; Oberste-Lehn, 1954a) (Fig. 9–8). This is especially plain in the verrucous lichen ruber (Oberste-Lehn, 1954a). Figure 9–8 shows closely packed, spheric elevations, which are most distinctly seen in two regions, lower left and upper right. Between these prominences there are rests of rete ridges bridging the gaps between the follicles. In other sections where the epithelial elevations are less dense, there is an occasional net of rete ridges. The elevations correspond to follicles filled with masses of keratin. This figure does not tell us anything about the state of the sweat glands, but this has been described in other places (Oberste-Lehn, 1954a). In the final stage, after the healing of the verrucous lichen, the scarring of the epithelium is also irreversible.

The preparations of a bullous drug eruption show completely different aspects (Fig. 9–9). The net of rete ridges is considerably atrophic, presumably because of the edema. Flattened epithelial ridges can be seen, which form a poorly demarcated net still clearly visible toward the right, in the region of the bulla. The appendages are preserved. The most essential alterations are four almost completely round areas with a sharply defined border. As can be seen in the lower left portion of the figure, the layer demarcating the lower part of the epithelium is destroyed in the affected areas. In these areas there is not even a trace of a net of rete ridges. The only structuring of the surface is provided by the skin fields. There is subepidermal bulla formation. In the left upper portion of the figure there is another large bulla, which has lost its roof, however. The aspect of the bulla in the righ upper portion is similar. In this case there is only circumscribed epidermolysis.

The epidermal-dermal interface of a bullous pemphigoid is different, although there are similar features (Fig. 9–10). Within the well-developed net of rete ridges and the normal hair follicles and sweat gland ducts, two round areas are sharply demarcated. They are character-

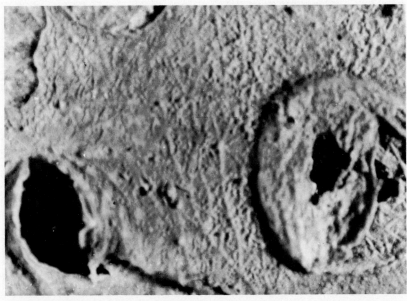

Figure 9–9 Bullous drug eruption. Skin fields showing through. Flattened net of rete ridges. Skin appendages are preserved. Four subepidermal bullae. ×20.

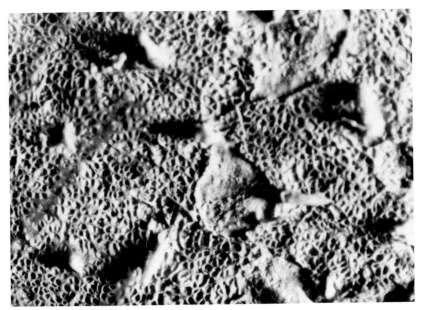

Figure 9–10 Bullous pemphigoid. Within the normal reverse side of the epithelium is a sharply demarcated area with the epithelial wall. Center almost without structure; roof of bulla. ×20.

ized by an epithelial wall. Within these areas there are considerable alterations of the rete ridges, which appear in the form of debris or are absent. The basal layer is partly dissolved. Those hair follicles or sweat glands which happen to be at the edge of the two areas are preserved. These alterations make the subepidermal bulla formation of bullous pemphigoid clearly appreciable in the epidermal-dermal interface. It ought to be stated, however, that dermatitis herpetiformis and malignant pemphigus vulgaris show different, although typical, structures on the reverse side of the epithelium, which make the differential diagnosis easily possible, even if the surface of the epithelium is viewed from below (Oberste-Lehn, 1957).

This survey of the features various diseases show at the epidermal-dermal junction illustrates that, after comparative studies, the differential diagnosis of dermatoses does not present any difficulties and that, on the basis of the morphogenetic principles discussed above, pathologic features can be correctly interpreted. This is the basis for a presentation of precancerous, pseudocancerous, and neoplastic alterations.

PRECANCEROUS KERATOSES, BOWEN'S DISEASE, AND KERATOACANTHOMA

Precancerous Keratoses

Senile Keratosis (Actinic Keratosis). The clinical and histologic diagnosis is based on well-known features and histologic as well as cytologic criteria. We shall try to show the development of this type of keratosis with the help of the representation of the epidermal-dermal interface.

When the partly parakeratotic, partly orthokeratotic lesions first appear on the skin with senile elastotic alterations, the epidermal-dermal interface does not show the reduced net of ridges that one would expect. The net of rete ridges, as well as the hair follicles and the excretory sweat gland ducts, is well developed (Fig. 9–11). At the upper edge of the figure there is a skin area with low rete ridges and reduced appendages. Toward the lower part the whole surface of the reverse side of the epidermis is covered with thickened hair follicles and sweat gland ducts. Prolonged (i.e., elevated) rete ridges part

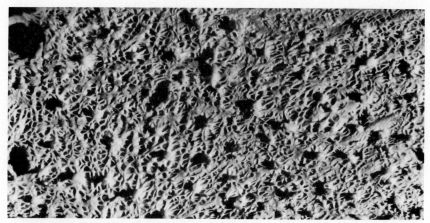

Figure 9–11   Recent senile keratosis. Thickened hair follicles and excretory sweat gland ducts. From these start elongated and narrowed rete ridges. ×*18*.

from the skin appendages and combine with others starting from neighboring appendages. The skin fields can partly be seen, a fact which means that the epidermis is relatively thin.

The reverse side of the epidermis shows similar alterations in a clinically frank actinic keratosis of a few weeks' duration (Fig. 9–12). The hair follicles form larger bulbs than the sweat gland ducts. The net of rete ridges is not as strongly marked as in Figure 9–11 and shows similar forms only at the lower edge of the figure. At the upper edge of the figure, an alteration of the structure is indicated by a coarsening of the epithelial ridges.

In a senile keratosis of many months' duration, the orderly structure of the epithelium, which can still be appreciated in Figures 9–11 and 9–12, is lost (Fig. 9–13). The rete ridges and appendages are considerably altered in a totally disorderly fashion. While at the lower edge of the figure the net of rete ridges still appears normal and there are normal appendages up to the zone of transition toward the pathologic alterations, an epidermal-dermal alteration spreads progressively from the bottom toward the top. Its features are such that they can no longer be properly described. At the lower border of the picture the ridges, starting from a still

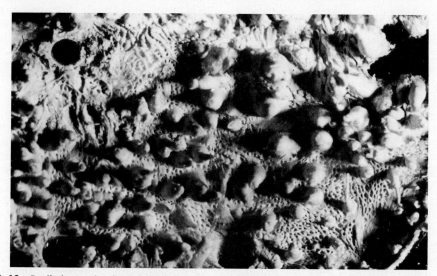

Figure 9–12   Senile keratosis of a few weeks' duration. Thickened hair follicles and excretory sweat glands. The net of rete ridges is less pronounced by comparison. Only the upper edge of the figure shows a coarser net of rete ridges. ×*25*.

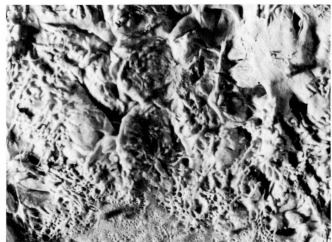

Figure 9-13 Senile keratosis of many months' duration with border region. Normal net of rete ridges and unchanged appendages only at lower edge of figure. From here toward the middle of the lesion there is progressive coarsening of rete ridges, until they form epithelial protrusions, which mostly consist of appendages, especially hair follicles. Normal excretory sweat gland ducts. ×20.

normal net of rete ridges, are becoming coarser and form a wide-mesh net, which disappears toward the upper part, in the direction of the center of the keratosis. Only isolated coarse ridges and cross-ridges are recognizable. They are located between coarse protrusions of the epithelium, mostly consisting of appendages, especially hair follicles. Distributed between these are many excretory sweat gland ducts of normal size. The transition between normal and thickened hair follicles is especially clear at the right side of the figure.

Figure 9–14, showing a clinically frank senile keratosis of several months' dura-

tion, has similar features at the epidermal-dermal interface. In the right upper part of the figure there are still traces of a net of rete ridges. The transition in the structuring of the senile keratosis is clearly visible. It can also be seen here that the blunt, cone-shaped, epithelial prominences are hair follicles, because the top is often broken off, so that the lumen becomes visible. The excretory sweat gland ducts are cone-shaped only in the vicinity of the epithelium, whereas the longer part of the duct which reaches the corium is still thin, that is, unchanged. Within the skin lesions the netlike distribution of the rete ridges can no longer be clearly distinguished (see

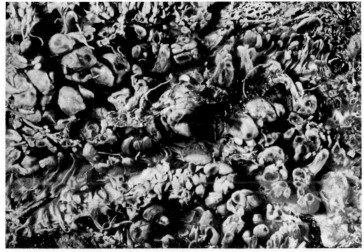

Figure 9–14 Senile keratosis of several months' duration. Indications of net of rete ridges at upper right. Blunt, cone-shaped protrusions are hair follicles. The excretory sweat gland ducts are thin and elongated and cone-shaped only in the vicinity of the covering epithelium. ×20.

Fig. 9–13). There are small leaf-shaped structures adjoining the appendages. It is possible that some of these are also located in the shadow of the blunt epithelial cones.

In summary, it has been possible to represent the full development of senile keratosis. In senile keratosis, the essential changes shown on the reverse side of the epithelium take place in the appendages, especially the hair follicles. These form coarse, sometimes large, masses. The pathologic process exerts little influence on the rete ridges. Some of these form small leaves in the vicinity of the appendages. The transition from the normal to the pathologic epithelium is continuously sharply marked, similar to the histologic section. The alterations of the appendages recall the umbrella-like changes shown by H. Pinkus (1967).

Bowen's Disease

The first example of Bowen's disease shows, in the lower half of the figure, a normal net of rete ridges (Fig. 9–15). The skin fields are evident on the reverse side of the epithelium. Coarse, roundish, partly parallel ridges enclose the tumor proper in a semicircle. From the rete ridges of the border structure of the tumor protrude cone- or button-shaped

elevations of the epithelium. These can become so monstrous that they can no longer be distinguished from thickened appendages. Isolated rete ridges can be distinguished between these epithelial tumor structures. Under the magnifying glass, the figure reveals no unaltered appendages. It is possible, though, that these may be hidden under the epithelial prominences. Figure 9–16, from another patient, gives the same impression. Here a greater part of the center of the lesion is represented. Similar to the features seen in Figure 9–15, the interface is dominated by coarse, roundish, epithelial elevations. When they are studied more closely, it becomes evident that the appendages do not participate in the formation of the prominences and that only the part of the appendages which adjoins the epithelium is thickened. The part facing the dermis is mostly unchanged. This means that there is considerable edema of the infundibulum of the appendages. The rete ridges form small lamellae and do not contribute to the growth of the epithelial portions. Their number is small, and they appear as a sort of connection between the appendages.

Although histologically and cytologically there is a difference between senile keratosis and Bowen's disease, the epidermal-dermal interface shows a relationship, because in both diseases the epithe-

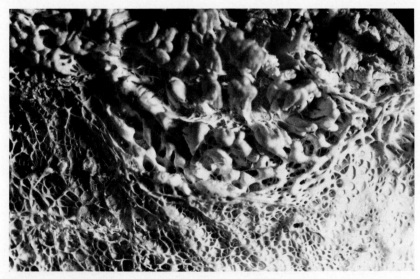

Figure 9–15   Border region of Bowen's disease. From the net of rete ridges cone- or button-shaped epithelial protrusions develop. Isolated narrow epithelial ridges are preserved. ×20.

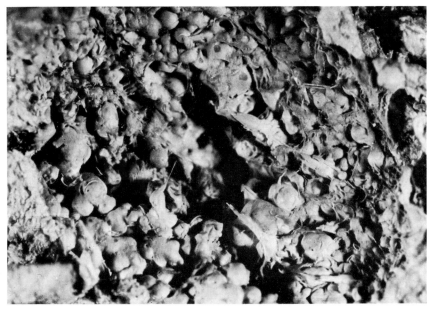

Figure 9–16 Center of lesion of Bowen's disease. Coarse, spheric, epithelial protrusions. Appendages are thickened only in the vicinity of the covering epithelium. Rete ridges are scarce and form narrow lamellae. ×25.

lium undergoes the same type of alteration, which leads to similar pathologic features (H. Pinkus, 1967). In a histologic section these features correspond to an acanthosis. The evaluation of the epidermal-dermal interface demonstrates once again that similar changes can be provoked by different processes.

Keratoacanthoma

It should be mentioned here that it is not possible to represent a spindle cell epithelioma, a keratoacanthoma, or a pseudoepitheliomatous hyperplasia in the interface. This is probably because of the fact that the tumoral tissue is no longer retractable, that the basal membrane and the basal cells are missing, and that there is a tendency to acantholysis similar to that in carcinoma. Consequently, only the border areas of the tumors are represented. These are identical in the case of the three above-mentioned diseases, so that the example of the keratoacanthoma will suffice for an illustration of all three (Fig. 9–17).

Figure 9–17 Border region of keratoacanthoma. The border runs from lower left toward upper right. The net of rete ridges increases in height from lower left toward upper right, i.e., the border region. In the border region there are smaller, parallel ridges. The coarsening of the rete ridges in the border region is accompanied by thickening of the appendages. ×20.

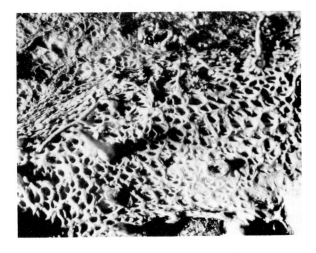

The border between the normal epithelium (lower right) and the transitional zone (upper left) runs from lower left to upper right. On the right side, the rete ridges are small and narrow. The impressions of the papillae of the connective tissue are relatively large. The appendages are normal. At the transition toward the border zone, the ridges are packed more closely and more parallel and give the impression of a graduated zone. The cross ridges are narrower and very small. From the top of the ridges in this zone there emerge blocklike, edematous rete ridges. The cross-ridges are also thickened to the degree of provoking a spongelike effect. This deepens and enlarges the spaces for the papillae of the connective tissue. It is remarkable that there is also a very considerable thickening of the hair follicles and of the epithelial portion of the sweat gland ducts. Moreover, there is not only an accentuation of the rete ridges, because of their increased height and width, but also a coarsening of the appendages. At the left upper edge of the figure, the transition of the interface between epithelium and corium into the tumor can no longer be followed, because the tumoral tissue could not be prepared. Only the border zone is represented. To judge by its structure, it shows the features of acanthosis, with the ends of the ridges turned toward the tumor as if to encircle it.

EPIDERMAL NEVI, BENIGN EPIDERMAL TUMORS, CIRCUMSCRIBED PRECANCEROUS MELANOSIS, AND MELANOMA

While the preceding section dealt with malignant epidermal tumors, we shall now consider the benign alterations of the epithelium. This will permit a comparison with the melanocytic neoformations. The representation of a melanoma in the interface will then follow.

Of the epidermal nevi, we shall discuss the nevus verrucosus (Fig. 9–18). The interface reflects the fact that the nevus verrucosus is a circumscribed hyperplasia of the epidermis with little alteration of its structure. A view of the reverse side of the epithelium shows that the structural changes affect above all the net of rete ridges. There are fine, coarse, and elongated rete ridges. The netlike distribution has been lost; instead, the impression is one of total confusion. Moreover, these rete ridges, which have become small lamellae, appear on elongated epi-

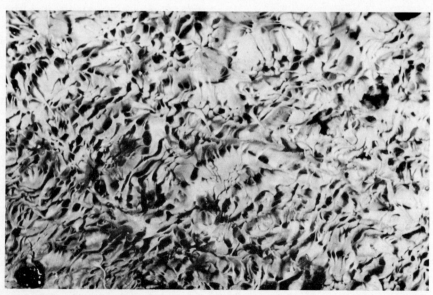

Figure 9–18   Nevus verrucosus. The rete ridges are narrow and elongated. They have lost their netlike distribution. ×25.

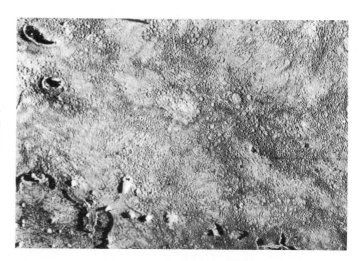

Figure 9–19 Syringoma. The epithelium covering a syringoma shows a fine-mesh net of rete ridges, which encloses thickened ends of excretory sweat gland ducts. ×20.

dermal protrusions of relatively great length. Fine cross-ridges connect the lamellated epithelial formations. This destroys the net effect and forms spaces of varying sizes into which the papillae of the connective tissue penetrate deeply. The depth of these crypts is not recognizable. The excretory sweat gland ducts are numerous and unchanged. There are no hair follicles, which suggests that these are hidden under the coarse, epithelial protrusions and the narrow, long, epithelial leaves. The fibroepithelial character of the nevi is evident in the transformation of the normal net of rete ridges in the direction of a papillary hyperplasia.

Among the tumors of the sweat gland apparatus, only the epithelium covering a syringoma can be represented (Fig. 9–19). It is occupied by a fine-mesh net of rete ridges of a singular tpe. This net includes the thickened ends of excretory sweat gland ducts, which are broken off just underneath the epithelium. At the lower edge of the figure, normal hair follicles are found.

Acanthosis Nigricans

This disease is being treated here because of its histologic similarity to some of the diseases treated in Chapter 10 (Fig. 9–20). Contrary to the nevus verrucosus, the epidermal-dermal interface preserves the original structure of the epidermal corium junction. Across the whole preparation, from the upper left to the lower right, there are strong, ridge-shaped epithelial formations, which run over long stretches. The cross-ridges are thin and connect the stronger epithelial ridges. At the reverse side of the epithelium, roundish epithelial prominences can be seen, which also form rows across the preparation. The smaller cross-ridges are lost on these prominences, so that their surface appears completely even. It is hard to say whether a penetration of the skin fields or keratotic cones are responsible for these flat areas of the interface. To judge by the histologic picture, it is possible that acanthotic and keratotic and, consequently, epithelial cones and ridges penetrate down to the corium and produce typical changes in the interface. The small, short epithelial ridges run toward these structures and disappear again at their level. The hair follicles are thickened, and there are no changes in the excretory sweat gland ducts. In summary, acanthosis nigricans is characterized by an accentuation of the net of rete ridges and coarse epithelial ridges, presumably formed because of marked acanthosis of the epithelium, covering long stretches of the epithelium and surface at the interface. Of the skin appendages, the hair follicles are thickened by keratosis. There are no changes in the excretory sweat gland ducts.

Seborrheic Keratosis

The prototype of the benign epidermoid tumors is seborrheic keratosis. Clinically, it is sometimes difficult to dif-

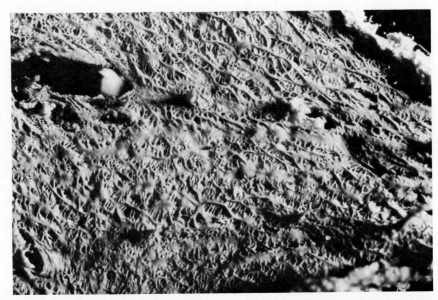

Figure 9–20 Acanthosis nigricans. The basic structure is preserved on the reverse side of the epithelium. We are struck by the penetration of round protrusions with a smooth surface. The rete ridges run toward them and disappear. The hair follicles are thickened. No alterations in the excretory sweat gland ducts. ×20.

ferentiate from a senile lentigo or the premalignant melanosis of Dubreuilh and the melanocytic melanoma developing from it. The histologic differentiation into a solid type and a papillomatous and reticulated type shall not be followed here in the interface, but we shall explain the formation of the common papillary type.

The first skin manifestations of a seborrheic keratosis, which histologically shows the usual papillomatous structure, appear on the reverse side of the epithelium, as represented in Figure 9–21. The net of rete ridges shows uniform changes. The ridges are elongated and slightly thickened. The cross-ridges, which are

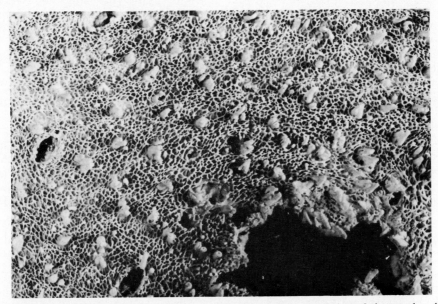

Figure 9–21 Recent seborrheic keratosis. Uniform net of rete ridges, consisting of elongated, only slightly thickened elements. The rete ridges connected with the appendages have not undergone these changes. Almost no changes in the appendages. ×20.

mostly smaller, show the same structure, so that the uniformity is general. Consequently the crypts for the papillae of the connective tissue are also more or less of the same size. These changes in the structure of the epithelial ridges often do not include those which are found in the immediate vicinity of the appendages, that is, those formations of ridges which have special importance (Horstmann, 1952; Oberste-Lehn, 1954a, 1964a, and 1964b). The so-called watch dial motif clearly consists of smaller ridges, which are just barely visible in the shadow which forms the higher surrounding net of ridges. This shows the nature of the papillary type of seborrheic keratosis and the development of its histologic structure. It further shows that Horstmann's motifs are special structures, which are not identical to the usual papillary ridge formations. The appendages are practically unchanged. The hair follicles are more strongly marked, but an evaluation will have to take into consideration that the specimen is from the temporal region with its terminal hair follicles.

The further development of the papillary seborrheic keratosis is represented in Figure 9–22. The preparation was made from a dark brown, pigmented, keratotic, seborrheic keratosis. The right border section of the figure includes the border of the seborrheic keratosis and the normal net of rete ridges. The transition from one structure to the other can also be seen. From the net of rete ridges epithelial proliferations have developed, which are mostly button-shaped and between which narrow ridge formations have been preserved. The epithelial portion of the hair follicles is thickened. There are no changes in the excretory sweat gland ducts, however. It should be stated that, because of the fixation process, the reverse side of the epithelium often does not show an existing pigmentation.

The true melanosis of Dubreuilh shows the criteria represented in Figure 9–23 in the epidermal-dermal interface. Within the normal structure of the interface with a net of rete ridges and hair follicles, as well as excretory sweat gland ducts, there is an almost round area, in which the rete ridges have lost their normal orientation. They are irregularly elevated, much scarcer than usual, and uneven in volume. Small zones have no rete ridges at all. The appendages are almost unrecognizable and can be found only upon very close examination. They seem to be scarcer. The reverse side of the epithelium itself ap-

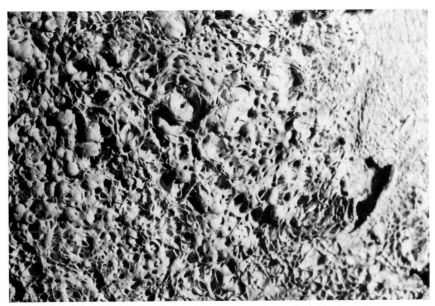

Figure 9–22 Border region of seborrheic keratosis of several months' duration. The net of rete ridges encloses round, epithelial protrusions, which cause a transformation of the reverse side of the epithelium. This structural change of the epithelium can be followed from the upper right corner of the preparation. ×20.

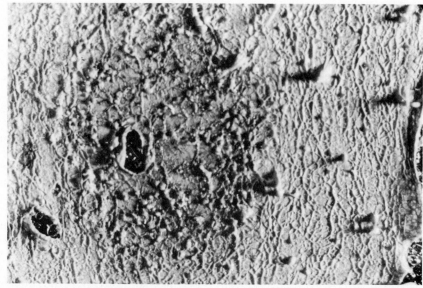

Figure 9–23   Circumscribed precancerous melanosis. Irregularly elevated, scarce rete ridges in a round area in the center and left portion of the figure. Within the lesion the number of appendages is diminished. ×20.

pears looser and coarser. The basal layer is no longer completely intact. This is a developmental stage of the melanosis of Dubreuilh, in which melanocytic nests have already appeared in the junction area, so that there is a transition to invasive melanocytic melanoma.

The tumor of the melanocytic melanoma can no longer be represented in the interface (Fig. 9–24). It cannot be prepared. Only the border region is represented

and characterized by a coarsening of the net of rete ridges (see lower half of figure). Each ridge appears elongated in comparison with the ridges in the neighboring zones, and the spaces for the papillae of the connective tissue are larger. This feature appears in all skin diseases which are accompanied by an "inflammation."

The nevocytic melanoma cannot be represented in the interface either, and for

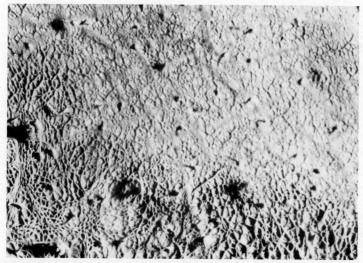

Figure 9–24   Border region of melanocytic melanoma. The melanoma is beyond the lower edge of the figure. The net of rete ridges is coarser in the border region. ×20.

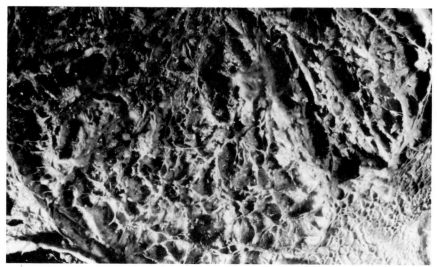

Figure 9–25   Papillomatous nevus cell nevus with border region. There is a structural change of the reverse side of the epithelium, i.e., a proliferation not involving the appendages, proceeding from the lower right corner of the figure. ×25.

the same reasons. The tumor as such is unpreparable; it succumbs to maceration.

This does not apply, though, to the papillomatous nevus cell nevus (Fig. 9–25). Here the reverse side of the epithelium is completely represented. There are no changes in the interface at the right lower edge of the figure. Then there follows, in a semicircle demarcation, a coarsening of the net of rete ridges. Each ridge is elongated and narrow. The space for the papilla of the connective tissue is so enlarged that it resembles a funnel. Small, short rete ridges run toward the larger ones, which are sometimes indented at their lower ends. Because of the proliferation of the rete ridges, the skin appendages are no longer prominent enough to protrude beyond the interface. They are found between the rete ridges in the form of buttons (hair follicles) or small plugs (excretory sweat gland ducts). The fields of the dermis can be seen on the reverse side of the interface.

BASAL CELL EPITHELIOMA, TRICHOEPITHELIOMA, AND ADENOCARCINOMA OF THE SKIN

Basal Cell Epithelioma

The basal cell epithelioma will be discussed in detail in other chapters of this book. Here we would like to show the features of this tumor in the interface. There has been a previous report on this subject (Oberste-Lehn, 1954b), and in the meantime the writer's views on the morphogenesis have changed little, although new investigations have changed our concepts of the etiology (Zackheim, 1963; and others). There is no doubt that the border zone of the basal cell epithelioma is the most interesting region (Fig. 9–26). While in the upper part of the figure and to the right the net of rete ridges is normal, in the middle and left parts pathologic alterations dominate. The net of rete ridges is much more marked in the border zone and then disappears completely. Only isolated rete ridges run from the border toward the atrophic epidermis. They run toward the appendages, around which they take the form of a sea anemone. These formations are found almost regularly around the appendages. Often they are connected by the rete ridges. Moreover, there are coarse, button-shaped, epithelial masses around the appendages, and the reverse side of the epithelium sometimes has a wavy aspect; that is, in some areas there are very small, parallel ridge formations.

The description of Figure 9–27, taken from a preparation of a basal cell epithelioma of the temple, is similar. The basal cell epithelioma in Figure 9–26 was taken from the forehead.

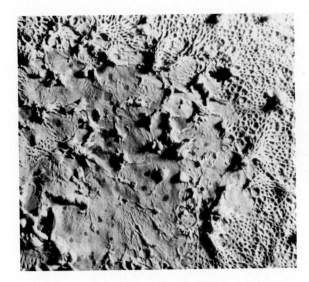

Figure 9–26 Border region of a basal cell epithelioma. A roundish, smooth area with a few appendages, around which the rete ridges are distributed in a sea anemone pattern is seen to develop from the normal system of rete ridges in the upper part and toward the right of the figure over a transitional border region. ×20.

Figure 9–27 shows clearly how the existing rete ridges are transformed into the above-described coarse, sea anemone-like formations which are found on the atrophic epidermis. Their interconnection can also be clearly seen. The sea anemone formations of the epithelium probably contain an appendage. From the interpretation of these formations one gets the impression that the epithelium of the epidermis and of the appendages gives rise to the tumoral masses, which then evolve into specific forms, owing to the formative influence of the appendages. No other dermatosis recognizable in the interface shows these features. The inhibiting or growth-producing effects of the appendages have been previously described (Oberste-Lehn, 1962, 1964a, and 1964b; see literature there).

Figure 9–28 of a basal cell epithelioma from the transition zone between the forehead (right side) and the hairy scalp (left side) again shows the sea anemone shape of the epithelial proliferation.

Experiences with other preparations have shown that the histologic variations of the basal cell epithelioma do not correspond to specific forms in the interface.

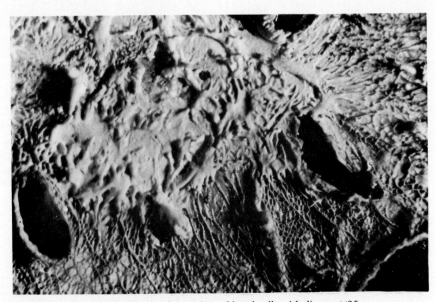

Figure 9–27   Border region of basal cell epithelioma. ×25.

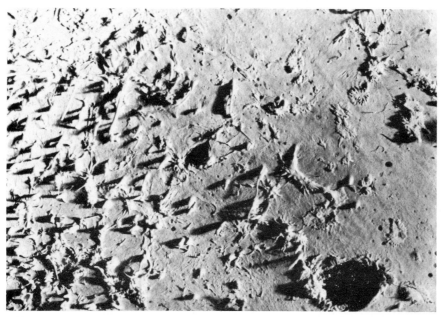

Figure 9–28 Center of basal cell epithelioma at hair line on forehead. Sea anemone–like formations of rete ridges around appendages on almost flat reverse side of epithelium. ×20.

The same basic structures are always repeated. It is possible that their variations suggest clinical and histologic variations, but here we would need further studies.

The superficial or pagetoid basal cell epithelioma has to be dealt with separately. First of all, the above-described epithelial structures are found here also, but we can make one additional observation: there are several basal cell epitheliomas within a few millimeters of each other (Fig. 9–29). We can distinguish beyond doubt a great number of tumor foci, which are all separate basal cell epitheliomas. This coexistence of several basal cell epitheliomas has led to the dis-

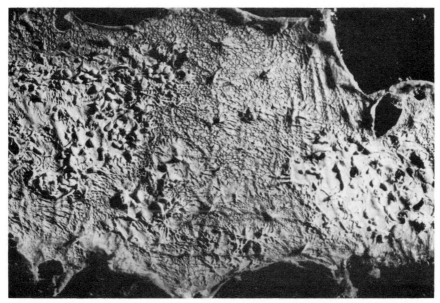

Figure 9–29 Superficial, pagetoid basal cell epithelioma. Four typical basal cell epitheliomas lying close together. ×18.

cussion of the question of multicentricity (Oberste-Lehn, 1954b; Sanderson, 1961; Madsen, 1965h; Pinkus, 1957 and 1967). The problem seems to be the definition of multiplicity and multicentricity. It is well known that superficial basal cell epitheliomas can appear in groups and close to each other in the same skin area. It is also well known that the different foci can become confluent and that it is not always possible to prevent a recurrence through an excision performed 1 to 2 mm. from the clinically distinguishable border of the basal cell epithelioma (see Menn et al., 1971). This purely clinical observation finds an explanation in the interface, where several basal cell epitheliomas are situated relatively close to each other. Growth very probably spreads from one single focus in each basal cell epithelioma. According to the ideas of Büngeler (1951) and under his influence, this has been interpreted as proliferation (hyperplasia, hypertrophy), and it was clearly understood that the outsized rete ridges of the border region were part of the parenchyma of the tumor. On the basis of cell and tumor biology, though, I fail to see how tumor material can reestablish contact with the epidermis beyond the border of the tumor (Madsen, 1965).

Trichoepithelioma (Adenoid Cystic Epithelioma)

In the systematic representation of tumors in this group, the trichoepithe-

lioma occupies a special place. This is reflected also in the epidermal-dermal interface (Fig. 9–30). Again the border zone is represented with part of the tumor. This shows the transition, and we can see that from the net of rete ridges of the surrounding skin another structure continuously develops, the characteristics of which are the dense epithelial elevations, which are interconnected by coarse, thickened rete ridges. The crypts of the papillae of the connective tissue are larger than normal and appear to be deeper also. The hair follicles are considerably enlarged. The excretory sweat gland ducts, although clearly visible in the border zone and in the vicinity of the tumor, have disappeared in the transformed epithelial proliferation. The interpretation of the features of the interface clearly shows that we deal with a tumor which is different from basal cell epithelioma.

Adenocarcinoma (Paget's Disease)

The preparation is from the areola and the surrounding skin of the left mamma of a 55 year old woman, who had been suffering from a moist skin condition for about one year. The lesion had started in the mamilla and spread over the lateral part of the areola.

The histology was typical for an epidermotropic adnexal carcinoma. The interface (Fig. 9–31) shows two epithelial alterations in the form of a semicircle and

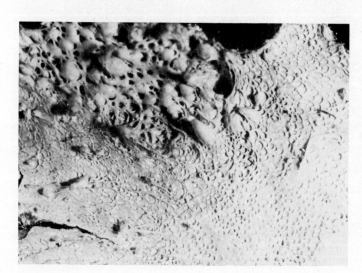

Figure 9–30 Border region of a trichoepithelioma. Continuous, closely packed epithelial protrusions interconnected by rete ridges are developing from the surrounding net of rete ridges. The hair follicles are coarser. ×20.

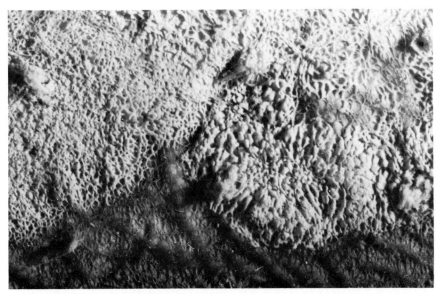

Figure 9–31 Paget's disease. Normal net of rete ridges in the lower portion of the figure. From this, two tumoral epithelial alterations in the form of a semicircle can be distinguished. The left portion if spongelike. The net of rete ridges is more distinctly marked, but fine. The right portion consists of irregular rete ridges and epithelial cones. ×20.

sharply delimited against the normal epidermis, which occupies the lower part of the picture. The net of rete ridges is diminished. The skin fields can be recognized in the form of rhombic ridges. The excretory sweat gland ducts are clearly visible. There are distinct differences between the two tumoral epithelial formations arranged in a semicircle. While the left part has a spongelike appearance, with an accentuated and finer net of rete ridges, the right part shows irregular, large, thick ridges resembling plugs. Although the epithelial ridges are coarser here also, they are much more irregular, so that the net structure has been lost. Isolated hair follicles can be seen toward the bottom and on the left side of the picture. It can no longer be determined whether the areola ends in the upper part of the picture, a fact which would explain the structural differences of the two parts of the tumor. It is also possible, though, that we are dealing with two different phases in the development of the tumor. As mentioned above, however, there is no doubt that the altered rete ridges contain nests of adenocarcinomatous cells.

LICHEN SCLEROSUS ET ATROPHICUS

In the interface, lichen sclerosus et atrophicus has the following characteristics as compared with the normal reverse side of the epithelium of the penis. The normal skin of the balanopreputial fold (Fig. 9–32) shows, in the middle of the preparation from the top toward the bottom, a reticular net of rete ridges. This continues on the dorsal side of the penis. Here the rete ridges are just somewhat more accentuated and continue over longer stretches, so that the aspect of the reverse side of the epithelium is changed. Toward the inner side of the prepuce (left side of the picture), the net of rete ridges develops into stronger, coarse, epithelial ridges in a parallel distribution from the bottom toward the upper right. The cross-ridges are relatively flat and have disappeared in large areas. The formation of the rete ridges is typical for the prepuce (Horstmann, 1952), although it can be found also in other skin regions which are poor in appendages. In comparison with these features, there is an alteration of the re-

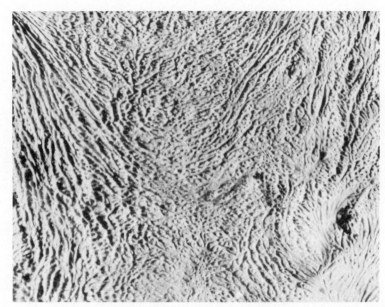

Figure 9–32   Prepuce. The balanopreputial fold cuts vertically through the center of the figure. ×*20.*

verse side of the epithelium in lichen sclerosus (Fig. 9–33). The lower third of the picture shows a fine net of rete ridges. The middle is occupied by flat areas of different sizes and configurations, between which there are still rete ridges in a reticular distribution. In the upper third of the picture, which shows the formation of a skin fold, there are also flat areas of epidermis situated in the upper right and in the center. Around them and in some spots at the edge of the pathologic foci we see more or less clearly developed rete ridges. The lichenoid character shows in the spotlike atrophy of the reverse side of the epidermis. There are no appendages.

In contrast, the aspect of circumscribed scleroderma in the interface is quite dif-

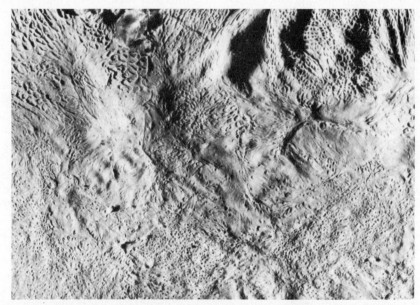

Figure 9–33   Lichen sclerosus and atrophicus of the prepuce. While the lower portion of the picture shows a normal net of rete ridges, there are, in the center of the preparation, flat areas of different configurations with remainders of rete ridges. The lichenoid character of the dermatosis shows in the foci of the flat areas. ×*20.*

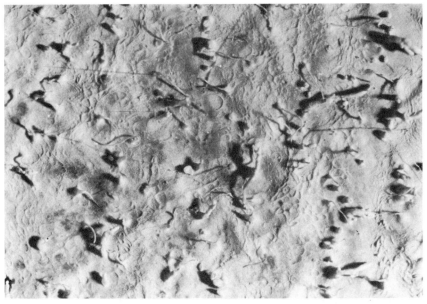

Figure 9–34   Circumscribed scleroderma. Apart from remainders of rete ridges, the reverse side of the epithelium is flat. Grouped hair follicles form loose rows. Between these are elongated excretory sweat gland ducts. ×25.

ferent (Fig. 9–34). There are only rests of rete ridges preserved. In some places weak, elevated stripes of the reverse side of the epithelium seem to be the only morphologic feature. The hair follicles, which are mostly grouped, are disposed in loose rows. Excretory sweat gland ducts are found between them. Atrophic acrodermatitis shows just such a change in the reverse side of the epithelium (Fig. 9–35), but in these lesions the atrophy is strictly limited to the appendages.

MESODERMAL TUMORS

Cutaneous Nodule and Fibroma Pendulum

The cutaneous nodule, as the prototype of a dermal fibroma, shows in the epidermal-dermal interface a circumscribed alteration of the rete ridge formation (Fig. 9–36). In a zone shaped like a semicircle, roundish, elevated rete ridges have developed. They are close together, and in the

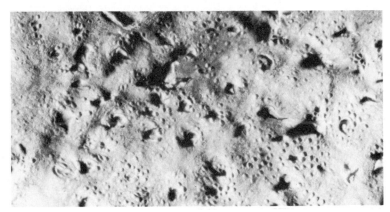

Figure 9–35   Atrophic acrodermatitis. Impressions of papillae of the connective tissue on the almost flat reverse side of the epithelium. Reduction of the rete ridges and of the appendages. ×25.

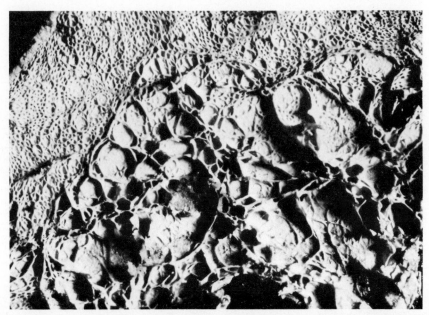

Figure 9–36   Cutaneous nodule. The normal net of rete ridges situated in the upper left of the figure limits an area shaped life a semicircle, which contains round fields formed by narrow, high rete ridges, enclosing the impressions of coarse papillae of the connective tissue. ×20.

background the net of rete ridges has been preserved in relatively large areas. Some smaller areas show only the impressions of the papillae of the connective tissue. The unchanged structure of the rete ridges of the surrounding skin forms a type of wall against this honeycomb structure. In this area the appendages are normal. The usual vertical section through such a skin area would probably correspond to Figure 378 in A Guide to Dermatohistopathology by Pinkus and Mehregan (1969).

The alterations found in a lenticular fibroma (histiocytoma) (Fig. 9–37) are more discrete. The normal structure of

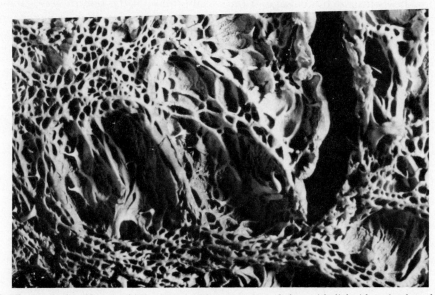

Figure 9–37   Lenticular fibroma (histiocytoma). The structure of the epithelial ridges is altered through coarse impressions of connective tissue with deformed rete ridges. ×30.

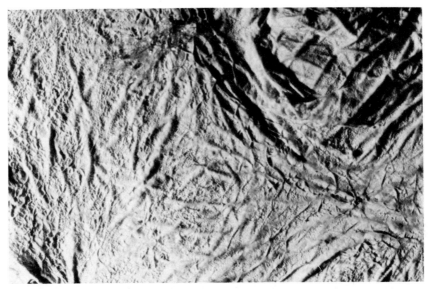

Figure 9–38 Fibroma pendulum. The skin fields show clearly on the reverse side of the epithelium. The net of rete ridges has been replaced by impressions of papillae of the connective tissue. ×20.

the rete ridges is characterized by several coarse impressions of connective tissue with a background in which rete ridges and appendages are preserved.

The fibroma pendulum shows no such change in the interface. The epithelium is elevated and folded because of the hardening which takes place after maceration, comparable to a deflated balloon (Fig. 9–38). The skin fields show very clearly on the reverse side of the epithelium, because the epithelium seems to be thinner. There is no net of rete ridges, which is replaced by a small impression of papillae of the connective tissue on the reverse side of the epithelium. No appendages are found in these areas.

Vascular Nevi and Kaposi's Sarcoma

In the preparation of a tuberous angioma in a 2 year old child the net of rete ridges is strongly marked. A similarly regular accentuation of this epithelial formation has been found in no other preparation (Fig. 9–39). The hair follicles are normal. They are equidistant from each other, and at the hair line we can see that they are distributed in rows. The rete ridges surrounding them are flatter than the other epithelial ridges. In many places the rosette formation of the rete ridges is clearly visible. Between the hair follicles we find excretory sweat gland ducts. One would think that the epithelium covering an angioma would be flat, as in the fibroma pendulum, but the angioma shows, on the contrary, a hypertrophy of the rete ridges. Kaposi's sarcoma (Fig. 9–40) does not show these features. We prepared the epithelium covering a tumor of the leg. The middle is flat with atrophic skin. This shows also in the fact that the epithelium tore a few times during preparation. In this specific area one excretory sweat gland duct has been preserved. It is round, and at its border, which is not sharply delimited, there are rete ridges with the usual net structure and hair follicles.

MESODERMAL MALIGNANT TUMORS

Mycosis Fungoides

The clinical and histologic picture of this cutaneous lymphoblastoma varies widely, and the epidermal-dermal interface is similarly uncharacteristic. In parapsoriasis en plaques, a precursor of mycosis fungoides, the reverse side of the epithelium shows the same alterations as a genuine psoriasis (Fig. 9–41). There is not

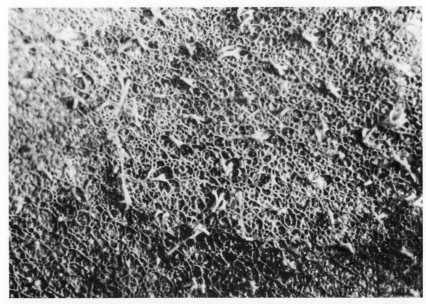

Figure 9–39 Tuberous angioma. Accentuated, fine net of rete ridges. Unchanged hair follicles grouped in loose rows. The special epithelial ridges surrounding them are lower than those in the vicinity. ×20.

much resemblance between these alterations and those of an eczema, in which the net of rete ridges is flatter and the ridges do not have the buttonlike appearance seen in psoriasis. The normal net of rete ridges with hair follicles and excretory sweat gland ducts (upper right in the figure) becomes increasingly accentuated toward the lower left. Each separate rete ridge becomes elongated and swells into a buttonlike shape at its extreme end. The hair follicles in the lower left corner of the figure appear plumper, but there are no changes in the excretory sweat gland ducts.

The view of an infiltrated focus on the

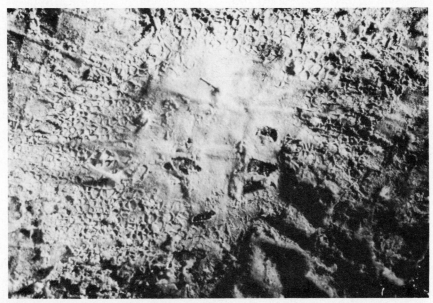

Figure 9–40 Multiple, hemorrhagic, idiopathic sarcoma. The epithelium covering the tumor is flat. One excretory sweat gland duct has been preserved. ×20.

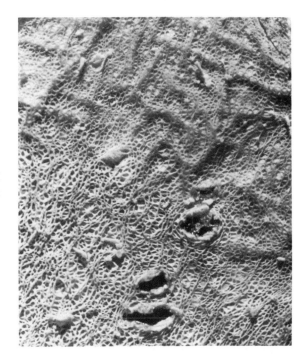

Figure 9–41 Parapsoriasis en plaques. Progressive changes of the net of rete ridges from the right toward the left edge of the figure. The restructuring of the epithelium is similar to that in eczema. ×20.

reverse side of the epithelium, which has already completed the parapsoriasis stage and can be considered mycosis fungoides en plaques even histologically, shows very similar features (Fig. 9–42). The acanthosis already represented in Figure 9–41 has become more marked. The crypts of the papillae of the connective tissue have become deeper, but not wider. Each rete ridge has become still more elongated, and its extreme end is more swollen and rounder. There are no changes in the hair follicles, nor in the excretory sweat gland ducts. In comparison with psoriasis the elongation of the rete ridges is more irregular, however, and the crypts for the papillae of the connective tissue are of different sizes.

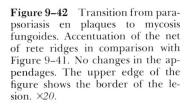

Figure 9–42 Transition from parapsoriasis en plaques to mycosis fungoides. Accentuation of the net of rete ridges in comparison with Figure 9–41. No changes in the appendages. The upper edge of the figure shows the border of the lesion. ×20.

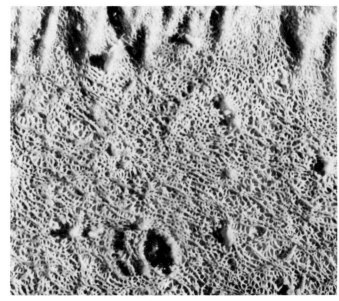

In comparison with this not very characteristic morphology, the atrophic vascular poikiloderma, which along with parapsoriasis en plaques is related to mycosis fungoides, presents a remarkable picture. The clinical characteristics, such as the foci of atrophy, the pigmentation, and the telangiectasis, actually explain the bizarre structures of the reverse side of the epithelium better than the histologic features, such as the variable thickness of the epidermis, the spotty basal pigmentation, the subepidermal macrophage pigmentation, the ecstatic vessels, and the occasional liquefaction of the basal cells (Fig. 9–43). The net of rete ridges appears mottled. The superficial skin fields, which normally form distinct, mostly rhombic figures, especially in senile skin, are irregular. These irregular skin fields show through at the reverse side of the epithelium. In some areas the bordering basal layer has lost its smoothness (liquefaction). There is no normal net of rete ridges. This makes the formations of rete ridges still more striking, with their equal distances and their distribution around the hair follicles, which can be seen under close observation. The hair follicles are generally disposed in rows and grouped and/or isolated (Oberste-Lehn and Nobis, 1963). In this body region, the hip, isolated hair follicles predominate. Around these, rests of the system of rete ridges have been preserved, even though the remainder of the covering epithelium has been atrophied. To me this suggests again the formative influence of the epithelium of the follicles or the covering epithelium in the vicinity of the follicles, respectively (Oberste-Lehn, 1954b, 1964a, and 1964b; H. Pinkus, 1957), which is exerted despite the atrophy of the epithelium caused by the pathologic process.

An erythroderma in mycosis fungoides shows still other features in the epidermal-dermal interface than the parapsoriasis en plaques or the poikiloderma. The interface shows the changes found in an eczema (Fig. 9–44). The skin fields can be seen on the reverse side of the epithelium. The net of rete ridges is coarser. Each ridge sits on the epithelium on a broad base, and its ends are sharp, not button-shaped as in parapsoriasis or psoriasis. The space for the papillae of the connective tissue has become a blunt cone. There are no changes in the appendages.

Reticulosarcoma

The skin of the patient from whom this preparation was taken was covered with

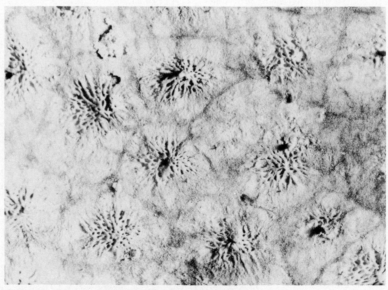

Figure 9–43   Vascular atrophic poikiloderma after parapsoriasis en plaques with mycosis fungoides. Irregular skin fields show on the reverse side of the epithelium, which has lost its system of rete ridges and looks rough. Equidistant formations of rete ridges around the hair follicles. ×20.

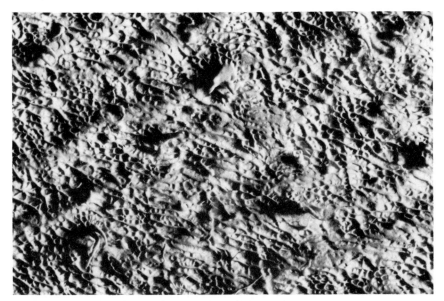

Figure 9–44   Erythroderma in mycosis fungoides. Coarsening of the net of rete ridges. ×25.

brownish, half-round tumors of moderate consistency. The histologic study revealed a reticulosarcoma. The interface (Fig. 9–45) shows roundish to oval impressions containing the rests of the system of epithelial ridges. The borders of these formations form elevated walls, whereas the spaces between them are almost flat.

The appendages have mostly disappeared or are atrophied, and only in one place can they still be clearly distinguished. In this place there is also still a well-outlined net of rete ridges. It is possible that the tumors located in the upper and middle corium have provoked these changes in the interface.

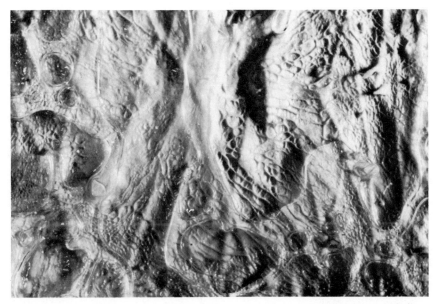

Figure 9–45   Reticulosarcoma. Round to oval impressions at the reverse side of the epithelium enclosing remainders of the system of rete ridges. The edges of the impressions are wall-shaped. The appendages have mostly disappeared.

SUMMARY

The method of preparation of figures of the epidermal-dermal interface has been described. The surface of the epithelium thus obtained shows the structures of the epithelium at the interface with the corium. A study of the figures of the epidermal-dermal interface in various dermatoses proves their diagnostic value. The present paper has described and compared normal skin and eczema, neurodermatitis, scar tissue, atrophy, discoid and chronic lupus erythematosus, verrucous lichen planus, drug eruption, bullous pemphigoid, senile keratosis, and acanthosis. The differential diagnosis of other dermatoses has been discussed in a number of earlier publications.

A study of the epithelial structures of dermatoses shows in the most diverse lesions repeated, identical alterations of general importance. These are parallel or radial rete ridges running toward the focus of the lesion, which is known to turn into a scar or atrophy in its final stage. Furthermore, the rete ridges which are found around the hair follicles and excretory sweat gland ducts (Horstmann's motives) are of special importance in various dermatoses. They represent the principle of a morphologic element of the skin (Oberste-Lehn, 1964a and 1964b). If the rete ridges and excretory sweat gland ducts, alone or together with the appendages, are destroyed, an irreversible skin alteration results. These specific epithelial ridges around the appendages usually do not participate in the formative changes undergone by the other rete ridges in the course of the pathologic process. If, on the other hand, the epithelium of the appendages is affected by the disease, the result is also a scarred or atrophic epithelium. It seems that growth or degeneration impulses start from the epithelium of the appendages or the specific rete ridges around them.

These basic rules have been applied to the dermatoses which form part of the subject matter of this book. Naturally, only those diseases could be represented in which the interface between the epithelium and the corium is not totally destroyed. Of the total material collected, isolated dermatoses can be studied, or the dermatoses can be discussed within the context to which they belong. In these discussions it is always helpful to recall the histologic features. The histologic structure of the dermatoses described finds its complement in the figures of the interface, which show basic aspects of the described affections.

REFERENCES

Blaschko, A.: Beiträge zur Anatomie der Oberhaut. Arch. Mikrosk. Anat., 30:495, 1887.

Büngeler, W.: Z. Krebsforsch., 58:72, 1951.

Colomb, D., Duncan, J. A., and Lartaud, J.: Individualisation anatomo-clinique d'une form inconnue de la peau Sénile: Les pseudo-cicatrices stellaires spontanées: Leur rapports avec le purpura de Bateman. Ann. Dermatol. Syph., 99:273, 1967.

Cowdry, E. V., and Nielson, P. S.: Cited by Pinkus, F.

Donders, B.: Enzyklopädie der mikroskopischen Technik. Bd. 2. Berlin, Urban u. Schwarzenberg, 1910.

Fleischhauer, K.: Über die Morphogenese des Haarstriches und der Papillarleisten. Z. Zellforsch., 38:50, 1953a.

Fleischhauer, K.: Über die Entstehung der Haaranordnung und das Zustandekommen räumlicher Beziehungen zwischen Haaren und Schweissdrüsen. Z. Zellforsch., 38:328, 1953b.

Greb, W.: Untersuchungen über die Gestalt des Papillarkörpers der menschlichen Haut. Z. Anat. Entwicklungsgesch., 110:245, 1940.

Hebra, H.: Beiträge zur Anatomie des Nagels. Wien. Med., Jb. 1880, p. 59.

Henle, J.: Die äussere Haut mit ihren Fortsetzungen. *In* Handbuch der systematischen Anatomie des Menschen. Bd. 2. Braunschweig, 1866.

Hoffmann, E.: Cited by Lehmensieck, R., and Horstmann, E.: Anatomische Untersuchung zur Form und Anordnung des Papillarkörpers. Hautarzt, 2:525, 1951.

Horstmann, E.: Über den Papillarkörper der menschlichen Haut mit ihren regionalen Unterschieden. Acta Anat. (Basal), 14:23, 1952.

Horstmann, E.: *In* Bargmann, W. (Ed.): Handbuch der mikroskopischen Anatomie des Menschen. Bd 3. Berlin, Springer-Verlag, 1957, pp. 56–63.

Kölliker, A.: Handbuch der Gewebelehre des Menschen. 6. Auflage, Band 1, Leipzig, 1889.

Kollmann, A.: Cited by Unna, P. G.

Lehmensieck, R.: Einfache Methode zur Darstellung der Wirbeltierepidermis und ihrer Anhangsgebilde. Z. Wiss. Mikr., 52:435, 1935–36.

Madsen, A.: Studies on basal-cell epithelioma of the skin. Acta Pathol. Mikrobiol. Scand., Suppl. 177, 1965.

Maurer, F.: Die Epidermis und ihre Abkömmlinge. Leipzig, Wilhelm Engelmann, 1895.

Medawar, P. B.: Sheets of pure epidermal epithelium from human skin. Nature (Lond.), 148:783, 1941.

Meijere, J. C. H. de: Über die Haare der Säugetiere. Morphologisches Jahrbuch, 21:312, 1894.

Menn, H., Robins, P., Kopf, A. W., and Bart, R. S.: The recurrent basal cell epithelioma. Arch. Dermatol., 103:628, 1971.

Oberste-Lehn, H.: Charakteristika der epidermalen Formelemente bei einigen Dermatosen. Hautarzt, 3:351, 1952a.

Oberste-Lehn, H.: Die Darstellung der Epidermisstrukturen durch Hyaluronidase-Maceration. Z. Mikrosk. Anat. Forsch., 60:463, 1952b.

Oberste-Lehn, H.: Die morphologische Abgrenzung des Lichen planus. Arch. Dermatol., 198:449, 1954a.

Oberste-Lehn, H.: Zur Histogenese des Basalioms. Z. Haut. Geschlechtskr., 16:334, 1954b.

Oberste-Lehn, H.: Die Bedeutung der Bündelhaare im menschlichen Haarkleid. Arch. Klin. Exp. Dermatol., 206:506, 1956.

Oberste-Lehn, H.: Die morphologischen Merkmale bullöser Dermatosen. Proceedings XI. International Congress of Dermatology. Acta Derm. Venereol. (Stockh.) 3:332, 1957.

Oberste-Lehn, H.: Dermoepidermal Interface. Arch. Dermatol., 86:114, 1962.

Oberste-Lehn, H.: Morphogenetische Studien an der menschlichen Haut an Hand des epidermocutanen Grenzflächenbildes. Studium Generale, 9:577, 1964a.

Oberste-Lehn, H.: Effects of aging on the papillary body of the hair follicles and on the eccrine sweat glands. *In* Montagna, W.: Aging. Oxford, Pergamon Press, 1964b.

Oberste-Lehn, H., and Nobis, A.: Die Haaranordnung beim Menschen und einigen Säugetieren. Z. Anat. Entwicklungsgesch., 123:589, 1963.

Philippson, L.: Über die Darstellung von Flächenbildern der Oberhaut und der Lederhaut. Monatsh. Prakt. Dermatol., 8:389, 1889.

Pinkus, F.: Die Entwicklungsgeschichte der Haut. *In* Keibel-Malls Handbuch der Entwicklungsgeschichte des Menschen. Bd. 1. Leipzig, Hirtzel, 1910, pp. 185–207.

Pinkus, F.: Die normale Anatomie der Haut. *In* Jadassohn's Handbuch der Haut- und Geschlechtskrankheiten. I, 1:378, Berlin, Springer-Verlag, 1927.

Pinkus, H.: The problem of multicentricity in skin cancer. Bull. Wayne State Univ. Coll. Med., 4:1, 1957.

Pinkus, H.: Malignant transformation of the epithelium. *In* McKenna, R. M. B.: Modern Trends in Dermatology. Vol. 3. London, Butterworth, 1966, p. 275.

Pinkus, H.: Modern Trends in Dermatology. London, Butterworth, 1966.

Pinkus, H.: The border line between cancer and noncancer. *In* Kopf, A. W., and Andrade, R.: Yearbook of Dermatology, 1966–67. Year Book Medical Publishers, Chicago, 1967, pp. 5–35.

Pinkus, H., and Mehregan, A. H.: A Guide to Dermatohistopathology. New York, Appleton-Century-Crofts, 1969.

Sanderson, K. V.: The architecture of basal-cell carcinoma. Br. J. Dermatol., 73:455, 1961.

Sappey, M. P. C.: Traité d'Anatomic. Ed. 3. Vol. 2. Paris, 1897.

Szabo, G.: The number of melanocytes in human epidermis. Br. Med. J., 1:1016, 1954.

Szabo, G.: Age changes in the human melanocyte system. *In* Montagna, W.: Aging. Oxford, Pergamon Press, 1965.

Unna, P. G.: Entwicklungsgeschichte und Anatomie der Haut. *In* Ziemssen's Handbuch der speziellen Pathologie und Therapie. Bd. 14/1. Leipzig, F. C. W. Vogel, 1883.

Unna, P. G.: Cited by Philippson, L.

Wilson, W.: Cited by Kölliker, A.

Zackheim, H. S.: Origin of human basal cell epithelioma. J. Invest. Dermatol., 40:283, 1963.

Zimmermann, K. W.: Über einige Formverhältnisse der Haarfollikel des Menschen. Z. Mikrosk. Anat. Forsch., 38:503, 1935.

10

Cytodiagnosis of Tumors and Reticuloses of the Skin

J. Piñol Aguadé, M.D.

HISTORY

Studies of cytologic smears in neoplasms and reticuloses of the skin are scarce, and research in this field of dermatology is not well advanced. It began with the work of Tzanck and his collaborators (Tzanck, 1947 and 1948; Tzanck and Melcki, 1951 and 1953; Tzanck et al., 1947, 1948, 1949, 1950, and 1952), but unfortunately the efforts of these dermatologists have not been followed up systematically. Nevertheless, there have been important contributions by Degos and Ossipowski (1957); Berardi (1966); Goldman et al. (1960); Knoth (1955); Haber (1954); Hauser (1960 and 1964); Lagerholm (1961); Renkin (1956); Wilson (1954); Hitch et al. (1951); Zoon and Mali (1950); and Andrade (1972), all on general aspects of cytodiagnosis in dermatology. Other articles have been published in reference to isolated aspects of cytology, such as those of Feldaker et al. (1954); Getz et al. (1956); Montgomery and Pease (1959); Brehmer-Anderson and Brunk (1967a and 1967b); Degos and Ossipowski (1957); Degos et al. (1957, 1959a, and 1959b); Kalamkaryan (1968); Swiller et al. (1953); Temime and Marchand

(1968); and Winer (1947) on cytodiagnosis of the malignant reticuloses, those of Coste and Piquet (1948); Goldman et al. (1958); Quero and Maso (1958); Scerrato (1956); Shklar et al. (1968); Sidi and Dobkevitch (1947); Temime (1951 and 1955); Temime and Costes (1969); Thibaut and Deniker (1949); Veronesi (1954); and Woodburne et al. (1960) on the cytology of some malignant tumors and precanceroses, and those on the cytologic aspects of the normal skin (Orbaneja and Castro, 1966).

In collaboration with Vilanova and Rueda, and also alone, I have published some articles on this subject (Piñol Aguadé, 1963, 1968, and 1969; Vilanova et al., 1962a, 1962b, 1963a, and 1963b; Vilanova and Piñol Aguadé, 1959 and 1967).

POSSIBILITIES OF CYTOLOGIC EXAMINATION

The small number of dermatologists dedicated to the study of cytology is striking if we consider that, at least in theory, it is extremely easy to obtain the necessary material for study. The modesty of the conclusions which they have reached contrasts with the very valuable research achieved in this field by other specialists, although in a great number of other kinds of study the material itself is more difficult to obtain.

Part of the explanation for this must be found in the fact that it is sometimes very difficult to obtain isolated cells in the cutaneous processes. This is because of the great cohesion provided by the desmosomes in the epidermis and the connective tissue of the dermis. It is not possible to obtain cells from most skin tumors by using puncture and aspiration, which is so easy in organs such as the spleen and lymph nodes, and it is even less practical to scratch with a stylet or a lancet, because this allows for only an incomplete examination which is therefore without any practical significance. The appearance of the prepared specimen is even acellular in many cases.

We can also explain the retarded development of cytodermatology by the refinement achieved by the histologic examination of the dermatoses, and the facility of skin biopsies in contrast to the difficulties of the biopsy of internal neoplasms. Finally, we must realize that, if under normal conditions identification of cytologic smears is complex, the difficulties logically increase if the abnormal cells under observation are mixed with the great variety of cellular elements which appear normally in the epidermis and the dermis.

In dermatology, most work on this subject has focused on the practical application of cytology to the immediate diagnosis of tumors. Very little has been done to investigate the possibilities of parallel cytohistologic research, but it is precisely in this field that we think cytology is most appropriate. The difficulties which exist in trying to solve in the mind's eye the cellular puzzle represented by the cutaneous smear in many cases prevent a positive diagnosis, and therefore cytology alone must be disqualified as a diagnostic method. Nevertheless, cytology supplies more detailed cellular patterns, and it can render a doubtful histologic diagnosis more convincing.

It is beyond doubt that one can obtain striking results by means of cytology when it is used for particular cases in which one technique is not sufficient. Histologic diagnosis of melanoma, Paget's disease, reticulosis, and fibrosarcoma can be checked, complemented, or corrected by the cytologic and cytochemical examination of the smears. We shall explain the cytologic aspects of the normal skin and of the different proliferative cutaneous processes, basing our discussion primarily on data accumulated through personal experience with thousands of smears.

TECHNIQUE

Various methods for the cytodiagnosis of lesions of the skin have been described: scraping of the lesions by Tzanck and colleagues (1947), the touch imprint by Degos and Ossipowski (1957) and by Montgomery and Pease (1959), and scarification and puncture of the lesions by Temime and Marchand (1968). In many cases we have found the quantity of cells so obtained too small to permit an accurate interpretation of the smears, and for the most part the elements were mixed with abundant blood. In 1962, the author, together with Vilanova and Rueda, proposed a simple technique explained below which does not require special instruments, a technique which we have continued to use with good results.

In the case of ulcerated surfaces, or when soft tissue lesions are available, the specimen for cytologic studies is obtained with a small curet, which in most instances provides enough material to permit the preparation of a satisfactory smear. Care must be taken to remove tissue from deeper levels so that a representative picture of the lesion will be obtained. Necrotic areas, crusts, scales, or debris must be avoided, and occasionally it is convenient to take specimens from different parts of the lesion or on successive days.

In the case of infiltrated lesions, hard tumors, and lesions situated deep in the dermis or in the hypodermis, examination requires a surgical specimen obtained from the lesion. Before fixing the tissue on the slide, it is advisable to remove all fatty tissue from the specimen with a small forceps and scissors, except when the lesion involves the hypodermis. In the latter instance the lesion must be carefully delimited, so that any excess of fat is eliminated. Crusts and blood should be washed away with gauze soaked in an isotonic solution of sodium chloride. As a general rule a piece of the lesion ranging in size from a lentil to a pea is sufficient.

Every detail in the preparation of the tissue is important. If these steps are not properly followed, the number of cells obtained will be too small, and adequate cytologic study will be difficult. When soft specimens are at hand, the whole material is crushed between two glass slides. The tissue will adhere to one of the slides, and as pressure is exerted, it is possible to cover most of the surface of the slide with an abundant number of cells, which produces an appearance comparable to that of a blood smear. Experience will tell how much digital pressure should be applied. Excessive compression will produce artifacts, and too little compression leaves an acellular imprint. Harder specimens must be teased apart with fine scissors or a blade prior to this procedure. If the section of the tissue is too slippery, blotting paper can be used on one of the slides. The procedure is carried out in the same manner, but only one slide is smeared at a time.

Satisfactory fixation is obtained by immersion of the slide in methyl alcohol for five minutes, or by exposure to dry heat. Then the slides are stained with May-Grünwald-Giemsa (MGG) stain in a solution containing two drops of dye per ml. of distilled water; this solution remains on the slide for 40 minutes. Hematoxylin-eosin or the Papanicolaou method can also be used routinely and special stains used when necessary. These include DOPA, tyrosinase, PAS, silver carbonate, Schmorl, Lillie, Masson-Fontana, and Ehrlich, all of them being used alone or in combination with the Giemsa stain. Equally, in specific cases, stainings of Sudan black, Nile blue, phospholipid staining, silver impregnation of reticulin with the Gomori stain, toluidine blue, silver methenamine for glycogen, alcian blue, or testicular hyaluronidase may be required. Procedures for the demonstration of nucleic acids can also be used, including the method of Feulgen, acid hydrolysis of Greig, methyl green–pyronine and methyl green, ribonuclease, and deoxyribonuclease. It is possible to stain for iron, zinc, and enzymes (Forteza, 1963).

The smears can also be used for the fluorescence examination with acridine orange according to Bertalanffy et al. (1956). On the other hand, direct examination can be done with a phase contrast microscope.

Examination of the Smear

A sufficient number of smears must be prepared since it is advisable to examine various smears from the same lesion in order to choose the one which has the most interesting fields or the greatest number of cells. Always use a low power lens when screening for malignancy, and alternate the lenses continually during the investigation in order to achieve a complete examination. It is also necessary to take into account that necrotic cells, including normal ones, can be confused with malignant cells.

NORMAL SKIN CYTOLOGY

Many authors have not paid much attention to the morphologic peculiarities of the different cellular components of the epidermis and dermis in smears, being concerned mainly with the diagnostic possibilities of the method. However, in order to make a confident statement about the abnormalities, we must first know the normal appearance of skin cells. It would be superfluous to describe the morphologic appearance of some cell types that are well known, such as lymphocytes, plasma cells and histiocytes. But dermatologic smears show cells with a slightly different picture from those we normally see in histology. Needless to say, this makes their recognition difficult in particular physiologic and pathologic conditions. We shall summarize the peculiarities observed with the most common stains, the May-Grünwald–Giemsa and the Papanicolaou methods.

Epidermal Cells

It is relatively easy to examine the epidermis from the roof of a bullous process with total detachment of the epidermis and with few cellular changes (Duhring's disease, pemphigus). Epidermis obtained from biopsies incubated in solutions of thioglycolate or trypsin can also be used, but in this case the picture is rather different because the cytoplasm is more visible and the number of cells is larger than in normal smears.

The stratum spinosum does not easily lose any cells, but it is possible to observe elements not only from the stratum spinosum but also from the stratum corneum by removing the roof of the bulla with scissors and squeezing it between two slides. Various cytochemical methods (PAS, enzyme stains) can be used to locate the strata to which the examined elements belong.

With the MGG method the cells of the lower layers of the stratum spinosum show rounded, oval, or slightly elongated nuclei devoid of cytoplasm, which are a little larger than a lymphocyte. The chromatin is rather compact and uniform with dense granules and an invisible or indistinct nucleolus. In more mature cells it is possible to observe the chromatin grain becoming progressively smaller and well designed, forming a very fine network. Sometimes the nuclear outline is reniform or shows indentations and therefore can be easily confused with the histiocyte. The bluish nucleolus becomes progressively more visible, one or two nucleoli usually being present. At the beginning of maturation there is only a fine cytoplasmic halo; later the cytoplasm becomes cuboidal and ends by becoming polygonal, pentagonal, or triangular, and in some cells showing very elongated angles. At first, it stains pale blue. Later this becomes deeper and oc-

casionally pink, and often it is finely vacuolar. The cells of the upper layers become transparent and their nuclei shrink until, in the horny layer, the cell is only a glistening lamella with or without punctiform nuclear residues.

In macerated regions and in ulcer edges the cells appear more voluminous and clearer than usual. It is not infrequent to find a perinuclear melanin deposit, sometimes only at one side of the nucleus or in other cells invading the whole of the perinuclear zone. In certain dermatoses (such as lichen planus) the melanin deposit of the cell is so abundant that this epithelial cell can be confused with a melanocyte or a melanophage. With the Papanicolaou method the cytoplasm is more visible and stains yellow. In keratinized cells the yellow can be of a deeper color.

Melanocytes

These cells have a characteristic nucleus which ranges in size from two to 15 times that of the erythrocytes. As a rule the nucleus of a melanocyte is oval or kidney-shaped with no indentation. The chromatin, arranged in a very fine network, is in some areas dustlike. A uniform, pale, single or double nucleolus is often seen within the chromatin. The size and shape of the cytoplasm vary infinitely but always preserve dendritic characteristics (Fig. 10–1). In exceptional cases the dentrites are almost absent (Fig. 10–2).

The cytoplasm itself has widely variable characteristics. In some cases it can be

Figure 10–1 Melanocyte. *Silver stain.*

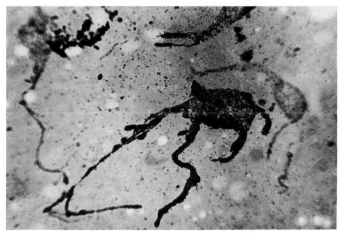

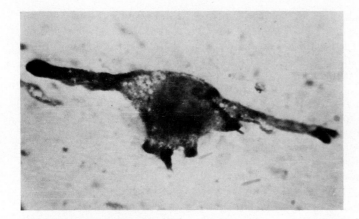

Figure   10–2   Melanocyte. *Dopa stain.*

uniformly pale blue or gray, in other cases colorless with a foamy appearance (Fig. 10–3), or there may be wider vacuolar spaces only in the perinuclear zone. The melanin granules, in greater or lesser amount, look like black dots in the MGG stain. They can either be spread uniformly in the cytoplasm or be found only at the periphery or in the dendritic endings. Their size ranges from a thin dust to the larger granules commonly found in the melanophages. In some melanocytes the granules are not black but grayish (premelanin?), or there may only be a smoky cytoplasm. By combining DOPA and MGG stains, we can obtain very clear pictures. Silver stains (silver carbonate, Masson-Fontana) produce very fine aggregates in some melanocytes, which can only be seen in the periphery of the cytoplasm. In other cases, the whole of the cytoplasm is stained. The melanic nature of these granules can be demonstrated with Schmorl

and Lillie stains. The bleaching of the melanin is more difficult in smears than in histologic sections; it can be obtained with sodium permanganate solutions, but many hours are needed for this process.

In some neoplastic skin processes (basal cell carcinomas, Paget's disease), giant melanocytes (macromelanocytes) can be found, but one can also observe dwarf or nevoid melanocytes (micromelanocytes) in basal cell carcinomas (Fig. 10–4) (Vilanova et al. 1962b). The achromic melanocytes in basal cell epitheliomas and melanomas can be identified only by the outline of their dendrites and the morphologic appearance of the nucleus. The cytoplasm contrasts with the pigmented background.

Melanophages

These are extremely abundant in the smears of some basal cell carcinomas,

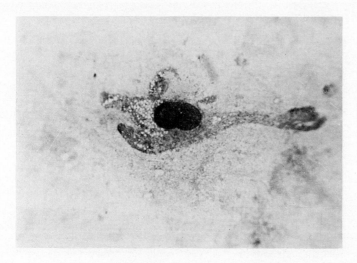

Figure 10–3   Melanocyte. Note the foamy aspect of the cytoplasm.

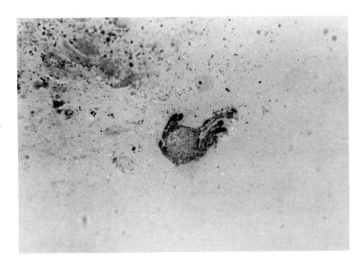

Figure 10–4 Micromelanocyte (nevoid melanocyte).

melanomas, and lichen planus. In most cases, they have a small ovoid or ellipsoid nucleus with the chromatin disposed in a loose network. The nucleus is surrounded by a transparent and a somewhat circular cytoplasm. The coarse melanin granules are conspicuous; there can be only a few or so many that they almost hide the nucleus. At times the cytoplasm is visible only because it is outlined by these melanin granules at the outermost periphery. The melanophage can attain great volume, and in the smears it is possible to see that some of the free melanin deposits observed histologically are in reality aggregates of voluminous melanophages completely filled with melanin.

In some smears the cytoplasm is not transparent but has a foamy appearance, as if it contained not only melanin but also fat. At times these foamy melanophages are bi- or multinucleated, giving in this last case a characteristic type of macrophagic giant cell (Fig. 10–5).

Fibroblasts

The typical fibroblasts with an elongated nucleus and a fusiform, pale blue, spoon-shaped, oval or indented cytoplasm are not always found in the smears. Almost the only way to recognize them is by the peculiar aspect of the parallel striped or triangular chromatin. Nevertheless, fibroblasts without any cytoplasm are frequent in the smears. The nucleolus is visible as a little spot. The size of the fibroblasts varies. Some are no larger than a lymphocyte; others can be twice as large as a red blood cell and can be confused with the epithelial cells of the deeper layers of the epidermis and with the endothelial cells.

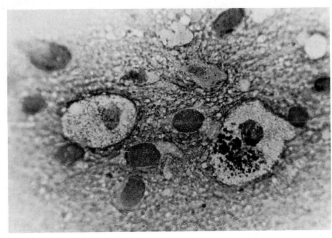

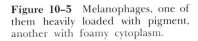

Figure 10–5 Melanophages, one of them heavily loaded with pigment, another with foamy cytoplasm.

Endothelial Cells

The characteristics of the adult endothelial cell are so typical that it can immediately be recognized. These cells abound in smears obtained from granulation tissue of skin ulcers, and they are the chief components of some tumors. Their size ranges from two or three times up to 15 times that of the erythrocyte, depending on the type of lesion in which they are found, but cells with very different sizes can coexist in the same smear. The nucleus stains pale violet with the MGG stain and is round, egg-shaped, or sometimes elongated with occasional indentations or protrusions. The chromatin grain is thicker than in the histiocytes and markedly netlike. In some smears the nucleoli can be easily seen as either dark or light blue spots. However, the most important characteristic is the wide, light blue or grayish, well-defined and angular cytoplasm. The cells are sometimes distributed in a mosaic pattern. Bi-, tri-, and multinuclear elements which constitute real giant endothelial cells can frequently be found (Fig. 10–6). Some of these cells keep the characteristic angular cytoplasm, while others are rounder. The nuclei can be in rows, in an irregular shape, or overlapping, and mitotic figures are not unusual.

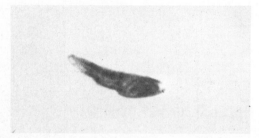

Figure 10–7   Smooth muscle cell.

Smooth Muscle Cells

Their nuclei are elongated or spoon-shaped, smaller and thinner than in the fibroblasts, with denser and more uniform chromatin. The very pale, almost invisible, cytoplasm is very thin, fusiform, and elongated (Figs. 10–7 and 10–61).

Sweat Gland Cells

It is not exceptional to find in the smears complete or almost complete sweat glomerules, which appear in clumps; their adenoid condition can easily be recognized (Fig. 10–8). The uniform nuclei are round and approximately the same size as a lymphocyte. The cuboidal cytoplasm stains pale blue. The ill-defined cytoplasm is slightly vacuolar.

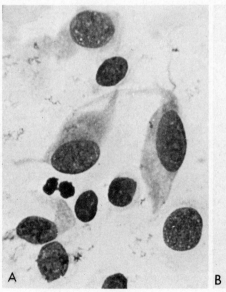

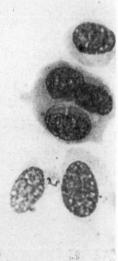

Figure 10–6 *A,* Characteristic cellular pattern of endothelial cells in different developmental stages. *B,* A trinuclear cell.

A

B

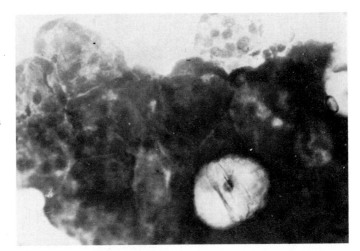

Figure 10–8 Sweat gland cells as seen on cytologic examination.

Sebaceous Cells

These are almost always found in lumps, distributed in a mosaic pattern, and are easily recognizable. Their nuclei are covered and in part hidden by fat deposits (Fig. 10–74).

Hair Follicle Cells

The hair follicle, formed by totally keratinized lamellae, is not suitable for cytologic study. The squeezing of hair roots produces scanty cells with an oval nucleus devoid of cytoplasm and a fine chromatin network; there are occasional melanocytes with fine grains of melanin (Fig. 10–9). In the background there is a great amount of brownish granulation. In alopecia mucinosa it is possible to study the characteristics of these cells.

Mastocytes

These are very easy to identify by their round outline, their oval or elongated uniform nuclei, and their metachromatic granules. These stain intensely red with MGG and cover the nucleus, which has no visible nucleolus. There are mastocytes with blunted or racket-shaped dendrites which can be confused with melanocytes (Fig. 10–10). In basal cell carcinomas and other inflammatory processes, and above all in the mastocytoses, the fragile cytoplasm easily releases these granules, which are then deposited in great quantities on the bottom of the smear. At times, however, the granules are so fine that the cytoplasm seems like a uniform eosinophilic mass. Finally, in some cells the nucleus is large with a narrow cytoplasmic rim.

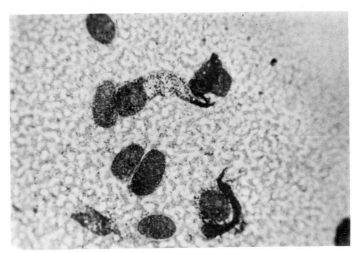

Figure 10–9 Hair sheath cells. Observe a melanocyte with pigmented cytoplasm. The granulation of the background of the smear is very evident.

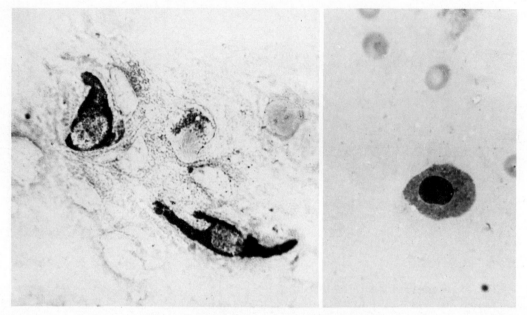

Figure 10–10   Different aspects of the mastocytes.

Chondrocytes

In some lesions located in the upper part of the cartilaginous zones in the nose or the external ear, it is possible to find chondrocytes, cells which in the smears reveal a dense round or irregular nucleus of variable size but which is generally bigger than that of normal dermal and epidermal cells (Fig. 10–11). The cytoplasm is generally not visible but can at times be transparent and cuboidal.

GENERAL CHARACTERISTICS OF CANCEROUS CELLS

The cellular characteristics which form the criteria of malignancy are well known. They are the same in the cells of the skin as in cells from other sources. The most important characteristic is that, with the low power lens, it is possible to see nests, masses, or sheets of cells whose features and organization are different from normal and which are dominant in the smear.

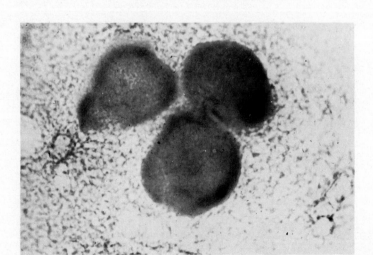

Figure 10–11   Chondrocytes.

They are frequent in basal cell and squamous cell carcinomas, melanomas and dermatofibrosarcomas.

Nuclear, nucleolar, and cytoplasmic pleomorphism is common. In some smears we find giant cells three times the normal size, together with small cells and elements with forms very different from the usual ones. There is loss of the nuclear-cytoplasmic ratio. Anisonucleosis is common: giant and small nuclei appear in the same field. Pleomorphism can be lacking in some cancers, such as basal cell carcinomas, but usually the disharmonic pattern is constant. Nevertheless, benign giant cells can be found in herpes and juvenile melanoma, and there may be pleomorphism in histiocytoma and telangiectatic granuloma. Nuclear anomalies and deformities are important (lobulation, detachment of chromatin portions, irregular outline, karyorrhexis). Nuclear anisochromasia is clearly visible in melanomas.

The chromatin is irregularly distributed. In sarcomas, melanomas, squamous cell carcinomas, and metastases, nuclei with excessively dense chromatin are frequent, together with others in which the chromatin forms loose meshes, and still other intermediate forms. The irregularity of chromatin distribution is the only cytologic suggestion of a nonkeratinizing small cell squamous cell carcinoma.

Hyperchromasia or polychromatophilia of the cytoplasm is a frequent finding in fibrosarcomas. In some smears there are syncytial elements forming multinucleated cells. They can be observed in fibrosarcomas, melanomas, epitheliomas, and other cancers of the skin. However, in some benign tumors, such as the calcifying epithelioma of Malherbe, telangiectatic granuloma, nevus, angioma, benign juvenile melanoma and epulis, there are also multinuclear cells, although in these cases the volume and form of the nuclei are generally uniform as opposed to cancers. Therefore polyploidy alone does not necessarily indicate malignancy.

Multiplicity and pleomorphism of the nucleoli and abnormal staining are common characteristics. In melanomas the nucleoli can reach enormous volumes and acquire bizarre forms. Multiplicity by itself does not mean malignancy. There are multiple nucleoli in many benign processes (nevi, hair follicle tumors, and others). The nucleoli of noncancerous tumors can also be voluminous and become intensely stained in some parts of the smears. Therefore, these two facts are of importance only when they occur in the same smear and in many cells. The structure of the abnormal nucleoli is clearly distinguishable from that of the vacuoles, which are completely transparent. They become clearer with Feulgen's stain, methyl green–pyronine, stains for fluorescence, hydrolysis with hydrochloric acid, α-chymotrypsin-deoxyribonuclease compound, or phase contrast microscopy.

There is an increase in the number of mitoses. Abnormal, multipolar, irregular mitoses with oversized or clumped chromosomes or with eccentric chromatin may be found.

Often a maturation sequence is absent. In squamous cell carcinoma the rate of keratinization is increased, and there is a high proportion of cells with a totally pyknotic nucleus and abnormal dyskeratotic cells. Whorls and horn pearls can also be observed (Fig. 10–37).

Cellular fragility and clumping of nuclei are minor factors. A great number of artifacts and clumping of the nuclei can be observed in reticulosis and fibrosarcomas, but they are also seen in benign processes. Other findings in the cytoplasm (inclusions, fibrillar structure) and in the nucleus (vacuolization, pyknosis, perinuclear halo) can be present.

CYTOLOGY OF SKIN TUMORS

Melanotic Tumors

Nevus. We shall summarize the cytologic features of junction nevi, compound nevi, and pigmented and non-pigmented intradermal nevi, since they present a similar morphology.

Good smears of nevus cells are easy to obtain, except in the fibrous nevi. The nevocytes form clumps and mosaics or remain isolated. The most notable peculiarity of the nevus cells is the isomorphism of the nuclei, which are round or oval

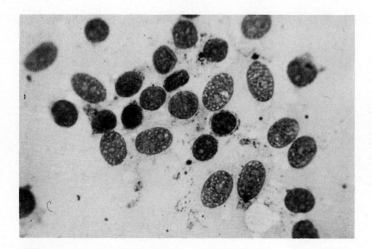

Figure 10-12 Sparsely pigmented nevus. Note the perfectly oval nuclear outline. The more mature cells are smaller and have denser chromatin.

and clearly outlined. Their size varies from 3 to 4 microns to double that of a lymphocyte (Figs. 10–12 and 10–13).

Normally the chromatin is finely grained, dense, and uniform and stains purple with MGG. The single nucleolus is clearly demarcated; in some nevi it is quite large and is pale blue or milky in color.

In many intradermal nevi most cells have no cytoplasm and show a striking isonucleosis and regularity of the nuclear outline. Nuclei of different sizes clump together in isomorphic fields. In lightly pigmented nevi the cytoplasmic outline of some cells generally stained blue or pale purple with MGG is discernible. Normally this is rounded or cuboidal and sharply demarcated. Occasionally one can see pseudopodic or dendritic processes (Figs. 10–4 and 10–14). In some nevi the cytoplasm can be discerned only as a perinuclear halo, and in others it has a foamy ap-

pearance. In these last cells there is often a variable number of melanin granules. In strongly pigmented nevi there is a greater quantity of visible cytoplasm because the melanin granules follow the cellular outline, even that of some short and blunt dendrites. In some cells there is such an abundance of pigment that it covers the nucleus.

Although the nevus cells often occur isolated or in small groups, an arrangement in *pairs* is characteristic (Fig. 10–13). There are also groups of mostly less than 12 nuclei. Often these small groups are situated on a syncytial cytoplasmic, normally basophilic, background, arranged in the form of a crown, or in tightly packed clusters with clumped nuclei. Typical *giant nevus cells* are formed like that and differ from the syncytia of some neoplasms by the regularity and uniformity of their nuclei (Fig. 10–15). Giant cells with visible

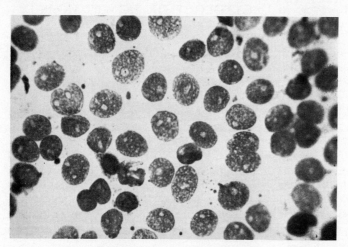

Figure 10-13 Intradermal nevus. Observe the monomorphism of the nuclei devoid of cytoplasm, the "paired cells," and the volume and regularity of the nucleoli.

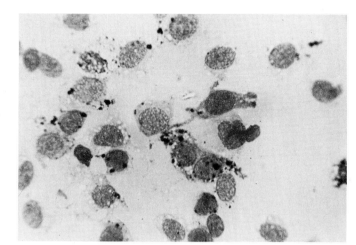

Figure 10–14 Pigmented nevus. Note the dendrites of the nevocytes.

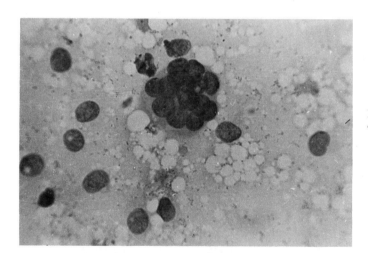

Figure 10–15 Nevus cells. A giant cell.

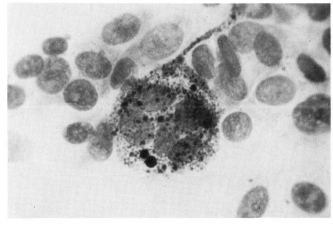

Figure 10–16 Intradermal and pigmented nevus. Giant cell with a unique elongated dendrite and heavily pigmented cytoplasm. The finding of pigmented giant cells is not frequent in the smears.

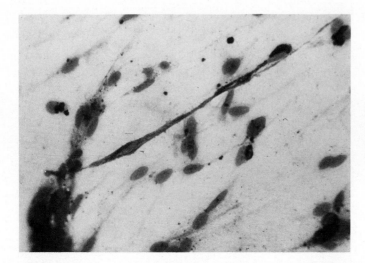

Figure 10–17   Blue nevus cells at a low magnification. Observe the extraordinary length of the bipolar dendrites of the nevocyte in the center of the field.

melanin are rare, and still rarer are cellular syncytia with dendritic prolongations (Fig. 10–16). In the junction nevi some cells without cytoplasm can be hypertrophic, but apart from their excessive volume, they are identical to the surrounding cells.

In many smears there are cells with coarse melanin granules which are possibly melanophages. The highly pigmented nevi have so much melanin that it escapes from the cells and accumulates in the background of the smear in the form of a film or thick clumps. There are also epithelial and keratinized cells which contain melanin in the cytoplasm arranged in an irregular form or accumulated at one of the nuclear poles. It is not infrequent to find sebaceous cells mixed with the nevocytes.

Blue Nevus.   There are few cells in the smear because of the firmness of the lesions and the adherence of the fibrous component. There are only accumulations of melanin together with an occasional isolated melanocyte or melanophage (Fig. 10–17).

By contrast, smears of *cellular blue nevi* are rich in cells. There are bipolar melanocytes with dendrites which sometimes are extraordinarily long. The cytoplasm is full of very fine melanin granules; the nucleus is oval and elongated, with granular, dense chromatin, and there are one or two transparent nucleoli. There are also pale blue, completely transparent nuclei without cytoplasm. Binuclear and multinuclear cells are numerous, but these giant nevus cells, in contrast to those of the normal nevus, possess very long bipolar dendrites, and their nuclei are often disposed in rows (Fig. 10–18).

The background of the preparation contains a great quantity of coarse melanin granules, either single or forming compact

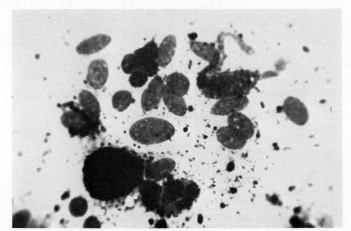

Figure 10–18 Cellular type of blue nevus. Nuclei devoid of cytoplasm. Adendritic nevocyte and melanophage filled with melanin.

masses. There is an abundance of melanophages.

Lentigo Maligna (Circumscribed Precancerous Melanosis of Dubreuilh). The smears should be made from the biopsy of the lesion. They are normally rich in cells. In the first stage of precancerous melanosis, the cellular components resemble the cells of pigmented nevi. The well-defined oval nuclei contain fine granules of chromatin, and a pale blue nucleolus is clearly demarcated and shows blunted dendrites. Most cells contain abundant melanin.

In contrast to the cells of the nevus, there are some abnormalities in these cells suggesting an early malignant transformation. There is marked hyperproduction and abnormal distribution of pigment. Melanin is not uniformly distributed in fine granules but lies in irregular masses. Also the anisocytosis which can be discerned in almost all fields is quite noticeable. Together with very voluminous cells, there are almost dwarf-sized cells in which, as opposed to those of the nevus, the nucleus is not devoid of cytoplasm but rather is visible and full of pigment. There are no bi- or trinuclear cells. Many cells are fusiform, and their dendrites are longer than those of nevus cells. There may be anisochromasia of the nuclei, and in some cells there are alterations in the outline and color of the nucleoli, although to a lesser degree than in melanomas. In this stage there are no irregularities in the nuclear outline (Fig. 10–19).

In the infiltrative phase of precancerous melanosis, the generally fusiform melano-

cytes become larger and there is distinct anaplasia. In the tumoral phase the smears are identical to those of primary melanoma. The cells lose their fusiform shape, and cell monstrosities and other signs of malignancy abound.

Melanomas. Cytologic examination constitutes one of the most useful techniques for the differential diagnosis of these tumors and complements the histologic examination. The appearance of the smears is variable and depends on the type of tumor. The smear from a fusiform melanoma is different from that of a melanoma with cuboidal cells or that of an amelanotic melanoma. Nevertheless, all slides are characteristic enough to permit an evaluation of the extreme malignancy of the picture (Fig. 10–20).

In *fusiform melanoma,* naked nuclei can be found next to cells with a visible cytoplasm. The nuclei are enlarged and oval or elliptical. The chromatin resembles that of the blue nevus, except that cells with a visible blue fusiform and pigmented cytoplasm are much rarer, and in most of the cells the cytoplasmic outline can only be discerned because of the pigment. The cells are fusiform, with uni- or bipolar dendrites, the melanin being arranged around one or both nuclear poles or only on the top of the dendrites. The melanophages are often loaded with free pigment. Fusiform melanoma presents numerous signs of malignancy that are absent in the blue nevus. The chromatin is denser and irregular; there are marked anisocytosis, giant nucleoli, irregularities in the nuclear outline, abnormalities in the

Figure 10–19 Precancerous melanosis (Dubreuilh). Hypertrophic melanocytes, fusiform in shape, with irregularly distributed melanin.

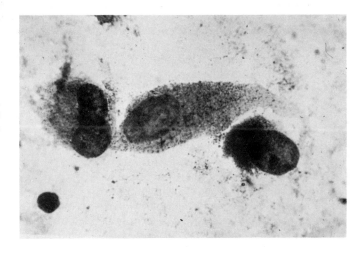

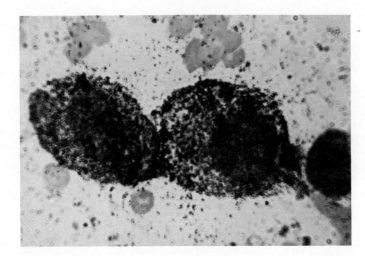

Figure 10–20 Malignant melanoma. Anaplastic cells.

distribution of pigment, and marked anisochromasia.

Pigmented melanomas do not generally present diagnostic difficulties. All accepted criteria of malignancy are present: anisocytosis, giant cells, abnormal nucleoli, irregular nuclei, atypical mitoses, and polyploidy, together with an abundance of melanin.

Amelanotic melanomas present greater difficulties. We have to distinguish preparations with cells devoid of cytoplasm in the MGG stain and those which present a clear cytoplasmic halo. The slides in the first case are normally extraordinarily rich in cells, which indicates lack of cohesion of the cells with the stroma and suggests the diagnosis of melanoma. The lumps of cells are so numerous in many fields that many nuclei appear to be superimposed in heaps or whorls. However, in other zones of the smear the slides may be uniform and comparable to those in a blood smear. In many cases malignancy is evident from the looseness of the chromatin, the multiplicity and abnormal form and size of the nucleoli, the marked anisocytosis and anisochromasia, and the large number of "clear" cells, all of which suggest an undifferentiated carcinoma. In these preparations there may be some individual cells with an intensely blue or foamy cytoplasm, and a few cytoplasms tattooed with fine or coarse melanin granules are frequent. The affinity of the MGG stain for this pigment permits staining of the melanin even in cases in which the melanoma is histologically completely amelanotic. In some cells

pigment is found not in the form of granules but as a grayish shadow.

In amelanotic melanomas with cells having visible cytoplasm, the general appearance is very similar to that of the histologic sections, since the cuboidal or pentagonal cytoplasms form an almost perfect mosaic. Anisocytosis and anaplasia are present, and most smears contain some isolated pigmented cells.

All types of melanoma show a tendency to form multinuclear cells. The nuclei of mononuclear cells are much larger than those of nevus cells; they are also more widely separated and irregularly distributed and show marked anisonucleosis.

Some melanomas abound in small cells which could be confused with nevus cells. Important for the differential diagnosis is that in melanoma the small cells have loose chromatin, whereas the chromatin of nevi is denser. Finally, the most important characteristic of melanoma is the frequency of monstrous nucleoli (Fig. 10–21).

In summary, then, we can say that with the MGG stain the diagnosis of melanoma is easier in smears than in histologic sections. Moreover smears have the advantage that in case of doubt they can easily be stained not only to show the melanin function but also to demonstrate nucleic acids and for phase contrast study. Thus it is possible to detect abnormalities in the distribution of nucleic acids with a low margin of error. So, for example, with Feulgen's method, characteristic features are obtained: ring nuclei, in which only a colored peripheral rim is visible while the whole of

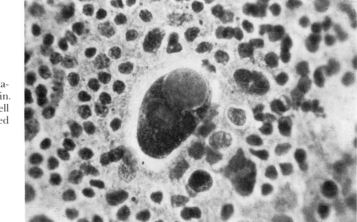

Figure 10–21 Malignant melanoma. Methyl green–pyronine stain. The enormous nucleolus of the cell in the center of the field is stained pink-red with this method.

the center is transparent; clear nuclei, because of disappearance of the DNA; fenestrated nuclei, with clearings in the form of a wide-mesh net; and multiperforated nuclei, because of the great number of nucleoli (Fig. 10–22). With acid hydrolysis the results are similar (Fig. 10–23). With methyl green–pyronine the parts of the nucleus which are stained pinkish red (RNA) occupy almost the whole of the nucleus in many instances and are also found in the cytoplasm of some cells. Fluorescent methods allow one to see areas of red fluorescence in the cytoplasm because of its RNA content. All these characteristics are found not only in melanomas with monstrous cells but also in the small cell melanomas and even in the first stages of the circumscribed precancerous melanosis of Dubreuilh. They explain the anisochromasia of the nuclei in

melanoma and also the difficulty in staining some *clear* nuclei with the MGG stain. These abnormalities are absent in nevi and benign juvenile melanoma.

Smears of *benign juvenile melanomas* are totally different from those of nevi and melanomas. The overall appearance of the smears and the cellular details seen with the immersion lens recall those of telangiectatic granuloma or angioma.

The cell of the benign juvenile melanoma is characterized by an abundance of cytoplasm, which sometimes stains intensely blue, and by its voluminous, round, irregular nucleus. The pasty or fine-grained chromatin is less uniform than in the nevi. The cytoplasm may be cuboidal or fusiform, but in both forms it shows sharp characteristic angles. Cells are often disposed in an angular mosaic form.

There are bi- or multinuclear cells. The

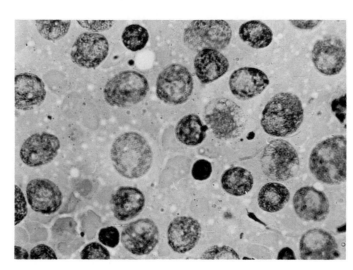

Figure 10–22 Malignant melanoma. *Feulgen stain.*

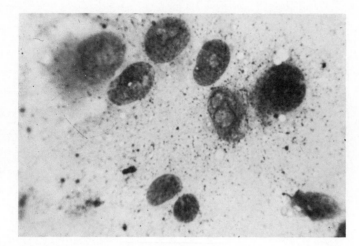

Figure 10–23 Malignant melanoma. Alterations of the nucleoli evidenced by the method of hydrolysis with hydrochloric acid.

nuclei form irregular lumps or vague lines and show differences in size. Often there are cells with more than a dozen nuclei. The nucleoli of some cells can be voluminous, and sometimes double, but they never approach the gigantism of melanoma cells.

In the smears one can find nuclei devoid of cytoplasm with the same appearance as those with visible cytoplasm, but the proportion of naked nuclei is less than in the vascular or melanotic tumors. Small-sized cells in the benign juvenile melanomas usually show a clear-cytoplasmic halo (Fig. 10–24).

PRECANCER, INTRAEPIDERMAL EPITHELIOMA, KERATOACANTHOMA, PSEUDOCANCER

Actinic Keratosis

Smears are not very useful for the diagnosis. As a rule the smear has a dirty background, is partly opaque and partly vacuolar and is often invaded by germs. One can see only a few cells and cellular fragments, naked nuclei, and anuclear scales of several shapes and sizes, isolated

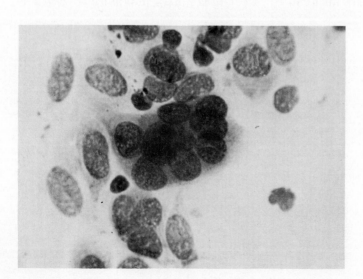

Figure 10–24 Benign melanoma. A giant cell surrounded by mononuclear elements.

or in clumps, which stain deep blue with the MGG stain and yellow with the Papanicolaou stain.

The cells with visible cytoplasm have a dense, pyknotic nucleus with an irregular outline. The naked nuclei are smaller and denser than those of the regular epithelial cells, and many of them are from cells whose cytoplasm has disintegrated and become diffused in the background of the smear. Dyskeratotic cells similar to those of squamous cell carcinoma are exceptional. The number of inflammatory cells is variable.

Leukoplakia and Erythroplasia

These lesions are not suitable for cytologic examination. For the most part only cells from the inflammatory infiltrate of the dermis are obtained.

Bowen's Disease

As in actinic keratosis, the background of the smear makes observation difficult because there are many cells in the process of disintegration. In very scaly lesions there are many keratinized cells which vary in size and shape. Nearly all smears contain large (sometimes gigantic) nuclei devoid of cytoplasm; some of these have an extremely large, bizarre nucleolus and a dense and pasty chromatin (Fig. 10–25). The cells with visible cytoplasm have lobu-

lated eccentric nuclei larger than those of normal epithelial cells and a transparent cytoplasm, which stains deep blue with the MGG stain and yellow with the Papanicolaou stain. Some smears show multinuclear cells resulting from atypical mitoses. Some cytoplasms still keep the pigment cap, and there may be isolated melanocytes. Occasionally we see small "ring cells" and "bird's eye cells." The inflammatory infiltrate consists mainly of lymphocytes.

The cytology as a whole is similar to that of keratinizing squamous cell carcinoma, but in Bowen's disease the anisocytosis can be more marked and the giant cells bigger.

Paget's Disease

Material for immediate cytodiagnosis is easy to obtain. Simple tapping and squeezing of the affected skin of the nipple, scrotum, or axilla yields sufficient material. Smears are usually rich in cells, and sometimes the diagnosis can be made after examination of the first microscopic field.

The characteristic Paget cells can be easily recognized by their extraordinary volume. They are isolated or disposed in clumps or in rows, and there is marked anisocytosis of the atypical cells. Usually the Paget cells are larger than 20 microns.

Some smears show only naked nuclei or cells with a sketchy cytoplasm, but normally the whole cell is visible. The most typical cells have a round or irregular, multilobulated, hump-shaped or indented

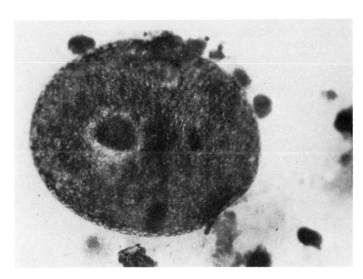

Figure 10–25 Bowen's disease. Monstrous cell with an enormous nucleolus. Compare with the surrounding lymphocytes.

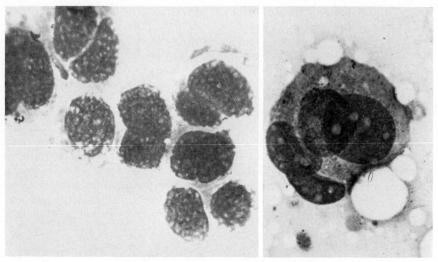

Figure 10–26   Different aspects of Paget cells.

nucleus. The chromatin is dense, sometimes forming a wide-meshed, loose net with numerous clear spaces within the nucleus. In some cells the chromatin forms irregular clusters, and sometimes there is marked anisochromasia of the neighboring nuclei. Many cells show large, sometimes monstrous or multiple nuclei which stain blue with MGG and are most striking in Feulgen's stain.

The cytoplasm is more visible in the clumps than in single cells and can be observed better with the Papanicolaou stain than with the Giemsa. With the Giemsa it stains pale blue or pink and is vacuolar or smoky with fine granulations inside. Its outline is cuboid, pentagonal, or polyhedral and larger than in regular epithelial cells (Fig. 10–26). The Paget cells of ex-

tramammary lesions are in general smaller and show more adenoid features than those obtained from lesions of the nipple.

Paget cells are fragile, and the nuclei are easily deformed and ruptured in the process of making the smear. The cytoplasm disintegrates easily with the protoplasmic substance, forming a granular background in some fields. Occasionally, what appear to be bi- or trinuclear cells are really superimposed nuclei and cytoplasm, but cells with two or more nuclei are not rare (Fig. 10–26). In lesions of long duration there are cells with signs of degeneration (deep blue cytoplasm, nuclei with pasty chromatin, faded cellular outlines).

The rare epithelial cells contain melanin granules and are irregularly scattered over

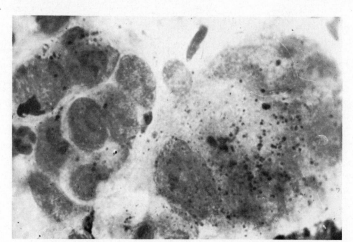

Figure 10–27   Paget's disease. Pigmented cells.

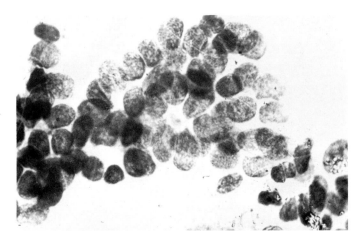

Figure 10–28   Intracanalicular dendritic adenoma of the nipple.

the cytoplasm. Nevertheless, the Paget cells can contain pigment (Fig. 10–27). In lesions affecting the skin around the nipple or in extramammary lesions, there is a great number of melanin granules in the neoplastic cells and an abundance of melanocytes, some of them dendritic, others round and so large as to suggest a melanoma.

Inflammatory cells and germs from secondary infections are common in the smears.

With the Papanicolaou stain, the cytoplasm, and in some Paget cells the nucleus as well, stains deep yellow, either partially or completely. Stains for mucopolysaccharides are less demonstrative and more difficult in the smears than in histologic sections.

In the metastatic adenopathies, puncture of the lymph node reveals neoplastic cells of enormous size, whose malignant features are more marked than in the primitive lesion. The cytoplasm of the metastatic cells is round or polyhedral, without vacuoles but finely granulated.

The differential diagnosis involves superficial melanoma, eczema of the nipple, and *intracanalicular papilloma* of the nipple. In smears of eczema there are only inflammatory cells and epithelial debris. In intracanalicular dendritic adenoma, the smears are characteristic and clearly different from those of Paget's disease. There is an abundance of cells, which occur isolated or in clusters. Their nucleus is slightly bigger than a lymphocyte, with dense chromatin and no visible nucleolus. The cells are monomorphous and round

or oval. The cytoplasm is cuboid, poorly demarcated, and pale blue in colour. There are adenoid features in some parts of the smear (Fig. 10–28).

Intraepidermal Epitheliomas

The cytologic picture is similar to that of Bowen's disease but without the cell monstrosities of the latter. There are naked, large, and atypical nuclei, together with normal ones. There is anisocytosis in some fields, and the dyskeratosis with advanced keratinization is less abundant than in Bowen's disease.

Keratoacanthoma

This tumor presents typical features. There is a large quantity of completely keratinized and anuclear cells, isolated or in clusters, which stain deep blue with the MGG stain and yellow with the Papanicolaou stain (Fig. 10–29). Together with these keratinized cells, there are uniform naked nuclei. The cells can sometimes be dyskeratotic with a transparent or refringent cytoplasm, which stains deep blue with the MGG stain and has voluminous nuclei. However, these dyskeratotic cells show a special characteristic: instead of decreasing and becoming pyknotic or anaplastic, the nuclei keep their primitive volume and disappear progressively. We have found this "frozen cell" several times in keratoacanthoma (Figs. 10–30 and 10–31).

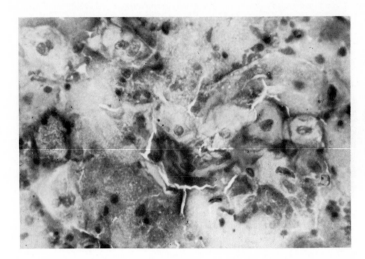

Figure 10–29 Keratoacanthoma. Typical cytologic picture. Almost completely keratinized elements in a mosaic distribution.

Figure 10–30 Keratoacanthoma. Frozen cell. In one element the nucleus has disappeared.

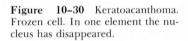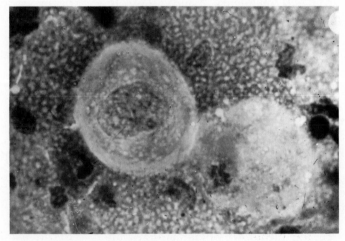

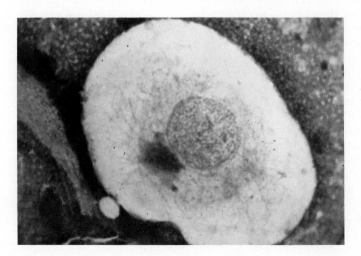

Figure 10–31 Keratoacanthoma. Frozen cell.

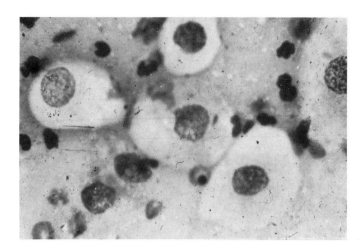

Figure 10–32 Pseudoepitheliomatous hyperplasia.

Anisokaryosis or marked nuclear deformities are rare. Anomalies in chromatin distribution are not discernible with Feulgen's method.

Pseudoepithelial Hyperplasia

The smears are nonspecific. There is an abundance of unremarkable epithelial cells. Many cells show a transparent cytoplasm and normal, round, monomorphous nuclei. Some cells are rounded, others polygonal, and the picture is generally harmonious (Fig. 10–32).

Infiltrating Papillomas of Buschke-Lowenstein

The smears show a monotonous pattern. The cells are typically epithelial, larger than average, and polyhedral or rectangular with a visible cytoplasm and show different stages of keratinization. The nuclei are monomorphous, dense, and oval. The cytoplasm stains blue or pink with the MGG stain. The cells are distributed uniformly without cluster formation. There is no anaplasia (Fig. 10–33). The cytologic picture is similar to that of pseudoepithelial hyperplasia, but the cells are more regular and smaller. The cytologic impression is benign.

Signs of secondary infection are frequent. We do not observe dense nuclei, as in some smears of verruca vulgaris.

EPITHELIOMAS

Squamous Cell Carcinoma

The Papanicolaou stain is most demonstrative since it gives almost histologic pic-

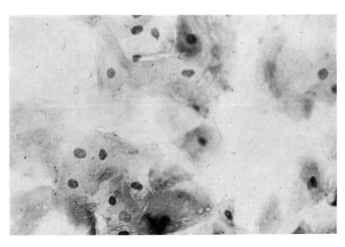

Figure 10–33 Venereal papillomas, Buschke-Löwenstein type. Regular keratinized cells.

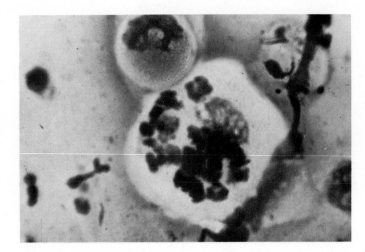

Figure 10–34 Squamous cell carcinoma. Abnormal mitosis. Dyskeratotic cells.

tures and brings out the cytoplasm of many cells, which remains invisible with MGG.

It is not difficult to obtain good smears with an abundance of cells. In most cases the curet is sufficient to obtain enough material, and the slides are almost perfect, especially if debris, necrotic zones, and blood are avoided.

Cytologically, squamous cell carcinomas are more varied than basal cell epitheliomas. Microscopic diagnosis is often easy with a low power lens, when either MGG or Papanicolaou stain is used.

We have to differentiate between carcinomas with variable amounts of dyskeratotic cells, corresponding to the keratinizing carcinoma of Broders' grades I, II, and III, and those without keratinization (Broders' grade IV). In the latter, cytodiagnosis is important for differentiation be-

tween a sarcomatous epithelioma and a true fibrosarcoma (Figs. 10–34 to 10–37).

Keratinizing Squamous Cell Carcinomas. These are the most frequent. Under low power we see a number of cells with a clear transparent, cytoplasmic halo, Under low power we see a number of cells with a clear transparent cytoplasmic halo, which with the MGG stain is sometimes refringent. Occasionally the · cytoplasm stains deep blue or purple. With the Papanicolaou stain these keratinized cells appear deep yellow. The cells are round like epithelial cells but not polyhedral, and they lack uniformity. Giant cells coexist with small ones. Despite the advanced keratinization, many cells preserve a large but deformed, round or irregular, and bizarre nucleus. It often stains excessively. The chromatin can be dense or loose. Some of the nuclei are monstrous and

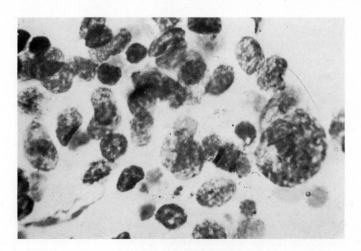

Figure 10–35 Squamous cell carcinoma. Grade IV of Broders.

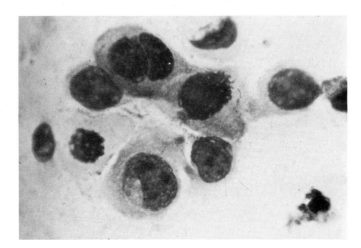

Figure 10–36 Squamous cell carcinoma, cuboidal cells.

multiple and show abnormal mitoses, pyknosis, and karyorrhexis. The cytoplasm sometimes contains reddish granules and traces of chromatin. There can be marked anaplasia.

Beside keratinized cells there are nuclei devoid of cytoplasm which sometimes, like the keratinized cells, show considerable anisonucleosis and marked anaplasia. The nuclei tend to overlap. There are also anuclear scales and incompletely keratinized cells. Instead of forming mosaics as in benign processes, they adopt an irregular pattern with a great diversity in size.

Bi- or trinuclear cells with irregular nuclei are not unusual. There are large syncytia with an enormous quantity of nuclei disposed in a half-moon or in an irregular form inside the cytoplasm, which stains intensely blue with the MGG stain and is refringent in the center. There is some

pyknosis. These syncytial formations, which can amount to some hundreds of microns, are the "epitheliomatous horn pearls."

Carcinomas on Epidermodysplasia Verruciformis. In constrast, the epithelioma that develops on epidermodysplasia verruciformis shows a special type of keratinization which makes it recognizable in the first low power fields. The slides are full of oversized cells, which stain intensely blue with the MGG stain and pale yellow with the Papanicolaou stain. The MGG stain shows uniformly distributed fine vacuoles, which can be vaguely seen also in cells whose cytoplasm appears "empty" in the Papanicolaou stain (Fig. 10–38). The nuclei are small, dense, elongated, and very uniform.

Squamous Cell Carcinomas With Incompletely Keratinized Cells. In other

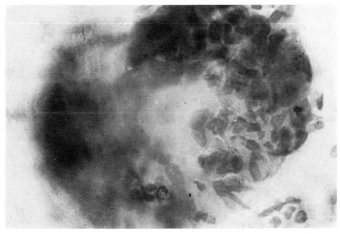

Figure 10–37 Squamous cell carcinoma. Epitheliomatous horn pearl.

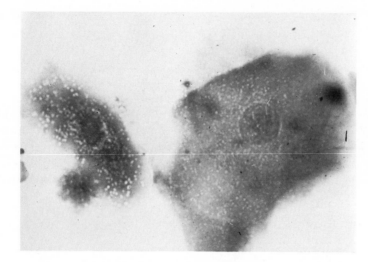

Figure 10–38   Squamous cell carcinoma on epidermodysplasia verruciformis. Note the peculiar vacuolar aspect observed in all the epithelial elements.

spindle cell epitheliomas one can only guess the epithelial origin of the neoplasm with the Papanicolaou method, which stains the cytoplasm yellow. In the MGG stain, most cells have naked nuclei or a cuboidal light blue cytoplasm, forming mosaics which are sometimes adenoid in appearance. Although signs of malignancy exist, such as anisonucleosis, irregularity in the distribution of the chromatin, abnormal nuclei, and occasional giant nucleoli, one cannot specify the type of neoplasia (Fig. 10–36).

Nonkeratinizing Carcinomas. These are the most difficult to diagnose since they are easily confused with basal cell epitheliomas. In most cases malignancy is evident because of the giant nuclei mixed with small ones and the undifferentiated appearance of the irregularly distributed pasty or loose chromatin. There are almost giant multiple or hyperchromatic nucleoli. In the cell clusters the nuclei overlap. The cells are fragile and subject to numerous artifacts, irregularities, or deformities of nuclei. There are necrotic or half-disintegrated cells with intranuclear vesiculation (Fig. 10–35).

In differentiating spindle cell carcinoma from sarcoma the following data should be considered:

1. With both the Papanicolaou and MGG stains, there usually is some isolated cell on the verge of keratinization in a spindle cell carcinoma.

2. The chromatin is normally much denser and the nucleoli more voluminous and more intensely stained in fibrosarcoma than in epithelioma.

3. Hyperchromasia of the cytoplasm is frequent in fibrosarcoma.

4. In the latter there tends to be a finely granulated mucoid background.

5. In fibrosarcoma isolated cells show the chromatin arranged in a "zebralike" fashion which is characteristic of the fibroblasts.

Carcinomas of the oral cavity are normally infected by bacteria and fungi. They have dense mucous filaments and a considerable inflammatory infiltrate. Superficial carcinomas of the mouth can provide smears in which confusion with pemphigus of the oral mucosa is possible.

The smears of *irradiated carcinomas* show an intensification of the characteristics of malignancy. The cells are swollen, and with the increase in size the peculiarities increase also. There is marked irregularity of the nuclei, variations in volume, a marked unevenness of the chromatin structure, giant nuclei, vacuolized and poorly delimited cytoplasm, and disintegration of the nuclei and nucleoli. In smears performed on successive days, one can follow perfectly the sequence of the progressive cellular disintegration.

Basal Cell Epithelioma

Clusters of closely packed cells are frequent and are characteristic of this type of tumor, but they are not pathognomonic (Fig. 10–39). One can find similar features in the smears of different neoplasms, such as fibrosarcoma and squamous cell carci-

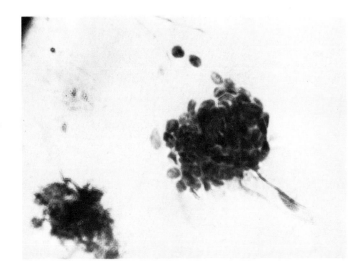

Figure 10–39 Basal cell epithelioma. Typical clumps.

nomas. Vilanova et al. (1962b) have described the following types of cells.

Small Cells. These cells have a naked nucleus, round or somewhat elongated, and closely packed chromatin. They are approximately twice the size of an erythrocyte. The nuclei are deformed, indented, and lobulated. This shows especially in the aggregates or "grapes" of clumped cells. The transparent cuboid or quadrangular cytoplasm is pale blue and visible only in isolated cells against the uniformly stained background of the smear. The morphology is similar to that of the epithelial cells of the basal layer and the deeper layers of the epidermis. The nucleoli are not recognizable.

Blue Cells. The most characteristic feature is the cytoplasm, which has a widely variable outline and is more or less well defined, but in all cases stains pale or intensely blue. Its size is variable, not only between different types of basal cell epithelioma but also within the same field. The oval or elongated nucleus has compact chromatin. Some cells are binuclear (Fig. 10–40). The nucleoli are not visible. There are cells devoid of cytoplasm which are recognizable by their nuclear structure.

Cells With a Clear Nucleus. These may constitute 60 to 80 percent of all cells in some smears, or they may be found only in isolated instances. The nuclei, always devoid of cytoplasm, resemble those of melanocytes. They are oval or kidney-shaped, with fine, dustlike chromatin and a uniform pale blue nucleolus. In other fields the chromatin is somewhat denser.

Cellular Syncytia. In general these formations are found in smears containing an abundant number of blue cells. They are visible under low power. These syncy-

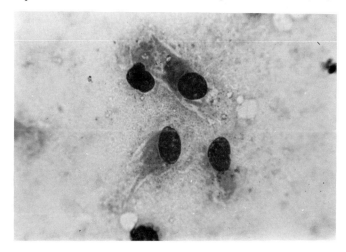

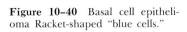

Figure 10–40 Basal cell epithelioma Racket-shaped "blue cells."

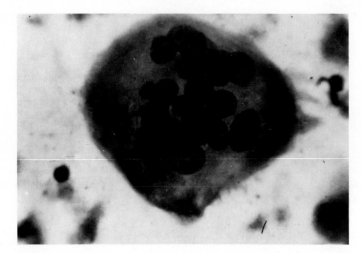

Figure 10–41 Basal cell epithelioma. Syncytium.

tia are oval or round, sometimes enormous, and sharply delimited (Fig. 10–41). They stain uniformly and intensely blue. Their outline can be angular or irregular. The syncytia contain a variable number of irregularly distributed nuclei. The nuclei are round or oval with a dense and pasty chromatin. The nucleoli can be seen.

It is difficult to determine whether these formations result from fusion of cells or multiplication of the nucleus of one cell. The tendency toward angulation in some parts of the cytoplasm would support the first possibility. The morphologic aspects of these syncytia with a small number of nuclei closely resemble those of the "blue cells" described above. They may be derivatives of those cells.

In some cases there is splitting between the different nuclei of these syncytia, or there may be a cell which is beginning to separate from the extensive cytoplasm, developing the clearer cytoplasm and denser, retracted nucleus characteristic of keratinizing cells. This fact would support the view that these syncytia correspond to the center of keratinization found in many basal cell epitheliomas.

Eosinophilic Cells. These cells are not characteristic of basal cell epitheliomas. They are dyskeratotic elements with an evenly colored, sometimes granular, round, intensely eosinophilic cytoplasm. The nucleus can be pyknotic or reduced to a dot.

Melanocytes. Some smears contain a great number of melanocytes. They are easily recognizable with the MGG stain, even under low power, and are variable in size and shape. Some of them are typical melanocytes, but some smears show nevoid melanocytes, macromelanocytes, and also the amelanotic melanocytes already described (see p. 238).

Cells From the Inflammatory Infiltrate. There is usually an inflammatory infiltrate in these smears, consisting of lymphocytes, plasma cells, melanophages, and fibroblasts. Melanocytes are abundant in some smears but scarce in others and sometimes have a foamy appearance. Mastocytes also may be found in great numbers.

Atypical and Nonconstant Cells. In smears of basal cell epithelioma the anaplasia seen in other tumors is rare. In some smears of basal cell epithelioma with histologic anisocytosis and monstrosities, we find large irregular nuclei with protrusions and multiple or giant nucleoli similar to those found in Bowen's disease or carcinoma in situ. There are also signs of degeneration, such as karyorrhexis, nuclear pyknosis, cellular "shadows," and a mucous or vesiculated cytoplasm. Many of these features are confusing and difficult to classify.

In the epithelial cells which have become completely keratinized, anuclear scales of quadrangular, pentagonal, or triangular shape are found; they may be isolated or massed together. There are also keratinocytes with a fusiform or rectangular outline and a blue, yellow, pink, or transparent cytoplasm.

In the morphea-like basal cell epithelioma it is difficult to classify the cell ele-

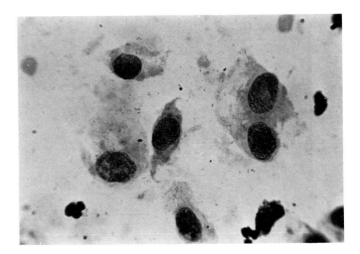

Figure 10–42 Angioma. Endothelial cells.

ments, since the chromatin of all the cells is too closely packed.

Background of the Smears. In some cases the acellular substance of the background of the smears has a granular aspect; in others it is rather mucoid or filamentous; in still others it stains uniformly. Naturally the amorphous substance is more abundant in cystic and cylindromatous basal cell epitheliomas. In these smears one can see round masses of a pasty and intensely eosinophilic substance. Some smaller masses appear to possess a structure and distribution similar to those of the degenerated cells. Some smears were literally filled with these formations. Frequently we have found these masses in basal cell epitheliomas of the eyelids.

In cases with an abundance of melanocytes, there are free melanin granules in the background of the smears.

TUMORS OF THE VASCULAR TISSUE

Angiomas

With the MGG stain the cytologic pattern varies according to whether one is considering a growing tumor or a stabilized angioma. In the first case, the smears show more angioblastic elements with naked nuclei, a lymphoid appearance, dense chromatin, and round or slightly indented outlines. In other angiomas or other fields, the angioblasts possess a cytoplasmic halo of a pale blue or grayish shade, with more of less delimited outlines, but generally round or polygonal. The most developed angiomas have a visible cytoplasm in most of their cells. The general cell picture shows many cells with the characteristics of adult endothelial cells and an abundant

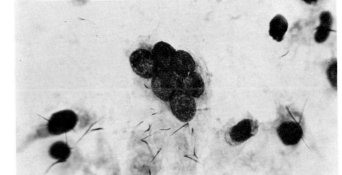

Figure 10–43 Angioma. Giant cell.

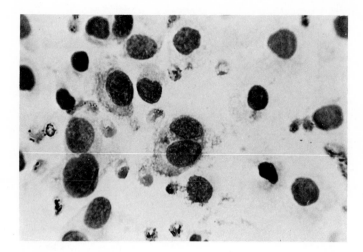

Figure 10–44 Telangiectatic granuloma. Typical appearance of the smear.

angular cytoplasm. Bi-, tri-, and multinucleated cells are found, with nuclei which preserve the characteristics of mononuclear cells. These cells are not so frequent here as in granuloma (pyogenicum). Figures 10–42 and 10–43 illustrate this cellular pattern.

Granuloma Pyogenicum

These lesions are demonstrative because the soft consistency of the tumor makes it possible to obtain smears rich in cells. For cytologic examination, the specimen must be washed with distilled water or physiologic saline to eliminate blood and fragments of epidermis.

The shape and arrangement of the cells in granuloma pyogenicum are similar to those of endothelial cells and therefore also to those of angiomas and granulation tissue from ulcers, but the cells are larger and more numerous. The cytoplasm is usually angular, but there are also cells with an abundant round or cuboidal bluish cytoplasm. In these cells, the nucleus is rounder than in fusiform cells (Figs. 10–44 and 10–45).

Frequently bi- or trinucleated cells are found, sometimes arranged in rows. The multinucleated cells form syncytia of considerable size (Figs. 10–46 and 10–47). A marked anisonucleosis can occur and can be seen in the cellular clusters, where the cells are sometimes arranged in a mosaic pattern with a perfectly visible cytoplasm and look like part of an already existent endothelium. Mitoses are not unusual.

It is normal to find polymorphonuclear leukocytes, lymphocytes, histiocytes, fibroblasts, epithelial cell fragments, and

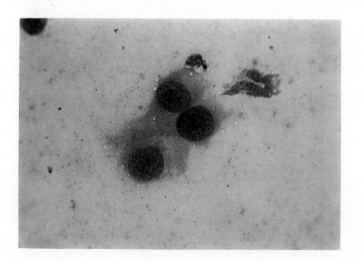

Figure 10–45 Telangiectatic granuloma. Typical cells.

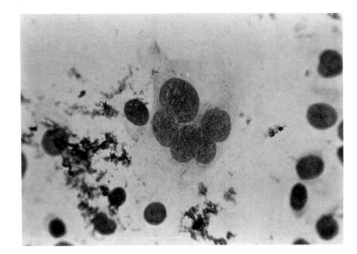

Figure 10–46 Telangiectatic granuloma. Giant cell.

bacteria mixed with endothelial cells. Some of the endothelial cells show phagocytosis of the erythrocytes and leukocytes.

Malignant Hemangioendothelioma

The abundant cells of these smears also resemble those of angioma and granuloma pyogenicum, for instance, in the abundance of the cytoplasm which stains bluish with MGG. However, the cytoplasm is round in almost all the cells, the nuclei are atypical with an irregular distribution of chromatin, and the nucleoli are more visible. There are abundant mitotic figures, and the anisocytosis is more sharply defined. Cells with a poorly delimited nucleus are frequent, and there are a great

many multinucleated cells with similarly anaplasic characteristics (Fig. 10–48).

Glomus Tumor

The tumors with mucoid degeneration of the stroma are the ones which present more characteristic cytologic pictures, because their cells are perfectly isolated and the cytoplasm stands out against the mucinous background.

The morphology of the glomus cells is typical. As a rule the nuclei are perfectly round, and their size varies from that of a lymphocyte to two or three times larger. Elongated nuclei seldom occur. The chromatin is dense and soft, and the nucleolus is hardly visible. The cytoplasm, either

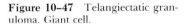

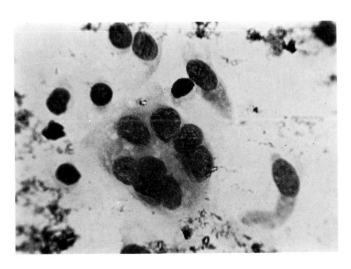

Figure 10–47 Telangiectatic granuloma. Giant cell.

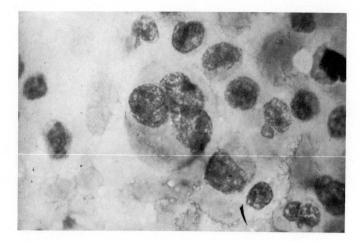

Figure 10–48 Hemangioendothelioma.

perfectly cuboidal or with short, blunted expansions, appears transparent against the background of the smear and sometimes stains light pink with the MGG stain. The cells occur isolated or in little clusters, and almost all are the same size (Fig. 10–49).

Hemangiopericytoma

In our single case, the cytologic characteristics were unremarkable. There were clumped and isolated nuclei with a dense chromatin and no visible nucleolus. They resembled glomus cells, but with an elongated or ovoid shape. The transparent cytoplasmic halo of the glomus cells was not evident (Fig. 10–50).

TUMORS OF THE CONNECTIVE TISSUE

Fibromas

To obtain suitable smears, the tumoral zone of the biopsy site must be defined by palpation and the unusable portions, especially the adipose tissue, cut off. Once the tumor is clean, we make several incisions in the surface in order to obtain the greatest number of cells.

The fibroblasts appear as elongated cells, some with a visible fusiform, irregular, pale blue cytoplasm, and naked round, oval, lobulated, or elongated nuclei. The dense chromatin is arranged irregularly, with clearer spaces which are sometimes vaguely parallel. The nucleoli are very small, hardly visible, or pale blue (Fig. 10–

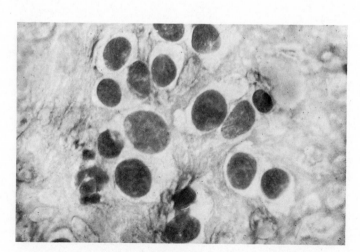

Figure 10–49 Glomus tumor. Typical cells.

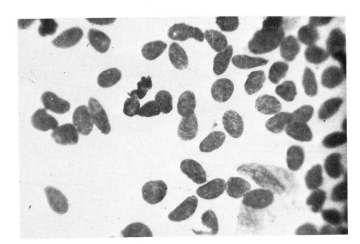

Figure 10–50 Hemangiopericytoma.

51). The background of the smears can contain a pink granular substance, which in some cases becomes very abundant (fibromyxomas). There is no evident anisocytosis, and generally the size of the cells is about two to three times that of a lymphocyte.

Fibrohistiocytoma and Xanthomatous Histiocytoma

The cytologic picture varies with the number of cells resembling fibroblasts and with the predominance of histiocytic cells. Generally it is possible to find all degrees of transition between both cellular types in the smears, which gives a false impression of anisocytosis. There is a considerable cellularity, and groups, clumps, or isolated cells can be observed.

The cells with fibroblastic appearance are more voluminous than the common fibroblasts. The cells with histiocytic appearance have an oval, round, indented nucleus. The chromatin is pasty and without the dusty appearance of the common histiocytes. In some cells one can observe uniform cytoplasmic rims, blue or pink in color and imprecise in outline, but in many cells the cytoplasm is vacuolar. In the xanthomatous fibrohistiocytoma the vacuoles are more numerous and not only fill the outline of the cytoplasm but also cover the nucleus as well. In the fully developed xanthoma the whole background of the smear is filled with vacuoles, which makes staining difficult. There are multinucleated cells, some of which can have more than a dozen nuclei and a completely foamy cytoplasm. (Fig. 10–52).

In the fibrohistiocytoma containing he-

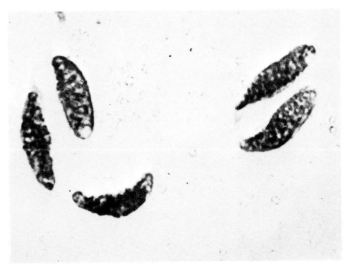

Figure 10–51 Typical fibroblasts with the characteristic chromatin pattern.

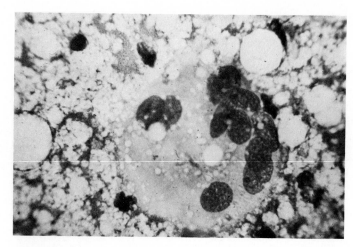

Figure 10–52   Histiocytoma. Giant cell.

mosiderin, this is found in the giant cells and some isolated mononucleated cells in coarse granulations varying in size and irregularly distributed. Adequate staining brings out the ferric pigment in the cells and in the free granulations in the background of the smear.

With the acridine orange stain, xanthomatous degeneration can be made clear not only in the giant cells but also in isolated cells, including those with a fibroblastic appearance. There is a characteristic perinuclear halo of yellow lipids.

Dermatofibrosarcoma (Darier-Ferrand)

The smears are rich in cells which are arranged in clusters or isolated. The cytologic diagnosis is easy in this case. The cells are larger than the common fibroblasts and are more monomorphous with a less elongated nucleus; the majority are oval, pear-shaped, or round.

Although the chromatin sometimes shows a "fibroblastic" arrangement, for the most part it is pasty and irregular (Fig. 10–53). The nucleolus is hardly visible. The cytoplasm appears like a halo with imprecise outlines, and with the MGG stain, a pale blue or pink cytoplasmic magma can often be observed, which fills the background of the clusters of nuclei. The cytoplasm of these cells is very fragile.

There is a slight anisokaryosis, with small or voluminous round nuclei. The anisochromasia of the nuclei is notable in some smears.

Exceptionally the MGG stain shows vesicular or granular cytoplasm with pink granules. In the lesions with mucoid degeneration, the background is completely filled with a pink granular sub-

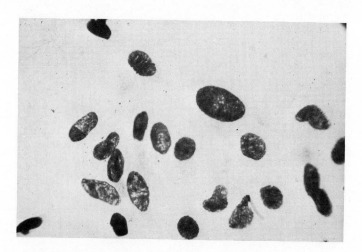

Figure 10–53   Darier-Ferrand's dermatofibrosarcoma. Some elements with the "fibroblastic" pattern of the chromatin.

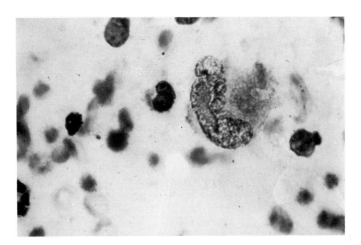

Figure 10–54 Fibrosarcoma. Monstrous cell.

stance or filaments. In these cases the outlines of the cytoplasm are not visible, and the nuclei, which are covered with the mucinous strands, stain badly with MGG. With the Gomori reticulin stain, the slightly wavelike reticulin fibers show clearly. The Gomori stain is useful in showing the "fibroblastic" arrangement of the chromatin with the characteristic clear spaces.

The Feulgen stain does not reveal great anomalies in the distribution of the nucleic acids. The Papanicolaou and hematoxylin-eosin stains are not adequate here.

Fibrosarcoma

The cytologic picture and the cellularity are variable, but generally the smears are less rich in cells than those of dermatofi-brosarcoma. The background mostly contains a lot of mucinous substance.

Some cells resemble the typical fibroblasts, but atypical cells with signs of malignancy are frequent. There are excessively large, deformed cells (Figs. 10–54 and 10–55); overlapping nuclei; syncytia of the cytoplasmic magma; pronounced anisokaryosis, with small pyknotic cells next to giant cells; cells with a badly distributed, irregular, coarse chromatin; abnormal, lobulated, polymorphous nuclei; and multiple, irregular, and sometimes giant blue or pink nucleoli. The volume of the nucleoli does not reach that in melanoma. There is marked hyperchromasia of the cytoplasm, which stains totally or partially blue or deep purple with the MGG stain. Bi- or trinucleated cells and partial necrosis of the nuclei can be found. It is not rare to find greenish granules (hemosiderin?) in-

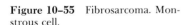

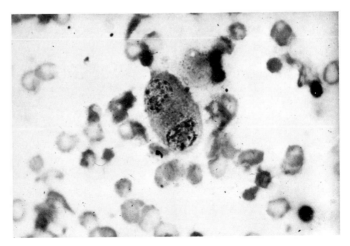

Figure 10–55 Fibrosarcoma. Monstrous cell.

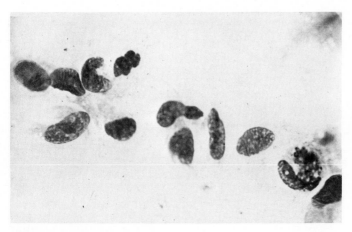

Figure 10–56 Fibrosarcoma. One element (right) with cytoplasmatic inclusions.

side the cytoplasm of these fibroblasts (Fig. 10–56).

In other fibrosarcomas there is less anaplasia, but in some smears the excessive atypia of the cells obscures their fibroblastic origin. Gomori's reticulin stain brings out the anisonucleosis. The cytoplasm looks like a violet halo, and the chromatin is folded, leaving clear spaces. The reticulin fibers form thick bundles or are delicate and wavelike with ramifications (Fig. 10–57). The Feulgen stain shows the change in the distribution of nucleic acids and anisochromasia.

Pseudosarcomatous Fascitis

Most of the cells resemble fibroblasts. There is substantial monomorphism, but there are also cells with a vesicular cytoplasm and clearer nucleus (histiocytoid) and occasional isolated, large, bi- or trinucleated cells. The background is mucoid, amorphous, or granular and sometimes finely vacuolar (Fig. 10–58). Cells with large abnormal nuclei are rare. Some fibroblasts show brownish granulations with the MGG stain. Usually the smears of these lesions are not rich in cells.

Kaposi's Angiosarcoma

The tumors and infiltrated plaques are not suitable for cytologic examination because of the great amount of connective tissue which is often present. All cases we examined were poor in cells. The smears were made up exclusively of cells resembling fibroblasts but with slight abnormalities (hypertrophy, anomalies of shape, and so forth). Some cells are round, have a denser chromatin, and are difficult to classify, and a great number of red blood cells are present.

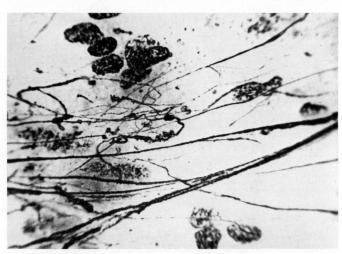

Figure 10–57 Fibrosarcoma. Gomori stain for reticulin.

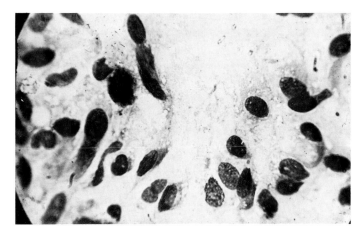

Figure 10–58 Pseudosarcomatous fascitis.

Giant Cell Epulis

These tumors resemble vascular tumors. The preparations contain mono- and multinucleated cells (Fig. 10–59). The mononucleated cells have a characteristically wide angular cytoplasm, which stains dark blue or purple with the MGG stain. Their nuclei are oval or round with a finely granular chromatin and a scarcely visible nucleolus. Morphologically these cells closely resemble endothelial cells, but frequently a coarse granular substance, reddish or brown in color, covers the cytoplasm of the epulis cells. There are free granules around the cell limits.

The mononucleated cells are found isolated, grouped in a mosaic fashion, or arranged in rows. There are mitoses and some cells are in a stage of disintegration.

Bi- and trinucleated cells with the same angular outlines as the mononuclear cells are frequent, but the most characteristic feature is the occurrence of multinucleated giant cells, whose size can reach 50 microns or more (Fig. 10–60). The cytoplasm of these cells has the same granular structure as in the mononucleated cells and also stains blue or purple. There can be more than a dozen irregularly arranged, overlapping, but uniformly sized nuclei. The cytoplasm is round or oval with angular projections. The morphology of the epulis cells does not favor the hypothesis of the fibroblastic origin of this tumor.

TUMORS OF MUSCULAR TISSUE

Leiomyomas

The smears are not characteristic and are poor in cells. The cells are elongated

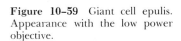

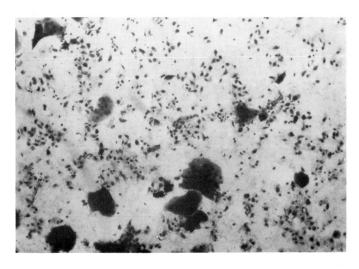

Figure 10–59 Giant cell epulis. Appearance with the low power objective.

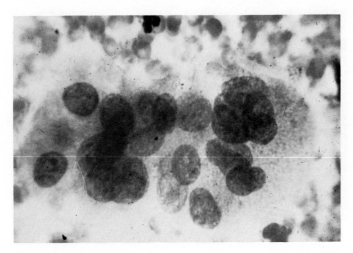

Figure 10–60 Giant cell of an epulis.

with a smoky, almost invisible cytoplasm, are smaller than fibroblasts, and have elongated or lanceolate naked nuclei with a dense chromatin (Fig. 10–61). The angioleiomyomas show a similar picture. In distinction to the fibromas, there is no background substance.

Granular Cell Myoblastoma (Abrikosov's Tumor)

This neoplasm offers a very peculiar picture which is more evident in the smears than in histologic sections. The smears would seem to favor the theory that these cells are derived from myoblasts. Some cells show an almost perfect striation of the very fine dark brownish granules in the enormous cuboidal or polygonal cytoplasm which stains blue or greyish with the MGG stain (Fig. 10–62). The nuclei are disproportionately small, with deep pink round or oval outlines. In other cells the granules condense, become thicker, and lose their striated arrangement. In some cells there are small vacuoles intermingled with the granules (Fig. 10–63). The few cells present have a poorly demarcated cytoplasm. Most cells form syncytia with small, more or less regularly distributed nuclei.

Leiomyosarcoma

Our only case showed a surprising picture, with an abundance of extraordinarily large cells with a fusiform or irregular pink cytoplasm, up to several hundred microns long, and with deformed nuclei, some of which covered almost the whole field of the oil immersion objective. The chromatin, uniform in some nuclei, was irregularly distributed in others. The nucleoli were hardly visible in spite of the evident cellular anaplasia (Figs. 10–64 and 10–65).

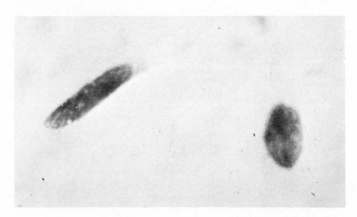

Figure 10–61 Leiomyoma. Two common aspects of the cells. An almond-shaped nucleus devoid of cytoplasm and another fusiform with barely visible cytoplasm.

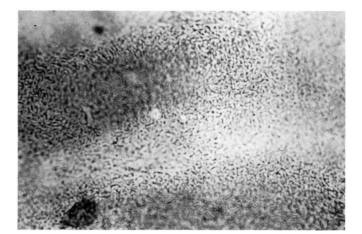

Figure 10–62 Granular cell myoblastoma. Cell showing the striated pattern of the granulation.

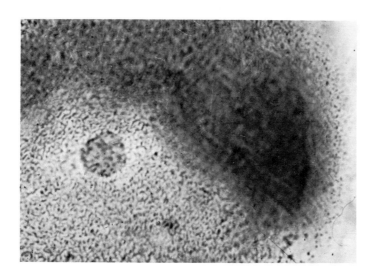

Figure 10–63 Granular cell myoblastoma. A characteristic cell.

Figure 10–64 Leiomyosarcoma. Monstrous cell.

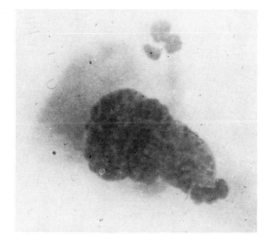

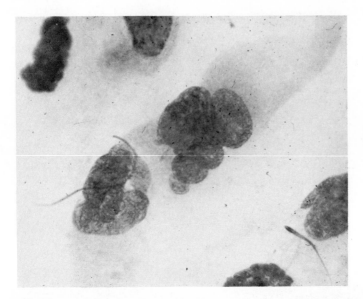

Figure 10–65 Leiomyosarcoma. Monstrous cells.

SOME TUMORS OF THE APPENDAGES OF THE SKIN

Nodular Hidradenomas

The smears, which are normally rich in cells, offer an appearance which varies with the histologic structure of the tumor. The most frequent cellular patterns are the following:

Solid Hidradenomas. There are numerous lumps of cells in irregular groups, cells arranged in rows, cells with a vaguely adenoid disposition and a clear space in the center, and many isolated cells. These are generally cuboid or polyhedral with a well-defined, bluish or pale purple, sometimes lightly vacuolar cytoplasm. The nuclei are round or oval, sometimes in-dented; the chromatin is finely grained, uniform, and without a visible nucleus. The background of the smear is finely granular or mucoid (Fig. 10–66).

Clear Cell Hidradenomas. The cytoplasm is more voluminous, more acidophilic, and less well defined, and also very fragile, since in many of the cells it has disappeared or only fragments of it can be seen. Many of the naked nuclei are chromophobic, so that to see them clearly the smears have to be overstained. In these cases the background is dense and granular, and in some fields becomes the principal element of the smear, which stains pink with MGG (Fig. 10–67).

With the periodic acid–Schiff stain the cytoplasm stains deep red with thick granulation (Fig. 10–68). In stains in which the

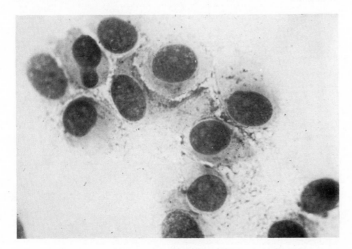

Figure 10–66 Nodular hidradenoma. Cells in a mosaic fashion with cuboidal cytoplasm.

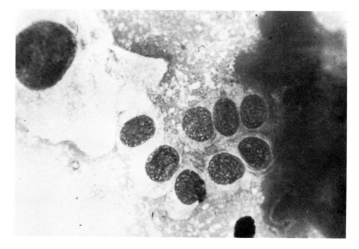

Figure 10–67 Nodular hidradenoma. "Clear cell" beside cuboidal elements. On the opposite side a mucoid mass.

naked nuclei are dominant, the granular background also stains intensely with PAS, which suggests that the granules which constitute it come from the destroyed cytoplasm.

Hidradenomas With Chondroid Degeneration (Mixed Tumors, Chondroid Syringomas). The appearance is still more peculiar than that of other types of hidradenoma and very characteristic. The preserved cellular elements have lost their cuboidal outline and have become round. The cells vary widely in size and are drowned out by the mucoid substance of the background of the smear (Fig. 10–69). Some cells show a yellowish, transparent, and progressively more hyaline cytoplasm in varying stages of degeneration. In the more degenerated cells the nucleus is in-

creasingly less visible, until it finally disappears completely, producing yellow hyaline spheres without structure (Fig. 10–70).

Salivary Gland Adenoma

The main cytologic features are similar to those of nodular hidradenomas. Chondroid degeneration can be present, and the background of the smears is more or less mucoid, finely granular, and sometimes stains intensely purple with the MGG stain. The cytoplasm is cuboidal, and the nuclei are more globular and richer in chromatin than those of the sweat gland cells. In the areas of chondroid transformation, the cytoplasm becomes round.

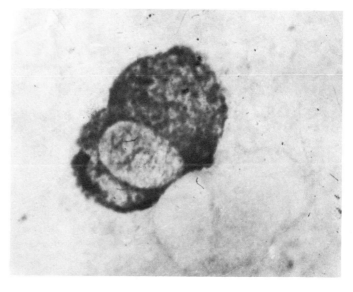

Figure 10–68 "Clear cell hidradenoma," PAS stain. Note the cytoplasmatic PAS-positive granules.

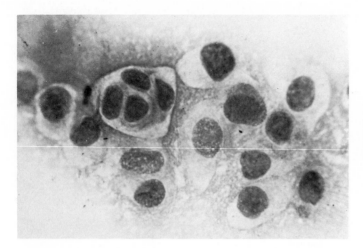

Figure 10–69 Nodular hidradenoma with chondroid degeneration. The cells are drowned and framed by the mucoid substance becoming rounded.

Calcifying Epithelioma of Malherbe

In the smears the following types of cells can be observed:

Cells With a Basophilic Nucleus. They are arranged in rows or in elongated sheets without a visible cytoplasm. The nuclei are oval or elongated with irregular chromatin, which forms dense clots. The cells are three times larger than a lymphocyte, although there are others about the size of lymphocytes with very dense chromatin (Figs. 10–71 and 10–72).

Cells With Visible Cytoplasm. Some isolated cells present a bluish, barely perceptible cytoplasmic halo. The outlines are well defined and polygonal with rounded angles. Other cells are eosinophilic with a vacuolar cytoplasm.

Syncytial Laminae. Syncytia made up of a great number of nuclei (as many as a score or more) are typical. They have a uniform, bluish, hardly visible cytoplasm which can also be vacuolar, with lumps of a denser, sometimes blackish substance (Fig. 10–73). Totally anuclear *laminae* of almost transparent cytoplasm can be present. There are *dense masses* which possibly correspond to calcium deposits.

Sebaceous Adenoma

There is an abundance of sebaceous cells which occur isolated or in small lumps of usually less than a dozen cells, together with a great number of nuclei whose cytoplasm has been destroyed by the handling of the smear. The lumps of cells form an irregular mosaic. (Fig. 10–74).

The lesions are easy to diagnose because of the great number of cells, their lack of uniformity, and the number of

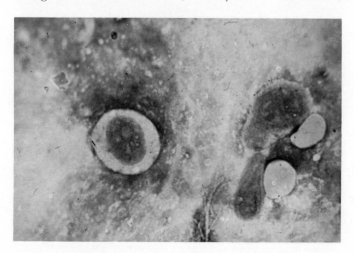

Figure 10–70 Progressive disappearance of the cells in nodular hidradenoma. The nuclear outlines become fuzzy, and the cells are transformed in the transparent and refringent spherules.

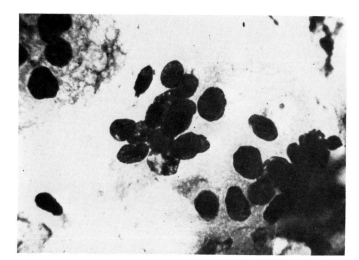

Figure 10–71 Calcifying epithelioma of Malherbe. Basophilic cells.

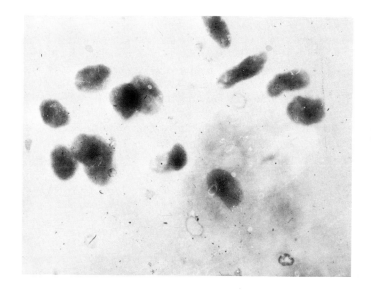

Figure 10–72 Calcifying epithelioma of Malherbe. "Shadow" cells.

Figure 10–73 Calcifying epithelioma of Malherbe. Syncytium.

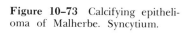
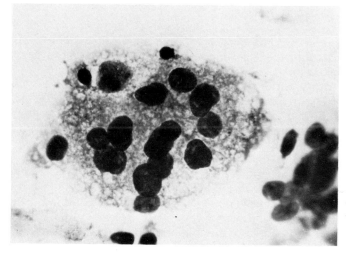

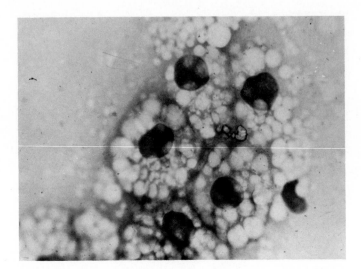

Figure 10–74 Senile sebaceous adenoma.

lumps. The cells which stand out above the foamy background stain purple and have a round or irregular, sometimes petal-shaped nucleus with chromatin of low density. Above this nucleus the cytoplasmic vesiculations are projected in the form of more pallid bluish spherules. In the smears one can see the process of sebum formation. The least mature cells are relatively small with grayish cytoplasm. The intermediate phase is composed of cells with a vacuolar cytoplasm. Finally there are cells with a punctiform nucleus whose cytoplasm contains a large drop of fat.

SOME BENIGN TUMORS OF THE EPIDERMIS

Verruca Seborrheica

The smears show a moderate number of cells with the following characteristics: (1) cells with naked, round, or somewhat irregular nuclei about the size of a lymphocyte, with a dense and pasty chromatin and without a visible nucleolus; (2) medium-sized, completely keratinized cells with a pyknotic nucleus and a bluish or transparent cytoplasm; (3) keratinized cells disposed in irregular clusters. The contrast between cells with cytoplasm and completely keratinized masses is typical. There are occasional isolated cells with a clear vacuolar cytoplasm resembling sebaceous cells. Some smears show small isolated melanocytes with short blunted dendrites.

Epithelial Nevus

The smears are characterized by their monotony. There is a great quantity of round nuclei, which are twice the size of a lymphocyte and have granular chromatin and a barely visible nucleolus; the uniformity is such that in some fields there is a certain resemblance to lymphoma. Keratinized cells without visible nuclei are also present.

Pilonidal Cysts

These are neoformations with very peculiar cytologic characteristics. Two cell types occur in the smears: isolated cells and cellular syncytia.

The *isolated cells* vary widely in size, some reaching the volume of a normal epidermal cell while others are much smaller. The cytoplasm is variable in its outline and intensely blue in color. The nucleus is dense and finely granular, and the sometimes voluminous nucleolus is not always visible. The cytoplasm contains two types of granulation, one fine, reddish or gray and the other diffuse and black, resembling melanin. Bi- or trinucleated cells are present.

Cellular Syncytia are very characteristic. They form great masses, sometimes with dozens of oval or round nuclei with a dense granular and uniformly distributed chromatin. The nucleoli, which can be double or triple, are very evident in these nuclei.

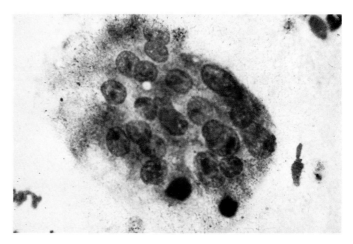

Figure 10–75 Pilonidal cyst. Syncytium.

The cytoplasmic portion of the syncytia can stain blue as in isolated cells but other syncytia show reddish, gray-brown, or even black pigmented granulations (Figs. 10–75 and 10–76). The background of the smear is also granular with the same reddish and black grains which are found in the interior of the cytoplasm.

LIPIDOSES

Histiocytosis X

In all forms of the disease, the characteristic cells are easy to distinguish.

In the *Abt-Letterer-Siwe syndrome*, the slides taken from the "papular" lesions reveal an abundance of cells, which resemble histiocytes, reticular cells, or monocytes. There is a noticeable anisocytosis, with some cells about the size of normal histiocytes and others two or three times larger. The nucleus is denser and more intensely colored than that of histiocytes, round or oval, or deeply indented. The scarcely visible nucleolus is single or multiple and generally small. Some cells have no visible cytoplasm; others have a large cytoplasm that stains bluish or grayish with the MGG stain (Figs. 10–77 to 10–79). There are lymphoid or lymphoblastic cells and some binucleated or huge multinucleated cells with a dense grayish or lightly eosinophilic cytoplasm. The nuclei are irregularly distributed, and whereas cells with foamy cytoplasm are rare in histologic slides of Abt-Letterer-Siwe syndrome, they are more frequent in the cytologic picture.

In *Hand-Schuller-Christian disease*, the cytologic characteristics are similar, and the characteristic cells described above occur in greater numbers.

In *eosinophilic granuloma of bone*, reticu-

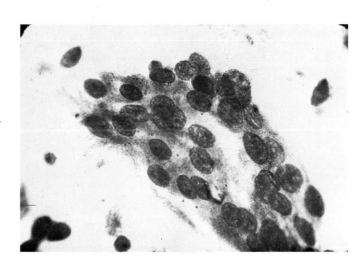

Figure 10–76 Pilonidal cyst. Cellular syncytium.

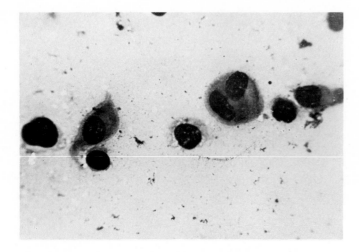

Figure   10–77 Abt-Letterer-Siwe disease. Abnormal histiocytes.

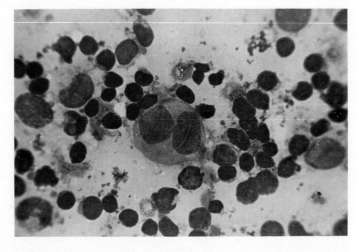

Figure   10–78 Abt-Letterer-Siwe disease. A binuclear cell.

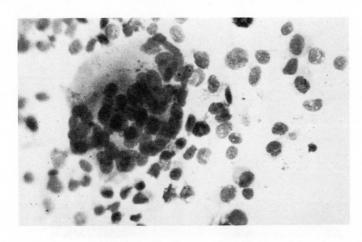

Figure   10–79 Abt-Letterer-Siwe disease. Giant cell surrounded by mononuclear elements.

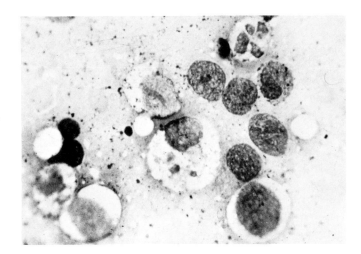

Figure 10–80 Eosinophilic granuloma of bone. Histiocytes with foamy cytoplasm and eosinophils.

lum or histiocytoid cells are found in abundance. They have globular or perfectly round nuclei. The cytoplasm is similarly round, abundant, transparent, or vacuolar in most cells and bluish in others (Fig. 10–80). Beside these, the smear shows many eosinophils, most of which contain only a few granules. One finds also a number of isolated osteoblasts, with their typical granular cytoplasm, which is dense and stains purple with MGG. The nuclei are uniform and irregularly distributed.

In all cases of histiocytosis X, the Sudan black stain shows the intracytoplasmic deposits in the form of small drops in the cells which contain lipids.

Nevoxanthoendothelioma (Juvenile Xanthogranuloma)

The cytologic picture varies considerably with the stage of development. Under low power the slides show an abundance of cells with an oval nucleus, evenly granular chromatin, and a clearly visible nucleolus with an abundant fusiform or lanceolate, pale blue cytoplasm. They can easily be confused with endothelial cells, but the cells are smaller in xanthogranuloma. Alongside these elongated cells there are others with a round cytoplasm, globular nuclei, and single or multiple nucleoli. Only a few cells have two, three, or four small oval nuclei and denser chromatin (Fig. 10–81).

Under higher magnification the cytology is characteristic. The background of the smear is filled with a substance which stains purple or blue with the MGG stain. There are also numerous mononuclear cells with a naked oval nucleus and granular chromatin, forming a thick mesh with other cells which show a visible dense blue or purple, sometimes smoky cyto-

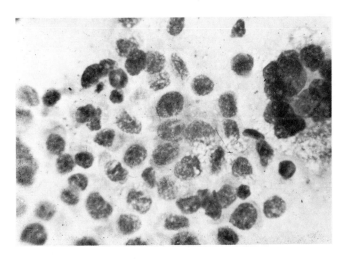

Figure 10–81 Nevoxanthogranuloma. Mononuclear cells showing a foamy cytoplasm.

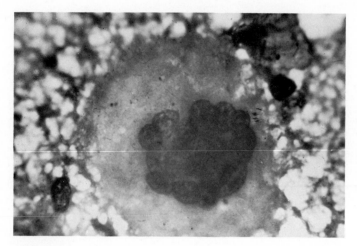

Figure 10–82 Nevoxanthogranuloma. Giant multinuclear cell showing the finely vacuolar cytoplasm and the nuclear clumping in the center.

plasm. The most typical finding consists of numerous, huge multinucleated cells which stand out in the smear under low power (Fig. 10–82). Sometimes these cells have more than a dozen nuclei which are disposed in the center of the cells in packed masses or in an irregular pattern. The cytoplasm is spread out, dense, and muddy, and it stains intensely purple or blue. In some mononuclear cells, transparent cytoplasmic vacuoles can be seen. Bi- or trinucleated cells with a vacuolar cytoplasm are rarer.

The Sudan black stain shows fatty deposits in the background of the smear and in the cytoplasm. The lipids stain diffusely or form tiny droplets.

Xanthomas

Smears from xanthomatous lesions are difficult to obtain. The cells are so fragile

that in the great majority of cases the smear shows only the naked nuclei isolated in the background of the smear which is made up of a vacuolar substance. This substance covers many of the nuclei and prevents their staining.

Occasionally the sequence of the formation of the xanthomatous cell can be seen in the smear. There are mononucleated cells loaded with fatty droplets next to multinucleated cells with a big vacuolar cytoplasm completely filled with fat (Figs. 10–83 and 10–84). Lipid stains show the fat not only inside the cytoplasm but also in the background of the smear.

LYMPHOMAS

Malignant Lymphomas

Together with melanoma, the malignant lymphomas constitute the processes in

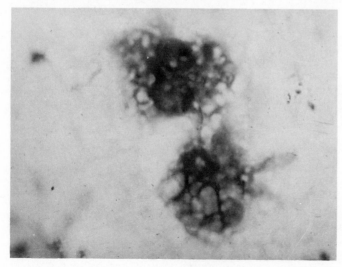

Figure 10–83 Xanthoma. A mononuclear and a binuclear cell containing lipid droplets.

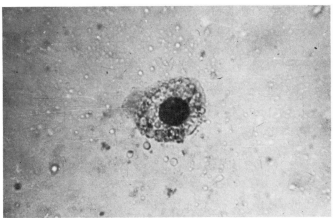

Figure 10–84 Xanthelasma. Cell with cytoplasm containing crystalline depots of cholesterol. Observe the crystals in the background of the smear.

which the examination of the smears proves most useful. In the lymphomas the infiltration is in general sufficiently important to provide the necessary quantity of cells for the smears.

Although morphologically it is almost impossible to classify the blasts in the cutaneous infiltrations, we have the advantage that the most frequent are the lymphocytic cells (lymphocytes, lymphoblasts, atypical or monstrous lymphoid cells), together with the reticulum cells (histiocytes, atypical or monstrous reticulum cells). Myeloid and other cells are rare. Therefore, cytochemical studies are usually not necessary, and the routine MGG, Feulgen, and Papanicolaou stains are sufficient. The smears show the following features:

Undifferentiated Reticulum Cell Sarcoma (Stem Cell Lymphoma). The smears show immature cells with pale round or oval nuclei, sometimes 10 times the size of a lymphocyte, a pasty or finely granular chromatin, and a bluish, oval, or polygonal cytoplasm of varying abundance. The nucleolus can be single or multiple and sometimes irregular and huge. Differential diagnosis with some metastases is difficult, and in fact some cases considered as stem cell lymphomas may well be metastases (Fig. 10–85). In some cases there are isolated cells resembling normal histiocytes. In these lesions the reticulin stain is negative.

Histiocytic Reticulum Cell Sarcoma (Reticulohistiocytic Lymphoma) (Fig. 10–86). These lesions can be of two types: with *small reticulum cells* and *large reticulum cells.*

In the first case, the reticulum cells are roughly the size of lymphocytes, but the chromatin is very different, much clearer and in a finer mesh. The nuclear outline

Figure 10–85 Lymphoma (stem cell).

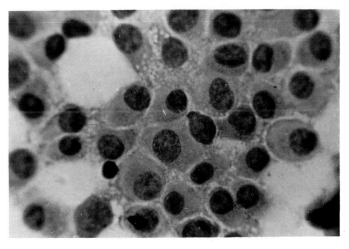

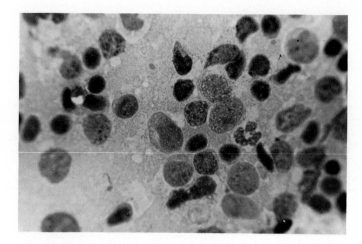

Figure 10–86 Lymphoma (reticulum cell). Smear showing the characteristic features of the reticulohystiocytic lymphoma.

frequently shows the same indentations or foldings as the histiocyte. In most of these cells no cytoplasm is visible, and if it does exist it is of a light blue color. The lymphocytic component always forms an important part of the cytologic picture.

In the *large reticulum cell* lymphoma, reticular and histiocytic elements predominate, although there is always also a mixture of lymphocytes and polymorphonuclear neutrophils and eosinophils. The histiocytic cells have a folded and indented nucleus. The chromatin is granular and distributed in a fine mesh with a scarcely visible nucleolus. The reticular cells are round or oval with a more visible bluish cytoplasm. There is marked anisocytosis, and histiocytosis with an excessively folded or irregular nucleus is frequent. There are some mitotic figures. The lymphoid

component is always important, and there are many intermediate stages between the reticulum and the lymphoid cells.

The Gomori stain for reticulin shows scarce, fine fibers in many fields of the smear. There are many transitional stages between this type of lymphoma and the lymphosarcoma. In cutaneous smears morphologically "pure" lymphomas are exceptional.

Lymphosarcoma (Lymphocytic Lymphoma, Lymphoblastic Lymphoma). In these lesions the lymphoid elements predominate. The cytologic picture is variable (Figs. 10–87 to 10–89).

In some smears *mature* cells predominate. The great majority of cells are small with a naked nucleus, dense chromatin, and the characteristics of the adult lymphocyte. There are no atypical cells, al-

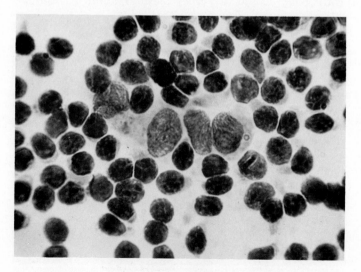

Figure 10–87 Lymphosarcoma (lymphocytic lymphoma). The lymphoid cells are the predominant elements in the smear. In the center of the field there are some somewhat atypical reticulum cells.

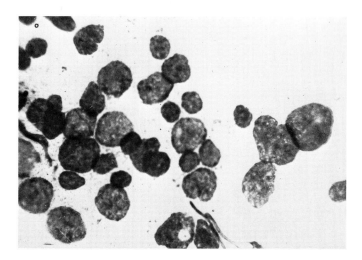

Figure 10–88 Lymphosarcoma with atypical cells.

though one can find some huge isolated cells, karyorrhexis, single cells with a monocytoid appearance, and some isolated eosinophils. The monotony of the cellular pattern is the only guide regarding the origin of the process. In some cases, the hemogram reveals a concomitant lymphatic leukemia. On rare occasions there are some more voluminous lymphoid cells resembling those of mycosis fungoides.

In other smears *immature* cells predominate. The nuclei are more voluminous. In a particular cell the cytoplasm may be visible in the form of a bluish halo. The chromatin is often disposed in a cartwheel arrangement (Strünge's aspect grumelé). This characteristic fissured aspect of the chromatin is accentuated with the Papanicolaou stain. The nucleoli are difficult to distinguish in spite of the juvenile or *lymphoblastic* appearance of the cells. Over-

lapping of the nuclei is frequent, and there are some transitional stages with reticulum and multinucleated cells. The mitotic figures can be numerous. Isolated reticulum cells and eosinophils are found occasionally. The smears resemble the adenograms of lymphoid leukemia. Some of the lymphoblastic elements possess a bluish cytoplasmatic halo.

In other lymphosarcomas the majority of cells are *atypical* and excessively voluminous. Some are deformed with badly distributed chromatin and marked nuclear irregularities. Most fields show features of malignancy. The anisocytosis is very marked. These lesions are indistinguishable from some metastases.

Some of these lymphosarcomas correspond to the last stage of mycosis fungoides, while others are primary lymphosarcomas.

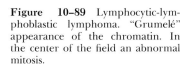

Figure 10–89 Lymphocytic-lymphoblastic lymphoma. "Grumelé" appearance of the chromatin. In the center of the field an abnormal mitosis.

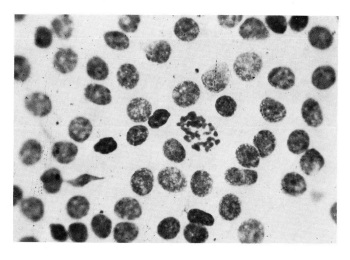

The Gomori stain is negative in all lymphosarcomas. The PAS stain shows some granular cytoplasmatic inclusions in isolated cells. The Feulgen stain reveals nucleolar abnormalities in some cases. Fluorescence microscopy after the acridine orange stain (Bertalanffy, 1962) reveals an intense fluorescence of the cells, indicating a considerable wealth of cytoplasmic RNA. The Sudan stain, alkaline phosphatase esterase, and peroxidase stain are all negative.

Mycosis Fungoides

In the *premycotic stage* the smears are not demonstrative. There are occasional isolated lymphoid cells, but with an excessive volume and abnormal shape. They sometimes have irregularly distributed chromatin or a blue cytoplasmic rim. Epidermal dyskeratosis is more frequent in the smears than in histologic slides.

In the *infiltrating stage* the smears are generally characteristic: there are mature lymphocytes and small pyknotic lymphocytes with a deformed outline; at the same time peculiar lymphomonocytoid cells are present, which are very voluminous with a dense, irregularly distributed chromatin and sometimes a bluish cytoplasmic halo. They can be up to 10 times the size of a normal lymphocyte. These may be *mycosis cells* (Figs. 10–90 and 10–91). Their nucleus is round or oval and in many cells deformed. Exceptionally there are bi- or trinucleated cells with barely visible bluish cytoplasm. Some cells are similar to reticulum cells. Karyorrhexis and mitoses are frequent. Together with these lymphoid and reticular components, one can see isolated polymorphonuclear neutrophils and numerous eosinophils, some with preserved granules in the cytoplasm and some with naked nuclei. In the background of the smear, granules are mixed with nuclear debris, which is also found in the cytoplasm of the lymphoid or reticular cells.

In the *tumoral stage* the cytologic picture is indistinguishable from that of atypical lymphosarcoma. Large lymphoid or monocytoid cells predominate. Some of the cells resemble the previously described *mycosis cells.*

The PAS stain is not demonstrative. There are some cells with PAS-positive granules or masses.

Hodgkin's Disease (Malignant Lymphogranuloma)

The smears of cutaneous lesions almost never contain typical Sternberg-Reed cells. The picture we have observed in the nodules was similar to that of reticulum cell sarcoma. Some cells showed a monstrous nucleus (Figs. 10–92 and 10–93).

Plasmacytoma (Fig. 10–94)

The characteristic atypical plasmablastic cells are easily found in the smears of the cutaneous nodules. The anisocytosis, the reddish cytoplasm, and the anisochromasia, together with the irregularity of the nuclei and other anaplastic features, help to establish the cytodiagnosis.

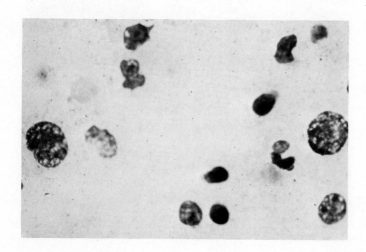

Figure 10–90 "Mycosis cells" in both sides of the field.

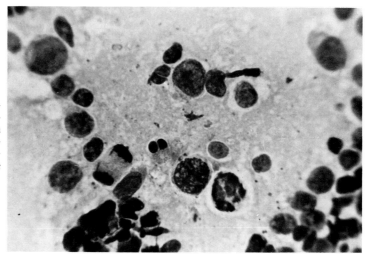

Figure 10–91 Mycosis fungoides. Infiltrative stage. Mycosis cells, one eosinophil, and a cell in mitosis. One element disintegrating and the characteristic granular background of the smear.

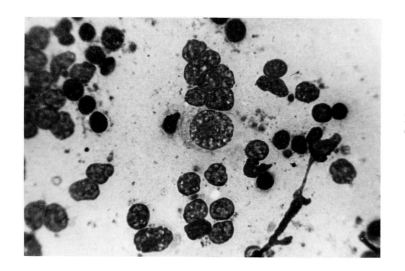

Figure 10–92 Hodgkin's disease. Sternberg-Reed cell.

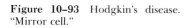

Figure 10–93 Hodgkin's disease. "Mirror cell."

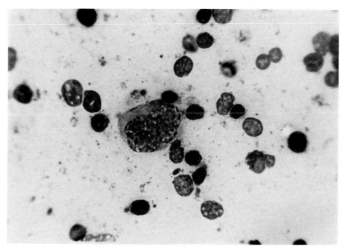

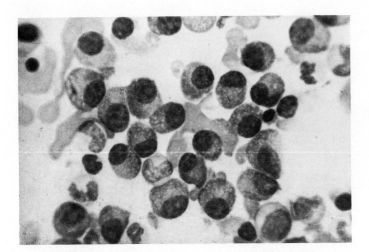

Figure 10–94 Plasmacytoma.

On the contrary, diagnosis is not possible in the smears of myeloid leukemia, macroglobulinemia with cutaneous lesions, and erythroleukemia. In the leukemias a cytochemical and cytoenzymologic investigation is necessary. In the *Sezary syndrome* some PAS-positive cells are found in the smears of erythrodermic skin, but the same is true for the infiltrates of other malignant reticuloses. The presence in the blood of cells with PAS-positive granules which are diastase-resistant and peroxidase-negative, alkaline phosphatase–negative, Sudan-negative, and contain only a few granules positive to nonspecific esterase, seems to be decisive (Moragas and Woesner, 1968).

Alopecia Mucinosa

In some patients with malignant reticuloses, the first skin manifestation is alopecia mucinosa. The smears of isolated hair follicles show polygonal cells with a granular cytoplasm which stains intensely red with MGG. Some of these cells have lost their nuclei. If the nucleus is preserved, it shows signs of degeneration. In the well preserved cells the nuclei are round or oval with a finely granular chromatin. Some areas of the smears show clusters of cells embedded in a mucinous substance with no visible cytoplasm. The background contains reddish granulations similar to those observed in the cytoplasm. The cytoplasm is angular and somewhat different from that of epidermal cells.

Benign Lymphocytoma

The smears show a variable amount of mature lymphocytes and reticulum cells, most of them devoid of cytoplasm, with

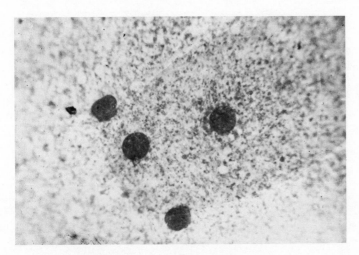

Figure 10–95 Mastocytosis. The cells have liberated their granules, which are seen in the background of the smear forming a thick film.

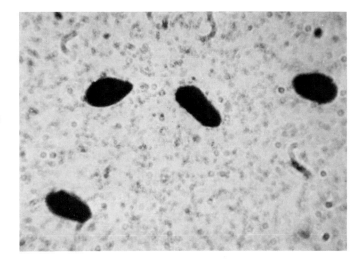

Figure 10–96 Neurofibromatosis (von Recklinghausen).

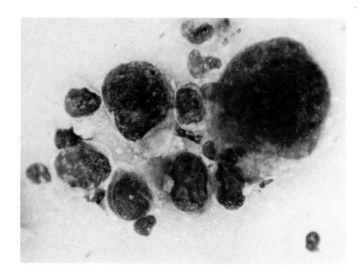

Figure 10–97 Cutaneous metastasis of rectal carcinoma. The anaplastic features are very visible.

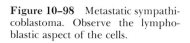

Figure 10–98 Metastatic sympathicoblastoma. Observe the lymphoblastic aspect of the cells.

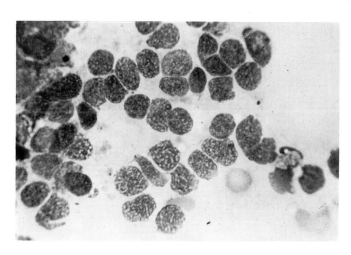

regular nuclear outlines. In some cases of histologically benign lesions we have found a confusing cellular picture in the smears, with anisokaryosis in the reticular cells.

Mastocytosis

The main feature in the smears is an enormous amount of metachromatic granules in the background. Some mastocytes are easily recognizable, but most of these cells have lost their cytoplasm and are seen as oval or round, dense nuclei in the dense film of granules (Fig. 10–95).

TUMORS OF THE NERVOUS TISSUE

Neurofibroma

The smears are poor in cells. One can see only isolated nuclei devoid of cytoplasm, very dense, and with a peculiar morphology (rice grain feature – Fig. 10–96).

CUTANEOUS METASTASES OF VISCERAL CANCERS

The cellular picture of the cutaneous metastases is widely variable. Most of the smears show abnormal cells with a pattern of high malignancy (Fig. 10–97). Their origin is unrecognizable, and some cases of metastatic mammary adenocarcinoma or metastasis of sympathicoblastoma are easily confused with malignant reticuloses (Fig. 10–98).

REFERENCES

Andrade, R.: Citodiagnóstico en Dermatología Clínica. Cortes, J. L. (Ed.): Mexico, D. F., 1972.

Berardi, P.: Contributo allo studio della citologia dermatologica. Arch. Ital. Dermatol., 34:87, 1966.

Bertalanffy, F. D.: Sobre el citodiagnostico del cancer: Microscopia fluorescente por coloración con naranja de acridina. Triangulo, 5:152, 1962.

Bertalanffy, L. von, and Bickis, I.: Identification of cytoplasmic basophilia (ribonucleic acid by fluores-

cence microscopy). J. Histochem. Cytochem., 4:481, 1956.

Bertalanffy, L. von, Masin, F., and Masin, M.: Use of acridine-orange fluorescence technique in exfoliative cytology. Science, 124:1024, 1956.

Brehmer-Andersson, E., and Brunk, U.: Tape-stripping method for cytological diagnosis of mycosis fungoides. Acta Derm. Venereol. (Stockh.), 47:177, 1967a.

Brehmer-Andersson, E., and Brunk, U.: Cytological diagnosis in mycosis fungoides. XIII Congressus Internationalis Dermatologiae, München, 1967. Vol. II. 1967b, pp. 735–738.

Burnham, T. K., Neblett, T. R., and Bank, P.: The immunofluorescent tumor imprint technique. Arch. Dermatol. Syph., 99:611, 1969.

Castelain, G., and Castelain, C.: Les frottis tissulaires. Méthode de diagnostic et d'étude cytologique. Presse Med., 59:1783, 1951.

Castelain, G., and Castelain, C.: Cyto-diagnostic et histodiagnostic des tumeurs. (A propos de 16,000 confrontations cyto-histologiques.) Presse Med., 72:3379–3382, 1964.

Coman, D. R.: Decreased mutual adhesiveness. Property of cells from squamous cell carcinomas. Cancer Res., 4:625, 1944.

Coste, F., and Piquet, B.: Maladie de Bowen. Cytodiagnostic non probant. Bull. Soc. Fr. Dermatol. Syphiligr., 55:22, 1948.

Cottini, J. B.: Aspects hématologiques et histopathologiques de trois cas de mycosis fongoide. Ann. Dermatol. Syphiligr. (Paris), 8:15, 1937.

Chadli, A.: La cellule cancéreuse. Presse Med., 71:2507, 1963.

Degos, R., and Ossipowski, B.: Le dermogramme. Dermatologica, 115:482, 1957.

Degos, R., Ossipowski, B., Civatte, J., and Touraine, R.: Réticuloses cutanées. (Réticuloses histiomonocytaires.) Ann. Dermatol. Syphiligr. (Paris), 84:125, 1957.

Degos, R., Lortat-Jacob, E., Ossipowski, B., Civatte, J., and Ruissant, A.: Erythrodermie leucosique (leucose lymphoïde) précédée de poussées eczématiformes. Opposition entre les aspects histologiques cutanées non spécifiques et les dermogrammes. Bull. Soc. Fr. Dermatol. Syphiligr., 66:40, 1959a.

Degos, R., Delort, J., Civatte, J., Ossipowski, B., and Puissant, A.: Réticulose histiocytaire maligne précédée d'une dermatose psoriasiforme évoluant depuis 28 ans. Signes de malignité cliniques et histologiques (dermogramme) plus précoces que les signes histologiques. Bull. Soc. Fr. Dermatol. Syphiligr., 66:44, 1959b.

Duperrat, B.: Etude anatomo-clinique des naevi melaniques cutanées chez l'adulte. Les tumeurs noires de la peau. Paris, L'Expansion, 1962.

Feldaker, M., Kierland, R., and Montgomery, H.: Cutaneous lymphoblastoma. Report of two unusual cases of reticulum cell sarcoma with emphasis on cutaneous touch smears. Arch. Dermatol. Syph., 70:583, 1954.

Forteza Bover, G.: Atlas de Citologie Sanguinea. Barcelona, Toray, 1963.

Getz, K., Pease, G. L., and Montgomery, H.: Evaluation of cutaneous smears in lymphoblastomas of the skin. Arch. Dermatol. Syph., 74:86, 1956.

Goldman, L., Preston, R. H., and Richfield, D. F.: Extruded basal-cell epithelioma nodules simulating molluscum contagiosum bodies. Arch. Dermatol. Syph., 77:331, 1958.

Goldman, L., McCabe, R. M., and Sawyer, F.: The importance of cytology technic for the dermatologist in office practice. Arch. Dermatol. Syph., 81:359, 1960.

Graham, J. H.: Papanicolaou smears and frozen sections on selected cutaneous neoplasms. J.A.M.A., 178:380, 1961.

Graham, R. M.: The Cytologic Diagnosis of Cancer. Philadelphia, W. B. Saunders Co., 1963.

Haam, E. von: Exfoliative cytology: Its role in the diagnosis of cancer. *In* Recent Advances in the Diagnosis of Cancer. Chicago, Anderson Hospital and Tumor Institute Year Bk. 1966, p. 126.

Haber, H.: Cytodiagnosis in dermatology. Br. J. Dermatol., 66:79, 1954.

Hartmann, P.: Möglichkeiten und Grenzen der Zytodiagnostik. Dtsch. Med. Wochenschr., 80:1839–1841, 1850, 1955.

Hauser, W.: Cytodiagnostik von Tumoren und Retikulosen der Haut. Arch. Klin. Exp. Dermatol., 210:339, 1960.

Hauser, W.: Die Cytodiagnostik in der Dermatologie. In Jadassohn's Handbuch der Haut- und Geschlechtskrankheiten. I., 2:783–829, Berlin, Springer-Verlag, 1964.

Heilmyer, L., and Begemann, H.: Atlas der klinischen Hämatologie und Cytologie. Berlin, Springer-Verlag, 1955.

Hitch, J., Wilson, T. B., and Scoggin, A.: Evaluation of a rapid method of cytologic diagnosis in suspected skin cancer. South. Med. J., 44:407, 1951.

Kalamkaryan, A. A.: Diagnostic importance of dermogram in patients with fungoid mycosis. Vestn. Dermatol., 42:12, 1968.

Knoth, W.: Die allgemeinen Probleme der Cytodiagnostik und ihre Bedeutung für die Dermatologie. Arch. Klin. Exp. Dermatol., 201:106, 1955.

Lagerholm, B.: Clinical cytodiagnosis as an aid to dermatology. Indian J. Dermatol. Venereol., 27:129, 1961.

Lopez Cardoso, P.: Clinical Cytology. Leyden, Stafleu, 1954.

Montgomery, H., and Pease, G.: Cutaneous smears as a diagnostic aid in mycosis fungoides and other lymphoblastomas. Proceedings of the XIth International Congress of Dermatology. Vol. 2. Lund, Hakan Ohlssons Bok, 1959, p. 103.

Moragas, J. M. de., and Woesner, S.: Cytoenzymologic study in the Sézary syndrome. Dermatol. Ibero Lat. Am. (Engl. Edit.), 3:149, 1968.

Niemi, M., and Mustakallio, K. K.: Fine structure of spindle cell in Kaposi's sarcoma. Acta Pathol. Microbiol. Scand., 63:567, 1965.

Orbaneja, J. G., and Castro Torres, A. de: Estudio citológico de la epidermis normal. Act. Dermosifiliogr. (Madr.), 57:125, 1966.

Papamiltiades, M., and Belezos, N.: Vaginal cytology in psoriatic women. Dermatologica, 136:160, 1968.

Peris Asins, J.: Citologia de algunos procesos cutaneos de origen melanomatoso. Tesis presentada para aspirar al grado de Doctor en medicina. Barcelona, Frontis, 1962.

Peris Asins, J.: Citologia de algunos procesos cuta-

neos de origen melanomatoso. Med. Clin. (Barcelona), 14:339, 1966.

Piñol Aguadé, J.: Estudio comparativo cito-histológico en las reticulosis malignas. Conferencia pronunciada en los Cursillos Previos al V Congreso Ibero-Latino-Americano de Dermatologia, Buenos Aires, 1963.

Piñol Aguadé, J.: Nuevos conceptos sobre las reticulosis malignas de la piel. Medicina Cut., 2:355, 1968.

Piñol Aguadé, J.: Citologia del epitelioma basocelular. Acta Ginecol. (Madr.), 20:237, 1969.

Quero, R., and Maso, C.: A rapid method useful in the differential diagnosis of Paget's disease of the nipple. J. Invest. Dermatol., 31:307, 1958.

Renkin, A.: Quelques années de pratique du cytodiagnostic. Arch. Belg. Dermatol., 12:18, 1956.

Rovin, S., and Lexington, K.: An assessment of the negative oral cytologic diagnosis. J. Am. Dent. Assoc., 74:759, 1967.

Sans Sabrafen, J.: Aplicación de algunas técnicas citoquímicas a la clasificación citológica de las leucemias agudas. Tesis presentada para aspirar al grado de Doctor en medicina, Barcelona, 1968.

Scheman, P., Lumerman, H., and Altchuler, L.: Improved oral cytologic sampling by means of deep suction abrasion. Oral Surg., 26:505, 1968.

Schumann, J.: Cytologische Befunde an lokal gefärbter lebender Haut. Arch. Klin. Exp. Dermatol., 232:66, 1968.

Scerrato, R.: Il cancro cutaneo. Gli epiteliomi. Perugia, Natali Simonelli, 1956.

Shklar, G., Meyer, I., Cataldo, E., and Taylor, R.: Correlated study or oral cytology and histopathology. Report on 2052 oral lesions. Oral Surg., 25:61, 1968.

Sidi, E., and Dobkevitch, S.: Maladie de Bowen. Cytodiagnostic immédiat. Bull. Soc. Fr. Dermatol., 57:447, 1947.

Stahl, S. S., Koss, L. G., Brown, R. C., Jr., and Murray, D.: Oral cytologic screening in a large metropolitan area. J. Am. Dent. Assoc., 75:1385, 1967.

Stormby, N. G.: Personal communication.

Stupel, H.: Die Wirkung von Waschmitteln auf die Haut. Heidelberg, Alf. Hüthig Verlag, 1957, p. 101.

Swiller, I. Feldman, F., and Morrison, M.: Mycosis fungoides: Diagnosis by aspiration technique; observations in skin and bone marrow. Arch. Dermatol. Syph., 67:403, 1953.

Temime, P.: Epithélioma spino-cellulaire post-traumatique avec adénite métastatique et suppurée. Intérêt du cytodiagnostic Bull. Soc. Fr. Dermatol. Syphiligr., 58:618, 1951.

Temime, P.: Sur la difficulté du diagnostic d'un épithélioma baso-cellulaire pigmenté du cuir chevelu. Bull. Soc. Fr. Dermatol. Syphiligr., 62:121, 1955.

Temime, P., and Costes, A.: Nouveau cas de mastocytome en tumeur unique confirmé par cyto scarification. Bull. Soc. Fr. Dermatol. Syphiligr., 76:435, 1969.

Temime, P., and Marchand, J. P.: Le cytodiagnostic sur scarification. La cyto scarification dans les hématodermies et affections voisines. Bull. Soc. Fr. Dermatol. Syphiligr., 75:357, 1968.

Thibaut, D., and Deniker, F.: Epithélioma spino-cellulaire de la main. Cytodiagnostic de Tzanck. Exérèse avec suture immédiate. Bull. Soc. Fr. Dermatol. Syphiligr. 56:476, 1949.

Treballs de la Societat Catalana de Biologia. Filial de l'Institut d'Estudis Catalans. Barcelona, 1967.

Tzanck, A.: Le cytodiagnostic immédiat en dermatologie. Bull. Soc. Fr. Dermatol. Syphiligr., 54:68, 1947.

Tzanck, A.: Valeur diagnostique respective des frottis et de la biopsie dans certaines affections cutanées. Presse Med., 10:112, 1948.

Tzanck, A., and Melcki, G. R.: Contribution à l'étude du cyto-diagnostic par le microscope à contraste de phase. Bull. Soc. Fr. Dermatol. Syphiligr., 58:533, 1951.

Tzanck, A., and Melcki, G. R.: Cyto-diagnostic de la maladie de Paget. Bull. Soc. Fr. Dermatol. Syphiligr., 60:226, 1953.

Tzanck, A., Aron, R., and Rozencweig, M.: "Cyto-diagnostic rapide:" Modification de la méthode de Papenheim. Bull. Soc. Fr. Dermatol. Syphiligr., 54:477, 1947.

Tzanck, A., Bourgeois-Gavardin, and Aron-Brunetière, R.: Le cytodiagnostic immèdiat en dermatologie. Ann. Dermatol. Syphiligr. (Paris), 8:205, 1948.

Tzanck, A., Aron-Brunetière, R., and Melcki, G.: Le cyto-diagnostic immédiat des métastases ganglionnaires des néoplasmes cutanés ou muqueux. Bull. Soc. Fr. Dermatol. Syphiligr., 56:503, 1949.

Tzanck, A., Aron-Brunetière, R., and Melcki, G.: Vue d'ensemble du cyto-diagnostic des tumeurs malignes. Presse Med., 58:681, 1950.

Tzanck, A., Melcki, G. R., and Wiel, R.: Découverte par la cyto-ponction ganglionnaire d'un épithélioma du gland associé à un chancre mixte. Bull. Soc. Fr. Dermatol. Syphiligr., 59:214, 1952.

Veronesi, V.: La diagnosi citologica nella malatia di Paget del capezzolo. Tumori, 40:204, 1954.

Viglioglia, P. A., and Viglioglia, J.: El citodiagnostico inmediato en Dermatologia. Prensa Med. Argent., 42:3422, 1955.

Vilanova, X., and Piñol Aguadè J.: Etude cyto-logique de l'epithelioma basocellulaire. Communication to the Xth Congress of Dermatol. and Syphiligr. Langue Francaise, Argel, 1959.

Vilanova, X., and Piñol Aguade, J.: Els acids ribonucleic i desoxiribonucleic en la discitologia del melanoma maligne. Treballs de la Soc. Catalana Biol. XXI, Barcelona, 1967.

Vilanova, X., Piñol Aguadé, J., Castells, A., and Moragas, J. M. de: Juvenile melanoma. A tumor of vascular origin? Dermatologica, 125:189, 1962a.

Vilanova, X., Piñol Aguadé, J., and Rueda, L. A.: The cytologic aspects of basal cell carcinoma. J. Invest. Dermatol., 39:123, 1962b.

Vilanova, X., Piñol Aguadé, J., and Rueda, L. A.: Cytopathologie du systeme endothélial vasculaire dans quelques lésions cutanées. Ann. Dermatol. Syphiligr. (Paris), 90:457, 1963a.

Vilanova, X., Piñol Aguadé, J., and Rueda, L. A.: Algunos aspectos poco conocidos de la citomorfologia cutánea. Vth Congreso Ibero Latino Americano de Dermatologia, Buenos Aires, 1963b.

Walker, J. C., and Sandison, A. T.: The cytological examination of nipple discharges as a diagnostic aid. Scott. Med. J., 3:297, 1958.

Wilson, G. T.: Cutaneous smears: A diagnostic aid in certain malignant lesions of the skin. J. Invest. Dermatol., 22:173, 1954.

Winer, L. H.: Mycosis fungoides. Benign and malignant reticulum cell dysplasia. Arch. Dermatol. Syph., 56:480, 1947.

Wolf, J.: Die innere Struktur der Zellen des Stratum desquamans der menschlichen Epidermis. Z. Mikr.-Anat. Forsch., 46:170, 1939.

Woodburne, A. R., Philpott, O. S., and Philpott, J. A.: Cytologic studies in skin cancer. Arch. Dermatol. Syph., 82:992, 1960.

Zimmer, S. Zytologische Diagnostik. Medico Boehringer. 5, 1961.

Zoon, J. J., and Mali, J. W. H.: Remarks on cell-diagnostics in normal and some pathological conditions of the skin. Dermatologica, 101:145, 1950.

11

Cutaneous Malignancy-Associated Changes in Cancer of the Skin and Other Sites

Herbert E. Nieburgs, M.D.

Dermatologic manifestations of occult malignant neoplasms have been reported by numerous investigators. Generalized pruritus of unknown etiology may be associated with Hodgkin's disease, lymphatic leukemia, and mycosis fungoides, whereas localized pruritus of the extremities and trunk may occur with internal carcinomas (Cormia, 1965). Dermatomyositis in adults over the age of 40 is associated with carcinoma in 50 percent of the cases (Arundell et al., 1960). The most commonly encountered carcinomas are those of the breast and lung. Dermatomyositis may appear simultaneously with the neoplasms but has been found two or three years before and after clinical evidence of cancer (Christianson et al., 1956). Successful treatment of the neoplasm may lead to remission of dermatomyositis, whereas relapse may indicate recurrence of the tumor. Dermatitis herpetiformis is often associated with choriocarcinoma and malignant tumors of the prostate, bladder, rectum, uterus, ovary, and breast (Davis, 1922; Elliott, 1938; Tobias, 1951). Pemphigoid eruptions of the skin and mucous membranes of unknown etiology were found in association with carcinoma of the lung and stomach and with melanoma (Marks, 1961). Urticaria and more often its variant, erythema gyratum repens, may accompany carcinoma of the lung, breast, and cervix (Gammel, 1952; Leavell et al., 1967). Palmar and plantar hyperkeratosis were found in association with carcinoma of the esophagus (Howel-Evans et al., 1958; McConnell, 1966; Shine and Allison, 1966). Lymphomas, leukemias, and mycosis fungoides are often reflected by exfoliative dermatitis. However, internal tumors, such as adenocarcinomas of the stomach, liver, and prostate, have also been found in association with exfoliative dermatitis (Graham and Helwig, 1959).

Acanthosis nigricans in the adult over the age of 40 is invariably associated with visceral malignant neoplasms (Curth,

281

1952; Curth et al., 1962). Acanthosis nigricans affects mainly body folds in the neck, axillae, antecubital spaces, and groin. The associated malignant tumor is usually an adenocarcinoma, which is highly malignant and occurs in 90 percent of the cases intra-abdominally and most commonly in the stomach (Curth, 1952 and 1955). Of the extra-abdominal carcinomas, the majority arise in the lung and breast (Ellenbogen, 1949; Spear, 1950; Marmelzat, 1955). Appearance of the dermatosis simultaneously with the tumor was observed in 60 percent of cases, and it preceded the clinical evidence of cancer by 5 to 18 years in 8 percent of the cases (Curth, 1955). Successful removal of the tumor may produce regression of the skin changes; their reappearance may reflect recurrence of the tumor. Persistence of acanthosis nigricans after tumor resection is usually associated with metastases. A high incidence of predominantly gastric carcinomas was reported in family members of patients with benign and malignant acanthosis nigricans (Curth and Aschner, 1959).

Conversely, a family history of cancer was found in 48 percent of patients with Bowen's disease of the skin (Graham and Helwig, 1961). Bowen's disease is associated with the eventual development of internal carcinomas, most frequently in the respiratory system, gastrointestinal system, and genitourinary tract (Graham and Helwig, 1959). The presence of Bowen's disease for an average period of 8½ years prior to clinical evidence of cancer may well constitute a cutaneous manifestation of systemic carcinogenic factors.

Identification of the cutaneous manifestations which either accompany or precede the clinical evidence of malignant tumors is based upon classic histopathologic criteria for the diagnosis of clinically evident skin lesions. However, systemic carcinogenic effects may also be identified in cells of the normal-appearing skin, which by traditional microscopic examination may not reveal significant histologic alterations. These systemic changes occur primarily in the cell nuclei, and may also be found in blood leukocytes (Nieburgs et al., 1965; Nieburgs and Goldberg, 1968) and in cells of the bone marrow Nieburgs and Goldberg, 1963; Nieburgs et al., 1967), buccal mucosa (Nieburgs et al., 1962; Finch, 1971; Finch and von Haam, 1971), lung (Nieburgs, 1967 and 1968), stomach (Nieburgs and Glass, 1963), liver (Elias et al., 1962; Nieburgs et al., 1965; Baccaglini and Preto, 1966), and various other sites.

Microscopic examination of these malignancy-associated changes (MAC) in skin tissue sections is made first by use of low power objectives and then by the highest magnification of the light microscope (×100 oil impression objective) for evaluation of the minute nuclear structures.

CLASSIFICATION OF NUCLEAR STRUCTURES

Nuclear MAC may be accurately identified solely by use of an oil immersion objective. To distinguish this alteration from other cellular changes, knowledge of all nuclear structures which may be evident at the highest magnification of the light microscope is a prerequisite.

Cells from benign tissue alterations as well as those from malignant neoplasms contain nuclei which are classified according to three major structural changes and are designated A, B, and C. In addition, combined structures AB, BC, and AC are often present (Nieburgs, 1970a, 1970b, and 1971; Nieburgs et al., 1970).

A: This nuclear structure consists of numerous pale, round, or slightly oval-shaped areas of almost uniform size surrounded by curved chromatin bands (Figs. 11–4,*B*, 11–7,*B*, 11–8,*B*, and 11–9,*B*).

B: Nuclear structure B is recognized by the presence of a prominent nucleolus. The remaining nuclear chromatin may either not be evident or have structure A or C (Figs. 11–5,*B*, 11–10,*B*, 11–11,*B*, and 11–12,*B*).

C: This structure consists of prominent chromocenters, which vary in size and have chromatin band attachments of varying number and length. The spaces between chromatin bands are of diverse shape and size (Figs. 11–6,*B*, 11–13,*B*, 11–14,*B*, and 11–15,*B*).

Each of these structures may be benign

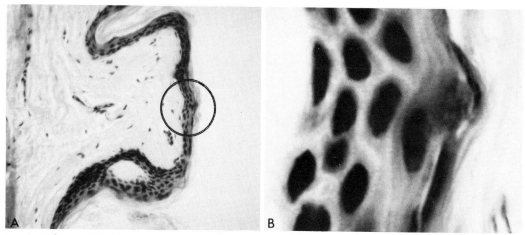

Figure 11-1 *A*, Skin biopsy from 74 year old female patient with diabetes. (×125). *B*, High magnification of epidermis in *A*. (×1250). Note the horizontal polarity of cells with oval-shaped nuclei. The chromatin has a homogeneous appearance.

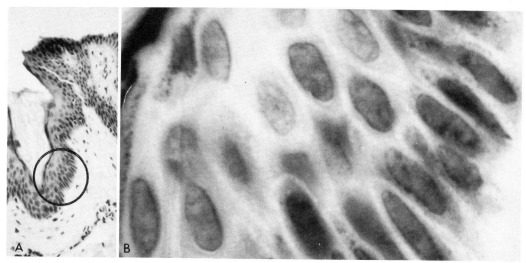

Figure 11-2 *A*, Skin biopsy from 22 year old female patient with phlebosclerosis of right leg. (×125). *B*, High magnification of epidermis in *A*. (×1250). Note the vertical polarity of the columnar and oval-shaped cells which have pale nuclei and a homogeneous appearance of the chromatin.

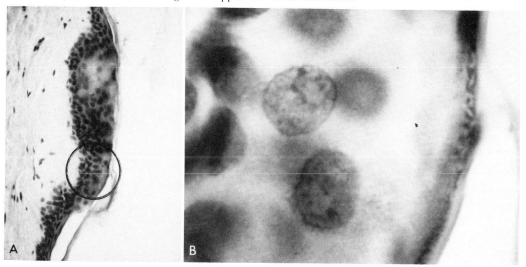

Figure 11-3 *A*, Skin biopsy from 74 year old female patient with diabetes. (×125). *B*, High magnification of epidermis in *A*. (×1250). Note the lack of uniform polarity of cells with round nuclei and pale chromatin.

or malignant, depending upon degree of chromatism, amount of chromatin, nucleolar/nuclear ratio, and nuclear/cytoplasmic ratio. Cells with MAC have increased chromatism and an increased amount of chromatin in a slightly enlarged nucleus. The interpretation of nuclear MAC is made solely when they are present in a well-differentiated cell with a low nuclear/cytoplasmic ratio; this interpretation must be distinguished from that of malignant tumor cells, which may have the same nuclear changes but with a high nuclear/cytoplasmic ratio.

NORMAL SKIN OF PATIENTS WITHOUT EVIDENCE OF CANCER

The cells of the epidermis may be arranged in a uniform manner with their long axes horizontal to the skin surface (Fig. 11–1) or perpendicular to the dermis (Fig. 11–2). In both cases, the cell nuclei are columnar or oval-shaped. Often, however, the nuclei of the cells are round and fail to display the uniform polarity of cells with columnar or oval-shaped nuclei (Figs. 11–3 and 11–6).

In tissue sections of the skin from patients without evidence of cancer, the nuclear chromatin of the cells may have either a homogeneous appearance (Figs. 11–1 to 11–3) or prominent structures A, B, or C (Figs. 11–4 to 11–6). Evidence of nuclear structures is usually found in round or oval-shaped cells which lack uniform polarity.

The normal epidermis rarely consists of cells with nuclear structure A (Fig. 11–4). The most commonly encountered cells are those with nuclear structure B (Fig. 11–5) and, less frequently, with nuclear structure C (Fig. 11–6).

CANCER CELLS AND NUCLEAR, MALIGNANCY-ASSOCIATED CHANGES

Abnormally altered nuclear structures A, B, and C may be encountered in cells of cutaneous malignant tumors and in the skin adjacent to the tumor, as well as in cutaneous manifestations of a variety of internal malignant tumors. These structures, however, differ from those in the skin of patients without evidence of tumor by their hyperchromasia of the nuclear chromatin and by their well-delineated spaces between chromatin bands.

Squamous cell carcinomas of the skin may have cells with either malignant neoplastic nuclear structure A (Fig. 11–7) or C (Fig. 11–13) and often with malignant structure B. In melanomas of the skin, the cells usually have nuclear structure B or combined forms AB and less frequently BC (Fig. 11–10).

Cutaneous MAC Adjacent to Skin Tumors

The skin adjacent to cutaneous malignant tumors but uninvolved by the tumor may have cells with either the same nuclear structure as those of the tumor (Figs. 11–8, 11–11, and 11–14) or other malignant neoplastic-like A, B, or C structures. The normally differentiating cells of the epidermis adjacent to cutaneous malignant tumors differ from the undifferentiated cancer cells by their low nuclear/cytoplasmic ratio. These cells with nuclear MAC, however, resemble those of the tumor by their often identical degree of nuclear hyperchromasia. In cases in which the skin adjacent to malignant tumors consists of cells with structure B, the nucleoli may have either the same or, more often, slightly smaller diameters than those of tumor cells. In the epidermis, the cells with MAC are occasionally of the same size as the cells in the adjacent tumor area, whereas the nuclei are usually smaller than those in the malignant tumor cells.

The cells with MAC in the epidermis adjacent to cutaneous malignant tumors differ by their increased nuclear hyperchromasia from cells with corresponding nuclear structures in the skin of patients without evidence of tumors. Although a slightly increased nuclear/cytoplasmic ratio may be evident in cells with MAC, no consistently significant differences of nuclear and cellular size exist between cutaneous cells adjacent to malignant tumors and those in the skin of patients without tumor.

Text continued on page 289

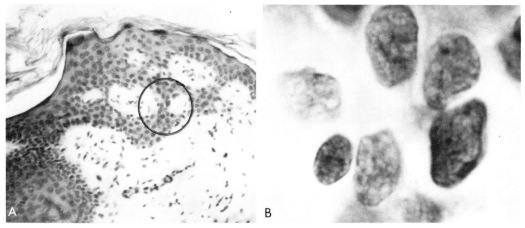

Figure 11–4 *A*, Skin biopsy from 54 year old male patient with aortic aneurysm. (×125). *B*, High magnification of area in *A*. (×1250). Chromatin structure A, with numerous round, pale areas of uniform size, is present in most of the cells but is most clearly evident in the small nucleus in the center of the photomicrograph.

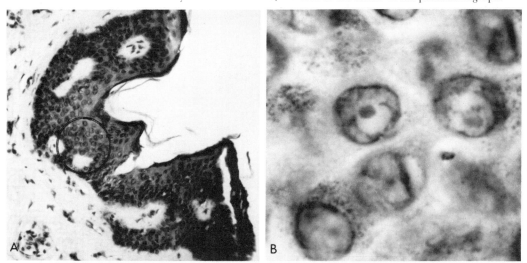

Figure 11–5 *A*, Skin biopsy from 50 year old male patient with chronic cholecystitis. (×125). *B*, High magnification of epidermis in *A*. (×1250). The cells have prominent nucleoli, and the nuclear chromatin is either absent or delicate and pale.

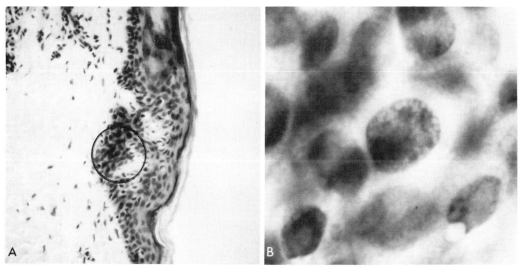

Figure 11–6 *A*, Skin biopsy from 33 year old patient with phlebosclerosis of left leg. (×125). *B*, High magnification of epidermis in *A*. (×1250). The nucleus in the center of the photomicrograph has a chromatin structure which consists of pale chromocenters and chromatin bands.

285

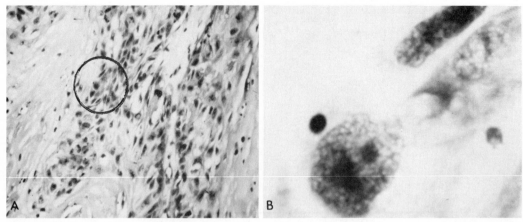

Figure 11–7 *A,* Skin biopsy of forehead with squamous cell carcinoma. (×125). *B,* High magnification of malignant tumor cells in *A.* (×1250). The nuclei have the malignant neoplastic structure A, which consists of numerous prominent, round, pale areas of uniform size. The chromatin bands which surround the pale areas are more deeply stained than in the benign structure A of Figure 11–4,*B.*

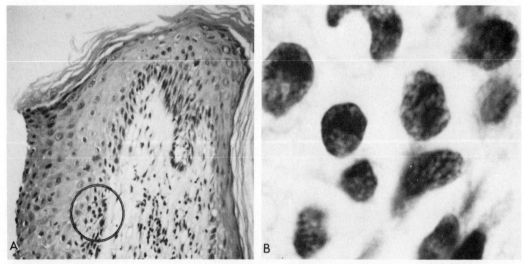

Figure 11–8 *A,* Skin adjacent to squamous cell carcinoma in Figure 11–7,*A,* but uninvolved by tumor. (×125). *B,* High magnification of area in *A.* (×1250). Nuclear structure A consists of hyperchromatic chromatin bands and pale, round areas.

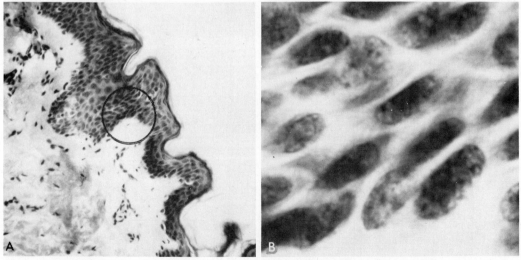

Figure 11–9 *A,* Skin biopsy from 38 year old male patient with adenocarcinoma of the head of the pancreas and with liver metastasis. (×125). *B,* High magnification of cells in the epidermis of *A.* (×1250). The cell nuclei have malignant structure A.

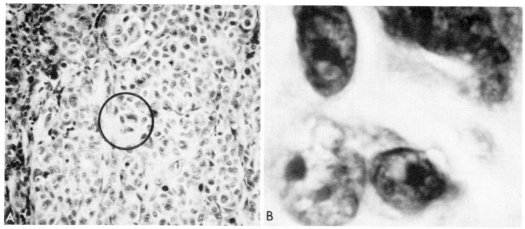

Figure 11-10 *A*, Skin biopsy with melanoma. (×125). *B*, High magnification of tumor cells in *A*. (×1250). The cells have nuclei with hyperchromatic chromocenters and chromatin bands and with prominently enlarged nucleoli and increased nuclear/cytoplasmic ratios.

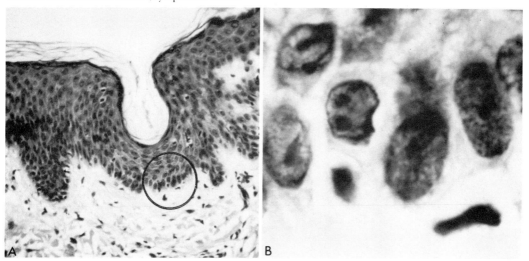

Figure 11-11 *A*, Benign-appearing skin section adjacent to melanoma in Figure 11-10,*A*. (×125). *B*, High magnification of epidermis in *A*. (×1250). The cells have malignant neoplastic-like nuclear structures B, AB, and BC.

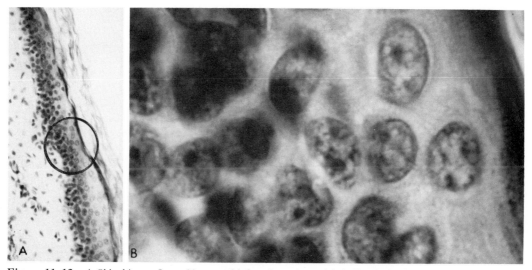

Figure 11-12 *A*, Skin biopsy from 60 year old female patient with infiltrating adenocarcinoma of sigmoid colon. (×125). *B*, High magnification of epidermis in *A*. (×1250). The cells have malignant neoplastic-like nuclear structures BC and AB.

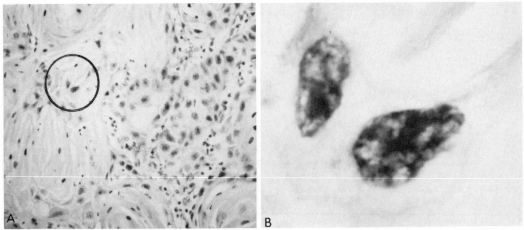

Figure 11-13 *A,* Squamous cell carcinoma of the skin. (×125). *B,* High magnification of tumor cells in *A.* (×1250). The nuclei have hyperchromatic malignant neoplastic structure C, which consists of chromocenters of varying size and chromatin bands. Compare with benign structure C in Figure 11–6*B.*

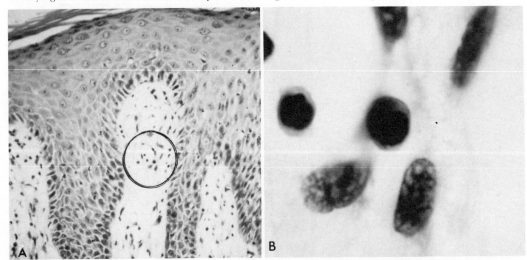

Figure 11-14 *A,* Uninvolved skin adjacent to squamous cell carcinoma in Figure 11–13, *A.* (×125). *B,* High magnification of area in *A. (×1250).* Note two fibroblasts with malignant neoplastic-like nuclear structure C in the dermis.

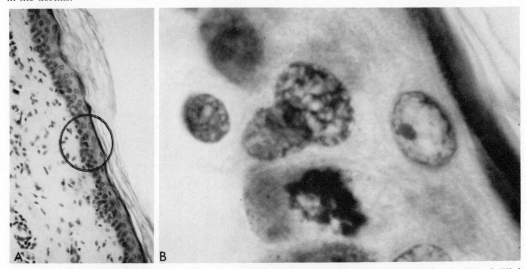

Figure 11-15 *A,* Skin biopsy from 60 year old female patient with adenocarcinoma of colon. (×125). *B,* High magnification of epidermis in *A.* (×1250). The cell in the center has malignant neoplastic-like nuclear structure C.

288

Cutaneous Cellular MAC as a Manifestation of Internal Malignant Tumors

At the usual low microscopic magnifications, the tissue sections of skin from patients with a variety of internal malignant tumors fail to reveal any feature which may differ from the skin of patients without evidence of tumor (Figs. 11–9,*A*, 11–12,*A*, and 11–15*A*). The epidermis is markedly thinner than in areas adjacent to malignant tumors (Figs. 11–8,*A*, 11–11,*A*,

and 11–14,*A*) and often slightly thinner than in the normal skin (Figs. 11–4,*A*, 11–5,*A*, and 11–6,*A*). The prominence of collagen bundles in the dermis and the amount of inflammatory cell infiltration may occasionally differ from those of the normal skin, but these features are subtle and not consistently evident.

Utilization of the highest magnification of the light microscope for examination of cells in the epidermis from patients with internal malignant neoplasms often permits identification of abnormally altered

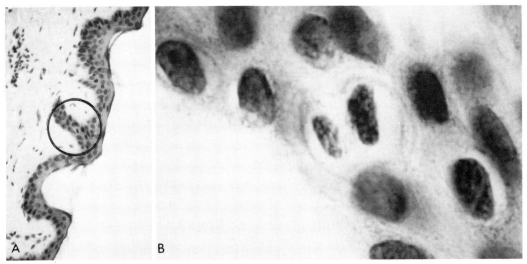

Figure 11–16   *A*, Skin biopsy from 20 year old male patient with clinical diagnosis of retroperitoneal lymphoma and histologic finding of metastatic carcinoma in excised lymph nodes. (×125). *B*, High magnification of epidermis in *A*. (×1250). The mitotic figure in the early telophase has malignant neoplastic-like structure A in both nuclei.

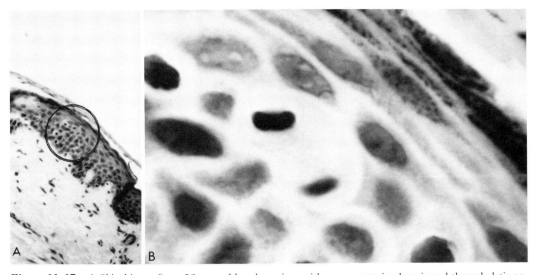

Figure 11–17   *A*, Skin biopsy from 56 year old male patient with severe arteriosclerosis and thrombolytic occlusion in left leg. (×125). *B*, High magnification of epidermis in *A*. (×1250). The nuclei of the dividing cell in the early telophase have homogeneous appearance of the chromatin.

nuclear structures (Figs. 11–9,*B*, 11–12,*B*, and 11–15,*B*). These differ markedly from the corresponding benign nuclear structures in patients without tumor (Figs. 11–4,*B*, 11–5,*B*, and 11–6,*B*).

In tissue sections of the skin that are associated with internal malignant tumors, the prominence of nuclear structures and the degree of hyperchromasia (Figs. 11–9,*B*, 11–12,*B*, and 11–15,*B*) are often either identical to or occasionally more clearly evident (Figs. 11–15,*B*) than those

in skin adjacent to cutaneous malignant tumors (Figs. 11–8,*B*, 11–11,*B*, and 11–14,*B*).

In comparison with normal skin, the nuclear structures in cells of the epidermis associated with internal tumor are more prominent and hyperchromatic than those in cells with corresponding benign structures. The slightly increased nuclear/cytoplasmic ratio of cells with MAC may not consistently differ from that of cells of the normal skin.

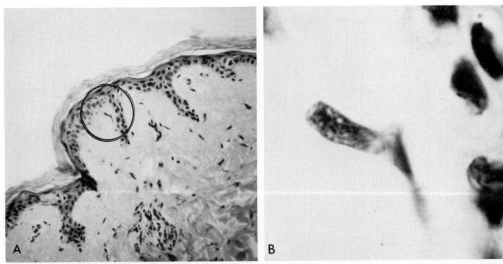

Figure 11–18   *A*, Skin biopsy from 44 year old male patient with metastatic carcinoma of the abdominal wall. (×125). *B*, High magnification of dermis and epidermis in *A*. (×1250). The fibroblast in the center has malignant neoplastic-like nuclear structure A.

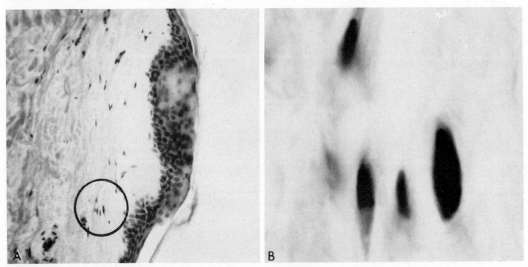

Figure 11–19   *A*, Skin biopsy from 74 year old female patient with diabetes and with severe arteriosclerosis and calcification with gangrenous ulceration of the toes of left leg. (×125). *B*, High magnification of dermis in *A*. (×1250). Note the fibroblasts with homogeneous pyknotic appearance of the nuclei.

Nuclear structure A, with its malignant neoplastic alteration, is most commonly associated with internal malignant tumors and occurs rarely in the benign form in normal skin sections. Nuclear structure B in the skin of patients with internal malignant tumors is often found together with either A or C, whereas in the normal skin, this nuclear structure is usually not encountered in association with other structures within the same nucleus.

Mitotic figures in the epidermis of patients without tumor and in those with malignant neoplasms are usually encountered in the late anaphase. When associated with internal malignant neoplasms, the nuclei of the dividing cells often have a hyperchromatic nuclear structure A (Fig. 11–16), which differs from the homogeneous nuclei in the mitotic figures of the normal epidermis (Fig. 11–17). Similarly, the fibroblasts with hyperchromatic nuclear structure C (Figs. 14*A,B*) or with structure A (Figs. 18*A,B*) in the dermis of patients with malignant tumors differ from fibroblasts with homogeneous nuclear chromatin in cases without evidence of tumor (Fig. 11–19).

Morphogenesis and Mitotic Aspects of Malignancy-Associated Changes

The nuclear alterations of cells in various mitotic phases are comparable to those that were designated as A, B, and C (Nieburgs, 1968a, 1968b, and 1969–70). Nuclear structure A is present in the late anaphase and telophase and towards the end of the S phase, whereas structure B occurs in the early interphase. Nuclear structure C is present in cells during the early prophase. Therefore, in MAC the presence of malignant nuclear structures A and C or their transitional forms may be interpreted as a mitotic arrest in differentiating cells, such as blood leukocytes, ciliated bronchial cells, superficial buccal mucosal cells, and cells of the epidermis, which have otherwise retained their ability to differentiate normally. Conversely, the presence of identical nuclear structures in tumor cells does not permit their interpretation as a mitotic arrest because they may occur in cells that are com-

mited to undergo mitosis. The occurrence of identical nuclear structures in cells distant from malignant tumors and in those of the tumor site points to some role of MAC in the biology of cancer.

Systemic MAC in cells of the host may either occur simultaneously with or precede the tumor growth as a result of carcinogenic effects. In cells of the host, the nuclear structure of the MAC in the telophase or prophase seems to represent an impairment of the nucleus to undergo the changes which are normally observed in differentiating cells. The malignancy-associated arrested mitotic phase in cells of the skin may reflect the systemic disease of cancer. The local manifestation of tumor growth may depend upon the tissue predilection of carcinogenic insults which lead to decreased cell differentiation with alterations in cell replication.

REFERENCES

Arundell, F. D., Wilkinson, R. D., and Haserick, J. R.: Dermatomyositis and malignant neoplasms in adults. Arch. Dermatol., 82,:722, 1960.

Baccaglini, G., and Preto, G.: Hepatic pathology in the course of distant malignancies. Arch. Pathol., 82:113, 1966.

Bluefarb, S. M.: Some nonspecific cutaneous lesions associated with internal cancer. Geriatrics, 11:387, 1956.

Caldwell, I. W.: A dermatomyositic symptom-complex associated with malignant disease. Br. J. Cancer, 9:575, 1955.

Christianson, H. B., Brunsting, L. A., and Perry, H. O.: Dermatomyositis. Unusual features, complications, and treatment. Arch. Dermatol., 74:581, 1950.

Christianson, H. B., Brunsting, L. A., and Perry, H. O.: Dermatomyositis. Arch. Dermatol., 74:581, 1956.

Cormia, F. E.: Pruritus, an uncommon but important symptom of systemic carcinoma. Arch. Dermatol., 92:36, 1965.

Curth, H. O.: Pseudo-acanthosis nigricans. Ann. Dermatol. Syphiligr. (Paris), 78:417, 1951.

Curth, H. O.: Significance of acanthosis nigricans. Arch. Dermatol. Syph., 66:80, 1952.

Curth, H. O.: Dermatosis and malignant internal tumors. Arch. Dermatol., 71:95, 1955.

Curth, H. O., and Aschner, B. M.: Genetic studies on acanthosis nigricans. Arch. Dermatol., 79:55, 1959.

Curth, H. O., Hilberg, A. W., and Machacek, G. F.: The site and histology of the cancer associated with malignant acanthosis nigricans. Cancer, 15:364, 1962.

Curtis, A. C., Blaylock, H. C., and Harrell, E. R., Jr.: Malignant lesions associated with dermatomyositis. J.A.M.A., 150:844, 1952.

Davis, H.: On two cases of exudative erythema associated with malignant disease of the uterus. Br. J. Dermatol., 34:12, 1922.

Dobson, R. L., Young, M. R., and Pinto, J. S.: Palmar keratoses and cancer. Arch. Dermatol., 92:553, 1965.

Elias, H., Sherrick, J. D., and Bouldin, R. F.: Reaction of normal liver parenchyma to metastatic carcinoma. Acta Hepatosplenol. (Stuttg.), 9:357, 1962.

Ellenbogen, B. K.: Acanthosis nigricans associated with bronchial carcinoma. Report of 2 cases. Br. J. Dermatol., 61:251, 1949.

Elliott, J. A.: Bullous dermatoses of toxic origin: report of a case involving an association with choriocarcinoma. Arch. Dermatol., 37:219, 1938.

Finch, R. R.: A classification of nuclear aberration in relation to malignancy associated changes (MAC). Acta Cytol. (Baltimore), 15:553, 1971.

Finch, R. R., and von Haam, E.: Malignancy associated changes in buccal smears. Acta Cytol. (Baltimore), 15:46, 1971.

Gammel, J. A.: Erythema gyratum repens. Arch. Dermatol., 66:494, 1952.

Graham, J. H., and Helwig, E. B.: Bowen's disease and its relationship to systemic cancer. Arch. Dermatol., 80:133, 1959.

Graham, J. H., and Helwig, E. B.: Bowen's disease and its relationship to systemic cancer. Arch. Dermatol., 83:738, 1961.

Hill, E. M.: Cutaneous manifestations of internal malignancy. Minn. Med., 43:838, 1960.

Howel-Evans, W., McConnell, R. B., Clarke, C. A., and Sheppard, P. M.: Carcinoma of the esophagus with keratous palmaris et plantaris (tylosis). Quart. J. Med., 27:413, 1958.

Leavell, U. W., Winternitz, W. W., and Black, J. H.: Erythema gyratum repens and undifferentiated carcinoma. Arch. Dermatol., 95:69, 1967.

Marks, J. M.: Pemphigoid with malignant melanoma. Proc. Roy. Soc. Med., 54:225, 1961.

Marmelzat, W. L.: Pachydermoperiostosis associated with acanthosis nigricans–like syndrome. Arch. Dermatol., 72:90, 1955.

McConnell, R. B.: The Genetics of Gastrointestinal Disorders. London, Oxford University Press, 1966, p. 40.

Morin, M., Graveleau, J., and Aillet, J.: Dermatomyositis and other paraneoplastic muscular syndromes. Bull. Soc. Med. Hôp. Paris, 76:115, 1960.

Nakanishi, A., Maeda, S., and Kawamura, J.: A case of Bowen's disease with cancer of the stomach. Clin. Dermatol. (Tokyo), 6:843, 1964.

Nieburgs, H. E.: Diagnostic Cell Pathology in Tissue and Smears. New York, Grune & Stratton, 1967.

Nieburgs, H. E.: Systemic cellular manifestations of malignant tumors. Proc. 1st Int. Symp. Detection of Cancer, 1:552, 1968a.

Nieburgs, H. E.: Recent progress in the interpretation of malignancy associated changes (MAC). Acta Cytol. (Baltimore), 12:455, 1968b.

Nieburgs, H. E.: Biologic aspects of systemic malig-nancy associated changes (MAC) in malignant neoplasias. Estr. Boll. ed Atti Acad. Med. Roma, 93:187, 1969–70.

Nieburgs, H. E.: Tissue and cell pathology in the classification of uterine cervix dysplasias and carcinoma in situ. Minerva Ginecol., 22:1135, 1970a.

Nieburgs, H. E.: Systemic aspects and manifestations of malignant neoplasias (MAC) and methods of early detection. Gassetta Sanitaria, XLI:289, 1970b.

Nieburgs, H. E.: Tissue and cell pathology of uterine cervix dysplasias and carcinoma in situ. Acta Cytol. (Baltimore), 15:513, 1971.

Nieburgs, H. E., and Glass, G. B.: Gastric-cell maturation disorders in atrophic gastritis, pernicious anemia, and carcinoma. Am. J. Dig. Dis., 8:135, 1963.

Nieburgs, H. E., and Goldberg, A. F.: Bone marrow karyo-morphology in benign conditions multiple myeloma and with distant carcinomas. 11th Ann. Meeting of the Am. Soc. Cytol., Columbus, Ohio, 1963.

Nieburgs, H. E., and Goldberg, A. F.: Changes in polymorphonuclear leukocytes as a manifestation of malignant neoplasia. Cancer, 22:35, 1968.

Nieburgs, H. E., Goldberg, A. F., Bertini, B., Silagi, J., Pacheco, B., and Reisman, H.: Cellular changes (MAC) in blood and bone marrow of patients with malignant tumors. Read before the 2nd Int. Congr. of Exfoliative Cytol., Paris, May 23, 1965.

Nieburgs, H. E., Goldberg, A. F., Bertini, B., Silagi, J., Pacheco, B., and Reisman, H.: Malignancy associated changes (MAC) in blood and bone marrow cells of patients with malignant tumors. Acta Cytol. (Baltimore), 11:415, 1967.

Nieburgs, H. E., Herman, B. E., and Reisman, H.: Buccal cell changes in patients with malignant tumors. Lab. Invest., 11:80, 1962.

Nieburgs, H. E., Levis, F., and Cappa, A. P. M.: The histopathologic basis of cell pathology for diagnostic cytology. Minerva Med., 61:4926, 1970.

Nieburgs, H. E., Parets, A. D., Perez, V., and Boudreau, C.: Cellular changes in liver tissue adjacent and distant to malignant tumors. Arch. Pathol., 80:262, 1965.

Shine, I., and Allison, P. R.: Carcinoma of the esophagus with tylosis (keratosis palmaris et plantaris). Lancet, I:950, 1966.

Spear, P. W.: Acanthosis nigricans associated with cancer of the lung. Report of a case. J. Thorac. Surg., 20:304, 1950.

Szendai, B.: Kraurosis vulvae and gastric cancer. Magy. Onkol., 8:53, 1964a.

Szendai, B.: Kraurosis vulvae and carcinoma of the stomach. Zentralbl. Gynaekol., 86:687, 1964b.

Tobias, N.: Dermatitis herpetiformis associated with visceral malignancy. Urol. Cutan. Rev., 55:352, 1951.

Williams, J. R. C.: Dermatomyositis and malignancy: review of literature. Ann. Intern. Med., 50:1174, 1959.

12

Electrometric Studies in Skin Cancer

N. Melczer, M.D.

On the basis of its electrical characteristics, the skin can be regarded as a system of insulators and semiconductors in which, at the interface of the barrier layers and extracellular fluid, *phase-boundary potentials* are produced. They arise either from the different mobilities and adsorptions of positive and negative ions on the surface of the electronegative and cation-permeable barriers (Beutner, 1920 and 1944) or from the differing penetration ability of these ions to permeate the barriers (Michaelis, 1925).

The *active* electrical phenomena of the skin, such as its own potential, and the *passive* phenomena of the skin, such as its polarizability, remain unaltered and characteristic only as long as the barrier layers are intact.

In malignant melanomas and in primary cancers of the skin, as well as after trauma, the electronegativity of the barrier layers decreases, and the measurement of the skin potential gives a voltage 30 to 35 percent lower than that of the normal neighboring skin.

In spite of this decrease, the measurement of skin potentials has not been used up to now for recognition of malignancy.

The changes are considerably greater and more significant during the polarization of the skin, when a weak direct current is conducted into it by means of nonpolarizable electrodes, and the *apparent resistance* caused by a countercurrent is measured.

More than a decade ago Melczer and Kiss (1957a, 1957b, and 1958) called attention to the fact that malignant melanomas and primary cancers of the skin cause, at the beginning of the malignant transformation, a partially irreversible hysteresis of the barrier. This results in a *diminution of the charging* and thus of the *polarizability* of the barrier. Moreover, the barrier membranes can become completely *nonpolarizable*. This is accompanied by an increased *ion permeability* of the barriers after malignant transformation of the skin.

During the last 15 years a large number of patients with malignant melanomas and primary cancers of the skin were investigated. In the case of the highly malignant melanomas and squamous cell carcinomas, it was almost always possible to establish, by means of a simple potentiometer method, the characteristic *hypopolarizability* or *nonpolarizability* (Melczer, 1958, 1960, 1961, and 1965) of these malignant

293

growths. Basal cell carcinomas, which are of lesser practical importance because of their relative benignity—especially in the case of the nodular or cystic type or in proliferations originating from the sebaceous glands when the barrier is probably damaged to a lesser extent—can be counted with false-negative results in 15 to 20 percent of the cases.

Hence, on the basis of the polarizability, an essential difference can be shown between the benign and malignant epithelial growths of the skin.

DATA ON THE PASSIVE PHENOMENA OF THE SKIN

Changes in the Conductivity of the Skin Influencing the Effect of Current

Weak direct current conducted into the skin by means of nonpolarizable electrodes comes up against considerable resistance. This so-called *apparent resistance* to the course of the flow of direct current into the skin is derived from two sources:

1. The major part originates from the capacitive charging of the double ionic layer situated on the surface of the cells composing the barrier membranes of the skin; this charging induces, however, a *polarization counterelectromotive force*, weakening the entering current.

2. The smaller part of the apparent resistance is caused by a *change in the electrolyte concentration* of the tissue fluid owing to the effect of the direct current passing through the skin. The negatively charged barrier membrane is cation-permeable and does not allow the permeation of anions. The flux and adsorption of cations caused by the direct current lead to an *alteration of the ion concentration* which, in turn, induces a *diffusion potential.* This diffusion potential builds up a countercurrent which adds to the polarization current induced by the double ionic layer.

Accordingly, in the course of passing a direct current when both the ion migration and adsorption are going in the same direction, the diffusion potential plays an essential part in the formation of the polar-

ization countercurrent.

Low-frequency alternating current (50 to 5000 Hz.) gives rise in the skin, just like direct current does, to an apparent resistance, the so-called *impedance,* because it induces a polarization countercurrent. However, in the formation of polarization counterelectromotive force by alternating current, it is only the capacitive charging of the double ionic layer that plays a part. For with alternating current, when the change in the direction of current occurs within fractions of a second, the relatively slow ion migration cannot cause an alteration in ion concentration, and therefore, diffusion potential and polarization countercurrent cannot be produced.

Voltage Changes in the Skin Upon Closing and Opening of a Weak Direct Current

Using either a string galvanometer or a cathode-ray oscillograph, a photographic record of the strength of the direct current conducted into the skin can be made, which reveals that the polarization countercurrent developing at closing of the current can increase, forming a spike up to 10 to 100 times the value of the original voltage (Garten, 1909). (See also Fig. 12–6.) The *ascending part* of the spike is caused by the rapid capacitive charging of the double ionic layers and hardly lasts longer than 1/10,000 msec.

At discharge its steep *descending part* continues within 14 to 22 msec. in a flatly protracted curve. The latter is the *marginal* or *residual current,* lasting 0.5 to 1.0 msec. and observable also by means of a slow galvanometer; the marginal current is generated by diffusion capacity. At cut-off of the polarization-inducing current, the condenser-like capacitance of the double ionic layers rapidly discharges; the diffusion capacitances originating from ion permeation do it more slowly. The rapid discharge of the double ionic layer indicates that it functions as an imperfect condenser. The two plates of condenser are composed of the inner and outer ionic layers, while the dielectric medium of the condenser is the extracellular fluid between them.

The Polarization Countercurrent

Polarization is possible only if the introduced direct current elicits changes in the ion concentration. If two electrolyte solutions are separated by a diaphragm, which impedes or retards the diffusion velocity and the permeation of certain ions while being permeable to others, the current flow elicits changes in the ion concentration on both sides of the diaphragm. Not only an accumulation of ions takes place on the one side, but also, correspondingly, the number of oppositely charged ions decreases on the other side of the diaphragm.

Boundary layers function like a diaphragm, and the speeds of migration of various ions in extracellular fluids are dissimilar. Accumulation of ions, however, means the accumulation of electrical charges which, in turn, leads to generation of potential. However, this potential is opposite in direction to the current causing the alteration of the ion concentration. Thus, the strength of the polarizing current will be diminished parallel to the increase in the concentration changes. At breaking of the polarizing voltage, the changes in ion concentrations begin to equalize; the ions migrate back and thereby give rise to the generation of a polarization current of opposite direction.

When direct current is conducted into the skin, the polarization is generally higher than it is with alternating current. With alternating current, the increase of the frequency diminishes the capacitances originating from the diffusion potential. At a frequency of 150 Hz., the change in direction of the current takes 3.3 msec., but at a frequency of 4800 Hz., it takes only 0.11 msec. Measurement of the resistance by means of alternating current reveals a gradual decrease up to a frequency of 20,000 Hz., after which one can obtain a constant value. In the case of high frequency, this constant value is already a *measure of the ohmic resistance.*

Permanent Changes in the Active and Passive Electrical Phenomena of the Skin

If potential is led from two neighboring skin areas by means of nonpolarizable electrodes with isophoretic KCl solution, one would think that the two sites would give identical values because of the vicinity, since the ion permeability of the bordering membranes of the skin and the electrolyte content of the cells are presumably the same. If this were the case, one ought to obtain from the two sites currents of identical magnitude but of opposite direction which would neutralize one another; thus, no potential would be measured at all. However, in Rein's opinion (1929) this occurs very rarely. In spite of the vicinity and the identical lead conditions, one generally does obtain a potential, a finding indicative of the functional dissimilarity of even the most closely adjacent skin areas.

The resting potential and also, of course, the polarizability of the skin are subjected to continuous alterations owing to the changes in ion permeability during the vital functions of the skin. In addition, the active and passive electrical phenomena of the skin show individual, regional, and diurnal alterations; thus only repeated investigation of the same region under identical conditions makes the determination of the mean values possible.

Keller (1929) has demonstrated that, because of the electrolyte solution used for the recording of potentials, Ca, Na, and K ions are washed out from the skin, causing an alteration of the skin potential. Previous washing of the skin with water or soap similarly can cause considerable changes. If the previous washing of the skin is performed with solutions of higher acidity, the concentration effect will be reversed and, in the case of recording by KCl solution of lower concentration, an increased negativity of the skin potential can be observed. On the other hand, previous washing with solutions of concentration higher than pH 3.0 to 4.0 augments gradually the positivity of the skin potential by leading it off with gradual dilution of KCl solution.

The continuous change of the potential and polarizability of the skin is demonstrated in the findings of Storz, Voelkel, and Krause (1954). They used a relatively perfect apparatus, the electropermeagraph, and performed measurements on 2000 individuals. The initial resistance of the skin was between 13 and 98 KΩ and the polarization resistance varied between 1.5 and 800 KΩ.

All these changes, however, *do not essentially influence the measurements* performed with the simple ammeter method recommended by Melczer and Kiss (1958) for the diagnosis of primary malignant epithelial tumors and malignant melanomas of the skin at the earliest stage.

The magnitude of the polarization current is influenced by *concentration* of the recording *electrolyte solution* (Ledouc, 1905). The more concentrated the KCl solution used in the electrodes, the smaller the polarization of the skin. In addition, the valences of the cations of the electrode solution also influence the potential.

Rein (1929) observed an acidification on the anode and an augmentation of the concentration of neutral salts on the cathode. Both processes diminish the ability for polarization. In the case of high capacitance, the apparent polarization resistance is low, and in the case of smaller capacitance it is higher. For electrophysiologic investigations, the alternating current seems to be more suitable (Schaefer, 1940). However, the necessary equipment is too expensive and too complicated. Thus, in medical practice, neither measurement of the impedance of the alternating current nor the electropermeagraph of Krause et al. (1954) is used. The latter equipment also gives the same data (such as apparent resistance, capacitances, ohmic resistance) in measurements with direct current.

Accordingly, the skin contains, against the electric current, a combination of different polarizable capacitances and nonpolarizable resistances which are connected partly in parallel and partly in series.

Circuit Models for the Explanation of the Electrical Phenomena of the Skin

Since the characteristics of polarizability and capacitance of the skin have been recognized, many attempts have been made to construct models to imitate and investigate the apparent resistance curves of the skin.

The model of Einthoven and Bijtel (1923) gave a curve resembling that of the skin at introduction of galvanic current flow. They connected, to a high-degree external resistance, a circuit corresponding to an imperfect condenser, which contained a second high resistance with serially connected condenser. The amplitude and the width of the polarization voltage changed in the model with the value of the series-connected condenser and resistance. The above-mentioned authors regarded the capacitance of the skin to be of dielectric character, and the polarization itself to be of minor importance only.

In contrast to the opinion of Einthoven and Bijtel, and mainly on the basis of Gildemeister's experiments (1928), it is now believed that the polarizability and polarization capacitance of the skin are of major importance in the explanation of the resistance curves obtained at the switching in of either direct current or low-frequency alternating current.

In accordance with Gildemeister's view (1928), the electropermeagraph of Krause, Storz, and Voelkel (1954) contains a nonpolarizable external resistance corresponding to the ohmic resistance of the skin. Then comes a small condenser connected in series and high resistance connected in parallel, which represent the capacitance of the double ionic layer. Similarly connected in series with this is a large condenser connected in parallel with low resistance, which corresponds to the diffusion capacitances of the skin. Since, in the model, the two capacitances had to be connected in series, they are probably connected in series also in the skin, i.e., the two capacitances should not necessarily be at the same place.

The electropermeagraph of Krause et al. (1954) works with 2 v., with a resistance of 1 KΩ, and uses 10 percent NaCl as electrode solution. With round electrodes 3 cm. in diameter placed at a distance of 8 cm. from each other, these authors found resistances between 13.8 and 6666 KΩ on the C-dermatome of the forearm, i.e., the resistances exhibited marked individual differences.

In alternating current measurements, the significance of diffusion capacitance is low. According to Gildemeister (1928), high-frequency alternating current gave individual values of the ohmic resistance between 100 and 165 ohms.

According to Keller (1964), the polarizability can be completely different on various regions of the body; even 50-fold differences can occur between various parts of the body. The skin of the forehead generally shows an apparent resistance of low polarization grade; the polarizability of the palms is greater, and that of the limbs and trunk is even higher.

With the exception of the forehead, it is the number of the eccrine sweat glands which plays a leading role in the greater polarizability of the above-mentioned regions.

The Boundary Layers of the Skin in General

From the investigations of Rein (1926), it may be concluded that there are several layers functioning as boundary membranes in the skin. He did not succeed in reversing the charge of the skin by the application of acid solutions on the surface of the skin; by this means, only a discharge, at most, could be achieved.

Also the electromotive thermoreaction of Rein (1929), as well as Keller's (1933) primary epidermic reaction to ultraviolet light, speaks for the existence of several layers. According to Rein (1929), the potential of the skin can be discharged by warming, because, up to a temperature of 35° C, the negative potential of the membrane on the fingers' skin reversibly becomes some 25 to 40 mv. more positive, as established by measurements performed with 1 N KCl electrode fluid. Keller (1964) observed an alteration due to heat effect in the negative potential of the barrier membrane in other parts of the body also, a fact making the existence of this reversible phenomenon indisputable.

In Keller's opinion (1964), the epidermal light reaction following irradiation with UV light is an irreversible process. The potential of the superficial barrier becomes 3 to 25 mv. more positive immediately after irradiation, depending on the dose used. This indicates that the irradiation induces a discharge of the electronegative potential of the protein walls composing the membrane. UV light is known namely for its ability to precipitate protein solutions and denature them in an irreversible way. This reaction can be observed also when the cold light of Kromayer's lamp is used, but the reaction is not identical with the thermoreaction.

It has been assumed already by Gildemeister (1928), Rein (1926, 1929), and Schaefer (1940) that the electrical characteristics of the skin can only be understood by accepting the existence of several polarizable membranes connected one after the other. Among these, the location of the membrane showing concentration effect was searched for by Rein (1929) in the stratum lucidum.

Keller (1931) looked for the most easily accessible superficial membrane undergoing charge alteration, which, because of the accumulation of cations, shows a concentration effect in the stratum disjunctum. According to him, the superficial barrier should lie immediately below this layer and should correspond to the stratum lucidum or to the barrier equal with it. According to Szakáll (1955), it is located in the stratum corneum conjunctum. This is the membrane which, upon superficial scraping or pin-pricking, loses its electromotive functional ability for a few hours.

The charging of the boundary membranes of the skin is dependent also on the perspiration, especially when the thickening of the sweat causes an increase of the cation content and leads to a decrease of the electronegativity of the membrane charge. After administration of pilocarpine, the originally electronegative barrier membrane can partially discharge.

The Electrical Charge of the Barrier Membranes. The protein-containing boundary membranes of the skin are generally negatively charged in the neutral extracellular fluids. This negativity becomes stronger in an alkaline milieu. On the other hand, an acid milieu can reverse the electrical charge of the most superficial membrane, and this so-called cationic membrane will become positive.

At the isoelectric point, around pH 3.0 to 4.0, the skin loses its electrical charge, with a simultaneous decrease of its polarizability.

Short Circuit in the Skin. Continuous loading of the skin with 20 v. direct current can cause short circuit.

The usual voltage which can be used in

electrophysiologic investigations without injury of the boundary membrane lies between 0.1 to 7 v.

In skin diseases accompanied by inflammation, when breaks in continuity develop on the barrier membranes, short circuit can occur. The conductivity of the horny layer decreases after desiccation, and this layer becomes an especially poor conducting dielectric.

The Three Boundary Membranes of the Skin. According to Keller (1963), there are three boundary membranes to be distinguished in the skin: (1) the cation-potential membrane; (2) the basal membrane or barrier, the function of which, however, is inseparable from that of the underlying epidermis; and (3) the tone-potential membrane, occurring only in the sweat glands of the hands and feet.

The cation-potential membrane is situated in the stratum disjunctum. The charge of this membrane is easily reversed. Its isoelectric point lies at pH 4.0. Above this point, in a medium of pH 4.0 to 7.0—which counts alkaline—its charge is negative, while in acid milieu, below pH 4.0, it is positive.

This membrane does not take part in the polarization and has no significance in the measuring of the polarizability of the skin.

The superficial membrane, or Szakáll's barrier, is situated in the stratum conjunctum of the horny layer. It has a negative charge. By means of alkaline electrode solution, the membrane can be brought to a discharge, at most, but the charge cannot be reversed. It is sensitive to heat and mechanical injuries, such as pricking, pressing, rubbing, and scraping, and becomes, upon such influences, electromotively unable to function for a few hours. Its most important characteristic is the generation, together with the underlying epidermis, of polarization countercurrent, in the case of both direct and low-frequency alternating current flow.

The tone-potential membrane is found exclusively in the sweat glands of the hands and feet. It is strongly electronegative and represents the site of origin of the galvanic reflex.

Keller (1963) measured the potential lead from the barrier with 1 N KCl electrode fluid by means of a Philips Nr. GM 6010-type valve voltmeter. He found that, if the first two or three adhesive tape strippings are disregarded, the potential irreversibly decreases following each new stripping, yet before the barrier would be reached. In the case of an intact horny layer, he obtained a current of −13 to −24 mv., but only −2 to −4 mv. after removing the horny layer. Accordingly, not only the barrier but also the middle lamellae of the horny layer figure in the development of barrier potential.

According to Szakáll (1955), the barrier lies immediately over the stratum granulosum. By using Wolf's method, he succeeded in removing the fine, fibrous, elastic barrier as an unbroken layer. The barrier had a pH value between 4.62 and 5.17 and consisted of 42 percent water-solube material and 58 percent water-insoluble horny material. 17.6 percent of the water-soluble material consisted of amino acids which, in his opinion, originated from the cells decaying during hornification and not from sweat.

The removal of the barrier by means of the adhesive tape method of Wolf (1939) renders impossible the charge build-up in the double ionic layer. Therefore, the polarizability of the barrier decreases, but still remains higher than the ohmic resistance measurable with high-frequency alternating current. The remaining polarization resistance is the consequence of the diffusion capacitance, the membrane of which is situated at a site other than that of the double ionic layer and is to be looked for in the deeper layers of the epidermis.

DIMINUTION OF THE POLARIZABILITY OF THE SKIN

Decrease of the Polarizability in Certain Diseases of the Skin

Rein (1929) has mentioned that psoriasis, eczema, trichophytosis, scars, and the covering of bullae exhibit a decreased polarization resistance.

The data of direct current polarization resistances vary to a great extent also, according to the errors involved in the measuring methods;

therefore, the older data of the pertaining literature can hardly be compared with one another.

Polarizability of Scars

Kiss (1970) investigated the electrical characteristics of the scar formations on 36 patients after third-degree burns, furunculosis, and ulcerations of various origins. He found a decreased electrolyte permeation in the scarred regions in every case. This finding is in contradiction to the previous statements of Rein (1929) and Keller (1963); Rein had observed a decreased polarization, i.e., a decreased polarization resistance of scars.

Effect of Trauma on the Skin Barrier

It is known that the charge build-up in the double ionic layer of the boundary membranes of the skin is rendered impossible by traumatization of the membranes. Such traumas include excoriation, erosion, ulceration, pin-pricking, and the adhesive-tape removal, according to Wolf (1939), of the horny layer of the skin. Therefore, the generation of the polarization countercurrent of the skin reversibly decreases, or ceases, depending on the extent of the injury. Then one can measure the ohmic resistance of the skin only with high-frequency alternating current.

The Local Galvanic Reaction of Ebbecke

Ebbecke (1922) recognized as early as the beginning of the third decade of this century that mechanical stimuli, such as touching, rubbing, scraping, and pressing, cause the skin to lose the ability to generate polarization countercurrent in a reversible way for a shorter or longer period of time, and that, for this reason, such events can cause erroneous results, i.e., hypopolarizability or apolarizability.

On the other hand, mechanical influences do not alter the real ohmic resistance of the skin, a feature which can be checked by measurement with high-frequency alternating current.

In Keller's explanation (1964), the barrier will be stretched by mechanical influences, making the pores wider and more permeable for ions. And since the barrier is an elastic one, stopping the pressure results in the reestablishment of the original state.

If, at investigation of the skin for malignant transformation, there is any suspicion about traumatization of the skin, the best procedure is to place an occlusive bandage on the region and to remove it 24 to 48 hours later, quite cautiously without pressing, rubbing, or washing the skin, prior to a new measurement.

Heat-Induced Diminution of the Polarizability of the Skin

The Electromotive Thermoreaction of Rein. The barrier of the skin can be discharged by warming. Up to a temperature of 35° C., the electronegative charge of the barrier in the skin of the fingers becomes 25 to 40 mv. more positive. These results were obtained by Rein (1926), who used 1 N KCl electrode fluid. Even though in Keller's (1964) opinion the skin of the fingers is not suitable for such investigation because of its richness in sweat glands in which tone-potential develops upon the influence of emotional excitation which can disturb the investigation, the existence of heat-induced change of the barrier membrane is indisputable. Keller observed this phenomenon on other regions of the body also.

Diminution of the Polarizability of the Skin After Ultraviolet and X-ray Irradiation

According to Keller (1931 and 1933), the potential of the barrier becomes 3 to 25 mv. more positive immediately after ultraviolet light irradiation. The extent of this change depends on the dose used. This finding indicates that irradiation causes a discharge of the potential of the protein walls composing the membrane. It is known that ultraviolet light can precipitate and even irreversibly denature protein solutions in vitro. The reaction is an irreversible one; it can also be observed after irradiation with the cold light of Kromayer's lamp and is not identical with the thermoreaction.

Ultraviolet light irradiation with erythema dose diminishes the polarization of the skin in the region of the erythema; after the disappearance of the erythema, an increased polarization develops.

The Irreversible Effect of X-ray Irradiation

Recently, Kiss (1970) dealt with the lesser known, long-lasting characteristics of x-ray irradiation causing permanently increased apparent resistance. A total of 80 patients (46 males and 34 females) were investigated. They had skin carcinomas and had been treated with contact x-ray irradiation according to Chaoul.

The measurements were performed seven years (24 cases), six years (5 cases), five years (9 cases), four years (8 cases), three years (9 cases), two years (10 cases), and one year (15 cases) after the irradiation, respectively.

The patients received the irradiation on the face, forehead, nasal region, and, in one case, on the back. The total dose of the irradiation applied in several fractions was between 4000 and 6000 R. (Chaoul's apparatus, 60 kv., 1.5 to 5.0 cm. skin-focus distance, 4 m.Å., 300 to 500 R. per day).

During development of radiation erythema and, especially, of epitheliosis, no polarization resistance could be demonstrated. On the other hand, during the months and years following the disappearance of the erythema, the initial and especially the polarization resistance *increased severalfold over the normal value.*

According to the investigations of Kiss (1962 and 1970), the decrease in the percentage ion permeability can be demonstrated as long as six months after the administration of 1000 or 1200 R.

Six months after the application of 800 R., the decrease in electrolyte permeation could no longer be demonstrated.

Kiss also investigated the effect of over-erythema doses of irradiation on the skin of dogs

possessing no sweat glands at all. He observed an increase in the apparent resistance resembling completely that of the human skin. From this finding it was concluded that the electrolyte permeation decreasing parallel to the increase of the apparent resistance is due to injury to the barrier membrane rather than to the sweat glands.

The results obtained in the investigations of Kiss are in accord with the data of Sulzberger et al. (1952).

According to the latter authors, a fractionated superficial irradiation treatment with a total dose of 1000 R. does not cause any x-ray damage. However, after a total dose of 1000 to 2650 R., a cosmetic damage was found in 1.5 percent of the cases. In patients treated for malignant skin tumors, the percentage of occurrence of late x-ray damage increased as high as 20 percent.

Pseudorecurrences After X-ray Irradiation

It is known that, after fractionated contact irradiation, pseudorecurrences can develop on the irradiated regions in 7 to 8 percent of the cases. These benignant and spontaneously reversible pseudorecurrences resemble the real malignant recurrences. Up to now, their identification was made by histologic investigations.

Kiss studied some years ago, with the aid of the electropermeagraph apparatus modified by him, whether the decreased or lacking polarizability characteristic of malignant transformations could be observed also in pseudorecurrences.

Pseudorecurrences were found in 11 (6.1 percent) of the 178 patients who received contact irradiation. The pseudorecurrences were also controlled histologically; at measurement with the electropermeagraph, not only the mere presence of polarization was stated but also there was a slight incline toward augmentation, showing that the ion permeability of the recurrences was diminished.

On regions treated with a total radiation dose of about 4000 to 6000 R., the increase of the polarizability is, according to the experiences, an irreversible one. This fact can probably account for the increased polarizability of pseudorecurrences originating in these regions. However, the exact answer to this question requires knowledge of the data on the polarizability of the real recurrences originating in these irradiated regions.

DEVICES FOR INVESTIGATION OF THE PASSIVE ELECTRICAL PHENOMENA OF THE SKIN

The Direct Potentiometer Method of Measuring Apparent Resistance Used By Melczer and Kiss

Determination of the polarizability of the skin can be performed even with the most simple potentiometer method. The determination of the polarizability is indispensable for the everyday practice of a dermatologist in the recognition of (1) beginning malignant transformation of various precancerous lesions; (2) primary malignant epithelial proliferations of the skin; and especially (3) pigmented nevi undergoing malignant transformation and malignant melanomas.

In these cases we conduct a known low-voltage current of a dry battery through a sensitive galvanometer by means of non-

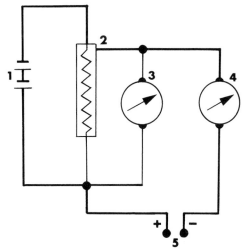

Figure 12–2 Diagram of an apparatus with the voltmeter-ammeter method. *1*, Dry batteries of 2 to 4 v. *2*, An adjustable potentiometer of 10 kilo-ohms. *3*, Voltmeter of 0 to 10 v. *4*, *Deprez-d'Arsonval* moving-coil ammeter with a sensitivity of 10^{-7}. *5*, Coupling of the nonpolarizable electrodes.

polarizable electrodes with the insertion of a high resistance (Figs. 12–1 and 12–2). In order to avoid changes in the potential by pressure and assure adequate electrode surfaces, we place on the skin a filter paper disk which has a surface of 0.3 to 0.5 cm.² and which is made by a punch and soaked with 0.1 N KCl solution. Under the indifferent electrode, we can also use a large strip with a surface of 7 to 9 cm.², and, with a change of the electrodes, we can separately determine the values of the anodic and cathodic polarizations.

Nonpolarizable Electrodes. Nonpolarizable metal electrodes immersed in solution containing cations of the same metal, e.g., Zn in $ZnSO_4$, Cu in $CuSO_4$, and so forth, can be used in the procedure.

A zinc plate 5 cm. in length and about 4 mm. in width is soldered to the end of a copper wire. Then the plate is put into a glass tube about 15 cm. in length and 6 mm. in inner diameter and is fixed with epoxy resin or a rubber stopper perforated in the middle. The site of the soldering and the end of the copper wire must be carefully insulated with nitrovarnish so that the zinc plate is in contact with the electrode fluid only. As electrode solution 0.1 N zinc sulfate solution (2.76 percent) was used. In the case of copper electrodes we applied, as electrode solution, a 0.1 N (2.5 percent)

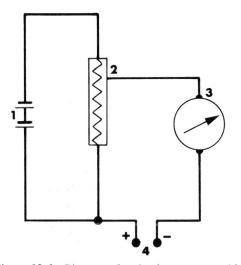

Figure 12–1 Diagram of a simple apparatus with the potentiometer method. *1*, Dry batteries of 2 to 4 v. *2*, An adjustable potentiometer of 10 kilo-ohms. *3*, *Deprez-d'Arsonval* moving-coil galvanometer with a sensitivity of 10^{-7}. *4*, Coupling of the two nonpolarizable electrodes.

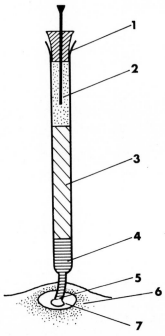

Figure 12–3 Diagram of a nonpolarizable Zn-ZnSO$_4$ electrode. *1*, Rubber cork perforated in the middle with a zinc plate soldered to the copper wire. *2*, 0.1 N (2.76 percent) zinc sulfate solution. *3*, Agar bridge [2 percent agar is added to 0.1 N potassium chloride (0.76 percent) solution]. *4*, 0.1 N potassium chloride solution. *5*, A cotton wool stopper through which a piece of cotton yarn passes or a few threads are pulled out for measurement. *6*, Skin. *7*, Filter paper disk.

copper sulfate solution to the end of the 5-cm. stripped copper wire (Fig. 12–3).

Thereafter, a 0.76 percent potassium chloride solution containing 2 percent purified agar swollen previously at room temperature, then dissolved by heating, was layered over the zinc sulfate or copper sulfate solution. After the hardening of the bridge, the electrode tube was closed with a cotton stopper from which a few threads were pulled out which could be used, after twisting, for the measurement.

When not in use, the electrodes should be kept short-circuited in 0.1 N (0.76 percent) KCl solution to ensure their discharge and to avoid their desiccation.

In order to avoid pressure potential, we place filter paper disks, 0.5 cm. in diameter and soaked with 0.76 percent KCl solution, on the places to be measured. These disks have to be brought into contact with the cotton thread pulled out (Fig. 12–4).

In determination of the zero point, in order to obtain average values, we perform several measurements on the neighboring intact skin areas, and this same procedure can be followed in determining the polarizability along the pathologic alteration.

The indifferent electrode is generally

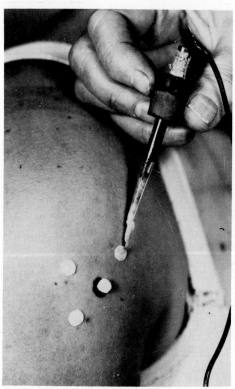

Figure 12–4 Mode of electrometric measurement. To avoid false potential by pressure of the electrode on the skin and to assure similar electrode surfaces, filter paper disks are placed on the surface of the lesion and the surrounding normal skin. The disks have a surface of 0.3 to 0.5 cm.² made by a hollow punch and soaked with 0.1 N potassium chloride solution.

Then a greater filter paper disk, about 3 cm. in diameter soaked with a 0.1 N (0.76 percent) potassium chloride solution, is placed into one palm of the patient, and the different electrode (using the simple ammeter method whichever is from the two electrodes) should be held in such a way that the cotton thread is in contact with the filter paper disk.

Now the current of the dry batteries is switched on, and the cotton thread of the different electrode is brought into contact with one filter paper disk of the surrounding normal skin for the determination of the zero point.

After registration of the zero point, the cotton thread of the different electrode is brought into contact with the paper disk of the lesion for the determination of its polarizability.

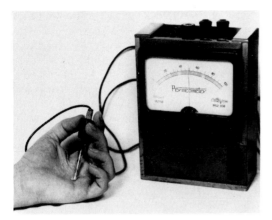

Figure 12–5 Mode of holding the indifferent electrode in the palm of the patient. On the right is a portable apparatus with a direct-reading galvanometer.

given to the patient, who should hold it in his palm (Fig. 12–5). The cotton thread pulled out of the electrode must be in contact with the filter paper disk and should be soaked with a 0.76 percent potassium chloride solution.

Since, in the case of filter paper disks of identical size, the polarization countercurrent developing at the different (anodic) electrode is opposite in direction to the polarization countercurrent developing at the indifferent (cathodic) electrode, the two currents neutralize each other to a great extent. It is therefore advisable to place a filter paper disk of larger diameter (3 to 4 cm.) in the palm of the patient under the indifferent electrode.

Adjustment of the Apparatus. A disk about 2 cm. in *diameter* and soaked with a 0.76 percent potassium chloride solution is placed into our left palm or into the one palm of the patient. The indifferent electrode should be held in such a way that the cotton thread is in contact with the filter paper disk (Fig. 12–5). Then a smaller filter paper disk, 0.5 cm. in *diameter* and soaked with KCl solution, is placed on the dorsal surface of the forearm. Thereafter, the current of the dry battery of the apparatus is switched on, and the cotton thread of the different electrode is brought into contact with the filter paper disk. Because of the normally high polarization countercurrent, the pointer of the ammeter shows only a slight deflection. Now the potentiometer is adjusted so that the pointer stands

at 2 to 3 μamp. This is taken for the zero point. Then we gently scarify the skin of the forearm with a sterile needle until mild bleeding occurs and, after placing the smaller filter paper disk soaked with KCl solution on the injured area, we bring the cotton thread of the different electrode into contact with the paper disk. Since the injured area scraped with the needle loses the majority of its polarizability owing to the injury of the barrier—just as is the case with malignant skin cancers or malignant melanomas—the pointer of the ammeter of the apparatus will show a maximum deflection. The extent of this deflection can be regarded in practice as roughly proportional to the grade of the malignant transformation. *Now, with the adjustment of the potentiometer, the apparatus is set in such a way that the intact skin area gives a minimum deflection and the injured one a maximum deflection.*

Since direct current of even a few volts can, after longer application, injure the barrier and thereby cause a diminution of the polarizability, the current is allowed to flow into the skin during the measurement for a few seconds only. On the other hand, the measurement can be repeated several times at 1-minute intervals.

Furch (1963) and Leonhardi and Furch (1964) took the average of four to five measurements made on the intact areas around the pathologic alteration and divided it by the average value obtained on several points of the alteration. These experiments clearly showed that the conductivity of the tumor region is much higher, i.e., the polarizability of the tumor part considerably decreases, and correspondingly, its permeability increases.

Storz et al. (1954), in their measurement of polarization resistance with the electropermeagraph, gave these values in terms of kilo-ohms, while Kiss expresses the hypo- or apolarizability of the pathologic region in terms of increased ion permeability.

Furch (1963), Leonhardi and Furch (1964), Kantner (1965), and Gulbert (1968) used a similar apparatus with direct potentiometer method. Furch (1963) and Leonhardi and Furch (1964) also connected a voltmeter to the apparatus in addition to the ammeter (Fig. 12–2).

The Electrodermatometer of Regelsberger

A similar apparatus, also commercially available, is the electrodermatometer constructed by the firm Siemens and Reiniger on the basis of Regelsberger's data (1950). This apparatus is mainly used in neurologic practice.

The electrodermatometer has a highly sensitive ammeter and functions with the current of a 2-v. dry battery and with two metal electrodes. The silver plates of the electrodes are covered with a felt layer which, according to the instructions, should be soaked with physiologic saline. Permanent gentle contact between the electrodes and the skin is ensured by means of a spring mechanism.

One of the disadvantages of the apparatus lies in the fact that the resistances corresponding to current intensities of 1×10^{-7} to 6×10^{-7} amp. do not augment linearly, and that, in the case of measuring higher resistances, the deflection of the pointer of the ammeter is small. No difference can be made between the resistance of the anode and cathode, and the difference between the opposite polarization currents of the two skin areas cannot be determined. A further drawback of the apparatus is that it can give rise to nondesirable diffusion potential, because it does not use isophoretic KCl solution.

The Electropermeagraph of Krause and His Coworkers

The drawbacks of the electrodermatometer were eliminated to a great extent by the electropermeagraph apparatus constructed by Krause, Storz, and Voelkel (1954). This apparatus gives reproducible data on the electrical characteristics of the skin and is indispensable in electrophysiologic research.

The apparatus consists of two circuits. One of these is a 2-v. current source with two nonpolarizable electrodes and an external resistance of 1.0 KΩ. The other one consists of a direct current amplifier connected to the two poles of the 1.0 KΩ external resistance and of a light-beam string galvanometer which fixes the current

curve on film. Because of the inertness of the apparatus, the curve of the polarization countercurrent is some 3 msec. late. For this reason, according to Keller (1963), it is necessary to extrapolate in order to determine the current value which can cause an error as high as ±25 percent. Of course, during one single series of investigations, this does not cause any essential trouble, for the error is a constant one.

The Modified Electropermeagraph-like Apparatus of Kiss

Since the abrupt rise of the Garten's spike of the polarization current induced by closing and opening of a direct current passes off within one-tenth of a msec., and since the value of polarization marginal current caused by the diffusion potential can be regarded as practically constant, the application of short impulses seems more suitable for investigations of the electrical characteristics of the skin. For the production of such direct current impulses, Kiss used a low-frequency cathode-ray oscillograph, to which a wide-band square-wave impulse generator of 0.03 to 0.1 v. and 50 Hz. was connected. The outer metal parts were carefully grounded, and the nonpolarizable electrodes were connected with shielded cables in order to eliminate electrical disturbances from outside.

One of the electrodes placed on the skin was connected to the output of the square-wave generator, and the other one to the input of the vertical amplifier of the cathode-ray oscillograph. Between the latter and the grounding, a resistance of 1.0 KΩ was inserted.

After synchronization of the oscillograph and the square-wave generator, the curve of the current fluctuations developing between the two poles of the 1.0 KΩ resistance appears on the screen and recorded in the form of a still-film picture. The oscillograph was calibrated in such a way that a 1-mv. current fed into the input caused a 10-mm. deflection on the screen. As nonpolarizable electrodes he used Ag-AgCl cotton-wicked electrodes. The outer walls of the glass tube had to be shielded. Both electrodes were of the same size.

The resistance of the electrode can be

measured by means of a Wheatstone bridge, and the actual change in resistance must be taken into account. The electrodes were stored in the dark, and great care was taken to prevent them from desiccation.

In order to eliminate the pressure-induced fluctuations of the potential, the cotton thread pulled out from the cotton stopper of the electrode was brought into contact with a filter paper disk with a surface of 0.5 cm.², which was soaked with a 0.1 N KCl solution and placed on the skin area to be investigated. It is advisable to perform several measurements on this area for determination of the average value.

The skin area serving as the place of the indifferent electrode was injured with a sharpened Francke's needle. The injury should reach the papillary layer; this is indicated by a slight bleeding.

At the moment of the closing of the current, its strength suddenly increases, corresponding to the ascending branch of the Garten's spike (S), and it can be measured in mm. Thereafter, it falls exponentially on the value of the marginal current (G). Upon switch-off we see a Garten's spike of opposite direction on the screen of the oscillograph (Fig. 12–6).

Determination of the value S was performed by comparison with a constant calibration current strength. Knowing the magnitude of S and G, as well as the value of the inserted 1 KΩ resistance (Rv) and the voltage of the current source, one can calculate, according to the method of Storz et al. (1954) and on the basis of Ohm's law, the initial resistance R appearing at the moment of the switch-on by the following equation:

$$R = \frac{Ue \cdot c \cdot Rv}{Uc} \cdot \frac{1}{S}$$

where Ue = voltage of the current source,
$\quad c$ = magnitude in mm. of the calibration voltage,
$\quad Rv$ = constant resistance of 1 KΩ,
$\quad Uc$ = 10 mv. calibration voltage,
$\quad S$ = magnitude in mm. of the charge build-up of the Garten's spike.

The total resistance Rg of the skin can be computed in a similar way:

$$Rg = \frac{Ue \cdot c \cdot Rv}{Uc} \cdot \frac{1}{G}$$

where G = length on the screen in mm. of the marginal current following the descending branch of the Garten's spike.

The difference between the two resistances is a measure of the polarization resistance r indicated in Figure 12–6 by the distance P.

The extent of the electrolyte permeation is

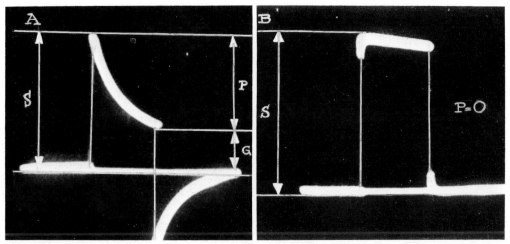

Figure 12–6 Oscillogram of the normal skin A and of a malignant lesion (basal cell carcinoma) B during square-wave impulses.

A, According to Krause et al. (1954), the true ohmic resistance S is equivalent to the initial resistance which corresponds to the ascending part of the Garten's spike. P, apparent resistance due to the polarizing counter-current, is equivalent to the descending part of the Garten's spike. The latter is continued in G, the marginal current caused by diffusion potential.

B, Lack of the Garten's spike indicates that the apparent resistance of this basal cell carcinoma has entirely failed.

obtained by means of the equation of Storz et al. (1954):

$$P \% = \frac{S - G}{S} \cdot 100$$

This number is the so-called percentage permeation.

S = Ascending branch in mm. of the Garten's spike.

G = magnitude in mm. of the marginal current,

P = magnitude in mm. of the polarization resistance.

The limit current, as well as the magnitude in mm. of the initial Garten's spike, is inversely proportional to the real ohmic resistance (R) and total resistance (Rg), and is in direct proportion to the polarization resistance (P).

Kiss (1970) is of the opinion that, in clinical investigations and also in research the determination of the *permeability* of the boundary membranes is more characteristic than the inhibition of permeability expressed in P %.

The apparatus of Kiss has advantages over the apparatus of Storz et al. Because of the lower measuring voltage, the injury of the barrier is less probable. In addition, the use of a cathode-ray oscillograph eliminates the inertness of the string galvanometer. A further advantage is the possibility of photofixation of the pictures.

The Whelan Apparatus of Midana and His Coworkers

Midana and Ormea (1960) investigated the effect of meteorologic factors on the skin in an air-conditioned room. According to Ormea (1959), the high-altitude climate influences the ability of the skin to generate polarization countercurrent. He used Whelan's measuring apparatus in his investigations.

The Malignometer of Kiss and Horváth

Because of the above-mentioned drawbacks of the electropermeagraph, Kiss and Horváth (1969) constructed a new apparatus for the recognition of malignancy in the different pathologic alterations of the skin which can be found in malignant primary carcinomas and melanomas of the skin. The apparatus, which is also commercially available, uses the impedance of alternating current. It works with 1600 Hz. alternating current and has the advantage that no nonpolarizable electrodes are needed, since, as a consequence of the use of alternating current, polarization cannot develop on the electrode surface.

In the malignometer, the current necessary for the measurement is derived from a dry battery, and the alternating current is produced by an oscillator. A cylindrical nickel-plated iron electrode with a surface of 80 cm.², placed into the palm of the patient, serves as the indifferent electrode. It is covered with deerskin and has to be moistened with 0.1 N KCl solution. The different electrode comes into contact with a filter paper disk soaked with 0.1 N KCl solution. During measurement, the disk is first placed on the surrounding intact skin. By turning the kilo-ohmic potentiometer of the equipment to the calibration mark, we can determine the impedance of the intact skin on the scale of the potentiometer.

The measurement on the pathologic skin areas is performed in the very same way.

The quotient of the superficial impedance values of the intact and pathologic skin areas is over 1.5 in the case of malignant transformation.

THE DIMINUTION OF POLARIZABILITY OF THE SKIN IN MALIGNANT GROWTHS

Decrease or Complete Failure of the Polarizability in General

The basic principles in the cases of amelanotic and melanotic malignant melanomas as well as of the primary cancers of the skin are *the recognition and treatment of the alterations as early as possible.*

For the diagnosis generally, it is the histologic investigation which plays the decisive part. However, in the case of a suspicion about primary malignant melanoma, it is forbidden to perform a biopsy. *The recognition of whether a malignant transformation is present or not is of utmost importance for judging the malignant transformation of precancerous lesions, especially for that of the amelanotic clinically recognizable cases and of pigmented nevi undergoing malignant transformation.*

In these cases the presence or absence of malignant transformation can be established by recognizing the decrease or complete failure of the polarizability by means of simple electric measuring equipment. Thus, we can avoid the hazard of a too-late diagnosis and also those tragic cases when the physician excises or cauterizes pigmented nevi already undergoing malignant transformation.

One of the greatest problems in dermatologic practice is generally caused by amelanotic melanoma and pigmented nevi undergoing malignant transformation. Malignant melanomas can cause, mostly after puberty or during pregnancy, subjective complaints, such as burning sensations, itching, and formication. The nevi can occasionally enlarge and become more pigmented — signs indicative of malignant transformation. In these cases excision is prohibited, for surgical trauma to a proliferation containing malignant segregated cells can promote, or even provoke regional or remote metastases.

The Jaksch test, i.e., detection by $FeCl_3 \cdot H_2O$ of the melanogen excreted in the urine, does not give satisfactory results, even after x-ray irradiation. In 33 percent of the 253 patients of Sinner (1962), the test was negative, even in the case of malignant transformation. Of 37 cases in which both the clinical findings and histologic examinations ascertained the presence of malignant melanoma, no melanogen in the urine could be detected in 35 percent.

It is known that the ^{32}P accumulation test is not reliable either. ^{14}C-labeled tyrosine gave positive results in only 37.5 percent of the melanoblastoma cases described by Poppe et al. (1954). For the diagnosis of melanoblastoma, Grupper (1954) suggested the investigation of the antityrosinase activity of the serum. As to the applicability of this test, there are few data at present.

Venkel and Bakos (1961) suggested that the thermodifference between benignant and malignant proliferations could be used in the recognition of the malignant skin proliferations.

The diagnostic method described and suggested by Melczer and Kiss (1957 and 1958) and is of great importance in the

recognition of malignant transformations, especially in cases of amelanotic malignant melanomas and pigmented nevi undergoing malignant transformation (Fig. 12–10). The procedure can be applied without any harm to the patient as many times as necessary, and it determines the presence or absence of malignant transformation.

Of course, in an injured or ulcerated area, we may try the measurements only several mm. from the edge of excoriation, erosion, or ulceration. On the injured area, we can obtain a false-positive result because of the demarcation potential.

The applicability of the procedure was confirmed by Furch (1963), Leonhardi and Furch (1964), Kantner (1965), and Gulbert (1968).

Leonhardi and Furch (1964) have stated that the method, which is relatively simple and completely harmless to the patient, makes the recognition of malignant skin proliferations easier.

The method involves an investigation of the polarizability of the pathologic alteration and plays a prominent part in the diagnosis of the early stages of malignant transformations and of malignant melanomas of the skin.

Diminution or Complete Failure of the Polarizability in Primary Cancers and Malignant Melanomas of the Skin

Along the malignant primary tumors of the skin the barrier is injured, and its polarizability diminishes or ceases completely, just as is the case with scarified or pin-pricked skin areas. Therefore, if one of the nonpolarizable electrodes of the measuring apparatus is placed into the palm of the patient, and the other one on the suspected alteration, and the 1- to 2-v. exosomatic current source is switched on, the pointer of the ammeter will show a considerable deflection relative to the value taken for the zero point of the adjacent intact skin area, since the polarization countercurrent weakening the introduced current is diminished or not present at all.

Results obtained from several thousand measurements have shown the possibility

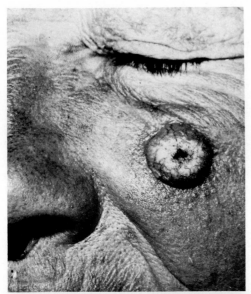

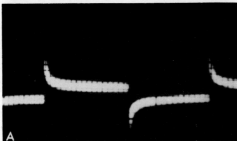

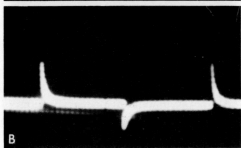

Figure 12–7 Keratoacanthoma faciei. According to the histologic examination, the neoplasm corresponds to a benign growth. *A*, Oscillogram of the normal skin surrounding the keratoacanthoma reveals a great polarizability (80 percent).

B, The skin over the keratoacanthoma also shows a great polarizability (60 percent), which is characteristic for normal skin.

of setting a sharp limit between benignant and malignant epithelial skin tumors on the basis of the diminution of or loss of the polarizability characteristic of intact skin.

Verrucae, fibromas, nevi, and keratoacanthomas (Fig. 12–7) show a potential of 1.0 to 3.0 mv. In contrast, precancerous areas undergoing malignant transforma-

tion (Fig. 12–8), basal cell carcinomas (Fig. 12–6), squamous cell carcinomas (Fig. 12–9), and malignant melanomas (Fig. 12–10) show a value of 20 to 40 mv. owing to the increased conductivity which causes the polarizability to decrease.

Also the malignant transformation of the mucous membrane in the neighborhood of the skin shows substantially increased conductivity when compared with that of the adjacent intact tissue. In carcinomas of the oral cavity, in intraepidermal carcinoma of the portio, or in malignant leukoplakia oris (Fig. 12–8), values between 20 and 30 mv. can be measured.

The apparatus is not suitable for exploring the sorts of malignant transformation which occur in proliferations independent of the barrier membranes of the skin, such as proliferations of connective tissue origin not injuring the barrier, or metastases.

When we want to recognize the potential for malignant transformation of eroded or ulcerated areas, we should perform the measurements at a few mm. distance from the injured region.

The Results of Kiss Obtained With His Electropermeagraph-like Apparatus

Kiss (1970) also performed experiments on the applicability of the electropermeagraph-like apparatus constructed by him.

Forty-six malignant proliferations (24 basal cell carcinomas, 19 squamous cell cancers, and 3 malignant melanomas), as well as 67 benign alterations (16 senile keratoses, 22 senile verrucae, 14 pigmented nevi, 10 fibromas, and 5 keratoacanthomas), were investigated. A decreased polarization resistance, i.e., increased electrolyte permeation, was found in both the different precancerous lesions with malignant transformations, i.e., at the beginning of the malignancy, and the already developed malignant proliferations.

The results of his measurements are shown in Table 12–1.

In 57 benign proliferations, the quotients, i.e., the grade of permeability of the adjacent intact areas divided by the grade of permeability of the proliferations, gave a value around 1.0. However, in the 47 malignant proliferations, the quotient was,

Figure 12–8 Leukoplakia of the lower lip (indicated by arrow). Microscopically the lesion proved to be an early squamous cell carcinoma.

Top right, the oscillogram of the adjacent normal skin; bottom right, the oscilloscopic representation of a leukoplakia undergoing malignant change.

Distance *S* indicates the initial resistance (in inverse ratio to the height). The distance *P* shows the size of the apparent resistance (in direct ratio to the height of the curve) due to the polarization electromotive force.

Owing to malignant transformation of the leukoplakia, the decrease of the initial resistance is 37.9 percent; that of the apparent resistance is 69.2 percent. (Courtesy of Dr. J. Kiss.)

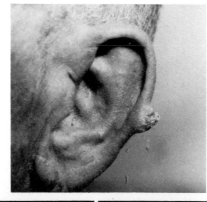

as a rule, many times higher than that of the intact skin. In basal cell carcinomas, and especially in the elevated forms in which, as it seems, the barrier membranes of the skin are injured but to a slight extent, he obtained a quotient of less than 1.0 (i.e., a negative value) in some 15 to 20 percent of the cases.

In squamous cell cancers, which are of greater importance, and especially in malignant melanomas and Bowen's disease, the quotient was always several times higher than 1.0.

In some cases of basal cell carcinomas, and especially in the outward-growing epithelioma elevatum, he occasionally found a value below 1.0; this finding has

Figure 12–9 Squamous cell carcinoma. Microscopically the growth proved to be an early squamous cell carcinoma.

A, Oscillogram of the adjacent normal skin of the lesion.

B, Oscillogram of the lesion's covering skin.

The initial resistance (ascending part of the spike) of the skin along the tumor is diminished 42.85 percent. Simultaneously the curve of the polarizing countercurrent (descending part of the spike) is completely eliminated, i.e., it is diminished 100 percent.

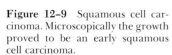

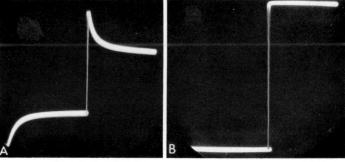

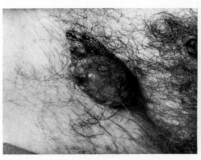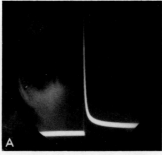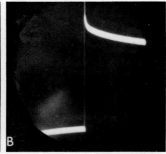

Figure 12–10 Malignant melanoma of the right inguinal region. After contact x-ray irradiation (Chaoul's apparatus, 60 kv., 3.0 cm. skin-focus distance, 4 milliamperes, total dose of 10,000 R.), the diagnosis was also confirmed by biopsy.

A, Oscillogram of the surrounding normal skin. Note the great polarizability of the adjacent normal skin.
B, The polarizability of the malignant growth (descending part of the spike) diminished 77.1 percent.

not yet been explained. Up to now, a *false negativity* has never been observed in malignant melanomas.

In benign tumorlike proliferations and in precancerous states in general, the apparent resistance caused by the polarization current is identical to the apparent resistance of the adjacent intact skin area (Fig. 12–7).

The electropermeagraph, however, is an expensive and complicated apparatus. For recognition of the malignant transformation of the skin, the small, portable apparatus, easily and inexpensively constructed, is completely suitable; this apparatus has a *Wheatstone* bridge or a directly connected potentiometer circuit and functions with a 2.0- to 4.5-v. dry battery.

Measurement Data Obtained By Kiss and Horváth (1969) With the Malignometer

A total of 65 patients were investigated. Out of them 28 persons had basal cell carcinoma, which only exceptionally causes metastases. If these cases are disregarded and only the squamous cell carcinomas and the most dangerous malignant melanomas are taken into account, the malignometer revealed the presence of malignant transformation in 100 percent of the cases.

However, in 5 of the cases with basal cell carcinomas, i.e., in 17.7 percent, they obtained false-negative results. In these cases histologic investigation of serial sections revealed basal cell carcinoma originating from the sebaceous glands.

Even if we take into account the false results obtained in a certain percentage of basal cell carcinomas, the apparatus gave correct results in 92.3 percent of 65 cases of skin carcinomas and malignant melanomas.

The reliability of the apparatus is shown by the finding that, in control measurements on benign proliferations in 157 patients, the extreme values of the quotient were between 0.55 and 1.35, which means that *in no case did the apparatus show a false-negative result.*

TABLE 12–1

Diagnosis	Number of Cases	Histo-logically Verified	Quotient	Extreme Values
Keratoacanthoma	5	5	1.1	0.5 – 1.4
Nevus pigmentosus	14	14	0.9 ± 0.2	0.5 – 1.2
Verruca senilis	22	13	0.8 ± 0.3	0.4 – 1.6
Keratoma senile	16	9	1.0 ± 0.3	0.5 – 1.4
M. Bowen	1	1	11.7	11.7
Basal cell carcinoma	24	24	2.1 ± 0.9	0.8 – 8.3
Squamous cell carcinoma	19	19	3.5 ± 1.1	1.8 – 6.2
Malignant melanoma	3	3	5.3	2.8 – 8.1

Diminution of the Initial Resistance in Primary Cancers and Melanocarcinomas of the Skin

According to Kiss and Horváth (1969), the initial resistance, i.e., the capacitance, of the barrier decreases in malignant tissues. They found, on the average, a 15 percent decrease in basal cell carcinomas (9 cases), a 31 percent decrease in squamous cell cancers (Fig. 12–8) (6 cases), and a 39 percent decrease in malignant melanomas (2 cases). At the same time the average diminution of the polarization resistance was around 60 percent.

Possible Causes of the Diminution of Initial and Polarization Resistance

It has long been known (Beebe, 1904; Clowes and Frisbie, 1905; Clowes, 1919) that the permeability of the malignant cells is higher than that of normal ones. The above-mentioned authors generally explained this phenomenon by the decreased calcium content of the malignant tissue. According to Waterman (1922), the diminished polarization ability and the diminished capacitive charging of excised tumor parts are to be accounted for by the increased permeability and decreased calcium content of the malignant cells. In in vitro experiments, he succeeded in normalizing the polarization ability of malignant tissue by keeping it in isotonic calcium chloride solution.

However, in the experiments of Melczer (1960), the bathing of excised parts of Guérin rat carcinoma in isotonic calcium chloride solution restored the diminished polarization ability of the in vitro tumor tissue to 30 to 35 percent at the most.

Carruthers and Suntzeff (1944 and 1946) investigated the ion content of human epitheliomas and of the methylcholanthrene-induced skin tumor of the mouse. When compared with intact tissue, a diminution of the calcium content but no change in the K, Na, or Mg content was observed Graffi and Pisarzewski (1959) described that, in his institute, Pisarzewski had found 6.5 times more potassium and sodium, calculated on the basis of the

nitrogen content, in rat hepatoma than in intact rat liver. According to him similar changes also occur in Flexner-Jobling carcinoma and Jensen sarcoma. The equivalent value of the four cations (K, Na, Mg, and Ca) was about 30 percent higher in the tumor tissue.

Kiss and Horváth (1969) established that the conductivity at 18°C of a solution containing calcium chloride, potassium chloride, and sodium chloride in 5 weight per volume each is about 0.200 ohm cm^{-1}. Increasing the amount of K and Na to 10 weight per volume, and leaving the amount of calcium unchanged, they observed an increase of the specific conductivity to 0.321 ohm cm.$^{-1}$, i.e., an increase of 60 percent in comparison with the initial value. One could think, on the basis of this model experiment, that the diminution of the polarizability and capacitive charging of tumor tissues is caused by the increase in number of K and Na ions in the malignant tissue at the expense of calcium ions.

False-positive and False-negative Results

If we see any signs of desquamation, excoriation, or erosion on the region of the alteration, especially if there is a suspicion of malignant melanoma, the best procedure is to put on an occlusive bandage for 24 to 48 hours. While removing this bandage we have to avoid any pressure, rubbing, or scraping of the skin since, as a consequence of Ebbecke's reversible galvanic reaction, slight trauma can cause a *diminution of the polarization* and thereby cause suspicion of a malignant transformation in the case of intact tissue.

Local application of a thermophore and bathing in warm water decrease the negative charging of the barrier membrane because of Rein's thermoreaction, rendering it more permeable for anions. Therefore, the polarizability of the skin decreases in a reversible way, which, for a short period of time, can give rise to states resembling malignant transformation.

Similarly, false positivity can be caused by mechanical traumatization of the skin, such as pressure, brushing, or rubbing, which can lead to a discharge of the electronegativity of the barrier and can render the membrane more permeable for ions.

According to Keller (1928), a hypopolarization can be caused by ultraviolet light irradiation. Immediately after the irradiation, the barrier becomes 3 to 25 mv. more positive. This process can go as far as causing the barrier to discharge. In his opinion, this state is an irreversible one.

After an erythema dose of ultraviolet light irradiation, the *hypopolarizability* under the inflammation turns, after about four days, into *hyperpolarizability*, which can give, on the region of the malignant skin transformation, a *false negativity*.

In practice the most important factors are the ionizing radiations. After irradiation with a total dose of 1200 R., an irreversible, increased polarizability, even after decades and even in cases in which the alteration itself had not been cured by the radiation treatment, can be found; in these cases we can observe a false negativity. Measurements performed following irradiation with the above-mentioned high doses can no longer be used for the determination of the presence or absence of malignant transformation.

Thus, in the diagnosis of recurrent squamous cell carcinoma or malignant melanoma, it is necessary to know the exact data from the occasional previous x-ray treatment, especially the total dose which was administered.

The apparatus can give false-negative results in the case of basal cell carcinomas, which, because of their benignity, are of lesser practical importance. Negative results can occur in cases of outward-growing epithelioma elevatum and basal cell carinomas originating from the sebaceous glands. In these cases the barrier is probably not injured to any great extent.

REFERENCES

Beebe, S. P.: The chemistry of malignant growth. Am. J. Physiol., 11:139, 1904.

Beutner, R.: Die Entstehung elektrischer Ströme im Gewebe. Stuttgart, 1913. *In* Glasser, L. (Ed.): Bioelectricity in Medical Physics. Vol. 1. Chicago, Year Book Medical Publishers, 1944, p. 35.

Beutner, R.: Die Entstehung elektrischer Ströme in lebenden Geweben. Stuttgart, F. Enke, 1920.

Beutner, R.: Bioelectricity in Medical Physic. Glasser, O. (Ed.) Vol. I, Chicago, Year Book Medical Publishers, 1944, p. 35.

Carruthers, C., and Suntzeff, V.: Chemistry of transformation of mouse epidermis by methylcholanthrene to squamous cell carcinoma. J. Biol. Chem., 155:459, 1944.

Carruthers, C., and Suntzeff, V.: Copper and zinc in epidermal carcinogenesis induced by methylcholanthrene. J. Biol. Chem., 159:647, 1946.

Clowes, G. H. A.: Preliminary note on the action exerted by antagonistic electrolytes on the electrical resistance of emulsion membranes. J. Cancer Res., 4:86, 1919.

Clowes, G. H. A., and Frisbie, W. S.: On the relationship between the rate of growth, age and potassium and calcium content of mouse tumors (adenocarcinoma, Jensen). Am. J. Physiol., 14:173, 1905.

Ebbecke, N.: Über elektrische Hautreizung. Pflügers Arch. Ges. Physiol., 195:300, 1922.

Einthoven, V., and Bijtel, J.: Über Stomleitung durch den menschlichen Körper. Pflügers Arch. Ges. Physiol., 198:439, 1923.

Furch, W.: Leitwertmessungen zur Diagnose maligner Hauttumoren insbesondere des malignen Melanoms. Inaug. Diss., Frankfurt/Main, 1963.

Garten, S.: Beitrage zur Kenntniss des Erregungsvorganges in Nerven und Muskel. Z. Biol. (München), 52:534, 1909.

Gildemeister, M.: Über elektrischen Widerstand, Kapazität und Polarisation der Haut. II. Mitteil, Menschliche Haut. Pflügers Arch. Ges. Physiol., 219:89, 1928.

Graffi, A., and Pisarzewski, A.: Effect of various supplements on respiration and oxydative phosphorylation in the mitochondria of normal and malignant tissues. Acta Biol., Med. Germ., 5:310, 1959.

Grupper, C. H.: Activité antityrosmasique du sérum Note preliminaire sur les possibilités d'un sérodiagnostic du mélanome malin. Bull. Soc. Fr. Dermatol. Syphiligr., 61:145, 1954.

Gulbert, A.: A melanoblastoma korai diagnosisának megerösitése thermodifferentia-, radioaktiv foszfor-és elektrometriás vizsgálatokkal. Börgyögy. Vener. Szle., 44:201, 1968.

Kantner, V.: Electrometry of Skin Tumours, as Described by Melczer, Compared with Histological and Fluorescence Examinations. Čess. Dermatol., 40:245, 1965.

Keller, P.: Über die Wirkungen des ultravioletten Lichtes auf die Haut. Strahlentherapie, 28:152, 1928.

Keller, P.: Untersuchungen an der gesunden und erkrankten Haut. Die Bedeutung des Konzentrationseffektes. Klin. Wochenschr., 8:1081, 1929.

Keller, P.: Grund- und Tonuspotentiale der menschlichen Haut. Arch. Derm. Syph. (Berl.), 162:581, 1931.

Keller, P.: Primäre und sekundäre Lichtreaktionen in der Haut. Klin. Wochenschr., 12:421, 1933.

Keller, P.: Elektrophysiologie der Haut (review). *In* Jadassohn, J.: Handbuch der Haut- und Geschlechtskrankheiten Ergänzungswerk. Normale und pathologische Physiologie der Haut. I/3. Berlin, Springer-Verlag, 1963.

Kiss, J.: Beitrag zur Pathogenese der Strahlenspätschädigungen. Strahlentherapie, 117:474, 1962.

Kiss, J.: A bör elektropermeatiojára ható tényezök. Esztergom. Dissertation for candidacy, 1970.

Kiss, G., and Horváth, I.: Elektromos mérömódszer és készülék a bör malignus burjánzásainak a kimutatására. Börgyögy. Vener. Szle., 45:164, 1969.

Krause, R. A., Storz, H., and Voelkel, A.: Modelluntersuchungen zum Ersatzschaltbild der menschlichen Haut bei Gleichstrommessungen. Ärztl. Wochenschr., 9:444, 1954.

Ledouc, S.: Die Ionen- oder elektrolytische Therapie, Leipzig, 1905.

Leonhardi, G., and Furch, W.: Hautwiderstandmessungen gegenüber Gleichstrom, eine Möglichkeit zur Unterscheidung von benignen und malignen Hauttumoren, insbesondere zur Erkennung des malignen Melanoms. Hautarzt, 15:308, 1964.

Melczer, N.: Melanoblastomák korai felismerése. MTA. V. Orvosi Oszt. Közl., 9:35, 1958.

Melczer, N.: Polarisationsminderung der Epithelzellen während der Carcinogenese. Abhandl. Dtsch. Akad. Wissenschaft. Berliner Symposion über Fragen der Carcinogenese. Klasse f. Med. 1960, 78.

Melczer, N.: Prä-cancerosen und primäre Krebse der Haut. Verh. Ungar. Akad. Wissenschaft. 1961.

Melczer, N.: Zur frühzeitigen Erkennung von Melanoblastomen und primären Hautkrebsen. Seminaire Européen sur la "Prophylaxie du cancer." Inst. Prevent. Profilattico Anti-Malatti Soc. Ed. Anti-canceroso Centro Soc. Studio Precancerosi. Roma. Documenti Di Lavoro, Rapport II., 19:1965.

Melczer, N., and Kiss, J.: Electrotest for detection of early cancerous growth of the skin. Nature (Lond.), 179:117, 1957a.

Melczer, N., and Kiss, J.: Elektrometrie zur frühzeitigen Erkennung der bösartigen epithelialen Umwandlungen der Haut und umgebender Schleimhäute. Hautarzt, 8:395, 1957b.

Melczer, N., and Kiss, J.: Zur frühzeitigen Erkennung von Melanoblastomen. Dermatologica, 117:342, 1958.

Michaelis, L., and Fujita, A.: Untersuchungen über elektrische Erscheinungen und Ionendurchlässigkeit von Membranen. II. Mitteil.: Die Permeabilität der Apfelschale. Biochem. Z., 158:28, 1925. IV. Mitteil.: Potentialdifferenzen und Permeabilität von Kollodiummembranen. Biochem. Z., 161:46, 1925.

Midara, A., and Ormea, F.: Untersuchungen von Haut funktionen in künstichen elektrischen Feld. Hautzart, 11:340, 1960.

Ormea, F.: Fattori meteorologici del bioclima e resistenza elettrica cutanea. Minerva Dermatol. (Torino), Suppl. 72, p. 34, 1959.

Poppe, H., and Frädrich, G.: Excision oder Strahlenbehandlung des Melanoblastoms? Langenbecks Arch. Klin. Chir., 278:50, 1954.

Regelsberger, H.: Der bedingte Reflex und die vegetative Rhythmik des Menschen dargestellt am Elektrodermatogramm. Acta Neuroveg. (Wien), Suppl. 1, 1950.

Rein, H.: Zur Elektrophysiologie der Haut. Z. Biol. (München), 84:118, 1926.

Rein, H.: Elektrophysiologie der Haut (review) 1929. *In* Jadassohn, J.: Handbuch der Haut- und Geschlechtskrankheiten. I/2. Berlin, Springer-Verlag, 1963, pp. 43–90.

Schaefer, H.: Elektrophysiologie. Vol. I.: Allgemeine Elektrophysiologie. Wien, Fr. Deuticke, 1940.

Sinner, W.: Die moderne Diagnostik und Therapie der malignen Melanome (Melanocytoblastoms). Praxis, 51:430, 1962.

Sinner, W.: Beitrag zur Klinik und Therapie der malignen Melanome. Zürcher Erfahrungen an 145 Fällen (1919–1961). Strahlentherapie, 117:18, 1962.

Storz, H., Voelkel, A., and Krause, R. A.: Zur Auswertung von Gleichstrommessungen an der menschlichen Haut. (Elektropermeagramm). Ärztl. Wochenschr., 9:617, 1954.

Sulzberger, M. B., Baer, L. R., and Borota, A.: Do Roentgen-ray treatments as given by skin specialists produce cancers or other sequelae? Follow-up study of dermatologic patients treated with low-voltage Roentgen-rays. Arch. Dermatol., 65:639, 1952.

Szakáll, A.: Über die Eigenschaften, Herkunft und physiologischen Funktionen der für die H-Ionenkonzentration bestimmenden Wirkstoffe in der verhornten Epidermis. Arch. Klin. Exp. Dermatol., 201:331, 1955.

Venkei, T., and Bakos, L.: A melanoblastoma korai felismerése a "thermodifferentia teszt" segitségével. Börgyögy. Vener. Szle., 39:101, 1961.

Waterman, N.: Physikalische-chemische Untersuchungen über das Karzinom. Biochem. Z., 133:535, 1922.

Wolf, J.: Die innere Struktur der Zellen des Stratum desquamativum der menschlichen Epidermis. Z. Mikr.-anat. Forsch., 46:170, 1939.

13

Biochemistry of Skin Cancer

Eliane Le Breton, M.D., and Arlette Jacob, Ph.D.

In a limited sense, the expression "biochemistry of cancer" designates first of all the study of the metabolism of the cells constituting the affected tissue in their precancerous and cancerous stages, comparing the results with those obtained from normal cells of the same type. Such a study obviously includes the constitution and activity of the enzyme systems, whose level of activity reflects the quantitative variations of their constituents.

Even though fundamental, such an outline is complex, reflecting the interactions between the cell layers of the dermis, the mesoderm, and the epidermis, which are particularly interesting in view of the embryonal development of the skin. In addition, we feel that we should go beyond this aspect of the biochemistry of skin cancer.

During the last 20 years a great many investigations and hypotheses have been published on the subject of the mechanism of malignant transformation. All these studies are essentially concerned with biochemistry. Besides, as Bernard, Loeb, and their students have remarked, each apparently static morphologic modification in fact represents corresponding changes in the chemical composition of the cells.

The aspects of general biology which bear upon a study of the process of car-cinogenesis concern for the most part cellular biochemistry and physiology. Studies of cell multiplication, the properties of biologic membranes, deletion of enzyme systems, somatic mutations, hybridization of normal and malignant cells, the relationship between carcinogenesis and embryonal development, and so on imply in general an evaluation of the role and function of nucleic acids or of the macromolecules which play an active role within the cell.

We should start with the impressive results of Jacob and Monod (1963), which marked an important forward step in the formulation and conception of the theories concerning the mechanism of carcinogenesis. Since 1961, the introduction of the concepts of molecular biology formulated with respect to bacteria has appeared to cancer researchers as crucial in bringing their theories up to date, notably those dealing with the "deletions" which had more often than not been held responsible for triggering the malignant transformation more or less directly.

Many cancer investigators have based their theories on the functioning of metabolic pathways, whose induction and regulation were believed to be dependent on operative and regulative genes. These

314

genes differ from structural genes. This theory has been studied particularly with reference to bacterial cells and could also be applied to the activity of animal cells, an hypothesis which Ephrussi favored in 1969, although he had remarked in 1965 that so far no experimental fact had turned up to prove this connection. At any rate, between 1963 and 1965, Pitot, Heidelberger, and Potter revised or abandoned their previous schemas concerning "deletions" in accordance with the facts and theories advanced by Jacob and Monod.

In the second half of this chapter we shall define what was understood by the term "deletion," a mechanism which is still frequently mentioned in an effort to explain carcinogenesis. When discussing the enzyme deletions we shall also deal with the most important aspects of the hybrid cells which have led to the rejection of the concept of deletions such as it had been formulated in 1965.

THE TWO STAGES OF MALIGNANT TRANSFORMATION

Two stages exist for all types of cancer, although they have been best studied and defined in skin cancer, a field in which numerous investigations and studies have been published during the last 30 years. We shall make some brief remarks on this aspect of neoplastic transformation, which is treated in detail in another chapter of this book.

Since the classic investigations by Berenblum (1941), Fridewald and Reus (1944), and Berenblum and Schubik (1947 to 1952) published in Berenblum's journal in 1954, it has been generally accepted that experimental application to animal skin of a carcinogenic polycyclic hydrocarbon leads to a process which can be divided into two separate, often independent phases.

Initiation

Initiation or induction is the result of the penetration and direct contact of the cells with the carcinogenic agent or one of its metabolites; this is a rapid, specific, irreversible phenomenon responsible for the primary lesion of the cell, which in various forms will lead to formation of the neoplasm. During this period of initiation the hydrocarbons first react with the macromolecules, the proteins, and above all the nucleic acids. Initiation can be accomplished with a great number of agents (chemical, physical, or biologic). It leads to the creation of dormant, latent neoplastic cells, which with our present means are indistinguishable from the surrounding normal cells.

Promotion

These latent cells undergo transformation following activation under the influence of endogenous and exogenous factors; the multiplication of cells gives rise to tumoral nodules, the number of which depends on the experimental conditions.

Thus, during the promotion stage, the dormant cell is transformed into a malignant cell. The duration of latency depends on the promoting agent—the most frequently used is croton oil or one of its components—and on the mode of application, as well as on the state of the tissue when the hydrocarbon was applied. There are variations between species and also intraspecific variations according to cell strain and generation, reflecting the intervention of genetic characteristics. Of the experimental species, rabbits and especially mice have given the best results. Within one generation of mice, however, the latency period varies according to age, sex, hormonal function, diet, and environment (whether the animal is kept isolated or in a group, the cage temperature, and the presence or absence of noise that could induce a state of "stress").

In the absence of an appropriate promoting agent and under certain conditions, the dormant cell can escape transformation for the duration of its life; the two stages have often been found to be independent of each other.

In 1969, Boutwell modified this schema and proposed another much more complicated one, which is almost impossible to understand. On the other hand, Hennings and Boutwell claimed in the same year that initiation is the result of an interaction between the carcinogenic hydrocarbon and the DNA molecules. We quote this publication here, because the authors agreed with the opinion of Frei and Ritchie (1964) that frank and lasting hyperplasia facilitates the transformation of latent cells into neoplastic cells. This relatively old theory has been defended by some investigators, whereas others (notably Berenblum and Schubik) consider the hyperplasia to be a secondary phenomenon. This problem is treated in another chapter of this book.

THE TWO SPECIFIC CHARACTERISTICS OF THE CANCER CELL

Once the transformation of the cancer cell is accomplished, it becomes manifest in two characteristic properties, the result of which is the formation of a malignant tumor: *autonomous multiplication* and *modification of the cell surface*, the plasma membrane.

Autonomous Cell Multiplication

This is not subject to the regulating mechanisms that apply to normal multiplication. This problem is more complex than it seems at first sight. Let us state, to begin with, that the tumoral multiplication process and the modification of the cell surface are two interacting phenomena which are difficult to separate. In fact, during embryonal development, growth, and regeneration, the formation of organized tissues is possible because of specific interactions between neighboring cells which regulate their growth and their movements through inhibition of contact, charge phenomena, and hormonal actions. Each factor causing a modification or lack of interaction between the cells will damage the maintenance of ordered structures. The structural changes occurring in tumoral tissues can be expressed in terms of alterations of the cellular surfaces, and the result would be the so-called "anarchical" multiplication of the neoplastic cells. They

are freed from the restraints which for normal cells play a functional role with respect to the level of activity which the cells are to reach.

These two specific characteristics of the transformed cell are, as we know, hereditary and are preserved during the multiplication of the cancer cell, independent of the carcinogenic agent (chemical, physical, or biologic) which caused them. This transformation includes somatic mutations, which we shall discuss in the second part of this chapter. These mutations can be the result of alterations of various metabolic pathways, but the final impact will always bear on the same group of genes. Consequently, independent of the agent, there are cellular alterations in certain structures, which will more or less rapidly give rise to these specific mutations, and which imply an involvement of DNA.

Cellular multiplication is always a dynamic phenomenon whose characteristics vary according to the type of multiplication. Each living cell, even in a state of rest, combines multiple syntheses whose rhythm and interdependence vary with the type of the cell and the conditions in which it is placed. There is a renewal of various constituents, which have a different turnover rate, but the result is always a stationary equilibrium or homeostasis of the adult cell. If the syntheses—anabolism—are more rapid than the catabolic reactions, the cell grows.

Although the growth of the cancer cell is not bound by the normal regulation processes, it is nevertheless linked to the growth of the cells surrounding the tumor. This fact has often been mentioned, and in certain cases the repercussions of the neoplastic growth on the whole organ have been established. In the liver of a rat with hepatoma, for instance, we find functional modifications and abnormal enzymatic activity in the lobes which macroscopically and microscopically appear normal: this is the stage which we can call "precancerous." These modifications are related to the hepatomegaly caused by the tumor through the inability of the neighboring lobes to take over the hepatic functions to the extent required by the organism. This means that the tumoral growth modifies the behavior of the entire organ. We shall not discuss this aspect of cancerous multiplication here, but we would like to stress two important features.

(1) Not all cell types show neoplasia. Let us briefly recall that those cells which have lost their division potential do not undergo cancerous transformation, as for instance neurons from the moment in which their number becomes fixed; they grow in size during the growth of the individual, but there is no division and no cancerization of these "eternal" cells (Bizzozero). The same applies to the striated muscle fibers. The cells which undergo cancerization are the *labile* cells of the epithelium and the *stable* cells of those organs which have preserved their division potential. There is no doubt that this problem is related to embryonal development and to cell differentiation. We shall take this up again later.

(2) It is often thought that cancerous growth evolves very rapidly and that tumors present a higher rate of cell multiplication. There are some types of neoplasms for which this is true, but there are also very rapid normal growths, whose rate of evolution is higher than that of the most rapidly multiplying cancers, such as the growth of embryonal tissues in certain stages of their development and especially the rate at which syntheses take place in the phenomenon called compensatory hypertrophy, which is provoked by the ablation of an important part of an organ. The best known example of this is hepatic regeneration in the rat, triggered by the ablation of two thirds of the lobes (Frayssinet, 1962); within 72 hours, the hypertrophy and hyperplasia of the cells reaches a rate much higher than that of rapidly growing neoplasms.

Specific Biochemical Characteristics of Normal and Malignant Growth. We shall refer again to the rat liver tissue, because this is the medium in which the separation of the cellular structures has been obtained with the greatest precision, and because hepatoma is one of the cancers that we know most about. The results presented are taken from Frayssinet (in LeBreton et al., 1963), who compared normal and cancerous growth rates of hepatic tissue, a study which could be made only under two conditions: (1) the studied tumors must be close to the original tissue, and they must be free from degeneration or necrosis due to secondary lesions; i.e., they must be hepatomas which are not undifferentiated and still consist of hepatocytes; (2) the investigator has to have access to normal growing tissue. Frayssinet worked with a liver affected by compensatory hypertrophy triggered by ablation of an important part of the organ, on one hand, and with fetal livers, in which apart from proliferative factors there is a progressive differentiation, on the other.

We mentioned above the quantitative importance and the rate of cell growth during compensatory hypertrophy: within 48 hours the tissue which remains in situ doubles its weight. The lobes increase in size; there is no formation of new lobules, but there is an increase in the volume of the lobes. The architecture of the whole is not modified, and each cell type evolves according to its own rhythm.

In the last analysis, compensatory hypertrophy is a rather pure mitotic process, in which neither differentiation nor organization play a role.

If hepatic nuclei are separated from cytoplasm, the part affected by cellular hypertrophy and hyperplasia becomes visible. Graphs of the evolution of the synthesis of the different elements plotted against time show that synthesis of nuclear RNA is rapid. It doubles before DNA synthesis even starts. It is possible to observe the size and number of the nucleoli before cell division.

On the basis of this information, let us examine the differences between these three types of growth. Variations of a cell constituent are expressed in relation to the fixed value of DNA content per cell, and we obtain the DNA content per cell by averaging the quantities contained in the different constituents. Ratios of interest are cytoplasmic RNA to total DNA and nuclear RNA to total DNA. RNA is linked directly to protein synthesis, through which it controls the presence and the activity of the enzyme systems which control the life of the cell. Variations in the first ratio reflect the synthetic ability of the cell and give an idea of the degree of cell differentiation and of the intensity of the work going on in cells with a given enzyme equipment. The relation of nuclear RNA to total DNA varies essentially with the mitotic activity of the cell.

In the liver of the normal adult rat (taken as a basis for comparison), the first of the two ratios varies between 2.5 and 3.5 to 1, and the second varies between 0.15 and 0.21 to 1. In order to separate the experimental facts and permit comparisons, Frayssinet established a graph on which we would like to comment briefly.

During compensatory hypertrophy, the two ratios increase simultaneously; the functional hepatic activity becomes ever greater, and there are numerous mitoses.

During fetal (and postnatal) development, when rapid multiplication and progressive differentiation take place, a regular elevation of the ratio of cytoplasmic RNA to DNA is found only during the developmental period, whereas the relation of nuclear RNA to DNA remains elevated during all of the growth period.

In the case of neoplastic *not undifferentiated* livers, there is an elevation of the second ratio, whereas the first remains the same.

Consequently, all normal or cancerous hyperplastic processes provoke an elevation of the nuclear RNA per cell, which is accompanied by an elevation of the cytoplasmic RNA only if cell divisions are the result of a stimulus of cytoplasmic origin. Multiplications occurring in a tumor depend only on *nuclear* phenomena (mitoses), a fact which coincides with the autonomous character of this type of multiplication, which is largely independent of functional factors.

We believe that this distinction between the growth of normal and cancerous cells is the only one that has been established until now and that it is capable of yielding much information.

Modifications of the Cell Surface (Plasma Membrane)

The modifications appear during malignant transformation owing to the more or less total disappearance of contact inhibition. This disappearance is related to a structural, architectural change of the membrane and implies the acquisition by the neoplastic cell of certain specific characteristics, whose importance has always been noted by cancer investigators. The absence of contact inhibition between the cells is one of the principal reasons why cancerous multiplication is not controlled by normal restrictions. This phenomenon has also been studied by embryologists, notably Piwein, since 1944. They found that at the beginning of embryonal development, during the first stages of cell differentiation, contact inhibition is reduced, but it evolves rapidly so we can observe simultaneously the establishment of contact inhibition and modifications of cell adhesion and of the histotypical aggregation of the cells, which becomes manifest after dissociation of the cells at the beginning of postembryonal life. In short, we find phenomena that are inverse to those characterizing cancerous transformation.

As far as the malignant cells are concerned, a diminution of normal cell adhesion develops and manifests itself in two ways: invasive character and transplantability, which leads to the formation of *metastases.* The cancerous cells abandon the tumor and through the bloodstream or the lymphatic system settle down in other tissues. After a variable period of time, the proliferation of these cells can give rise to secondary tumors. This characteristic of transplantability has been chosen as a malignancy test; after a graft or an injection of cultured cells, there is a characteristic multiplication. In this context the studies by Toolan (1957) on cellular compatibility and the effects of radiation and cortisone should be mentioned, for they have permitted the creation of specific conditions necessary to avoid defensive immune reactions in the case of heterogenous grafts.

Weiss (1951) and Andrew have isolated a fact which ought to be mentioned here, because it clearly outlines the differences in the behavior of cultured normal and cancerous cells. When injected into an embryo, normal cells diffuse and fix themselves through the circulatory system *exclusively* at the level of a tissue homologous to that of their origin; cancer cells, on the contrary, fix themselves at the level of various tissues and organs, without evidence of any specific tropism.

In their now classic publications (1950 to 1966) Abercrombie, Ambrose, and their collaborators summarized their observations on cultures of fibroblasts and epithelial cells, in comparison with the behavior of homologous cells from sarcomas or carcinomas: monocellular layers on one hand, and agglomerations of round cells, on the other. There is a definite suppression of contact inhibition, but these phenomena are more complex, since even during the mitoses of normal cells contact inhibition is suppressed; this would favor a relation between cell division and contact inhibition.

Malcolm and Steinberg have also studied the properties of the membranes of cultured cells and have found the decrease in adhesion and the increase of inhibition to be parallel.

Coman and his associates obtained interesting results between 1944 and 1960. From the beginning of his experiments, he focused his attention on the adhesion of cell surfaces after the separation and dispersion of cells from malignant or benign tumors or normal tissues. He found that the force necessary to obtain this separation is two times weaker for *malignant* tumors. This reduced adhesion constitutes the physical basis for malignancy and its manifestations. He theorized that the reduced adhesion may be due to the low Ca^{++} content of the cancerous cells, which would reduce the force of attraction between the cells.

Of direct importance in the field of skin cancer are the findings of Coman (1960), that one hour after application of 7,12-dimethylbenzanthracene to the ear of a rabbit, the cells of tissues affected by the hydrocarbon show reduced adhesion, whereas there is no modification of adhesion if the polycyclic carbon applied is not carcinogenic. Measurements in an electrophoretic field show that cancerous cells are more mobile than their normal homologues. According to the author this brings to mind the role of sialic acid and the phospholipids in these phenomena at the level of the membranes. Coman also states that the permeability by large molecules is greater in cancerous cells.

We agree with a number of authors that the modifications found in the pericellular membrane concern in reality all intercellular membranes. This fact has been demonstrated for the membranes of the mitochondria, whose permeability has been studied in normal and neoplastic hepatic cells. DeRobertson studied the continuity of the microsomal membranes (endoplasmic network) with the plasma membrane; it seems improbable that during the course of cancerization the microsomal membranes would not undergo the same changes as the plasma membrane. The biochemical and biophysical study of these membranes is difficult, but the investigations under way should furnish important results.

Weiss (1951) believed that better information on the alterations of the membranes due to the loss of contact inhibition, evasion, and transplantability of neoplastic cells would be important to help us understand the mechanism of cancerization. This opinion is borne out by the results mentioned above and strongly supported by findings on the architecture of the biologic membranes made during the last few years.

Present Concepts Regarding the Membranes. The biologic membranes separate the media and isolate the cellular compartments in which metabolic reactions corresponding to definite functions take place. In order for a cell to live, its membranes must be permeable to permit exchanges of metabolites in both directions. The membranes must have a certain flexibility, since they are subject to a number of movements, and at the same time a stability and permanence apart from the sites which show a controlled permeability.

There are, as a matter of fact, two types of membranes which are totally different in their structural and functional characteristics. The first are stable, lamellar membranes, which have been thoroughly studied by Danielli and Davson since 1935. Their stability has been confirmed by electron microscopic findings. These studies of the static membranes concerned the myelin sheath of the Schwann cells, which serves as electrical insulation against the nerve impulse in the axon. Their constitution explains their rigidity: they consist of an association of proteins and lipids, phospholipids, and cholesterol in equimolecular quantities. The characteristics of the molecules suggest compact associations with a high energy of interaction. This energy varies with the nature of the fatty acids of the phospholipids; it is high for those with a long, saturated chain.

Nevertheless, this type of membrane and this concept do not agree with the metabolic activity and the role that most of them fulfill, notably the pericellular, microsomal, mitochondrial, and nuclear membranes. Investigations carried out during the last couple of years have led to a completely different dynamic concept, based on the existence of globular structures or a micellium, postulated by Sjostrand (1959), Lucy (1968), Pascaud (1964–1970), and others. At the same time, Emmelot and Benedetti used the term "mosaic membrane" to sum up their experimental observations. This concept favors a functional specialization of the various globular or mosaic units and a great plasticity both on the surface and in the deep portions of the membrane, which is reflected in its movements and enzyme activity.

The phospholipids and the proteins are obligatory components, and the cholesterol is a constant component. Without entering into detail let us just restate that the phospholipids have a double polarity—hydrophilic and hydrophobic—and that their negative and positive groups establish an interaction with the protein-charged groups. Their role in connection with the mitochondrial membranes has been thoroughly studied. Pascaud explained in 1964 the transfer of fatty acids through the membranes, describing the specialization of the units in the different selective transfers. The discontinuity between the lipoprotein units has led researchers to a simple concept of pores and their functioning. The role of bivalent ions and especially of Ca^{++} is essential in the maintenance of associations of connections between the units, in which the phospholipids play an important role. Due to the calcium bridges, these connections would be reversible.

Since the units that make up the mosaic membranes are susceptible to movement and to renewal, the membranes could probably acquire different structures according to physiologic needs and go from a globular, dynamic architecture to one similar to the inert lamellar architecture.

As Pascaud wrote in 1970, the functional adaptation would then be the result of a dynamic equilibrium between these diverse structures in which the lipids participate in a definite molecular ecology setting and associate with the proteins.

We have insisted on these concepts regarding the membranes because of their close connection with the phenomena of the alteration of cell surfaces in the course of malignant transformation.

OTHER SPECIFIC GENERAL CHARACTERISTICS OF THE NEOPLASTIC CELL

Cancer researchers have been trying for a long time to understand the various phenomena linked with malignant transformation. These slowly develop during cancerization under the influence of the carcinogenic agent, until they finally lead to lesions which are cytologically and biochemically characteristic. In 1961, it was impossible to say that there were any special characteristics of neoplastic cells, according to Oberling and Bernhard (1961), who discussed the problem in two articles on the cancer cell. They concluded that, even with the most modern techniques, it was impossible to establish "a morphological characteristic which would be truly specific for cancer cells," but distinguished nevertheless a tendency of tumor cells toward a more simple organization ("dedifferentiation" or anaplasia). Le Breton and Moulé (1966) affirmed in an article on the biochemistry that as long as investigations dealt with cancers whose cells present multiple secondary lesions provoked by a variety of agents and covering up the characteristic modifications of the neoplastic transformation, it would be impossible to find out which of these modifications were crucial. Since 1951, Le Breton and associates have been trying to separate lesions provoked by an unbalanced diet, not adapted to the total needs of the rat. Great care has had to be taken to avoid not only infections but also conditions that might disturb the hormonal equilibrium. The toxicity of the carcinogenic agent used also had to be taken into consideration. In short, studies could be made exclusively on "pure" cancers which were exempt from all concomitant lesions, and for biopsies tumoral nodules had to be used whose homogeneity was guaranteed by their size.

The above gives an idea of the theoretic and practical importance which would be attributed to any evidence of a specific initial lesion.

Under these conditions, the researchers obtained well-differentiated nodules with a functional parenchyma similar to that of the livers of control rats. If the results presented in the literature were so widely divergent, it is because this principle was not respected. Since 1963, research done by Morris and associates has obtained numerous graftable hepatomas capable of giving rise to metastases according to the prototype of hepatoma No. 5123, classified as a hepatoma with "minimal deviations." An analysis of the properties of this neoplasm revealed that, morphologically and biochemically, the cells were well differentiated and very close to normal hepatocytes. We thought it necessary to restate this conclusion briefly, because even today many authors believe that dedifferentiation is a specific characteristic of cancerization.

This attitude was built on two dogmas which had resisted all technical progress for decades: the theory of Warburg on the mechanism of carcinogenesis, on the one hand, and the theory of Greenstein on the numerous deletions occurring in all types of cancers, on the other. It is because of the predominance of the thoughts of these two investigators that in 1968–70 numerous deletions and dedifferentiation are mentioned as attributes of the cancer cell.

The theory formulated by Warburg in 1924 concerning the *origin* of cancer can be explained in short as follows: an irreversible alteration of cell respiration leads to a significant increase in *aerobic glycolysis* in order to maintain the energy level of the cell. This glycolysis has to be significant, because *oxidation* of the glucose molecule leads to the formation of 38 ATP molecules, whereas glycolysis creates only 2. This process ends either in the death or the cancerization of the cell. This theory has been prevalent for a long time, as many authors could observe the decrease in respiration and the increase in glycolysis. Nevertheless, after 1932 a trend of contrary opinions began to take hold, and in 1956 Weinhouse presented an explanatory constructive critique of the phenomenon.

At the same time, laboratory experiments by Jacob and LeBreton showed that, in the normal liver and in hepatoma, glycolysis is the same. During the precancerous stages, aerobic glycolysis of the nucleus increases and makes up a more important part of the total glycolysis.

In our opinion, the experiments of Morris and associates described below with the slow growth hepatoma No. 5123 presented conclusive evidence that the *increase in aerobic glycolysis is not a characteristic of the neoplastic cell.*

According to the theory of Greenstein (1954), morphologic dedifferentiation represents a biochemical, enzymatic dedifferentiation. According to this author, a comparison of the enzymatic equipment of cancerous tissue and its normal homologue shows the disappearance of a certain number of functional activities, which leads to suppression of the differentiation characteristics that were present in the original tissue. Moreover, in a given enzyme system, the variations between the various types of tumors are always less marked than those present in normal tissue. Biochemically speaking, one would tend to believe that there is one type of enzyme system that all the different tumors have in common. Greenstein and many others have shown, for instance, that in liver tumors a great number of functional systems are lost. This was remarkably well demonstrated in the hepatoma of Nonkoff (1957), which was subsequently studied by a number of authors; an examination of ultrafine sections of this hepatoma shows, however, that many structures are quantitatively diminished. This example is contrary to the type 5123 hepatomas of Morris. An analysis by the biochemists collaborating with Morris established that the disappearance of enzymes and biochemical and morphologic dedifferentiation are concepts in need of being revised, and that apart from some metabolic enzymes especially studied by Pitot, few deviations can actually be demonstrated. We feel that we should not forget the fact that all these determinations were made on grafted hepatomas. Pitot and Morris arrive at the conclusion that there is "no lesion in any of these systems, and that the alterations in activity observed might be explained by representative mechanisms, which are partly or totally inoperative in neoplastic cells."

The above shows that some of these approaches are inconclusive, and in the second part of this chapter we shall see the importance of the intervention of the nucleic acids in triggering the cancerization process; we still have to discover the stages in which their metabolism is irreversibly upset for certain genes. At any rate, it is absolutely necessary that research be done on tumors as exempt as possible from nonspecific lesions if the results are to have any meaning. In this case the tumors do not consist of dedifferentiated cells.

SKIN CHEMISTRY AND METABOLISM

The skin is a tissue important because of its mass, and complex as to its origin and its constitution. It makes up 8 percent of the total mass of the body; quantitatively it is surpassed only by the muscles (50 percent of the body weight) and the skeleton (16 percent). The functions of the skin are regulation of body temperature, production of vitamin D and, above all, protection against the external physical and chemical environment.

Among the components of the skin, collagen, which quantitatively is the most important, representing 70 percent of the dry weight, and the mucopolysaccharides (7 percent of the dry weight) have the capacity to capture or reject water, which explains the importance of the cutaneous tissue to water metabolism. Moreover, the skin retains from 18 to 40 percent of the body water. Thus the skin intervenes in thermal regulation as well as in the elimination of numerous components: water at the rate of 50 g. per sq. cm. per minute, proteins at the rate of 0.1 g. per sq. cm. per minute, and salts at the rate of 10 to 20 mg. of potassium chloride per day. The loss of nitrogen is negligible.

The skin consists of several parts distributed in three layers, which are, from the innermost to the exterior, the hypodermis, the dermis, and the epidermis. The *hypodermis* is a fatty tissue which separates the subcutaneous tissue from the dermis.

It is subdivided by areas of connective and elastic tissue which demarcate lobules filled with adipose cells, and it is irrigated by blood vessels which are more voluminous than those of the dermis. There are also sweat glands and hair follicle roots in the hypodermis.

The *dermis* is of mesodermic origin and furnishes physical and nutritional support for the epidermis. It is formed by a gelatinous base substance which envelops the connective tissue fibers (collagen, reticulum, and elastin) between which blood and lymph vessels and nerves are disposed. The dermis is connected with the epidermis through a zone of dermoepidermal junction of mesodermic origin.

The *epidermis* is 0.1 to 0.3 mm. thick, of ectodermic origin, and epithelial in nature. It consists of four layers, the three lowest of which form the living epidermis. The uppermost or horny layer constitutes the dead epidermis. The nerve fibers terminate in the lower epidermis. There are no blood vessels in the epidermis, which is nourished through diffusion of nutritives from the underlying dermis.

During their migration toward the exterior, the epidermal cells penetrate the overlying malpighian layer. Here they become subject to the action of enzymes which leaves them dehydrated and flattened to form the dead horny layer. We have to distinguish between the lower, compact horny layer, which is strongly joined to the underlying layer, and the upper horny layer, in which the dead cells lose their adhesion and desquamate. In man it takes the cells 27 days to pass from the basal layer to the desquamating horny layer. There are also appendages belonging to the epidermis: the hair follicles, sebaceous glands, and eccrine and apocrine sweat glands.

Morphologic Constitution

In order to better understand the metabolism of the normal and neoplastic cutaneous tissue and its functions, we shall have to deal in some detail with its morphologic constitution.

The *dermis* is a connective tissue, which represents a barrier against infectious agents and plays an important role in wound healing.

The dermis is not homogeneous and consists from the interior toward the outside of (1) the *deep dermis* or reticular layer, consisting of large horizontal bundles of collagen fibers and penetrating into the hypodermis; (2) the *middle dermis* with oblique or horizontal collagen bundles; and (3) the *superficial or papillar dermis*, which has a loose texture and is relatively rich in cells.

The structure of the dermis is formed by three types of interlacing fibers characterized by their components. *Collagen fibers* make up the most important part of the dermal connective tissue. They are arranged in bundles forming crisscrossing undulating strands; they consist of fibrils and the fibrils again are constituted by protofibrils. Thin and sinuous *elastic fibers* are the second type, and finally there are *reticulin fibers*, which form a fragile net and are colored through silver impregnation. They are found near the surface of the dermis, close to the zone of the dermoepidermal junction and around vessels and sudoriparous coils.

The cells disseminated throughout the dermis are of two types: dermal connective cells (fibroblasts, histiocytes, and some mast cells) and a very small number of cells of blood origin (lymphocytes, polymorphonuclear leukocytes, and plasmacytes).

The *zone of dermoepidermal junction* appears in the form of an undulating line. It assures adhesion and metabolic exchange between the dermis and the epidermis. It consists of two elements of dermal origin, netlike reticulin fibers, and mucopolysaccharides, and it is traversed by the appendages of the epidermis.

The *epidermis* is a stratified squamous epithelium protecting the tissues against the external physical and chemical environment through a continuous proliferation of living epidermal cells which die to form the external horny keratin layer.

The epidermis consists of several layers which from the interior toward the outside are (1) the thin *germinative layer*, in which cell divisions and melanogenesis take place; (2) the *stratum spinosum* or malpighian layer with polyhedric cells which are rich in tonofibrils. The tonofibrils consist of a fibrous protein, or prekeratin, which is rich in sulfhydryl groups but does not contain cystine, and which is formed by peptides rich in glycine (30 percent) and in serine (20 percent); (3) the *stratum granulosum*, the cells of which are charged with *keratohyaline*. In this layer, the —SH groups increase and —S—S groups appear; and (4) the *stratum corneum*, formed by dead cells which have lost their nucleus and their cytoplasm; they practically consist of nothing but *keratin* surrounding lipidic deposits. This layer is rich in —S—S groups. Only the first three layers constitute the living epidermis. In the epidermis we find two types of cells: melanocytes and keratinocytes.

Chemical Constitution and Metabolism

The complexity of the cutaneous tissue and the existence of the different layers, which differ in their chemical constitution and function, suggest that there are metabolisms corresponding to the dermis and to the epidermis, respectively, so that we would do well to study them separately. Since metabolism depends on the chemical constitution of the tissue, however, we shall briefly examine the latter before concentrating on the metabolism.

THE DERMIS

Taken as a whole, the dermis consists, in terms of its dry weight, of 70 percent collagen, 7.1 percent mucopolysaccharides, and 2 percent elastin; it contains important quantities of proteins, water (18.4 percent of the total body water), and electrolytes. Let us examine the components of the dermis successively:

Fiber Components of the Connective Tissue. *Collagen* is a scleroprotein and makes up the fibrillar portion of the connective tissue. It constitutes 72 percent of the dermis or 75 percent of the dry weight of human skin and 18 to 30 percent of its volume (6 g. of collagen/g N). The volume of collagen in the skin increases with age, although the mass of collagen per unit of surface area diminishes.

Collagen is characterized by its high content of glycine (32 to 35 percent), proline (11 to 14 percent), hydroxyproline (10 to 13 percent), and hydroxylysine; the percentages of the other amino acids are relatively low, particularly those of tyrosine, histidine, and methionine, and collagen does not contain any cystine. The amino acids are arranged on three chains of polypeptides forming a triple helix around a common axis and linked by transverse H bridges between the $-NH_2$ of the glycine and the $-COOH$ groups of the other amino acids.

Collagen contains a high proportion of water, 79 percent of which is free water and 21 percent is strongly bound. This water is bound through the mucopolysaccharides present in the dermis and associated with the collagen, a fact which explains the strong mobilization of water through the connective tissue and especially through the dermis. This water movement is associated with the movements of Na^+, K^+, Ca^{++}, and Mg^{++}.

During the formation of collagen, lysine and proline are hydroxylated only after their incorporation into the peptide chain of the collagen through a specific hydroxylase, which is contained in the fibroblasts and uses dissolved atmospheric oxygen. This oxygen is activated through a transfer of electrons in the presence of a cofactor containing Fe^{++} and ascorbic acid which yields electrons (Vitto, 1970). This explains the lesions of the connective tissue observed in scurvy patients. Barnes and his collaborators (1970) found that in scorbutic guinea pigs the elastine and the collagen were deficient in hydroxyproline and that there was an accumulation of peptides of low molecular weight, rich in proline and deficient in hydroxyproline.

In its original form or organized in fibers, the collagen is not degraded by a proteolytic enzyme with the exception of *collagenase*, a specific protease. Some of the epithelial cells in the skin synthesize this collagenase by degrading the collagen into amino acids and peptides, which are eliminated through the urine; part of the amino acids are used again, whereas the hydroxyproline is degraded and used as a source of energy.

Collagen is quite stable, with a half-life of 20 days in adult skin. This rate of molecule renewal is much higher in growing organisms and during tissue changes (metamorphosis or cicatrization).

During aging and under prolonged sunlight exposure, the dermal collagen degenerates and the skin slackens.

Reticulum represents only 0.4 percent of the dry weight of human skin and consists of fine, undulating fibers with few anastomoses in contrast to the collagen fibers. These fibers stain with silver and are located especially around blood vessels and hair follicles close to the epidermis. Collagenous reticulin fibers can be found also in the basal membrane and in regenerating connective tissue. Some authors believe that these reticulin fibers are the true precursors or young forms of collagen; they do not represent a permanent structure in the mature collagen bundles like the persisting reticulum. It is nevertheless difficult to distinguish the permanent reticulum fibers and the transitory reticulin of the young connective tissues, since both are argyrophilic because of the large quantities of sugar associated with them.

Reticulum and collagen have the same amino acid composition, but they differ in their content of polysaccharides (4.2 percent and 0.55 percent, respectively), of lipids (10.9 percent and traces), and of sulfur (2 percent and 0.5 percent, respectively). Several collagenases digest both the reticulum and the reticulin.

Elastin is responsible for the elasticity of normal skin, although in man it represents only 4 percent of the dry weight and 1 percent of the fresh weight of the skin. It is a yellow, retractable substance, with a fibrillar, membranous, or fibrillomembranous structure that is arranged in the form of a net with tridimensional meshes and without loose ends.

Elastin is a scleroprotein which is difficult to dissolve completely in neutral solvents. The principal amino acids constituting elastin are glycine, which is by far the most abundant (20 to 23 percent), alanine, valine, proline, and leucine; elastin differs from collagen in its lesser content of arginine, lysine, glutamic and aspartic acids, and especially of hydroxyproline, which accounts for only 2 percent of the amino acids in elastin. This protein contains two lysine derivatives: desmosine and isodesmosine, which are tetra-amino acid–tetracarboxylics.

It is generally supposed that the fibroblast at first forms a soluble proelastin, which is subsequently incorporated into the transverse binding structure of the elastic fibers.

Ground Substance. Collagen and elastin fibers as well as cells are embedded in this substance, which is one of the most important components of the hematoparenchymatic barrier which regulates the flow of simple (salts, water) or complex (hormones, bacterial toxins) substances.

The ground substance is a porous jelly of variable consistency, which contains water, all mineral ions, most plasma proteins, and polysaccharides in solution: hyaluronic acid, and compounds of mucopolysaccharide-protein and chondroitin sulfate. The two major components of polysaccharides are hyaluronic acid and dermatan sulfate, the absolute concentrations of which in the human dermis are on the order of 0.05 percent of the fresh weight each.

Thanks to histochemistry it has been possible to isolate hyaluronic acid in the intercellular and interfibrillar spaces of the dermis and to demonstrate that dermatan sulfate is associated with the collagen fibers of the connective tissue. This is the reason why hyaluronic acid is more abundant in the lax connective tissue of the subpapillar layer of the dermis than in the reticular layer, whereas the concentration of dermatan sulfate grows with the degree of penetration into the skin. It is associated with the coarse collagen fibers, which explains why the ratio of hyaluronic acid to chondroitin sulfate diminishes in cases of myxedema, while the fibrous elements of the skin increase.

Quantitatively, it has been shown that human skin contains 43 to 75 mg. of mucopolysaccharides per 100 g. of fresh weight. This concentration decreases with age. Actually, the concentration of hexosamine in the skin is 2 mg. per g. of dry weight in a 6-cm. fetus, and 6.7 mg. per g. of dry weight in an adult up to 50 years; after that there is a progressive decrease down to the lowest value of 0.4 mg. per g. in a 90 year old man. The same decrease can be observed for the hexuronic acid content of the mucopolysaccharides, which is 8 mg. per g. of dry weight for a 7-cm. embryo, 4 mg. per g. at birth, and 1 mg. per g. at age 90.

This variation in the content of the components is not limited to man; it has been observed also in pigs, where the ratios of these components are modified in the course of the animal's development (Meyer et al., 1956; Loewi and Meyer, 1958):

	embryo	*adult*
hyaluronic acid	78 percent	30 percent
chondroitin-6-sulfate	17 to 20 percent mucopolysaccharides	0
dermatan sulfate	4 to 12 percent	64 percent

The hyaluronic acid content probably diminishes in all connective tissues in the course of maturation and aging, contributing in this manner to the decrease in water content and the turgescence of the tissues. This decrease is explained by the fact that the polysaccharides are formed in the mastocytes of the connective tissue, which decrease with age.

Since many studies have been done on rat skin, it has been possible to determine its components. In 1961, Schiller found a heparin content of 25 mg. per 100 g. of dry skin and found that the rat was the only animal that contained heparin in its cutaneous tissue. Apart from this, all known sulfated mucopolysaccharides are found, with hyaluronic acid and dermatan sulfate present in major proportions (Schiller, 1966).

In the embryo skin an α_2-glycoprotein has been isolated which is very similar to fetuin. It is rich in glucides and occurs in a quantity of 5 mg. per 100 g. of fresh skin.

In day-old rats (Hardingham and Phelps, 1970) the glycosaminoglycans of the skin contain 56 percent hyaluronic acid, 15.6 percent dermatan sulfate, and 9.1 percent chondroitin-6-sulfate, plus small quantities of chondroitin-4-sulfate, heparan sulfate, and heparin. Prodi (1963 and 1966) found that the total glycosaminoglycans extracted from rat skin between two and nine months of age amount to 300 g. per g. of dry skin.

Hardingham and Phelps (1968) showed that after parturition the precursors of glycosaminoglycans are already to be found in mouse skin. The rates of synthesis per gram of dry weight are 1.5 and 0.24 millimicromoles per minute for UDP-N-acetylhexosamine and UDP glucuronic acid, and the average time of the turnover of the total tissue mucopolysaccharides is about five days.

The permeability of the large molecule connective tissue is modified by treating the perfused tissues with substances which act on the components of the ground substance. The mucopolysaccharides of the connective tissue have a very active metabolism, which is slowed down in diabetics, a fact which might be responsible for the greater susceptibility of these patients to infection and for the slowdown in cicatrization. This slowdown is due to an insulin insufficiency.

There are also other hormones which act on the metabolism of mucopolysaccharides. An injection of estradiol, for instance, given to mice at the rate of 5 mg. per g. during 12 days, raises the hexosamine content from 50 mg. to 110 mg. per 100 g. of dry weight. Testosterone activates the synthesis of hyaluronic acid but does not influence chondroitin sulfate. In cases of hypothyroidism, these two components are more or less doubled.

Vitamins also act on the metabolism of mucopolysaccharides. Certain vitamin deficiencies affect the components which contain the hexosamine. In the scorbutic guinea pig, for instance, the uronic acid content is 22.4 mg. per 100 g. of fresh skin instead of 27.2 Ross and Benditt observed in animals with scurvy an accumulation of mucoproteins and a marked decline in collagen synthesis during wound healing. The fibroblasts of these animals do secrete mucoproteins, but they are unable to elaborate the essential polypeptide chains of collagen. Collagen synthesis picks up again after ingestion of vitamin C.

Vitamin A deficiency is associated with hyperkeratosis. Treatment with vitamin A is accompanied by a thickening of the epidermis, especially of the granular layer, and by a slowdown in keratin formation.

Lipid Metabolism. According to Brooks and coworkers (1963, 1966), the dermis is characterized by a specific, active lipogenesis. Fibroblasts and mast cells synthesize 18-carbon fatty acids or those with a shorter chain and certain monoenes. The synthesis of fatty acids with a chain of 18-C or less and of those with chains of 20-C or more and the diene synthesis (eicosanoic acid and a dienoic acid which is not linoleic acid) take place in the papillary reticulum. Moreover, the papillary reticulum is the only place where there is an important synthesis of squalene, from which the sterols are derived.

Different bodies are synthesized, depending on the presence or absence of dermal cells in the papillary reticulum: if there is no epidermis, more squalene is formed, whereas in the presence of epidermis, acetate incorporates in the sterols, particularly Δ^7-cholesterol, rather than in the squalene.

Modifications Observed in Tumor Growths. Various authors have pointed out the importance of collagenase in tumor growth. Strauch and collaborators (1968) observed that, in cultures of cells from higher animals or of HeLa cells, collagen and collagenase activity are inversely proportional.

Collagenase activity increases in young populations in the multiplication stage and is equally increased in cancers of the mammary gland, where it favors tumor growth by digesting collagen (Langer et al., 1968). Seilern-Aspang et al. (1969) also found a marked collagenase activity in epithelium after painting with benzene and a carcinogen; according to these authors, the upset of the equilibrium between dermal collagen synthesis and collagenase synthesis in the epidermis and the resulting increase of collagenase synthesis are the cause of the malignant growth of the epidermal cells.

Similarly, a decrease in collagen synthesis brought about by corticosterone implants would be responsible for the skin cancers produced in 50 percent of the salamanders treated (Seilern-Aspang, 1969). The ascorbic acid deficiency which reduces collagen synthesis, also favors the formation of skin cancers (Wirl and Seilern-Aspang, 1970).

These experiments confirm that the proliferation and differentiation of the epidermis during embryogenesis and re-generation depend on the structure of the connective tissue; this depends on the collagen synthesis, which in turn is dependent on the ascorbic acid.

As far as the modifications of the ground substance of the dermis are concerned, when painting rabbit skin with 9,10-dimethyl-1,2-benzanthracene (DMBA), Prodi (1963) observed that (1) the hexosamine content of the mucopolysaccharides is little modified in relation to tissue weight, but notably modified in relation to skin surface area; (2) hyaluronic acid is clearly increased and chondroitin sulfate is markedly decreased; there is an increase in the ratio of glucosamine to galactosamine in the mucopolysaccharides; and (3) the fibrous structures of the dermis are totally modified. If the animal is treated only with croton oil, an increase in hyaluronic acid can be observed, which is smaller than with DMBA, and there is little change in the fibrous structure. Croton oil maintains a relative integrity in the deeper portions of the dermis, despite the hyperplasia and the increased thickness of the skin.

Consequently, the changes in the mucopolysaccharides which occur during carcinogenesis in the dermis are not specific, since they are found also in hyperplasia, but they are indispensable for the neoplastic process, because they create the environment which permits epithelial proliferation. The large proportion of hyaluronic acid in comparison with chondroitin sulfate, which has also been observed in the fetus and newborn, is a sign of immaturity. All these modifications of the mucopolysaccharides occur in the promotion stage, which takes place in the dermis.

Epidermis

The amino acid composition of the epidermis varies depending on whether we consider the epidermis as a whole or the horny layer. This is especially clear in the case of cystine and hydroxyproline, two amino acids which play an important role in the keratinization process. Cystine content jumps from 399 μg. per g. of epidermis to 757 μg. per g. in the stratum corneum, whereas hydroxyproline goes down

from 393 to 0. Methionine content is the same (130 μg. per g.) in both tissues.

Flesch and Esober have extracted from the horny layer a glycoproteolipid which contains hexosamine.

The total amino sugars reach 1.3 and 0.7 mg. per g. of dry weight of the skin in the epidermis and the stratum corneum, respectively. The amounts of glucosamine and galactosamine are 0.90 and 0.25 mg. per g. for the epidermis, and 0.30 and 0.14 mg. per g. for the stratum corneum.

In the living skin and its appendages, glycoproteins and mucopolysaccharides are found. Whereas glycogen, the glycoproteins, and the glycosaminoglycan sulfates are found in the horny layer, hyaluronic acid is present in the superficial portion.

The total quantity of lipids extractable with ether in the horny layer is on the order of 2 to 4 percent, which is sufficient to fill the intercellular spaces. The greater part of these are glycerides, sterols, waxes, and hydrocarbons. Some fatty acids with a very long chain and very few phospholipids are also present.

Matoltsy and Sinesi (1955) and Montagna (1956) showed that there is a "keratogenic" zone in the epidermis. In 1958, Flesch suggested that thiol compounds and enzymes could accumulate in this zone to consolidate the keratin, the formation of which was accompanied by an important captation of sulfurated aminoacids.

Keratin is a fibrous protein which is rich in cystine; therefore —S—S bonds permit numerous transverse linkages between the neighboring polypeptide chains, a fact which renders keratin resistant to chemical agents. Keratin constitutes a barrier against the harmful agents of the environment and protects the higher vertebrates against the stress of life.

Process of Keratinization. A study of the keratinization process in the skin of the newborn rat shows that it consists of several stages, which take place in the various layers of the epidermis. Small protein filaments, together with particles of ribonucleoprotein, appear in the basal cells of the germinative layer. During their passage into the stratum spinosum, these filaments increase in diameter and bundle together in tonofibrils, which undergo chemical changes. These filaments are associated with keratohyalin granules, which are free of —SH and —S—S radicals and are surrounded by ribonucleoprotein particles. These granules are synthesized by epithelial cells and are present in the stratum spinosum from which they pass into the stratum granulosum, where they grow in size while the nuclei and mitochondria of the cells degenerate.

When the cell reaches maturity, the keratohyalin granules disintegrate by themselves, and their material mixes with the fibrous compounds of the cell to form the soft keratin in the horny layer. In the human epidermis, the cell matures in 200 days, and the half-life of mature cells is between 7 and 20 days. This keratinized cell is thin, flat, and hexagonal. Each cell consists of keratin and a nonkeratinous membrane, and the cells are connected to one another by desmosomes.

The keratinization process depends on the presence of the dermis and is regulated by the local vitamin A content: an excess of vitamin A can suppress keratinization, while a vitamin A deficiency can provoke follicular hyperkeratosis (Kusaba, 1970). This process starts a whole series of reactions. Corresponding to the morphologic modifications which were observed during the differentiation leading from the cell of the stratum spinosum to the cell of the stratum corneum are numerous biochemical phenomena: The lysosomal enzymes and the numerous hydrolases which are present in human skin (Ockermann, 1969) participate in the disappearance of the cell. In the skin of the rat, Cashman and collaborators (1969) found a hyaluronidase activity which assured the renewal of 0.23 mg. of hyaluronate per day per g. of skin. The disappearance of the nucleus is accompanied by a liberation of purines, ribose, and ribodesose. When the mitochondria disappear, the phosphatides decrease considerably. The phosphatide content falls from 2.6 percent of dry weight in the deeper portions of the epidermis to 0.15 percent in the cells of the stratum corneum. The cell becomes strongly dehydrated. The globular proteins of the cells produce amino acids through proteolysis and thus increase the number of —SH groups at the beginning of keratinization.

The constant renewal of the epidermal cells and the constant shifting of the cellular components of the epidermis lead to an active protein synthesis. Bernstein (1970) showed that the biogenesis of the tonofilaments and the keratohyalin takes place in the stratum spinosum and the stratum granulosum, respectively, after which the two elements combine in the stratum corneum to form keratin fibers.

In the cells of the granular layer a particular protein is found, which is rich in histidine; this "histidine protein" would be synthesized in the cytoplasm of the granular cells and would then associate with the keratohyalin. The fact that in psoriasis we see a simultaneous deficiency in the synthesis of this protein and of keratohyalin would favor the above hypothesis.

According to Baden and collaborators (1967 and 1968), adult epidermis contains little histidine but a lot of urocanic acid, its deaminated derivative; the same is true for benign epidermal tumors (seborrheic keratoses) and keratoacanthomas. In contrast, the basal cells and squamous cells contain a normal amount of histidine and only traces of urocanic acid because of lack of histidase; this disappearance of urocanic acid was also observed by Carruthers (1968) during the cancerization process in mouse skin. Cancers of the human epidermis contain nicotinamide, which is absent in normal epidermis.

For the biosynthesis of keratin another factor is needed: energy in the form of ATP. This ATP is furnished by active glycogenolysis during the keratinization process of the epidermis in the first half of fetal life. In the adult there is little epidermal glycogen, and the energy is furnished by aerobic and anaerobic glycolysis.

Lipid metabolism also plays a role in the epidermis. Gaylor (1963) and Gaylor and Sault (1964) observed an intense cholesterol formation in the sebaceous glands and in the malpighian layer, where cholesterol and its precursors, Δ^7-cholesterol and 7-dehydrocholesterol or provitamin D, are found. Nicolaides (1965) showed that in the sebaceous glands the cholesterol comes in an esterized form, accompanied by squalene, triglycerides, and free fatty acids, and that free sterols form in the keratinizing epidermis. It is noteworthy that, in patients suffering from psoriasis, an affection characterized by excessive keratinization, cholesterol esterification slows to one-tenth of the rate observed in normal skin. There is an active lipid formation, and the numerous open chain fatty acids which are characteristic for cutaneous lipids in man and animals have as precursors the open chain amino acids valine, isoleucine, and leucine (Wheatley et al., 1967 and 1971). Lipids are used in the membrane architecture of the cells which are constantly being renewed. When degradation of the cellular components occurs during keratinization, the lipids of the cell membranes are also degraded and constitute a source of energy beside glucose.

Melanogenesis. Burnett and co-workers (1967) found that melanogenesis takes place in the melanosomes, melanin-containing bodies, which are formed by the melanocytes in the basal layer of the epidermis in the zone of dermoepidermal junction; their precursors are the melanoblasts. The melanocytes occur in constant numbers and are different from the malpighian cells. Their number is not changed by sun irradiation. In pathologic alterations, the increase of melanin concentration in the skin is due to modifications of the rate of melanogenesis and not to an increase in the number of melanocytes. In the vertebrates, the melanocytes are derived from the neural crest and migrate toward the epidermis during embryonal life. They are specialized cells which synthesize tyrosinase and contain light brown or dark brown cytoplasmic melanin granules. These granules consist of a complex aggregate of pigment, tyrosinase, succinodehydrogenase and cytochrome C, beside RNA and heavy metals, especially copper. The melanin granule is enclosed in a protein matrix.

Melanogenesis is a combination of processes which lead from tyrosinase to melanin. This transformation consists of five stages, of which only the first two are catalyzed by tyrosinase. The latter, which is localized exclusively in the skin, catalyzes the hydroxylation of tyrosine into dihydroxyphenylalanine or DOPA, as well as the dehydrogenation of DOPA into DOPA-quinone. This is then spontaneously transformed into hallachrome, which after decarboxylation and oxydation

forms indole-5,6-quinone, which is polymerized into melanin. During the hydroxylation of monophenol into diphenol, tyrosinase activates the O_2 molecule and incorporates one oxygen atom into the substrate, while the other is reduced to water.

In the initial stage of tyrosinase activation, there is a reduction of the enzyme from the cupric to the cuprous form, a reduction in which the DOPA acts as substrate and as activator. Consequently, the tyrosinase can exist in vivo both in a reduced form, acting on tyrosine and DOPA, and, because of a high oxidation-reduction potential, in an inactive, oxidized form, which may, however, become active with respect to the tyrosine, and which may rapidly act on the DOPA.

Even though tyrosinase catalyzes the two above-mentioned reactions, the oxidation of DOPA into DOPA-quinone and then into melanin is also catalyzed by a number of enzymes and oxidizing systems other than tyrosinase, since the hydroxylation of tyrosine depends on the presence of tyrosinase in the cytoplasm of the melanocytes. This specific enzyme consequently plays a key role, and its absence impedes pigment formation (albinism). On the hands of people working with tannic acid, we observe unpigmented zones due to the presence of a tyrosinase inhibitor in the protective glove.

The tyrosine derivatives which combine with tyrosinase impede the oxidation of tyrosine and consequently the formation of melanin. Phenylalanine also inhibits tyrosinase through competition with tyrosine for the fixation site on the enzyme. Compounds with an —SH group, hydroquinone, ascorbic acid, and cyclic amines also inhibit tyrosinase.

Avitaminosis C is accompanied by melanodermia, and hypervitaminosis A provokes a localized depigmentation; a deficiency in sulfhydryl compounds produces hyperpigmentation following increased tyrosinase activity.

It has been observed that when tyrosinase concentration is weak, as for instance in the melanocytes in the human epidermis, the time of induction of tyrosine oxidation into DOPA is very much prolonged, whereas DOPA oxidation and its transformation into melanin are rapid. After UV irradiation this activity becomes evident, which suggests that epidermal tyrosinase exists in the melanocytes in an inactive or inhibited form, whereas tyrosinase in the melanosomes occurs in an active form.

Normal and neoplastic tissues contain an inhibitor of the auto-oxidation of DOPA into melanin which is much stronger in normal than in neoplastic tissue. This inhibition seems due to compounds which are closely bound to copper or other ions necessary for the auto-oxidation of DOPA. This inhibitor is destroyed by x-rays and UV rays.

Alterations Observed During Tumor Growth. Im (1968) compared glucose metabolism in normal and cancerous skin of rhesus monkeys. In normal tissue, a great part of the glucose is transformed into lactate, and only a small quantity enters into the Krebs cycle; an important part of the glucose is metabolized through the shunt, thus contributing to the metabolism of nucleic acids and fatty acids. In papillomas formed after eight months of painting with 7,12-dimethylbenzanthracene, Im observed a marked increase in glucose-6-phosphate dehydrogenase activity and 6-phosphogluconate dehydrogenase activity (four and five times greater, respectively), and in the glyceraldehyde-3-phosphate dehydrogenase and isocitrate dehydrogenase activities (both three times greater). This result has been confirmed by Halprin and coworkers (1968) in epitheliomas, and by DiBella and coworkers (1968) in experimental cancers in rats, provoked by 9,10-dimethyl-1,2-benzanthracene, with which the authors also observed an increased citrate and isocitrate oxidation. Zador (1969) studied the modifications of oxygen consumption and lactate formation during the cancerization process of the cutaneous tissue of the mouse produced by painting with DMBA and demonstrated very clearly a sharp increase in respiration and lactate formation at the time of the appearance of the tumors. We can conclude from these studies that the appearance of the tumor is accompanied by an increase in glucose metabolism with respect to both energy production (glycolysis and respiration) and pentose phosphate shunting.

Riley (1968) found that malignant blue nevi, in contrast to other tumors of the skin, have a very weak cytochrome oxidase and succinoxidase activity.

All authors have reported a marked increase in lysosomal hydrolase activity during the cancerization process. Schamberger and Rudolph (1967) observed a marked increase in cathepsin, β-glucuronidase, and acid phosphatase activity in the lysosomes of skin tumors, which would favor the destruction of normal tissue. Hewitt and collaborators (1970) found a strong β-glucuronidase activity in malignant melanoma, and Atsushi (1968) found an increase in serum β-glucuronidase in patients with carcinoma and in animals with tumors. Sulfatase activity, which is present in five layers of the epidermis, increases in malignant epithelial tumors and in melanotic tumors, according to Vezekenyi (1968).

Other observations have been made regarding the cancerization of cutaneous tissue. Voorhess in 1968 described an increase in urinary excretion of DOPA during the growth of transplanted melanomas. This excretion decreased with a slowdown of tumor growth. Menon and Habermann (1970a and 1970b) found tyrosinase in the melanocytes of the B_{16} melanosome and a tyrosinase activity in the serum of mice with melanomas, a fact already observed by Takahashi in 1964; according to these authors, there is even a relationship between the size of the tumors and the tyrosinase activity of the serum. Menon and Haberman (1970a) located this tyrosinase in the microsomes of B_{16} melanomas, where it is present in an inactive form but can be activated through various treatments (freezing-thawing, influence of deoxycholate or digitonin).

The blue nevi, in contrast, are characterized by a very weak tyrosinase and DOPA-oxidase activity compared with malignant melanomas, as shown by Riley in 1968.

Conclusion

As the present study shows, the complex cutaneous tissue has a very active metabolism. Cancerization is accompanied by collagen destruction following a marked collagenase activity, an alteration of the fibrous structure, and an increase in hyaluronic acid. Moreover, the utilization of energy-producing glucose is increased, as is the shunt. The total reorganization of the tissue is furthered by an increase in the hydrolase activity of the lysosomes. Cancerization is accompanied by a modification of the metabolism, which, however, remains very active.

LINKAGE BETWEEN NUCLEIC ACIDS AND POLYCYCLIC HYDROCARBONS

Nowadays all cancer biologists agree that all carcinogenic agents will eventually act on the genes and modify their structure. We shall study this problem in the following pages. For many years, the linkage between nucleic acids and polycyclic carcinogenic hydrocarbons has been studied predominantly in vitro. In vivo studies remained indirect, the linkage being viewed in terms of modifications of the rate of RNA and especially DNA synthesis after application of hydrocarbons to the skin.

In Vitro Studies of the Linkage

Boyland and Green (1962) were the first to present solid experimental arguments in favor of a union between the carcinogenic polycyclic carbons and DNA. The importance of this discovery warrants a review of their conclusions here. In previous publications, Boyland and Sims (1965a and 1965b) showed that plane molecules united with the heteroatoms or groups capable of offering specific linkage sites for nucleic acids. The special interest of the carcinogenic polycyclic hydrocarbons resides in the fact that they do not present groups of this type.

Working with carcinogenic benzo(a)pyrene and noncarcinogenic pyrene, the authors developed the following facts: an aqueous solution of deoxyribonucleic acid links with these two hydrocarbons, increases their solubility, and suppresses their fluorescence. There is also a modification of the wavelength of the DNA absorption maximum in ultraviolet. The double helix of DNA is necessary for the link to occur. Thermal denaturation suppresses these phenomena. The authors thought that there was an interspersion of hydrocarbon molecules between the base pairs of DNA, producing molecular distortion without modifying the sugarphosphate chains.

Following the findings of Ts'O and Lu, Boyland thought in 1964 that there was no distortion of the rigid helix, but that hydrocarbons were introduced into certain loci of the chain, which was stretched during DNA replication or RNA transcription in vivo. These are the facts arrived at with precise methods and by now established beyond criticism.

In 1964, Giovanella and his collaborators (among them Heidelberger) published an article questioning the findings of Boyland and Green, but this minor controversy was settled when Heidelberger stated in 1970 that "Boyland, whose studies on hydrocarbon metabolism (were) conducted with imagination and patience, has provided most of the fundamental information that we have on this subject."

Tissue Studies In Vivo

A number of studies have been carried out, either in the mouse or in cell cultures, and published; all proved more or less directly the presence of a linkage between nucleic acids and carcinogenic polycyclic hydrocarbons. Davenport et al. (1961) used radioactive markers; Brookes and Lawley (1964) used mouse skin and marked hydrocarbons, tracking their linkage with the nucleic acids. Noteworthy is the study of Brookes (1966) concentrating on the quantitative aspects of the problem. He showed that there is a union between the nucleic acids of alkylating nitrosamine agents, azoic stains, lactones, and polycyclic hydrocarbons. He pays special attention to the role of cell alkylation. In 1969, Brookes and Heidelberger used 7,12-DMBA (marked with ^{14}C) and found on the one hand a covalent type of linkage with the nucleic acids of mouse skin, and on the other, that these phenomena remain unchanged if cultured fibroblasts are used. They maintain that the hydrocarbon is linked to the proteins and to the nucleic acids, the covalent linkage being established by the nucleotides and free bases.

All these studies yield an interesting fact concerning the alkylation of the nucleic acids in position 7 of the guanine, which renders the linkage of this base and sugar labile (Lawley and Brookes, 1963). Magee and Farber (1962) had detected methylation in position 7 of the RNA guanine in the course of their in vivo experiments with dimethylnitrosamine.

Pitot in 1970 considered guanine as a molecule that could be involved in deletions; we shall revert to the subject of this mechanism, which is considered as one of those leading to cancerization.

Proteins

We shall not consider here the studies by J. A. Miller and his collaborators, who have concerned themselves since 1942 with the union between proteins and hepatocarcinogenic agents, and will mention only the publication by E. C. Miller (1950). The linkage with proteins can be considered as a source of "deletions;" it would attain the crucial and decisive target represented by the nucleic acids in an indirect manner. Miller studied the linkage formation between the proteins of epidermal cells and 3,4-benzpyrene or its metabolites. The carcinogenic polycyclic hydrocarbon is applied to mouse skin, from which a gross protein extract is obtained subsequently; Miller finds that, at the level of the epidermis, there are fluorescent substances with a greater polarity than the hydrocarbon itself.

These derivatives are specific for the epidermis; they are absent from other layers of the skin and from other organs studied by the author. The quantity of the carcinogenic agent (or its derivatives) increases between the third and the 24th hour and then decreases; it increases also with the number of applications to the skin and especially if the mouse is kept in a dark place. Miller is convinced that this strong HC-protein linkage plays a role in carcinogenesis, just as linkage between

azoics and microsomal proteins of the hepatocyte is involved in the origin of cancer of the liver. Since 1950, and after a review of the question published by Miller and Miller in 1952, the team of these two authors has continued the studies of azoic stains. The results obtained by Miller were confirmed in 1953 by Heidelberger and his collaborators, who used hydrocarbons marked with the ^{14}C isotope.

MODIFICATIONS OF THE SYNTHESIS AND TURNOVER RATE OF NUCLEIC ACIDS UNDER THE INFLUENCE OF POLYCYCLIC HYDROCARBONS

Once the linkage between carcinogenic hydrocarbons and nucleic acids had been established, the biochemists began to research the modification of the metabolism of the nucleic acids in the case of hydrocarbons. The carcinogenic agent was applied to mouse skin either through an injection or by simple painting. Specific radioactive precursors were used, and the rate of their incorporation during neoplastic transformation was measured.

Although the notions explained in the following appear in other chapters, we thought it might be useful to repeat them here, especially since this very short review may help in understanding the last section of this chapter.

As far as the DNA is concerned, since the stable molecule is not renewed during the life of a cell, there will be an incorporation of the radioactive precursor indicating synthesis only if multiplication has taken place, including duplication of the molecule of DNA. The specific precursor here is tritiated thymidine, whose incorporation into the DNA molecules we shall follow.

All other cell components are subject to a constant turnover, the rate of which influences their metabolism. Here again the introduction of radioactive isotopes into the molecules of specific precursors enables us to follow the rate of their progressive incorporation during the different stages of carcinogenesis by measuring the specific activities of the synthesized molecules. In the case of RNA, the precursor is orotic acid marked with ^{14}C.

Studies of the isotopes can be qualitative or quantitative in character, according to the specific goal. A study of the isotopes is a potent means of observation which has yielded important results, but the use of radioactive isotopes is a delicate matter, and the pitfalls awaiting an investigator not well versed in the techniques are manifold, especially in quantitative investigations. The biochemist uses complicated techniques adjusted to his own mode of investigation.

The cytologist, it should be briefly recalled here, is able to obtain an autoradiograph of an organ, a cell, or a cell structure through the localization of the marker, which emits radiation onto a special photographic film. In the case of tritiated thymidine, in which the energy emission of tritium is feeble, radiation stops in the proximity of the marked molecules, so that the DNA can be localized. Autoradiography permits both qualitative and quantitative studies.

We would like to review chronologically some of the investigations concerning modification of the renewal of nucleic acid molecules through application of the carcinogenic agent to the mouse, either by painting of the skin or through subcutaneous injection. The carcinogenic agent most frequently used was 7,12-DMBA; comparison of the results is difficult because of wide variations in the conditions under which the animals were placed and even in the course of the experiment. Thymidine is usually used as a marker, and deoxyribonucleic acid is the cellular target.

In 1963, Jensen and coworkers found the incorporation rate of thymidine clearly diminished but not completely suppressed after administration of 7,12-DMBA. They localized the phenomena at the level of the nuclei of the germinal epithelium, using autoradiography. Their conclusion was that the incorporation is inhibited but that the mechanism cannot be determined, the question being whether the relationship between this inhibition and carcinogenesis is really evident, since there is inhibition in intact tissues not undergoing cancerization.

In 1965, McCarter used the same carcinogen and the same marker and observed tritiated thymidine inhibition in the hair follicles. At the same time, he introduced polycyclic hydrocarbons into a culture of *E. coli* and observed their effect on the ratio of DNA to RNA. His conclusion was that DMBA and also 3-methylcholanthrene damage some cells of the hair follicle permanently in a specific way. The mechanism of carcinogenesis that is thus set in motion could be checked through the manifestations it produces on the *E. coli* and the phages.

In the same year, Epstein and Maibach carried out an interesting experiment in man. They injected tritiated thymidine with a special technique which allowed them to follow it from the basal cells into the epidermis and to note how long it took to reach different zones of the epidermis, a procedure which marked the DNA of the new cells. In all it takes 10 to 12 days to reach the granular layer. We feel that this study is worth mentioning because it concerns human skin, although it does not permit a simple deduction concerning the influence of hydrocarbons on the renewal rate.

In 1966, Flamm and coworkers also studied an interesting problem, although one that takes us away from our general theme. They investigated the parallelism between the effects of DMBA and actinomycin D on mouse skin, as well as the interactions between these two substances. They wanted to measure synthesis of the RNA, especially the RNA-DNA dependence. The mode of action of actinomycin D is well known, and it is precisely because of this that it is so interesting. The authors noted first of all an inhibition of carcinogenesis. Using orotic acid labelled with ^{14}C, they were able to show that actinomycin does not inhibit RNA synthesis at the moment the DMBA is applied, but 24 hours later if only hydrocarbon is used or if actinomycin C is injected 24 hours after DMBA. The authors felt that this probably is not the irreversible phenomenon of tumor formation, despite the inhibition of RNA synthesis through the hydrocarbon.

We should further mention the studies by Giovanella et al. (1964) and by Goshman and Heidelberger (1967). In 1965 an ingenious technique was devised to permit the isolation of basal cells of mouse epidermis after injecting tritium-marked hydrocarbons. Enough cells were obtained to proceed with the biologic and biochemical determinations (autoradiographs and measurement of a specific activity.) Goshman and Heidelberger first isolated the hydrocarbon-marked DNA and then plotted the evolution graphs against the interval of specific DNA activity for a total of four hydrocarbons; the most active and the most bound is 1,2,3,4-DBA; the others are also bound but not so strongly, with the exception of the MCA. (Note that the hair cycle has been taken into consideration). Other aspects of these studies are interesting, as well as the authors' comments on the subject, but they do not warrant a delay in our discussion, especially since we shall explain in detail some of the results of Heidelberger (1970) with regard to the transformation mechanisms.

In a publication that appeared in 1969, Paul studied the interactions of the effects of cancerization-promoting agents on modifications of the rate of synthesis of nucleic acids in DMBA-treated mice.

In 1970, Hennings and Boutwell used the same hydrocarbon (DMBA), also gearing their experiments to the influence of the promoting agent, croton oil, on the rate with which their tritiated precursors were incorporated into the macromolecules of mouse skin. The authors took the hair cycle into consideration. After different intervals, the macromolecules were extracted in order to measure the incorporation. These authors observed an inhibition of DNA synthesis followed by acceleration later on. The synthesis of proteins and of RNA is highly sensitive to the application of promoting agents together with the carcinogen, and the authors think that the stimulation of RNA synthesis by croton oil may play an important role in the promotional phase.

Alexandrov et al. (1970) published a study on the evolution of RNA content in the skin during the formation of epitheliomas. These are provoked by painting mouse skin with DMBA or benzpyrene. In another series of experiments, these authors provoked sarcomas by injecting the same hydrocarbons under the skin. They measured the ratio of RNA to DNA, which increases in epitheliomas, reaches a maximum after two weeks which persists during the appearance of the tumor, and then decreases by about 40 percent. In sarcomas the ratio is low at first, increases progressively, and then decreases by 50 percent when the sarcoma is visible. The marking is obtained with tritium-labelled orotic acid as a radioactive body, and RNA synthesis can be followed by inducing cancer with DMBA. The authors measured the radioactivity of two RNA fractions: 4S and 5S. They also showed that variations in the rate of synthesis do not modify electrophoretic separations. They concluded that "the mechanism of RNA synthesis remains unknown along with the interaction of the carcinogenic carbons with this constituent." They feel that their experiments favor the theory according to which the carcinogen acts directly on cell macromolecules and thus causes an irreversible transformation of the cell. Obviously, this conclusion agrees with the established facts.

From these various types of experiments we can draw the general conclusion that the covalent linkages between the molecules of carcinogenic hydrocarbons and nucleic acids, which have been proved by biochemists, are always accompanied by a depression and subsequent inhibition of macromolecule synthesis, slowing down the turnover of these molecules.

MECHANISMS OF CARCINOGENESIS

Present Theories

By now the concept of the mechanism of carcinogenesis has been unified. The three prevalent theories invoke the results of genetics and molecular biochemistry obtained in bacteria by Jacob and Monod (1963). These theories are the following:

(1) The theory maintaining that the "deletions" are the determining mechanism, which has been much studied since the work of Greenstein and which cannot be discarded since many enzymatic deletions affect the cell constituents and can thus be responsible for the transformation. They may be due to alterations of the operating genes, which regulate the metabolic cir-

cuits (Jacob and Monod, 1963). These genes are independent from the structural genes, which for a long time were the only ones studied by the classical geneticists. The regulating genes can act as repressors or derepressors of enzymes.

(2) The theory based on somatic mutations — i.e., modifications of the structural genes. The final target of the carcinogen must always be DNA, but in the case of the deletion theory, this is reached indirectly, whereas through the somatic mutations, the target is reached directly.

(3) After about two decades, a number of observations have led to the theory that a number of cancers are caused by anomalies in embryonic development. This mechanism can also be expressed in genetic terms. At some stage in development, certain cells do not undergo the evolution followed by the other cells of the same type surrounding them. In their case, the operating genes of the genome are repressed. In a later, sometimes much delayed stage, there would be a derepression, and the repressed, silent cells would be found to be liberated and manifest.

All three theories are based on intervention of the genes and the macromolecules constituting them, the former controlling the synthesis of the latter.

Let us briefly explain here the theory of *cell transformation* formulated by Heidelberger, who was not quite satisfied with the concepts of molecular biology and spent a number of years carrying out experiments on cultured cells.

In order to make these theories quite clear, let us recall first of all the essential facts. Among the changes which forcibly accompany the transformation of a normal into a malignant cell are the following: (1) faster synthesis of cell DNA; (2) uncontrolled cell multiplication; (3) loss of contact inhibition; (4) acquired "immortality" through inheritance of changes under (2) and (3); (5) appearance of new antigens; and (6) appearance of a neoplastic characteristic defined by the crucial test of tumor production in immunologically compatible hosts.

We would like to quote here the opinion of Dulbecco, formulated in 1962 during the Cold Spring Harbor Symposium:

It seems most likely, and essentially necessary, that the mechanism of transformation involves an alteration of some genetic component of the cell, because the transformation appears to be hereditary and probably irreversible. Thus a knowledge of the genetic properties of the somatic cells is required before an intimate understanding of the process of transformation can be gained; extensive information on the genetics of these cells is therefore urgently needed.

Two years later, this author wrote the following in an article on cancerization through an oncogenic virus; ". . . it is conceivable that transformation is the consequence of a transient action of the virus, and the persistence of the genes (viral) is purely a consequence of the fact that the cells were originally infected" (Dulbecco, 1964).

Ephrussi remarked in 1970 that, at the time of his 1962 communication, Dulbecco understood an "alteration of some genetic component" to be a somatic mutation, whereas we know today that a genetic mutation does not produce stable cell changes because epigenetic changes (i.e., changes in the functional state of the genome) can also be clonally inherited.

In the same vein, Ephrussi wrote in 1970 that because of the complexity of the interactions between the parameters of the cancerous cell, the mechanism of differentiation and of neoplasia would for a certain time be more accessible to genetic analysis than to any other means of analysis. This is particularly important, since in 1965 this author thought that the application to the cells of superior animals of the genetic discoveries of Jacob and Monod regarding the existence and functioning of genes regulating metabolic chains, as demonstrated in bacteria, apart from the structural genes was a long time off. In view of recent developments, he felt in 1970 that these results of molecular genetics on one hand, and the admirable tool furnished by the hybrid cells on the other, would make it possible in the near future to establish the genetic bases regulating the functioning of normal and neoplastic cells in superior animals, but under one condition: that all investigators pool their efforts toward this goal.

In view of the above-mentioned importance of the hybrid cells for this fundamental research, we will point out the essential facts concerning these cells. They have been studied for a very long time, but the important discoveries concerning them were made between 1960 and 1970.

Barski and collaborators (1961) and Ephrussi and Sorieul (1962) showed that the hybridization of two cells, belonging to two different lines of C3H inbred mice, yields a hybrid cell layer, which in a pure culture has the capacity of growing indefinitely, a fact which permits the study of their karyotype and phenotype. These pure cultures of hybrid cells are more likely to produce transformed cells after a time than the cultures of the two parent cells. Barski and collaborators (1960–62) found that in a hybridization of a normal and a neoplastic cell, the characteristics of the cancerous cell predominate and that the more active the hybridized cancerous cell, the greater the carcinogenic activity of the hybrids. In the case of hybridization of two neoplastic cells, the hybrids have the characteristics of the cell with the greatest neoplastic activity (tested through inoculation and subsequent tumor formation in an appropriate host). The attention of researchers has been focused on the plasticity of hybrid cells. Ephrussi (1970) thought that the absence of contact inhibition was the precondition for hybridization if one cell is cancerous. He was convinced that contacts between cells permit the exchange even of indiffusible substances from one cell to another. On the other hand, the same author showed the effects of a lowering of the temperature of the culture medium (from 37° to 29° C.). At 29° C, the pure culture of hybrids is more easily obtained, and the union and viability of new cells increase.

As for the "deletions," it was thought for a number of years that they were incompatible with the results obtained with hybrids. Hybridization itself was used to test the possibility of the existence of such a type of deletion. But Ephrussi had insisted since 1965 on the fact that hybrid cells with metabolic anomalies had been isolated which corresponded to the modern form of "deletions" described in 1963 by Pitot and Heidelberger, where carcinogenesis would be the result of an alteration of the genetic regulating mechanism rather than a mutation of the structural genes. This type of deletion could be the result of a diffusion of a substance through the special membranes of the hybridized cells.

Before going on to the principal facts resulting from errors in embryonal development, we would like to recall some fundamental notions with regard to cell differentiation linked to embryonal development. Each cell of a superior organism, independent of its ultimate specialization, contains a complete set of genetic information; consequently, differentiation is one of the mechanisms of stable restriction of the expression of one or more genes during the course of embryonal development.

In a unicellular organism, the nuclei are identical in genetic content, and these monocellular units, such as ciliated protozoa, can assume various stable functional states of vegetative reproduction. In pluricellular organisms, the potential development of the various cell strains depends on the structural genes and on epigenetic changes—i.e., on portions of the genome which, under the appropriate conditions, can express themselves even if the rest remains silent. This implies that the global term of differentiation designates two different types of mechanisms regulating the genes: *determination,* which selects a particular segment of the genome, which subsequently could express itself in a cell strain excluding all others, followed by *differentiation* in the strict sense of the term, a terminal process which should be based on rather simple factors similar to those inducing enzyme biosynthesis in bacteria.

The normal and neoplastic development presupposes epigenetic changes, and in order to understand embryonic carcinomas it is necessary that we review the regulating mechanisms underlying determination and differentiation.

Developmental Errors Leading to Carcinogenesis

The facts under this heading can be divided into four groups:

1. Existence of antigens of fetal origin found in carcinomas of the adult. The two best known of these carcinoembryonic an-

tigens are the following: In 1963 Abelew and in 1967 Grabar and collaborators found in the hepatoma of the adult (rat or man) an antigen (fetuin) identical with one of those found in embryo liver but absent in the liver of the normal adult and studied it with enzymatic and immunochemical methods. In 1965 Gold and Freedman also identified a specific antigen in embryonic carcinomas of the adult human digestive system. Burton and collaborators (1970) studied this antigen in cancers of the human digestive system; they were maintained in an organotypical culture for seven to eight years following the technique of Etienne and Emilienne Wolf. The immunochemical study is conclusive. In these cases, there is a derepression of previously silent genes in the adult.

2. On the other hand, a number of investigations involving the hormone secretion of certain glandular carcinomas have been carried out. The presence of malignant cells in the form of little islets or nodules coincides with hypersecretion: insulin secretion in the pancreas, thyroxine in the thyroid, pituitary hormone in the hypophysis. The process suggests the alteration of the control mechanism of these secretions by means of an activating substance. This anomaly can be compared to one produced by an operating gene (Jacob and Monod, 1963). This is also true for osteochondrosarcomas, in which the fibroblasts of the connective tissue synthesize an excess of cartilage. Still more interesting is the case of carcinomas in which the differentiation and the hormone secretion do not correspond to the normal homologous tissue, as for instance bronchogenic carcinomas secreting a parathyroid hormone (Sherwood and collaborators, 1966). For the cancer researcher, the term "metaplasia" takes these facts into account, whereas the embryologist sees them as an interruption of the normal embryonal development, a transdetermination.

3. Another case is the teratoma studied and described by Markert in a 1968 article with the title, "Neoplasia, a Disease of Cell Differentiation." This tumor is a chaotic arrangement of different types of cells, which are often organized like the normal corresponding tissues. In the teratoma, the neoplastic phenomenon seems to occur very early at the beginning of development and before any clear sign of differentiation. This suggests the existence of a unique base mechanism for programming the genes. Once the "teratoma" stage is passed, a normal differentiation of specific cell types takes place. The anomaly depends on epigenetic mechanisms which produce a neoplastic model of the metabolism, in which all individual components are normal.

4. To round off this review of facts with regard to the intervention of embryonic development in carcinogenesis, we would mention the modifications of the (plasmic) cell surface described by Weiss (1951). This author maintained that in the first stages of embryonic development there is no contact inhibition between the cells, that this inhibition develops later. In contrast, it disappears progressively during transformation. Weiss believed that a knowledge of these two processes is very helpful in understanding the mechanisms of cancerization. In this context we might mention recent findings in electron microscopy on ultrathin sections of normal cells. They show sheets of cells with reduced intercellular contact, a fact which shows that during cell division, the membranes of this zone are more fragile and more labile and independent. This is confirmed by the behavior of normal cultured fibroblasts: during mitosis there is a loss of contact inhibition, and the fibroblasts move around freely over the other cells. If cortisone is introduced into the culture, the contacts are restored and inhibition of cell growth occurs, which suggests that certain hormones can influence the structure of plasmic membranes and partly control cell proliferation.

Weiss thought that the absence of contact inhibition in the initial stages of development favors diffusion, a transfer of inducive substances. It has often been said that during the course of differentiation of a multicellular region of the embryo, this region undergoes alterations because of an interaction between cell groups, an observation which is basic for embryonic induction. The capacity of a given tissue to induce or obey a stimulus is in general limited to a few specific developmental stages, and we ignore the chemical substances which are responsible for these changes in reactivity.

There remains the question as to the eventual role of the growth factors studied by Cohen (1964) and some other biologists and biochemists. Cohen isolated and purified (on the basis of a salivary gland extract) two specific growth factors, the nerve growth factor and the epidermal growth factor. These have a spectacular effect on embryos or very young animals. Future studies will show whether they play a role in development or not.

Tiedemann (1965) studied the initial effects of the mesodermic factor, which quickly leads to changes in the mutual affinity of the cells; the endoderm spreads in a thin layer over the ectoderm at the onset of gastrulation, and there is an alteration of the cell membranes. We still know little about the mechanism linking these changes to modifications of the ectoderm or the mesoderm.

In discussing the importance of these surface phenomena, we should bear in mind the observations of Ephrussi and collaborators on the role of intercellular contacts, which are necessary for hybridization.

Theory of Somatic Mutations

The two most quoted theories concerning the mechanism of the cancerization of cells and their transformation in their modern form both refer to the role of either the structural genes (classic genetics) or the operating genes influencing the functional metabolic expression (Jacob and Monod, 1961). The opinions of cancer investigators are divided on this subject. One of the principal arguments against the theory of deletions concerns the difficulties we encounter in trying to explain the hereditary and permanent character of the modifications. Ephrussi (1970), however, has expressed the opinion that the modifications which are epigenetic in origin exhibit the same hereditary and permanent characteristic. We cannot give the complete history of these theories based on the macromolecular mechanisms here, but we would like to repeat the following stages: the theory of somatic mutations was for-

mulated for the first time by Boveri (1907 and 1929); Smith in 1907 wrote that the transformation is accompanied by a permanent and irreversible modification of the genome due to mutations. A series of investigators have taken positions for or against this theory, and while space does not permit a discussion here, let us quote the opinion Kark expressed in 1966, which sums up the basis for accepting the somatic mutation: "If normal cells are transformed into cancerous cells, there must be one or more mutations during this transformation. If a somatic mutation represents a permanent change in the integrity of the genetic information of the normal cell, then this term designates a modified karyotype of the structural genes." Evidently, in the case of a mutation, all information is transmitted to the macromolecules by transcription.

This theory of somatic mutations can also rely heavily on research, for Boyland has proved the union between the chemical carcinogens (especially the polycyclic hydrocarbons) and the DNA molecules; in fact, these form the basis for the synthesis of all cellular macromolecules. We have described some of these investigations above, and we shall later discuss a number of publications which have appeared since 1965 and are concerned more particularly with the linkage of the carcinogens or their active metabolites with the nucleotides or the purine bases of the DNA and RNA molecules. This union of carcinogens with DNA is accompanied by an alteration of the structure of one or more genes, and once the replication and transcription of information of this part of the DNA chain are modified, there emerges in the course of the transformation a new cell type: the malignant cell.

Obviously, the somatic mutation implies a direct effect on the structural genes, and it is surprising that clinical investigators and biochemists like Heidelberger, who has published research backing up this mechanism (especially together with Brookes) could have concluded as late as 1970 that there was no conclusive proof in favor of any one of the theories based on the intervention of either the structural or the operating genes.

It would seem logical to admit that,

among the very numerous types of cancers affecting different organs, some are due to a somatic mutation and others to the functional, genetic expression of the operating genes. In fact, a connection between these two theories is already established if one or the other of the mechanisms leads to stable and hereditary characteristics of transformed cells, be it by attaining the target (DNA) directly or through phenomena availing themselves of various metabolic channels before affecting the genes.

It is true that some of the arguments Boveri uses as a basis for the somatic mutation and the origin of malignant change do not always correspond to the facts: the chromosomal anomalies often found by this outstanding biologist are not a constant factor, and the karyotypes observed during the evolution of the normal cell toward the neoplastic cell might be a consequence and not a cause of transformation. On the other hand, the objection against the mutational theory on the basis of the rarity of spontaneous mutations of somatic cells and the need for various mutations to accomplish a transformation seems rather ill founded to us, since the frequency of mutations can increase considerably either with x-rays or with chemical carcinogenic agents, especially in cells with numerous mitoses. We also have to bear in mind that alterations of genes at the level of the DNA molecules can be provoked by the modification of the qualities of certain molecules. Let us just mention in passing that carcinogenic molecules are not always mutagenic and that the correlation between these two properties is far from being constant.

Genetic mutations which occur at the level of the structural or operating genes, independent of the carcinogen used, necessarily lead to an alteration of the mechanism which controls cell multiplication.

In our opinion, all recent studies invariably present results in favor of somatic mutations as the origin of transformation.

LINKAGE OF THE CARCINOGENS WITH THE COMPONENTS OF NUCLEIC ACID MOLECULES: THE CASE OF GUANINE

Ever since the linkage between carcinogens and nucleic acids was first demonstrated, many researches have tried to specify the nature of this linkage and the location in the macromolecule where it is produced. Without dwelling on this interesting problem in detail, we would like to point out some facts concerning a particular purine base, guanine.

(1) In 1962, Magee and Faber showed that dimethylnitrosamine (a hepatocarcinogen) could methylate certain soluble RNA's in vivo, and that it marks guanine nuclei in position 7. Other authors found that ethionine ethylates guanine nuclei in the same position. These experiments proved that macromolecules other than proteins can be alkylated and react in a covalent manner with carcinogens or their active metabolites.

(2) In 1964, Lawley and Brookes demonstrated chemically that the alkylation of position 7 of the guanine labilizes the linkage between this base and its sugar, a fact which leads to depurinization and then scission of the implicated nucleic acid chain in this place; this phenomenon is frequent with DNA. On the other hand, the esterification of the phosphoryl group of the RNA can also lead to scission of the chain (1963–1967). Besides, we know that, at the level of the microsomes, the RNA messengers are agents of the synthesis of the amino acids and therefore the proteins (Krick et al., 1967).

Since DNA is the genetic material, it was important to study especially the effect of carcinogens on this material. In 1967, Krick and collaborators, among them J. A. Miller, found that the most active derivative of the acetyl aminofluorene (A.A.F.) metabolism unites with guanosine to form a derivative, 8-(N-2 fluorenylacetamido)-guanosine. The union occurs in position 8 of the base nucleus. These same authors isolated and identified the products, and in the case of several hepatocarcinogens, this furnished direct proof of the incorporation of the carcinogen used into the DNA molecule.

In 1969, Miller and Miller published a very interesting article on the nature of the active products derived from the metabolism of a series of carcinogens and showed that, in the case of azoics, the most active are the N-hydroxylated esters which react with the nucleophilic sites. The union of these derivatives with the DNA molecules or structural genes was an important finding. For the most part radioactive A.A.F. and its radioactive derivatives were studied; this was the first demonstration of the incorporation of carcinogenic molecules into the genetic molecules of hepatic cells. We have to point out that the union in position 8 of the guanine nucleus does not have the instability of the union in position 7. The importance of the findings with respect to guanine is evident, but we feel that they are particularly important insofar as they open the way for delicate research which may be able to specify which of the two molecular mechanisms involved is the true one: somatic mutations or deletions. Such studies might bring us the proof required by some cancer investigators.

Theory of Deletions

Even the definition of the term "deletion" implies a wide range of phenomena which can be considered as a cause of cancerization through this mechanism: the modifications, alterations, or suppressions which influence the components of the normal cell or its enzymatic activity. On the whole, however, there is much more conjecture than proof to show that such a deletion is carcinogenic. Investigators have often had to admit that the deletions found in tumor cells may be a consequence of the tumor rather than a determining factor.

It has to be admitted, nevertheless, that since the publications of Monod and Jacob in 1961, which we discussed above, the theory of deletions has acquired a solid basis. We explained at the beginning of this chapter why the ideas of Warburg and Greenstein, which were the starting point for the "deletions," have had to be abandoned, as their bases no longer correspond to the facts.

Let us briefly review here our present knowledge of the theory of deletions: (1) The first and at the time the most important findings were those of Miller and Miller (1947 and 1966). In the case of the hepatoma induced by azoic dye in the rat, transformation occurred because of a permanent alteration of the proteins which are essential for the regulation of cell multiplication; in the tumor itself this protein has disappeared. Sorof et al. (1951) confirmed and specified this finding; he designated this protein as h.2. After the application of carcinogenic hydrocarbons, Abell and Heidelberger (1962) found in mouse skin a protein analogous to h.2., the concentration of which is greatly diminished in epidermal carcinoma.

(2) Potter, writing between 1950 and 1958 saw modifications of the enzymatic activity as determining factors, especially in the case of catabolic rather than anabolic enzymes. In a joint study with Morris on the enzymology of hepatoma No. 5123 "with a minimum of deviations," he was forced to abandon his hypothesis according to which the modifications of enzymatic activity were considered as a cause of transformation.

It ought to be pointed out here that, with the exception of the enzyme-forming systems which are ribonucleins and which, when dormant, might even influence the operating genes, it is difficult to view the modification of enzymatic activities as a factor in carcinogenesis. In most cases, the enzymatic activities are modified by the presence of metabolites, cofactors, and ions which can act either as activators or as inhibitors. It follows that the disappearance of enzymatic activity cannot be seen as a deletion, since a simple modification of the content in its metabolites or cofactors, or even the intervention of hormones, suffices to set the enzymatic activity in motion again (Jacob, 1970).

On the basis of the preceding explanations, we can understand the position of leading scientists in the field of the mechanism of carcinogenesis without further details.

(3) Pitot (1970), who has devoted much study to the problem of deletions, summed up his views in an article on the hepatoma. There is one fact which stands out as especially important: namely, the publication of this author in collaboration with Heidelberger, which appeared in 1963 and called a theory based on the investigations of Jacob and Monod a "purely intellectual game." Carcinogenesis might be the result of an alteration of the operating genes

governing the metabolic circuits; an outline similar to that of these two geneticists illustrates their thought.

Pitot never alluded to that publication again, at a time when other cancer researchers defended outlines of the same type. This is the more surprising as in the meantime the theory concerning the operating genes as the basis of certain types of transformation had been defended and further developed. The two valid objections against epigenetic mutations had been refuted since 1965: according to the first objection, epigenetic modifications resulting from "deletions" or mutations of the operating genes could not be considered as hereditary or permanent. The heredity of the neoplastic characteristics, however, constitutes the necessary basis for the adoption of any theory. According to Ephrussi, though, a biologist whose opinion carries much authority, epigenetic changes—i.e., changes of the functional stage—can be hereditary.

The second objection (Braun, 1970) maintained that the results of studies on the hybridization of normal and cancerous cells are contrary to the theory of deletions. As we have pointed out above, though, the hybrid cells show metabolic anomalies which are compatible with deletions based on epigenetic mutations (Ephrussi).

It is noteworthy that Pitot and Heidelberger (1963) were the first to consider the application of the genetic concepts of Jacob and Monod to deletions.

The results obtained by Morris on certain types of rat hepatomas constitute an important stage in the evolution of the theory of deletions as a mechanism of carcinogenesis (Morris, 1965; Morris and Wagner, 1968).

HEPATOMA OF MORRIS NO. 5123 "WITH MINIMAL DEVIATIONS": BEARING OF HIS STUDY ON THE THEORY OF DELETIONS

It has been said in the introduction that the characteristics of cancerous cells should be studied only in well-differentiated tumors, which have shown no dedifferentiation in the course of the transformation process. Morris induced slowly evolving, clearly differentiated hepatomas in the rat under excellent conditions and with carcinogenic agents of minor toxicity. One of them, No. 5123 with minimal deviations, is highly differentiated and morphologically and biochemically consists of cells strongly resembling normal hepatocytes. This affirmation is based on a detailed study carried out by Morris and a number of his collaborators, including Pitot, Potter, and Sorof. The study by Sorof, Morris, and collaborators (1966) pointed out that h.2. protein—the deletion of which was considered as the cause of the carcinogenesis—exists in the same quantity in normal rat liver and in hepatoma No. 5123. From then on, it would have been difficult to invoke the deletion of enzymes and constituents as the mechanism responsible for neoplastic transformation. This hepatoma contrasts with others, which are highly dedifferentiated and constituted by cells which have lost their hepatocytic aspect more or less completely. This is true for the hepatoma of Novikoff, which had often been studied and of which the author, after his collaboration with Morris, himself became critical.

Nevertheless, a detailed study of transplant hepatomas based on No. 5123 has shown some modifications with regard to certain enzyme systems and the behavior of these systems toward corticosteroid hormones. Examples are tyrosine transaminase and threonine and serine dehydrogenases, the regulation of which changes. Tryptophan pyrrolase disappears; it has been shown that the activity of this enzyme responds to various factors, especially hormones, and depends on whether the rat is prenatal or postnatal. We do not believe that these deletions have any significance for the theory whose mechanism we are discussing, since they clearly present as an evolutionary consequence of the tumor; on the other hand, we cannot ignore the irrigation differences between the transplants and the hepatoma that developed on the liver.

Since the first publications of Morris in 1961–63, enzyme systems in the various more or less differentiated hepatomas induced by this author have been studied. Criss and collaborators (1970) studied adenylate kinase (phosphotransferase ATP-ADP) in particular and found that the content of this enzyme is the greater the more differentiated the hepatoma (on the basis of gram/tumor it has come down from 128 to 16 units). Its concentration also varies with the state of nutrition. Jost and Pitot (1970) examined the metabolic adaptations in the 5123 hepatoma for serine dehydrogenase in the presence of glucose or amino acids.

These examples have cautioned investigators, since many modifications of enzymatic activity do not correspond to the mechanism of carcinogenesis and are only consequences of transformation. Theoretically, we can also affirm that hepatoma No. 5123 should result in a series of somatic mutations; the carcinogenic agent should combine with the DNA of the structural genes and give rise to alterations and to cancerization. In the last section we shall discuss the hepatoma induced by aflatoxin, for which we know the alterations in detail, but ignore the component of the macromolecule with which it combines (guanine?).

Investigation of the Neoplastic Transformation of Cultured Cells

We have seen from the preceding pages that Heidelberger and his associates contributed greatly to the solution of the problem of the linkage of carcinogenic hydrocarbons with cellular macromolecules. The important publication by Monod and Jacob (1961) promoted Heidelberger to write in 1963, together with Pitot, on "the two general molecular mechanisms concerning somatic mutation and the modifications of genetic expression, including repression and derepression." For Heidelberger, the problem of chosing between these two mechanisms is not yet resolved, each of them presenting its pros and cons. Both he and Ephrussi, writing in 1965, find it difficult to transfer to animal cells the results obtained in bacteria and based on the existence of two types of genes with different roles. Heidelberger decided to momentarily abandon the studies of neoplastic transformation at the molecular level and to concentrate on the cellular aspects of this vast problem, using cultured cells.

A number of investigators had previously studied the transformation of normal cells in cultures, with and without the addition of a chemical carcinogen (polycyclic hydrocarbon). We shall sum up the most important conclusions of these investigations before discussing the most recent, very rigorous deductions of Heidelberger. The investigation was carried out with the aim of showing under which conditions normal cultured cells undergo transformation, and if this transformation can be produced spontaneously. In a series of publications between 1941 and 1956, summed up in The Harvey Lectures in 1956, Gey and collaborators described their work on isolated systems and their observation of cell anomalies and neoplastic transformation during the aging of the cultures. We find the experiments of Earle and associates, carried out between 1943 and 1952, more convincing; they show the cancerous transformation of four strains of fibroblasts of the mouse without the addition of dimethylcholanthrene. From one of these cells they obtain eight strains, six of which are injected into mice and produce sarcomas. The cells present one or another of the anomalies described by Gey. These experiments are considered as proof that the cancerous transformation of a single cell can be observed in vitro. In 1958 Sanford obtained from one cell two strains with a malignant activity of differing intensity and characterized biochemically by their arginase content. Beside the test of tumor production in the mouse after subcutaneous injection of transformed cells, Sachs and collaborators demonstrated that loss of contact inhibition resulted in the culture filling up with transformed cells.

It seemed, consequently, an established fact that spontaneous transformation could be observed in cell cultures without using carcinogenic hydrocarbons. Heidelberger felt, however, that there was a serious objection to the conclusion that there is spontaneous transformation, a phenomenon he had observed, together with Iype in 1967 and 1968, as far as he was concerned, the conditions under which cultured cells are obtained, taking the characteristics of mouse cells into consideration, do not exclude a preceding transformation.

For these reasons he tackled the problem again on a new basis, with all the precautions that he found to be necessary. He took advantage of the studies of Prehn (1964) and of the fact that this author, in a culture based on a clone of cells, found that the chemical carcinogen sought out cells which were latently precancerous in the sense defined by Boutwell. From the beginning of his experiments, Heidelberger saw three alternatives: (1) transformation of normal into malignant cells due to the action of the chemical agent; (2) selection of precancerous cells by the carcinogenic agent; and (3) activation by the polycyclic hydrocarbon under the influence of a latent oncogenic virus.

Heidelberger obtained convincing results only between 1967 and 1970. His aim was to establish an adequate system for studies of chemical carcinogenesis which were not only qualitative but also quantitative (as in virology). He also felt that until his very last experiments, there had been no evidence favoring one of the three alternatives. Together with his associates, he used prostate cells of inbred C3H mice; in culture, these showed profound morphologic alterations but no other changes. In 1966, he and Iype obtained permanent strains from a culture of adult mouse prostate cells, using pronase for cell dispersion. Using dimethylbenzanthracene on some strains but not on others, the authors obtained two types of cultures: untreated controls died, but treated cells yielded persistent permanent strains, which when injected into the adult mouse produced growing, transplantable tumors. These tumors are mostly sarcomas, but the authors obtained also two anaplastic carcinomas. They concluded that in vitro they had produced a malignant transformation of prostate cells with a carcinogenic hydrocarbon as chemical agent. The authors wonder, though, whether this is just a process of transformation.

Heidelberger believed that his experiments were not perfect yet. That was why, in 1969, Chen and Heidelberger prolonged the growth time of the cells under observation, arguing that the period of latency for a spontaneous transformation might be long; after 70 days, though, the test of subcutaneous injection did not yield any tumor. When methylcholanthrene was added in the center of the culture, however, growth ensued, the monocellular layer was transformed, and the cultured cells piled up. In another observation the authors found again that without the carcinogen the cells did not pile up, but that colonies of piled up, malignant cells formed in the presence of the carcinogenic agent. Both tests evolved in a parallel manner, depending on the hydrocarbon used.

Finally, organ cultures treated with hydrocarbons show degeneration of the connective tissue and a proliferation of epithelial cells. One might think that isolated cells put in an organ culture actually derive from epithelial cells, whose morphologic aspect they imitate, but these cells yield strains which, after transformation and injection, produce mostly sarcomas. After attempts at identification, the authors thought that the cultured cells would be fibroblasts.

A last, truly crucial experiment was carried out by Mondal and Heidelberger (1969), thanks to a remarkable technique. On the basis of one single cell the authors showed unequivocally that the process is a transformation of the normal into a neoplastic cell and not a selection from among the cells of the culture. That was the first time such a demonstration was made for chemical carcinogenesis.

There obviously remains one question: instead of resulting from an interaction between the hydrocarbon and some critical cellular target, could the transformation be the result of the activation of a carcinogenic virus? Whatever the answer, Heidelberger (1970) thinks that his cell system will permit new studies of the linkage between the hydrocarbons and the macromolecules and a true explanation of the mechanism of carcinogenesis in the future.

Contribution to the Mechanism of Carcinogenesis

EXAMPLE OF INTERACTION BETWEEN NUCLEIC ACIDS AND CARCINOGENESIS OF THE CELL STRUCTURES IN VIVO

Many cancer investigators and biochemists accept the union between the chemical carcinogen and the DNA as a fact but think that the experimental proof of the union in vivo is not convincing and that in many cases it is impossible to decide in favor of one of the two theories: deletion or somatic mutation. In most cases we certainly ignore the series of events that take place between the moment the carcinogen is introduced into the organism and the moment of induction of the neoplastic transformation.

The interactions between the nucleic acids and the carcinogen often require a modification of the latter, and the union then takes place with a product of its metabolism. But is the result really due to a mutational process? There are some rare examples in which, because of the radioactive precursors used, the experimental proof might be considered as favoring one theory or the other.

We think that there is one particularly demonstrative case in which the stages of the union between the two nucleic acids have been clearly shown: the case of aflatoxin, the potent hepatocarcinogen, synthesized by *Aspergillus flavus*, a mold which in certain climates pollutes cereals, particularly peanut grains. Aflatoxin has been thoroughly studied by a number of European biologists (British and French) and then by American and Indian specialists. They concentrated especially on barnyard fowl and rats.

Since 1960–62, some of the associates of Le Breton, especially Frayssinet, LaFarge, and de Recondo, have studied carcinogenic doses in the rat and particularly the mode of action of this toxin. In the field of mechanisms of carcinogenesis, a study cannot be too complete, and the results obtained by these investigators finally led to an explanation of the mechanism of canceration of the rat liver cell. Let us briefly review the results.

(1) Since 1962, the lethal dose (LD_{50}) had been found to be high for this species if the animals were on a balanced protein-vitamin diet. The dose varies with age, sex, diet, and the cell strain used. On the contrary, the dose inducing cancerization is very low, and here age is an important factor. It has been established that at weaning the administration of a toxin dose of 2 μg.

per 100 g. of rat weight per day for six to seven weeks induces a hepatoma which becomes discernible after one year or later, the animal having been on a control diet without addition of any carcinogen during this long period of latency. In the oldest rat (about two months) the daily administration of 0.5 μg. per 100 g. for 14 to 16 months produces hepatomas.

(2) With the intraperitoneal administration of aflatoxin, rapid inhibition and synthesis of nucleic acids have been demonstrated. The inhibition is more important the higher the dose, the younger the animal, and the more intense the liver growth. Experiments were carried out on rats showing a compensatory hypertrophy of the lobe that remained in situ after partial ablation (hypertrophy of the hepatocytes followed by hyperplasia). The results obtained by Frayssinet (1962) concerning compensatory hypertrophy permitted determination of inhibition.

Moreover, the synthesis and inhibition can be followed with precision using radioactive precursors (orotic acid and thymidine), which are incorporated into the synthesized nucleic acids.

The investigation was carried out at the level of the cell structures. Contrary to what might be expected of a carcinogen, a low dose of toxin was found to produce an inhibition of the compensatory hypertrophy, resulting from the inhibition of the syntheses of nucleic acids necessary for cell multiplication and not from an action on the mechanisms of cell division itself. Let us examine first the case of RNA and then that of DNA.

Ribonucleic Acid. With a dose of aflatoxin corresponding to the dose inducing hepatic cancer, it is possible to produce progressive effects and to demonstrate specific sensibilities according to the localization of the RNA. Within 30 to 60 minutes after intraperitoneal injection, total inhibition of cell RNA is on the order of about 80 percent. Eighty percent of cell RNA is found in the ribosomes and 5 percent in the nucleus.

When the nucleoli are isolated, it becomes clear that 90 percent of the inhibition of nucleolar RNA occurs after 20 minutes, while at that moment inhibition for the nucleus totals only 35 percent. It is interesting that at the moment of minimal nucleolar synthesis, the morphology of the nucleolus is profoundly modified: there is total segregation of the content. This is important because the nucleolus is a solid cell organelle without a membrane, resistant to energy pressure like that of ultrasound, so that the presence of a few molecules of aflatoxin were actually sufficient to upset its architecture totally. All these biochemical and morphologic modifications are reversible within 24 hours, while the reversibility for the nuclear ribonucleic acid is complete within 12 hours. LaFarge and Frayssinet (1970) analyzed ribonucleic acids in gradients of saccharose after breaking up the nuclei with ultrasound and found that the heavy molecules (45S and 35S) with a long chain—i.e., those synthesized in the nucleolus—are the first and most intensely affected, while at that moment there is still marking and consequently synthesis of light 18S molecules.

In the cytoplasm there is an important diminution of ribosomes and temporarily of the enzyme systems under the influence of the toxin.

Deoxyribonucleic Acid. De Recondo and associates (1966) obtained some results which are important because of their bearing on the mechanisms of carcinogenesis. DNA synthesis is strongly inhibited in liver cells during compensatory hypertrophy. In vivo this inhibition occurs progressively and more slowly than in the case of ribonucleic acids: after one hour there is 65 percent inhibition and after 12 hours 95 percent. One injects 100 μg. of aflatoxin into the rat and tritiated thymidine one hour before killing the animal. Autohistoradiography shows that the percentage of marked nuclei is the same as in controls without aflatoxin, but the number of grains is severely diminished. Reversibility is complete but starts only after 48 hours. During all this time the DNA content of the hepatocytes is not modified, and there is neither synthesis nor catabolism.

When examining the activities of the enzyme systems of the DNA metabolism, De Recondo found in vitro, using DNA of calf thymus as a primer, that the enzyme activity of the synthesis is still great (phosphokinases, polymerases, and the activating factor of the native DNA); the deoxyribonucleases are hardly affected. These results suggest that aflatoxin acts directly on the DNA molecules (as does actinomycin D), thus inhibiting its primer activity.

This union has two consequences: it blocks the replication of DNA in the occupied sites, and it makes it impossible for the dependent RNA polymerase–DNA to fulfill its role of transcribing the information given by the DNA.* Experiments in vitro have shown that the activity of this enzyme is very much diminished and that the nucleotide transcript of the RNA is modified. These experiments have also shown that in order to block the DNA polymerase, the quantity of toxin needed is ten times greater. They equally suggest that in vivo one of the metabolites of aflatoxin would be the active substance.

The union of aflatoxin (or its active derivative) with DNA is important. This reaction would be in direct relation to its highly carcinogenic activity. In fact, the transformation of a normal cell into a neoplastic cell is always translated into specific, hereditary characteristics. These characteristics obviously presuppose mutations, which in this case would be the result of the repression of certain fractions of the DNA chains. When the rat is given very weak daily doses of the mycotoxin, the repression cannot be reversible, and after a certain time cancer of the liver is induced by the somatic mutations described above.

Obviously, this gene blocking effect of aflatoxin has been qualified by some as a "deletion," while in fact it is genetic information from the structural genes. But at this point the term "deletion" loses its original significance, since it no longer applies exclusively to the intervention of the operating genes controlling the choice of metabolic channels.

---

*Shortly after this publication, in 1966, J. L. Clifford and collaborators demonstrated the union of aflatoxin with DNA molecules by following the modifications of the spectrum of the toxin.

REFERENCES

Abell, C. W., and Heidelberger, C.: Interaction of carcinogenic hydrocarbons with tissues. VIII. Binding of tritium-labeled hydrocarbons to the soluble proteins of mouse skin. Cancer Res., 22:931, 1962.

Alexandrov, K., Vendrely, R., and Vendrely, C.: A comparative study of the action of carcinogenic substances on the RNA synthesis in mouse skin. Cancer Res., 30:1192, 1970.

Abercrombie, M.: General review of the nature of differentiation. *In* De Reuck, and Knight, J. (Eds.): Cell Differentiation. Vol. 3. London, Churchill, 1967.

Atsushi, N.: Changes in the serum β-glucuronidase activity of tumor-bearing hosts and the mechanism of glucuronidase inhibition by glucuronic acid and related compounds. Sapporo Igaku Zasshi, 28:387, 1968.

Baden, H. P., Mittler, B., Sviokla, S., and Pathak, M. A.: Urocanic acid in benign and malignant human epidermal tumors. J. Natl. Cancer Inst., 38:205, 1967.

Baden, H. P., Sviokla, S., Mittler, B., and Pathak, M. A.: Histidase activity in hyperplastic and neoplastic rat epidermis and liver. Cancer Res., 28:1463, 1968.

Barnes, M. J., Constable, B. J., Morton, L. F., and Hodicek, E.: Studies in vivo on the biosynthesis of collagen and elastin in ascorbic acid–deficient guinea-pigs. Biochem. J., 119:575, 1970.

Barski, G.: Symposium international. Cell Biol., 3:1, 1964.

Barski, G., and Belehradek, J.: Etude microcinématographique du mécanisme d'invasion cancéreuse en cultures de tissu normal associé aux cellules malignes. Exp. Cell Res., 37:464, 1965.

Barksi, G., Sorieul, S. C., and Cornefert, F. C.: Hybrid type cells in combined cultures of two different mammalian cell strains. J. Natl. Cancer Inst., 26:1269, 1961.

Berenblum, I.: Carcinogenesis and tumor pathogenesis. Advances Cancer Res., 2:129, 1954.

Berenblum, I., and Shubik, P.: A new quantitative approach to the study of the stages of chemical carcinogenesis in the mouse's skin. Br. J. Cancer, 1:383, 1947.

Bernstein, I. A.: Chemical differentiation in the epidermis. J. Soc. Cosmot. Chem., 21:583, 1970.

Bernstein, I. A., Chakrabarti, S. G., Kumaroo, K. K., and Sibrack, I. A.: Synthesis of protein in the mammalian epidermis. J. Invest. Dermatol., 55:291, 1970.

Bock, F. G.: Early effects of hydrocarbons on mammalian skin. Progr. Exp. Tumor Res., 4:126, 1964.

Boutwell, R. K.: Some biological aspects of skin carcinogenesis. Progr. Exp. Tumor Res., 4:207, 1964.

Boveri, T.: Zellstudien Heft 6. Jena, G. Fischer, 1907.

Boveri, T.: The origin of malignant tumors. (Translation by Marcella Boveri.) Baltimore, Williams and Wilkins, 1929.

Boyland, E., and Green, B.: The interaction of polycyclic hydrocarbons and nucleic acids. Br. J. Cancer, 16:507, 1962.

Boyland, E., and Sims, P.: The metabolism of 7,12-dimethylbenzanthracene by rat liver homogenates. Biochem. J., 95:780, 1965, and Biochem. J., 97:7, 1965a.

Boyland, E., and Sims, P.: The metabolism of benzanthracene and dibenzanthracene and their 5,6-epoxy-5,6-dihydro derivatives by rat-liver homogenates. Biochem. J., 97:7, 1965b.

Braun, A. C.: The Cancer Problem. New York, Columbia University Press, 1969.

Braun, A. C.: On the origin of the cancer cells. Am. Sci., 58:309, 1970.

Brookes, P.: Quantitative aspects of the reaction of some carcinogens with nucleic acids and the possible significance of such reactions in the process of carcinogenesis. Cancer Res., 26:1994, 1966.

Brookes, P., and Heidelberger, C.: Isolation and degradation of DNA from cells treated with tritium-labeled 7,12-dimethylbenzanthracene: Studies on the nature of the binding of this carcinogen to DNA. Cancer Res., 29:157, 1969.

Brookes, P., and Lawley, P. D.: Evidence for the binding of polynuclear aromatic hydrocarbons to the nucleic acids of mouse skin. Relation between carcinogenic power of hydrocarbons and their binding to deoxyribonucleic acid. Nature (Lond.), 202:781, 1964.

Brooks, S. C., Godefroi, V. C., and Simpson, W. L.: Specific sites of fatty acid and sterol synthesis in isolated skin components. Fed. Proc., 22:589, 1963.

Brooks, S. C., Godefroi, V. C., and Simpson, W. L.: Specific sites of fatty acid and sterol synthesis in isolated skin components. J. Lipid Res., 7:95, 1966.

Bullough, W. S., and Laurence, E. B.: Tissue homeostasis in adult mammals. *In* Montagna, W., et al. (Eds.): Advances in Biology of Skin. Vol. 7. Carcinogenesis. New York, Pergamon Press, 1967, p. 105.

Burnet, M.: Clonal Selection Theory of Acquired Immunity. Nashville, Vanderbilt University Press, 1959.

Burnett, J. B., Seiler, H., and Brown, J. V.: Separation and characterisation of multiple forms of tyrosinase from mouse melanoma. Cancer Res., 27:880, 1967.

Burton, P., Buffe, D., von Kleist, S., Wolff, E., and Wolff, E.: Mise en évidence de l'antigène carcinoembryonnaire spécifique des cancers digestifs des tumeurs humaines entretenues en culture organotypiques. Int. J. Cancer, 5:88, 1970.

Carruthers, C.: Urocanic acid in epidermal carcinogenesis. J. Invest. Dermatol., 50:41, 1968.

Cashman, D. C., Laryea, J. V., and Weissmann, B.: The hyaluronidase of rat skin. Arch. Biochem. Biophys., 135:387, 1969.

Champion, R. H., Gillman, T., Book, A. T., and Sims, R. T. (Eds.): An Introduction to the Biology of the Skin. Oxford, Blackwell Scientific Publications, 1970.

Chen, T. T., and Heidelberger, C.: In vitro malignant transformation of cells derived from mouse prostate in the presence of 3-methylcholanthrene. J. Natl. Cancer Inst., 42:915, 1969a.

Chen, T. T., and Heidelberger, C.: Quantitative studies on the malignant transformation of mouse prostate cells by carcinogenic hydrocarbons in vitro. Int. J. Cancer, 4:166, 1969b.

Clayson, D. B.: Chemical Carcinogenesis. London, Churchill, 1962.

Clifford, J. I., and Rees, K. R.: The action of aflatoxin B_1 on the rat liver. Biochem. J., 102:65, 1967.

Clifford, J. I., Rees, J. R., and Stevens, E.: The effect of aflatoxin B_1, G_1 and G_3 on protein and nucleic acid synthesis in rat liver. Biochem. J., 103:258, 1967.

Cohen, S.: Isolation and biological effects of an epidermal growth-stimulating protein. Natl. Cancer Inst. Monogr., 13:21, 1964.

Criss, W. E., Litwack, G., Morris, H. P., and Weinhouse, S.: Adenosine triphosphate: Adenosine monophosphate phosphotransferase isozymes in rat liver and hepatomas. Cancer Res., 30:370, 1970.

Davenport, G. R., Abell, C. W., and Heidelberger, C.: The interaction of carcinogenic hydrocarbons with tissues. VII. Fractionation of mouse skin proteins. Cancer Res., 21:599, 1961.

Davidson, R. L., and Ephrussi, B.: A selective system for the isolation of hybrids between L cells and normal cells. Nature (Lond.), 205:1170, 1965.

Dechambre, R. P.: Effet de groupe et évolution des tumeurs ascitiques chez la souris. Thèse de Doctorat Fac. des Sciences, Paris, 1970.

Di Bella, S., Panazzolo, A., Scarpa, F., and Cacciari, P.: Carbohydrate metabolism in experimental and human neoplasia. I. Experimental study of neoplasias induced in rats by 9,10-dimethyl-1,2-benzanthracene. Cancro, 21:267, 1968.

Dipple, A., Lawley, P. D., and Brookes, P.: Theory of tumour initiation by chemical carcinogens: Dependence of activity on structure of ultimate carcinogens. Eur. J. Cancer, 4:493, 1968.

Dulbecco, R.: The induction of cancer by viruses. Sci. Am., 216:28, 1967.

Eagle, H.: Amino acid metabolism in mammalian cell cultures. Science, 130:432, 1959.

Earle, W. R., and Nettleship, A. J.: Production of malignancy in vitro; results of injections of cultures into mice. J. Natl. Cancer Inst., 4:213, 1943.

Ephrussi, B.: *In* Developmental and Metabolic Control Mechanisms and Neoplasia. University of Texas M.D. Anderson Hospital and Tumor Institute, Houston, Texas. 19th Annual Symposium on Fundamental Cancer Research, 1965, 486. Baltimore, Williams and Wilkins, 1965.

Ephrussi, B.: *In* Somatic hybridization as a tool for the study of normal and abnormal growth and differentiation. 23rd Annual Symposium on Fundamental Cancer Research. Baltimore, Williams and Wilkins, 1970, p. 9.

Ephrussi, B., and Sorieul, S. C.: Nouvelles observations sur l'hybridisation in vitro de cellules de souris. C. R. Acad. Sci. (Paris), 254:184, 1962.

Epstein, W. L., and Maibach, H. I.: Cell renewal in human epidermis. Arch. Dermatol., 92:462, 1965.

Flamm, W. G., Banerjee, M. R., and Counts, W. B.: Topical application of actinomycyn D on mouse skin: Effect on the synthesis of ribonucleic acid and protein. Cancer Res., 26:1349, 1966.

Frayssinet, C.: Etude chez le rat de l'hypertrophie compensatrice du foie après ablation partielle. Mise en évidence d'une caractéristique du tissu hépatique selon le type de croissance. Thèse de Doctorat, Fac. des Sciences, Paris, 1962.

Frei, J. V., and Ritchie, A. C.: Diurnal variation in the susceptibility of mouse epidermis to carcinogen and its relationship to DNA synthesis. J. Natl. Cancer Inst., 32:1213, 1964.

Gaylor, J. L.: Biosynthesis of skin sterols. III. Conversion of squalene to sterols by rat skin. J. Biol. Chem., 238:1643, 1963.

Gaylor, J. L., and Sault, F. M.: Localization and biosynthesis of 7-dehydro cholesterol in rat skin. J. Lipid Res., 5:422, 1964.

Gelboin, H. V.: A microsome-dependent binding of benzopyrene to DNA. Cancer Res., 29:1272, 1969.

Georgiev, G. P.: A hypothesis regarding the structural organization of the operon and regulation of RNA synthesis in the animal cell. (Translation by Molekulyarnay Biologiya.) 4:17, 1970.

Gey, G. O.: Some aspects of constitution and behavior of normal and malignant cells maintained in continuous culture. Harvey Lect., 50:154, 1954–55 (1st publication 1941).

Giovanella, C., McKinney, L. E., and Heidelberger, C.: On the reported solubilization of carcinogenic hydrocarbons in aqueous solutions of DNA. J. Mol. Biol., 8:20, 1964.

Gold, P., and Freedman, S. O.: Specific carcinoembryonic antigens of the human digestive system. J. Exp. Med., 122:467, 1965.

Gordon, M. (Ed.): Pigment Cell Biology. New York, Academic Press, 1959.

Grabar, P., et al.: Immunochemical and Enzymatic Studies on Chemically Induced Rat Liver Tumors (in UICC monograph series). Copenhagen, R.I.C. Harris, 1967.

Haddow, A., Scott, C. M., and Scott, J. D.: Influence of certain carcinogenic and other hydrocarbons on body growth in the rat. Proc. R. Soc. [B], 122:477, 1937.

Halprin, K. M., Ohkawara, A., and Fukui, K.: Enzymatic characteristics of human basal cell epithelioma. Arch. Dermatol., 98:80, 1968.

Hardingham, T. E., and Phelps, L. F.: The tissue content and turnover rates of intermediates in the biosynthesis of glycosaminoglycans in young rat skin. Biochem. J., 108:9, 1968.

Hardingham, T. E., and Phelps, L. F.: The glycosaminoglycans of neonatal rat skin. Biochem. J., 117:813, 1970.

Heidelberger, C.: Studies on the cellular and molecular mechanism of hydrocarbon carcinogenesis. Eur. J. Cancer, 6:161, 1970.

Heidelberger, C., and Giovanella, B. C.: Studies on the molecular and cellular mechanisms of hydrocarbon cancerogenesis. *In* Montagna, W., et al. (Eds.): Advances in Biology of Skin. Vol. 7, Carcinogenesis. New York, Pergamon Press, 1967, p. 105.

Heidelberger, C., and Iype, P. T.: Malignant transformation in vitro by carcinogenic hydrocarbons. Science, 155:214, 1967.

Heidelberger, C., Iype, P. T., Roller, M. R., and Chen, T. T.: Study of hydrocarbon carcinogenesis in organ and cell culture. *In* Proliferation and Spread of Neoplastic Cells. University of Texas M.D. Anderson Hospital and Tumor Institute. Baltimore, Williams and Wilkins, 1968.

Hennings, H., and Boutwell, R. K.: The inhibition of DNA synthesis by initiators of mouse skin tumorigenesis. Cancer Res., 29:510, 1969.

Hennings, H., and Boutwell, R. K.: Studies on the mechanism of skin tumor promotion. Cancer Res., 30:312, 1970.

Hennings, H., Smith, H. C., Colburn, N. H., and Boutwell, R. K.: Inhibition by actinomycin D of DNA and RNA synthesis and of skin carcinogenesis initiated by 7,12-dimethylbenzanthracene or β-propiolactone. Cancer Res., 28:543, 1968.

Hewitt, J., Guigon, M., Bolubasz, J., and Masson, C.: Activité de la β-glucuronidase dans les tumeurs pigmentaires de la peau humaine. Etude histochimique et biochimique. Rev. Eur. Etud. Clin. Biol., 15:416, 1970.

Horton, A. W., Van Dreal, P. A., and Bingham, E. L.: Physicochemical mechanism of acceleration of skin carcinogenesis. *In* Montagna, W., et al. (Eds.): Advances in Biology of Skin. Vol. 7. New York, Pergamon Press, 1967, p. 165.

Im, M. J. C.: Glucose metabolism in skin tumor and hyperplasia induced in the rhesus monkey by 7,12-dimethylbenzanthracene. J. Natl. Cancer Inst., 41:73, 1968.

Iverson, O. H.: Discussion on cell destruction and population dynamics in experimental skin carcinogenesis in mice. Progr. Exp. Tumor Res., 4:169, 1964.

Iype, P. T., and Heidelberger, C.: Characteristics of murine prostatic acid phosphatase: Comparison with other tissues and species. Arch. Biochem. Biophys., 128:434, 1968.

Jacob, A.: Modification du métabolisme glucidique dans le foie en voie de cancérisation par le diméthylaminobenzène. III. Recherches au niveau de la voie des pentoses phosphates. Int. J. Cancer, 5:111, 1970.

Jacob, F., and Monod, J.: *In* Locke, M. (Ed.): Cytodifferentiation and Macromolecular Synthesis. New York, Academic Press, 1963, p. 30.

Jensen, E. V., Ford, E., and Huggins, C.: Depressed incorporation of thymidine-H³ into deoxyribonucleic acid following administration of 7,12-dimethylbenzanthracene. Proc. Natl. Acad. Sci. USA, 50:455, 1963.

Jost, J. P., and Pitot, H. C.: Metabolic adaptations in rat hepatomas: Altered regulation of serine dehydratase synthesis by glucose and amino acids in hepatocellular carcinomas. Cancer Res., 30:387, 1970.

Krick, E., Miller, J. A., Juhl, V., and Miller, E. C.: Biochemistry (Wash.), :6, 1967.

Kusaba, K.: Light and electron microscopic studies on lesions of the skin in experimental vitamin A deficiency. Vitamin 42:118, 1970.

LaFarge, C., and Frayssinet, C.: The reversibility of inhibition of RNA and DNA synthesis induced by aflatoxin in rat liver. A tentative explanation for carcinogenic mechanism. Int. J. Cancer, 6:74, 1970.

LaFarge, C., Frayssinet, C., and de Recondo, A. M.: Inhibition par l'aflatoxine de la synthèse du RNA hépatique chez le rat. Bull. Soc. Chim. Biol., 47:1724, 1965.

Langer, E., Keiditsch, E., Strauch, L., and Hannig, K.: Activity of collagenase in the simple, solid carcinoma of the breast. Verh. Dtsch. Ges. Pathol., 52:438, 1968.

Le Breton, E., and Moule, Y.: Biochemistry and physiology of the cancer cell. *In* Brachet, J., and Mirsky, A. E. (Eds.): The Cell. Vol. 5, Part 2. New York, Academic Press, 1966, p. 497.

Le Breton, E., Frayssinet, C., and Boy, J.: Sur l'apparition d'hépatomes spontanés chez le Rat Wistar. Rôle de la toxine de l'Aspergillus flavus. Intérêt en pathologie humaine et cancérologie expérimentale. C. R. Acad. Sci. (Paris), 255:784, 1962.

Le Breton, E., Boy, J., Chany, E., Frayssinet, C., Jacob, A., Moule, Y., and de Recondo, A. M.: L'hépatome expérimental du rat. *In* Tumeurs Malignes du Foie. Journées de Gastroentérologie. Paris, Masson, 1963, p. 2.

Le Breton, E., Frayssinet, C., LaFarge, C., and de Recondo, A. M.: Aflatoxine, mécanisme d'action. Food Cosmet. Toxicol., 2:675, 1964.

Loewi, G., and Meyer, K.: The acid mucopolysaccharides of embryonic skin. Biochim. Biophys. Acta, 27:453, 1958.

Lynch, H. T.: Hereditary Factors in Carcinoma. New York, Springer, 1967.

Menon, I. E., and Habermann, H. F.: Activation of tyrosinase in microsomes and melanosomes from B16 and Harding-Passey melanomas. Arch. Biochem. Biophys., 137:231, 1970a.

Menon, I. E., and Habermann, H. F.: Tyrosinase activity in serum from normal and melanoma bearing mice. Cancer Res., 28:1237, 1970b.

Meyer, K., Davidson, E., Linker, A., and Hoffman, P.: The acid mucopolysaccharides of connective tissue. Biochim. Biophys. Acta, 21:506, 1956.

Miller, E. C.: Studies on the formation of protein bound derivatives of 3,4-benzopyrene in the epidermal fraction of mouse skin. Cancer Res., 10:100, 1950.

Miller, E. C., and Miller, J. A.: Presence and significance of bound aminoazo dyes in livers of rats fed p-dimethylaminoazobenzene. Cancer Res., 7:468, 1947.

Miller, E. C., and Miller, J. A.: Mechanisms of chemical carcinogenesis: Nature of proximate carcinogens and interactions with macromolecules. Pharmacol. Rev., 18:805, 1966.

Miller, J. A., and Miller, E. C.: The metabolic activation of carcinogenic aromatic amines and amides. Progr. Exp. Tumor Res., 11:273, 1969.

Mondal, S., and Heidelberger, C.: Malignant transformation of single prostate cells *in vitro* with methylcholanthrene. Proc. Am. Assoc. Cancer Res., 10:61, 1969.

Monod, J., and Jacob, F.: General conclusions: Teleonomic mechanisms in cellular metabolism, growth and differentiation. Cold Spring Harbor Sympos. Quant. Biol., 26:389, 1961.

Montagna, W., et al. (Eds.): Advances in Biology of Skin. Vol 7, Carcinogenesis. New York, Pergamon Press, 1967.

Morris, H. P.: Biology of experimental hepatomas. Advances Cancer Res., 9:227, 1965.

Morris, H. P., and Wagner, B. P.: Induction and transplantation of rat hepatomas with different growth rate (including "minimum deviation hepatomas"). *In* Methods in Cancer Research. New York, Academic Press, 1968, pp. 4–125.

Moulé, Y., and Frayssinet, C.: Action of aflatoxin on

transcription in liver cell. Nature (Lond.), 218:93, 1968.

Nicolaides, N.: Skin lipids. IV. Biochemistry and function. J. Oil. Chem. Soc., 42:708, 1965.

Oberling, C., and Bernhard, W.: *In* The Cell. New York, Academic Press, 1961.

Ockermann, P. A.: Acid hydrolases in human skin. Acta Derm. Venereol. (Stockh.), 49:139, 1969.

Ove, P., Jenkins, M. D., and Laszlo, J.: DNA polymerase patterns in developing rat liver. Cancer Res., 30:535, 1970.

Paul, D.: Effects of carcinogenic, noncarcinogenic and cocarcinogenic agents on the byosynthesis of nucleic acids in mouse skin. Cancer Res., 29:1218, 1969.

Paul, D., and Hecker, E.: On the biochemical mechanism of tumorigenesis in mouse skin. *In* Early effects in the biosynthesis of nucleic acids induced by initiating doses of DMBA and by promoting doses of phorbol-12-13 diester TPA. Z. Krebsforsch., 73:149, 1969.

Pitot, H. C.: Some biochemical aspects of malignancy. Ann. Rev. Biochem., 35:335, 1966.

Pitot, H. C.: *In* Paton, A. (Ed.): Liver Disease. Vol. III. Philadelphia, J. B. Lippincott, 1970, p. 77.

Pitot, H. C., and Heidelberger, C.: Metabolic regulatory circuits and carcinogenesis. Cancer Res., 23:1964, 1963.

Potter, V. R.: Enzymes, Growth and Cancer. Springfield, Ill., Charles C Thomas, Publisher, 1950.

Potter, V. R.: The biochemical approach to the cancer problem. Fed. Proc., 17:691, 1958.

Potter, V. R.: Biochemical perspectives in cancer research. Cancer Res., 24:1085, 1964.

Prehn, R. T.: A clonal selection theory of chemical carcinogenesis. J. Natl. Cancer Inst., 32:1, 1964.

Prescott, D. M., and Goldstein, L.: Nuclear-cytoplasmic interaction in DNA synthesis. Science, 155:469, 1967.

Prodi, G.: Acid mucopolysaccharides of the dermis ground substance during skin treatment with 9,10-dimethyl-1,2-benzanthracene and with croton oil. Br. J. Cancer, 17:504, 1963.

Prodi, G., and Romeo, G.: The metabolism of acid mucopolysaccharides of the dermis ground substance during skin treatment with 9,10-dimethyl-1,2-benzanthracene. Br. J. Cancer, 20:852, 1966.

De Recondo, A. M., Frayssinet, C., LaFarge, C., and Le Breton, E.: Action de l'Aflatoxine sur le métabolisme du DNA au cours de l'hypertrophie compensatrice du foie après hépatectomie partielle. Biochim. Biophys. Acta, 119:322, 1966.

Riley, V.: Some enzymic and metabolic characteristics of malignant pigmented tissue. Adv. Biol. Skin, 8:581, 1968.

Roth, J. K.: Histones in development, growth and cancer. Nature (Lond.), 207:599, 1965.

Rubin, H.: *In* Locke, M. (Ed.): Major Problems in Developmental Biology. New York, Academic Press, 1966, p. 315.

Sanford, K. K.: Natl. Cancer Inst. Monogr., 26:387, 1958.

Sanford, K. K., Earle, W. R., et al.: Production of malignancy in vitro; further transformations of mouse fibroblasts to sarcomatous cells. J. Natl. Cancer Inst., 11:351, 1950.

Sanford, K. K., Likely, G. D., Bryan, W. R., and Earle, W. R.: Production of sarcomas from cultured tissues of hepatoma, melanoma, and thyroid tumors. J. Natl. Cancer Inst., 12:1057, 1952.

Schamberger, R. J., and Rudolph, G.: Increase of lysosomal enzymes in skin cancer. Nature (Lond.), 213:617, 1967.

Schiller, S.: Isolation of heparin sulfate from skin of normal rats. Biochim. Biophys. Acta, 124:215, 1966.

Seilern-Aspang, F.: Auslösung eines Carcinoms bei lokaler Einwirkung von Corticosteron. Naturwiss, 56:564, 1969.

Seilern-Aspang, F., Mazzucco, K., and Christian, I.: Der Einfluss von Methylcholanthren auf Synthese, Vernetzung and Abbau des Kollagens der Mäusedermis und die mögliche Bedeutung dieses Abbaues für malignes Wachstum. Z. Naturforsch. [B], 24:894, 1969.

Sherwood, I. M., et al.: Parathyroid Hormone Production by Bronchogenic Carcinomas. Forty-Eighth Meeting of the Endocrine Society. Philadelphia, 1966, p. 29.

Shubik, P.: Some biological implications of chemical carcinogenesis. *In* Montagna, W., et al. (Eds.): Advances in Biology of Skin. Vol. 7, Carcinogenesis. New York, Pergamon Press, 1965, p. 89.

Sorof, S., Cohen, P. P., Miller, E. C., and Miller, J. A.: Cancer Res., 2:383, 1951.

Sorof, S., Young, E. M., Luongo, L., Kish, V. M., and Freed, J. J.: Inhibition of cell multiplication *in vitro* by liver arginase. Wistar Inst. Sympos. Monogr., 7:25, 1967.

Strauch, L., Vencelj, H., and Hannig, K.: Kollagenase in Zellen höher entwickelter Tiere. H.S. Z. Physiol. Chem., 349:171, 1968.

Temin, H. M.: *In* Defendi, V., and Stoker, M. (Eds.): Growth Regulating Substances for Animal Cells in Culture. Philadelphia, Wistar Institute Press, 1967, p. 103.

Toolan, H. W.: The potentialities of normal cells implanted in cortisonized and/or X-radiated hosts. Guest Editorial. Cancer Res., 17:248, 1957.

Tregear, R. T.: Physical Functions of Skin. New York, Academic Press, 1966.

Umeda, M., Diringer, H., and Heidelberger, C.: Inhibition of the growth of cultured cells by arginase and the soluble proteins from mouse skin. Israel J. Med. Sci., 4:1216, 1968.

Van Scott, E. J.: Reaction patterns of normal and neoplastic epithelium. *In* Montagna, W., et al. (Eds.): Advances in Biology of Skin. Vol. 7, Carcinogenesis. New York, Pergamon Press, 1967, p. 75.

Vezekenyi, K.: Sulfatase activity in human epidermis and various tumors. Acta Morphol., 16:237, 1968.

Vitto, J.: A method for studying collagen biosynthesis in human skin biopsies in vitro. Biochim. Biophys. Acta, 201:438, 1970.

Voorhess, M. L.: Effect of d-methyl-p-tyrosine on 3,4-dihydroxyphenylalanine excretion of hamsters with melanotic melanoma. Cancer Res., 28:452, 1968.

Weiss, P.: A general mechanism of differentiation based on morphogenetic studies in Ciliates. Am. Nat., 85:203, 1951.

Wheatley, V. R., Lipkin, G., and Woo, T. H.: Lipogenesis from amino-acids in perfused isolated dog skin. J. Lipid Res., 8:84, 1967.

Wheatley, V. R., Hodgins, L. T., Coon, W. M., Kumarasiri, M., Berenzweig, H., and Feinstein, J. M.: Cutaneous lipogenesis: precursors utilised by guinea pig skin for lipid synthesis. J. Lipid Res., 12:347, 1971.

Wirl, G., and Seilern-Aspang, F.: Beziehungen zwischen Induzierbarkeit eines Hautkarzinoms, dem Kollagengehalt der Haut und der Synthese der Askorbinsäure bei Triturus cristatus. Arch. Geschwulstforsch.. 35:36, 1970.

Wolff, E.: *In* Cell Differentiation and Morphogenesis. International Lecture Cours Wageningen, The Netherlands. Amsterdam, North-Holland, 1966.

Wright, S.: The physiology of the gene. Physiol. Rev., 21:487, 1941.

Zador, S.: Simultaneous respiratory and histological studies on mouse skin during carcinogenesis with DMBA. Virchows Arch. [Zellpathol.], 4:71, 1969.

14

Fine Structure of Skin Neoplasms

Leonard P. Merkow, M.D., Ph.D.,
and Hernando Salazar, M.D., M.P.H.

Benign Neoplasms

INTRADERMAL NEVUS (NEURONEVUS)

By electron microscopy, the neval elements appear to be organized into small groups of rounded neoplastic cells of uniform size surrounded by bundles of collagen fibers. Frequently they are seen organized around nonmyelinated nerves, forming a distinct neuroneval unit. The relationship between neval cells and cellular elements of the perineurium is not apparent. Fibroblasts, however, are identifiable as such in the connective stroma of the tumor.

The neval cells may or may not contain melanin inclusions. The majority of cells are devoid of pigment granules. These cells are generally rounded, with a large ovoid nucleus sometimes displaying indentations and/or large nucleoli. Occasionally, spheroidal nuclear bodies are seen. In general, the cytoplasm is relatively clear, with ovoid mitochondria bearing transverse cristae, large Golgi complexes, and occasional lysosomes. The endoplasmic reticulum is usually formed by scattered short channels of granular

membranes intermingled with cytoplasmic filaments and other organelles.

In areas where neval cells are closely apposed to each other, leaving narrow intercellular spaces, it is not unusual to observe pseudovillous projections of the plasmalemma. Cilia are occasionally seen. The pigmented cells contain typical melanosomes and premelanosomes of variable size and shape, either organized toward the periphery of the cytoplasm or polarized in one area of the cell.

LEIOMYOMA CUTIS

The fine structural features of this neoplasm conform to the classic characteristics of leiomyomas in other organs. The tumor is essentially composed of bundles of smooth muscle cells embedded within a collagenous stroma.

The neoplastic smooth muscle cells are of variable size and shape, but in general they appear elongated or fusiform, with longitudinal axes parallel to each other within the bundle. The external margins of the cells are fairly regular, and the ex-

Text continued on page 355.

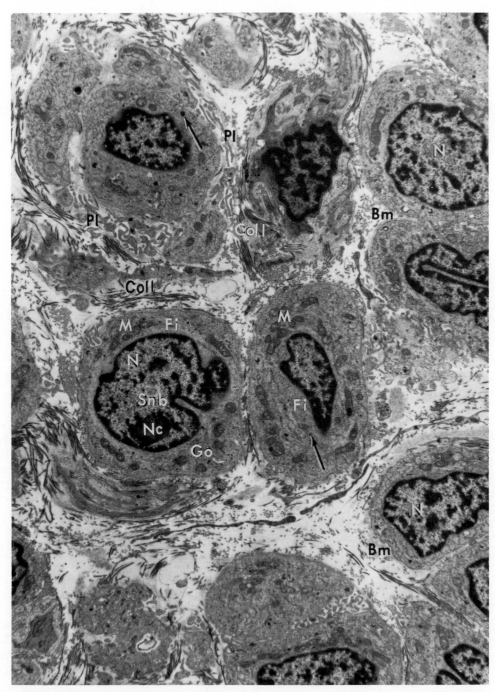

Figure 14–1 *Neuronevus.* Numerous neval cells are grouped in a cluster with intervening strands of collagen (Coll). The nuclei (N) are prominent and may display a nucleolus (Nc) or spheroidal nuclear body (Snb). Some of these neval cells contain delicate filaments (Fi), especially circumscribing the nucleus. Mitochondria (M), Golgi complexes (Go), and a few dense bodies (arrows) are evident. Premelanosomes and melanosomes are not evident in this power field. Basement membrane–like material (Bm) surrounds the plasmalemma (Pl). The latter sometimes forms pseudovillous projections. ×7,000.

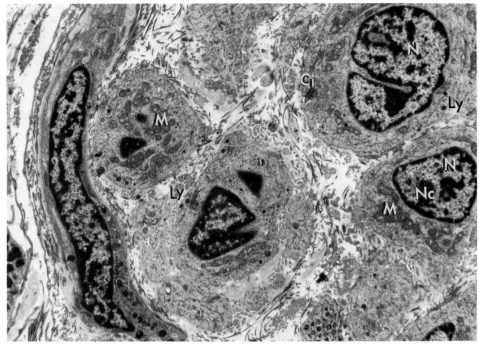

Figure 14–2 *Neuronevus.* Neval cells display prominent nuclei (N) and nucleoli (Nc). A cilium (Ci) consisting of a rootlet and basal body is evident near the surface of one neval cell. Other neoplastic cells contain mitochondria (M), lysosomes (Ly), and a granular cytoplasm. ×6,500.

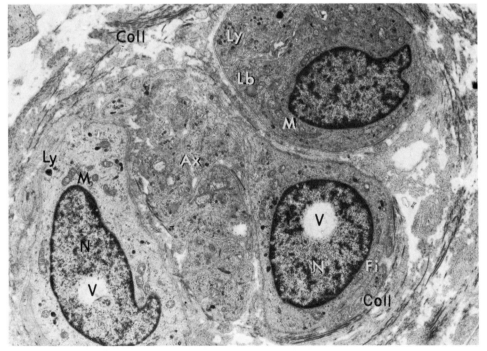

Figure 14–3 *Neuronevus.* Several neval cells are clustered about an axon (Ax). Note that these tumor cells have intranuclear (N) vacuoles (V). Their cytoplasm contains lipid bodies (Lb), mitochondria (M), lysosomes (Ly), and delicate filaments (Fi). The tumor cells are circumscribed by bundles of collagen (Coll) forming the neval nest. The close relationship between the neural tissue (axon) and neval cells is demonstrated here. ×7,000.

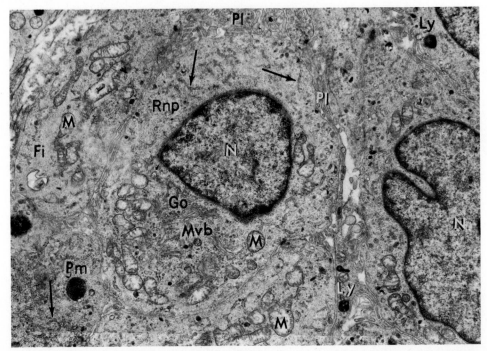

Figure 14-4 *Neuronevus.* Neoplastic cells show nuclei (N) surrounded by a prominent group of cytoplasmic organelles. Large Golgi complexes (Go), mitochondria (M), lysosomes (Ly), free ribosomes (Rnp) as well as vesicles or short cisternae of rough endoplasmic reticulum (arrows), a multivesicular body (Mvb), delicate filaments (Fi), and prominent microvillous projections of the plasmalemma (Pl) are evident. A premelanosome (Pm) is discernible at lower left. ×9,000.

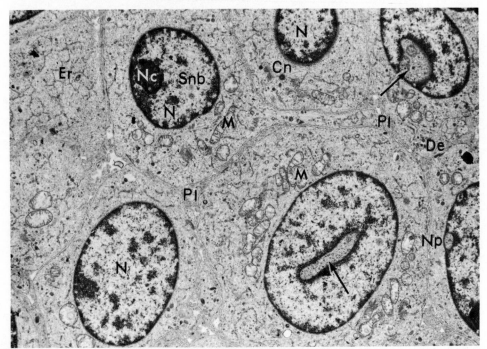

Figure 14-5 *Neuronevus.* Numerous neval cells show quite uniform nuclei (N), occasionally displaying a groove or fold actually representing an invagination (arrows). In addition, these nuclei contain nucleoli (Nc), spheroidal nuclear bodies (Snb), or nuclear projections (Np). The cytoplasm in these cells contains a reticular background consisting of endoplasmic reticulum (Er), mitochondria (M), a centriole (Cn), and prominent pseudovillous projections of the plasmalemma (Pl). A desmosome (De) is present on the right. ×7,500.

tremes or tips are blunted or rounded. Each individual cell is surrounded by a distinct delicate "basement lamina" of medium electron density, closely apposed to the plasmalemma. Rows of micropinocy-totic vesicles are frequently observed at the cell border.

The cytoplasm of these cells is abundant and completely filled by myofilaments following the long axis of the cell.

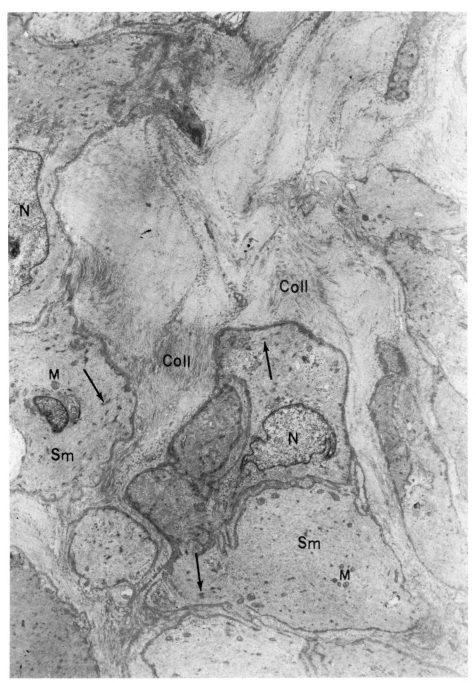

Figure 14-6 *Leiomyoma.* Embedded within abundant collagen (Coll) are numerous smooth muscle cells containing a nucleus (N) and cytoplasm with numerous myofilaments representing immature smooth muscle (Sm), dense regions within the smooth muscle (arrows), and a few small mitochondria (M). ×7,000.

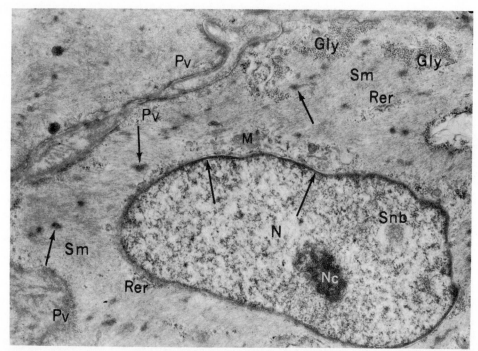

Figure 14–7 *Leiomyoma.* At higher magnification, a smooth muscle cell shows a cytoplasm filled with myofilaments of smooth muscle (Sm), infrequent cisternae of rough endoplasmic reticulum (Rer), a few clusters of glycogen (Gly), a paucity of mitochondria (M), focal dense regions within the abundant smooth muscle (arrows), and pinocytotic vesicles (Pv). The nucleus (N) displays a prominent internal nuclear membrane (arrows), a coiled nucleolus (Nc), and a spheroidal nuclear body (Snb). *×17,000.*

They present the characteristic features of smooth muscle filaments, including the presence of distinct "dense bodies" irregularly distributed within the cytoplasm and at the level of the cell membrane. Clusters of small mitochondria associated with glycogen deposits and free or membrane-bound ribosomes are usually seen in a juxtanuclear location but also may be found in the vicinity of the cell margins. The Golgi apparatus is generally seen adjacent to the nucleus.

The nucleus is usually elongated, with smooth outlines and rounded ends, but it is not uncommon to observe indentations and deep infoldings. The chromatin is finely granular and well dispersed. Spheroidal nuclear bodies are occasionally seen. Nucleoli are constantly seen in most cells and frequently display a honeycomb appearance of dense nucleolonemal reticula and clear granular interstices.

It is not unusual to observe occasional neoplastic cells with a very dense cytoplasm, showing multiple vacuoles and marked increase in the number and size of pinocytotic vesicles. They are interpreted as degenerated or necrotic cells.

The intercellular space and the interfascicular stroma of the neoplasm are composed of large amounts of densely packed collagen fibers (640 Å periodicity). Occasional fibroblasts and small stromal blood vessels are also present.

CAPILLARY HEMANGIOMA

Although efforts have been made to try to differentiate normal capillaries from the proliferating capillaries of hemangiomas or other neoplasms, they have been fruitless, and it is accepted that the structure of normal and abnormal terminal vasculature is practically identical.

The fine structure of the vascular elements in capillary hemangiomas confirms the histologic findings. These elements represent true capillaries composed of an intimal lining of continuous endothelium supported by a delicate endothelial basement lamina, which separates the endothe-

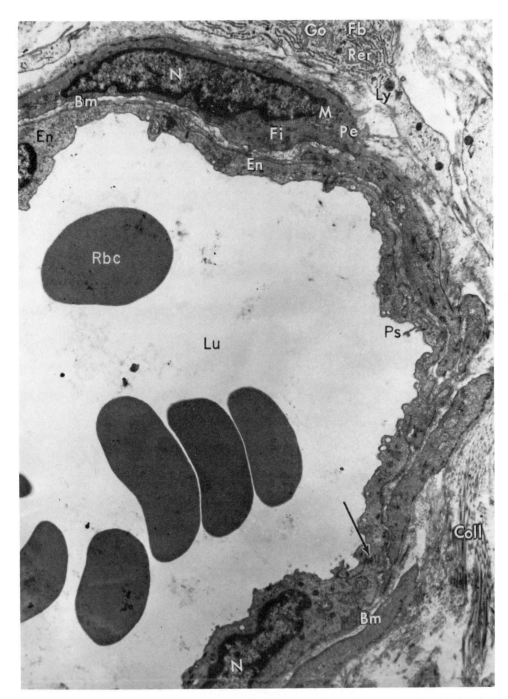

Figure 14–8 *Capillary hemangioma.* A capillary consists of endothelial (En) lining cells with intraluminal pseudovilli (Ps) and adventitial pericytes (Pe) beneath fibroblasts (Fb). Note the basement membrane (Bm) on the external side of the endothelial cells. Pericytes (Pe) contain delicate filaments (Fi) and mitochondria (M). The fibroblasts display Golgi complexes (Go), abundant rough endoplasmic reticulum (Rer), and lysosomes (Ly). Tight junctions (arrow) are present between adjacent endothelial cells and serve as a locus wherein the cellular elements slip through to the tissue. The lumen (Lu) contains red blood cells (Rbc). ×7,500.

lium from the perivascular connective tissue space. Frequently, pericytes are observed adjacent to the external aspect of the basement lamina.

The endothelial lining is formed by flat, irregular cells, unperforated or nonfenestrated, which circumscribe the luminal space and rest upon a continuous external basement lamina. Usually, only two or three portions of endothelial cells are seen in a given section. Most are devoid of a nucleus in the plane of section; the cytoplasm is usually rich in ribosomes, mitochondria, endoplasmic reticulum, and lysosomes, as well as containing numerous pinocytotic vesicles along the luminal and basal margins and intracytoplasmic bundles of fine filaments. In the areas about the endothelial nuclei, a well-developed Golgi complex, centrioles, and lipid inclusions are frequently observed. In association with the pinocytotic vesicles of the luminal border, the endothelial cells commonly present cytoplasmic digitations or microvilli of variable size and shape; these structures are related to the transport of

fluids across the endothelium. At the site of junction, adjacent endothelial cells seem to imbricate and interlock in "jigsaw puzzle" fashion by interdigitating processes which close the narrow intercellular space; distinct tight junctions are present at the luminal end of this space, making it impermeable. However, this intercellular space is the site through which the blood-formed elements escape in case of need.

The pericytes of capillaries and venules are cells located outside the basement lamina and are surrounded by a coat of amorphous material of medium electron density which is continuous with the endothelial basement lamina. These pericytes have characteristics similar to those of smooth muscle cells, namely an elongated shape, an irregular nucleus with blunted ends, a cytoplasm rich in filamentous bundles with dense bodies, marginal pinocytotic vesicles, and the already mentioned peripheral basement lamina–like coat.

The perivascular space between capillaries is rich in collagen fibers and fibroblasts. In addition, histiocytes and mast

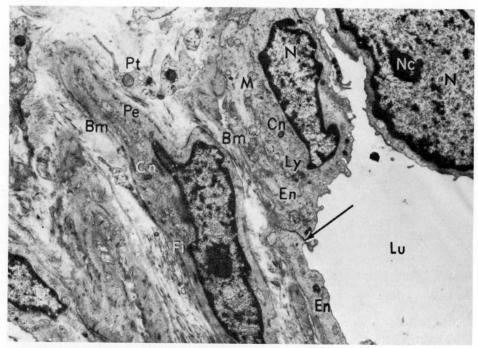

Figure 14–9 *Capillary hemangioma.* An endothelial cell (En) displays a nucleus (N) and nucleolus (Nc). The cytoplasm contains a centriole (Cn), small mitochondria (M), and lysosomes (Ly). A tight junction is present (arrow) between adjacent endothelial cells. The external pericyte (Pe) also contains a centriole (Cn) and delicate filaments (Fi). Basement membrane (Bm) material is noted along the external surface of the endothelial cells and the pericyte. The lumen (Lu) is in the lower right. A platelet (Pt) is near top. ×7,000.

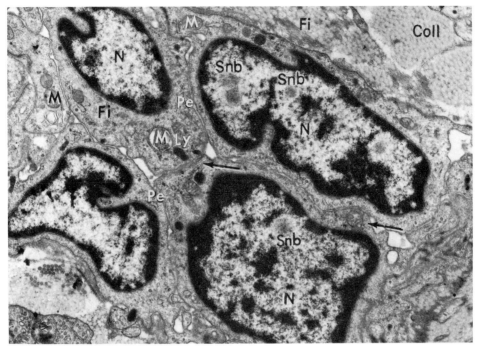

Figure 14–10 *Capillary hemangioma.* Several pericytes (Pe) display prominent nuclei (N) and spheroidal nuclear bodies (Snb). Pinocytotic vesicles (arrows) are evident, as well as mitochondria (M), delicate filaments (Fi), and an occasional lysosome (Ly). Abundant collagen (Coll) is present on the external or peripheral surface. ×11,000.

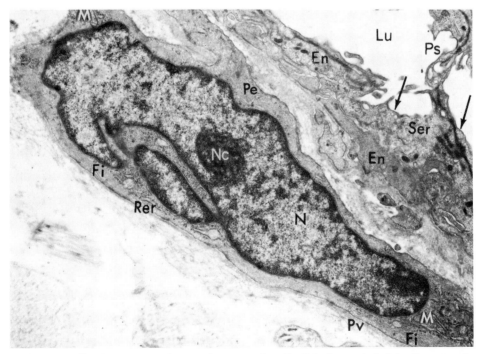

Figure 14–11 *Capillary hemangioma.* The prominent pseudopodia (Ps) of an endothelial cell are noted on the lumen (Lu) side of a capillary. The cytoplasm of this endothelial cell (En) contains numerous vesicles originating from pinocytotic vesicles (arrows). The larger cell represents a pericyte (Pe) displaying a lobular nucleus (N) containing a nucleolus (Nc). The cytoplasm contains mitochondria (M), delicate filaments (Fi), and rough endoplasmic reticulum (Rer). Pinocytotic vesicles (arrow) are aligned at the internal plasmalemma at right. ×11,000.

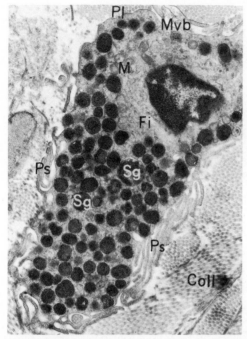

Figure 14–12 *Capillary hemangioma.* A mast cell within the collagenous region (Coll) of the adventitia. This tissue cell also shows prominent pseudopodia (Ps) of the plasmalemma (Pl), delicate filaments (Fi), an occasional mitochondrion (M), a multivesicular body (Mvb), and many secretory type granules (Sg) filling the cytoplasm. ×10,000.

cells containing the characteristic large, dense, cytoplasmic secretory granules are observed in these neoplasms.

FIBROUS XANTHOMA

The fibrous xanthoma is a fairly common skin neoplasm composed of two types of neoplastic cells. The more prominent is the histiocyte or foam cell, which is the hallmark of this tumor. These "xanthoma cells" contain a floppy, relatively translucent nucleus with occasional spheroidal nuclear bodies (SNB) and a large cytoplasm with clear intracytoplasmic vacuoles, which display frequent herniations into one another. Occasional crystalloids surrounded by myelin figure material are often seen associated with rough endoplasmic reticulum, ribosomes, mitochondria, and lysosomes within these histiocytic cells.

The usually less frequent fibroblast-like cell component of fibrous xanthoma displays a cytoplasm containing more numerous and closely packed organelles, including small mitochondria, dilated cisternae of rough endoplasmic reticulum, delicate filaments, and prominent Golgi complexes. Unusual occurrences within these tumor cells are myelin figure material showing numerous condensed laminations about lipid, intranuclear lipid bodies, and occasional nuclei containing multiple spheroidal nuclear bodies.

NEUROFIBROMATOSIS

The fine structural characteristics of the peripheral neurofibromas in von Recklinghausen's disease confirm the histologic features ascribed to them. Essentially, the tumoral masses are formed of intricate bundles of fibroconnective tissue and nerve elements intermixed in a random fashion.

The neural component consists of myelinated nerves and Schwann cells, which are fairly numerous and disorganized. The axons contain scant organelles and are surrounded by a thick complete coat of regularly arranged myelin lamella. The myelinated axons are usually seen within the cytoplasm of the neoplastic Schwann cells. The cytoplasm of these cells is abundant and well endowed with free and membrane-bound ribosomes, occasional lysosomes, and a distinct Golgi apparatus. The plasmalemma frequently presents redundant infoldings depicting an intricate system of cytoplasmic digitations in the intercellular space.

The fibroconnective tissue component is represented predominantly by numerous and prominent bundles of mature collagen (~ 640 Å periodicity), frequently seen in association with fibers of the long-spacing variety (1,500 to 2,500 Å periodicity). Fibroblasts and small blood vessels are also seen.

KERATOACANTHOMA

The fine structural features of neoplastic cells in keratoacanthoma cannot be

Text continued on page 365.

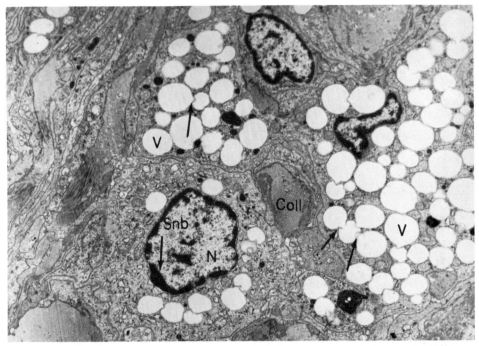

Figure 14–13 *Fibrous xanthoma.* In this benign fibroxanthoma (Fx), numerous xanthoma cells are present between histiocytes, each associated with collagen (Coll). The xanthoma cells contain numerous clear to light osmiophilic cytoplasmic vacuoles (V) displaying frequent herniations of one vacuole into another (arrows). Nuclei (N) contain spheroidal nuclear bodies (Snb) and display a peripheral condensation of chromatin adjacent to the internal nuclear envelope (arrow). ×7,000.

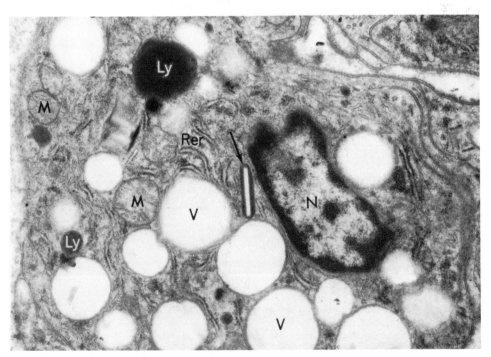

Figure 14–14 *Fibrous xanthoma.* Within a xanthoma cell, there are numerous vacuoles (V), a prominent crystalloid (arrow) surrounded by a myelin figure adjacent to rough endoplasmic reticulum (Rer), mitochondria (M), lysosomes (Ly), and nucleus (N). ×21,000.

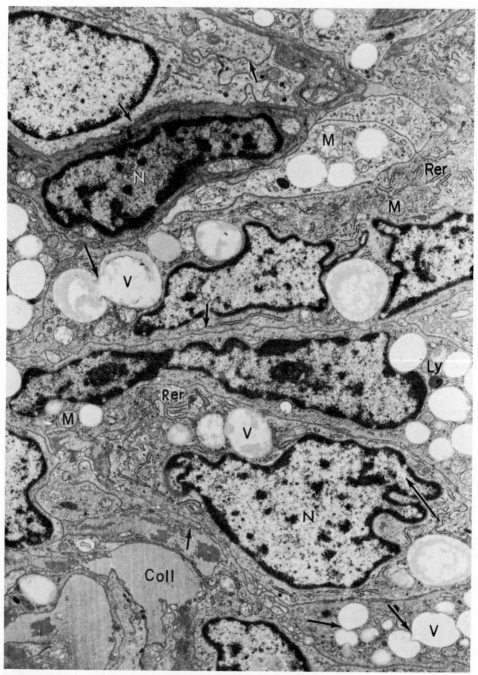

Figure 14–15   *Fibrous xanthoma.* Neoplastic cells are of two types. One histiocytic-like tumor cell displays a more translucent, floppy-shaped nucleus (N) containing relatively translucent nucleoplasm (arrows). These cells contain cytoplasmic rough endoplasmic reticulum (Rer) and vacuoles (V) with frequent herniations (arrows), thus imparting characteristics of xanthoma cells. Pinocytotic vesicles are present along the internal plasmalemma (short arrows) in several areas. Mitochondria (M) and lysosomes (Ly) are present. The intercellular collagen (Coll) is considerable. ×*10,000.*

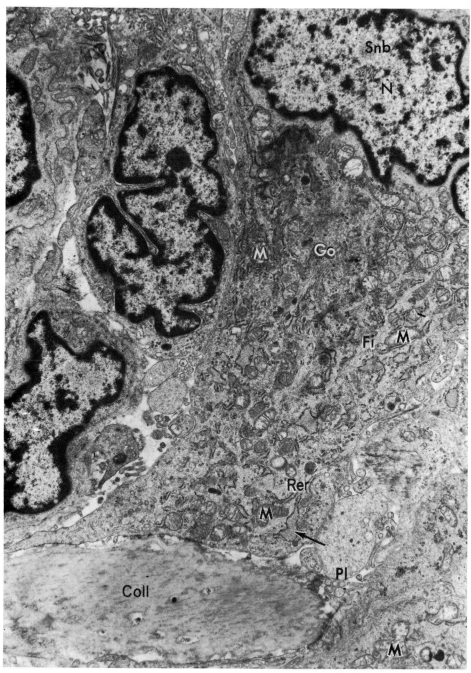

Figure 14–16 *Fibrous xanthoma.* The second type of neoplastic cell is fibroblastic-like in appearance and displays numerous cytoplasmic organelles and a prominent nucleus (N) containing a spheroidal nuclear body (Snb). The cytoplasm contains numerous small mitochondria (M), cisternae of rough endoplasmic reticulum (Rer), the latter occasionally dilated with osmiophilic material (arrow), a prominent Golgi complex (Go), and delicate filaments (Fi) comprising the background. Abundant collagen (Coll) is evident at bottom and interdigitates with the plasmalemma (Pl) of adjacent cells. ×*10,000.*

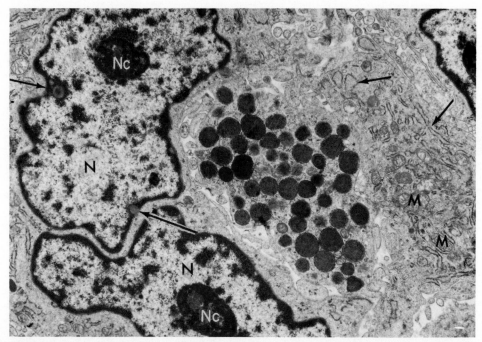

Figure 14–17 *Fibrous xanthoma.* In these neoplastic cells, the nuclei (N) contain prominent nucleoli (Nc) and several nuclear projections (arrows). The central cell contains many double membrane-bound dense bodies nearly filling the cytoplasm and representing a mast cell. The adjacent fibroblasts contain small mitochondria (M) and cisternae of dilated and nondilated rough endoplasmic reticulum (arrows). ×10,000.

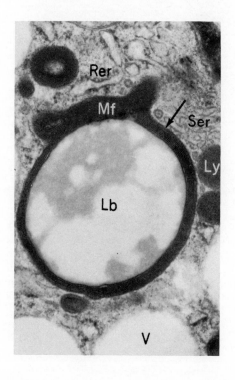

Figure 14–18 *Fibrous xanthoma.* A large cystically dilated lipid body (Lb) is surrounded by a myelin figure (Mf) with several smaller satellites. Lysosomes (Ly) are evident adjacent to numerous vacuoles (V) and rough and smooth endoplasmic reticulum (Rer, Ser). The myelin figure shows numerous condensed laminations of densely osmiophilic double membranes (arrows). ×38,000.

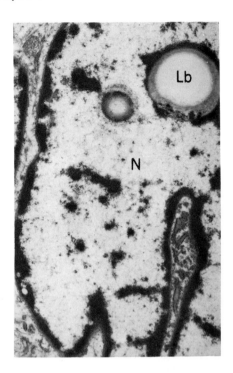

Figure 14-19 *Fibrous xanthoma.* The nucleus (N) contains prominent lipid bodies (Lb) adjacent to invaginations of the nuclear membrane. The nuclear chromatin has condensed along the internal nuclear envelope, leaving the nucleoplasm relatively clear. ×11,500.

considered characteristic of this entity but rather are unspecific modifications of squamous keratinizing cells similar to those seen in other lesions of rapidly proliferating squamous epithelia.

The neoplastic squamous cells appear pleomorphic, with irregular outlines and dense, convoluted nuclei. The cells are usually attached to each other by numerous well-preserved desmosomes to

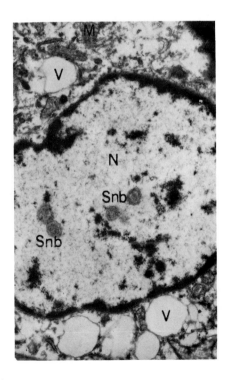

Figure 14-20 *Fibrous xanthoma.* Within the nucleus (N), four spheroidal nuclear bodies (Snb) are present in the relatively translucent neoplasm. The cytoplasm contains numerous vacuoles (V) and small mitochondria (M). ×11,000.

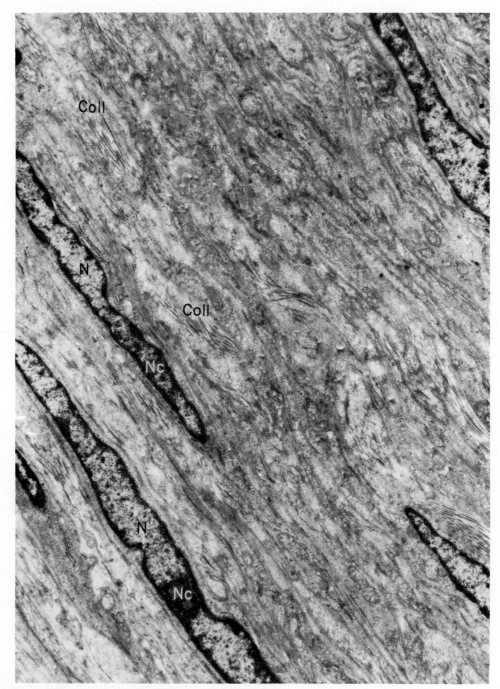

Figure 14–21 *Neurofibroma.* A low-power view shows numerous, slender, neural, spindle-shaped cells alternating with intercellular collagen (Coll). Note that nuclei (N) are also quite elongated and contain a coiled nucleolus (Nc). ×10,000.

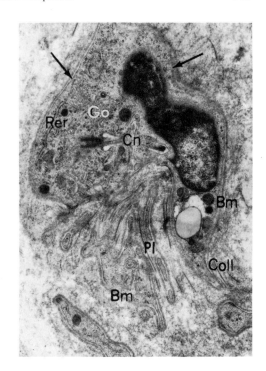

Figure 14–22 *Neurofibroma.* This neurofibroma neoplastic cell displays a nucleus adjacent to a dividing centriole (Cn) and Golgi complex (Go). A cisterna of rough endoplasmic reticulum (Rer) is parallel to the plasmalemma (Pl). The external surface of the plasmalemma shows a basement membrane (Bm) associated with collagen fibers (Coll). In addition, pinocytotic vesicles (arrows) are evident. These cytoplasmic organelles, *as a group*, characterize a neural type cell. ×*12,000*.

which dense bands of tonofilaments are inserted. The intercellular spaces are frequently dilated and present numerous pseudovilli protruding from adjacent cells.

The cytoplasm of the cells of the acanthomatous component is relatively abundant and contains numerous tonofilament bundles, RNP particles, mitochondria, lysosomes, and glycogen pools. The clumped chromatin toward the margins

Text continued on page 374.

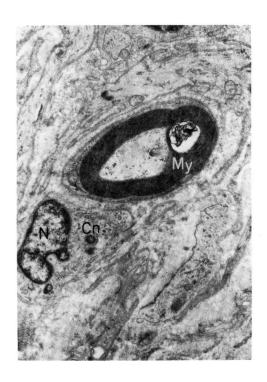

Figure 14–23 *Neurofibroma.* A Schwann cell displaying prominent myelin (My) within its cytoplasm. Note that, as the mesoaxon forms, the delicate filaments tend to aggregate and form a dense laminated structure which eventually forms the myelin. The adjacent nucleus (N) and a centriole (Cn) have just divided. ×*9,000*.

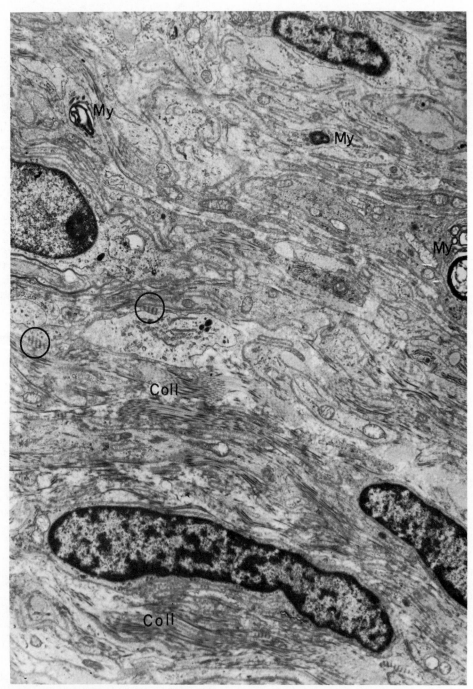

Figure 14–24 *Neurofibromatosis.* Survey view showing numerous myelin figures (Mf) present within several Schwann cells can be seen. Two foci of collagen show long-spacing variety with a periodicity ranging from 1,500 to 2,500 Å (circles). Interspersed between the tumor cells is collagen (Coll), with the characteristic periodicity of 640 Å. ×8,000.

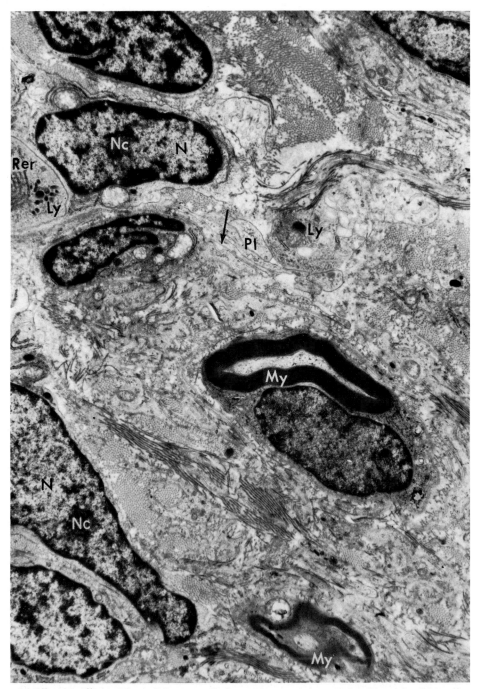

Figure 14–25 *Neurofibromatosis.* A Schwann cell shows characteristic cytoplasmic myelin (My) adjacent to the plasmalemma. The nuclei (N) of these neoplastic cells are mottled, and some contain nucleoli (Nc). A few cells contain rough endoplasmic reticulum (Rer) and lysosomes (Ly). The plasmalemma (Pl) displays some redundancy, as well as an association with a basement membrane (arrows). ×10,000.

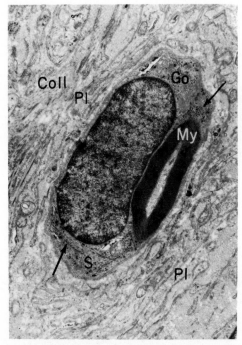

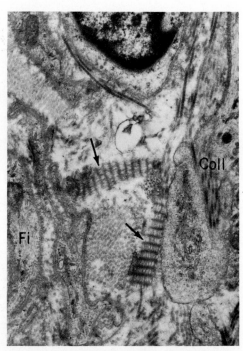

Figure 14–26 *Neurofibromatosis.* Myelin (My) is associated with the plasmalemma (Pl) of a Schwann cell (S). The cytoplasm contains a Golgi complex (Go), ribosomes (arrows), and a few cisternae of rough endoplasmic reticulum (arrows). The surrounding neural tissue displays redundancy of the plasmalemma (Pl) and abundant collagen (Coll). ×8,000.

Figure 14–27 *Neurofibromatosis.* At higher magnification, the long-spacing variety of collagen fibers (arrows) can be seen, especially in comparison to adjacent collagen fibers (Coll) displaying the characteristic 640 Å periodicity. Note the delicate filaments (Fi) in an adjacent cell. ×15,000.

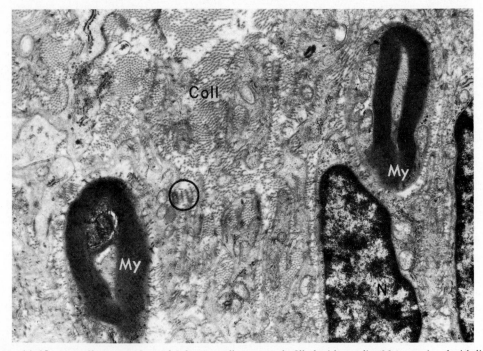

Figure 14–28 *Neurofibromatosis.* Several Schwann cells are nearly filled with myelin (My) associated with little, if any, cytoplasmic organelles in the plane of section. Abundant collagen (Coll) is present between neoplastic cells, as well as a focus of long-spacing collagen (circle) and nuclei (N). ×12,000.

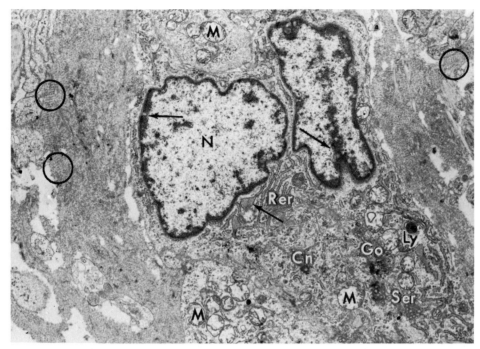

Figure 14–29 *Keratoacanthoma.* Amid amorphous collagenous material which displays long spacing in some regions (circles), there is a neoplastic cell showing slightly dilated cisternae of rough endoplasmic reticulum (Rer), containing osmiophilic material (arrows), a prominent Golgi complex (Go), a centriole (Cn), and numerous mitochondria (M). In addition, a lysosome (Ly) and branched cisternae of smooth endoplasmic reticulum (Ser) are evident. Nuclei (N) display a prominent margination of chromatin along the internal nuclear membrane (arrows). ×5,000.

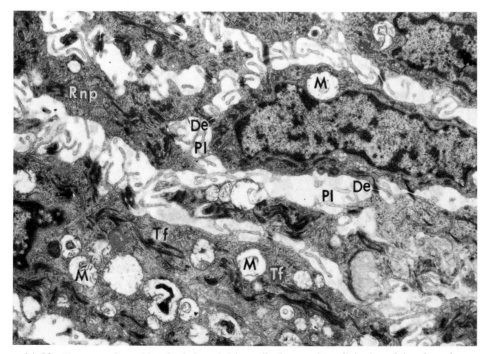

Figure 14–30 *Keratoacanthoma.* Neoplastic keratinizing cells show an interdigitating of the plasmalemma with probable artifactual space formation between cells. Desmosomes (De) are quite prominent and are usually located at the mid or distal portion of the fingerlike projections of the plasmalemma (Pl). Numerous tonofilaments (Tf) are present in the cytoplasm, along with mitochondria (M) and ribosomes (Rnp). ×10,000.

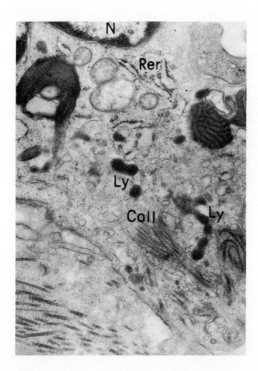

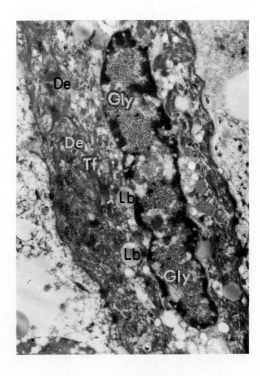

Figure 14–31   *Keratoacanthoma.* Several cytoplasmic bodies sectioned in two planes show the long spacing of collagen associated with myelin figure material in a formed body. Rough endoplasmic reticulum (Rer), lysosomes (Ly), and collagen (Coll) are present, as well as a nucleus (N). *×19,500.*

Figure 14–32   *Keratoacanthoma.* A nucleus of a squamous neoplastic cell shows clusters of glycogen (Gly) within the nucleoplasm. Chromatin material is aggregated along the internal nuclear membrane. Lipid bodies (Lb) are seen within the cytoplasm in association with abundance of tonofilaments (Tf) and disorganized desmosomes (De). *×10,000.*

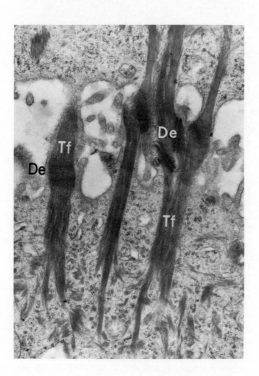

Figure 14–33   *Keratoacanthoma.* Several desmosomes (De) attached to adjacent cells are shown in contiguity with tonofilaments (Tf) extending deep into the cytoplasm of the cells. *×18,000.*

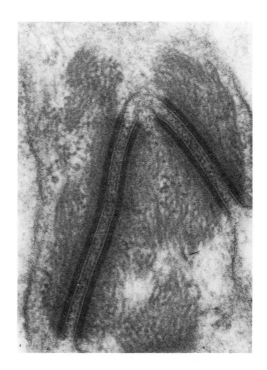

Figure 14–34 *Keratoacanthoma.* A desmosome at higher magnification shows tonofilaments contiguous with plates, extending deep into the cytoplasm of adjacent cells. The desmosome displays a trilaminar structure. A dense, amorphous, osmiophilic material forms a thick plate against the inner layer of the plasmalemma of each cell. Cementing material is present between the external layer of the plasmalemma within the desmosome. This cementing matrix is divided equally by a thin, dense, central lamina extending the length of the desmosome. ×37,000.

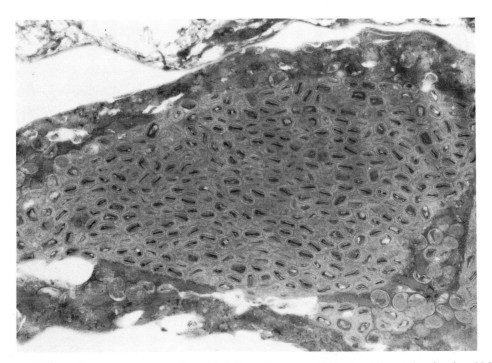

Figure 14–35 *Molluscum contagiosum.* The epithelial papular tumor of human skin contains the virus *Molluscum contagiosum.* Within the epidermis an egg-shaped lesion contains numerous oval-shaped particles replacing the epithelial cells. Myriad uniform virus particles replicate within specific lesions as closely packed units. This is a DNA virus which belongs to the family of pox viruses. ×27,000.

and intranuclear aggregates of glycogen particles.

Toward the keratinizing layers of the lesion, the epithelial cells become more elongated, desmosomes decrease in number, and large, dense, intracytoplasmic inclusions of variable electron density appear, recognized as keratohyaline granules. The number of lysosomes seems to increase in these more superficial cells, but the other organelles decrease in number.

Toward the basal regions of the lesion, the proliferating squamous cells are identical to those described in the acanthotic regions. However, in some areas they seem to become embedded within the underlying connective tissue of the upper dermis formed by collagen bundles, both mature (short-spacing) and immature (long-spacing striations), and large fibroblasts actively synthesizing collagen.

MOLLUSCUM CONTAGIOSUM

Molluscum contagiosum is caused by a DNA virus of the poxvirus group that measures approximately $300 \times 200 \times 100$ mμ in its mature form. The DNA dense viral core has a biconcave dumbbell configuration, and it is covered by a thick protein capsule and two or more enveloping membranes.

The most characteristic ultrastructural feature of this distinct egg-shaped epidermal lesion is the presence of myriad viral particles within infected cells of the stratum spinosum. Assembling and replication of virions apparently occur within the cytoplasm of these cells in independent foci of fine particulate material of medium electron density called "viroplasm." From this material, immature viral particles are formed and can be observed as amorphous electron-dense nucleoids surrounded by membrane envelopes. The mature virions present a typical dumbbell-shaped central core or nucleoid surrounded by a thick wall and assemble in large groups within cytoplasmic vacuoles. Trabeculae of preserved cytoplasmic structures containing ribosomes, mitochondria, and endoplasmic reticulum are seen between virion-filled vacuoles, but

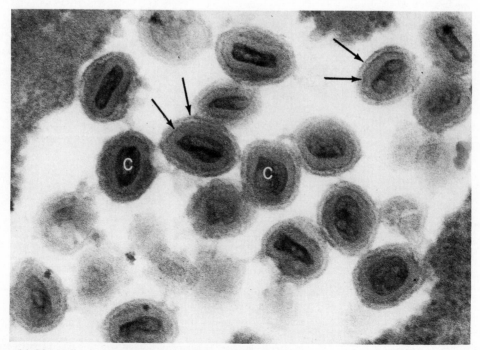

Figure 14–36 *Molluscum contagiosum.* At higher magnification, the molluscum contagiosum shows a dense DNA core (C) and the classic pox virus type of envelope consisting of two or more circumscribing membranes (arrows). The matrix between the envelope and viral core is dense. ×*88,000.*

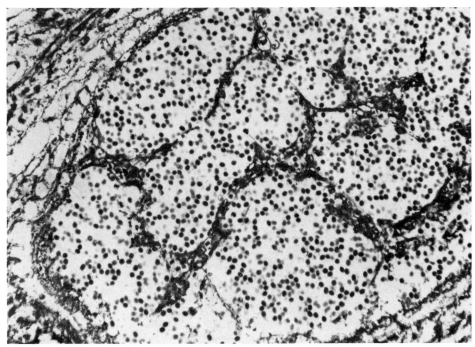

Figure 14–37 *Molluscum contagiosum.* An egg-shaped lesion within the epidermis contains myriad virus particles representing molluscum contagiosum. The replicating virions are separated by fibrous septa of remaining necrotic epidermal keratin. ×9,500.

those portions of cytoplasm are most frequently seen directed towards the periphery of the cells.

Infected cells do not keratinize, although keratinization occurs in adjacent noninfected superficial cells. Peculiar clumps of electron-dense material are seen within the nuclei of basal epidermal cells, but virions do not seem to differentiate in these cells.

Malignant Neoplasms

SQUAMOUS CELL CARCINOMA

The ultrastructural features of invasive squamous cell carcinoma of the skin are identical to those of the same type of tumor in other organs.

The epithelial neoplastic cells, either isolated or forming small groups or nests, appear loosely immersed within a connective tissue stroma. The cells are polygonal, with irregular outlines separated from each other by wide intercellular spaces containing a complicated mesh of interdigitating cytoplasmic microvilli. At points of contact, adjacent tumor cells are attached by typical trilaminar desmosomes associated with dense bundles of cytoplasmic tonofilaments.

The squamous neoplastic cells have large nuclei with irregular outlines, densely clumped chromatin, and large, irregular nucleoli. The cytoplasm is not very abundant relative to the size of the nucleus and contains large numbers of organelles, including pools of glycogen and irregularly distributed bundles of tonofilaments.

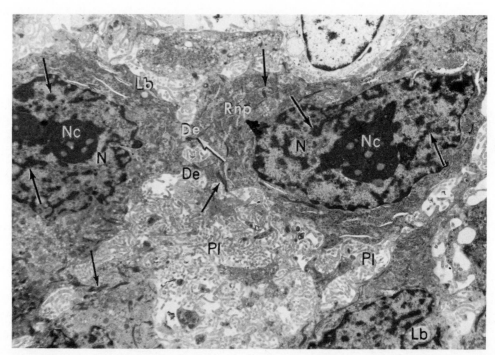

Figure 14–38 *Squamous cell carcinoma.* Several neoplastic squamous cells show a prominent large nucleus (N) with well-delineated nuclei (Nc) and considerable parachromatin material (arrows). The cytoplasm contains clusters of ribosomes (Rnp) and groups of tonofilaments (arrows) in addition to prominent desmosomes (De). Even at this low magnification, the connection of tonofilaments to desmosomes is discernible (white arrow). The plasmalemma (Pl) is arranged in voluminous folds of pseudovilli. An occasional lipid body (Lb) is evident. ×6,500.

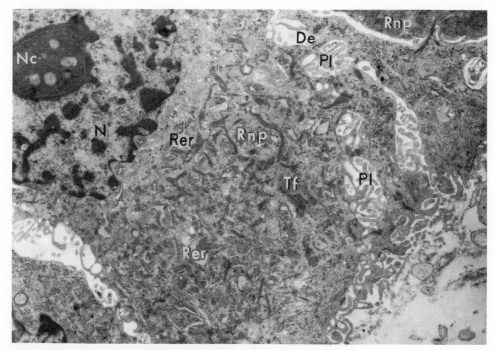

Figure 14–39 *Squamous cell carcinoma.* The neoplastic squamous cells display prominent clusters of tonofilaments (Tf) within the cytoplasm in association with small clusters of ribosomes (Rnp) and dilated cisternae of rough endoplasmic reticulum (Rer). Desmosomes (De) are quite prominent and characteristic of neoplastic squamous cells. The plasmalemma (Pl) displays many undulations and interdigitating projections between adjacent cells. The nucleus (N) is mottled and shows a prominent coiled nucleolus (Nc). ×9,500.

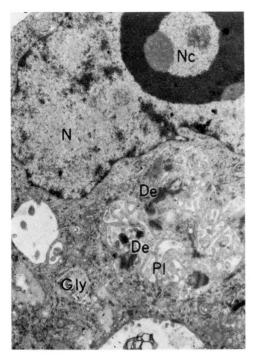

Figure 14–40 *Squamous cell carcinoma.* Nucleus (N) displays a quite prominent nucleolar (Nc) region composed of chromatin and parachromatin material varying in density. The cytoplasm contains clusters of glycogen (Gly) granules; a plane of section through adjacent cells reveals the prominence of the plasmalemma (Pl), which is contiguous with desmosomes (De). ×*11,000.*

Occasional macrophages containing vast numbers of lysosomes, cytophagosomes, and amorphous inclusions can be seen among the neoplastic cells.

MELANOCARCINOMA (MALIGNANT MELANOMA)

The histogenesis of the neoplastic elements in malignant melanoma is still a matter of controversy, and although electron microscopic studies have provided important data in this respect, the origin of the melanoma cells is not clear as yet. There is a current tendency to believe that they originate from epidermal melanocytes rather than from pigmented cells of the upper dermis.

The neoplastic cells are usually arranged in large groups, closely packed and related to each other either by apposition of plasma membranes or by interdigitation of cytoplasmic pseudovilli that project within the narrow intercellular spaces.

The melanoma cells are either rounded or angulated, with large nuclei and relatively scant cytoplasm. The nuclei are pleomorphic, the majority displaying irregular and bizarre configurations, with peripheral clumping of chromatin toward the inner lamina of the nuclear envelope. Large nucleoli and intranuclear inclusions (spheroidal nuclear bodies) are frequently observed.

Various types of neoplastic cells can be distinguished according to the content of cytoplasmic pigment inclusions. Neoplastic cells devoid of any recognizable pigment inclusion are infrequent but can be seen within groups of pigmented cells. The amelanotic cells have more abundant cytoplasm and a more regular nucleus. The cytoplasm contains numerous variably shaped mitochondria, free ribosomes and polyribosomes, a small Golgi appara-

Text continued on page 382.

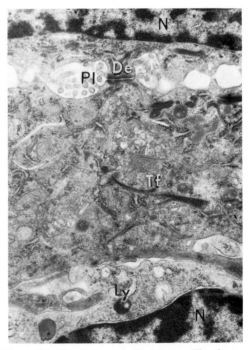

Figure 14–41 *Squamous cell carcinoma.* The desmosome (De) is contiguous with microvilli of the plasmalemma (Pl) between two adjacent cells, resembling a bile canaliculus. Lysosomes (Ly), tonofilaments (Tf) and nuclei (N) are evident. ×*12,000.*

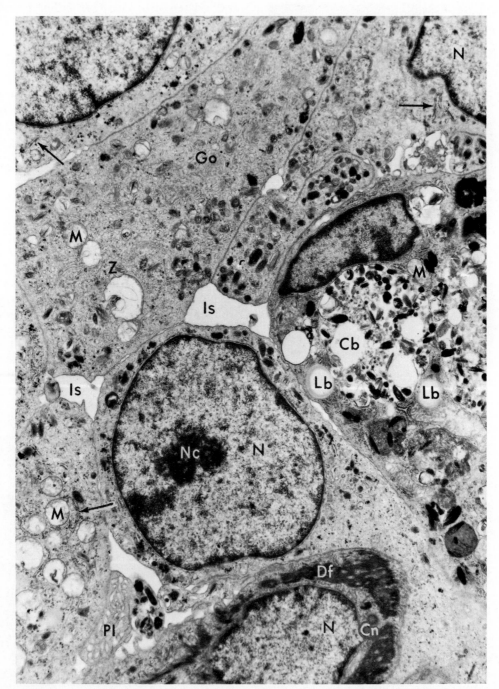

Figure 14–42 *Melanocarcinoma.* Survey view showing numerous melanoblasts containing many melanosomes of various stages. Note the presence of compound bodies (Cb) wherein many different-staged melanosomes and premelanosomes are present and surrounded by a delimiting membrane. The cytoplasm contains abundant Golgi complexes (Go), and these organelles are closely associated to melanin synthesis. Mitochondria (M), lipid bodies (Lb), and dense fibrillar (Df) structures are also noted within this cytoplasm. Only occasionally are cisternae of rough endoplasmic reticulum observed (arrows). A centriole (Cn) is present; nuclei (N) with prominent internal nuclear membranes may contain a nucleolus (Nc). The plasmalemma (Pl) is occasionally arranged in numerous folds and is associated with apparent intercellular spaces (Is) between juxtapositioned cells. ×*11,000.*

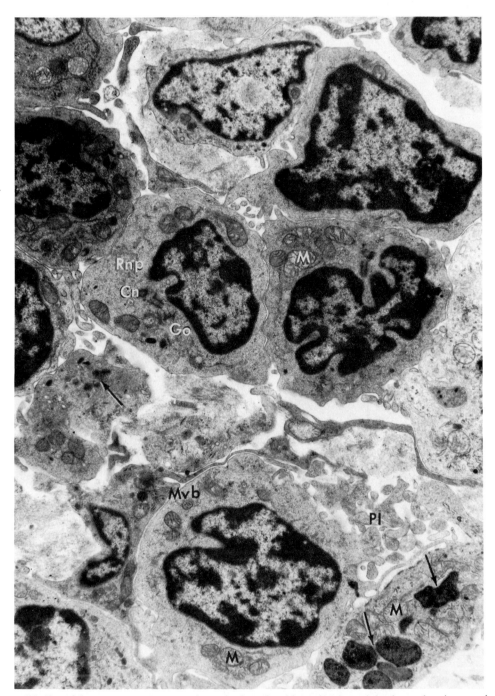

Figure 14–43 *Melanocarcinoma.* An area of neoplastic melanoblasts showing minimal cytoplasmic premelano-somes (arrows). Note that in these cells the cytoplasm contains abundant ribosomes (Rnp), mitochondria (M), centrioles (Cn), a Golgi complex (Go), and multivesicular bodies (Mvb). The plasmalemma (Pl) shows numerous redundant interdigitating folds. This area of the tumor is relatively undifferentiated and appears to be associated with a higher index of mitoses. ×*10,000.*

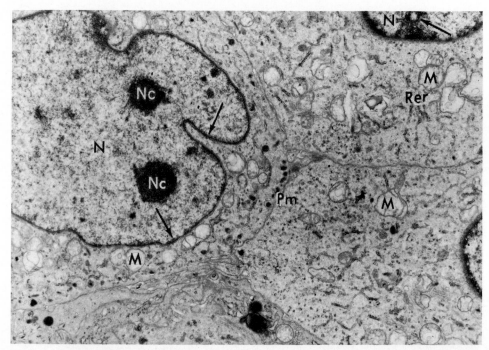

Figure 14–44 *Melanocarcinoma.* One of several neoplastic cells shows a large nucleus (N) with two noncoiled nucleoli (Nc). Note the dense internal nuclear membrane (arrows). The cytoplasm contains mitochondria (M), short cisternae of rough endoplasmic reticulum (Rer), and a paucity of premelanosomes (Pm). A nuclear invagination (arrow) is evident in the smaller upper nucleus (N). ×10,000.

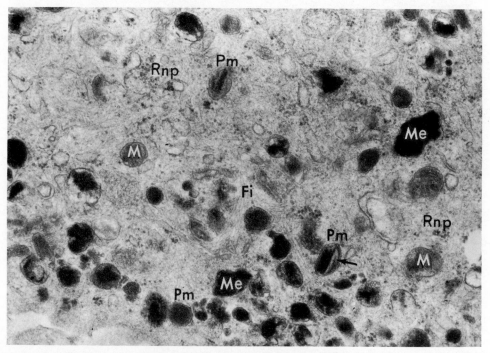

Figure 14–45 *Melanocarcinoma.* Numerous premelanosomes (Pm) and melanosomes (Me) at various stages of development. The premelanosomes are surrounded by a single delimiting membrane and contain protein lamellae displaying a beaded appearance (arrow). As the premelanosome matures, excessive melanin protein fills the vesicle and obscures the beaded appearance. Delicate filaments (Fi), ribosomes (Rnp), and mitochondria (M) are evident. ×33,000.

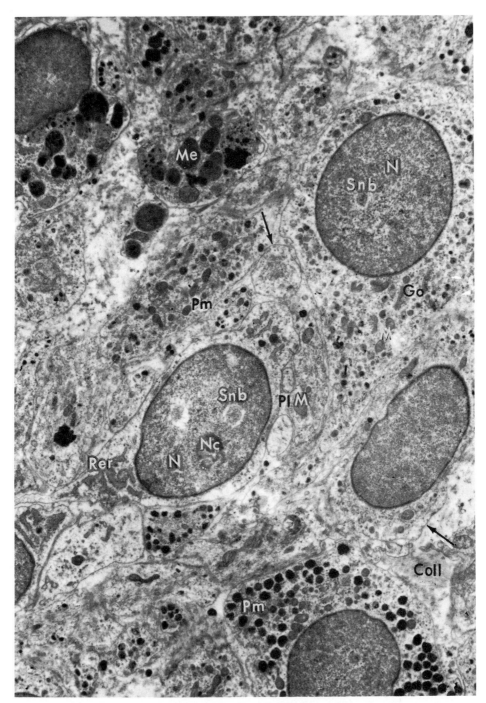

Figure 14–46 *Malignant blue nevus.* A low-power survey view shows numerous neoplastic cells with prominent oval to round nuclei (N), an occasional nucleolus (Nc), and spheroidal nuclear bodies (Snb). The central portion of this photograph has an arrangement of neoplastic cells in a transverse plane, suggesting the appearance of an axon (arrows). Note that premelanosomes (Pm) are present in all cells, including the axonlike cells. In addition, melanosomes (Me) are present in some cells. The former display more frequent but less dense granular material delimited by a surrounding membrane. Within the cytoplasm of neoplastic cells, numerous Golgi complexes (Go), mitochondria (M), infrequent branching cisternae of rough endoplasmic reticulum (Rer), pinocytotic vesicles (arrows) on the internal side of the plasmalemma (Pl), and intercellular collagen (Coll) are evident. ×8,000.

tus, short ergastoplasmic lamellae, and, very occasionally, dense bodies. They appear closely apposed to each other and to neighboring pigmented cells.

The most frequently observed neoplastic cells are the pigmented cells which contain dense cytoplasmic inclusions. Two kinds of pigmented cells can be distinguished: those containing only dispersed, small melanotic inclusions and those with large, irregular pigment granules.

The first type includes the classic neoplastic melanocytes with irregular indented nuclei and large nucleoli, surrounded by abundant cytoplasm containing variable numbers of small ovoid or fusiform membrane-bound inclusions, representing melanosomes and premelanosomes. Premelanosomes reveal parallel striations and folds within the moderately dense matrix of the central core. Melanosomes are more homogeneous and electron-dense, but they are also surrounded by a single limiting membrane.

The second type of cells containing pigment in these tumors is represented by phagocytic neoplastic cells with irregular and eccentrically located nuclei and abundant cytoplasm containing large, dense inclusions of variable size and shape. These inclusions are actually large lysosomes which contain the melanin pigment granules, probably in the process of digestion. The pigment granules appear as darker particles within the finely granular phagolysosomes. The remainder of the cytoplasm of these cells is rich in organelles.

MALIGNANT BLUE NEVUS

The malignant blue nevus (MBN) is a rare melanotic neoplasm of the skin. It

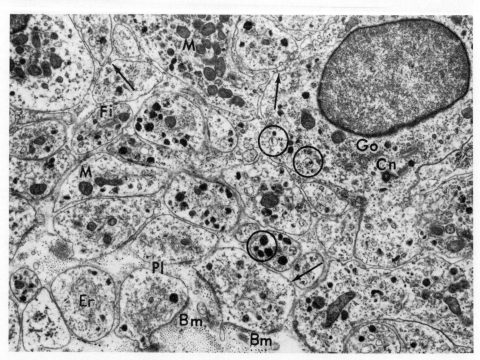

Figure 14–47 *Malignant blue nevus.* A group of neoplastic cells in a transverse plane present an appearance of an axon. These cells contain vesicles of endoplasmic reticulum (Er), small mitochondria (M), pinocytotic vesicles (arrows), and basement membrane–like material (Bm) along the external surface of the plasmalemma (Pl). Certain tumor cells have a Golgi complex (Go), delicate filaments (Fi), and a centriole (Cn). The presence of premelanosomes and melanosomes (circles) within these neoplastic cells indicates that these cells are not a portion of a normal nerve trunk but rather neoplastic cells of Schwann cell derivation. ×8,000.

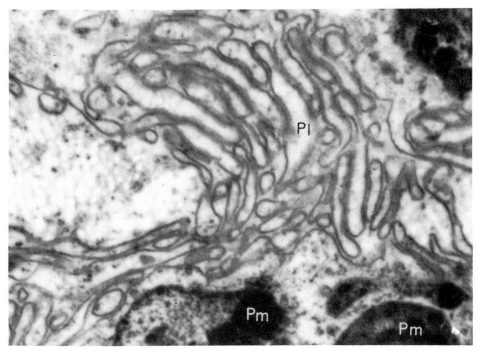

Figure 14–48 *Malignant blue nevus.* The plasmalemma of two adjacent neoplastic cells assumes many interdigitating folds to form fingerlike projections. This modification of the plasmalemma (Pl) mimics the mesoaxon region of Schwann cells. The cytoplasm contains several premelanosomes (Pm) displaying more frequent but less dense granular material surrounded by a limiting membrane. ×33,000.

closely resembles the more common cellular blue nevus (CBN) described by Allen and Spitz (1953). Pleomorphism of the tumor cell pattern from one area to another appears to be the hallmark of this neoplasm (Merkow et al., 1969). Since a malignant blue nevus is usually associated with a coexisting cellular blue nevus, differentiation is frequently a problem. The diagnostic criteria, such as necrosis, mitotic figures, pleomorphism, enlarged hyperchromatic nuclei, vacuolization of neoplastic cells, and residual evidence of CBN, are helpful in the differential diagnosis.

Figure 14–49 *Malignant blue nevus.* Branching cisternae of rough endoplasmic reticulum (Rer) are associated with premelanosomes (Pm), mitochondria (M), delicate filaments (Fi) within the cytoplasm, a nucleus (N), and extracellular collagen (Coll). ×10,000.

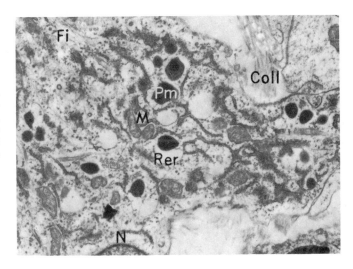

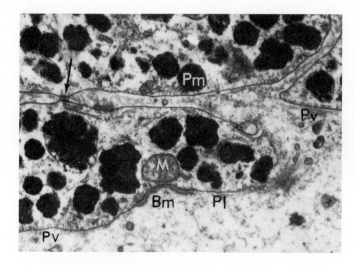

Figure 14–50 *Malignant blue nevus.* Adjacent to numerous premelanosomes (Pm) and a mitochondrion (M), there is a focally dense plasma membrane (Pl) associated with a basement membrane (Bm), a tight junction (arrow), and numerous pinocytotic vesicles (Pv). ×15,000.

Electron microscopy has been contributory in determining not only the degree of malignancy but also its derivation. The plasmalemma of some MBN cells is quite redundant and forms very elongated interdigitating folds. Large numbers of melanosomes varying in size are usually located adjacent to the Golgi complex and/or centriole. Premelanosomes and melanosomes vary from 135 to 5,500 mμ in size and shape. The nuclear envelope frequently displays a triple-layered effect, and desmosome-like structures form focal attachment sites between cells. The presence of basement membrane–like material circumscribing neoplastic cells, desmosome-like structures, interdigitations of a redundant plasmalemma, enclosed unmyelinated nerve fibers, and a triple-layered nuclear envelope indicates that this is a neoplasm derived from Schwann cells. Some neoplastic cells resemble unmyelinated nerve fibers in transverse section. These axonlike tumor cells display intracellular pigment granules and pinocytotic vesicles.

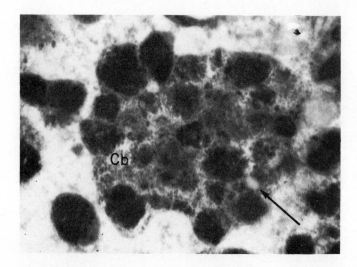

Figure 14–51 *Malignant blue nevus.* A compound body (Cb), composed of ingested aggregates of melanosomes, displays a lighter staining matrix background and numerous irregularly shaped, dense structures. Vacuoles (arrow) are noted within some compound bodies. Some of the largest compound bodies attain a diameter of 5,500 millimicrons. ×25,000.

REFERENCES

Allen, A. C., and Spitz, S.: Malignant melanoma, a clinicopathological analysis of the criteria for diagnosis and prognosis. Cancer, 6:1, 1953.

Banfield, W. G.: Dense granule in the elementary body of molluscum contagiosum. J. Biophys. Biochem. Cytol., 5:513, 1959.

Calap Calatayud, T., et al.: Ultraestructura del molusco contagioso. Investigacion Experimental Actas Dermosifilograficas, 64:595, 1973.

Cesarini, J. P.: Recent advances in the ultrastructure of malignant melanoma. Rev. Eur. Etud. Clin. Biol., 16:316, 1971.

Dourmashkin, R., and Bernhard, W.: A study with the E. M. of the skin tumor of molluscum contagiosum. J. Ultrastruct. Res. 3:11, 1959.

Epstein, W. L., Conant, M. A., and Krasnobrod, H.: Molluscum contagiosum: Normal and virus infected epidermal cell kinetics. J. Invest. Dermatol.,46:91, 1966.

Jukubowica, K., et al.: Comparative study on the ultrastructure of malignant melanoma and pigmented nevi. Acta Med. Pol., 12:107, 1971.

Kimura, M., et al.: E. M. Study on the tumor of von Recklinghausen's neurofibromatosis. Acta Patol. Jap., 24:79, 1974.

Lutzner, M. A.: Molluscum contagiosum, verruca and zoster viruses. Arch. Dermatol., 87:436, 1963.

Mann, P. R.: Leiomyoma cutis: An EM study. Br. J. Dermatol., 82:463, 1970.

Maul, G. G., et al.: Ultrastructural comparison of two human malignant melanoma cell lines. Cancer Res., 30:2782, 1970.

Merkow, L. P., Burt, R. C., Hayeslip, D. W., Newton, F. J., Slifkin, M., and Pardo, M.: A cellular and malignant blue nevus: A light and electron microscopic study. Cancer, 24:890, 1969.

Middelkamp, J. N., and Munger, B. L.: Ultrastructure and histogenesis of molluscum contagiosum. J. Pediatr., 64:888, 1964.

Timbow, K., et al.: Ultrastructure of giant pigment granules (macromelanosomes) in the cutaneous pigmented macules of neurofibromatosis. J. Invest. Dermatol., 61:300, 1973.

15

The Borderline Between Cancer and Noncancer: Interrelationships Between Stroma and Epithelium

Hermann Pinkus, M.D.

INTRODUCTION

The expression "borderline between cancer and noncancer" can have four different connotations to physicians concerned with the diagnosis and treatment of skin cancer. It can simply mean: Where is the edge of the cancerous lesion? It can also mean: Of the large number of neoplastic entities in the skin, which are benign and which are malignant? It can mean: Is the lesion under consideration still benign or is it already malignant? And finally, it can mean: Is the lesion a true cancer, or is it pseudocancer, a reactive process mimicking neoplasia? All four questions have to be answered in every case before proper therapy can be decided on.

The general principles for the treatment of skin cancer were outlined in Chapter 2, and carcinogenesis was discussed in Chapter 6. Before entering into a consideration of the four facets of this chapter, however, we have to define carefully what cancer is. This might seem superfluous in-

asmuch as every layman can tell us that cancer is a dread disease which starts at one point in the body, sooner or later becomes generalized and ends in the death of the patient. Most clinicians would accept a similar definition, including local origin of an invasive and destructive growth, metastasis, and a fatal outcome. The pathologist (especially the dermatopathologist), on the other hand, is confronted with a more difficult task when he examines a biopsy specimen (Pinkus, 1967). He cannot judge the clinical course under the microscope, and he may be dealing with initial stages of the cancerous process. Consultation of textbooks of pathology confirms these difficulties.

THE DEFINITION OF CANCER

In Anderson's well-known text, Shields Warren (1961) defines a neoplasm as an uncontrolled new growth of tissue. Cancer

386

is a malignant neoplasm, and carcinoma specifically is a malignant tumor of epithelial origin. Warren points out that from a clinical standpoint cancer is not one disease, but many. He uses as extreme examples carcinoma of the breast, which may develop, spread widely, and kill in a matter of months, and basal cell carcinoma of the skin, which may be present for many years and may remain localized throughout its course. According to Warren, malignant tumors have four general characteristics that differentiate them from benign tumors. However, no one criterion of malignancy is absolute. At least two are needed for diagnosis. Warren's four criteria are : (1) Malignant tumors tend to be anaplastic, i.e., less differentiated than the normal cells from which they are derived. They resemble embryonic forms of cells. (2) Malignant tumors infiltrate and destroy normal tissue, whereas benign tumors grow by expansion and push aside normal tissue. (3) Malignant tumors in general grow more rapidly and have higher mitotic counts and abnormal mitoses. (4) Malignant tumors have the power of metastasis, whereas benign tumors remain localized.

It should be noted that, by requiring at least two of the four criteria in the diagnosis of cancer, Warren broadens the border line into a border zone. This is emphasized by Robbins (1962), who states that the majority of tumors can be assigned to either benign or malignant categories, but that some fall into an intermediate zone: "Every tumor does not have to be either benign or malignant." We shall return to this fascinating thought later.

Warren's definitions and criteria are the classic ones of the practical pathologist. Hopps (1964) introduces a modern biologic note. He points out that proliferative growth of cells is the most fundamental characteristic of living beings. If regulative capacity is lost, the result is cancer. Cancer is a cellular disease in which a new race of cells develops as the result of some intracellular phenomenon. It begins in a single cell or a small focus of cells. The abnormal capacity for growth is transmitted to the progeny. Cancer can be cured by complete destruction of all cancer cells. As they grow, cancer cells invade and destroy normal tissue.

Hopps admits that a good definition of cancer is not possible at present but defines neoplasia in general as "a new growth of tissue, autonomous in nature, serving no useful purpose, obeying its own laws without respect for the organism as a whole, and growing at the expense rather than for the benefit of the body." He lists characteristics of malignant neoplasia on two levels. At the tissue level, there is altered organization, destructive invasion, often heterotopia, proneness to ischemic necrosis, frequent stimulation of nonseptic inflammatory reaction, and abnormal function. At the cellular level, there is anaplasia, pleomorphism, hyperchromatism, increased nuclear-cytoplasmic ratio, increased nucleolar-nuclear ratio, abnormal and increased mitoses, and abnormal function.

The length of this excerpt, from a considerably more lengthy discourse, and the multiplicity of criteria indicate the difficulties encountered by biologically oriented pathologists as well as by those of the descriptive school when they try to define and diagnose cancer.

In the skin even more than in other tissues, we encounter gray areas, border zones between benign and malignant, and we shall discuss in this chapter neoplasms which are "benign, malignant, not-so-benign, and not-so-malignant" (Fig. 15–1). We have to consider two situations, mentioned already in the first paragraph: (1) When we follow the course of one neoplasm, we must try to decide when it is still benign and when it becomes malignant. (2) When we compare a series of tumors, we must try to decide which are benign and which are malignant. These two situations are illustrated in two diagrams devised by Rous (1960); although the drawings illustrate carcinogenesis in rabbit skin, they are well applicable to human skin if we substitute "actinic keratosis", "premalignant melanoma", or "prelymphomatous reticulosis" for his "benign papilloma." Figure 15–2 shows how, in a skin exposed to a carcinogen, various members of the population undergo changes which give rise either to benign tumors or to cancers of greatly varying degrees of malignancy. Figure 15–3 illustrates how originally benign tumors may progress to more or less malignant ones in stages.

In the definition of cancer, one meets

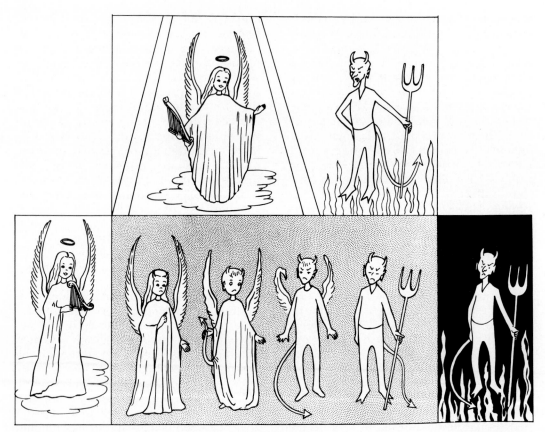

Figure 15–1 Tumors "benign, malignant, not-so-benign, and not-so-malignant." (*Adapted from* Hamperl, 1968.)

several terms which themselves have to be defined. The concepts of "progression," "anaplasia," "undifferentiated cells," "uncontrolled growth," and "somatic mutation" are examples. Some of these terms have been current for a long time; others are of recent coinage. They express an hypothesis, and some of the older ones have changed their meaning as the hypothesis about cancer changed. In a discussion aimed at clarification of shadowy territories, every term must be examined and defined. It may be unavoidable that some definitions do not meet with general approval, but at least the reader will know that the author has given thought to the matter and will know where he stands.

Anaplasia

"Anaplasia" was coined by von Hansemann (1897) to express the view that adult cells become tumor cells by developing in reverse and by becoming similar to, though not identical with, embryonic cells. This was in contrast to Cohnheim's theory (1877) that tumor cells are embryonic cells, arrested embryonic material. It has long been recognized that most tumor cells, although they may share certain morphologic and metabolic characteristics of embryonic cells, are quite different from them in other respects. More will have to be said about this later. Here, it is of interest to note that many books in their definitions of "anaplasia" refer to the old concept by characterizing anaplastic cells as having lost morphologic differentiation, specific function, and organization and then go on to say that these changes usually are associated with pronounced atypical changes of morphology. Actually, under the microscope, "anaplasia" in epithelial tissue is recognized by variability of size and shape of cells, loss of polarity in arrangement, unusual nuclei, and atypical mitoses—in short, by those characteristics (Fig. 15–4)

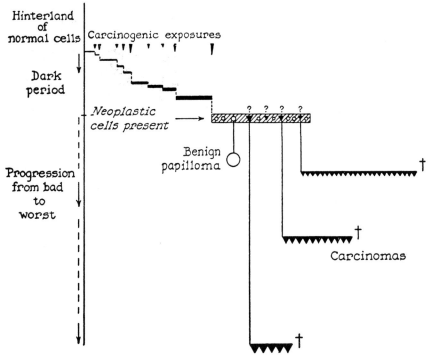

Figure 15–2 Primary epidermal carcinogenesis in rabbit skin according to Rous. Multiple carcinogenic exposures lead to the presence of variously altered cells, some of which give rise to benign and malignant tumors of varying degrees of virulence. (*From* Rous: Cancer Res., 20:672, 1960.)

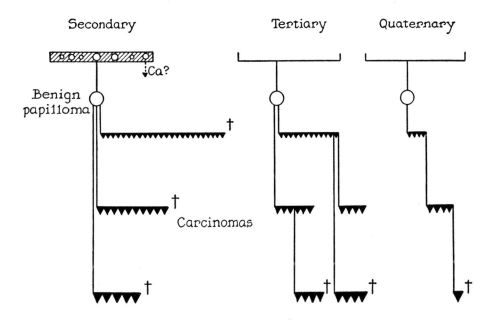

Figure 15–3 Sequential epidermal carcinogenesis in rabbit skin according to Rous. Progressive changes in steps. (*From* Rous: Cancer Res., 20:672, 1960.)

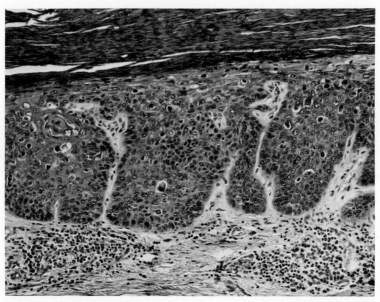

Figure 15–4   Bowen's precancerous dermatosis exhibiting dysplasia and dyskeratosis. *H&E*, ×*135*. (*From* Pinkus and Mehregan: A Guide to Dermatohistopathology, 1969. Courtesy of Appleton-Century-Crofts, Publishing Division of Prentice-Hall, Inc., Englewood Cliffs, N.J.)

which the dermatologist knows in Bowen's precancerous dermatosis as dyskeratosis. A tissue of this type does not resemble embryonic tissue, even morphologically. Inasmuch as dyskeratosis, in the strict sense of Darier (1925), is almost a synonym for individual cell keratinization, the more general term "dysplasia" may be a good substitute for "anaplasia."

Differentiation and Maturation

In almost any discussion and definition of malignancy, the terms "undifferentiated cells" and "loss of differentiation" are used. Thus Anderson (1964) says that malignant tumors are usually composed of more embryonic or poorly differentiated cells. However, he also quotes Berenblum as follows: "A tumor is composed of cells derived from one that has undergone an abnormal type of irreversible differentiation." There seems to be inconsistency in one author stating that a tumor cell is "poorly differentiated" and another insisting that it has "undergone an irreversible differentiation." The explanation for this paradox which has caused a good deal of confusion in oncologic hypothesizing lies in the fact that the word "differentiation" is used with two completely unrelated meanings by pathologists and embryologists.

To the pathologist, lack of differentiation means absence of morphologic, histochemical, or, perhaps, biochemical evidence of function. An undifferentiated cell in this sense is an immature cell, and if we call a tumor "well-differentiated" or "poorly differentiated," we refer to the larger or smaller proportion of tumor cells that show morphologic signs of maturity.

On the other hand, differentiation in the embryologic sense (Weiss, 1949) refers to a cell's being determined to develop in a certain direction, to form a certain organ or tissue. A "differentiated" cell in this sense may be completely immature morphologically, that is, it may be absolutely "undifferentiated" in the sense of the pathologist. It is of the utmost importance to be aware of this duplicity of meaning of the word "differentiation."

Differentiation in the embryologic sense means loss of potency. The egg is totipotent and completely undifferentiated. As the organism develops, parts become determined, that is, differentiated for a certain task, and conversely, they lose their potency for other tasks (Hamilton et al., 1962). In the skin, the germinal cells of the various epithelia are differentiated as skin cells but are not irrevocably committed to their specific tasks of forming epidermal, sebaceous, or other adnexal cells (Montagna, 1962). They can be modulated (Argyris, 1956) under conditions of stress, such as wound healing. They retain some pluripotentiality and are equipotential with germinal cells of other parts of the cutaneous epithelial system.

A tumor cell, on the other hand, may be completely immature, undifferentiated in the pathologist's sense, and yet it has no residual potency for developing into anything else; it will only form more tumor cells of the same type, perhaps exhibiting some maturation along specific lines. The cells of squamous cell carcinoma, for instance, usually undergo keratinization, which effectively removes them from the germinative pool. This process, as Broders (1925) pointed out, is a means of self-control in a cancer, but it does not mean that the maturing cells have reverted to normal: they are dying carcinoma cells. The cell of a skin cancer, therefore, is actually more highly differentiated than its normal prototype, the pluripotential adult ectodermal cell.

Among the various definitions of cancer in current textbooks, this state of affairs is expressed only by Berenblum, as quoted by Anderson (1964): "A tumor is an actively growing tissue, composed of cells derived from one that has undergone an abnormal type of irreversible differentiation: its growth is progressive, due to a persistent delay in maturation of its stem cells." Here, the two terms "differentiation" (in the sense of determination) and "maturation" are clearly separated. I recommend that every time one reads or writes "differentiation," one should use the test of substituting "determination" or "maturation." Many statements in oncologic literature become clearer if this test is applied, and some become absurd.

Autonomy

The next term to be defined is "autonomous" or "uncontrolled" growth. Warren (1961) quotes, with approval, Ewing's simple definition of neoplasia: "A neoplasm is an uncontrolled new growth of tissue."

Hopps (1964) makes a similar statement. It would seem that this expression must be taken with a grain of salt. A certain degree of escape from the regulative influences of the organism is a feature of all tumors; otherwise no mass would be formed. However, the degree of autonomy varies widely, and there are probably few tumor cells whose growth can be described as completely uncontrolled or autonomous. Many malignant tumors obey hormonal regulations. Really uncontrolled cells in tissue culture are apt to double their number every 24 to 48 hours. Therefore, the growth of even the wildest cancer in the body appears to be restrained to some extent.

Progression

The next two terms, "progression" and "somatic mutation," are of much newer vintage and express modern concepts of oncology.

"Progression" (Foulds, 1957) means that a benign or relatively nonmalignant tumor changes into one of higher malignancy. The concept is illustrated in Figure 15–3. Some textbooks state that this event is rare. In the skin, both in clinical experience and in experimental carcinogenesis, it seems to be common, as will be discussed in the section Border Lines and Border Zones in Neoplasia.

Somatic Mutation and Other Mechanisms of Carcinogenesis

Somatic mutation, as the basic mechanism of the origin of cancer cells, has been a much-discussed hypothesis for a number of years (Bauer, 1963). It has been championed and belittled by many competent authors (Burdette, 1953; Brues, 1958; Rous, 1959; Burch et al., 1964). It seemed to lose ground when viral causation of cancer became an undeniable possibility. However, the very similarity of viruses and genes and the evidence that viruses interfere with the genetic mechanism of cells have led to rapprochement of the viral and somatic mutation hypotheses (Potter, 1964; Graffi, 1964; Temin, 1966), which at first seemed incompatible.

For the purposes of this discussion, we need not confine the theory of somatic mutation to the strict concept of a gene mutation. It is sufficient to agree that cancer originates when one cell undergoes some heritable change of its biologic functions (Weiss, 1949). The change may be due to any one of a number of mechanisms (Burdette, 1953; Brues, 1958; Rous, 1959; Pitot and Heidelberger, 1963; Burch et al., 1964; Potter, 1964; Graffi, 1964; Temin, 1966). It sets the affected cell apart from normal neighbors in certain ways. If the cell remains viable, it will pass its changed properties to its progeny. Malignant transformation is not a commonplace event (Pinkus, 1966a). Even in an animal skin painted with carcinogens, only a limited number of tumors develop, and each one enlarges from a point source. Similarly, it has been shown that a single DNA virus particle acts on a single cell to transform it into a cancer cell and that this event is rare, even in an infected tissue culture (Stoker, 1966).

Conversely, the concept of carcinogenesis being a singular event in one cell argues against the continual transformation of normal cells around the original cancer cell as a means of tumor growth. These issues were thoroughly debated by pathologists early in the 20th century. The experience that cancers are able to metastasize, bolstered by transplantability of animal and human cancers, by tissue culture, and particularly by propagation of cancers from single cells (cloning), has practically laid to rest the idea of continuous peripheral conversion of normal cells into cancer cells. Most modern oncologic publications presuppose without question that the cell of any cancer is a genetically fixed cell and will reproduce its own type unless it undergoes another heritable change.

Reversibility

The question arises whether this second change always means progression to greater malignancy or may at times initiate reversion to normal. In the discussion of differentiation, we quoted Berenblum as calling the process of cancerization an irreversible differentiation. While this concept is true for all practical purposes in dealing with human cancer, neuroblastoma of children perhaps being an exception, some recent experiences in other animal species have produced a glimmer of hope that carcinogenesis may not be completely irreversible. Considerable attention was paid to the so-called embryonal carcinoma of mice, a highly malignant transplantable tumor (Kleinsmith and Pierce, 1964). Cells of this teratocarcinoma will differentiate and mature into tissues of various types. The neoplasm can be transplanted to a new animal by a single malignant cell. In each case tumors develop which contain, in addition to the immature cell type, as many as 15 types of differentiated cells. These differentiated cells, which must have descended from the single transplanted cell, have lost their malignancy and are not transplantable, even in large numbers. In this very exceptional case, cells of a highly malignant strain revert to normal, but the stem cell is pluripotential rather than unipotential as most other cancer cells seem to be.

More significant are experimental data in the field of cancer virology and molecular genetics. The recent report of a National Panel (Schmidt and Farber, 1970) lists several avenues of research. Cells transformed into cancer cells by oncologic viruses in tissue culture have been observed to revert to a more normal growth pattern either spontaneously or by certain experimental influences. In all cases, the loss of neoplastic growth characteristics in vitro was accompanied by loss of malignancy on reimplantation into animals. The multipotentiality of certain cancer cell nuclei was demonstrated by implanting nuclei of a frog kidney tumor into eggs from which their own nuclei had been removed. The reconstituted frog eggs were capable of normal division and developed into normal larvae. These experiences argue against the principle of the irreversibility of cancer and suggest that the mechanisms responsible for the malignant state are involved with gene expression rather than gene mutation. The report points out that this line of thinking is supported by recent reinterpretation of the differentiation process of the normal embryo. When the fertilized egg divides, each daughter cell receives an identical set of genes through the equal division of the chromosomes, and this process continues into adult life. The differences in enzymes, other proteins, and the metabolites produced under enzymatic control are now believed to be due to the fact that not all genes function in all cells at the same time. Molecular biology strongly supports the view that genes are not lost during differentiation, but are masked or repressed, and that they may be unmasked under certain circumstances. Application of these concepts to the field of cancer raises hopes that we may be able in the future to revive the normal expression of genes in cancer cells and thus control the tumor instead of destroying it. For the present, however, standard methods of treatment must be used.

Carcinoma in situ and Precancerosis

Inasmuch as invasiveness is one of the basic properties of malignant neoplasms, the concept of carcinoma in situ is paradoxical. Without going into its historical development in detail, we may mention that the first example was described in the skin by Bowen (1912) who, however, chose to call it a precancerous dermatosis (Fig. 15–4). Recently, the questions of carcinoma in situ and precancerous dysplasia have been discussed in great detail in the gynecologic literature in connection with cancer of the cervix uteri.

The concept of precancerous lesions (Andrade, 1964) has met the objection that it involves prognostication and is not a proper pathologic term. Precancerosis is indeed basically a statistical concept and is applied to conditions which progress to cancer in a high proportion of cases, 20 per cent or more having been chosen by Montgomery (1939) in his discussion of precancerous dermatoses and epithelioma in situ. The pathologist has the obligation to state prognosis in many situations, and the use of the term "precancerous" may be justified with a quip, attributed to Pusey (Rattner, 1937), that he had known many premedical students who never became physicians. In practice, we call a skin lesion precancerous or premalignant either if it

presents cellular morphology of the type ordinarily seen in cancer without exhibiting invasiveness, or if statistical experience has shown that cancer develops in this type of lesion in at least 10 per cent of cases. Under this definition, the precancerous lesion may be either a neoplasm of noninvasive (benign) nature or a non-neoplastic condition, such as chronic x-ray dermatitis.

In the latter case, "precancerous" is synonymous with "preneoplastic"; in the former it may or may not coincide with carcinoma in situ. Thus, the carcinogen-induced papilloma of mouse skin is precancerous but is not carcinoma in situ, while Bowen's precancerous dermatosis meets all requirements of carcinoma in situ.

A diagnosis of carcinoma in situ is appropriate in a tissue section when we see a stretch of epithelium (in three-dimensional view, an island) which has cytologic characteristics of dysplasia but is confined within the basement membrane. The epithelium may be that of the cervix uteri, of a bronchus, of a milk duct, or of the epidermis. Dysplasia ("anaplasia") is expressed by the presence of unevenly sized cells in disorderly arrangement and especially by hyperchromatic nuclei and atypical mitoses. Presence of a PAS-stainable basement membrane shows that the deranged epithelial cells are still capable of interacting with mesodermal elements to form and maintain the membrane (see Chapter 17).

Multiple and Multicentric Cancers

It was mentioned previously that malignant transformation is not a commonplace event. Yet we know that many patients have multiple cancers either in different organs or in the skin itself. Farmer's skin with multiple keratoses and squamous cancers, arsenicism, and basal cell epitheliomatosis are well-known examples. Multiple cancers are the result of strong genetic or external influences, and the number of cells that will transform into cancer in any one skin is after all a tiny percentage of the available germinal precursor cells.

The term "multicentric," however, implies a different concept. It is applied

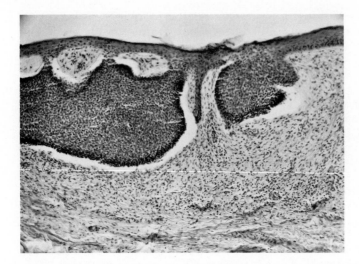

Figure 15–5 Superficial basal cell epithelioma of the so-called multicentric type. The seemingly isolated nest at the right can be shown to be connected with the others by the examination of serial sections. The multiple connections with the epidermis do not represent points of origin but points of collision and adherence. *H&E,* ×*60.*

mainly to superficial basal epithelioma and says that each plaque represents a field of skin in which neoplastic transformation takes place in numerous closely aggregated centers. The concept is obviously based on the appearance of these tumors in histologic sections (Fig. 15–5) which usually show several separate epithelial nests attached to the lower surface of the epidermis. Madsen (1965) has shown convincingly, by means of three-dimensional reconstruction from serial sections of such tumors, that they represent fenestrated plates (Fig. 15–6) and spread peripherally from one center. Only larger lesions may indeed show isolated epithelial islands (Fig. 15–7) within the advancing ring of epithelium. If one focuses attention on the stroma rather than on the epithelial portion of superficial basal cell epitheliomas, it

becomes obvious that they represent a fibroepithelial plate (Fig. 15–8) replacing the pars papillaris of the dermis and extending peripherally along the epidermal-dermal interface. The concept of multicentricity in the sense of a field of skin predisposed to the spawning of many epitheliomas should lead to wide excision or destruction of even small lesions. Yet practical experience shows that superficial basal epitheliomas do not recur if they are removed with only a few millimeters of margin. The concept of multicentricity is obsolete, and it may be hoped that the term will disappear from use.

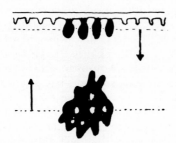

Figure 15–6 Diagrammatic representation of vertical (above) and horizontal (below) sections of a small plaque of superficial basal cell epithelioma. The dotted lines indicate the location of the other section. The appearance of multicentric nests results from the presence of holes in a unicentric plate. (*From* Madsen: Arch. Dermatol., 72:29, 1955.)

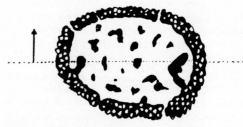

Figure 15–7 Diagrammatic representation of vertical (above) and horizontal (below) sections of a large plaque of superficial basal cell epithelioma. The periphery continues spreading as a fenestrated plate (see Fig. 15–6). The center has broken up into multiple islands owing to partial regression. The dotted line indicates the location of the vertical section. (*From* Madsen: Arch. Dermatol., 72:30, 1955.)

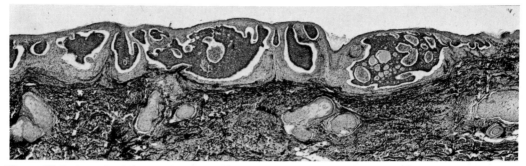

Figure 15–8 Superficial basal cell epithelioma. *Acid orcein and Giemsa ×20.* This stain emphasizes the fact that the epithelial portions are embedded in a solid plate of stroma which stains lighter than the underlying reticular dermis because it does not contain elastic fibers. The fibroepithelial tumor occupies and distends the stratum papillare. Note the persistence of pilosebaceous complexes beneath the tumor.

BORDER LINES AND BORDER ZONES IN NEOPLASIA

Progressive Cancerization

The progression from an innocuous to a malignant lesion is most frequently and most easily observed in actinic keratoses, less frequently in similar lesions caused by arsenic and in Bowen's dermatosis. Comparable processes occur in the development of precancerous melanosis of Dubreuilh (lentigo maligna) or cellular nevus into malignant melanoma, and in the transformation of parapsoriasis into mycosis fungoides. These topics will be discussed in detail in Chapter 17 under the respective headings.

Here, we are concerned with the basic principles underlying the progression. Why do any keratoses and Bowen lesions remain "in situ" for long periods of time? It is unlikely that purely mechanical factors prevent them from becoming invasive. Breaks in the basement membrane occur probably every day. The membrane certainly is destroyed when we curet or fulgurate. Yet, quite often, an incomplete-

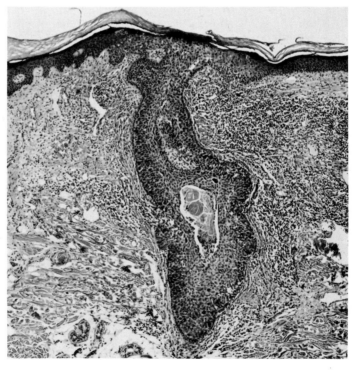

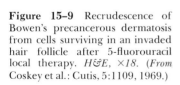

Figure 15–9 Recrudescence of Bowen's precancerous dermatosis from cells surviving in an invaded hair follicle after 5-fluorouracil local therapy. *H&E, ×18.* (*From* Coskey et al.: Cutis, 5:1109, 1969.)

ly removed keratosis recurs as a keratosis and not as an invasive cancer. It seems that the cells of the keratosis are biologically unable to break the basement membrane or even to take advantage of a break. A very interesting example of this fact was observed by Coskey et al. (1969) in a case of Bowen's dermatosis treated topically with 5-fluorouracil. The lesion healed clinically. In a followup biopsy specimen, it was found that indeed the dysplastic epidermis had been replaced by a normal one. Dyskeratotic cells, however, had replaced most of a hair follicle, still confined within the basement membrane. These more deeply situated cells had not been destroyed and were seen (Fig. 15–9) to retrogradely move upward into the epidermis and cause a recrudescence of the lesion. Yet, there was no sign of dermal invasion.

Just as the origin of an actinic keratosis or a Bowen lesion is a cellular event, so apparently is the progression from carcinoma in situ to invasive carcinoma. Actually, a number of steps may be involved. Figure 15–10 is an attempt to illustrate the process. A cell that is heritably deranged in only one or a few of its metabolic functions is neoplastic but may be benign or at least not fully malignant. It may progress at any time closer to malignancy; for instance, it may take the step of becoming invasive. Even among "malignant" cells—those that do invade and destroy other tissues—there

is gradation which we express in histopathologic classification.

The concept of focal progression was beautifully demonstrated by Peyton Rous in a series of experiments (Rous and Henderson, 1964). Small pieces of carcinogen-induced mouse papillomas, the precancerous lesion in that species, were implanted subcutaneously into young mice. There they grew and formed keratinizing cysts, which could again be chopped up and serially transplanted. In some of the cysts, either of the first or a later generation, a focus of invasive cancerous growth will develop. It is difficult to think of a more striking demonstration of the concept that a carcinogen induces cellular change, which is maintained in successive generations of precancerous cells, until, in one of many, a second change takes place. It is the second change that initiates the growth of fully malignant cancer. Similar mechanisms probably are involved in progressive changes in melanotic and reticuloendothelial lesions.

A promising new method has been introduced into the differential diagnosis of precancerous and cancerous states of a tissue by Jordon et al. (1970). The sera of pemphigus patients contain antibodies against cell surface antigens, while those of patients having bullous pemphigoid contain antibodies against basement membrane. Using indirect immunofluorescent

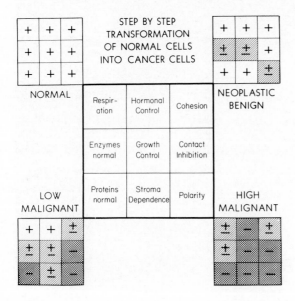

Figure 15–10 Diagram illustrating stepwise progression from normal to benign neoplastic and malignant. Nine representative biologic characteristics of a cell are indicated. Others may be added or substituted. All systems are plus in the normal cell. Partial loss or deviation of some functions characterizes a benign tumor cell. Additional disturbances or losses give the cell the character of lower or higher grades of malignancy. (*From* Pinkus: The borderline between cancer and non-cancer. *In* Year Book of Dermatology 1966/67. Chicago, Year Book Medical Publishers, 1967.)

methods, the authors demonstrated loss of both types of antigens in "anaplastic" squamous cell carcinoma, while cell surface antigens persist in well-differentiated tumors. This method is likely to become a valuable tool in the investigation of cellular changes associated with progressive cancerization.

While the histologic and cytologic criteria vary, depending on the type of neoplasia, we must keep in mind the focal origin of the more malignant tissue and the possibility that we may encounter lesions in which benign or less malignant cells are present side by side with more malignant cells. While the latter are apt to outgrow and obliterate the precursor cells after a while, we must insist on examination of the entire lesion, or at least of a significant sample, before ruling out malignancy if histologic examination of a small biopsy specimen of a recently growing lesion shows no malignant cells. Actinic keratoses and Bowen's dermatosis may exhibit invasion in small foci, and so may Dubreuilh's precancerous melanosis and the superficially spreading (pagetoid) melanoma of McGovern (1969) and Clark (1967). A compound nevus may contain malignant cells at the epidermal-dermal junction, while benign nevus cells persist deeper in the dermis. In parapsoriasis, only one plaque may exhibit progression to mycosis fungoides. There is indeed a broad border zone in the cancerization process of the skin, and there may be honest disagreement between experts in individual cases.

Benign and Malignant Tumors, and Those In Between

We shall now consider the other border zone, the one separating categories of tumors which are either frankly malignant or definitely benign. In the field just discussed, there is no question that the condition started as benign, or at least not very malignant, and progressed to full-blown malignant disease. The main question was, when did the change occur? Now we approach the question, given a certain tumor and, in particular, a histologic section thereof, is this tumor malignant and does it require radical treatment, or is it benign and can it be handled conservatively?

Refinement of Diagnostic Criteria. This border zone, of relatively minor concern not so many years ago, has assumed major significance owing to several developments, but mainly because more clinicopathologic material and better follow-up of cases have revealed discrepancies between histologic diagnosis and clinical course. Well-known examples of this dilemma, and how the answer depends on concepts outside the scope of strict histopathology, are keratoacanthoma versus squamous cell carcinoma (Baer and Kopf, 1963) and juvenile melanoma of Spitz versus malignant melanoma (Kopf and Andrade, 1966). In both instances, clinical experience (in the first case supported by experimental evidence) forced the histopathologist to refine and, to some degree, alter his criteria for malignancy. Details will be found in Chapter 17.

The difficulty with these lesions is twofold. Not only does the histologic picture suggest a malignant process, but also this suspicion is supported by the initial clinical course, which usually includes rapid growth and not infrequently ulceration as a sign of destructiveness. Keratoacanthoma fulfills at least two of Warren's criteria: rapid growth and destructive invasiveness: in addition, it often has atypical cells, a third criterion. The fourth criterion, metastasis, of course is absent. Juvenile melanoma also fulfills at least two of the criteria: highly atypical cells and invasiveness. Growth also is usually fairly rapid. Again, the fourth criterion, metastasis, is absent.

Somewhat different is the case of dermatofibrosarcoma protuberans. This tumor grows slowly and does not exhibit cellular dysplasia. Its claim to malignancy was based on infiltrating growth and the frequency of recurrence (Preaux and Texier, 1970). It is now recognized, however, that total excision, including the peculiar subdermal shelf, which may extend much farther than the visible tumor, practically guarantees cure. Metastasis is rare and usually occurs only late in ineffectively treated cases.

The Significance of Metastasis. All these examples show that metastasis is the one decisive proof of malignancy in skin tumors as it is in all other organs. It humbles the pathologist that this criterion actually is a clinical or biologic one. The microscope is needed only to see the metastases that are yet too small to be apparent clinically or to identify the source of the metastatic lesion when the primary lesion is not obvious. In the case of an early cancer, the pathologist can make only an educated guess whether it will metastasize or not.

The emergence of metastasis as the sole, secure criterion of malignancy has some other implications which seem revealing and important. Metastasis demonstrates the ability of single tumor cells (or perhaps very small aggregates of tumor cells) to establish themselves in foreign surroundings, to multiply independent of local tissue factors, and to induce the host tissue to supply a nourishing stroma. On the other hand, these cells must be sufficiently inoffensive so as not to provoke an inflammatory response that would kill them.

The existence and the mode of growth of metastatic cancer prove better than any other clinical experience that cancer consists of irrevocably determined (differentiated) cells which pass on their heritable characteristics to their progeny. Tissue culture, implantation of human tumors into animals, and a large body of evidence in experimental cancer research fully support these conclusions.

Basal Cell Epithelioma. Thus, metastasis is not only clinical but also biologic proof of malignancy. Warren states that "benign tumors remain localized and do not metastasize." Yet, in the same chapter, he mentions basal cell carcinoma of the skin as a form of "localized cancer," acknowledging the fact that it metastasizes only under exceptional circumstances. Indeed, a review of the literature reveals only about 60 cases of metastasis, and many of these were due to massive implantation of tumor in the lung of patients having longstanding and highly destructive facial tumors. In other cases, one wonders whether the basal cell cancer diagnosed in a routine section may not have had unusual biologic properties from the beginning. Such differences need not show up in a hematoxylin and eosin-stained paraffin section. If one also considers the possibility of progression, which is not too uncommon in the development of basal cell can-

cer from benign adnexoid tumors, it is actually astounding that this common cutaneous neoplasm does not acquire full malignancy in a much higher proportion of cases. In spite of Cotran's (1961) estimate of 0.1 per cent on the basis of his highly selected material, the actual incidence of metastasis in run-of-the mill material of the practicing dermatologist, surgeon, and radiologist is probably less than 0.001 per cent. In fact, all therapy of basal cell epithelioma is predicated on the assumption that eradication of the local lesion equals cure.

The record speaks for an unusual stability of this class of tumor. Yet there is no doubt that basal cell cancers are formidable tumors. They do invade and destroy. They will recrudesce unless completely removed. They are not benign. Terms such as "locally malignant" or "aggressive" have been used. On another occasion (Pinkus, 1966b), I have called them "not-so-benign." They are decidedly occupants of the border zone and remind one of Robbins' statement (1962): "Every tumor does not have to be either benign or malignant." Several attempts have been made to find a good name for basal cell cancer that expresses its peculiar biologic position. Foot's (1947) designation "adnexal carcinoma" is objectionable because it includes the word carcinoma, and because true adnexal carcinomas exist in the skin in the form of adenocarcinomas of eccrine, apocrine, and sebaceous glands. Belisario (1959) proposed "rodent carcinoma" based on the old name of Jacob's rodent ulcer for this type of lesion. Many American dermatologists follow Lever's (1948) lead of calling the tumor "basal cell epithelioma," and this is the term used in this volume. It has the advantage of telling the surgeon that he does not have to fear the dread implications of the carcinoma concept, and similarly it reassures the patient that no danger to his life exists. German usage had coined the word "basalioma," which is perhaps the best term because it avoids the controversy concerning cancer and noncancer and puts the tumor into a niche by itself. "Basalioma" also has the advantage that one can use "basaliomatous" to express the specific attributes of the neoplasm.

Although basal cell epithelioma will be

discussed in detail in Chapter 17, it seems appropriate to examine here the nature of this common tumor, which is the principal occupant of the border zone between cancer and noncancer. The nature of basalioma has provoked frequent discussions before and after Krompecher (1900) recognized its epithelial nature. Dubreuilh (1892) and Darier (1922) in France, Adamson (1914) and others in Great Britain, and Krompecher (1903), Borrmann (1904), and Jadassohn (1914) in Germany are among many contributors to the discussion. In more recent times, Lever (1948) pointed out convincingly the close relationship of basal cell epithelioma to the large group of benign adnexal tumors. He and Pinkus (1966b) devised tables to express these relations in graphic form. Much of the discussion had to remain somewhat speculative because no experimental models existed.

Tumors with the characteristics of human basaliomas have been produced only recently in animals. As a result of the findings of some earlier workers, Zackheim (1962) and Dobson (1963a and 1963b) investigated the earliest stages of basalioma in rat skin, and Zackheim (1963) investigated them also in human skin.

It is now generally agreed that human basaliomas can follow the same carcinogenic stimuli that produce squamous cell cancers. However, the possibility cannot be ruled out that these carcinogens act only to trigger the growth of hidden predisposed cells and that human basaliomas are, after all, "provoked hamartomas." The probability of this hypothesis is lessened by the experience that similar tumors can be produced in rat skin by common chemical carcinogens, inasmuch as spontaneous basaliomas are extremely rare in rats.

Interrelationship Between Stroma and Epithelium. Basaliomas seemingly can arise from epidermis as well as from the infundibulum and other parts of the hair follicle. Epithelial proliferation is accompanied, and perhaps preceded, by changes in the dermis. The morphology of the very earliest basalioma closely resembles the fetal hair follicle, which is from the start a fibroepithelial structure (Pinkus, 1958), never a purely epithelial germ. For years, there has been good reason to believe that

mesoderm and ectoderm interact and influence each other in the production of the hair follicle. This view is based, in part, on experimental work with other fibroepithelial organs (see Grobstein, 1964), which would lead us too far afield to discuss here. The most convincing proof for the primacy of mesodermal action in the development of hair follicles in the mouse was published by Kollar (1970). He separated and recombined fetal epidermis and dermis from the snout, the dorsum, and the hind foot pad and implanted the fragment into the anterior chamber of the eye of adult animals. Snout mesoderm induced histotypical development of hair follicles from foot pad epidermis, which normally would have remained hairless.

It is, then, not unreasonable to assume that a basalioma also needs the interaction of epithelium and stroma for its origin and continued existence. It seems logical to assume that this coordination of two tissues prevents metastasis, because it would be an extremely rare occurrence for competent cells of both tissues to disseminate together. The experiments of Van Scott and Reinertson (1961) with unsuccessful autotransplantation of either "parenchyma" or "stroma" of human basaliomas support this theory.

What does this mean in relation to the thesis of irrevocable transformation of a single cell as the origin of basalioma? Where is this cell: in the epithelium or in the dermis? Three possibilities exist. The epithelium may be altered and may respond in a faulty manner to influences from the mesoderm, or the mesodermal cells may supply faulty stimuli to normal ectoderm, or both parts may be deranged.

One conclusion seems to be safe on the basis of present evidence. A basalioma probably does not arise because a break in the basement membrane permits a normal basal cell to enter the dermis. The histochemically demonstrable basement membrane often is thought of as a rigid wall thrown up by the mesoderm to contain the epithelium. This concept must be revised in the light of recent evidence (Hay, 1964) that it seems to be a joint product of both tissues, the expression of orderly organization. In human fetal skin, a PAS-positive membrane first appears wherever a fibroepithelial hair germ is differentiated (Pinkus, 1958). The disappearance of the membrane at the time of malignant transformation in a precancerous keratosis (Cawley et al., 1966) would seem to be the consequence of order lost rather than the precondition of invasion. Dobson's data (1963a and 1963b) on the earliest stages of basal cell epithelioma in rat skin are amenable to similar interpretation. Furthermore, breaks in the basement membrane occur in psoriasis (Pinkus and Mehregan, 1966) and other simple inflammations. The ability of the epidermis to form pseudoepitheliomatous proliferations in granulomatous inflammatory disease and to return to its normal boundaries when the exciting lesion heals is a good argument for the stability of normal epithelial cells. Another instance is the basalioma-like proliferation often found above histiocytomas. This mimics superficial epithelioma closely in histologic sections (Halpryn and Allen, 1959; Steigleder et al., 1962; Cramer and Cramer, 1963; Schoenfeld, 1964), but only two published cases (Yanowitz and Goldstein, 1964; Caron and Clink, 1964) are available in which there was fair clinical suspicion of a growing tumor.

These examples and the spectrum of maturity (Pinkus, 1966) exhibited by the epithelia of the benign organoid tumors make it likely that it is indeed the epithelial cells that are permanently altered, that they respond in an abnormal manner to stimulating and regulating influences from the mesoderm and perhaps also exert abnormal effects on the mesoderm. The epithelial alteration may be conceived of as any form of heritable change. Loss of enzyme systems or faulty expression of enzymes are favorite modern explanations for so-called minimal deviation cancers (Potter, 1964). It has been shown by Rothberg and Van Scott (1964) that a specific normal protein antigen of epidermis is absent in basal cell epithelioma. Jordon et al. (1970) found no significant amount of epidermal cell surface antigens in basalioma. The same, however, was true for benign hidradenomas. The results of both investigations may only mean that the basalioma is indeed "adnexoid" rather than "epidermoid."

Great clinical and histologic differences

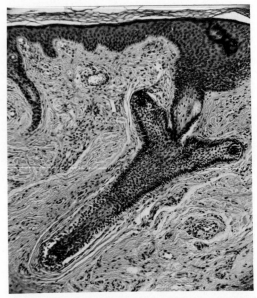

Figure 15–11 Tripartite hair follicle in facial skin of a patient who had multiple trichofolliculomas. The two accessory hair roots "invade" the dermis in an abnormal direction. *H&E, ×90. (From* Pinkus: Adv. Biol. Skin, 7:255, 1966.)

exist within the group of basaliomas. Why are some tumors "benign" in a clinical way, and why are others destructive, invasive—in short, locally malignant? In this connection, we may remember that each hair follicle possesses some degree of invasiveness. The first embryonic hair germs grow through the developing dermis into the subcutaneous fat tissue. With every hair change, the new anagen follicle burrows its way downward (see Chapter 4). Accessory hair roots make new and abnormal paths into the surrounding dermis (Fig. 15–11). From there, it is only a step to the behavior of a trichofolliculoma or a trichoepithelioma. It is said that these benign tumors grow by expansion rather than by invasion. However, there usually is little evidence of compression of normal structures; rather, the dermis seems to be replaced by the tumor (Fig. 15–12). Thus, step by step, we can go a long way toward explaining invasiveness of adnexal tumors as a monstrous exaggeration of normal fibroepithelial growth processes. The one feature that separates true basalioma from all its benign congeners is of quite different character. It is the reactive inflammatory infiltrate that seems to be an in-

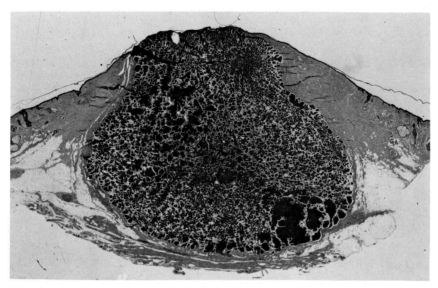

Figure 15-12 Solitary trichoepithelioma of bald scalp. The tumor protrudes through the dermis and sub-cutaneous tissue as a solid fibroepithelial mass analogous to a monstrous pilar apparatus. The lower pole rests on the fascia. *H&E*, ×9. (*From* Pinkus: Arch. Dermatol., 91:24, 1965.)

dicator that the body recognizes a malignant tumor as "nonself" (see Chapter 17 and Pinkus et al., 1963). And this leads us again to the view that the epithelial cells are basically deranged and are indeed malignant cells which are restrained by their dependence on stroma.

The Spectrum of Fibroepithelial Tumors. Table 15–1 illustrates the concept that there is a spectrum of more or less organized tumors in the skin, which may originate anywhere in the germinal cell pool of the pluripotential ectodermal epithelium and may express differentiation along one or several lines, always in association with specific stroma. The most highly organized and mature lesions are stable malformations, the organoid nevi, which represent a localized excess of either epidermis or any of the adnexa or a combination of several of these. Farther away from the "cool blue" end of the spectrum,

TABLE 15-1 ADNEXOID NEVI AND TUMORS

Level of Maturation		Direction of Differentiation		
		Pilar Apparatus		*Eccrine Apparatus*
Normal structure	sebaceous gland	hair and follicle	apocrine gland	
Malformation	nevus sebaceus	hair nevus	apocrine nevus	eccrine nevus
Adenomatous	sebaceous adenoma	trichofolliculoma trichoadenoma follicular poroma trichilemoma	cystadenoma syringocystadenoma papilliferum hidradenoma papilliferum of vulva	hidrocystoma syringocystadenoma papilliferum poroacanthoma dermal duct tumor syringeal hidradenoma nodular hidradenoma eccrine spiradenoma
Epitheliomatous	sebaceous epithelioma	pilomatrixoma trichoepithelioma	cylindroma syringoma (debated)	hidroacanthoma simplex poroepithelioma mixed tumor of skin clear cell hidradenoma
Basaliomatous		basal cell epithelioma		

we find benign neoplasms. If they are relatively well organized, we call them adenomas or acanthomas; the less mature ones often are called benign (cystic) epitheliomas. At the "red hot" end of the spectrum, all adnexoid tumors merge in the pool of complete morphologic immaturity. We call these tumors basal cell epitheliomas but should remember that they too preserve an organoid relationship to their mesodermal stroma, which is as much a part of the tumor as the fibrous root sheath is a part of the hair follicle.

The Topographical Border Line

We have seen that the general pathologic concepts of benign and malignant have to be reexamined and evaluated carefully to account for the great variety of cutaneous neoplasms and to devise adequate therapy on the basis of their biologic behavior. There remain two other practical questions: Where is the topographical boundary of a given tumor, and how far do we have to go beyond the clinical lesion to achieve cure by surgery or irradiation? These questions also require a somewhat different consideration in the skin, because we usually do not deal with amputations or other radical surgery or with saturation radiotherapy of large segments of the body. The reason for a relatively conservative approach is based on the knowledge that, with the exception of malignant melanomas, skin cancer is not apt to metastasize early. This knowledge enables the therapist to take the cosmetic end result of his activities into consideration and reinforces the wish to remove or irradiate as little tissue as is compatible with achievement of cure.

Determination of the physical border between the cancer and normal tissue is based on two opposed facts: the border line is sharp because each cancer grows from a point source, and we do not have to worry about diffuse or multicentric cancerization of a predisposed field. On the other hand, the peripheral extension of a cancer may be far beyond the clinically obvious border.

Thus, the superficial type of basal cell epithelioma (Figs. 15–5 and 15–8), which often is called multicentric but actually is a thin and often fenestrated plate (Figs. 15–6 and 15–7), rides on and does not invade the reticular portion of the dermis. It does not require excision of the full thickness of the dermis, and cure can be achieved by curettage and cautery extending a few millimeters beyond the visible border. On the other hand, some types of sclerosing basal cell epitheliomas may extend for several centimeters beyond the visible border and may grow unexpectedly deep, as the chemosurgical method of controlled excision has amply demonstrated (see Chapter 70). Cooperation between the clinician and the pathologist is required to delineate therapy in each individual case.

PSEUDOCANCER

The last border line to be discussed in this chapter is that between true cancerous neoplasia and pseudoneoplasia in the sense of a reactive process that mimics cancer — clinically or histologically. The history of pseudocancer is long, but the term has gained prominence in dermatology only recently. Possibly, keratoacanthoma or self-healing squamous cell carcinoma may belong in this group rather than under the heading of nonmalignant neoplasms. Pseudocarcinomatous hyperplasia of epidermal and adnexal epithelium in response to such diverse stimuli as deep fungous infection (blastomycosis), sensitivity to halogens (bromoderma), or underlying benign mesodermal tumors (histiocytoma, granular cell myoblastoma) has long been known. Giant condyloma acuminatum of the Buschke-Loewenstein type is an epithelial reaction to virus infection that may simulate carcinoma. In the field of mesodermal lesions, pseudosarcomatous fasciitis and atypical fibroxanthoma, granuloma pyogenicum, and pseudolymphoma present diagnostic challenges.

With all these lesions, however, there is no conceptual gray zone. Cooperation between clinician and pathologist, sufficient material for histologic examination, and, perhaps, repeated biopsy should enable the diagnostician to decide the question of cancer versus pseudocancer in every case.

SUMMARY

The discussions in this chapter should serve as a reminder to the clinician that in the field of skin cancer he cannot expect to make a diagnosis without the assistance of the pathologist. He also cannot expect to get a final answer from the pathologist in every case, and particularly cannot expect this answer if he sends a piece of tissue to the laboratory without rather detailed clinical information. In many cases, because of technical and theoretical difficulties, close cooperation between clinician and pathologist is required to insure maximum benefit to the patient.

REFERENCES

Adamson, H. G.: On the nature of rodent ulcer. Lancet, 1:810, 1914.

Anderson, W. A. D.: Synopsis of Pathology. Ed. 6. St. Louis, C. V. Mosby Company, 1964.

Andrade, R.: Die praecanceröse und canceröse Wucherung von Epidermis und Anhangsgebilden. *In* Jadassohn, J.: Handbuch der Haut-und Geschlechtskrankheiten Ergänzungswerk. I,2:344, Berlin, Springer-Verlag, 1964.

Argyris, T. S.: The effect of wounds on adjacent growing or resting hair follicles in mice. Arch. Pathol., 61:31, 1956.

Baer, R. L., and Kopf, A. W.: Keratoacanthoma. *In* Year Book of Dermatology. Chicago, Year Book Medical Publishers, 1962–1963, p. 7.

Bauer, K. H.: Das Krebsproblem. Ed. 2. Berlin, Springer-Verlag, 1963.

Belisario, J. C.: Cancer of the Skin. London, Butterworth & Company, Ltd., 1959.

Borrmann, R.: Die Entstehung und das Wachstum des Hautcarcinoms. Z. Krebsforsch., 2:1, 1904.

Bowen, J. T.: Precancerous dermatoses: A study of 2 cases of chronic atypical epithelial proliferation. J. Cutan. Dis., 30:241, 1912.

Broders, A. C.: Cancer's self control. Med. J. Rec., 121:133, 1925.

Brues, A. M.: Critique of the linear theory of carcinogenesis. Science, 128:693, 1958.

Burch, P. R. J., Burwell, R. G., and Rowell, N. R.: Autoimmunity and chromosomal aberrations. Lancet, 1:720, 1964.

Burdette, W. J.: The significance of mutation in relation to the origin of tumors. Cancer Res., 15:201, 1953.

Caron, G. A., and Clink, H. M.: Clinical association of basal cell epithelioma with histiocytoma. Arch. Dermatol., 90:271, 1964.

Cawley, E. P., Hsu, Y. T., and Weary, P. E.: The basement membrane in relation to carcinoma of the skin. Arch. Dermatol., 94:712, 1966.

Clark, W. H., Jr.: A classification of malignant melanoma in man correlated with histogenesis and biologic behavior. *In* Advances in Biology of Skin. VIII. The Pigmentary System. 621. New York, Pergamon Press, 1967.

Cohnheim, J.: Vorlesungen über allgemeine Pathologie. Berlin, A. Hirschwald, Publisher, 1877, p. 634.

Coskey, R. J., Mehregan, A. H., and Bryan, H. G.: Bowen's disease. II. Unsuccessful response to topical 5-fluorouracil therapy. Cutis, 5:1109, 1969.

Cotran, R. S.: Metastasizing basal cell carcinomas. Cancer, 14:1036, 1961.

Cramer, R., and Cramer, H. J.: Über die pseudobasaliomatöse Epithelhyperplasie der Haut. Arch. Klin. Exp. Dermatol., 216:231, 1963.

Darier, M. J.: Des épithéliomes primitifs de la peau. Br. J. Dermatol., 34:145, 1922.

Darier, M. J.: Note sur la dyskeratose, en particulier la maladie de Paget. Bull. Soc. Fr. Dermatol. Syphiligr., 32:1, 1925.

Dobson, R. L.: Anthramine carcinogenesis in the skin of rats. I. The epidermis. J. Natl. Cancer Inst., 31:841, 1963a.

Dobson, R. L.: Anthramine carcinogenesis in the skin of the rat. II. The pilosebaceous apparatus. J. Natl. Cancer Inst., 31:861, 1963b.

Dubreuilh, W.: De l'ulcus rodens. Proc. 2nd Int. Congr. of Dermatology, Vienna, 1892, p. 377.

Fleischmajer, R., and Billingham, R. E. (Eds.): Epithelial-Mesenchymal Interactions. Baltimore, The Williams & Wilkins Company, 1968.

Foot, N. C.: Adnexal carcinoma of the skin. Am. J. Pathol., 23:1, 1947.

Foulds, L.: Tumor progression. Cancer Res., 17:355, 1957.

Graffi, A.: A review of theories of carcinogenesis. Arch. Geschwulstforsch., 22:13, 1964.

Grobstein, C.: Cytodifferentiation and its controls. Science, 143:643, 1964.

Halpryn, H. J., and Allen, A. C.: Epidermal changes associated with sclerosing hemangiomas. Arch. Dermatol., 80:160, 1959.

Hamilton, W. J., Boyd, J. D., and Mossman, H. W.: Human Embryology. Ed. 3. Baltimore, The Williams & Wilkins Company, 1962.

Hamperl, H.: Lehrbuch der allgemeinen Pathologie und der pathologischen Anatomie. Ed. 28. Berlin, Springer-Verlag, 1968.

Hay, E. D.: Secretion of a connective tissue protein by developing epidermis. *In* Montagna, W., and Lobitz, W. C., Jr. (Eds.): The Epidermis. New York, Academic Press, 1964, p. 97.

Hopps, H. C.: Principles of Pathology. Ed. 2. New York, Appleton-Century-Crofts, 1964.

Jadassohn, J.: Die benignen Epitheliome. Arch. Dermatol. Syphiligr. (Berl.), 117:577, 705, 833, 1913/1914.

Jordon, R. E., Winkelmann, R. K., and De Moragas, J. N.: The study of skin tumors by indirect immunofluorescence using antibodies to basement-membrane and cell-surface antigens. J. Invest. Dermatol., 54:352, 1970.

Kleinsmith, L. J., and Pierce, G. B., Jr.: Multipotentiality of single embryonal carcinoma cells. Cancer Res., 24:1544, 1964.

Kollar, E. J.: The induction of hair follicles by embryonic dermal papillae. J. Invest. Dermatol., 55:374, 1970.

Kopf, A. W., and Andrade, R.: Benign Juvenile Melanoma. Year Book of Dermatology, 1965–1966. Chicago, Year Book Medical Publishers, 1966, p. 7.

Krompecher, E.: Der drüsenartige Oberflächen-Epithelkrebs. (Carcinoma epitheliale adenoides.) Beitr. Pathol. Anat., 28:1, 1900.

Krompecher, E.: Der Basalzellenkrebs. Jena, Gustav Fischer, 1903.

Lever, W. F.: Pathogenesis of benign tumors of cutaneous appendages and of basal cell epithelioma. I and II. Arch. Dermatol., 57:679, 709, 1948.

Madsen, A.: The histogenesis of superficial basal-cell epitheliomas; unicentric or multicentric origin. Arch. Dermatol., 72:29, 1955.

Madsen, A.: Studies on basal cell epithelioma of the skin. Acta Pathol. Microbiol. Scand., Suppl. 177, 1965.

McGovern, V. J., and Lane Brown, M. M.: The Nature of Melanoma. Springfield, Ill., Charles C Thomas, Publishers, 1969.

Montagna, W.: The Structure and Function of Skin. Ed. 2. New York, Academic Press, 1962, p. 425.

Montgomery, W.: Precancerous dermatosis and epithelioma in situ. Arch. Dermatol., 39:387, 1939.

Pinkus, H.: Embryology of hair. *In* Montagna, W., and Ellis, R. A. (Eds.): The Biology of Hair Growth. New York, Academic Press, 1958, p. 1.

Pinkus, H.: Epithelial and fibroepithelial tumors. Arch. Dermatol., 91:24, 1965.

Pinkus, H.: Malignant transformation of epithelium. *In* Mackenna, R. M. B.: Modern Trends in Dermatology. Series 3:275. London, Butterworth & Company, Ltd., 1966a.

Pinkus, H.: Adnexal tumors, benign, not-so-benign and malignant. *In* Montagna, W.: Advances in Biology of Skin. Vol. 7:255. London, Pergamon Press, 1966b.

Pinkus, H.: The borderline between cancer and noncancer. *In* Year Book of Dermatology, 1966/1967. Chicago, Year Book Medical Publishers, 1967, p. 5.

Pinkus, H., and Mehregan, A. H.: The primary histologic lesion of seborrheic dermatitis and psoriasis. J. Invest. Dermatol., 46:109, 1966.

Pinkus, H., Jallad, M., and Mehregan, A. H.: The inflammatory infiltrate of precancerous skin lesions. J. Invest. Dermatol., 41:247, 1963.

Pitot, H. C., and Heidelberger, C.: Metabolic regulatory circuits and carcinogenesis. Cancer Res., 23:1694, 1963.

Potter, V. R.: Biochemical perspectives in cancer research. Cancer Res., 24:1085, 1964.

Preaux, J., and Texier, M.: Quelle est la gravité du dermatofibrosarcome de Darier et Ferrand? Que penser de sa malignité? Ann. Dermatol. Syphiligr. (Paris), 97:49, 1970.

Rattner, H.: William Allen Pusey at close range. Arch. Dermatol., 35:25, 1937.

Robbins, S. L.: Textbook of Pathology with Clinical Application. Ed. 2. Philadelphia, W. B. Saunders Company, 1962.

Rothberg, S., and Van Scott, E. J.: Absence of normal epidermal protein in basal cell tumor. J. Invest. Dermatol., 42:141, 1964.

Rous, P.: Surmise and fact on the nature of cancer. Nature (Lond.), 183:1357, 1959.

Rous, P.: Opening remarks: Symposium on the possible role of viruses in cancer. Cancer Res., 20:672, 1960.

Rous, P., and Henderson, J. S.: The spread from uniformity to diversity when benign tumors become malignant. Am. J. Pathol., 44:19a, 1964.

Schmidt, B. C., and Farber, S.: Report of the National Panel of Consultants on the Conquest of Cancer. Washington, D.C., U.S. Government Printing Office, 1970.

Schoenfeld, R. J.: Epidermal proliferations overlying histiocytomas. Arch. Dermatol., 90:266, 1964.

Steigleder, G. K., Nicklas, H., and Kamei, Y.: Die Epithelveränderungen beim Histiozytom, ihre Genese und ihr Erscheinungsbild, Dermatol. Wochenschr., 146:457, 1962.

Stoker, M.: Viral carcinogenesis. Endeavour, 25:119, 1966.

Temin, H. M.: Genetic and possible biochemical mechanisms in viral carcinogenesis. Cancer Res., 26:212, 1966.

Van Scott, E. J., and Reinertson, R. P.: The modulating influence of stromal environment on epithelial cells studied in human autotransplants. J. Invest. Dermatol., 36:109, 1961.

von Hansemann, D. P.: Die mikroskopische Diagnose bösartiger Geschwülste. Berlin, A. Hirschwald, Publisher, 1897.

Warren, S.: Neoplasms. *In* Anderson, W. A. D.: Pathology. Ed. 4. St. Louis, C. V. Mosby Company, 1961.

Weiss, P.: The problem of cellular differentiation. Proc. 1st Natl. Cancer Conference, 50, 1949.

Yanowitz, M., and Goldstein, M.: Basal cell epithelioma overlying a dermatofibroma. Arch. Dermatol., 89:709, 1964.

Zackheim, H. S.: The origin of experimental basal cell epitheliomas in the rat. J. Invest. Dermatol., 38:67, 1962.

Zackheim, H. S.: Origin of the human basal cell epithelioma. J. Invest. Dermatol., 40:281, 1963.

16

Worldwide Epidemiology of Premalignant and Malignant Cutaneous Lesions*

Douglas Gordon, M.B., B.S., F.R.A.C.P., F.A.C.M.A., F.R.A.C.G.P., and
Harold Silverstone, M.A. (N.Z.), Ph.D. (Edin.)

"The mainspring of epidemiological study is curiosity."

D. Snow

Methods Used in Epidemiologic Investigations

There are three main ways of advancing medical knowledge: by clinical observation, by epidemiologic investigation, and by experimental research.

Epidemiology in essence is an observational method of research concerned with the study of disease and disability in numbers of people rather than in single individuals; it carries the implication that the data so gathered will be recorded systematically and, when indicated, subjected to techniques of statistical assessment. Any type of disease — or its absence — is an area of legitimate epidemiologic investigation. Hence it is fitting that epidemiologists should study skin cancer.

The "clinical observer" and the epidemi-

ologist, of course, tend to merge. Nevertheless, there are important differences in the modern setting. As we all know, clinical observation not only has added much to medical knowledge but also has stimulated much experimental research. Yet clinical observation is at the mercy of individual prejudices, emotional aberrations, current social pressures, and ideologic beliefs. In theory at least, the epidemiologic method is designed to overcome as far as is humanly possible the effect of such factors

---

*In this chapter "skin cancer," unless otherwise stated, has a restricted meaning, namely that group of skin cancers which is composed of squamous cell carcinomas, basal cell carcinomas, and variations of these. It does not include lip or anal cancer or other cancers of mucocutaneous surfaces. From time to time we will refer to solar keratoses (hyperkeratoses). "Melanoma" means all types of malignant melanoma of the skin. Less common types of skin malignancy have been excluded because, from an epidemiologist's viewpoint, there is insufficient data to warrant discussion. The term "head and neck" is used in its anatomic sense to include face. Special attention has been paid to the effect of sunlight.

which so often appear when human beings draw conclusions from their own "observations." In epidemiology the accent is on planning, recording, deductive reasoning, and the employment of statistical techniques to help in planning and in the assessment of the results collected. It is a form of organized observation with built-in safeguards.

If this concept of modern epidemiologic method is accepted as correct, then we must agree with Urbach et al. (1971) and Higginson (1963) that up to the present time epidemiology, with a few notable exceptions, has not played a large part in the investigation of skin cancer.

We would suggest as well that the epidemiologic investigations which have so far been carried out have raised almost as many problems as they have solved.

The modern day medical graduate, nurtured by a system of medicine which has taken most of its scientific basis from the experimental laboratory, may on the one hand have misgivings about the validity of "observation" as a research tool, and on the other, be repelled by methods which reduce human patients to mere "numbers."

These views can be readily refuted, but it will suffice to say here that there are situations in human skin cancer research in which the experimental method has almost insurmountable deficiencies. It is relevant to quote Blum (1966):

Direct quantitative comparison cannot be drawn between experimental induction of cancer in laboratory animals with ultraviolet light and the hazard of skin cancer in man resulting from this agent.

He went on to say that UV radiations penetrate more deeply in mice than in man; that there are indeterminable biologic differences between man and experimental animals; and that reliable statistics giving information about the incidence of skin cancer correlated with the amount of exposure to ultraviolet B are scarce and difficult to obtain.

Now that we are more readily adverting to the fact that most diseases have multifactorial causes, we are once again perceiving the usefulness of epidemiologic methods of study.

Lilienfeld et al. (1967) remarked:

That epidemiology should have been neglected for so long in relation to cancer is particularly surprising when we consider how much of our knowledge of carcinogenesis has stemmed directly from isolated observations that were essentially epidemiological in character.

In other words, well-planned epidemiologic investigations should receive support. To date, much of the information of an epidemiologic nature which we have collected about skin cancer has come from study of records of patients carried out almost as an afterthought some time subsequent to the clinical management of these patients. The information so gained has been not only useful but also a lasting monument to the zeal and intellectual curiosity of many hard-working clinicians. Nevertheless, this approach usually reveals that some of the facets in which we have become interested cannot be investigated because the facts in the clinical record which would have enabled us to do this are missing.

However, in the last decade or so it is noteworthy that clinicians, particularly in certain departments of dermatology, are compiling clinical records of skin cancer in a planned way so that such records can be used later to answer specific questions which have excited the investigators. In addition to this, the characteristics of groups of patients who have skin cancer have been contrasted with the characteristics of groups of people who have not had skin cancer. Thus, in one or two clinical situations, the use of the control group has emerged.

Finally and more recently there have been two or three epidemiologic surveys into skin cancer specifically for the purpose of garnering knowledge quite apart from clinical management.

All in all, therefore, epidemiology is on the move in this area, and probably our initial pessimism as expressed above could be greatly modified.

In this chapter we will try to describe in broad terms the epidemiologic information about skin cancer and melanoma which is so far available. In the case of skin cancer, we will look first at prevalence and incidence, then at the causes of skin cancer, and finally discuss some miscella-

PLATE I

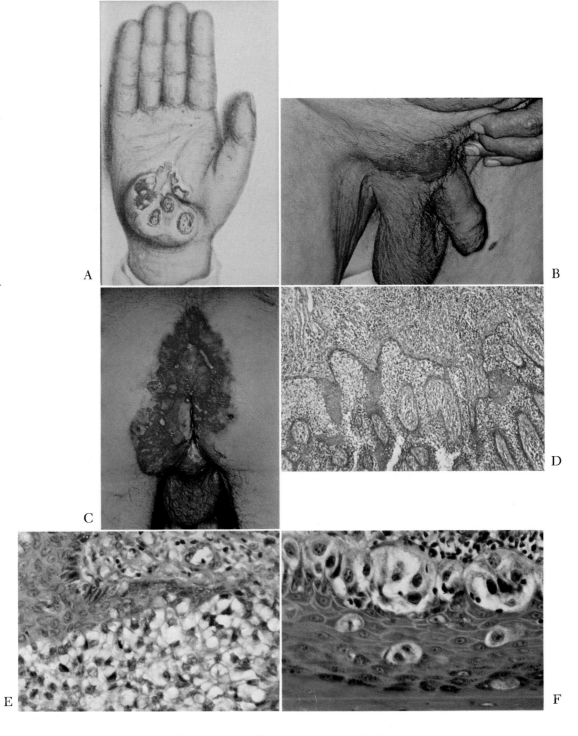

A, Arsenical keratoses and squamous cell carcinoma (Fig. 19–4).
B, Extramammary Paget's disease (Fig. 28–1).
C, Extramammary Paget's disease (Fig. 28–2).
D. Extramammary Paget's disease: biopsy from patient shown in B (Fig. 28–4).
E. Vacuolar cytoplasm of the Paget cell complex (Fig. 28–8).
F. Malignant melanoma with pagetoid structure (superficial spreading type) (Fig. 28–10).

PLATE II

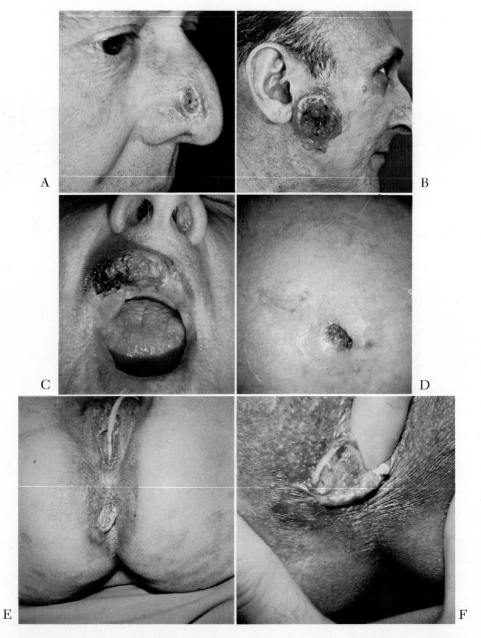

A, Basosquamous carcinoma (Fig. 38–1).
B, Squamous cell carcinoma mistaken for keratoacanthoma (Fig. 38–2).
C, Squamous cell carcinoma of upper lip (Fig. 38–6A).
D, Recurrent squamous cell carcinoma of scalp (Fig. 38–7A).
E, Squamous cell carcinoma in old burn scar (Marjolin's ulcer) (Fig. 39–3).
F, Perianal squamous cell carcinoma in a patient with Fanconi's anemia (Fig. 39–1).

PLATE III

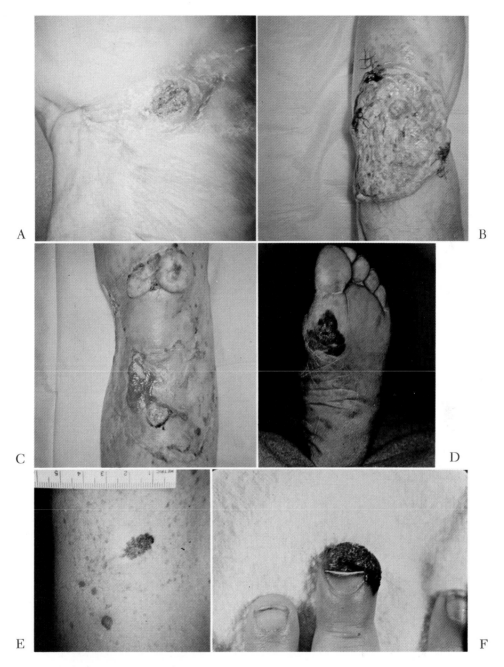

A, Close-up view of Plate II-F (Fig. 39–2).

B, Ulcerating squamous cell carcinoma in osteomyelitis of leg (Fig. 39–4).

C, Postoperative recurrence in lesion shown in B (Fig. 39–5).

D, Melanoma of sole of foot (Fig. 42–1).

E, Melanoma of previous smallpox vaccination site (Fig. 42–3).

F, Melanoma of fingertip in infant at birth and at 12 months (Fig. 42–4).

PLATE IV

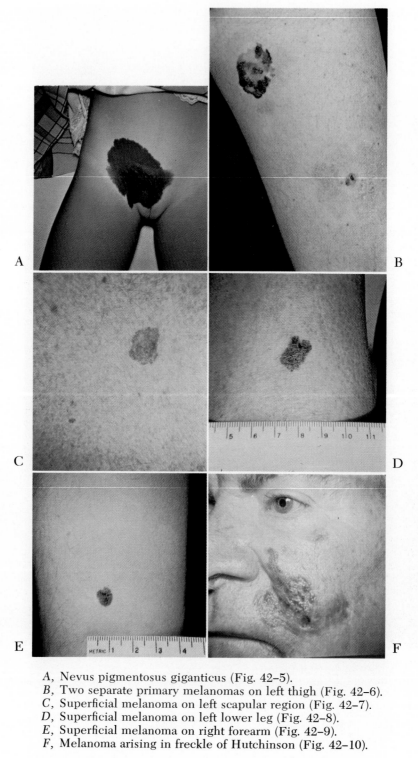

A, Nevus pigmentosus giganticus (Fig. 42–5).
B, Two separate primary melanomas on left thigh (Fig. 42–6).
C, Superficial melanoma on left scapular region (Fig. 42–7).
D, Superficial melanoma on left lower leg (Fig. 42–8).
E, Superficial melanoma on right forearm (Fig. 42–9).
F, Melanoma arising in freckle of Hutchinson (Fig. 42–10).

PLATE V

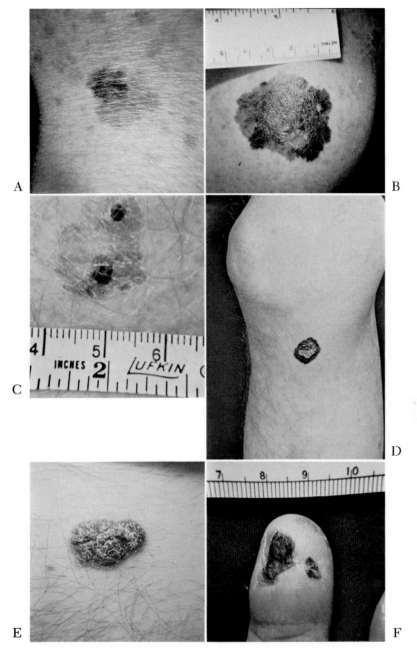

A, Melanoma arising in freckle of Hutchinson (dorsum of right hand) (Fig. 42–11).
B, Invasive melanoma of left shoulder (Fig. 42–12).
C, Invasive melanoma of left thigh (Fig. 42–13).
D, Invasive melanoma of right leg (Fig. 42–14).
E, Invasive melanoma of abdomen (Fig. 42–15).
F, Subungual melanoma of left middle finger (Fig. 42–16).

PLATE VI

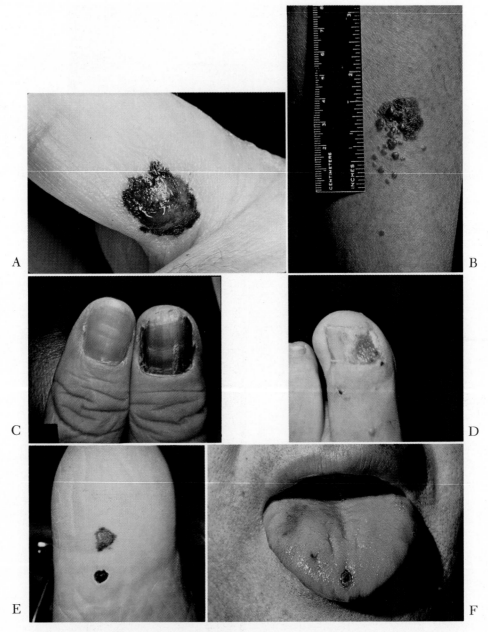

A, Invasive melanoma of right middle finger (Fig. 42–17).
B, Melanoma and satellitosis of left lower leg (Fig. 42–23).
C, Subungual melanoma of right thumb (Fig. 42–27).
D, Amelanotic melanoma and satellitosis under left great toenail (Fig. 42–29).
E, Melanoma of right heel (top lesion) (Fig. 42–30).
F, Melanoma of tip of tongue (Fig. 42–32).

PLATE VII

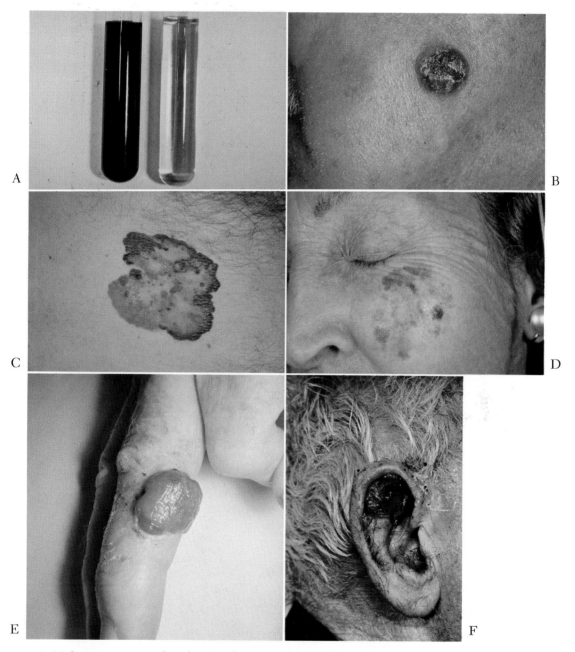

A, Melanuria compared with normal urine specimen (Fig. 42–34).
B, Nodular malignant melanoma. (Courtesy of Dr. E. S. Lupton.)
C, Superficial spreading malignant melanoma. (Courtesy of Dr. E. S. Lupton.)
D. Lentigo maligna melanoma. (Courtesy of Dr. E. S. Lupton.)
E. Postirradiation pseudosarcomatous ulcerated lesion of lateral aspect of finger (Fig. 47–6).
F. Atypical fibroxanthoma of the external ear (Fig. 47–1).

PLATE VIII

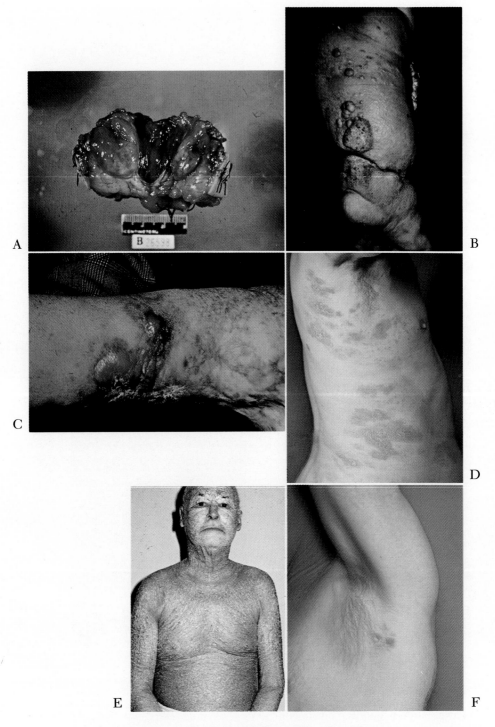

A, Pseudosarcomatous fasciitis of shoulder (Fig. 47–10).
B, Lymphangiosarcoma of leg (Fig. 48–7).
C, Postmastectomy lymphangiosarcoma (Fig. 48–9).
D, Psoriasiform lesions in premycotic stage (Fig. 53–2).
E, Erythroderma in patient with Sezary syndrome (Fig. 53–9).
F, Nodular lesions of lymphocytoma cutis (Fig. 53–36).

PLATE IX

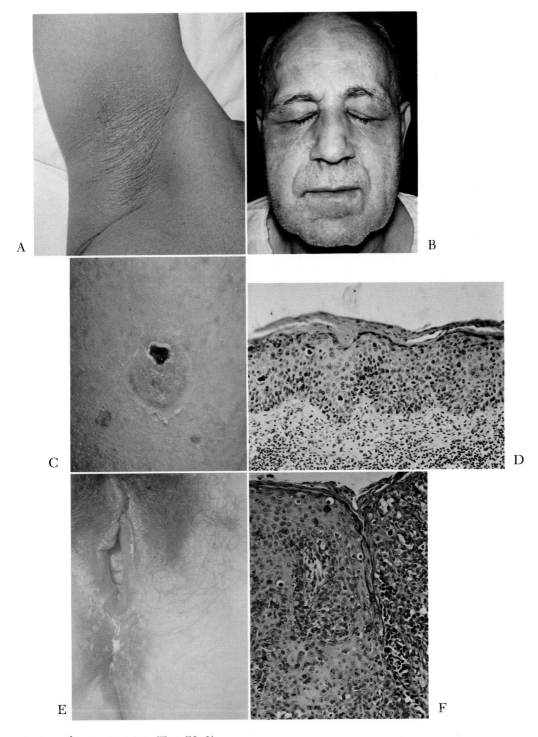

A, Acanthosis nigricans (Fig. 56–2).
B, Dermatomyositis and carcinoma of nasopharynx (Fig. 56–6).
C, Bowen's disease of trunk (Fig. 56–23). (Courtesy of Dr. Lewis Shapiro.)
D, Bowen's disease (Fig. 56–24). (Courtesy of Dr. Lewis Shapiro.)
E, Extramammary Paget's disease (Fig. 56–25). (Courtesy of Dr. A. N. Domonkos.)
F, Extramammary Paget's disease of scrotum (Fig. 56–26). (Courtesy of Dr. Lewis Shapiro.)

PLATE X

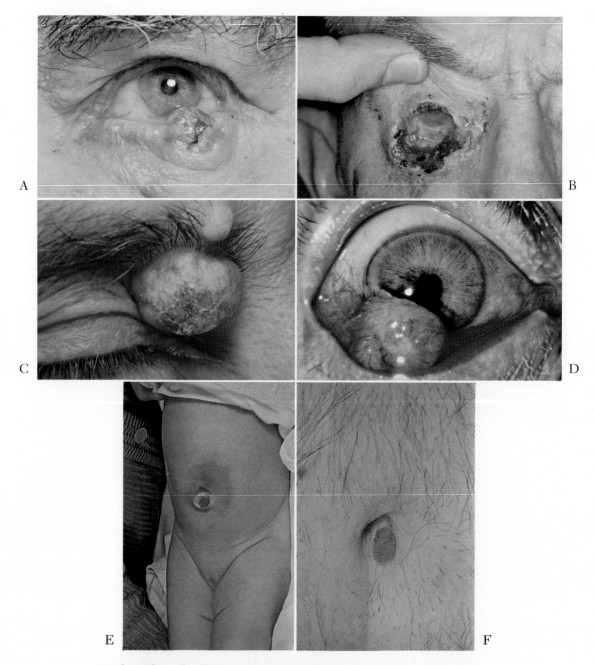

A, Polypoid basal cell epithelioma (Fig. 57–5).
B, Far advanced basal cell epithelioma (Fig. 57–7).
C, Keratoacanthoma (Fig. 57–15).
D, Malignant melanoma arising at limbus of right eye (Fig. 57–24).
E, Adenoidal diverticular tumor with enzymatic oozing dermatitis (Fig. 59–1).
F, Benign nevus of navel (Fig. 59–4).

PLATE XI

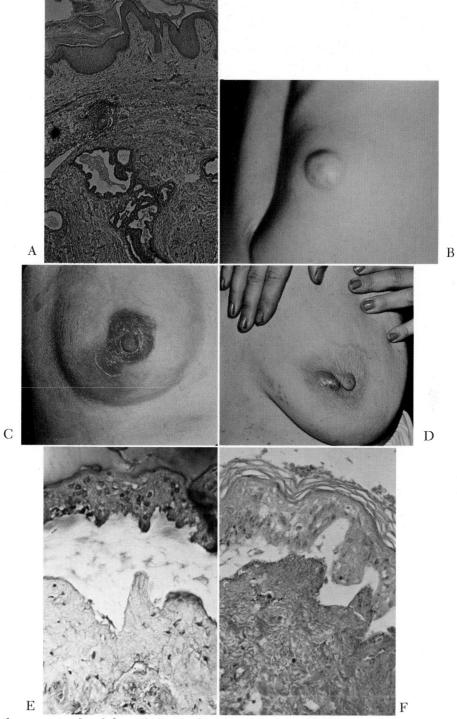

A, Endometriosis of umbilicus (Fig. 59–6).

B, Intraductal papilloma (Fig. 63–12).

C, Eczema (Fig. 63–18).

D, Periductal mastitis (Fig. 63–19).

E, Flat, pigmented nevus 24 hours after freezing (Fig. 72–5). (Courtesy of Dr. Farrington Daniels, Jr.)

F, Twenty-four hours after freezing (Fig. 72–6). (Courtesy of Dr. Farrington Daniels, Jr.)

PLATE XII

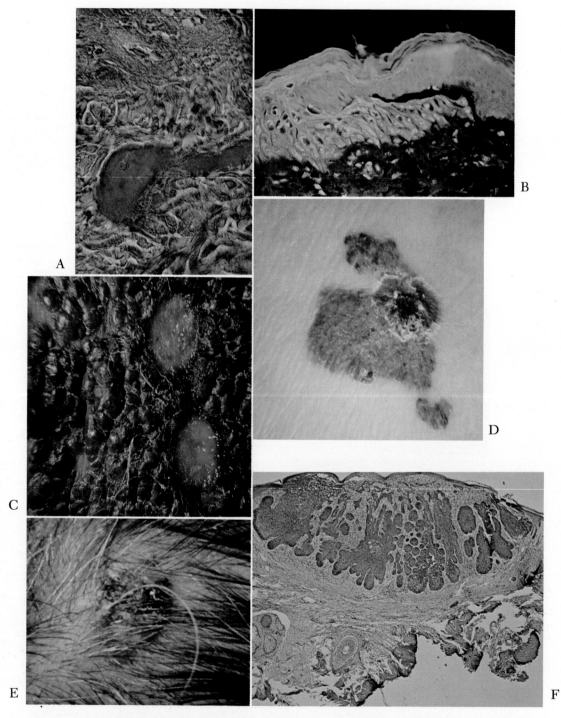

A, Red cell thrombus 24 hours after freezing (Fig. 72–7). (Courtesy of Dr. Farrington Daniels, Jr.)

B, Epithelial regrowth at margin of cryoinjury at 48 hours (Fig. 72–8). (Courtesy of Dr. Farrington Daniels, Jr.)

C, Metastatic melanoma of thigh five days after laser treatment (Fig. 76–4).

D, Melanoma of lower leg with skin metastases before laser treatment (Fig. 76–5A).

E, Pigmented basal cell epithelioma of scalp before laser treatment (Fig. 76–7A).

F, Bloodless excision of basal cell epithelioma by CO_2 laser (Fig. 76–9).

neous topics, such as metastases rates, prognoses, accuracy of diagnoses, and multiplicity of primary cancers.

Broad Historical Trends

In the temperate climate of Europe "skin cancers" were traditionally associated with neoplasms caused by chemical carcinogens. (This commenced with Pott in 1775 and persisted until this century.) This view came about because workers in certain occupations were seen to have a noteworthy incidence of skin cancers, particularly scrotal cancers. We now know, of course, that sunlight-induced neoplasms, certainly basal cell carcinoma, would have been occurring even more frequently among fishermen, farmers, and the like, even in those temperature climates. Nevertheless, historically the accent was on the new urban occupational groups of the Industrial Revolution. It was only when large numbers of migrants from Northern Europe spread down into the New World, to the southern areas of the United States, Australia, New Zealand, and South Africa, that it came to be commonly realized that the most important causal factor was excessive sunlight. For most of this century that has been abundantly apparent.

What we knew originally of skin cancer came from isolated clinical observations and from descriptions furnished by pathologists who were essentially morbid histologists.

Neither the experimentalist nor the professional epidemiologist had been prominent in furnishing new knowledge. It was not until 1928 that Findlay produced a skin cancer on an animal by using UV light, and organized epidemiology was even later in the field. Furthermore, it was not until 1932 that the first pure substance known to produce cancer was prepared, namely 1, 2, 5, 6–dibenzanthracene. In the next year 3, 4–benzpyrene was discovered (Lilienfeld et al., 1967). However, even before we had realized the nature of these specific carcinogens, a good deal of successful prevention had been practiced empirically in occupational situations. Contact with soot and tar had been greatly reduced; refined "white oils" had replaced the harmful shale oils in the cotton manufacturing industry. This kind of thing has occurred rather frequently in the history of medicine, for example, the prevention of scurvy before anything was known of vitamins, smallpox vaccination before we knew anything of viruses, and so on.

At the present time research is mainly concerned with those skin malignancies which have a causal association with sunlight. It is this aspect of skin cancer which has always been important in New World countries and which will be stressed here.

SKIN CANCER

Prevalence and Incidence of Skin Cancer

WORLDWIDE DISTRIBUTION OF SKIN CANCER

Incidence data for skin cancer, other than melanoma, must be treated with considerable reserve. The most comprehensive set of figures are those published in *Cancer Incidence in Five Continents*, Vol. II (Doll et al., 1970). Discussing the registration of neoplasms other than melanomas, the editors point out that "many registries do not register these neoplasms as they are often treated in a consulting room, frequently without histological verification of diagnosis. When skin cancer is not registered, the overall cancer incidence is of course substantially reduced. On balance, it is probably better not to register . . . cancers (except melanoma) than to publish unreliable and incomplete figures."

In presenting a summary of the global distribution of skin cancer other than melanoma, it is preferable, therefore, to work only within broad subdivisions of the range of incidence. The analysis in Table 16–1 uses the age-standardized rates ("world population" standards) for 37 countries or regions, mostly from the data of *Cancer Incidence in Five Continents* but also including some independently collected data from Australia (Carmichael and Silverstone, 1961). In order to demonstrate something of the correlation between skin cancer and geographic latitude,

TABLE 16–1   GLOBAL DISTRIBUTION OF SKIN CANCER INCIDENCE OTHER THAN MELANOMA; MALE DATA WITH CORRESPONDING FEMALE TO MALE RATIOS (F/M)

Average Incidence of Skin Cancer per 100,000 (both sexes)	Zone°				
	A	B	C	D	E
0.0–4.9			Japan F/M = 0.80	S.A. Cape Bantus S. A. Cape Colored Natal Africans Natal Indians Bulawayo Africans F/M = 1.27	Bombay Nigeria F/M = 1.49
5.0–19.9	Sweden** F/M = 0.48	Poland Rumania Denmark F/M = 0.84†	Yugoslavia F/M = 0.56	Texas (Latin) F/M = 1.01	Jamaica F/M = 0.94
20.0–29.9	Finland F/M = 0.88	United Kingdom German Dem. Rep. Hungary F/M = 0.72§	New York State†† F/M = 0.66		
30.0–49.9		Canada F/M = 0.67	Nevada F/M = 0.64		Colombia Puerto Rico F/M = 0.95
50.0–99.9			Victoria (Australia) Tasmania (Australia) F/M = 0.49		
100 and over				S. A. Cape (whites)‖ Texas (non-Latin)¶ Queensland (whites)‡ F/M = 0.59	

*Zonal latitudes are: A, above 60°; B, 45°–60°; C, 35°–45°; D, 20°–35°; E, 0°–20°.
**Zoning based on male rates only.
†Poland = 0.84; Rumania = 1.09; Denmark = 0.59.
††Excluding New York City.
§U.K. = 0.58; G.D.R. = 0.70; Hungary = 0.88.
‖Males, 133.0; females, 72.2.
¶Males, 168.2; females, 106.1.
‡Males, 265.1; females, 155.8.

the results are shown in the form of a cross classification of skin cancer rates against latitudinal "zone." The tabulation is based on data for males, but in each cell of the table a figure is given for the average ratio of female to male rates for the countries listed in that cell. (For more complete details as to the regions of the respective countries which are represented in the data, the reader should consult the original sources mentioned above.)

Some indication of the correlation between latitude and skin cancer incidence is obtained by observing the "diagonal" pattern made by the group of ethnically similar peoples starting with Sweden at "top left" and running right down to Queensland at "bottom right." On the other hand, the more pigmented groups tend to be concentrated at the top right of the table. The other distinguishing feature is that, for the former groups (lightly pigmented), the ratio of female to male incidence rates is only about one-half of its value in the heavily pigmented groups. This table demonstrates a general trend; there are some obvious exceptions.

As we shall see later, much the same trend is observed with the incidence of

melanoma, but the correlational pattern is more diffuse.

AGE-SPECIFIC INCIDENCE RATES

Full details (for most of the regions concerned) of age-specific incidence rates are given in *Cancer Incidence in Five Continents*. For comparative purposes and for the presentation of data for Queensland (the region of highest incidence), graphs are given of both male and female incidence rates (skin cancer, excluding melanoma) for each of four regions, namely, Queensland, Texas, South Africa (Cape Province), and southwest England. The first three have high incidence rates for white populations (male standardized rates being 265, 169, and 133 per 100,000 population, respectively, with corresponding rates of 156, 106, and 72 for females), while southwest England, with male and female rates of 28 and 15, respectively, offers an interesting contrast. Figure 16–1 contains the data for males and Figure 16–2 the data for females.

The graphs are recorded on a double logarithmic scale (log of incidence against log of age).

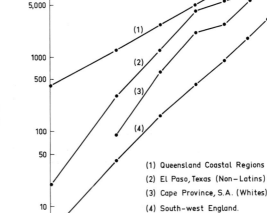

Figure 16–1 Age-specific incidence rates/ million for skin cancer, excluding melanoma, in 4 countries (males).

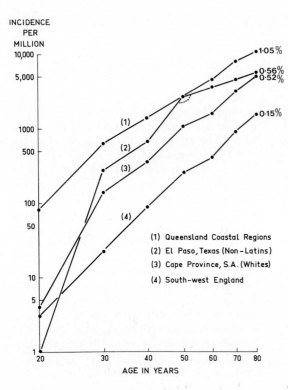

Figure 16–2   Age-specific incidence rates/million for skin cancer, excluding melanoma, in 4 countries (females).

(1) Queensland Coastal Regions
(2) El Paso, Texas (Non-Latins)
(3) Cape Province, S.A. (Whites)
(4) South-west England

If the graphs for the various countries were parallel, this would mean that their relative incidence rates were independent of age. While the graphs for skin cancer for Texas, South Africa, and southwest England are roughly parallel, the graph for Queensland has a distinctly more shallow slope, indicating a relatively greater spread of skin cancer into the younger age groups. Later we will show that in the case of melanoma this nonparallelism is less marked.

CORRELATION WITH ULTRAVIOLET SOLAR RADIATION

While much remains to be done in correlating skin malignancy rates with solar radiation levels in relatively limited geographic areas, it is nevertheless possible to demonstrate the correlation over wider (global) areas. It should be remarked, however, that on the global scale a correlation between latitude and incidence would serve almost as well as one between UV levels and incidence. A further complication is introduced by the necessity to obtain information only for genetically similar

populations in the various latitudes so that the correlation is unimpaired by "nuisance factors."

The global distribution of annual UV solar radiation is given by Schulze and Gräfe (1969). Figure 16–3 shows the results of plotting the logarithm of the age-standarized incidence rate for males against the annual UV radiation for eight groups approximately similar in respect to skin pigmentation.

It will be seen that it is possible to fit a straight line effectively to the data (r for linearity $= 0.983$, $P < 10^{-4}$), a fact which

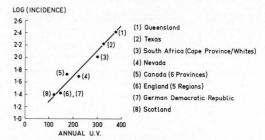

Figure 16–3   Logarithms of incidence rates for skin cancer, excluding melanoma, per 100,000 male population for eight regions (see text) against annual UV solar radiation in watt seconds per cm.² (10 mμ). Equation of fitted line is log (rate) $= 0.00419$ (UV) $+ 0.8508$.

would support a hypothesis that skin cancer incidence increases exponentially with UV levels. From the slope parameters of the fitted curve it is estimated that, on the exponential hypothesis, the skin cancer incidence rate doubles with every increase of 72 units of UV. Translated roughly into terms of latitude, this would mean a doubling of the incidence rate for every decrease of about 10° in latitude. This is in general agreement with known rates for north and south Queensland (relative rates approximately 2:1), but differs from the results given by Auerbach (1961), who estimated that within the United States the incidence rate doubled for every 3.8° of latitude (a result which could not, however, be extrapolated onto a global scale). In any case, the exponential hypothesis must, in the present state of knowledge, be regarded as extremely tentative. A more recent survey in the United States—the Third Cancer Incidence Survey (National Cancer Institute, 1974)—indicates that the incidence of skin cancer doubles with every 8° of latitude.

HISTOLOGIC TYPES OF SKIN CANCER

Direct estimations of melanoma incidence rates proceed according to standard techniques, but in regard to the other histologic types, such as basal cell and squamous cell carcinomas, it is practically impossible to obtain separate series, for reasons that must be obvious from the remarks made above by the editors of the volume on *Cancer Incidence in Five Continents*. The only practical alternative to direct estimation would appear to be the indirect method, whereby estimated incidence rates for all skin cancers (excluding

TABLE 16-2 RATIO OF THE NUMBERS OF BASAL CELL CARCINOMAS TO SQUAMOUS CELL CARCINOMAS FROM 21 DIFFERENT STUDIES (BOTH SEXES)

Country or Region	Source of Information	Ratio of B.C.C.'s to S.C.C.'s
Philadelphia, U.S.A.	Urbach et al., 1971	9.8:1
Queensland tropical coast	Silverstone and Gordon, 1966	5.2:1
New Zealand	Eastcott, 1963	4.9:1
New York State (excluding New York City)	Haenszel, 1963	4.6:1
Brisbane, Queensland	Silverstone and Smithurst, 1971	4.2:1
Transvaal (whites)	Findlay, 1964	4.1:1
Sydney (Australia)	Belisario, 1959	3.1:1
Texas (El Paso and Harlingen, non-Latin)	Macdonald, 1970	3.0:1*
Tasmania (Australia)	Wardale-Greenwood, 1964	2.3:1
Perth (Australia)	ten Seldam, 1963	2.0:1
Galway County (Ireland)	O'Beirn et al., 1970	1.3:1
Honolulu County (whites)	Quisenberry, 1963	1.0:1
Jakarta (Indonesians)	Pringgoutomo and Pringgoutomo, 1963	0.85:1
Singapore (Chinese)	Shanmugaratnam and La'Brooy, 1963	0.84:1
Philippines (Filipinos)	Pantangco et al., 1963	0.58:1
Japan	Miyaji, 1963	0.37:1
Bangkok	Tansurat, 1963	0.32:1
Taiwan (Chinese)	Yeh, 1963	0.26:1
Bantu (pigmented)	Oettlé, 1963	0.10:1
Bantu (albino)	Oettlé, 1963	0.07:1
New Guinea natives	Atkinson et al., 1963	0.04:1

*An earlier result for a similar region is given by Macdonald and Bubendorf (1964) as 1.8:1.

melanoma) are obtained by ordinary actuarial techniques, and the incidence of the separate types estimated by the analysis of their respective proportions in planned ad hoc surveys, in which special efforts are made to have all lesions in a clinical series subjected to histologic examinations.

A further difficulty is that frequently it is impossible to relate the clinical data to any relevant body of actuarial data. In other words, is the particular clinical series really representative in a demographic sense of any particular population? Nevertheless, since the recording of histologic types is the first stage of any comparative epidemiology of the different types, it will be of some value to record here a selection of the data, mainly recorded from clinical series, which are available.

Table 16–2 gives estimates of the ratio of the number of basal cell carcinomas (B.C.C.'s) to squamous cell carcinomas (S.C.C.'s) in 21 different studies, arranged in descending order of the ratio. All 1963 references are from the report of the Conference on Biology of Cutaneous Cancer (Urbach, 1963). Others are given separately.

When the ratios are arranged in descending order of magnitude, it is seen that all the "white" populations have a ratio at least equal to 1.0, while the "pigmented" populations have lower ratios. Within the former groups, however, no regularity is apparent. The Australian series, estimated for Queensland tropics, Brisbane, Perth, Sydney, and Hobart (in increasing order by latitude), shows ratios of 5.2, 4.2, 2.0, 3.1, and 2.3, respectively.

With the exception of Perth, this might lead to the conclusion that among genetically similar types the B.C.C.:S.C.C. ratio increases as latitude decreases. Against this, however, we have the extremely high ratio recorded for Philadelphia, as well as the high rate for New Zealand, whose latitudes correspond to those of Sydney and Hobart rather than those of Queensland. From what is said later about variations of the B.C.C.:S.C.C. ratio with anatomic site, it might be thought that the solution to the problem would emerge from an analysis by site of lesion. Table 16–3 shows a crude site analysis for four Australian regions and for Philadelphia. Clearly the dilemma is not resolved by this expedient. Some results are also given for three Asian and Pacific groups.

The anatomic distribution of B.C.C.'s and S.C.C.'s is in itself of considerable interest, as it is possible that the histologic type depends at least in part on the manner in which different cells in the skin respond to attack by the ultraviolet light.

Epidemiologic Information About the Causes of Skin Cancer

In a great number of disease states, the causes are multifactorial, and this certainly applies to many cancers and especially to skin cancer. Hence the word "cause" is here used with this concept in mind. Though indeed we will cite certain things as specific causes of skin cancer, this nevertheless is done with the clear understanding that quite a number of other factors

TABLE 16–3   ANATOMIC DISTRIBUTION OF B.C.C.'S AND S.C.C.'S IN
EIGHT STUDIES (BOTH SEXES)

Geographic region	Ratio of B.C.C.'s to S.C.C.'s			
	Head and Neck	*Trunk*	*Limbs*	*Trunk or Limbs*
Queensland	4.94	12.06	1.88	2.62
Sydney	4.76	1.14	0.07	0.14
Tasmania	4.58	–	–	0.12
Perth	2.52	1.16	0.60	0.72
Philadelphia	11.71	–	–	3.58
Bangkok	0.93			0.09
Philippines	0.79			0.14
Singapore (all groups)	2.01			0.25

will influence the development of skin cancer in any single individual. Conventionally the causes of skin cancer are stated to be chemical carcinogens, exposure to sunlight, ionizing radiations, and a miscellaneous group of causes which include cancers arising in scars and in chronic ulcers. Let us look at these in turn.

CHEMICAL CARCINOGENS

Chemical carcinogens have played a part, but never a prominent one, in the causation of skin cancer in "New World" countries, or, if they have, their occurrences have not been reported. However, we always have to accept the possibility that some cutaneous neoplasms of apparently unknown etiology may arise from this cause. Nevertheless one would not expect these to be numerous. In the United Kingdom, however, the reverse has applied. There skin cancers due to chemical carcinogenesis have received major attention.

The main chemical carcinogens are found in (1) arsenic and (2) the products arising from combustion and distillation of coal (black and brown), bituminous shales, and petroleum.

These three substances are used in a great variety of industries and occupations, but the carcinogens involved are for the most part identical; that is, they are polycyclic aromatic hydrocarbons of benzpyrene and benzanthracene compounds, arising from combustion and distillation of carbonaceous matter. [Other aromatic and aliphatic compounds might possibly be involved in addition to these (Hueper, 1963).]

The history of skin cancer until this century was the history of exposure to these distillation and combustion products. The main trends of this can be simplified. After Pott's original observation concerning skin cancer in chimney sweeps, other workers with exposure to soot and, later, to coal tars were seen to be at risk (Bell, 1794; Butlin, 1892). The gradual introduction of more humane methods of cleaning the tortuous English chimneys improved the position somewhat. (Nevertheless even today exposure to coal products such as tar still continues to cause some skin cancers.) Then from the middle of the 19th century,

mineral oil, including shale oil, replaced animal fats as lubricants in the machines of 19th century industry, and as a result another large group of workers—"mule spinners" in the cotton industry—became exposed to shale oil. The inguinal region particularly was contaminated (Bell, 1876; Southam and Wilson, 1922; Potter, 1963). However, from about 1928 the number of these operatives developing skin cancer has markedly decreased owing to greater cleanliness, greater personal protection, and particularly to using "white oil" refined in such a way that the aromatic fractions have been removed (Cancer from mineral oil, 1969; Hunter, 1969).

In more recent times a third group of workers was found to develop skin cancer due to industrial exposure to mineral oils—derivatives of petroleum. These were men employed in the engineering industry, particularly in the vicinity of what are known as automatic bar lathes, making commonplace articles such as nuts and bolts. These "tool setters" were exposed to a fine spray of oil used for cooling purposes (Cruickshank and Squire, 1950; Hunter, 1969).

The incidence of skin cancers arising from occupational exposures is influenced not only by the use of chemical carcinogens but also by industrial techniques which may vary from country to country, traditions of personal cleanliness, and the speed with which protective devices are adopted in various occupations. Needless to say, measures have been taken to overcome the hazard due to mineral oils, and one would think that in the future skin cancers due to chemical carcinogens will be an even smaller proportion of all skin cancers than they are today. It is difficult to make sure predictions about hazards in the petroleum industry, but any data we have suggest that these are minimal (Wade, 1963).

In occupational situations in which oil folliculitis, warts, and ulcers are occurring, obviously the men at risk should have regular medical examinations at six-month intervals at least. Under modern industrial conditions, the incidence of these lesions is certainly much less than it was. However, the small, dirty work-place often escapes official surveillance, and the awareness and vigilance of the practicing medical profession must always constitute the final warning system.

Records are available in the United Kingdom which give us reliable information about chemical carcinogenesis in that country. This is so because surveillance of industrial diseases is entrusted to a central authority there—the inspectorate of factories, which has been in existence since 1833. (This centralization is unusual in public health activities, since as a rule power is vested in local bodies, such as states, counties, municipalities, and so forth.) As a result, reasonably good records are available.

A study by Henry (1946, 1947a, and 1947b) of occupational skin cancers notified to the Factory Inspectorate (U.K.) between the years 1920 to 1945 (inclusive) gives some idea of what the extent and nature of the problem was. (As might be expected, the following statistics represented some degree of under-reporting.)

There were, in addition to the above, a variety of occupations in which only a few cancers occurred.

Latent period: The greatest number of men reported after 20 to 24 years in the case of mineral oil exposure.
: The greatest number of men reported after 50 to 54 years in the case of shale oil exposure.

There was, however, great variation between "a little under one year" to 75 years. In these occupations squamous cell cancer is the usual type of lesion produced, but some basal cell cancers also are recorded.

The continuing contemplation of chemical carcinogenesis of the skin, which the English have carried out so successfully for so long, should not blind us to the fact that the majority of skin neoplasms, even in that country, are not due to any obvious exposure to chemical substances. Harnett (1952), in a survey of cancers in London, discussed 1080 patients with primary skin cancers presenting for the first time. (Admittedly London does not have the concentration of engineering industries found in some other parts of the United Kingdom.) Only 11.4 percent of the males and 1.1 percent of females gave a history of exposure to known chemical carcinogens, whereas 25 percent of males and 3.1 percent of females gave occupational histories involving sustained outdoor work. Furthermore, Sweet (1964) in discussing surveys of skin cancer in four areas in England noted that the incidence of B.C.C.'s was much higher than the incidence of S.C.C.'s. This hardly suggests that chemi-

Percentage of Each Site Affected—Industrial Cancers—United Kingdom, 1920–45

	Head and Neck (%)	Upper Limb (%)	Scrotum (%)	Other (%)
Coal products: pitch, tar, and tar products: 2363 cancer sites	53.7	22	21.3	3
Shale oil and mineral oil: 1535 cancer sites	12.2	18.4	59	10.4

Thus lesions of the head and neck (1456) and lesions of the scrotum (1409) had much the same numerical representation.

Principal Occupations

Coal Products		*Shale and Mineral Oil*	
Patent fuel (briquettes)	640	Cotton industry	1419
Pitch loading (wharves)	55	Refining of shale and mineral oil	57
Manufacture electrical equipment	34	Metal working	40
Cable making and laying	25		
Net fixing	21		
Making of roads	23		
Tar distilling	1001		
Gas works	331		
Coke ovens	113		
Creosote storing and timber proofing	27		

cal carcinogens are the major cause numerically of these lesions. Collateral evidence of this comes from Winternitz (1947), who, in describing the histology of 124 chemically induced skin cancers of industrial origin, stated that 79 were well differentiated S.C.C.'s, 42 were S.C.C.'s (early stages), and only 3 were basosquamous cancers.

However, considering the relative smallness of their numerical representation, skin cancers produced by chemical carcinogens have played an inordinately important part in stimulating research into cancer. Pott's observation showed for the first time that there was a real cause of at least one type of new growth. This took cancer out of the realm of philosophic speculation and provided a major impetus to a search for other causes, which has been going on ever since (Potter, 1963).

ARSENIC AS A CAUSE OF SKIN CANCER

Skin cancers induced by arsenic are brought about by (1) industrial exposure to arsenic, (2) arsenic used as an ingredient of medicine, and (3) drinking water containing excessive amounts of arsenic.

Skin cancer due to arsenic may be preceded by arsenical hyperpigmentation, arsenical dermatitis, and hyperkeratosis. These keratoses are often observed on the palms and soles. However, this does not always occur. The skin cancers have a predilection for the unexposed parts of the body and for the fingers and toes. Inorganic arsenic is probably the simplest chemical agent known to produce multiple cancers in man.

Cancers arising from industrial exposure are rare but do occur in those who mine and treat the ore, in those who make pesticides and herbicides, and in those who use such substances. The use of arsenic in rural industries has markedly decreased with the introduction of a variety of new pesticides and herbicides since World War II (Hueper, 1963). In this area (Queensland), a great deal of arsenic formerly was used in banana plantations, in cattle dips, and to kill unwanted vegetation. Acute skin lesions and pigmentation were frequently seen, but cancer was a rarity.

Arsenical cancers due to the use of Fowler's solution, usually over long periods of time, to treat psoriasis, in particular, and a number of other skin conditions as well, used to be relatively common. Currie (1947) stated that over 50 percent of known skin cancers due to arsenic had occurred in people treated for psoriasis. In this situation it is the medical profession which determines the extent of the incidence.

A marked incidence of skin cancer (and other effects) has occurred in populations drinking water contaminated with arsenic in Silesia, in Argentina, and more recently in Taiwan. The incidence in the latter country has been well documented and occurs in a population of 160,000 people who drink artesian water containing arsenic. Certain systemic lesions occur, and about 10 percent of the population over 60 years of age develops skin cancer from this cause. It used to be said that arsenic produced only S.C.C.'s, but it is now known that B.C.C.'s occur as well (Yeh, 1963; Yeh et al., 1968). Arsenic, of course, also produces cancers in organs other than the skin.

ULTRAVIOLET LIGHT AS A CAUSE OF SKIN CANCER

History. The concept that sunlight is a cause of skin cancer is not new. Unna (1894), Hyde (1906), Cleland in the same year, Dubreuilh (1907), Lawrence (1912 and 1929), Paul (1918), and Molesworth (1927) had all put forward the hypothesis that exposure to sunlight played a major part in the etiology of skin cancer. It would be strange if anyone disputed this now.

As we have already noted, in 1928 an S.C.C. was produced on the skin of an experimental animal by using UV radiation. However, up to the present time, no one has produced a B.C.C. by using an UV source, in spite of the fact that this has been done with x-rays and with chemical carcinogens.

Evidence. The evidence which supports the theory that ultraviolet radiation in sunlight is a cause of skin cancer can be summarized under five main headings (Miedler, 1961):

1. Experimentally it has been shown that UV light of specific wavelengths (wave-

lengths shorter than 3200 Angstrom units) will produce a variety of tumors in animal skin.

2. Incidence and prevalence correlate with geographic latitude.

3. The amount of skin pigmentation affects incidence and prevalence.

4. Over 90 percent of skin cancers are on exposed parts of the body.

5. Skin cancers are seen more commonly in people in outdoor occupations: fishermen, sailors, ranchers, farmers.

The evidence in four out of five of these categories is based on epidemiologic observations and therefore concerns this chapter. Let us look at these four areas of evidence one by one.

DISTRIBUTION OF SKIN CANCER BY GEOGRAPHIC LATITUDE. The data which support this have already been supplied in our discussions on prevalence and incidence and need not be considered further now.

EFFECT OF SKIN PIGMENTATION. Some data concerning this have already been presented. Nevertheless a little more detailed treatment is warranted.

South Africa provides a very useful workshop to study the effect of skin pigmentation on the incidence of skin cancer. In South Africa, there is a sizeable "white" population, as well as the Bantu, who have markedly pigmented skins and live not only in urban surroundings but also under relatively primitive tribal conditions. Just for good measure, albinism is not uncommon among these people; the incidence is about 1 in 3759. Thus we can observe what happens in three different groups of Bantu as well as among "whites." Furthermore, in South Africa medical services are of a high standard, and hence there are facilities for making correct diagnoses and for the keeping of the necessary records.

Oettlé (1963) of Johannesburg summarized this South African experience. In "whites" of European extraction, the expected happens. Basal cell carcinomas are the most common tumors, followed by squamous cell carcinomas and melanomas. The effect of sunlight is obvious. Exposed areas are chiefly affected, and people who sunburn easily are the most common victims.

What happens among the Bantu?

1. The overall incidence of skin cancer is low, in fact slightly lower than among Negroes in the United States. (The Johannesburg Bantu are said to be more darkly pigmented.)

2. S.C.C.'s are the most common skin neoplasms.

3. Melanomas follow these in order of numerical importance.

4. B.C.C.'s are rare. The few that do occur are probably associated with exposure to sunlight.

5. A very high proportion of S.C.C.'s (about 60 percent) are on the lower limbs. These are often obviously associated with preexisting and predisposing chronic conditions: the effects of trauma, burn scars, and chronic ulcers (tropical, traumatic, and syphilitic). In heavily pigmented ethnic groups, one suspects that the proportion of solar-induced S.C.C.'s must be extremely small.

6. Melanomas are frequently found on the lower limbs, particularly on the soles of the feet. (Women are in the majority.) These are thought to be related to trauma in those who never use footwear. (However, the true position may not be so simple, since younger women in all countries tend to develop melanomas on the leg between knee and ankle.)

7. In general, the rural Bantu exhibit a greater number of these precursors of skin cancer than do their urban counterparts. (More of the city dwellers wear footwear.) Not surprisingly, therefore, the incidence of skin cancer would seem to be higher in rural Bantu than among those in cities. Such skin cancers are seen especially on the lower limbs.

8. Among "albino Bantu," S.C.C.'s occur very readily on exposed sites. These people probably have an increased susceptibility to melanoma as well. It is suggested that the incidence of skin cancer is a thousand times higher among albino Bantu than among their pigmented counterparts (Higginson and Oettlé, 1960). One would expect that these albinos would develop B.C.C.'s very readily, but for some unknown reason this does not happen. For every one B.C.C., there are perhaps 14 S.C.C.'s (Oettlé, 1964).

9. Xeroderma pigmentosum predisposes to skin cancer just as readily in the pigmented Bantu as it does among

"whites." On the other hand, skin cancer might be expected to develop frequently in patches of vitiligo, which are common, but this does not occur. The reason for this is unknown.

Thus Africans show the importance of "mechanical" conditions which cause chronic damage to the skin, namely, the effects of injury, burns, and chronic ulcers. On the other hand, "whites" demonstrate the importance of chronic injury to the skin due to UV radiation: so-called "senile elastosis." (The term "senile" is here used inappropriately.) S.C.C.'s may develop at the site of tropical ulcers in two to four years, which is surely an extremely short latent period, and tropical ulcers are particularly prone to develop such malignancies. However, in Nigeria, though a large proportion of S.C.C.'s are found on the lower limbs, only a small percentage (7 percent) are associated with ulcers, and here perhaps the chronic aftereffects of trauma are more important as causal factors. [In "western" clinical experience, S.C.C.'s are known to develop at the site of a chronic cutaneous sinus or fistula but rarely on a varicose ulcer (Humphrey et al., 1969).]

South African experience can be taken as a fair guide to the effect of dark skin pigmentation on the occurrence of skin cancer; the added complication of the influence of a social habit, namely, of not protecting the lower limbs and feet, must be taken into account. While on the subject of environmental factors, it might be noted that middle-aged and old Africans have a much lower incidence rate of all types of cancer when compared with their aged counterparts in "western" communities. This augments the theory that many of our cancers (perhaps 80 percent) have an environmental factor(s) in their cause (Davies et al., 1962).

We can sum up by saying that the overall pattern with respect to skin cancer among darkly pigmented peoples is one of low incidence, complete reversal of the usual B.C.C.:S.C.C. ratio, and no particular predilection for exposed areas (Oluwasanmi et al., 1969). In peoples with dark skin pigmentation, male preponderance in the incidence of skin cancer would seem to disappear to a great extent (Oettlé, 1963; Macdonald, 1959).

In the United States (all areas combined) it has been estimated that white males have seven or eight times the incidence of skin cancer compared with Negro males (Dorn, 1944). Southern areas, of course, would show an even greater difference. In Negroes skin cancers are only a small percentage of all malignancies found, whereas in American "whites," depending on the latitude, the corresponding percentage ranges from 99 percent to 50 percent (Cutaneous cancer, 1948; White et al., 1961). [For Australia as a whole, skin cancers constitute at least 50 percent of all cancers diagnosed. In areas nearer the equator, the proportion is even higher. At the Queensland Radium Institute, Cooper (1955) claimed that 70 percent of all patients presenting had skin cancer.]

The ethnic groups of Asia have a low incidence of skin cancer but would seem to be slightly more prone to develop it than are indigenous Africans. They exhibit more S.C.C.'s than B.C.C.'s, and exposed areas are not the most important sites numerically. [A number of contributions in Conference on Biology of Cutaneous Cancer (Urbach, 1963) deal with this subject.] Ethnic differences in Hawaii, a convenient "melting pot," have been studied by Quisenberry (1963). He gives the following incidence rates for skin cancer per 100,000 of population by ethnic origin: Caucasian, 138; Korean, 17.8; Chinese, 4.8; Japanese, 3.5; and Hawaiian and part-Hawaiian, 1.6.

At the other end of the spectrum of pigmentation, Macdonald (1959) and Urbach et al. (1971) have confirmed the clinical impression that those of Celtic extraction are particularly prone to suffer from skin cancer. They develop skin cancer very readily. The relatively high incidence of skin cancer among a population of Celts in County Galway, Southern Ireland, is perhaps the strongest evidence to support the importance of this genetic susceptibility (O'Halloran, 1967; O'Beirn et al., 1970). Galway is at 53° N. latitude, yet the prevalence of skin cancer among males aged 75 was approximately 10.5 percent, as compared with 26 percent in Southern Queensland (27° S.) and 3.5 percent in El Paso, Texas (32° N.). In Galway and Queensland the data suggested that the population was susceptible, whereas in El

Paso the population contains many of Latin stock (O'Beirn et al., 1970).

Silverstone and Searle (1970) have shown that in Queensland for any given latitude the most influential determinant is this genetic constitution. This outweighs other relevant factors, such as type of occupation, clothes worn, and sports played.

SKIN CANCER AND ANATOMIC AREAS EXPOSED TO SUNLIGHT. It was Dubreuilh (1907) who noted that among vineyard workers the women developed skin cancer on their faces, which received little protection from their scarf headgear, whereas the men developed lesions on the backs of their necks as they bent over tending the vines.

In the ensuing years a wealth of sound data has been recorded which has shown that, in those with poorly pigmented skin, namely, in those who are prone to skin cancer, most S.C.C.'s occur on the head and neck and exposed extremities, and that practically all B.C.C.'s (80 to 95 percent) occur on the head and neck (Bray, 1939; Macdonald, 1959; Howell, 1960; Carmichael and Silverstone, 1961; Lynch et al., 1970).

However, the subject has some complexities. Urbach (1966) has demonstrated that S.C.C.'s developing on the head and neck occur in areas which receive maximum UV radiation. Yet a third of the B.C.C.'s of the head and neck occur in areas which do not receive maximum UV radiation; in fact, they occur in areas receiving only 20 percent of maximum UV radiation. Brodkin et al. (1969) have reviewed the distribution of B.C.C.'s on the face and have carefully documented these inconsistencies. Their final conclusion was that sunlight still remains a most important cause of B.C.C.'s, even though other ill-understood determinants may also operate.

As a general finding it can be said that, among lightly pigmented people, the closer to the Equator and the more rural the area, the greater the male risk, compared with the female one, of developing skin cancer. However, there is less difference in risk between the sexes for skin cancers occurring on the trunk and lower extremities (Haenszel, 1963). This, of course, is consistent with our concepts about etiology.

OCCUPATION AND THE INCIDENCE OF SKIN CANCER. Unna's original observation (1894) that sunlight was a determinant of skin cancer was prompted by observing what happened to the skin of sailors. Professional fishermen are another exposed group of men who traditionally have excited the same speculation. Subsequently in all countries the added risk run by farmers and other rural workers has been almost universally noted (Phillips, 1941; Macdonald, 1959; Howell, 1960).

However, it is of interest to note that Haenszel (1963) in investigating incidence in urban and rural dwellers in New York State found a higher incidence of B.C.C.'s in the urban dwellers. This is, of course, a very indirect form of measurement. Nevertheless his careful analysis tended to cast doubt on our cherished traditional ideas on this subject. Silverstone and Searle (1970) found in inland tropical Queensland, which is sparsely populated, where there are no waterways for recreational purposes, and where isolation decreases sporting opportunities, that there was a higher prevalence of skin cancer in those engaged in outdoor jobs. But on the tropical and subtropical coastal areas, though there were still these differences engendered by occupation, they now failed to achieve statistical significance. Thus in the populated coastal areas occupation had ceased to be a determinant of any great strength. However, in this kind of epidemiology, though reasonably reliable occupational histories can be recorded, it is difficult to put any quantitative value on sporting activities.

As our urban populations have gained more leisure, dressed more scantily, and on the whole enjoyed higher standards of living in areas where the sea, lakes, and rivers are available, their exposure to sunlight has increased. Conversely rural occupations have become more mechanized, and this may have reduced exposure to the sun. At all events this is a subject to be approached with an open mind.

The age at which exposure to the sun occurs may also be of importance. Does exposure in childhood have a more marked influence? We should remember that, as a result of a survey among personnel in the armed forces, Sigismond Peller (1948) showed that, though exposure to sunlight while in the services could be assumed to be the same on the average for all personnel, men born in the southern United States developed a much greater proportion of skin cancer. "According to these figures, exposure to dermotropic agents in childhood is more effective in changing the distribution of cancer in a population than is exposure in later life."

This is yet another area which requires further investigation. The large scale migration to Australia after World War II might provide groups suitable for epidemiologic study in this regard. These people spent their childhood and youth in temperate climates.

In passing, it might be noted that Peller's other suggestion that skin cancer gave protection against the development of other forms of cancer has not stood up to investigation.

To date we have considered separately the principal causal associations of importance with respect to sunlight and skin cancer. Unfortunately, when this is translated into life situations, it is obvious that the various causes operate in conjunction. To try to estimate the strength of these combined effects is not easy.

Only a few studies have attempted to estimate the absolute or relative risk of skin cancer associated with factors such as those listed above. A study by Urbach et al. (1971) took the form of a controlled clinical survey in which the personal characteristics of 456 patients presenting with basal or squamous cell carcinomas were compared with those of a control group of 281 other dermatology patients with no known history of skin cancer. The two groups were similar in age and sex structure.

Table 16–4 shows the relative frequency with which a number of (presumably) high-risk factors occurred in the skin cancer group as compared with the control group. (For example, people of Irish descent were five times as common in the cancer group as in the control group.) It was also found that patients with basal and squamous cell carcinomas had significantly greater sunlight hour exposure than controls. (In the table the results for B.C.C.'s and S.C.C.'s have been combined.)

A different approach to the problem is

TABLE 16–4 RELATIVE FREQUENCY OF VARIOUS PERSONAL CHARACTERISTICS WITHIN A SKIN CANCER GROUP AS COMPARED WITH A CONTROL GROUP (DATA FROM SKIN AND CANCER HOSPITAL, PHILADELPHIA)

Characteristic	Relative Frequency in Cancer Group as Compared With Control Group
Blue or green eyes	1.52
Fair complexion	1.38
Fair hair	1.79
Inability to tan	1.67
Easily sunburned	1.71
Suffered severe sunburn	
(a) at least once	1.26
(b) more than once	3.06
Irish origin	5.00

presented in a Queensland study by Silverstone and Searle (1970). Field studies were used to obtain lifetime histories of skin cancer in various regions of the state, and the data are presented in the form of the risks associated with various factors or combinations of factors (the risk being that of having a history of skin cancer). Absolute risks are presented in the original paper. In Table 16–5 some results are given in terms of relative risks for high versus low levels of the individual factors and for some combinations of multiple factors. For example, among males over 60 there are 6.47 times as many persons with positive histories as among males under 40; positive histories are 2.45 times as common among males who sunburn easily as among males who tan readily, and so on.

It should be fairly obvious that such methods, as used by epidemiologists, are not precise tools for predicting what will happen in individual cases.

MISCELLANEOUS CAUSES OF
SKIN CANCER

Radioactivity. In 1895 Röentgen discovered x-rays. Within three months the first untoward side effect had been reported—conjunctivitis. By the time Frieben had recorded the first case of skin cancer radiologically induced, in 1902, a variety of other distressing results had been noted. In 1911 Hesse was able to document no less than 94 cancers, over half of which were in doctors or technicians

TABLE 16–5   RELATIVE FREQUENCY OF HISTORIES OF SKIN CANCER IN PERSONS
DISTINGUISHED ACCORDING TO VARIOUS PERSONAL CHARACTERISTICS
(DATA FROM QUEENSLAND FIELD SURVEYS)

Groups Compared			Relative Risk in First-named Group	
			Males	*Females*
Age over 60	vs.	age under 40	6.47	3.87
(ancestral lines both Scotch or Irish)	vs.	(lines both British or North European but not Scotch or Irish)	1.37	1.68
Fair complexion	vs.	dark complexion	1.69	1.67
Light eyes	vs.	dark eyes	1.44	1.37
Sunburns	vs.	tans	2.45	3.98
Outdoor occupation	vs.	indoor occupation	1.25	0.60
Tropical residence	vs.	subtropical residence	2.18	2.44
History of keratoses	vs.	no history of keratoses	4.14	5.34
Male	vs.	female	1.73	—
(Over 60, sunburns, works outdoors)	vs.	(over 60, tans, works indoors)	2.55	—
(Over 60, sunburns, works outdoors)	vs.	(under 40, tans, works indoors)	10.55	—

(Hunter, 1969). The lamentable story of the next couple of decades is well known.

Perhaps not realized are the regrettable results which occurred at a somewhat later period in this century as a result of a therapeutic fashion to treat a number of benign skin conditions with ionizing radiations.* A report by Martin et al. (1970) documents this. In their series 368 patients developed skin cancer following ionizing radiations for lesions such as acne and hirsutism. There was a tendency to develop multiple lesions. There were approximately four S.C.C.'s for each B.C.C. S.C.C.'s produced as the result of ionizing radiation have a much greater tendency to metastasize. The case-fatality rate in this type of cancer is usually 10 to 12 percent.

Most of the patients were irradiated prior to 1930, and medical specialists had produced twice as many of these cancers as had nonmedical therapists of various kinds. The authors noted that a survey of dermatology practice, as late as 1964, had revealed that ionizing radiations were still being used to treat some 26 percent of patients who suffered from acne.

In the survey carried out by Martin et al. (1970), a control group showed that the median age for development of radiation-induced skin cancer was 47 years, compared with 57 years for those with skin cancer who had not received radiation. There was, however, great variation in latent periods. The median interval for this was 21 years, but it ranged up to 64 years.

Radiodermatitis is not a condition to be treated lightly. In one investigation skin cancer developed in 24 percent of people with radiodermatitis (Pack and Davis, 1965). However, the modern problem has to be kept in perspective. In a Texas series of 4704 squamous cell cancers, only 2 had arisen in a radiation scar (Macdonald, 1967).

Scars and Burns.   The increased propensity to develop skin cancer at sites of ulcers, scars, and burn scars has already been mentioned. As we have seen, it is particularly important as a determinant of skin cancer in developing countries. However, against the general background of skin cancer among ethnic groups susceptible to UV radiation, this "cause" is not numerically important. Scars resulting from thermal burns deserve special notice. Lawrence (1952) reviewed 93 patient-reports which at that time he had been able to find in the literature. He was of the opinion that on general principles skin grafting, where indicated, was a preventative.

In the M.D. Anderson Hospital series reported by Macdonald (1967), three pa-

---

*One of us received quite lengthy courses of radiotherapy during the 1920's for the treatment of acne and later while in the service in World War II.

tients developed cancers on the scars of smallpox vaccinations; one was a B.C.C., one a S.C.C., and one a melanoma in a woman. However, other authors also have noted this happening (Goncalves, 1966; Marmelzat, 1968; Reed and Wilson-Jones, 1968).

Heat-induced Kangri cancer among the Kashmiris, and Dhoti cancer among Deccani Maharashtrians due to pressure of the loin cloth which they wear tightly are other examples of chronic skin damage leading to cancers (Mulay, 1963). The "Kang" cancer occurs in skin over the trochanter among Chinese who sleep on heated brick beds (Laycock, 1948), and erythema ab igne on the shins of people constantly heating themselves before fires may be a precursor of skin cancer (Peterkin, 1955). Cancer of the genitalia is not uncommon in parts of Asia, particularly among lower socioeconomic groups. It often follows phimosis, venereal disease, and poor personal hygiene (Miyaji, 1963; Tam et al., 1963; Tansurat, 1963.) Thus the less common causes of skin cancer exhibit great variety. The foregoing constitutes a résumé of the more important epidemiologic observations made with respect to the causes of skin cancer. There still remain a few other subjects of a varied nature on which the epidemiologic method has thrown some light.

Other Topics

ACCURACY OF DIAGNOSIS

It is a paradox not altogether unexpected that, in areas where the incidence of skin cancer is highest, a much smaller proportion of skin cancers may be submitted for histologic diagnosis (Dorn, 1944). It is certainly true of Australia. Moreover, some clinicians are convinced that the differentiation between S.C.C.'s and B.C.C.'s can be made without recourse to histology, provided that the observer is experienced (Payne, 1930). This may be so in the case of certain exceptional individuals, but the little epidemiologic evidence available does not support this contention as a general rule.

Lightstone et al. (1965) pointed out that,

in the clinical diagnosis of B.C.C.'s, almost one in four was subsequently shown to be in error. Ten Seldam (1963) supports these findings. In this department Silverstone and Smithurst (1971) have recently produced similar results in a small pilot survey. (Of 41 S.C.C.'s which were diagnosed by histology, 17 had previously been diagnosed as B.C.C.'s on clinical appearance.) Another matter of importance is to distinguish between solar hyperkeratoses and cancer. We can find no evidence on this point. However, in areas of high incidence, the academic researcher has to take some cognizance of the clinician's reluctance to carry out unnecessary biopsies, especially on the facial region. The number of patients with solar keratoses is huge. In this part of the world, for instance, almost the whole population of northern European extraction would at some time or another require a biopsy. For many aging adults it would be a frequent experience. When results of treatment are already so satisfactory one hesitates to be dogmatic, considering the inconvenience to the patients and the burden it places on medical resources. A feasible compromise might be to aim for 100 percent biopsies in the case of ad hoc surveys undertaken for specific purposes.

METASTASES

There is general agreement that squamous cell carcinomas arising in skin damaged by sunlight do not metastasize readily. Lund (1965) in North Carolina reported on 3700 S.C.C.'s confirmed histologically and collected during 12 years of *office* practice. He considered that 780 of these were what he termed "aggressive" in type. The rate of metastases for all S.C.C.'s was 0.1 percent, and for those considered "aggressive" it was 0.5 percent. However, this would seem to be low in the light of other reports. Macdonald (1967), studying approximately 4700 patients with S.C.C.'s, stated that "less than 10 percent metastasize." In New York State a study of 393 patients with 577 S.C.C.'s showed that over a five-year period 2.6 percent metastasized (Katz et al., 1957).

On the other hand, there would also be general agreement that S.C.C.'s with antecedents other than actinic ones, for example, cancers produced by chemical carcinogens or arising on scars and the like, have a higher rate of metastases.

It is accepted now that basal cell carcinomas do occasionally metastasize. Beerman (1969) found a record of about 50 cases in the literature.

Primary cancers in sites other than skin seldom metastasize to the skin. Surveys have shown ranges from 0.1 percent of all primary cancers (nonskin) to 2.7 percent in an autopsy series (Beerman, 1969; Macdonald, 1970).

MULTIPLE PRIMARY CANCERS OF THE SKIN

The chances of developing multiple skin cancers are, of course, very real. Katz et al. (New York State, 1957) estimated that, of males with a single lesion, 14 percent would develop a second lesion by the end of the fourth year, and of females, 5 percent would develop a second lesion by the end of the third year. If a patient had both an S.C.C. and a B.C.C., then the chance of developing a further lesion would be greatly increased.

In Texas the probability of developing a second primary lesion would seem to be even greater. In Macdonald's series (1967), 46.8 percent of the males who had skin cancer had multiple primary lesions, and 31.4 percent of the females. Of every 100 persons with a single primary lesion, 12 annually would develop a second primary cancer of the skin. The incidence rate of second primary cancers of the skin was at least 140 times the incidence rate of first primaries. In 1939 it was found at the Sydney Hospital Radium Clinic that, of every 100 patients who had had skin cancer and who were coming back after a period of time for a check-up, 30 required treatment for new lesions (Bray, 1939).

DEATHS

In areas of the world which have a relatively high incidence of skin cancers, that is, in areas where most of the skin cancers are solar-induced, the case-fatality rate is now so gratifyingly low that it is a rather futile exercise to draw any conclusions from the mortality rates of skin cancer. It

would be wiser to ignore their existence. In addition to this, deaths officially attributed to "skin cancer" are found to contain quite a high proportion of deaths due to a variety of skin conditions, but particularly due to secondary skin manifestations from primary tumors elsewhere.

It is estimated that in Queensland (Australia) a population of approximately 1.75 million of predominantly northern European ethnic extraction develop some 7000 to 8000 new primary skin cancers each year. In a five-year period (1960 to 1964), 99 people died from either S.C.C.'s (72) or B.C.C.'s (22) or "multiple lesions" (5). An effort was made to determine why these deaths occurred. No less than 40 either had failed to come to treatment or had not returned for treatment — and this in an area where the general population is markedly conscious of, and cautious about, skin blemishes. This neglect was associated particularly with extreme old age; 29 were 80 years or older at time of death. At the other end of the spectrum were 17 deaths in cases in which the lesion had exhibited "atypical histology." These were squamous cell tumors which were undifferentiated to an extreme degree or basal cell tumors which metastasized in the manner of an undifferentiated S.C.C. These atypical, highly malignant cancers were prominent in the ten people who died under the age of 50. In a larger series of tumors (4250) which were not lethal, there were 3.8 B.C.C.'s for every 1 S.C.C., but in neoplasms which caused death there was only 0.3 B.C.C. to every 1 S.C.C. In the larger series 5.3 percent of S.C.C.'s were in the vicinity of the ear, whereas among the S.C.C.'s which were lethal 18.1 percent were in the vicinity of the ear. Thus S.C.C.'s are certainly more dangerous than B.C.C.'s, and a lesion in the vicinity of the ear must be viewed with circumspection.

"Disturbed personality" contributed to death in the case of seven of the patients (this led to neglect of treatment), multiplicity of lesions in eight (literally "running out of skin" on the face after numerous treatments), and clinical misjudgment in seven (Gordon and Silverstone, 1969).

In California a population of some 15 million produces an estimated 6000 new cases of skin cancer each year. Between 40 and 50 deaths occur annually as a result of such malignancies. Here again failure to seek treatment associated in many cases with extreme age was the main reason for the fatal outcome. Over half the patients were 75 years or more (Dunn et al., 1965).

In Victoria (Australia) in 1958 100,000 people were estimated to have skin cancer or to have had it; this was the prevalence in a population of 2.8 million. Yet only 20 patients died that year from skin cancer (ten Seldam, 1963). All in all it would be difficult to reduce these low case-fatality rates much further, though indeed in theory many of these deaths both in California and in Australia were avoidable. By contrast the five-year survival rate of patients with S.C.C.'s of the skin in southwest England was only about 60 percent (Walker, 1968).

This is fairly typical of the discrepancies which are sometimes found when an attempt is made to compare results of treatment at an international level. No doubt a higher proportion of the English S.C.C.'s are not solar-induced, and hence the prognosis would be slightly worse. The important fact is that, in areas of higher incidences of skin cancers, case-fatality rates of less than 1 percent are the norm.

MALIGNANT MELANOMAS

History

Melanomas have been recorded back to Hippocratic times. "Black tumors" are mentioned in European medical literature in the 17th and 18th centuries. The great John Hunter left us a good description of the "black cancer"; Laennec discussed "la mélanose" in the early 19th century. In fact, black moles used to be considered beautiful. Bones of Incas 2400 years old show diffuse melanotic metastases, particularly in the skull and extremities (Urteaga and Pack, 1966; Bodenham, 1968). Indeed we travel a fairly well-worn track.

There would be general agreement that melanoma is a relatively uncommon neoplasm with an incidence which ranges from less than 1 per 100,000 among heavily pigmented ethnic groups up to 16 per 100,000 in Queensland (Doll et al., 1966;

Davis et al., 1966; Macdonald, 1967 and 1970; Bodenham, 1968; Lee and Merrill, 1970).

Incidence of Melanoma

In Table 16–6 we have correlated the incidence of melanoma with zones of latitude as we did for skin cancer (see Table 16–1).

The trend in both tables is somewhat similar; that is, among lightly pigmented ethnic groups, lower latitudes produce higher incidences. Nevertheless, the correlational pattern is more diffuse (as we have noted previously). Moreover, there appears to be no distinct dichotomy of the "female:male" ratios between heavily pigmented groups and lightly pigmented groups as was shown in skin cancer. For the lightly pigmented groups this ratio (unlike the ratio for skin cancers) exceeds unity. For the more heavily pigmented groups also, the ratio for melanoma exceeds unity; furthermore, it does not appear to differ much from its value for skin cancers where, as we have seen, it is greater than unity.

A general idea of the correlation between the incidence rates of melanoma and of skin cancers may be obtained by an inspection of the published data for 40 countries or regions from sources mentioned earlier. As we have seen, the range for skin cancer incidence in susceptible ethnic groups subdivides conveniently into four or five groups, each containing a "cluster" of regions when arranged in order of magnitude of incidence rates. For each stratum a rough (unweighted) average of age-standardized incidence rates is calculated, and the results are shown in Table 16–7 using the data for males.

It will be remembered that for lightly pigmented groups the order of magnitude of incidence rates for skin cancer correlated well with zones of latitude, so that here we are in effect indirectly attempting to correlate the incidence of melanoma with zones of latitude.

In a more detailed analysis, 42 regions were simultaneously classified into five skin cancer groups, as in Table 16–7, and

TABLE 16-6 GLOBAL DISTRIBUTION OF MELANOMA INCIDENCE; MALE DATA WITH CORRESPONDING FEMALE TO MALE RATIOS (F/M)

Average Incidence of Melanoma per 100,000 (both sexes)	Zone*				
	A	B	C	D	E
0.0–0.9		Rumania (Banat) F/M = 0.50	Japan F/M = 0.83	S.A. Cape Colored Natal Indians Bulawayo Africans California Negroes Hawaiian F/M = 1.92	Bombay Puerto Rico F/M = 1.81
1.0–1.9		United Kingdom Poland Hungary F/M = 1.51	Yugoslavia F/M = 1.47	S.A. Cape Bantu Natal Africans Texas Latins** F/M = 2.84	Jamaica Nigeria F/M = 1.24
2.0–2.9	Finland F/M = 0.83	Canada Denmark German Dem. Rep. F/M = 1.32	New Zealand Maoris New York State† F/M††	Israel (Native News) F/M = 1.55	Colombia F/M = 0.45
3.0–3.9	Norway Sweden F/M = 1.12		Nevada Connecticut Victoria (Australia) F/M = 1.28	Texas (non-Latin) California (whites) S.A. Cape (whites) F/M = 1.30	
4.0–4.9				Hawaii (Caucasian) F/M = 0.78	
5.0 and over			New Zealand§ (Europeans) F/M = 1.47	Queensland (whites)‖ F/M = 1.22	

*Zonal latitudes are: A, above 60°; B, 45°–60°; C, 35°–45°; D, 20°–35°; E, 0°–20°.
**S.A. Cape Bantus = 4.71; Natal Africans = 3.00; Texas Latins = 0.80.
†Excluding New York City.
††N.Z. Maoris = 4.38; N.Y. State = 1.13.
§Males, 6.2; females, 9.1.
‖Queensland is half in zone D and half in zone E; males, 14.3; females, 17.4.

TABLE 16–7 RELATIONSHIP BETWEEN
INCIDENCE RATES FOR MELANOMA AND
FOR SKIN CANCER (MALE DATA FROM 40
COUNTRIES OR REGIONS)

Skin Cancer Incidence/ 100,000	Number of Regions	Average Melanoma Incidence/ 100,000
0 and under 10	10	0.71
10 " " 20	7	1.21
20 " " 40	16	1.59
40 " " 80	5	2.30
80 and over	2*	3.15

*Excluding Queensland because of an unduly
high incidence of melanoma.

five melanoma groups (incidence 0 and
under 1, 1 and under 2, 2 and under 3, 3
and under 4, 4 and over respectively).
Kendall's "rank correlation coefficient" for
this classification system was estimated as t
= 0.62 (roughly equivalent to an ordinary
correlation coefficient of r = 0.8 for "normal" data). This was a highly significant
correlation (chi-square = 22.83 with 1 degree of freedom; $p < 10^{-5}$).

Therefore it would be difficult to avoid
the conclusion that the incidence of melanoma is strongly associated with latitude.

Mortality from Melanoma

Comprehensive series of age-specific
death rates on a global scale are difficult to
obtain, as in many cases no separation is
made between melanoma and skin
cancers. The following graph (Fig. 16–4) is
based on data for 1955–1957 published by
the World Health Organization (1960)
and, in the case of Queensland, official statistics from the Australian Bureau of
Census and Statistics (Solomon, 1956–
1958). The graphs comprise male data for
6 of the 11 regions available from the
above sources.

Except for the case of Japan, the graphs
are reasonably parallel up to age 60 (using
a logarithmic scale), so that the relative
mortality rates do not vary much with age
within this range. After age 60 there is,
however, a marked convergence of the
death rates. The results for Australia deserve some consideration. The graphs for
Queensland and for Australia as a whole

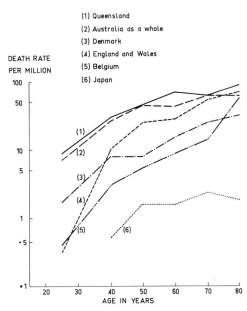

Figure 16–4 Age-specific death rates of males from
melanoma, 1955–57 averages in six different countries.

are very close. The overall death rate for
Queensland in the period concerned was
25.4 per million, as compared with 20.6
per million for the rest of Australia. In
other words, the mortality rate for
Queensland was only 25 percent in excess
of that for the rest of Australia. The excess
death rate for Queensland thus appears to
be much less than the excess incidence rate
for the state.

Although female incidence rates are
generally higher than the male rates, mortality among females is frequently somewhat lower. Some (crude) death rates per
million for males and females respectively
were: Canada, 7.2 and 5.2; United States
(whites), 13.2 and 10.9; United States
(nonwhites), 2.9 and 2.0; Japan, 0.4 and
0.3; Belgium, 5.6 and 5.8; Denmark, 14.1
and 15.6; Ireland, 4.5 and 4.9; Norway,
12.9 and 11.4; Netherlands, 6.2 and 6.4;
England and Wales, 7.4 and 9.2; Scotland,
8.4 and 7.7; Italy, 3.0 and 2.5; Australia,
21.3 and 18.9.

From the Queensland studies of Davis et
al. (1966) and from the official Statistics of
the State of Queensland (Solomon, 1964–
1968), graphs have been constructed to
show the relationship between age-specific

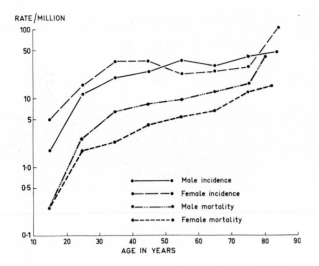

Figure 16–5 Age-specific rates per million for incidence and mortality for melanoma in Queensland (annual average for period 1963 to 1968).

incidence rates and age-specific mortality rates from melanoma for each sex during the period 1963–1968 (Fig. 16–5). This demonstrates points already mentioned, namely, the higher incidence rates and lower mortality rates among females. It also illustrates the gradual worsening of both rates with advancing age. Other aspects of this problem emerge from the work of McLeod et al. (1971), who present some results from a five-year follow-up study of 169 male and 192 female patients who formed part of the Queensland Melanoma Project. The percentage of patients dying from melanoma within five years in various age groups is shown (in condensed form) in Table 16–8.

The data in Table 16–8 show the remarkably good prognosis in females up to the age of 60 for at least five-year survival. (The case-fatality rate during this period in women between 20 and 39 years is only

5 percent.) On the other hand, the prognosis for both males and females 60 years and over is much the same. Approximately four out of every ten patients diagnosed will die from melanoma within five years. Having said this, nevertheless it should be noted that the prospects of five-year survival for the male aged 20 to 39 years, 73 percent, indicate improvement in recent years and engender hope.

In general, case-fatality rates for melanoma have markedly decreased in the last 20 years (Macdonald, 1967; End Results Group, 1968). Nevertheless, the outlook for many patients is still extremely serious. Indeed the result in any individual lesion is difficult to predict even though a prognosis based on statistical averages is often reassuring.

It must be accepted also that five-year survival rates can be very misleading in the case of melanomas. Texas experience led

TABLE 16–8 5-YEAR FATALITY RATES AMONG THE FIRST 361 PATIENTS IN THE QUEENSLAND MELANOMA SURVEY

Age	Number in Group		Percentage Dead Within 5 Years	
	Males	*Females*	*Males*	*Females*
10–19	3	8	33.3	12.5
20–39	45	59	26.7	5.1*
40–59	68	76	41.2	15.8**
60 & over	53	49	66.0	55.1†
All ages	169	192	45.0	22.4††

*Female rate is significantly less than male rate ($p < 0.01$ on chi-square test).
**Female rate is significantly less than male rate ($p < 0.001$ on chi-square test).
†No significant difference between male and female rates.
††The five-year case mortality rates for males and females differ at a high level of significance ($p < 10^{-5}$).

to the conclusion that at the end of five years all but 13 percent of those who will eventually produce metastases will have done so, and all but 5 percent within 7½ years (Macdonald, 1967). However, at the end of five years a number will still be alive who are already suffering from metastases, though they appear as "alive" in a five-year survival rate. In a few cases metastases have been known to become manifest as long as two to three decades after removal of the "primary" lesion.

Younger women have a tendency to develop melanomas between the knee and the ankle, and these have a relatively better prognosis. This may be a true biologic difference. [However, this happier prognosis does not apply to thigh lesions (Beardmore et al., 1969).] In men about two-thirds of melanomas are on head, neck, and trunk and one-third on limbs. Contrariwise, in women about two-thirds are on limbs (End Results Group, 1968). Melanomas on the trunk, particularly on the back, have the worst prognosis in either sex.

Other factors apart, a melanoma in a male has a worse prognosis than in a female. In the survey of melanoma in southwest England, females (all ages combined) had a 15 percent better prognosis (Bodenham, 1968). In the United States the End Results Group (1968) showed differences of about 6 to 8 percent in survival rates in favor of the female. However, melanomas are diagnosed on the average at an earlier stage among women than among men, and this would influence the prognosis.

In geographic regions of higher incidence, one would expect that a much higher proportion of melanomas would be on exposed surfaces, whereas in fact the *proportion* on exposed areas—approximately two-thirds—tends to remain much the same in all geographic areas (allowing for a few obvious exceptions which show no logical pattern) (Lee and Merrill, 1970).

For 50 years at least it has been realized that the clinical entity termed melanoma in its pathology and histology is not a homogeneous entity. (Further discussion of this subject might well be left to the pathologists.) Seventy to 80 percent of all melanomas would seem to be invasive of the reticular layer of the dermis (Petersen et

al., 1962; Davis et al., 1966; Lee and Merrill, 1970).

Heavy skin pigmentation obviously provides a degree of protection, but not as efficiently as for skin cancer. In Africans, the less pigmented areas tend to be affected, particularly the soles of the feet, palms of the hand and nail folds, conjunctiva, and genitalia. Intraoral, intranasal, and anal canal sites occur relatively frequently; intraocular sites on the other hand occur hardly at all, whereas in Norway a third of the melanomas are intraocular. As we have already mentioned, trauma was suggested to account for the relatively high incidence of melanomas on the lower limb, particularly in African women (Belisario, 1959; Lee and Merrill, 1970).

As we have seen, melanoma would seem to be causally associated with some factor in sunlight (McGovern, 1952; Lancaster, 1954 and 1955; Cooper, 1955; Lancaster and Nelson, 1957; Belisario, 1959; Gordon and Silverstone, 1969). The difficulty has been to explain why, in areas of low latitude and higher incidence, the proportion of tumors on exposed surfaces does not markedly increase. Lee and Merrill (1970) have recently and very persuasively postulated the presence of a "solar circulating factor." Thus sunlight would stimulate the body to produce this factor, and in turn the factor would initiate the development of a certain type of melanoma (nodular) in any part of the body irrespective of exposure. (This concept of a systemic agent was first put forward by Clark and Macdonald in 1953.) Such a factor would vary directly with sunlight and inversely with skin pigmentation.

Most would consider that, on the average in any single geographic locality, the people who develop melanoma have lighter complexions and spend more time out of doors than do members of a suitable control group (Lancaster, 1956; McGovern, 1957; Belisario, 1959; Gellin et al., 1969). In Sweden and Norway, for instance, the incidence is higher than their latitudes would suggest, and this might be explained by degree of skin pigmentation.

Trauma is said to be causally associated with the incidence of melanoma (Oettlé, 1964; Macdonald, 1967). Many, however, would doubt this. On the other hand, there is stronger support for the theory that existing melanomas are aggravated by trauma rather than caused by it (Lea, 1965; Bodenham, 1968).

The following factors worsen the prognosis in any melanoma (apart from being male and being aged and being on the trunk): lesions larger than 2 cm. at time of diagnosis; nodular tumors, particularly pedunculated tumors; ulcerated tumors and bleeding tumors; metastases at time of presentation. [Beardmore et al. (1969) discuss these various adverse factors and furnish an extensive and relevant bibliography.]

In some patients genetic influences are important (Cawley, 1952; Macdonald, 1967); that is, there are familial tendencies.

Moreover, pregnancy has been suggested as predisposing towards the development of melanomas, particularly in the lower limb. All in all the evidence is probably against this (Lee, 1969).

Discussion

Comparisons of survival rates in the international sphere have to be undertaken with caution, since not all series include the same pathologic entities—tumors arising on Hutchinson's melanotic freckles, for example. In this chapter, Hutchinson's freckle, lentigo maligna, and "mélanose circonscrite précancéreuse of Dubreuilh" mean the same thing. It is a precursor of a specific type of melanoma. There is controversy as to whether or not all such lesions inevitably become malignant and as to whether or not the prognosis in the resulting malignancies is relatively benign.

Lee and Merrill (1970) in a review article considered that end results (prognoses) were much the same in the high incidence areas (Queensland and New Zealand) as in England and the United States. Under the best conditions of treatment now prevailing, one would expect 75 to 80 percent of people with localized lesions at time of diagnosis to survive for five years, and 60 to 70 percent to be alive at the end of ten years. For those with regional lymph node involvement, the survival rates would be about half the above. These estimates are,

however, approximate and based on varying findings in different countries (Watson, 1963; Bodenham, 1968; McLeod et al., 1968; End Results Group, 1968).

The End Results Group data (1968) are an indication of what is happening:

% of Patients Surviving	Localized Tumor		Regional Involvement	
	M	F	M	F
Five years	75	79	44	42
Ten years	61	73	23	36

Obviously diagnosis while the tumor is still localized makes a major difference to prognosis.

Deaths from other causes have to be considered as well. In a prospective survey carried out by the Queensland Melanoma Project, of the 219 deaths which occurred within five years of histologic diagnosis, only 73 percent were due to melanomas (Beardmore et al., 1969). This is because melanoma incidence tends to rise with age, and in the aged the risk of dying from the common causes of death markedly increases.

Death rates from melanomas have been rising slightly but steadily each year during the last decade or so in countries such as the United States, England, Wales, Australia, and so forth. This is true in all age groups. Is this a real increase? Or is it due to some artifact, such as the doctors' only recently writing "malignant melanoma" rather than "skin cancer" on death certificates. Gordon and Silverstone (1969) suggested that this was the case. Lee and Carter (1970) doubted it. This is obviously an important problem which should receive further attention.

The Queensland Melanoma Project is posing another question. This survey began in 1963. The prospective portion of the study is showing an incidence of 16.3 per 100,000 of general population. This is so greatly in excess of anything that has been found elsewhere that one has to speculate about its cause. Even allowing for the fact that 30 percent of this incidence relates to types of melanoma not regarded as such in other places, namely those which do not invade the reticular layer of the dermis, the Queensland incidence is still three times as high as the incidence recorded in the non-Latin population of Texas and twice as high as the incidence in New Zealand, which produces the next highest incidence rate in the world. The Queensland incidence represents such a marked increase over anything as yet recorded that it is obviously a matter for concern when coupled with an increasing tendency to wear less and less clothing in a warm climate.

As well as increased incidence, other areas with respect to melanoma are worthy of epidemiologic investigation: schedules of treatment; the effect, if any, of changing modes in dress; and the effect of skin pigmentation and sex on a number of other variables, such as type of lesion, site, and outcome. Most of these are already the subject of inquiry by the local Melanoma Project.

Data gathered by the Queensland Melanoma Project show, as elsewhere, that case-fatality rates (prognosis) worsen with age. However, melanomas arising on Hutchinson's freckles contribute substantially to the incidence of melanoma in late middle age and in old age, whereas in younger age groups they are rare. To date, it has been the convention to regard such cases of melanoma as having a better prognosis. However, in view of this increased risk of a fatal outcome in older people at a time when such melanomas are more common, surely we should now look at this traditional concept with some degree of suspicion (Davis, 1971).

THE FUTURE FOR THE EPIDEMIOLOGIST

We have just outlined problems in the field of melanoma which might be studied by epidemiologic methods. There is little doubt that, in a disease such as this, in which the case-fatality rate is still high, as much research as possible should be undertaken. Few would argue about this.

But what of skin cancer? Here the situation is quite different. The case-fatality rate is now so low that many clinicians, who, after all, are the ones who have to record and supply much of the necessary data, might consider that further epidemiologic research, which would consume much in the way of staff time, facilities, and money, is hardly justified.

This is, of course, one of those questions about which honest men of good will might quite justifiably differ. Perhaps we might sum it up this way. If we are interested in the therapeutic problem of skin cancer only, then further complex investigations are probably not warranted. If, however, we look at skin cancer as a suitable and unique research tool which might eventually help us to elucidate the general problem of human carcinogenesis, then obviously we should press on.

Where does the epidemiologist fit into this?

Contemplation of skin cancer is bound to fill any professional epidemiologist with certain misgivings. On the one hand the criteria for diagnosing the various entities—S.C.C., B.C.C., and so forth—are reasonably definite. On the other hand it is difficult in practice to persuade some clinicians to undertake histologic examinations which will enable them to make these precise diagnoses. (We have already suggested a compromise which might help here.)

A second difficulty is the variety of medical practitioners who treat skin cancers, often without recourse to a pathologist and often, consequently, leaving little trace in medical records. A globe-trotting epidemiologist quickly comes to realize this, since his contacts are spread over a number of clinical groups. General practitioners, surgeons, dermatologists, plastic surgeons, and radiotherapists are all involved in various parts of the world. A colleague informs us, for instance, that in one area in Europe where he practiced, the general practitioners tended to send patients with lesions thought to be B.C.C.'s to dermatologists, those with S.C.C.'s to radiotherapists, and those with melanomas to surgeons. These considerations make it difficult to find reliable incidence or prevalence rates.

The third difficulty is fairly obvious. The stand-by of the medical demographer, when all other sources fail, is the death rate. In diseases such as skin cancer which kill only infrequently, mortality rates not only fail to be informative but also may be definitely misleading. On the other hand, in the case of malignant melanomas, study of death rates is very useful. Thus these factors all present difficulties.

Future Methods

To meet these difficulties we have to look at our methods more critically.

Clinical Records. To facilitate epidemiologic investigations, either present or future, clinical records relating to skin cancer should include the following: age, sex, ethnic particulars, summary of places of residence, summary of occupational history, clothing habits, recreational activities, clinical history, site of lesion (marked on a standard diagram), length of time since first noticed, changes observed in nature of lesion, histologic type (if possible), macroscopic appearance, treatment, and recurrences.

Control Groups. In a number of clinical departments, control groups might be used to further investigations of certain aspects of skin cancer. This has been done effectively in New York (Gellin et al., 1966 and 1969) and Philadelphia (Urbach et al., 1971).

Field Work. In a number of cases it may become necessary to go outside the clinical situations to measure long-term UV radiation, to gather demographic information about the proportion of various ethnic and occupational groups in a population, and to assess clothing and recreational habits and changes therein.

The problem facing Macdonald (1970) with respect to the incidence of skin cancer in two areas of Texas — El Paso County and Harlingen region — is an example of why these latter investigations may become necessary. Harlingen (26°) is 6 degrees of latitude nearer the equator than El Paso (32°), and it has a slightly larger proportion of its population in rural sites; nevertheless, the age-adjusted incidence of skin cancer in the non-Latin population is slightly higher in El Paso. This is certainly contrary to what we might expect. However, there are climatic differences. For instance, El Paso has longer average annual hours of sunshine than has Harlingen; it is a drier climate, and there is reason to believe that a higher proportion of its non-Latin population is of Celtic origin. Obviously here is a situation in which information of a nonclinical nature has to be gathered.

Moreover, in areas of higher incidence, it may sometimes be rewarding to undertake surveys of samples of the general population in order to assess prevalence and to collect other data.

Problems Which Might Be Studied

Though the overall aim of epidemiologic studies of skin cancer would be to throw light on the general problem of human carcinogenesis, in practice we obviously have to be more specific.

Basal Cell Carcinomas. This type of skin cancer poses some intriguing questions. Here we have a tumor which, in ethnic groups with light skin pigmentation, is always more numerous than the S.C.C., whereas in deeply pigmented ethnic groups the reverse applies. Yet the incidence in albinos is low. Furthermore, only a small proportion of B.C.C.'s are found on sites other than the head and neck, but on the face, at least 30 percent of B.C.C.'s occur in areas receiving relatively low solar radiation. It is believed by some that the greater the exposure to UV radiation, the higher the proportion of B.C.C.'s as compared with S.C.C.'s. On the other hand, some experts would not agree with this. Further, it has been noted that B.C.C.'s which have been solar-induced are different morphologically from those produced by other carcinogens (Brodkin et al., 1969). Are there only a limited number of cells which will produce B.C.C.'s? We do not know.

Compared with this, S.C.C.'s would seem to behave relatively simply. Their incidence bears some kind of direct relationship to the degree of carcinogenic stimulation, and they appear on the areas most exposed to such chronic stimulation.

Hyperkeratoses (solar). The relationship between solar keratoses and the subsequent development of skin cancer is by no means clear, though from time to time dogmatic statements about this are made.

Basic Considerations. Does the effect of UV radiation in the development of skin cancer depend on simple cumulative factors of dosage, or do the deleterious effects occur at a much faster rate after a certain threshold of UV dosage has been exceeded (Blum, 1959 and 1969)? Does the length of rest period between doses of UV have any effect on outcome? Are youthful skin cells more susceptible to solar damage than older ones, or vice versa? What is the effect of "fractioning" UV dosages by a climate which interposes a sunless winter between summers characterized by almost continual sunshine?

These are all questions which may prove to be important to our basic inquiry about carcinogenesis. The epidemiologist should play his part here in helping to find answers to these questions, if for no other reason than that we do not quite know how relevant the results of animal experiments are to human beings. In other words, observation of what actually happens in human beings becomes necessary, and epidemiologists can provide planned observation. Finally, in the cancer field, skin cancer is really the only human cancer which can be readily observed and which poses little threat to the patient's life. It therefore provides rather unique opportunities for observational research.

REFERENCES

Atkinson, L., Farago, C., Forbes, B. R. V., and Ten Seldam, R. E. J.: Skin Cancer in New Guinea Native Peoples. U.S. National Cancer Institute Monograph No. 10, 1963, pp. 167–179.

Auerbach, H.: Geographic variation in incidence of skin cancer in the United States. Public Health Rep., 76:345, 1961.

Beardmore, G. L., Davis, N. C., McLeod, R., Little, J. H., Quinn, R. L., and Burry, A. F.: Malignant melanoma in Queensland: a study of 219 deaths. Australas. J. Dermatol., 10:158, 1969.

Beerman, H.: Some aspects of cutaneous malignancy. Ruben Nomland Memorial Lecture. Arch. Dermatol., 99:617, 1969.

Belisario, J. C.: Cancer of the Skin. London, Butterworth & Company, Ltd., 1959.

Bell, B.: A Treatise on the Hydrocele on Sarcocele, or Cancer and Other Diseases of the Testes. Edinburgh, 1794.

Bell, J.: Paraffin epithelioma of the scrotum. Edinb. Med. J., 22:135, 1876.

Blum, H. F.: Carcinogenesis by Ultraviolet Light. Princeton, Princeton University Press, 1959.

Blum, H. F.: On hazards of cancer from ultraviolet light. Am. Ind. Hyg. Assoc. J., 27:299, 1966.

Blum, H. F.: Quantitative aspects of cancer induction by ultraviolet light: including a revised model. *In* Urbach, F. (Ed.): The Biologic Effects of Ultraviolet Radiation. Oxford, Pergamon Press, 1969, p. 543.

Bodenham, D. C.: A study of 650 observed malignant melanomas in the South-West region. Ann. R. Coll. Surg. Engl., 43:218, 1968.

Bray, S.: Work of Sydney Hospital Radium Clinic from 1911 to 1938 and analysis of cutaneous neoplasms treated. Br. J. Radiol., 12:303, 1939.

Brodkin, R. H., Kopf, A. W., and Andrade, R.: Basal-cell epithelioma and elastosis: a comparison of distribution. *In* Urbach, F. (Ed.): The Biologic Effects of Ultraviolet Radiation. London, Pergamon Press, 1969, p. 581.

Butlin, H. J.: Three lectures on cancer of the scrotum in chimney sweeps and others. Br. Med. J., 1:1341; 2:1, 66, 1892.

Cancer from mineral oil. Br. Med. J., 4:443, 1969.

Carmichael, G. G., and Silverstone, H.: The epidemiology of skin cancer in Queensland: the incidence. Br. J. Cancer, 15:409, 1961.

Cawley, E. P.: Genetic aspects of malignant melanoma. A.M.A. Arch. Dermatol. Syph., 65:440, 1952.

Clark, R. L., and Macdonald, E. J.: The natural history of melanoma in man. *In* Gordon, M. (Ed.): Pigment Cell Growth. Proceedings of the Third Conference on the Biology of Normal and Atypical Cell Growth. New York, Academic Press, 1953, p. 139.

Cleland, J. B.: Some remarks on the causes of cancer. Aust. Med. Gaz., 25:279, 1906.

Cooper, A. G. S.: Reflections on Cutaneous Malignancy in Queensland. Summary of paper presented at Section of Radiology and Radiotherapy, Ninth Australian Medical Congress (British Medical Association), held in Sydney, August 20–27, 1955. Med. J. Aust., 2:666, 1955.

Cruickshank, C. N. D., and Squire, J. R.: Skin cancer in the engineering industry from the use of mineral oil. Br. J. Ind. Med., 7:1, 1950.

Currie, A. N.: The role of arsenic in carcinogenesis. Br. Med. Bull., 4:402, 1947.

Cutaneous cancer. Br. Med. J., 1:986, 1948.

Davies, J. N. P., Wilson, B. A., and Knowelden, J.: Cancer incidence of the African population of Kyadondo (Uganda). Lancet, 2:328, 1962.

Davis, N. C.: Personal communication, 1971.

Davis, N. C., Herron, J. J., and McLeod, G. R.: Malignant melanoma in Queensland: analysis of 400 skin lesions. Lancet, 2:407, 1966.

Doll, R., Payne, P., and Waterhouse, J.: Cancer Incidence in Five Continents: A Technical Report. Geneva, UICC. Berlin, Springer-Verlag, 1966.

Doll, R., Muir, C. S., and Waterhouse, J. A. H. (Eds.): Cancer Incidence in Five Continents. Vol. 2. Geneva, UICC. Berlin, Springer-Verlag, 1970.

Dorn, H. F.: Illness from cancer in the United States. Public Health Rep., 59:33, 1944.

Dubreuilh, W.: Épithéliomatose d'origine solaire. Ann. Dermatol. Syphiligr. (Paris), 8:387, 1907.

Dunn, J. E., Jr., Levin, E. A., Linden, G., and Harzfeld, L.: Skin cancer as a cause of death. Calif. Med., 102:361, 1965.

Eastcott, D. F.: Epidemiology of Skin Cancer in New Zealand. U.S. National Cancer Institute Monograph No. 10, 1963, pp. 141–151.

End Results Group: End Results in Cancer Report No. 3. Washington, U.S. Department of Health, Education, and Welfare, 1968, p. 141.

Findlay, G. H.: Skin cancer in the Transvaal, South Africa. *In* Blum, H. F., and Urbach, F. (Eds.): Conference on Sunlight and Skin Cancer. National Cancer Institute, National Institutes of Health, Department of Health, Education, and Welfare, Bethesda, Maryland, 1964, p. 67.

Findlay, G. M.: Ultraviolet light and skin cancer. Lancet, 2:1070, 1928.

Gellin, G. A., Kopf, A. W., and Garfinkel, L.: Basal-cell carcinoma—a controlled study of associated factors. *In* Montagna, W. (Ed.): Advances in Biology of Skin. Vol. VII. Carcinogenesis. Oxford, Pergamon Press, 1966, p. 329.

Gellin, G. A., Kopf, A. W., Garfinkel, L.: Malignant melanoma. A controlled study of possibly associated factors. Arch. Dermatol., 99:43, 1969.

Goncalves, J. C.: Malignant change in smallpox vaccination scars. Arch. Dermatol., 93:229, 1966.

Gordon, D., and Silverstone, H.: Deaths from skin cancer in Queensland, Australia. *In* Urbach, F. (Ed.): The Biologic Effects of Ultraviolet Radiation. Oxford, Pergamon Press, 1969, p. 625.

Haenszel, W.: Variations in skin cancer incidence within the United States. *In* Urbach, F. (Ed.): Conference on Biology of Cutaneous Cancer. National Cancer Institute Monograph No. 10, Washington, U.S Department of Health, Education, and Welfare, 1963, p. 225.

Harnett, W. L.: British Empire Cancer Campaign: A Survey of Cancer in London. Report of the Clinical Cancer Research Committee. London, Br. Empire Cancer Campaign, 1952.

Henry, S. A.: Cancer of the Scrotum in Relation to Occupation. London, Oxford University Press, 1946.

Henry, S. A.: Occupational cutaneous cancer attributable to certain chemicals in industry. Br. Med. Bull., 4:389, 1947a.

Henry, S. A.: *In* Symposium—Industrial skin cancer, with special reference to pitch and tar cancer. Chemical aspects of industrial skin cancer caused by pitch and tar. Br. J. Radiol., 20:149, 1947b.

Higginson, J.: Techniques and methods in statistics and epidemiology of skin cancer. *In* Urbach, F. (Ed.): Conference on Biology of Cutaneous Cancer. National Cancer Institute Monograph No. 10, Washington, U.S. Department of Health, Education, and Welfare, 1963, p. 649.

Higginson, J., and Oettlé, A. G.: Cancer incidence in the Bantu and "Cape Colored" races in South Africa: report of a cancer survey in the Transvaal (1953–55). J. Natl. Cancer Inst., 24:589, 1960.

Howell, J. B.: The sunlight factor in ageing and skin cancer. Arch. Dermatol., 82:865, 1960.

Hueper, W. C.: Chemically induced skin cancers in man. *In* Urbach, F. (Ed.): Conference on Biology of Cutaneous Cancer. National Cancer Institute Monograph No. 10, Washington, U.S. Department of Health, Education, and Welfare, 1963, p. 377.

Humphrey, L. J., Playforth, H., and Leavell, U. W., Jr.: Squamous cell carcinoma arising in hidradenitis suppurativum. Arch. Dermatol., 100:59, 1969.

Hunter, D.: The Diseases of Occupations. Ed. 5. London, The English Universities Press, 1969.

Hyde, J. N.: On the influence of light in the production of cancer of the skin. Am. J. Med. Sci., 131:1, 1906.

Katz, A. D., Urbach, F., and Lilienfeld, A. M.: The frequency and risk of metastases in squamous-cell carcinoma of the skin. Cancer, 10:1162, 1957.

Lancaster, H. O.: The mortality in Australia from cancers of the alimentary system. Med. J. Aust., 1:744, 1954.

Lancaster, H. O.: The mortality in Australia from cancer for the period 1946 to 1950. Med. J. Aust., 2:235, 1955.

Lancaster, H. O.: Some geographical aspects of the mortality from melanoma in Europeans. Med. J. Aust., 1:1082, 1956.

Lancaster, H. O., and Nelson, J.: Sunlight as a cause of melanoma; a clinical survey. Med. J. Aust., 1:452, 1957.

Lawrence, E. A.: Carcinoma arising in the scars of thermal burns with special reference to influence of age at burn on length of induction period. Surg. Gynecol. Obstet., 95:579, 1952.

Lawrence, H.: Remarques particulières aux maladies de la peau en Australie. Trans. Intl. Dermatol. Congr., Rome, April, 1912.

Lawrence, H.: The relatively low humidity of the atmosphere and much sunshine as a causal factor for the great prevalence of skin cancer in Australia. Health Bull. (Aust.), 17:561, 1929.

Laycock, H. T.: The "Kang Cancer" of North-West China. Br. Med. J., 1:982, 1948.

Lea, A. J.: Malignant melanoma of the skin: the relationship to trauma. Ann. R. Coll. Surg. Engl., 37:169, 1965.

Lee, J. A. H.: Sunlight, sex, and site—factors in melanoma? *In* Summaries of Selected Papers from the 96th Annual Meeting of the American Public Health Association and Related Organizations, Detroit, Mich., Nov. 11–15, 1968. Public Health Rep., 84:227, 1969.

Lee, J. A. H., and Carter, A. P.: Secular trends in mortality from malignant melanoma. J. Natl. Cancer Inst., 45:91: 1970.

Lee, J. A. H., and Merrill, J. M.: Sunlight and the aetiology of malignant melanoma: a synthesis. Med. J. Aust., 2:846, 1970.

Lightstone, A. C., Kopf, A. W., and Garfinkel, L.: Diagnostic difficulty—a new approach to its evaluation; results in basal cell epitheliomas. Arch. Dermatol., 91:497, 1965.

Lilienfeld, A. M., Pedersen, E., and Dowd, J. E.: Cancer Epidemiology:Methods of Study. Baltimore, Johns Hopkins Press, 1967, p. 4.

Lund, H. Z.: How often does squamous cell carcinoma of the skin metastasize? Arch. Dermatol., 92:635, 1965.

Lynch, F. W., Seidman, H., and Hammond, E. C.: Incidence of cutaneous cancer in Minnesota. Cancer, 25:83, 1970.

Macdonald, E. J.: The epidemiology of skin cancer. J. Invest. Dermatol., 32:379, 1959.

Macdonald, E. J.: Some epidemiologic factors of skin cancer. J. Am. Med. Wom. Assoc., 22:235, 1967.

Macdonald, E. J.: Relation of Environment and Ethnic Group to Skin Cancer in Texas. 1970 (in press).

Macdonald, E. J., and Bubendorf, E.: Some epidemiologic aspects of skin cancer. *In* Tumors of the Skin. A Collection of Papers Presented at the Seventh Annual Clinical Conference on Cancer, 1962, at The University of Texas M.D. Anderson Hospital and Tumor Institute, Houston, Texas. Chicago, Year Book Medical Publishers, 1964.

McGovern, V. J.: Melanoblastoma. Med. J. Aust., 1:139, 1952.

McGovern, V. J.: Melanoma. Clin. Bull. R. Prince Alfred Hospital, Sydney, 1:45, 1957.

McLeod, R., Davis, N. C., Herron, J. J., Caldwell, R. A., Little, J. H., and Quinn, R. L.: A retrospective survey of 498 patients with malignant melanoma. Surg. Gynecol. Obstet., 126:99, 1968.

McLeod, G. R., Beardmore, G. L., Little, J. H., Quinn, R. L., and Davis, N. C.: Results of treatment of 361 patients with malignant melanoma in Queensland. Med. J. Aust., 1:1211, 1971.

Marmelzat, W. L.: Malignant tumours in smallpox vaccination scars: a report of 24 cases. Arch. Dermatol., 97:400, 1968.

Martin, H., Strong, E., and Spiro, R. H.: Radiation-induced skin cancer of the head and neck. Cancer, 25:61, 1970.

Miedler, L. J.: Skin cancer and occupation. A review of newer concepts of carcinogenesis based on animal experimentation with potential occupational skin carcinogens. Arch. Environ. Health, 3:276, 1961.

Miyaji, T.: Skin cancers in Japan: a nationwide 5-year survey, 1956–1960. *In* Urbach, F. (Ed.): Conference on Biology of Cutaneous Cancer. National Cancer Institute Monograph No. 10, Washington, U.S Department of Health, Education, and Welfare, 1963, p. 55.

Molesworth, E. H.: Rodent ulcer. Med. J. Aust., 1:878, 1927.

Mulay, D. M.: Skin cancer in India. *In* Urbach, F. (Ed.): Conference on Biology of Cutaneous Cancer. National Cancer Institute Monograph No. 10, Washington, U.S. Department of Health, Education, and Welfare, 1963, p. 215.

National Cancer Institute: Report of Third Cancer Incidence Survey, 1974 (in press).

O'Beirn, S. F., Judge, P., Urbach, F., MacCon, C. F., and Martin, F.: Skin Cancer in County Galway, Ireland. 1970 (in press).

Oettlé, A. G.: Skin cancer in Africa. *In* Urbach, F. (Ed.): Conference on Biology of Cutaneous Cancer. National Cancer Institute Monograph No. 10, Washington, U.S. Department of Health, Education, and Welfare, 1963, p. 197.

Oettlé, A. G.: Cancer in Africa, especially in regions south of the Sahara. J. Natl. Cancer Inst., 33:383, 1964.

O'Halloran, M. J.: Skin cancer in Ireland. J. Ir. Med. Assoc., 60:209, 1967.

Oluwasanmi, J. O., Williams, A. O., and Alli, A. F.: Superficial cancer in Nigeria. Br. J. Cancer, 23:714, 1969.

Pack, G. T., and Davis, J.: Radiation cancer of the skin. Radiology, 84:436, 1965.

Pantangco, E. E., Canlas, M., Basa, G., and Sin, R.: Observations on the incidence, biology, and pathology of skin cancer among Filipinos. J. Philipp. Med. Assoc., 39:259, 1963.

Paul, C. N.: The influence of sunlight on the production of cancer of the skin. London, H. K. Lewis & Company, 1918.

Payne, R. L.: Epidermoid carcinoma. Surg. Clin. North Am., 10:913, 1930.

Peller, S.: Epidemiology of skin cancer. J. Invest. Dermatol., 2:73, 1948.

Peterkin, G. A. G.: Malignant change in erythema ab igne. Br. Med. J., 2:1599, 1955.

Petersen, N. C., Bodenham, D. C., and Lloyd, O. C.: Malignant melanomas of the skin. A study of the origin, development, aetiology, spread, treatment, and prognosis. Br. J. Plast. Surg., 15:49, 97, 1962.

Phillips, C.: The relationship between skin cancer and occupation in Texas: a review of 1569 verified lesions occurring in 1190 patients. Texas State J. Med., 36:613, 1941.

Pott, P.: Chirurgical Observations Relative to the Cataract, the Polypus of the Nose, the Cancer of the Scrotum, the Different Kinds of Ruptures and the Mortification of the Toes and Feet. London, Hawes, Clarke and Collins, 1775, p. 63.

Potter, M.: Percival Pott's contribution to cancer research. *In* Urbach, F. (Ed.): Conference on Biology of Cutaneous Cancer. National Cancer Institute Monograph No. 10, Washington, U.S. Department of Health, Education, and Welfare, 1963, p. 1.

Pringgoutomo, S., and Pringgoutomo, S.: Skin Cancer in Indonesia. U.S. National Cancer Institute Monograph No. 10, 1963, pp. 191–195.

Quisenberry, W. B.: Ethnic differences in skin cancer in Hawaii. *In* Urbach, F. (Ed.): Conference on Biology of Cutaneous Cancer. National Cancer Institute Monograph No. 10, Washington, U.S. Department of Health, Education, and Welfare, 1963, p. 181.

Reed, W. B., and Wilson-Jones, E.: Malignant tumours as a late complication of vaccination. Arch. Dermatol., 98:132, 1968.

Schulze, R., and Gräfe, K.: Consideration of sky ultraviolet radiation in the measurement of solar ultraviolet radiation. *In* Urbach, F. (Ed.): The Biologic Effects of Ultraviolet Radiation. Oxford, Pergamon Press, 1969, p. 359.

Shanmugaratnam, K., and La' Brooy, E. B.: Skin Cancer in Singapore. U.S. National Cancer Institute Monograph No. 10, 1963, pp. 127–140.

Silverstone, H., and Gordon, D.: Regional studies in skin cancer: second report. Wet tropical and subtropical coasts of Queensland. Med. J. Aust., 2:733, 1966.

Silverstone, H., and Searle, J. H. A.: The epidemiology of skin cancer in Queensland: the influence of phenotype and environment. Br. J. Cancer, 24:235, 1970.

Silverstone, H., and Smithurst, B. A.: Survey of Queensland Radium Institute patients. Unpublished data, 1971.

Solomon, S. E.: Statistics of the State of Queensland for the Years 1955–1956, 1956–1957, 1957–1958, 1963–1964, 1964–1965, 1965–1966, 1966–1967, 1967–1968. Part A. Population and Vital. Brisbane, Government Printer, 1956–1958; 1964–1968.

Southam, A. H., and Wilson, S. R.: Cancer of the scrotum; the etiology, clinical features, and treatment of the disease. Br. Med. J., 2:971, 1922.

Sweet, R. D.: Skin cancer in England. *In* Blum, H. F., and Urbach, F. (Eds.): Conference on Sunlight and Skin Cancer. National Cancer Institute, National Institutes of Health, Department of Health, Education, and Welfare, Bethesda, Maryland, 1964, p. 69.

Tam, P. B., Hoanh, D. D., Chu, N. X., and Can, N.

H.: Some etiopathologic aspects of skin cancer in South Vietnam. *In* Urbach, F. (Ed.): Conference on Biology of Cutaneous Cancer. National Cancer Institute Monograph No. 10, Washington, U.S. Department of Health, Education, and Welfare, 1963, p. 75.

Tansurat, P.: Regional incidence and pathology of skin cancer in Thailand. *In* Urbach, F. (Ed.): Conference on Biology of Cutaneous Cancer. National Cancer Institute Monograph No. 10, Washington, U.S. Department of Health, Education, and Welfare, 1963, p. 71.

ten Seldam, R. E. J.: Skin cancer in Australia. *In* Urbach, F. (Ed.): Conference on Biology of Cutaneous Cancer. National Cancer Institute Monograph No. 10, Washington, U.S. Department of Health, Education, and Welfare, 1963, p. 153.

Unna, P. G.: Die Histopathologie der Hautkrankheiten. Berlin, A. Hirschwald, 1894.

Urbach, F. (Ed.): Conference on Biology of Cutaneous Cancer. National Cancer Institute Monograph No. 10, Washington, U.S. Department of Health, Education, and Welfare, 1963.

Urbach, F.: Ultraviolet radiation and its relationship to skin cancer in man. *In* Montagna, W. (Ed.): Advances in Biology of Skin. Vol. VII. Carcinogenesis. Oxford, Pergamon Press, 1966, p. 581.

Urbach, F., Rose, D. B., and Bonnem, M.: Genetic and environmental interactions in skin carcinogenesis. 1971.

Urteaga, O., and Pack, G. T.: On the antiquity of melanoma. Cancer, 19:607, 1966.

Wade, L.: Observations on skin cancer among refin-

ery workers. Limited to men exposed to high-boiling fractions. Arch. Environ. Health, 6:730, 1963.

Walker, R. M.: Cancer in south-west England. Ann. R. Coll. Surg. Engl., 42:145, 1968.

Wardale-Greenwood, I. J.: Epidemiology of Skin Cancer in Tasmania. Project for degree of M.B., B.S., University of Queensland, Australia—No. P.359, Department of Social and Preventive Medicine, 1964. Unpublished.

Watson, E. C.: Melanoma: a ten-year retrospective survey in New Zealand. Aust. N.Z. J. Surg., 33:31, 1963.

White, J. E., Strudwick, W. J., Ricketts, N., and Sampson, C.: Cancer of the skin in Negroes. A review of 31 cases. J.A.M.A., 178:845, 1961.

Winternitz, J. G.: *In* Symposium—Industrial skin cancer, with special reference to pitch and tar cancer. Chemical aspects of industrial skin cancer caused by pitch and tar. Br. J. Radiol., 20:158, 1947.

World Health Organization: Mortality from malignant neoplasms of the skin. W.H.O. Epidemiological and Vital Statistics Report, 13:426, 1960.

Yeh, S.: Relative incidence of skin cancer in Chinese in Taiwan: with special reference to arsenical cancer. *In* Urbach, F. (Ed.): Conference on Biology of Cutaneous Cancer. National Cancer Institute Monograph No. 10, Washington, U.S. Department of Health, Education, and Welfare, 1963, p. 81.

Yeh, S., How, S. W., and Lin, C. S.: Arsenical cancer of skin. Histologic study with special reference to Bowen's disease. Cancer, 21:312, 1968.

Part

II

Special Subjects

17

Actinic Keratosis — Actinic Skin

Hermann Pinkus, M.D.

DEFINITION, SYNONYMS, AND HISTORY

Actinic keratoses are circumscribed, rough, epidermal lesions developing on the skin under the influence of irradiation. In the widest sense, they include changes produced by all types of radiation emanating from radioactive elements, x-ray sources, and the sun. In a narrower sense, actinic keratosis is synonymous with solar keratosis and refers to certain more or less hyperkeratotic lesions found on the sun-exposed skin of susceptible individuals as part of the complex of "actinic skin."

Actinic keratoses are epidermal neoplasms in the sense that they consist of heritably altered epidermal keratinocytes (see under Etiology and Pathogenesis). They often do not cause clinical tumor formation; as a matter of fact, in some of them the epidermis is rather atrophic. Clinically and histologically, they are sharply defined islands replacing an area of epidermis. Statistically, they are classified as precanceroses because a considerable number of them, estimated as high as 20 percent by Montgomery (1939), transform into invasive squamous cell

carcinoma. Biologically, they may be considered carcinoma in situ.

Inasmuch as other hyperkeratotic lesions, such as seborrheic verrucae, senile freckles, Bowen's dermatosis, and discoid lupus erythematosus, may be found in actinic skin, we must narrow the definition by clinical and histologic criteria, which will be discussed in the following pages. A negative aspect of the definition, however, is obvious: a lesion occurring on ordinarily covered parts of the skin cannot be a solar keratosis.

The name "actinic keratosis" is relatively new. It was proposed by the committee on nomenclature of the American Academy of Dermatology and Syphilology (Becker, 1959). "Solar keratosis" is a synonym for the lesion we consider in this chapter. The older terms "senile keratosis" and "senile keratoma" have been abandoned as clinical designations because the age of the individual is not essential. Solar keratoses may occur in highly susceptible individuals in the second or third decade. The Latin name *keratosis senilis*, however, retains its value in histologic diagnosis as defined by Pinkus (1958). Lay terms such as "liver spot" or "old age freckle" are practically meaningless. "Precancerous keratosis" or "precancerosis" is not a true synonym. It implies prognostication and is equally applicable to x-ray keratosis and Bowen's dermatosis (see under Prognosis).

Actinic keratoses were known to physicians and laymen alike in olden times. Unna (1894) included them in his description of "seamen's skin." They are mentioned in practically all textbooks of dermatology as senile or precancerous lesions. It is to the merit of Freudenthal (1926) that he gave an exact description of histologic changes and separated once and for all "keratoma senile" (actinic keratosis) from "verruca senilis" (seborrheic keratosis, seborrheic verruca). Later authors (Montgomery, 1939; Portugal and Rocha, 1950; Caro and Szymanski, 1951; Pinkus, 1958; Braun-Falco and Langner, 1966) supported his conclusions. Unna's "seamen's skin" was complemented by the concept of "farmer's skin" of Dubreuilh (1907). Now, one speaks more generally of "actinic skin" (see Chapter 9).

EPIDEMIOLOGY AND INCIDENCE

The number of actinic keratoses seen in a certain population varies widely because it depends on three factors: the amount of insolation in a given locality, the susceptibility of the population at risk which reflects mainly a lack of natural pigmentation and inability to tan, and the habit of individuals to expose their skin to the sun. Incidence thus is extremely high in Australia (Belisario, 1959; ten Seldam, 1963), where a predominantly English-Scottish-Irish population, notorious for its poor pigmenting ability, has come to live in a semi-tropical or tropical climate without adopting the precautions of Europeans with darker complexions, who have always used wide-brimmed hats and protective clothing in similar climates.

Data from the United States confirm the importance of these three factors. In Michigan, in the writer's experience, actinic keratoses are never seen in Negroes and rarely in brunet Caucasians. A person seeking treatment for actinic keratoses and the ensuing skin cancer will usually be of Celtic or otherwise fair-skinned stock and will have had an out-of-doors occupation, or he may be an ardent fisherman or similar outdoors enthusiast, possibly a retiree who has been spending much time in Florida or another place with a sunny climate. Although most of the published statistical data refer to fully developed cancer rather than to actinic keratoses, they are germane to our discussion. Auerbach (1961) reported that skin cancer incidence rates in the white population are doubled for each 265 miles going south. Statistics from the New York Skin and Cancer Unit, although dealing mainly with basal cell epithelioma, confirm the importance of genetic complexion in sun-induced cutaneous neoplasia (Gellin et al., 1965). Instructive data on the incidence of skin cancer in the different ethnic groups of Hawaii were presented by Quisenberry (1963). They bear out the much higher incidence of sun-induced lesions in Caucasians living alongside Japanese, Hawaiians, and other ethnic groups with better pigmentary protection. Quisenberry relates a skin cancer rate of 138 per 100,000 Caucasians in Honolulu for 1955-56. Comparable yearly rates were 109 for Dallas, 90 for San Francisco, and 39 for Philadelphia. If one accepts the premise that all actinic carcinomas arise in keratoses but only a small percentage of actinic keratoses progress to carcinoma, one has to multiply these figures by at least a factor of 10 to obtain the local incidence of keratoses (see under Prognosis).

ETIOLOGY AND PATHOGENESIS

The preceding remarks and the name of the lesion incriminate the rays of the sun as the etiologic agent of solar keratosis, a thesis proposed by Dubreuilh as early as 1907. The cutaneous effects of sunlight are discussed in detail in Chapter 9. It is the ultraviolet part of the spectrum which has been implicated in carcinogenesis ever since the work of Blum (1948, 1959).

There are differences of opinion concerning the pathogenetic mechanism by which ultraviolet rays produce actinic keratoses. These differences concern the question of whether there is a direct effect on the epidermis or an indirect effect mediated through the dermis. The considerations favoring either mechanism were discussed by Mackie and McGovern (1958) and Pinkus (1966). A definite answer is important not only for theoretic reasons but also for practical prophylactic therapy (see under Treatment). Is it necessary to remove the actinically changed dermis in order to prevent the development of future keratoses and cancers? Or is it sufficient to destroy the precancerous epidermis and permit it to be replaced by new epithelium from the adnexa? We have to discuss this matter in some detail.

Inasmuch as carcinogenesis is considered a cellular event by experimental oncologists, direct carcinogenic action of ultraviolet rays on the genetic apparatus of epidermal germinative cells would seem to be a good possibility. There are two major objections. First, the incubation period for the formation of actinic keratoses is very long. It requires many years of cumulative exposure, and a single sunburn does not seem to cause keratoses or cancer. On the other hand, the epidermis continuously renews itself, cells being formed by mitotic division and eliminated by keratinization with a turnover time of about a month (see Chapter 4). The cells and particularly the fibers of the dermis have a much longer life span, and visible changes, increasing with time and exposure, are easily demonstrated in the form of actinic elastosis. Secondly, melanin pigment, which has such an obvious protective effect, is localized mainly in the deepest epidermal layer and is a sun screen for the dermis rather than for the epidermis. Negro skin indeed shows practically no changes of actinic elastosis. Mackie and McGovern (1958), in a very thorough quantitative morphologic study of actinic skin in Australia, therefore concluded that the sun exerts its effect on the dermis, the epidermis being secondarily affected by metabolic and nutritional changes.

This view, however, does not explain the fact that dermal actinic changes are diffuse and evenly developed over large areas, while keratoses are discrete, focal, and comparatively few. Many persons with pronounced actinic skin have only an occasional keratosis, and even those who have many develop them in focal fashion. In most cases, the therapist can be content to destroy individual lesions, and by doing so repeatedly at intervals (see under Treatment) can sanitize the patient's skin for prolonged periods. Even the topical application of 5-fluorouracil, while it brings out many more lesions than are visible to the naked eye, acts in a focal manner. It actually provides excellent proof of the fact that a severely and diffusely sun-damaged skin carries only a limited number of epidermal precancerous foci.

Furthermore, the two premises on which objections to direct effect of sunlight on the epidermis have been based are not entirely convincing. First, while the epidermal cells are continuously formed and eliminated, the germinal stock of basal cells remains, and its gene pool survives for the life of the individual. Minor genetic changes must not manifest themselves and may accumulate over the years (see Chapter 16) until a threshold is reached which makes an individual basal cell the stem cell of a visible lesion. It has been shown that actinic skin retains its epidermal alterations for as long as four years after transplantation to a nonexposed site (Papa et al., 1970). Secondly, the melanin granules have long been known to form a supranuclear cap in the basal cells and therefore to protect the gene material in the nuclei of germinal epidermal cells just as much as the underlying dermis. In addition, non-Caucasian skins, even of relatively light-complexioned people, contain quite a number of pigment granules in higher epidermal layers (see Chapter 4). Recent investigations on the genetic defect in xeroderma pigmentosum (Cleaver, 1968 and 1970; Reed et al., 1969) (see Chapter 19) have thrown additional light on the pathogenesis of actinic induction of keratoses and cancer. It has been shown that epidermal cells sustain chromatin damage through the direct ionizing effect of ultraviolet light and that normal cells can repair the damage. The tissues in xeroderma patients are unable to do so. Defective cells originate, some of which have the characteristics of malignancy. In these patients, all sun-exposed tissues undergo these changes, and sarcomas and melanomas as well as epidermal carcinomas develop. It is quite conceivable that, in normal individuals, ultraviolet-induced chromatin damage is not properly repaired on occasion and that, over many years, repeated "hits" produce cumulative changes of the same order that take xeroderma pigmentosum cells only a few years to develop. Because epidermal basal cells far outnumber melanocytes in poorly pigmented persons, it is not surprising that actinic keratoses are far more common than malignant melanomas, although there is a definite influence of sun susceptibility on the latter (Belisario, 1969).

It shall not be denied that actinic changes in the dermis contribute to epidermal vulnerability, in view of the close biologic interrelation of the two tissues. It is, however, more difficult to deny direct action of ultraviolet rays on the epidermis, and it is likely that epidermal and dermal changes parallel each other rather than one being completely secondary to the other. In view of the convincing results of experimental oncology that a cancer begins with the transformation of a single cell and that neoplasms result from the multiplication of individual transformed cells, it seems most likely that each actinic keratosis is the product of neoplastic transformation of a single basal cell, a concept (Pinkus, 1967a) which is illustrated in Figure 17–1.

Another highly important factor in the pathogenesis of actinic keratoses is the symbiotic composition of the epidermis, which was explained in Chapter 4. While the epidermis itself is maintained by mitotic division of its basal cells, it is traversed by epithelial tubes, the intraepidermal portions of eccrine ducts and pilosebaceous infundibula, which are maintained as separate biologic units by division of their own subepidermally located matrix cells. When the epidermis undergoes neoplastic transformation as a consequence of actinic exposure, the adnexal units generally remain healthy because their matrix cells are sufficiently remote from the surface. Symbiotic cooperation, however, between epidermal and adnexal keratinocytes is disturbed. To use Weiss's expression (1950), the normal and the neoplastic cells do not recognize each other, and contact inhibition is diminished. The adnexal (normal) keratinocytes try to do what they ordinarily do when the epidermis has been lost (see Chapter 5). They become hyperplastic and cover the surface in an attempt to establish a new epidermis. The dysplastic epidermal keratinocytes, on the other hand, tend to creep along the dermal-epidermal interface and may form collars around the adnexal structures (Halter, 1952). These phenomena are diagrammatically shown in Figure 17–2 (Pinkus, 1958). Their histologic expression will be discussed under Pathology.

CLINICAL DESCRIPTION

Actinic keratoses (Fig. 17–3) are sharply circumscribed lesions ranging from pinpoint size to more than 2 cm. in diameter, but they usually measure a few mm. Their outstanding feature is roughness, and small ones are often better recognized by palpation than by inspection. Roughness is due to adherent parakeratotic scale, and it is of diagnostic value that attempts to remove the scale by scraping usually elicit tenderness or pain. The color of actinic keratoses ranges from that of the surrounding skin to tan, brown, gray, or almost black, but it often includes a factor of

SOLAR KERATOSIS

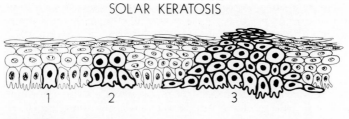

1   2   3

Heavy outline
denotes cancer cell

Figure 17–1 Diagram illustrating the concept that every actinic keratosis develops from one heritably deranged basal cell and represents a slowly enlarging island of carcinoma in situ. (*From* Pinkus: The borderline between cancer and non-cancer. *In* Year Book of Dermatology 1966/67. Chicago, Year Book Medical Publishers, 1967, p. 5.)

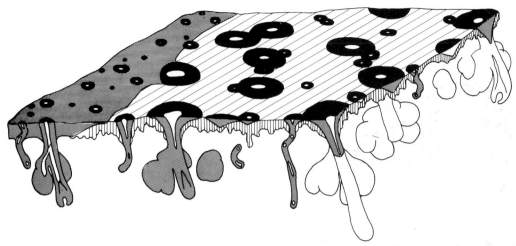

Figure 17–2 Diagram illustrating the relations of adnexal epithelium, normal epidermis, and dysplastic epidermis in three-dimensional view. Normal keratinocytes of epidermis and adnexal ostia live in close symbiosis and are morphologically similar. Dysplastic epidermal keratinocytes live in uneasy balance with normal epithelium. They undergrow normal epidermis and extend as collars around pilar and eccrine ostia. The keratinocytes of *acrotrichium* and *acrosyringium* become hyperplastic and form umbrellas on the surface. Some of these merge and submerge the dysplastic epidermis. The front cut shows how these biologic phenomena are expressed in a single vertical section. Compare with the photomicrographs in Figures 17–6 to 17–10. (*From* Pinkus: Am. J. Clin. Pathol., 29:193, 1958.)

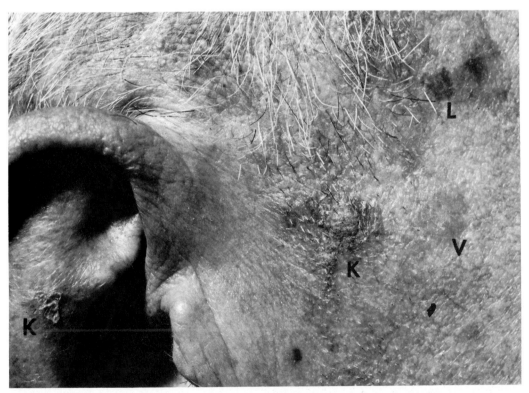

Figure 17–3 Right ear and preauricular skin of an elderly light-skinned man. Actinic keratoses are present on the anthelix and in the preauricular area (K). A seborrheic verruca (V) and senile lentigo (L) are seen near the right border of the field. Hyperplasia of sebaceous glands, telangiectasia, and mottled atrophy complete the picture of actinic skin.

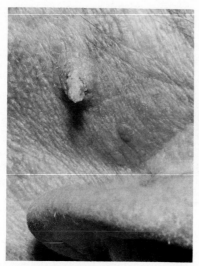

Figure 17–4 Actinic keratosis with hyperkeratosis resembling a small cutaneous horn in the post-auricular skin of an elderly man.

slightly elevated due to the thickened horny layer and a variable amount of inflammatory infiltrate. They do not ordinarily have an elevated rim. In rare instances, they may be verrucous through epidermal hyperplasia. More commonly, their horny layer becomes excessively thick (Fig. 17–4), and they begin to resemble tiny cutaneous horns. True cutaneous horns, even of great size, may have an actinic keratosis at their base (see Chapter 19).

Most actinic keratoses are dry and dull, and close examination with a magnifying glass does not reveal a particular pattern (Fig. 17–5*A*). These features contrast with those of seborrheic keratoses, which, true to their papillomatous nature (seborrheic verrucae), often have a definite pattern of tiny, round depressions and grooves or have a greasy or shiny surface. They also have substance (Fig. 17–5*B*) which remains after all horny matter has been removed, while the actinic keratosis owes its elevation to the horny covering, and the remo-

redness which may be so pronounced that the clinical picture resembles a patch of discoid lupus erythematosus. Actinic keratoses may be macular but usually are

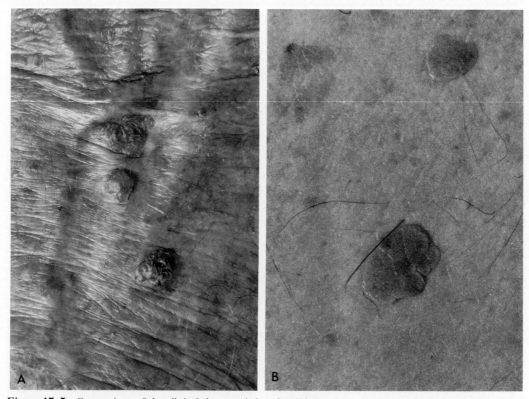

Figure 17–5 Comparison of the clinical characteristics of actinic keratoses (*A*) on the dorsum of the hand and seborrheic verrucae (*B*) on the neck of an elderly man. Both photographs also show pigmentary changes of actinic skin.

val of this leaves an oozing or bleeding area level with the surrounding skin. When lesions are not dry, they may be oozing or crusting due to superimposed bacterial infection (impetiginization). More often, this feature indicates beginning progression to invasive squamous cell carcinoma.

This description covers mainly the most common type of actinic keratosis which corresponds to the histologic picture of keratosis senilis. It also applies, however, to the few lesions which are histologically different and which will be mentioned under Pathology.

It may be worth repeating that solar keratoses cannot be expected on covered skin, and other diagnoses must be considered for clinically similar lesions in areas which do not show the general characteristics of actinic skin. These characteristics are redness due to telangiectasia and a yellow tinge contributed by the increased elastic tissue, the natural yellow color of which may be intensified by a high content of lipids (Urbach, 1934). The skin usually is less flexible and shows accentuated folds and furrows, which give the face and neck a characteristic pattern. The nape often has the aspect of cutis rhomboidalis nu-

chae (see Chapters 4 and 9). Other frequent features are irregularities of pigmentation, either in the form of freckles or in a reticulated pattern resembling poikiloderma. This aspect is enhanced by large sebaceous glands, so common on the sides of the neck. The peculiar picture resulting from telangiectasia, sebaceous glands, and reticular epidermal pigmentation has been described under a variety of names. Perhaps the most acceptable one is "erythromelanosis colli" (see Mishima and Rudner, 1966).

PATHOLOGY

Definite diagnosis of actinic keratosis must be made under the microscope (Lund, 1957; Lever, 1967; Allen, 1967; Montgomery, 1967; Pinkus and Mehregan, 1969). The lesion must be differentiated from inflammatory diseases, mainly seborrheic dermatitis and discoid lupus erythematosus, from certain epidermal nevi and noninvasive neoplasms, and particularly from invasive carcinoma. Diagnosis is relatively easy (Pinkus, 1958) if one keeps in mind the biology of the lesion, which was discussed under Etiology

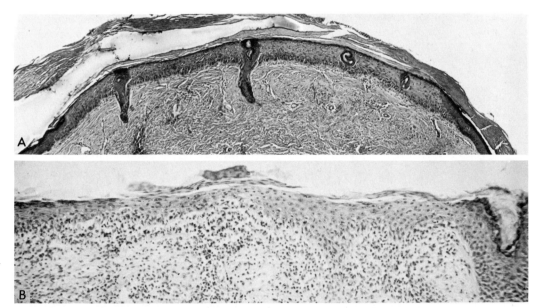

Figure 17–6 Keratosis senilis as an island of light-staining parakeratotic epidermis.

A, Lesion on the back of the hand. Sharp borders against normal epidermis and acrosyringia. Almost complete absence of inflammatory infiltrate is an exceptional feature of this keratosis. *H&E*, × *45*.

B, Lesion from the face showing sharp borders, slight downward budding, and dermal infiltrate of lymphocytes and some plasma cells. *H&E*, × *45*.

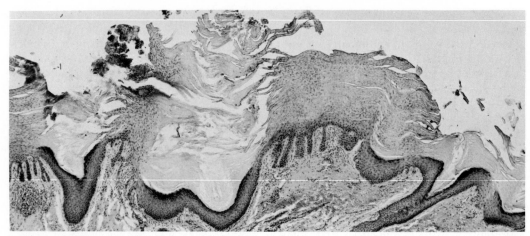

Figure 17–7   Keratosis senilis with compact parakeratotic layer sharply set off from the orthokeratotic horny plugs in hair follicles. Atypical budding of the dysplastic epidermis. Basophilic change (actinic elastosis) and reactive inflammatory infiltrate in the dermis. *H&E, × 45.*

and Pathogenesis, and takes into consideration the peculiar phenomenon that practically all precancerous epidermal lesions are associated with reactive cellular infiltrate in the dermis (Pinkus et al., 1963).

It must be realized, however, that there are rare variants of actinic keratosis which differ considerably from the pattern to be described now, which we designate as keratosis senilis (Pinkus, 1958) because it represents the prototype described by Freudenthal (1926). More than 99 percent of actinic keratoses follow this pattern. The rare exceptions will be described below as lichen planus–like keratoses and large cell acanthomas. Other light-induced

lesions are lentigo senilis and disseminated superficial actinic porokeratosis.

Keratosis Senilis

In its simplest expression (Fig. 17–6), keratosis senilis consists of an island of epidermis, in which the cells stain lighter and more eosinophilic and produce a nucleated (parakeratotic) horny layer without formation of a granular layer. The parakeratotic horny layer may be relatively thin or may be piled up to form thick, coherent masses (Fig. 17–7). Extreme degrees of this phenomenon approach the features found in cutaneous horn (see Chapter 19).

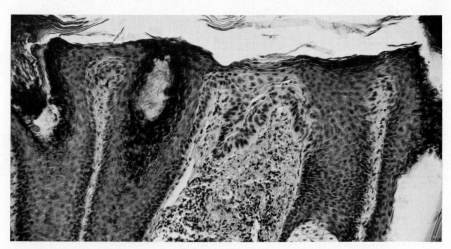

Figure 17–8   Cell-sharp borders between dysplastic epidermis and hyperplastic follicular ostia. Follicular keratinocytes merge in the left half of the field and submerge the epidermal keratinocytes. Compare with the diagram in Figure 17–2. *H&E, × 135.* (*From* Pinkus and Mehregan: A Guide to Dermatohistopathology, 1969. Courtesy of Appleton-Century-Crofts, Publishing Division of Prentice-Hall, Inc., Englewood Cliffs, N.J.)

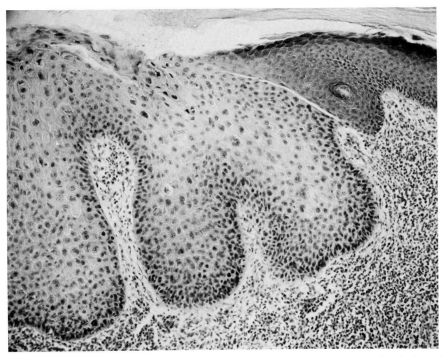

Figure 17–9   Bowenoid hyperplastic keratosis senilis. Slanting border and cleft between dysplastic and normal epithelium. Heavy lymphocytic and plasmocytic infiltrate in dermis. *H&E, ×135.*

The use of the word "island" implies that the altered epidermis is sharply limited and distinct from the surrounding normal epidermis (Figs. 17–6 and 17–9). It is also sharply distinct from adnexal keratinocytes of sweat ducts and hair follicles (acrosyringium and acrotrichium, see Chapter 4) which pass through it (Figs. 17–6 and 17–8). The border between normal and abnormal epithelium is so sharp (Figs. 17–8 and 17–9) that a trained eye has little difficulty in assigning each cell to one side or the other.

The border between epidermis and dermis may be straight and smooth (Fig. 17–6A) or may exhibit irregular budding projections (Figs. 17–6B and 17–8) different from the normal pattern of rete ridges. The PAS-positive basement membrane is present but may be of uneven thickness (Cawley et al., 1966). The thickness of the altered epidermis may be equal to the surrounding normal tissue, or it may be thinner or thicker. In some cases, it is quite atrophic (Fig. 17–13B); in others it becomes hyperplastic (Fig. 17–9) and, in rare cases, almost verrucous. The cells and their nuclei often are a little more variable in size and shape, and the regular stratification of the normal rete Malpighi may be

disturbed. Higher degrees of these cellular abnormalities (Fig. 17–9) are found in the so-called bowenoid variant of keratosis senilis.

A highly characteristic feature is the slanting direction of the cell-sharp border (Figs. 17–6 and 17–9) between dysplastic and normal epidermis and between dysplastic and adnexal keratinocytes. While it is not ascertainable in every section, it should be looked for. The direction of the slant is always as depicted in the diagrams in Figures 17–1 and 17–2: normal keratinocytes extend farther on the surface, dysplastic cells at the base of the epidermis. While the border may be almost vertical (Fig. 17–7), it may be so oblique in other cases that the umbrella-like disks of normal adnexal epithelium join on the surface and produce the paradoxical appearance that the epidermis consists of dysplastic lower layers and normally keratinizing upper layers. This deceptive appearance is illustrated in the diagram in Figure 17–2 and in the photomicrograph in Figure 17–8. Vertical paraffin sections exhibiting this feature can be interpreted correctly if the three-dimensional nature of the process is kept in mind. The incongruous stratification is caused by normal epidermis or ad-

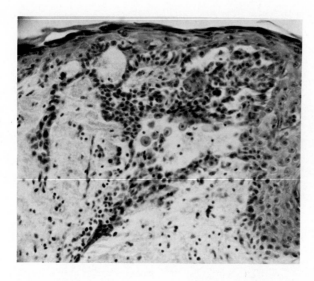

Figure 17–10 Darier-like keratosis senilis with beginning invasive downgrowth of the dysplastic epithelium. Acantholytic cells resembling corps ronds in the cleft between the submerged epithelium of the keratosis and the new epidermis formed from adnexal epithelium. *H&E, ×135.*

nexal epithelium overriding the dysplastic epidermis of the keratosis. The cells of the two populations may be in desmosomal connection, or they may be separated by a cleft (Pensley and Sims, 1961). Occasionally, individually keratinizing or degenerating cells float in the cleft and produce a picture similar to that of Darier's keratosis follicularis (Jablonska and Chorzelski, 1961). In extreme cases, the dysplastic epithelium is cut off from the surface and submerged for long distances, producing the histologic variant of Darier-like keratosis senilis (Fig. 17–10).

Another feature resulting from the lateral movement of dysplastic cells along the basement membrane is the perifollicular collar (Figs. 17–8 and 17–11*B*) previously mentioned. Neoplastic cells interpose themselves between the acrosyringeal or acrotrichial keratinocytes and the PAS-positive basement membrane, usually as a single sheet. They may creep down to the level of the sebaceous gland duct. In later stages, the adnexal umbrella is reduced, and the follicular epithelium may just reach the surface as a narrow lip (Figs. 17–7 and 17–11*C*). Still later, the territory of the infundibulum is occupied by dysplastic epithelium, but this does not mean that follicular epithelium has become dysplastic. It simply means a shift of the boundary

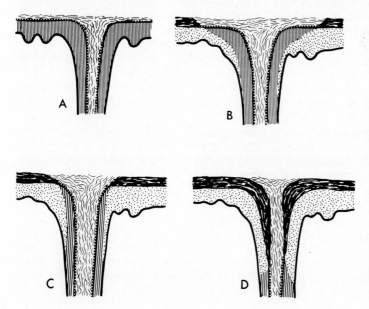

Figure 17–11 Diagram illustrating the shifting balance between dysplastic epidermis and follicular epithelium in actinic keratosis. *A,* The two types of keratinocytes are morphologically indistinguishable in normal skin. *B,* Adnexal epithelium forms an umbrella on the surface; dysplastic epidermis forms a perifollicular collar. *C,* Dysplastic epidermis begins to repress the adnexal epithelium, which reaches the surface as a narrow lip around the central core of normal keratin. *D,* Dysplastic epidermis and parakeratotic horny material have occupied infundibular territory. Normal epithelium persists deeper in the follicle. (*From* Pinkus: Malignant transformation of epithelium. *In* McKenna (Ed.): Modern Trends in Dermatology. Ed. 3. London, Butterworth & Company, Ltd., 1966, p. 275.)

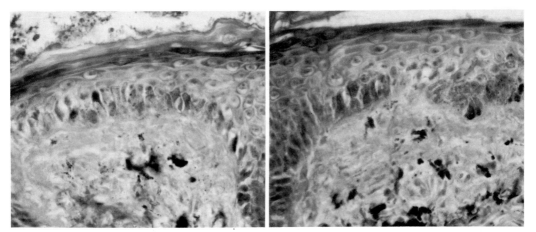

Figure 17–12 Pigmented keratosis senilis. Large melanocytes in the basal layer of the dysplastic epidermis. *H&E, ×370.*

line (Fig. 17–11*D*). The keratin plug filling the follicular lumen remains orthokeratotic (Figs. 17–7 and 17–14) because it derives from normal adnexal epithelium.

Melanocytes usually are not conspicuous in actinic keratoses and generally are completely absent (Niebauer, 1968). Occasionally, however, in the rare keratoses developing in dark-complexioned individuals, they may be prominent and may pose the problem of differentiating a pigmented actinic keratosis (Fig. 17–12) from precancerous melanosis of Dubreuilh.

Dermal alterations assist in the diagnosis of actinic keratosis. There is actinic elastosis varying from mild to severe. While it is only a concomitant feature (see under Etiology and Pathogenesis), its complete absence practically rules out a diagnosis of solar keratosis. As in otherwise normal skin, the elastotic changes occupy the upper third or half of the pars reticularis

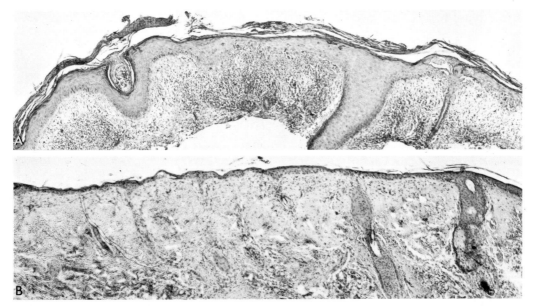

Figure 17–13 Atrophic forms of keratosis senilis. *A,* Similarly to discoid lupus erythematosus is produced by a combination of relatively thin epidermis, hyperplastic hair follicles with keratinous plugs, and heavy, dermal, round cell infiltrate which invades the epidermis in several places. The diagnosis must be made at higher magnification by identifying parakeratotic dysplastic epidermis bordering on orthokeratotic follicular umbrellas. *H&E, ×45.*

B, Severely atrophic parakeratotic epidermis above a broad layer of actinic elastosis with spotty round cell infiltrate. *H&E, ×45.*

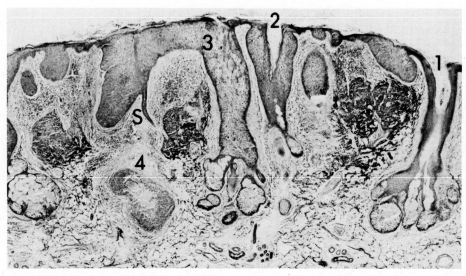

Figure 17–14 Replacement of follicular epithelium in keratosis senilis in facial skin. Follicle 1 outside the lesion is normal. Follicle 2 is surrounded by a broad collar of dysplastic epidermis; follicular epithelium barely reaches the surface but produces normal flaky keratin in the infundibular lumen. Follicle 3 is occupied by dysplastic epidermis down to the level of the sebaceous gland, which is not visibly affected. Follicle 4 is completely occupied by dysplastic epithelium; only the hair shaft remains in the center. The invasive epithelium is surrounded by fibrous root sheath and inflammatory infiltrate. A sweat duct (S) extends through dysplastic epidermis to the surface. Actinic elastotic material is present in clumps in the upper dermis. *Orcein and Giemsa,* × *30.*

but always spare the immediate subepidermal layer which corresponds to the atrophic pars papillaris. Of equal significance is the presence of cellular infiltrate (Pinkus et al., 1963), which is absent only in very early lesions (Fig. 17–6A). The infiltrate (Figs. 17–6B and 17–9) consists mainly of small, round cells, presumably lymphocytes, but includes few or numerous plasma cells in about 37 percent of cases. Some eosinophils may be present. Mast cells usually are neither decreased nor increased in number. This infiltrate, which resembles that found in Bowen's and Paget's dermatoses, perhaps represents a tissue immune response to intraepidermal malignancy. It may be minor and focal, mainly arranged around small vessels of the subpapillary plexus, or it may be dense and form an almost continuous band. Where such heavy infiltrate is associated with a relatively atrophic epidermis, the picture (Fig. 17–13A) may resemble discoid lupus erythematosus (see under Differential Diagnosis). The intradermal portions of pilosebaceous complexes and sweat glands usually show no significant changes.

Progression from actinic keratosis to invasive malignancy may take three different routes, and the resulting cancer is in all cases a squamous cell carcinoma. The irregular budding seen in many keratoses may increase and penetrate deeper into the dermis (Figs. 17–9 and 17–10), the periadnexal collars may finally penetrate the basement membrane, or the repression of adnexal epithelium by the dysplastic epidermis may lead to follicular atrophy and replacement by invasive epithelium (Fig. 17–14).

Lichen Planus–like Keratosis

Only a few years ago, Shapiro and Ackermann (1966), Lumpkin and Helwig (1966), and Hirsch and Marmelzat (1967) independently called attention to peculiar lesions on sun-exposed skin; Helwig cautiously called them solitary lichen planus, while Shapiro called them lichen planus–like keratosis. These are single, flat plaques, often occurring in skin bearing other actinic keratoses or showing other effects of weathering. Histologically, they are almost indistinguishable from true lichen planus. In contrast to the parakeratotic keratosis senilis, they show orthokeratotic hyperkeratosis. The malpighian layer

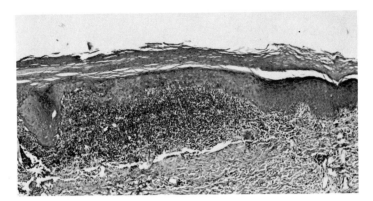

Figure 17–15 Lichen planus-like actinic keratosis. *H&E*, ×45.

consists of hypertrophic cells, and there may be some liquefaction necrosis of basal cells. There is a dense subepidermal zone of round cell infiltrate (Fig. 17–15). To my knowledge, no cases have been reported in which this type of lesion progressed to invasive carcinoma. It is important, however, to be aware of it, because biopsy usually is done under the clinical diagnosis of actinic keratosis vs. carcinoma, and the patients have no other lesions of lichen planus.

Large Cell Acanthoma

Occasionally (Pinkus, 1967 and 1970), lesions biopsied as actinic keratoses present an orthokeratotic epidermis, which consists of unusually large cells with unusually large nuclei which stain about the same density as normal nuclei and therefore are probably hyperchromatic. The involved stretches of epidermis have a cell-sharp border against surrounding epidermis and enclosed adnexa (Fig. 17–16). The epidermis either is of fairly normal thickness or is thickened in a papillomatous manner. While the nuclei often are somewhat uneven in size, the gross abnormalities of Bowen's dermatosis are absent, and the nuclear-cytoplasmic ratio is not altered in favor of the nuclei. Mitoses are uncommon and are of normal configuration, although they are considerably larger than normal mitotic figures. Inflammatory infiltrate is absent or minor. Photometric measurements have confirmed increased DNA content of the nuclei (Fand and Pinkus, 1970). The lesions seem to represent the establishment of an unusual strain of hyperploid, but presumably benign, keratinocytes in sun-exposed skin. More than 20 such lesions have been collected over a number of years, almost all of them in female patients.

Lentigo Senilis

Lentigo senilis is discussed here briefly because it is a not uncommon lesion in sun-exposed skin, most commonly found on the back of the hands, and because it seems to be able to progress either to squamous cell carcinoma or to the Dubreuilh melanosis type of malignant melanoma (Pinkus and Mehregan, 1969).

Clinically these lesions, often called liver spots by laymen, are gray or brown and rough and usually do not exceed 1 cm. in size. Histologically (Cawley and Curtis, 1950; Schnitzler et al., 1968) they are orthokeratotic. The epidermis (Fig. 17–17) has peculiar bulbous buds projecting into the dermis, their lower ends often deeply pigmented and exhibiting an increase of junctional melanocytes. Inflammatory infiltrate usually is absent, and its presence should make one suspect malignant transformation. This may take the form of increased budding, the buds penetrating deeper (Fig. 17–18) and showing central keratinization. True invasive squamous cell carcinoma may supervene. In other cases, the number and size of junctional melanocytes increase, they become atypical, and the picture merges into that of Dubreuilh's precancerous melanosis (lentigo maligna).

Disseminated Superficial Actinic Porokeratosis

While typical porokeratosis of Mibelli may occur anywhere on the body and has

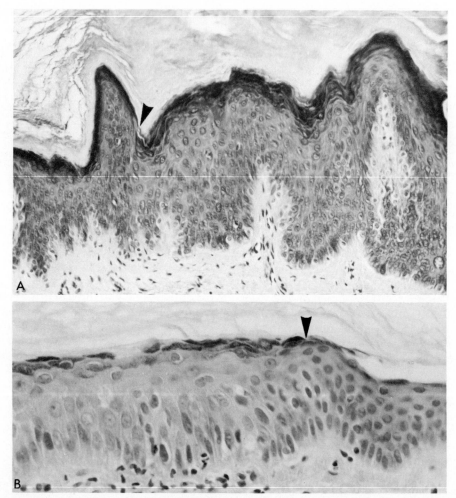

Figure 17–16   Large cell acanthoma. *S,* Slightly papillomatous lesion. *H&E,* ×*135.* B, Flat lesion. *H&E,* ×*180.* The borders between normal and abnormal epidermis are indicated by arrows. Note the accentuation of the granular layer and thicker horny layer in the acanthoma. (*From* Pinkus: Acta Dermatol. (Kyoto), 65:53, 1970.)

distinctive clinical features, there has been described a flat, scaly, rather inconspicuous lesion which may be present in considerable profusion on the sun-exposed skin of predisposed individuals and which is characterized histologically (Fig. 17–19) by a "cornoid lamella" of rather small depth. It therefore has been given the name "disseminated superficial actinic porokeratosis" (DSAP) by Chernosky and Freeman (1967). It has not been implicated as a precancerous lesion.

Actinic Skin

In between definite lesions, actinic skin has special histologic features which per-

mit the observer to make a diagnosis of solar effect, even if the biopsy is submitted for other purposes. These features must be identifiable in a section in order to permit a diagnosis of actinic keratosis as distinct from Bowen's dermatosis or arsenical keratosis.

The epidermis usually is slightly thinner than average and may show flattening of the rete ridges. It should be remembered that ridges are flat or absent in facial epidermis, even in youthful skin. Minor cytologic changes can be identified by electron microscopy (Mitchell, 1969; Everett, 1974). The upper third or half of the dermis has a gray or bluish appearance in hematoxylin and eosin–stained sections; it shows the change that old texts used to

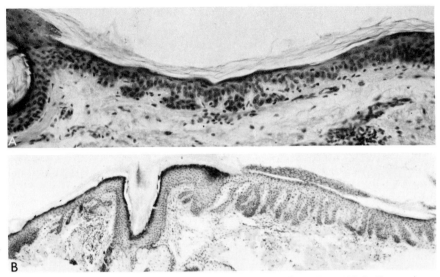

Figure 17–17 Lentigo senilis. *A,* An early lesion with short basal buds. *H&E, ×180. B,* Comparison of ortho-keratotic lentigo senilis to the left of the hair follicle with parakeratotic keratosis senilis to the right. The latter preserves some of the features of lentigo senilis. *H&E, ×60.*

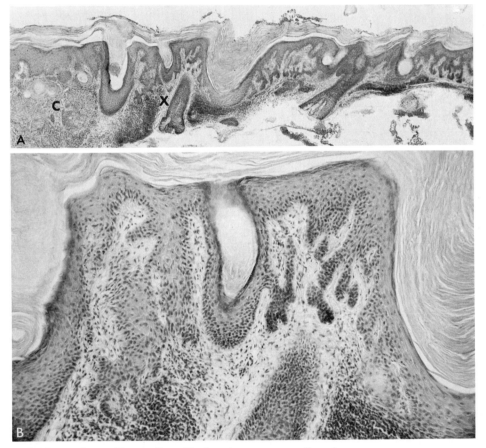

Figure 17–18 Lentigo senilis complicated by invasive squamous cell carcinoma.

A, Orthokeratotic epidermis with branching, pigmented, basal buds. At left border, full-blown invasive squamous cell carcinoma (*C*) with horn pearls is present in the dermis. At *X,* beginning invasion of nonpigmented epithelium is visible. Fairly heavy inflammatory infiltrate is present. *H&E, ×30.*

B, The area near *X* at higher magnification; photograph of a neighboring section. *H&E, ×135.*

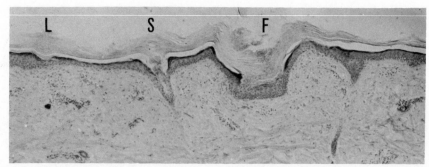

Figure 17–19   Actinic porokeratosis. Cross section of the peripheral parakeratotic lamella *(L)* and parakeratotic plugs in the sweat duct *(S)* and a hair follicle *(F)* within the disk of altered epidermis. *H&E, ×60.*

describe as "basophilic degeneration of collagen." We now use the expression "actinic elastosis" or "solar elastosis." Much has been written about the histogenesis of this feature—whether the alteration is a modification of collagen or new formation of elastic tissue. The latter view appears to be more likely (Lansing et al., 1953; Braun-Falco, 1956).

A narrow zone below the epidermis always remains free of elastotic changes. If elastic fiber stains are used, preferably the acid orcein-Giemsa combination (Luna, 1968), mild degrees of sun-induced changes appear as an increase of coarse elastic fibers in fairly normal arrangement in the reticular dermis. More pronounced stages exhibit curling and clumping of fibers, which may be merged into amorphous masses. At the same time, they are apt to lose their affinity to orcein and to stain blue with the basic component of the Giemsa mixture. The presence of silver-stainable reticulum fibers in the areas of solar elastosis speaks for active formation of new fibers. The everyday experience that actinic skin withstands ordinary trauma well and heals just as fast as normal skin after surgery has been confirmed experimentally by Serri and Cerimele (1967). To consider actinic elastosis an adaptation of the skin is probably closer to the truth than to consider it a degenerative process.

The eccrine and pilosebaceous apparatuses are not specifically affected in actinic skin, although the latter may vary from atrophy to hyperplasia. Small blood vessels often are ectatic.

DIFFERENTIAL DIAGNOSIS

Actinic keratoses must be differentiated from inflammatory lesions, benign nevi

and neoplasms, other precancerous dermatoses, and invasive skin cancer. Expert clinical examination can accomplish a great deal, but histologic confirmation is required in many cases.

Inflammatory Lesions

Clinical differentiation from chronic eczematous dermatitis, lichen simplex, and psoriasis or seborrheic dermatitis is relatively easy if one keeps in mind that the scale of actinic keratosis is neither branny nor lamellated, that it is firmly adherent, that its removal is usually associated with disagreeable tenderness or pain, and that after it has been removed a fragile bleeding or oozing surface remains. All these features, however, do not help in differentiation from a plaque of discoid lupus erythematosus (LE) or from lichen planus (LP), and some actinic keratoses of the atrophic type or the LP-like variety may be clinically indistinguishable from LE.

Histologically, none of the inflammatory lesions has the cell-sharp borders between normal and abnormal epithelium. Especially in lupus erythematosus, the atrophic orthokeratotic epithelium of the epidermis is continuous with the similarly involved epithelium of the follicles. One should not be confused by heavy round cell infiltrate, which may be almost as heavy in keratosis senilis as in LE. The differentiation, however, of the LP-like keratosis from true LP or a LP-like plaque of LE may be extremely insecure.

Benign Nevi and Neoplasms

Palpation and close clinical inspection, assisted by a magnifying glass, reveal many useful differential features. Actinic keratosis is rough and dry and rarely has any substance except for piled-up horny material. Epidermal nevi and seborrheic keratoses (seborrheic verrucae) are papillomas; their epidermis is thickened and often gives them a "stuck-on" appearance (Fig. 17–5*B*). Removal of their horny layer by scraping or soaking leaves behind an elevation consisting of the hyperplastic living portion of the epidermis, while most actinic keratoses, after removal of the keratinized portion, are flush with the surrounding skin. Actinic keratosis has few surface markings, while epidermal nevi and seborrheic verrucae show tiny round, elongated, or curved depressions due to their papillomatous character. Nevus cell nevi of junction type usually have a smooth, shiny surface, while intradermal nevi may have either a normal or a papillomatous surface pattern.

Histologic differentiation is accomplished by the features described on the preceding pages.

Porokeratosis of Mibelli may be considered here. The typical lesion is a slightly atrophic, rarely verrucous, disk. Close inspection reveals the characteristic rim bearing a parakeratotic fringe inserted in a groove. This feature, however, may be so inconspicuous in the actinic form (see pp. 449, 450) that it can be recognized only by histologic examination.

Other Precancerous Conditions and Intraepidermal Neoplasms

These disorders include Bowen's dermatosis, Paget's dermatosis, and the various types of intraepidermal epitheliomas discussed in Chapter 19. Actinic cheilitis, xeroderma pigmentosum, and cutaneous horn are so closely related to actinic keratosis that differentiation is based on location and other circumstances rather than on morphologic criteria. The same is true for keratoses due to x-ray, radium, tar, and arsenic. Bowen's dermatosis (BD) may occur on covered or sun-exposed areas of the body. Actinic keratoses may have histologic features closely resembling BD. The question arises whether definite

differential diagnosis can be established in exposed skin, and also whether distinction has practical value. The latter question may be answered by saying that actinic keratoses are more likely to become invasive than is BD, while BD may be associated with internal cancer. Therefore, distinction is of some value. Clinically, both lesions are very similar, but BD may attain larger size and often is a solitary plaque. If the patient also has lesions on covered parts of the body, then the one on the exposed skin probably is part of the disease.

Histologically, minor degrees of bowenoid dyskeratosis (Fig. 17–9) are so common in actinic keratosis that one should require a very typical picture of BD before considering that diagnosis. The presence of orthokeratotic portions speaks against keratosis senilis, the outstanding feature of which is parakeratosis. The nuclear-cytoplasmic ratio also should be taken into account. Relatively small size of the cell bodies shifts it in favor of the nucleus in BD (Clark and Watson, 1961). The dysplastic epidermis is more apt to overpower the adnexal epithelium in BD and to lead to loss of adnexal umbrellas and downgrowth of dyskeratotic cells into the infundibulum.

Paget's disease of the extramammary type (Paget's dermatosis) very rarely develops in sun-exposed areas. Clinically, it is more apt to be crusting or oozing rather than hyperkeratotic. Histologically, differential diagnosis is simple (see Chapter 19). Other lesions exhibiting intraepidermal nests of neoplastic cells occasionally become a factor in differential diagnosis, because they have a peculiar preference for the skin of the lower legs, an area definitely exposed to sun in women. These intraepidermal epitheliomas of the Jadassohn or Smith-Coburn type (see Chapter 19) form flat, scaly plaques easily confused with the lesions in actinic keratosis or Bowen's disease. Histologic distinction is based on the presence of intraepidermal islands of atypical cells surrounded on all sides by normal keratinocytes. This is in sharp contrast to keratosis senilis, in which the entire thickness of the epidermis is replaced by dysplastic cells, or dysplastic cells form a solid layer below normal upper strata.

Invasive Carcinomas and Epitheliomas

Actinic keratoses are precursors of squamous cell carcinoma and may be found associated with basal cell epitheliomas, many of which seem to be related to sun exposure.

It may be quite difficult to clinically differentiate actinic keratoses from those very superficial basal cell epitheliomas which spread along the lower surface of the epidermis and are not nodular or pearly. These basaliomas are rarely hyperkeratotic, although they may present occasional crusts and tiny ulcers. There is no proof that actinic keratoses give rise to basal cell epitheliomas, although they may occasionally develop into small-celled squamous cell carcinomas, which may be mistaken for basaliomas if one considers cell size and stainability alone and does not pay attention to epithelial-mesenchymal organization.

One of the most important problems is the differentiation of an actinic keratosis in the precancerous or carcinoma in situ stage from one which has transformed into invasive squamous cell carcinoma. Clinically, this process may be heralded by the subjective symptom of tenderness or pain. It is not unusual to have a patient point out one of several keratoses as the one he wants to have removed because it is "acting up." Objectively, these lesions may show increased redness, piled-up keratin, or crusting above an oozing surface. The histologic features of early invasion were described under pathology. The question remains, however, as to at what point the pathologist should give the clinician a diagnosis of squamous cell carcinoma rather than actinic keratosis with atypical budding. Several considerations complicate the answer. The invasive process usually starts at one or several small points which may be missed unless multiple sections are examined. It is objectively difficult to determine true invasion with loss of PAS-positive basement membrane and destruction of dermal elements unless special stains are employed. A good criterion is production of isolated nests associated with central keratinization. Multiple sections may be required to ascertain this feature.

Beyond the difficulties of objective evaluation of pathologic criteria, there are difficulties of communication between medical people of different training and philosophy. It must be realized that a lesion which fulfills all objective criteria of histologic invasion but is restricted to the upper third of the dermis may not require any more treatment than a preinvasive keratosis. To give the diagnosis of squamous cell carcinoma to a therapist to whom the word carcinoma means the necessity for major surgery or high doses of irradiation may expose the patient to increased morbidity and expense. On the other hand, a lesion that is not truly invasive but in which dysplastic epithelium has crept relatively far down around the adnexa will require more thorough treatment than superficial curettage and cautery. As in many other situations, the pathologist is well advised to have personal contact with the clinicians he serves, to be acquainted with their therapeutic philosophies, and to acquaint them with the exact significance of his diagnostic terms. Sometimes it is preferable to render a diagnosis of "actinic keratosis with early invasive budding" rather than "early invasive squamous cell carcinoma arising in actinic keratosis."

PROGNOSIS

Since rational treatment of actinic keratoses depends on a full understanding of their biologic potential, prognosis will be considered next. Actinic keratoses may progress to invasive squamous cell carcinoma (Montgomery, 1939; Woringer, 1961). We must ask how often this happens and how dangerous the carcinomas are.

Lund (1965) recently championed the view that carcinomas arising in actinic keratoses rarely metastasize. If this is correct, then treatment can be conservative. It is my opinion that Lund's teaching is applicable to modern practice and particularly to city practice. If actinic carcinomas remain untreated for many years, as may happen in rural populations under primitive conditions, I would not doubt that they do metastasize.

The question of the percentage of keratoses progressing to carcinoma is difficult to answer. There is little doubt that some actinic keratoses disappear spontaneously. They consist of diseased epithelium which is in precarious balance with healthy epithelium of the adnexa. Minor trauma or infection may damage the dysplastic epithelium and cause it to be cast off. This mechanism probably explains the good results of some relatively ineffective therapeutic procedures. It may play a large role in the beneficial effects of topical 5-fluorouracil (5-FU).

Montgomery (1939) estimated that 20 per cent of actinic keratoses progress to carcinoma. This figure appears to be high. Many patients have a great number of keratoses and develop only one or a few carcinomas. It has even been said that, while solar keratoses are found roughly in the same distribution as carcinomas, this may be a parallel development rather than a sequential one (Carmichael, 1961). Application of topical 5-FU has shown that there may be dozens or even hundreds of subclinical keratoses in skin which presents only a limited number of clinical lesions. The percentage of keratoses undergoing progression is further decreased by modern preventive therapy. All in all, actinic keratoses should not be trifled with, but they are no cause for undue alarm and heroic forms of therapy.

TREATMENT

On the basis of the preceding discussion, recommended treatment is conservative. The risk of dire consequences from malignancy should be carefully measured against avoiding morbidity and cosmetic disfigurement.

Available modalities are irradiation, surgery, and chemosurgery. X-radiation or radium usually are contraindicated in actinically damaged skin unless invasive carcinoma definitely complicates the case. Surgical procedures can use the knife or the curet. Full-thickness excision of the skin is not necessary in a noninvasive process but may be indicated if excision and suture promise the best cosmetic result.

Generally, actinic keratoses can be completely removed by sharp curettage, which usually is followed by electrodesiccation to ensure hemostasis and destruction of possibly remaining viable cells. Healing generally is prompt from adnexal epithelium remaining in the wound. Scars are pliable and inconspicuous except where their pale color contrasts with the telangiectatic redness of the surrounding skin.

Chemical agents have been used for a long time. The old ones remain effective in expert hands, and a new one, 5-FU, is producing dramatic results. Among the old remedies, trichloroacetic acid and bichloroacetic acid are very effective for strictly intraepidermal lesions. Liquefied phenol may be used. Other caustics are obsolete. The topical application of 5-FU, pioneered by Dillaha and his group (1963 and 1965), has found wide acceptance among dermatologists. Its rate of action can be increased by ultraviolet exposure (Kostel, 1970). Most recently, retinoic acid (vitamin A acid) has been advocated (Barranco et al., 1970). Its place in the therapy of actinic keratoses will have to be evaluated. Therapeutic methods are discussed in more detail in Chapter 24.

One point should be stressed. While it may not be necessary to do a biopsy on every noninfiltrated, quiescent keratosis, histologic confirmation should be sought whenever possible and certainly when crusting, inflammation, and thickening suggest the possibility of invasive cancer. This requirement need not delay treatment. Any excised tissue should, of course, be sent to the laboratory. If curettage is used, a forceful first stroke of the curet will usually obtain enough material to enable an experienced pathologist to make a diagnosis. Any lesion that recurs after initial treatment must be biopsied.

The author's practical approach to the management of a patient who has severely weather-beaten skin and numerous keratoses follows. Thorough inspection and palpation of all exposed areas will determine how many lesions are frank or suspected carcinomas. These should be biopsied and treated as indicated. If carcinoma has been treated or ruled out, 5-FU may be used to treat the entire face. If this is not feasible or not indicated, one should select a half dozen or more lesions which appear active and destroy them by curettage and electrodesiccation. A one-half per cent solution of gentian violet is then applied to the treated areas, using a fairly dry, small, cotton applicator. This seems to prevent infection and to promote healing. More lesions may be treated at a return visit a week or two later, or the patient may be asked to return after three to six months for reevaluation and treatment of any lesions that have acted up. At the same time, he is instructed to avoid unnecessary sun exposure and to wear a wide-brimmed hat. The use of protective creams is a two-edged sword. If the patient is careless once, he will burn severely. The conservative approach is usually effective and sanitizes the skin without excessive morbidity or cosmetic disturbance.

There remains the question of preventive therapy. Prevention, to be truly effective, should be practiced early in life by those individuals prone to develop actinic skin and keratoses. Generally, however, the patient seeks advice only when damage has already been done. Even then, protection from more insolation should be advocated vigorously. Protective clothing and sun screening lotions and creams should be prescribed in addition to the advice to stay out of the sun as much as possible. Beyond these measures, the question has been raised whether removal of damaged but not definitely diseased tissue and its replacement by "new skin" can prevent further development of keratoses and cancer for a prolonged period. The answer to this question is affirmative. The next question naturally follows: how much must be removed in order to achieve a beneficial effect? The answer touches the previously discussed controversy of whether the epidermis is damaged directly by the sun or secondarily by alterations in the dermis. It has been shown that dermabrasion, which removes not only epidermis but also the major portion of the elastotic dermis, is definitely beneficial (Epstein, 1970), and it was inferred that the effect is due to the removal of the dermis. The similarly beneficial effect of 5-FU, which destroys only diseased epithelium, supports the view that all that is needed is a new epidermis arising from sun-protected healthy adnexal epithelium. Application of 5-FU certainly has provided a technically easier and less disabling means of preventive therapy (Dillaha et al., 1965).

REFERENCES

Allen, A. C.: The Skin. Ed. 2. New York, Grune & Stratton, 1967.

Andrade, R.: Die prëcanceröse und canceröse Wucherung von Epidermis und Anhangsgebilden. *In* Jadassohn's Handbuch der Haut- und Geschlechtskrankheiten Ergänzungswerk. I,2:344, Berlin, Springer Verlag, 1964.

Auerbach, H.: Geographic variation in incidence of skin cancer in the United States. Publ. Health Rep., 76:345, 1961.

Barranco, V. P., Olson, R. L., and Everett, M. A.: Response of actinic keratoses to topical vitamin A acid. Cutis, 6:681, 1970.

Becker, S. W.: Dermatological nomenclature. Arch. Dermatol., 80:778, 1959.

Belisario, J. C.: Cancer of the Skin. London, Butterworth & Company, Ltd., 1959.

Belisario, J. C.: Epidemiology of the commoner skin cancers, solar keratoses, and keratoacanthomas. *In* Simons, R. D. G. P., and Marshall, J. (Eds.): Essays on Tropical Dermatology. Amsterdam, Excerpta Medica Monograph, 1969.

Blum, H. F.: Sunlight as a causal factor in cancer of the skin of man. J. Natl. Cancer Inst., 9:247, 1948.

Blum, H. F.: Carcinogenesis by Ultraviolet Light. Princeton, Princeton University Press, 1959.

Braun-Falco, O.: Über das Wesen der senilen Elastosis. Dermatol. Wochenschr., 134:1021, 1956.

Braun-Falco, O.: Pathologische Veränderungen an Grundsubstanz, Kollagen und Elastica. *In* Jadassohn's Handbuch der Haut- und Geschlechtskrankheiten Ergänzungswerk. I,2:519, Berlin, Springer-Verlag, 1964.

Braun-Falco, O., and Langner, A.: Zur Histochemie und Histogenese der Keratosis senilis. Arch. Klin. Exp. Dermatol., 226:336, 1966.

Carmichael, G. S.: The epidemiology of skin cancer in Queensland. The signficance of premalignant conditions. Br. J. Cancer, 15:425, 1961.

Caro, M. R., and Szymanski, F. J.: Symposium on diseases of skin; seborrheic and senile keratoses. Med. Clin. North Am., 35:419, 1951.

Cawley, E. P., and Curtis, A. C.: Lentigo senilis. Arch. Dermatol., 62:635, 1950.

Cawley, E. P., Hsu, Y. T., and Weary, P. E.: The basement membrane in relation to carcinoma of the skin. Arch. Dermatol., 94:712, 1966.

Chernosky, M. E., and Freeman, R. G.: Disseminated superficial actinic porokeratosis. Arch. Dermatol., 96:611, 1967.

Clark, W. H., Jr., and Watson, M. C.: The comparative study of normal human epidermal cells and the cells of carcinoma in situ (Bowen's disease) by planimetry. Proc. Am. Soc. Cell Biol., 1961.

Cleaver, J. E.: Defective repair replication of DNA in xeroderma pigmentosum. Nature (Lond.), 218:652, 1968.

Cleaver, J. E.: DNA damage and repair in light sensitive human skin. J. Invest. Dermatol., 54:181, 1970.

Dillaha, C. J., Jansen, G. T., Honeycutt, W. M., and

Bradford, A. C.: Selective cytotoxic effect of topical 5-fluorouracil. Arch. Dermatol., 88:247, 1963.

Dillaha, C. J., Jansen, G. T., Honeycutt, W. M., and Holt, G. A.: Further studies with topical fluorouracil. Arch. Dermatol., 92:410, 1965.

Dubreuilh, W.: Epithéliomatose d'origine solaire. Ann. Dermatol. Syphyligr. (Paris), 8:386, 1907.

Epstein, E.: Skin Surgery. Ed. 3. Springfield, Ill., Charles C Thomas, Publisher, 1970.

Everett, M. A.: Actinic degeneration of skin; a clinical histologic correlation. Brit. J. Dermatol., 1974.

Fand, S. B., and Pinkus, H.: Polyploidy in benign epidermal neoplasia. J. Cell Biol., 47:52a, 1970.

Freudenthal, W.: Verruca senilis und Keratoma senile. Arch. Dermatol. Syph. (Berl.), 152:505, 1926.

Gellin, G. A., Kopf, A. W., and Garfinkel, L.: Basal cell epithelioma; a controlled study of associated factors. Arch. Dermatol., 91:38, 1965.

Halter, K.: Über ein wenig beachtetes histologisches Kennzeichen des Keratoma senile. Hautarzt, 3:215, 1952.

Hirsch, P., and Marmelzat, W. L.: Lichenoid actinic keratosis. Dermatol. Internatl., 6:101, 1967.

Jablonska, S., and Chorzelski, T.: Epitheliomas presenting features of Darier's type dyskeratosis. II. Dyskeratotic epithelioma (carcinoma). Przegl. Dermatol., 48:195, 1961.

Kostel, J., Jr.: Treatment of actinic keratosis. Arch. Dermatol., 102:351, 1970.

Lansing, A. I., Cooper, Z. K., and Rosenthal, T. B.: Some properties of degenerative elastic tissue (senile elastosis). Anat. Rec., 115:340, 1953.

Lever, W. F.: Histopathology of the Skin. Ed. 4. Philadelphia, J. B. Lippincott Co., 1967.

Lumpkin, L. R., and Helwig, E. R.: Solitary lichen planus. Arch. Dermatol., 93:54, 1966.

Luna, L. G.: Manual of the Histologic Staining Methods of the Armed Forces Institute of Pathology. Ed. 3. New York, McGraw-Hill Book Company, 1968.

Lund, H. Z.: Atlas of Tumor Pathology, Section 1, Fascicle 2: Tumors of the Skin. Washington, D.C., Armed Forces Institute of Pathology, 1957.

Lund, H. Z.: How often does squamous cell carcinoma of the skin metastasize? Arch. Dermatol., 92:635, 1965.

Mackie, B. S., and McGovern, V. J.: Mechanism of solar carcinogenesis. Arch. Dermatol., 78:218, 1958.

Mishima, Y., and Rudner, E. J.: Erythromelanosis follicularis faciei et colli. Dermatologica, 132:269, 1966.

Mitchell, R. E.: Chronic solar dermatosis; an electron-microscopic study of the epidermis. Australas. J. Dermatol., 10:75, 1969.

Montgomery, H.: Precancerous dermatosis and epithelioma in situ. Arch. Dermatol., 39:387, 1939.

Montgomery, H.: Dermatopathology. New York, Hoeber Medical Division, 1967.

Niebauer, G.: Keratosis senilis (actinica) and carcinogenesis. Ann. Ital. Derm. Clin. Speriment., 22:375, 1968.

Papa, C. M., Carter, D. M., and Kligman, A. M.: The effect of autotransplantation on the progression or reversibility of aging in human skin. J. Invest. Dermatol., 54:200, 1970.

Pensley, N., and Sims, C. F.: Keratosis senilis with epidermal splits. Arch. Dermatol., 83:951, 1961.

Pinkus, H.: Keratosis senilis; a biologic concept of its pathogenesis and diagnosis. Am. J. Clin. Pathol., 29:193, 1958.

Pinkus, H.: Malignant transformation of epithelium. *In* McKenna, R. M. B. (Ed.): Modern Trends in Dermatology. Ed. 3. London, Butterworth, 1966, p. 275.

Pinkus, H.: The borderline between cancer and noncancer. Year Book of Dermatology 1966/67. Chicago, Year Book Medical Publishers, 1967a, p. 5.

Pinkus, H.: Large cell acanthoma. Presented at University of Kyoto (Japan), April, 1967b.

Pinkus, H.: Epidermal mosaic in benign and precancerous neoplasia. Acta Dermatol. (Kyoto), 65:53, 1970.

Pinkus, H., and Mehregan, A. H.: A Guide to Dermatohistopathology. New York, Appleton-Century-Crofts, 1969.

Pinkus, H., Jallad, M. S., and Mehregan, A. H.: The inflammatory infiltrate of precancerous skin lesions. J. Invest. Dermatol., 41:247, 1963.

Portugal, G. H., and Rocha, L.: La queratosis senil y las disqueratosis desde el punto de vista histológico. Act. Dermo-sifiliogr. (Madr.), 41:408, 1950.

Quisenberry, W. B.: Ethnic differences in skin cancer in Hawaii. *In* Conference on Biology of Cutaneous Cancer. National Cancer Institute Monograph No. 10, 1963, p. 181.

Reed, W. B., Landing, B., Sugarman, G., Cleaver, J. E., and Melnyk, J.: Xeroderma pigmentosum; clinical and laboratory investigation of its basic defect. J.A.M.A., 207:2073, 1969.

Schnitzler, L., Degos, R., and Civatte, J.: Tâches pigmentées séniles du dos des mains; étude histologique de 50 cas. Bull. Soc. Fr. Dermatol. Syphiligr., 75:550, 1968.

Serri, F., and Cerimele, D.: Le comportement des fibres élastiques dans la réparation des plaies cutanées provoquées sur la peau sénile exposée ou non exposée à la lumière. Ann. Dermatol. Syphiligr. (Paris), 94:491, 1967.

Shapiro, L., and Ackermann, A. B.: Solitary lichen planus–like keratosis. Dermatologica, 132:356, 1966.

Ten Seldam, R. E. J.: Skin cancer in Australia. *In* Conference on Biology of Cutaneous Cancer. National Cancer Institute Monograph No. 10, 1963, p. 153.

Unna, P. G.: Die Histopathologie der Hautkrankheiten. Berlin, August Hirschwald, 1894.

Urbach, E.: Imbibitio lipoidica telae elasticae degeneratae. Acta Derm. Venereol. (Stockh.), 15:69, 1934.

Urbach, F.: The Biologic Effects of Ultraviolet Radiation. New York, Pergamon Press, 1969.

Weiss, P.: Perspectives in the field of morphogenesis. Quart. Rev. Biol., 25:177, 1950.

Woringer, F.: De la kérotose sénile à l'épithélioma. Dermatologica, 122:349, 1961.

18

Chronic Radiodermatitis and Skin Cancer

Paulino L. Getzrow, M.D.

HISTORY

In November, 1895, Roentgen discovered so-called x-rays. Seven years later, Frieben (1902), in Germany, reported the first malignant neoplasm of the skin attributable to x-rays. This occurred in a technician who for four years had been blithely demonstrating Roentgen tubes by holding his hand under them while activated; he then developed a squamous cell carcinoma on the dorsum of that hand and later metastases to the cubital and axillary lymph nodes. Fourteen years later, in 1909, Cecil Rowntree in his Hunterian lecture referred to nine American and 11 English cases of cutaneous carcinoma caused by x-rays, the earliest case in England being in 1904 (Henry, 1950). In the same year Wolbach (1909) did the first extensive histopathologic study of cancer of the skin following x-radiation.

The earliest experimental sarcoma in animals caused by x-rays was produced in a rat in 1920 by P. Marie, J. Clunet, and G. Rulet-Lapointe (Glucksmann, 1958); the earliest carcinoma was produced in rabbits in 1924 by Block (Goodwin, 1952).

Kalz (1959) was the first to report malig-

nant degeneration of the skin in man after exposure to grenz rays alone. Shapiro et al. (1961) demonstrated experimentally in animals that grenz rays are carcinogenic.

GENERAL CONCEPTS

Radiodermatitis, according to Leider and Rosenblum (1968), designates all degrees of inflammation of the skin resulting from excessive exposure to electromagnetic energy of wavelengths less than 2 Å (radium, gamma or x-rays).

Chronic radiodermatitis may be a sequel to acute radiodermatitis, following shortly or delayed in its appearance by one or many years. It may also occur after exposures that have been insufficient to cause a clinically evident reaction, such as erythema or reactions of the acute type, but that have eventually been in excess of the ability of the skin to repair itself perfectly.

The mechanisms by which radiation induces neoplasia are as poorly understood as are the mechanisms of other carcinogens. Furth and Upton (1953) have studied extensively the carcinogenic effects of ionizing radiation in different tissues and in different species. They state that particle radiation, i.e., alpha and beta rays, produces the same changes as electromagnetic radiation: both are ionizing. However, whereas susceptibility to acute injury by ionizing radiation of any type and source is directly related to the rate of mitosis, liability to tumor induction is not dependent on the rate of cellular replication alone. Glucksmann (1958) says that irradiation seems to create environmental conditions for malignant changes in regenerating cells rather than to induce directly a malignant change in the irradiated cells themselves and in their descendents. According to Gofman and Tamplin (1970), "carcinogenic transformation" caused by radiation is not reversible, is not time-dependent, and is not subject to a dose threshold. They presume that the mechanisms involve certain kinds of injury to chromosomes and that this "carcinogenic transformation" of chromosomes caused by radiation is permanent; that the probability of such a transformation will depend simply on how much radiation is absorbed, not when; and that any amount of radiation, no matter how small, carries with it a certain possibility of carcinogenesis.

Before reviewing some specific statements made about the causal relationship between cutaneous cancer and ionizing radiation, it should be emphasized that ionizing radiation definitely has been shown, experimentally and circumstantially, to be carcinogenic in the skin. Occupational neoplasms in the skin, mainly squamous cell carcinomas, have been well-known since the introduction of x-ray therapy.

Sometimes there are difficulties in establishing a causal relationship between irradiation and cutaneous cancer. That is why malignancies as a result of therapeutic irradiation have been the subject of debate. Sulzberger et al. (1952) stated that no dangerous sequelae are produced when doses of "superficial" x-rays up to 1400 R. are used. In a study done by Epstein (1962), little difference was found with respect to previous history of x-ray therapy in groups of patients with (513) and without (525) epitheliomas at the time of examination.

However, epitheliomas appear to occur more often than can be accounted for by chance in areas which have been previously irradiated (Ridley, 1962). Martin et al. (1970) found that, of 457 patients who did not have skin cancer, only 23 (5 percent) had previously received irradiation, whereas of 192 patients, 36 (18.7 percent) who had skin cancer of the head and neck also had a history of previous irradiation of these areas for benign conditions. The study done by Macomber et al. (1959) also points to the same conclusion: in 853 lesions of cutaneous epitheliomas, when all possible causative factors were listed, association with radiation was found most frequently (29 percent of the cases; a figure of 53 percent of the cases having such an association was found in another study mentioned in the same publication). In the study done by Totten et al. (1957) of 105 patients with skin cancer, 20 (19 percent) had preexisting roentgenray dermatitis due to occupational exposure during radiotherapy for a benign condition. Shafer et al. (1949) studied 28 patients with skin cancer among a group of 85 patients with chronic radiodermatitis and stated that in this series neoplasms developed in persons of a younger age group than is ordinarily affected; moreover, they occurred more than twice as frequently among women than among men, which is the reverse of the usual phenomenon.

The role of grenz rays as carcinogenic agents is still being debated. Cipollaro and Crossland (1967) presented several cases as proof that grenz ray dermatitis is also precancerous. However, Epstein (1962) considers that, for this to be the case, the dosage must have grossly exceeded the recommended levels, or the sufferers must have been exposed to conventional x-radiation in addition to the borderline rays.

MATERIAL USED IN THIS STUDY

The cases of 79 patients with chronic radiodermatitis from the files of the Oncology Section of the Department of Dermatology of the New York University Medical Center were reviewed (Table 18–1).

Thirty (38 percent) of these patients did not develop keratoses, ulcers, or malignancies. The average time of observation of

TABLE 18-1   SUMMARY OF FINDINGS IN 79 PATIENTS WITH CHRONIC RADIODERMATITIS[*]

	Chronic Radio-dermatitis: 30 Cases	Chronic Radio-dermatitis With Radiation Kera-toses: 11 Cases	Chronic Radio-dermatitis With Ulceration: 10 Cases	Chronic Radio-dermatitis With Skin Malignancy: 28 Cases
Sex of Patients				
Males	9	5	6	5
Females	21	6	4	23
Cause for Radiation				
Internal malignancy	6	0	3	1
Skin malignancy	8	4	3	5
Benign skin tumor	8	0	4	0
Benign skin condition	8	7	0	22
Average Age:	46 years	58 years	56 years	60 years
Average Time of Observation	21 years	22 years	23 years	– – –
Average Time of Latency:	– – –	– – –	– – –	25 years

*From the files of the Oncology Section of the Department of Dermatology of the New York University Medical Center.

these patients was 21.5 years, and their average age was 46. If we accept the opinion that, after development of radiodermatitis, malignant skin changes will inevitably ensue if the patient lives long enough (Macomber et al., 1957), it follows that carcinomas did not develop in this group of patients because not enough time had passed. However, a closer examination of the facts makes such an assumption too pat.

According to some studies, the average latent period for malignancies in areas of radiodermatitis is 21 (Martin et al., 1970) to 28 years (Cannon et al., 1959). Pack and Davis (1965), in studying the latent period, take into consideration the type of irradiation, whereas Conway and Hugo (1966) make much of the type of carcinoma. In our material there are cases in which 30 years or more elapsed after irradiation, and still no carcinoma had appeared. Some of these patients were 40 years old or more. It is also significant that in 15 patients the radiodermatitis was situated on the face and neck, that is, in a place where neoplasms of the skin are more prone to develop spontaneously. This points to the fact that there are individuals with chronic radiodermatitis in whom cancer will not appear in the area of radiodermatitis "regardless of the amount of irradiation given, the extent of radiation sclerosis evi-

dent, or the amount of time which has elapsed" (Martin et al., 1970).

Our cases of chronic radiodermatitis showed defined areas of atrophic scarring with prominent telangiectasia. Hyperpigmentation, mainly at the periphery, and hypopigmentation, usually more marked in the center, were common. According to Miescher (1954), patients with radiodermatitis of the trunk and extremities have a considerably greater predisposition toward telangiectasia.

Eleven (14 percent) of the patients developed keratoses in the areas of chronic radiodermatitis, six of them on the extremities, sites which are predominantly affected by radiation keratoses (Saunders and Montgomery, 1938). Epstein (1962) has stated that radiation keratoses are more apt to occur following repeated small doses than following one or more large doses of radiation. Seven of our 11 patients showed this type of change as a result of irradiation of a benign condition. Kalz (1959) says keratoses are very rare after therapeutic grenz rays. The development of radiation keratoses in patients with chronic radiodermatitis and the subsequent development of cancer are not clearly established. Epstein (1962) considers radiation keratoses to be "the first definite step on the road to cancerous changes." For Montgomery (1967), keratoses must first develop before a carcinoma appears in patients with chronic radiodermatitis. Cipollaro and Crossland (1967) think that radiation keratoses are not inevitably premalignant, but they also state that malignant changes take place most frequently in relation to keratoses. Our patients with keratoses were followed for an average of 22 years, and there was no evidence of carcinoma. Lagrot (1966), in his

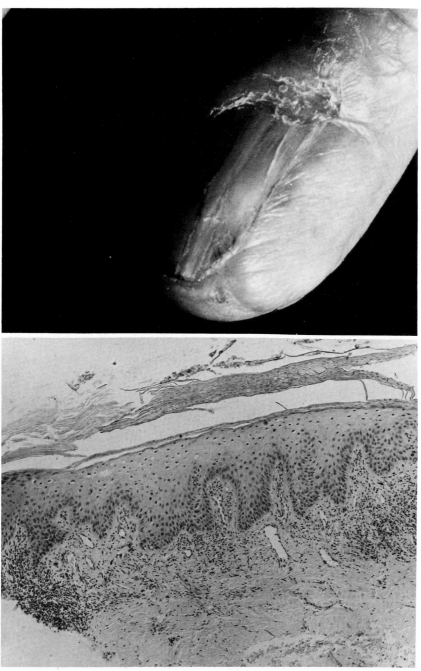

Figure 18–1 (Case No. 56.) Radiation keratosis. The patient is a 60 year old veterinarian who had been using a fluoroscope without protection for the past five years. (From the collection of the Dermatology Department of the New York University Medical Center.)

study of occupational radiodermatitis of the fingers, found that carcinomas developing in keratoses were superficial.

The radiation keratoses of our patients were moderately elevated, hard, usually brownish lesions of rather small size (Fig. 18–1). It is clinically difficult to determine when a radiation keratosis has transformed into cancer. A biopsy must be done to determine if such a transformation has or has not taken place.

Ten (12.6 percent) of our patients developed ulcers in the sites of chronic radiodermatitis. The ulcers usually appeared several years after irradiation. This was the only group of cases in which the number of males exceeded that of females (six to four). According to Cipollaro and Crossland (1967) and Saunders and Montgomery (1938), hands and feet are more prone to ulcer formation. There was no such tendency in the cases presented here. The relationship of ulcers and malignancies in areas of chronic radiodermatitis has been stressed by Duperrat and Andrade (1958), Totten et al. (1957), and Martin et al. (1970). Again it must be noted that our patients had been followed for a long period of time (23 years, on the average) without signs of a skin malignancy showing. Lagrot (1966) thinks that, when carcinomas of the fingers develop on ulcerations in patients with occupationally acquired radiodermatitis, they have infiltrative features. In general, there is clinical difficulty in differentiating between ulcers that have and those that have not gone on to malignant degeneration. Biopsies are essential. Specimens should be taken from the edge of ulcers that have developed in chronic radiodermatitis.

Of our 79 patients with chronic radiodermatitis, 28 (35 percent) had malignant skin neoplasms. Other studies in the literature report percentages that vary from 10 percent (Saunders and Montgomery, 1938; Duperrat and Andrade, 1958) to 55 percent (Mason, 1951). It should be noted that Mason's study was of radiodermatitis of the hands exclusively.

In our 28 patients, the average time between the irradiation and the diagnosis of the malignancy, the so-called latent period, was 25 years. Duperrat and Andrade (1958) in a review of the literature and from their own experience considered four years as the shortest possible latent period. The longest latent interval recorded in the literature is 64 years (Martin et al., 1970).

Twenty-two of the 28 malignancies were situated in areas of chronic radiodermatitis that followed irradiation of benign conditions, and 26 of them were on the face.

None of the patients in our series showed evidence of metastasis, but it has been reported in the literature. Hartwell et al. (1964) reported four cases of metastases out of a total of nine cases.

In one of our cases (case No. 27) death resulted from spreading of the tumor to neighboring areas. There is a mortality for roentgen carcinoma of 25 percent, according to Porter (1909) and Saunders and Montgomery (1938), and of 12 percent, according to Pack and Davis (1965). Duperrat and Andrade (1958) think that the chances of metastasis and the percentage of mortality are similar in radiogenic and spontaneous skin malignancy.

CLASSIFICATION

Meaningful conclusions are not easy to draw from a review of the literature. While some authors have studied the relationship between radiodermatitis and skin cancer from a general point of view, most have restricted their study to more specialized aspects. The problem becomes complex when one realizes that some authors deal only with lesions of the head and neck (Martin et al., 1970), while others deal with lesions of the hands (Hartwell et al., 1964) or of the head following x-ray epilation of the scalp (Albert and Omiran, 1968; Ridley, 1962).

One aspect of this problem, namely the type of radiation given, is considered in several reports. Hartwell et al. (1964) suggest that the type and depth of radiation and the dose and time span through which the radiation is received may determine the character of radiation injury. Pack and Davis (1965) and Teloh et al. (1950) indicate specifically that repeated smaller doses appear to induce skin cancers more readily than massive single doses. According to Glucksmann (1958), the depth of the initial radiation burn in relation to the thickness of skin structures influences the eventual effect.

Technical factors of x-ray quality and potential for malignancy have not been well studied using large, statistically significant samples and adequate controls. The main problem is lack of reliable information regarding technical factors, especially when several years have elapsed since x-ray procedures took place. The patient, of course, is not qualified to give such information with accuracy. I will try to overcome this problem in our series by grouping cases according to the reason for radiation being given. In this way similarity of technical factors may be assumed, because it is likely that radiation dosages were the same for each group of conditions cited, and therefore conclusions are likely to be valid.

I have cast our 79 cases into four groups, according to the reason for radiotherapy: treatment for (1) internal malignancies (10 cases), (2) skin malignancies (20 cases), (3) benign skin tumors (12 cases), and (4) benign, nontumorous conditions (37 cases).

Some patients have been followed in our Oncology Section for long periods of time, but the age stated in the tables corresponds to that at the time of the first consultation.

Chronic Radiodermatitis Resulting from Treatment of Internal Malignancies (Table 18–2)

Only in our case No. 10 (Fig. 18–2) did malignant degeneration to a basal cell carcinoma occur in an area of chronic radiodermatitis on the chest due to irradiation of a breast tumor. The remaining nine cases of chronic radiodermatitis resulting from irradiation of internal malignancies showed no cutaneous malignancies, although three of them had ulcer formation.

Other authors have noted the same low incidence of skin neoplasms in areas damaged as a result of irradiation of a deep malignancy. Conway and Hugo (1966) describe only two cases of cutaneous malignancies out of 58 cases of chronic radiodermatitis caused by irradiation of internal malignancies; Neuman et al. (1963) report 2 out of 45, and Cade (1957) reports 4 out of 34. In contrast, Conway and Hugo (1966) showed 24 skin neoplasms in 68 cases of chronic radiodermatitis resulting from irradiation for causes other than deep malignancies; Neuman et al. (1963) reported 43 in 70 cases. It is apparent that penetrating and intensive x-radiation for deep malignancies does not often cause cutaneous carcinomas (Teloh et al., 1950).

TABLE 18–2 CASES OF CHRONIC RADIODERMATITIS RESULTING FROM TREATMENT OF INTERNAL MALIGNANCIES

Case No.	Age	Sex	Localization	Cause for Radiation	Observation Time (Years)	Latency Time (Years)	End Result
1	61	F	face	mouth tumor	33	—	chronic radiodermatitis
2	35	F	neck	thyroid tumor	4	—	chronic radiodermatitis
3	61	F	chest	mammary tumor	1	—	chronic radiodermatitis
4	65	F	chest	mammary tumor	4	—	chronic radiodermatitis
5	62	F	chest	mammary tumor	9	—	chronic radiodermatitis
6	56	F	chest	Hodgkin's disease	44	—	chronic radiodermatitis
7	65	F	face (mandibular area)	parotid tumor	35	—	ulcer in chronic radiodermatitis
8	59	M	lumbar region	testicular tumor	26	—	ulcer in chronic radiodermatitis
9	78	F	lumbar region	hypernephroma	35	—	ulcer in chronic radiodermatitis
10	70	F	chest	mammary tumor	—	36	basal cell epithelioma in chronic radiodermatitis

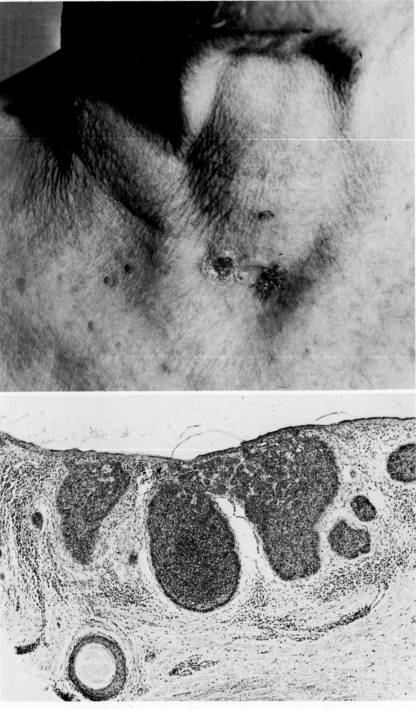

Figure 18–2   (Case No. 10.) Basal cell carcinomas in patient with chronic radiodermatitis of the chest. The patient is a 70 year old woman who had a mastectomy and radiotherapy of the left breast for a malignancy 36 years ago. (From the collection of the Dermatology Department of the New York University Medical Center.)

Our patients with chronic radiodermatitis in this group have remained without malignant changes for an average period of 21 years after irradiation. In the single patient who developed a basal cell carcinoma, the malignancy appeared 36 years after the area was irradiated.

It is apparent from a review of the literature that, no matter how long after irradiation a neoplasm appears, it is considered to be related to the therapeutic procedure. In elderly persons with carcinomas in areas known to be susceptible to spontaneous malignant degeneration, some doubt must be entertained about such a relationship. As I mentioned before, the longest interval recorded in the literature is 64 years (Martin et al., 1970). Considering the age of the patient and the location of the carcinoma on the face, it is likely that the neoplasm

TABLE 18–3 CASES OF CHRONIC RADIODERMATITIS RESULTING FROM TREATMENT OF SKIN MALIGNANCIES

Case No.	Age	Sex	Localization	Cause for Radiation	Observation Time (Years)	Latency Time (Years)	End Result
11	43	M	face (inner canthus)	basal cell epithelioma	26	—	chronic radiodermatitis
12	60	F	face (nose)	squamous cell carcinoma	13	—	chronic radiodermatitis
13	67	M	face (nose)	basal cell epithelioma	2	—	chronic radiodermatitis
14	61	M	face (nose)	basal cell epithelioma	10	—	chronic radiodermatitis
15	59	F	face (nose)	basal cell epithelioma	14	—	chronic radiodermatitis
16	45	M	face (cheek)	basal cell epithelioma	22	—	chronic radiodermatitis
17	74	M	face (lip)	basal cell epithelioma	10	—	chronic radiodermatitis
18	83	M	face (ear)	basal cell epithelioma	20	—	chronic radiodermatitis
19	70	M	face (nose)	basal cell epithelioma	4	—	ulcer in chronic radiodermatitis
20	69	M	face (nose)	squamous cell carcinoma	11	—	ulcer in chronic radiodermatitis
21	73	M	face (lip)	squamous cell carcinoma	8	—	ulcer in chronic radiodermatitis
22	50	F	face (nose)	basal cell epithelioma	25	—	keratosis in chronic radiodermatitis
23	65	M	face (lip)	squamous cell carcinoma	6	—	keratosis in chronic radiodermatitis
24	64	M	face (lip)	basal cell epithelioma	17	—	keratosis in chronic radiodermatitis
25	62	M	hand	squamous cell carcinoma	19	—	keratosis in chronic radiodermatitis
26	72	F	face (below eye)	basal cell epithelioma	—	2	keratoacanthoma in chronic radiodermatitis
27	86	M	face (ear)	basal cell epithelioma	—	1	squamous cell carcinoma in chronic radiodermatitis
28	71	M	face (forehead)	basal cell epithelioma	—	3	basal cell epithelioma in chronic radiodermatitis
29	55	F	face (forehead)	basal cell epithelioma	—	7	basal cell epithelioma in chronic radiodermatitis
30	64	F	face (nose)	basal cell epithelioma	—	13	basal cell epithelioma in chronic radiodermatitis

could have appeared even if no radiodermatitis had been induced in the area.

Chronic Radiodermatitis Resulting from Treatment of Skin Malignancies (Table 18–3)

Five of the 20 cases in which chronic radiodermatitis developed as a result of treatment of original skin cancer showed a malignant neoplasm in the area after treatment. This percentage is quite like that of Conway and Hugo (1966), who in five cases of irradiated basal cell epithelioma found one that developed squamous cell carcinoma in the area 26 years after the irradiation.

In considering this type of malignant development after irradiation of an original malignancy, a pertinent question arises: Is the new neoplasm really new? When a carcinoma of the same type develops in an area where a malignancy was present before, it is at least debatable whether the second carcinoma might not represent a failure to eradicate the original malignancy. Even when a different type of neoplasm evolves, it could be argued that one is dealing with a recrudescence of the original malignancy which changed its character because of the radiation. This could have been the event in our case No. 27.

Robinson and Masters (1960) state that very few malignancies develop within 10 years after irradiation. I already mentioned that Duperrat and Andrade (1958) consider four years as the shortest latent period. Of our five cases in which a "new" malignancy developed after irradiation, three had a latent period of three years or less; of the remaining two, one appeared after seven years, the other after 13.

Although radiodermatitis is inherently precancerous, its role in cases of skin cancer in which the "second" malignancy appears after a very short period of time is in doubt, and the possibility of a recurrence from treatment failure must be entertained.

With this in mind it appears, as in the series of cases in which radiation was given for treatment of internal malignancies, that the radiation as it is used for skin carcinomas causes few new malignancies.

Because the case of keratoacanthoma in an area of radiodermatitis (case No. 26) is the only one among all 79 cases, no prophetic conclusion can be drawn from it.

Chronic Radiodermatitis Resulting from Treatment of Benign Skin Tumors (Table 18–4)

The main feature in this group of cases is that none of these patients developed

TABLE 18–4 CASES OF CHRONIC RADIODERMATITIS RESULTING FROM TREATMENT OF BENIGN SKIN TUMORS

Case No.	Age	Sex	Localization	Cause for Radiation	Observation Time (Years)	Latency Time (Years)	End Result
31	16	F	face (forehead)	angioma	16	—	chronic radiodermatitis
32	9	F	face (cheek)	angioma	8	—	chronic radiodermatitis
33	40	F	chest	keloid	33	—	chronic radiodermatitis
34	58	F	chest	keloid	40	—	chronic radiodermatitis
35	11	M	chest	angioma	11	—	chronic radiodermatitis
36	18	F	chest	angioma	25	—	chronic radiodermatitis
37	22	F	abdomen	angioma	22	—	chronic radiodermatitis
38	17	F	arm	angioma	23	—	chronic radiodermatitis
39	11	M	face (cheek)	angioma	12	—	ulcer in chronic radiodermatitis
40	47	M	face (cheek)	angioma	35	—	ulcer in chronic radiodermatitis
41	31	F	thigh	angioma	38	—	ulcer in chronic radiodermatitis
42	59	F	sole	fibroma	6	—	ulcer in chronic radiodermatitis

malignancy. It is difficult to draw firm conclusions from the fact, because the patients constitute a young population. Moreover, they have only been followed for approximately 17 years.

In 9 of the 12 cases, the benign tumor treated with radiation was an angioma. Conway and Hugo (1966) mention three angiomas with subsequent radiodermatitis which did not develop malignancy and one which did. Of the 368 patients with radiation-induced skin cancer of the head and neck studied by Martin et al. (1970), 11 patients received irradiation for an angioma.

Chronic Radiodermatitis Resulting from Treatment of Benign, Nontumorous Conditions (Table 18–5)

I consider this group of cases the most important because it is the largest of the series (37 cases) and because it shows the highest percentage of malignant degeneration (22/37=60 percent). It should also be noted that 21 of the 22 malignancies occurred in the face, and that 20 of the 22 were basal cell carcinomas.

It was this group that decided me to group the cases of chronic radiodermatitis as I did. It is in this group that the reason for irradiation seems to play an important role in the development of malignant degeneration following radiotherapy. In 13 cases radiotherapy was administered for hirsutism (Fig. 18–3) and in six cases for acne. There may be argument about the representative character of this group because of its limited size, but correlation with other reports in the literature is suggestive of certain reasonable conclusions.

Acne and hirsutism were the reasons for which irradiation was given in 62 percent of the 368 patients with radiation-induced skin cancer of the head and neck in the series of Martin et al. (1970). Previous irradiation for acne is specifically mentioned in the patients with skin neoplasms by Totten et al. (1957), Cannon et al. (1959), and Robinson and Masters (1960). Cipollaro and Einhorn (1947) warned "that superfluous hair can not be permanently removed with radiation of any kind without permanent injury to the skin."

Even though the face is a common site for spontaneous development of skin cancer, it is worth noting that in this group all of the irradiated acne patients developed malignancies, and all but three patients irradiated because of hirsutism developed malignant skin neoplasms. In the previous groups of cases in this series, when irradiation was given to the face for internal malignancies (two cases) or for benign skin tumors (four cases), no skin malignancy developed. In the group in which chronic radiodermatitis resulted from irradiation of skin neoplasms, 14 patients did not develop a second cancer; five did, and I already noted that, in some of these, the distinction between a "second" malignancy and a recurrence is rather difficult to make.

I have mentioned the possibility that some of the cutaneous neoplasms appearing in areas where natural malignancies are frequent in elderly persons may not be related to chronic radiodermatitis. Such reasoning is not cogent in a group in which the percentage of cases with malignant degeneration in areas of chronic radiodermatitis is so high.

Contradictory statements can be found in the literature as to which of the malignant epitheliomas—basal cell or squamous cell—is the most frequent skin malignancy in areas of chronic radiodermatitis. Again it should be remembered that there are several factors to be considered when analyzing some statistics. In most publications that consider squamous cell carcinomas as the most frequent radiation-induced skin neoplasm, many cases are occupational (Leddy and Rigos, 1941), which means a special type of exposure and a particular localization. When the tumors reported were situated on the face, basal cell epitheliomas were usually the most frequently found (Anderson and Anderson, 1951). These differences due to anatomic localization have been specifically mentioned by Totten et al. (1957), Cannon et al. (1959), Robinson and Masters (1960), and Martin et al. (1970).

I have found no case of chronic radiodermatitis eventuating in a sarcoma, and this appears to be the experience of most authors, except Bloom-Ides (1950), Jones (1953), Pettit (1954), Anderson (1956), and Russell (1959). Whether some of these

TABLE 18–5 CASES OF CHRONIC RADIODERMATITIS RESULTING FROM TREATMENT
OF BENIGN CONDITIONS

Case No.	Age	Sex	Localization	Cause for Radiation	Observa-tion Time (Years)	Latency Time (Years)	End Result
43	65	M	scalp	tinea	57	—	chronic radiodermatitis
44	54	F	face (chin)	mumps	43	—	chronic radiodermatitis
45	55	F	face	hirsutism	37	—	chronic radiodermatitis
46	62	M	shoulder	bursitis	22	—	chronic radiodermatitis
47	32	F	arm	x-ray ex-aminations	19	—	chronic radiodermatitis
48	21	F	hand	x-ray ex-aminations	13	—	chronic radiodermatitis
49	37	F	hands and feet	dermatitis	47	—	chronic radiodermatitis
50	42	F	sole	warts	15	—	chronic radiodermatitis
51	38	F	face	hirsutism	24	—	keratosis in chronic radiodermatitis
52	67	F	face	hirsutism	35	—	keratosis in chronic radiodermatitis
53	61	F	shoulder	bursitis	27	—	keratosis in chronic radiodermatitis
54	47	F	hand	dermatitis	39	—	keratosis in chronic radiodermatitis
55	56	F	hand	dermatitis	39	—	keratosis in chronic radiodermatitis
56	60	M	hand	occupational	5	—	keratosis in chronic radiodermatitis
57	43	M	hand	occupational	7	—	keratosis in chronic radiodermatitis
58	70	F	face	hirsutism	—	33	squamous cell carcinoma in chronic radio-dermatitis
59	64	M	hand	dermatitis	—	30	squamous cell carcinoma in chronic radio-dermatitis
60	63	F	face	lupus vulgaris	—	12	basal cell epithelioma in chronic radio-dermatitis
61	68	M	face	dermatitis	—	4	basal cell epithelioma in chronic radio-dermatitis
62	70	F	face	hitsutism	—	10	basal cell epithelioma in chronic radio-dermatitis
63	45	F	face	hirsutism	—	20	basal cell epithelioma in chronic radio-dermatitis
64	65	F	face	hirsutism	—	25	basal cell epithelioma in chronic radio-dermatitis

TABLE 18–5 CASES OF CHRONIC RADIODERMATITIS RESULTING FROM TREATMENT OF BENIGN CONDITIONS (*Continued*)

Case No.	Age	Sex	Localization	Cause for Radiation	Observa-tion Time (Years)	Latency Time (Years)	End Result
65	46	F	face	hirsutism	—	30	basal cell epithelioma in chronic radio-dermatitis
66	46	F	face	hirsutism	—	30	basal cell epithelioma in chronic radio-dermatitis
67	55	F	face	hirsutism	—	30	basal cell epithelioma in chronic radio-dermatitis
68	72	F	face	hirsutism	—	30	basal cell epithelioma in chronic radio-dermatitis
69	56	F	face	hirsutism	—	32	basal cell epithelioma in chronic radio-dermatitis
70	64	F	face	hirsutism	—	32	basal cell epithelioma in chronic radio-dermatitis
71	72	F	face	hirsutism	—	35	basal cell epithelioma in chronic radio-dermatitis
72	69	F	face	hirsutism	—	39	basal cell epithelioma in chronic radio-dermatitis
73	64	F	face	hirsutism	—	43	basal cell epithelioma in chronic radio-dermatitis
74	40	F	face	acne	—	24	basal cell epithelioma in chronic radio-dermatitis
75	43	F	face	acne	—	24	basal cell epithelioma in chronic radio-dermatitis
76	57	F	face	acne	—	30	basal cell epithelioma in chronic radio-dermatitis
77	60	F	face	acne	—	30	basal cell epithelioma in chronic radio-dermatitis
78	66	M	face	acne	—	30	basal cell epithelioma in chronic radio-dermatitis
79	57	F	face	acne	—	36	basal cell epithelioma in chronic radio-dermatitis

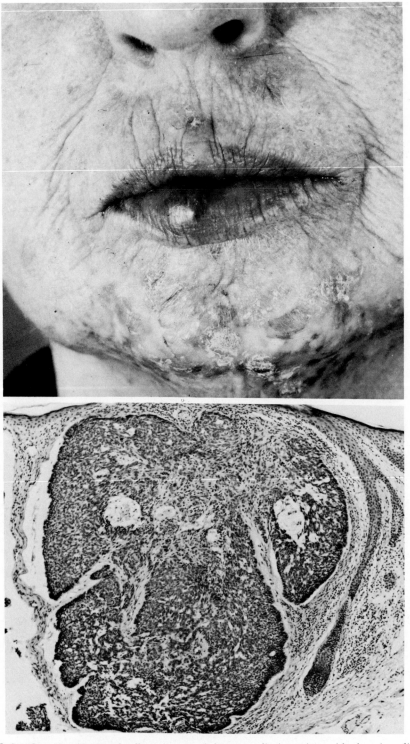

Figure 18–3 (Case No. 65.) Basal cell carcinoma of the upper lip in patient with chronic radiodermatitis of the face. The patient is a 46 year old woman who received x-ray treatment for hirsutism 30 years ago. (From the collection of the Dermatology Department of the New York University Medical Center.)

"sarcomas" were really undifferentiated squamous cell carcinomas (Martin and Stewart, 1935; Sims and Kirsch, 1948; Martin et al., 1970) or "pseudosarcomas" due to hyperplastic proliferation of connective tissue (Rachmaninoff et al., 1961; Samitz, 1967) is open to debate.

TREATMENT OF CHRONIC RADIODERMATITIS

The treatment of otherwise uncomplicated chronic radiodermatitis is based on two main principles: (1) the tissues are permanently damaged and therefore irritation of any type should be avoided, and (2) the lesion is potentially carcinogenic and therefore changes should be watched for suggestion of malignant degeneration in order to detect and treat it as early as possible. No detailed rules can be established. The common sense of the physician and the cooperation of the patient are critical.

Small keratoses can be destroyed by electrodesiccation and curettage or with liquid nitrogen. Small ulcers can be treated locally, keeping in mind that irritation should be avoided. If the ulcer does not heal, surgical excision of the entire area damaged by the radiation should be considered. When there are recurring or painful ulcerations or spreading keratoses, the lesions may have to be treated surgically, as in cases of malignant degeneration.

When malignancy has evolved in the area of chronic radiodermatitis, surgical excision must be performed. Again it must be stressed that the surgeon is going to deal with chronically damaged skin. Early detection is all the more important, and it is advisable to remove all the radiation-injured tissue if feasible. It is obvious that ionizing radiation is ordinarily contraindicated for malignancy within radiodermatitis.

CONCLUSIONS

Radiation-injured skin must be considered potentially carcinogenic. Those who deny that there is carcinogenic potential under acceptable medical use of ionizing radiation (Epstein, 1965) have the burden of proof of their contention.

Not all cases of chronic radiodermatitis will develop cancer. I have tried to emphasize some of the circumstances that favor malignant degeneration in chronic radiodermatitis. Until we know more about the mechanisms of carcinogenesis, no predictions can be made as to the outcome of particular cases of radiodermatitis. Caution and judicious use of ionizing radiation are the correct prophylactic approaches to the problem of chronic radiodermatitis.

I conclude from my study that particular consideration in the use of radiotherapy should be given to (1) the type of radiation used, (2) the site on the body where radiation is going to be used, and (3) the condition for which the radiation is going to be used.

Small doses of radiation over long periods of time, such as those used for benign, nontumorous conditions or those involved in occupational exposures, appear to be more dangerous than large, single-dose radiation, such as that customarily used to treat malignant conditions.

Ionizing radiation for the treatment of conditions in areas of the body known to be naturally susceptible to the development of malignancies should be carefully weighed and, if possible, replaced by other therapeutic measures.

Finally, whereas treating a malignancy with radiation may outweigh any conceivable contraindication, the presumptive benefits of the roentgen treatment of a benign condition should be carefully weighed against the known and possible radiation injuries (The hazards of X-ray, 1948; Love, 1955).

REFERENCES

Albert, R. E., and Omiran, A. R.: Follow up study of patients treated by X-ray epilation for tinea capitis. Arch. Environ. Health, 17:899, 1968.

Anderson, L. P., and Anderson, H. E.: Development of basal cell epithelioma as a consequence of radiodermatitis. Arch. Dermatol. Syph. (Berl.), 63:586, 1951.

Anderson, V.: Roentgen sarcoma. Acta Radiol. (Stockh.), 45:155, 1956.

Bloom-Ides, C.: Sarcoma in roentgenderma. Acta Derm. Venereol. (Stockh.), 30:47, 1950.

Cade, S.: Radiation induced cancer in man. Br. J. Radiol., 30:393, 1957.

Cannon, B., Randolph, J. G., and Murray, J. E.:

Malignant irradiation for benign conditions. New Engl. J. Med., 260:197, 1959.

Cipollaro, A. C., and Einhorn, M. B.: The use of X-rays for the treatment of hypertrichosis is dangerous. J.A.M.A., 135:349, 1947.

Cipollaro, A. C., and Crossland, P. M.: X-rays and Radium in the Treatment of Diseases of the Skin. Philadelphia, Lea and Febiger, 1967.

Conway, H., and Hugo, N. E.: Radiation dermatitis and malignancy. Plast. Reconstr. Surg., 38:255, 1966.

Duperrat, B., and Andrade, R.: Radiodermite et cancer. Presse Med., 66:59, 1958.

Epstein, E.: Radiodermatitis. Springfield, Ill., Charles C Thomas, 1962.

Epstein, E.: Dermatologic radiotherapy 1965. Arch. Dermatol., 92:307, 1965.

Frieben, E.: Demonstration eines Cancroids des rechten Handruckens, das sich nach langdauernder Einwirkung von Roentgenstrahlen entwickelt hatte. Fortschr. Roentgenstr., 6:106, 1902.

Furth, J., and Upton, A. C.: Vertebrate radiobiology: histopathology and carcinogenesis. Ann. Rev. Nuclear. Sci., 3:303, 1953.

Glucksmann, A.: Carcinogenesis of skin tumors induced by radiation. Br. Med. Bull., 14:178, 1958.

Gofman, J. W., and Tamplin, A. R.: Radiation, cancer, and environmental health. Hosp. Practice, 5:91, 1970.

Goodwin, J. T.: Carcinogenic effects of ionizing radiation. Internatl. Rec. Med. Gen. Pract. Clin., 165:355, 1952.

Hartwell, S. W., Huger, W., and Pickrell, K.: Radiation dermatitis and radiogenic neoplasms of the hands. Ann. Surg., 160:828, 1964.

The hazards of X-ray. (Editorial.) J.A.M.A., 138:214, 1948.

Henry, S. A.: Cutaneous cancer in relation to occupation. Ann. R. Coll. Surg. Engl., 7:425, 1950.

Jones, A.: Irradiation sarcoma. Br. J. Radiol., 26:273, 1953.

Kalz, F.: Observations on grenz ray reactions. Dermatologica, 118:357, 1959.

Lagrot, F.: Que peut-on attendre de la chirurgie dans le traitement des radiodermites professionelles des doigts? Presse Med., 74:2923, 1966.

Leddy, E. T., and Rigos, F. J.: Radiodermatitis among physicians. Am. J. Roentgenol., 45:696, 1941.

Leider, M., and Rosenblum, M.: A dictionary of dermatological words, terms and phrases. New York, McGraw-Hill Book Company, 1968.

Love, J.: Dermatologic problems in practice of radiology. Am. J. Roentgenol., 74:1123, 1955.

Macomber, W. B., Wang, M. H., Trabue, J. C., and Kanzler, R.: Irradiation injuries, acute and chronic, and sequellae. Plast. Reconstr. Surg., 19:9, 1957.

Macomber, W. B., Wang, M. H., and Sullivan, J. G.: Cutaneous epithelioma. Plast. Reconstr. Surg., 24:545, 1959.

Martin, H., Strong, E., and Spiro, R. H.: Radiation-induced skin cancer of the head and neck. Cancer, 25:61, 1970.

Martin, H. E., and Stewart, F. W.: Spindle-cell epidermoid carcinoma. Am. J. Cancer, 24:273, 1935.

Mason, M.: Radiation injuries of the hand. Quart. Bull., Northwestern Univ. M. School, 25:51, 1951.

Miescher, G., Pluss, J., and Weber, B.: Die Rontgentelangiektasie als spatsymptom. Strahlentherapie, 94:223, 1954.

Montgomery, H.: Dermatopathology. New York, Harper & Row, 1967.

Neuman, Z., Ben-Hur, N., and Shulman, J.: The relationship between radiation injury to the skin and subsequent malignant change. Surg. Gynecol. Obstet., 117:559, 1963.

Pack, G. T., and Davis, J.: Radiation cancer of the skin. Radiology, 84:436, 1965.

Pettit, V. D., Chunness, J. T., and Ackerman, L. V.: Fibromatosis and fibrosarcoma following irradiation. Cancer, 7:149, 1954.

Porter, C. A.: The surgical treatment of X-ray carcinoma and other severe X-ray lesions. J. Med. Res., 21:357, 1909.

Rachmaninoff, N., McDonald, J. R., and Cook, J. C.: Sarcoma-like tumors of the skin following irradiation. Am. J. Clin. Pathol., 36:427, 1961.

Ridley, C. M.: Basal-cell carcinoma following X-ray epilation of the scalp. Br. J. Dermatol., 74:222, 1962.

Robinson, D. W., and Masters, F. W.: Surgery for radiation injury. A. M. A. Arch. Surg., 80:946, 1960.

Russell, B.: Fibrosarcomata of the skin and subcutaneous tissues. Trans. St. John's Hosp. Derm. Soc. London, 42:15, 1959.

Samitz, M. H.: Pseudosarcoma. Arch. Dermatol., 96:283, 1967.

Saunders, T. S., and Montgomery, H.: Chronic roentgen and radium dermatitis. J.A.M.A., 110:23, 1938.

Shafer, J. C., Braestrup, C. B., and Fisher, J. K.: Relation of exit dose and other dosage factors to roentgen injuries. Arch. Dermatol. Syph. (Berl.), 59:472, 1949.

Shapiro, E. M., Knox, M. J., and Freeman, R. G.: Carcinogenic effect of prolonged exposure to grenz ray. J. Invest. Dermatol., 37:291, 1961.

Sims, C. F., and Kirsch, N.: Spindle cell epidermoid epithelioma simulating sarcoma in chronic radiodermatitis. Arch. Dermatol Syph. (Berl.), 57:63, 1948.

Sulzberger, M. B., Baer, R. L., and Borota, A.: Do roentgen-ray treatments as given by skin specialists produce cancers or other sequellae? Arch. Dermatol. Syph. (Berl.), 65:639, 1952.

Teloh, H. A., Mason, M. L., and Wheelock, M. C.: A histopathologic study of radiation injuries of the skin. Surg. Gynecol. Obstet., 90:335, 1950.

Totten, R. S., Antypas, P. G., Dupertuis, S. M., Gaisford, J. C., and White, W. L.: Pre-existing roentgen-ray dermatitis in patients with skin cancer. Cancer, 10:1024, 1957.

Wolbach, S. B.: The pathological histology of chronic X-ray dermatitis and early X-ray carcinoma. J. Med. Res., 21:415, 1909.

19

Arsenic and Skin Cancer

Kenneth V. Sanderson, M.D.

INTRODUCTION

Until recently the proof that arsenic caused cancer rested mainly on clinical case reports. A considerable number of animal experiments had been fruitless, and epidemiologic studies had produced conflicting results. The published clinical data were sufficient to convince most physicians that liquor arsenicalis was a remedy to be avoided, and it is unlikely ever to become popular again. Case reports are, however, vulnerable to critical attack, and some writers have disputed the evidence that arsenic is a carcinogen. It might be thought that this is not a practical question now that arsenic therapy has been given up and more potent pesticides are largely displacing arsenicals in agriculture and industry. It is possible, however, that the use of the newer industrial poisons will be restricted because they are too effective for the safety of the environment. Arsenicals might then come back into widespread use, and, if the errors of the past are to be avoided, this must be done with full knowledge of their long-term dangers. It is therefore important to establish the fact of their carcinogenic potential beyond doubt.

Frost (1967) ended his review of arsenicals in biology with the statement, "arsenicals appear remarkably free of carcinogenicity." He dismissed the evidence of the clinical cases with the suggestion that the skin lesions were due to exposure to tar, mineral oils, or other agents of fossil origin. This ill-informed idea will be discussed later with the differential diagnosis. Frost ignored the epidemiologic evidence from Córdoba, Burgundy, and the Moselle in favor of arsenic cancer but stressed the absence of changes in workers exposed to arsenic dusts in some smelting and refining works.

Since the review was published a decisive epidemiologic study from Taiwan (Tseng, et al. 1968; Yeh, et al., 1968) has shown a prevalence of skin cancer occurring in a population not normally affected by it which increases with the concentration of arsenic in the drinking water and with the age of the patient. This and other smaller published and unpublished epidemiologic studies define the skin response to inorganic arsenic salts, taken in small doses over a long period, and vindicate the large volume of clinical evidence. There are no adequate data on the prevalence of visceral malignancy in a large population exposed to arsenic, and there probably never will be.

The patients now being seen in American, British, or European clinics with arsenic cancer are most likely to have been given arsenic medicinally. Apart from its use in orthodox therapy for skin and atopic disorders, in bromide mixtures and tonics, arsenic has been the basis of many proprietary medicines, and its presence may not be known until the carcinogenic effect becomes obvious. For instance, many patients have been seen in the Newcastle, England, area with profuse keratoses and Bowen's disease in recent years. Enquiry showed they had all taken a skin remedy which had been sold in the market for many years and which was found to contain liquor arsenicalis (Shuster, personal communication). It took vigorous representations from the dermatologists to have the commerce stopped.

It is not surprising that previous arsenic ingestion is known to only a minority of patients whose clinical condition suggests that arsenic is the cause of their skin cancer, when all the hidden sources of arsenic, its long latent interval, and the weakness of human memory are considered. A knowledge of the patient's previous occupations and his ailments in childhood or early life, coupled with an awareness of the uses of arsenic at that time, helps greatly in establishing the presumption of arsenic ingestion. It is inevitable, therefore, that the emphasis in this chapter must be as much on the origins of the disease as on its clinical features.

HISTORY

The credit given to Paris (1820) as the first to describe arsenic cancer is unjustified (Kennaway, 1942). There is no historical or experimental substantiation for his account of animals with cancer from arsenic, and his description of scrotal lesions in men has the quality of village gossip rather than clinical observation. By contrast, the account given by Hutchinson (1888) relied on precise observation and reasoned argument from a small series of cases. His key patient, a physician from Boston, Massachusetts, who had treated his own psoriasis with liquor arsenicalis, developed corns on his palms which later progressed to ulcerating tumors and spread to the axillary

lymph nodes (see Fig. 19–4). The patient died with tumors in the lung whose microscopic picture differed from the cornifying squamous cell carcinoma of the palm. He may therefore have had multiple primary cancers. White (1885) had previously described the same patient as demonstrating the sequence "psoriasis, verruca, epithelioma" without linking it to arsenic treatment. Arsenical keratoses of the palms and soles had been recorded earlier by Erasmus Wilson (1873). Of the descriptions of arsenic cancer since Hutchinson, many are case reports, often with inadequate details, some are of a particular lesion, such as Bowen's disease or superficial basal cell epithelioma, and others are based on environmental poisoning of one type or another. A committee of the Medical Research Council in Britain reviewed the evidence (Neubauer, 1947) and accepted 167 cases to that date. It is likely that published cases examined by the Committee represent only a small proportion of the patients suffering from, or recognized as having, arsenic cancer. For instance, a series of 10 cases (Sanderson, 1963) could now be more than doubled by new cases seen at one hospital in London in the last eight years, but there is no justification for publishing an additional series without a new angle.

Although the skin is usually the first organ affected, there is an increased incidence of cancer of other tissues in groups such as the Moselle vintners, who have been exposed to arsenic for a considerable time (Roth, 1956; Denk et al., 1969), and series of cases of multiple skin and internal malignancies have been recorded in patients given arsenic (Sommers and McManus, 1953; Berlin and Tager, 1962). The apparent correlation of internal malignancy with palmar keratoses (Dobson et al., 1965) has, however, not been confirmed in other areas (Bean et al., 1968; Rhodes, 1970; Stolman, 1970).

There have been numerous endeavours to justify the diagnosis of arsenic cancer by demonstrating abnormal amounts of arsenic in the tissues. The earlier analyses of the skin used unsatisfactory methods (Osborne, 1925 and 1928; Montgomery and Waisman, 1941). Neutron-activation analysis provides a precise and sensitive measure of arsenic in biologic tissues (Smith, 1959), but most of the reports of its use (Scott, 1958; Domonkos, 1959; Ferguson, 1960) can be criticized for not allowing for the varying affinity of arsenic for the different tissue constituents. The varying proportions of collagen, epithelial, and other structures in different biopsies are certain to produce considerable variation from site to site in the same patient, as has indeed been shown (Domonkos, 1959). Until the source of variation is eliminated, the technique can give only a rather rough idea of whether the patient has been exposed previously to arsenic, as in the series of patients with Bowen's disease (Graham and Helwig, 1961). Indeed it is not necessary for arsenic to accumulate in the tissues in order to exert a cumulative effect.

The sources of arsenic consumed by humans will be discussed in the section on epidemiology, but reference may be made here to the history of its use in therapy in the last two centuries. Fowler (1786) suggested that arsenic was useful in treating ague and remitting fevers, and Paris (1820) reported that one of the effects of arsenic contamination of the land in Cornwall was to eliminate the ague. In the early nineteenth century arsenic was thought to be as effective in treating malaria as quinine, though less rapid in action. When Hutchinson (1888) wrote about arsenic cancer, it was a well established treatment for anemia and Hodgkin's disease, as well as for a variety of common skin disorders. These included psoriasis, eczema, lichen planus, and lupus erythematosus, and in one widely read book (Hunt, 1847) its use was recommended for almost any chronic skin disease. Hebra (1868), in his critical manner, would not allow that arsenic was of any benefit in eczema but used it for psoriasis, lichen planus, and lupus erythematosus in long courses of substantial dosage. It was later used as the only effective remedy for dermatitis herpetiformis until sulfapyridine was introduced. Its use in dermatology persists in some countries, and Knoth (1966) found 591 dermatologists using arsenic in Germany in 1963. Arsenic was widely used in nervous disorders and was originally thought to be helpful in cases of epilepsy and chorea. It was a constituent of the bromide mixture of the Na-

tional Hospital for Nervous Diseases and of the British National Formulary until 1939 and was probably prescribed unwittingly by many British physicians who used the mixture. It has been employed for a long time in treating asthma and hay fever, and its continued use in the Gay regime has been the subject of controversy (Harters and Novitch, 1967; Bleiberg, 1968; Taub, 1970). In a personal communication to the writer (Gay, 1965) it was claimed that no case of cancer attributable to arsenic had been found in over 50,000 patients. Hyperkeratotic lesions had, however, been noticed. This large number of patients would provide a population of considerable epidemiologic value if the individuals could be followed through their lifetimes.

EPIDEMIOLOGY AND ETIOLOGY

Natural Sources of Arsenic

Because of its transitional position in the periodic table, arsenic can react to produce a variety of compounds, as well as acting as a metalloid in alloys with metals.

In the primary rocks it is present mainly in the form of the sulphides—orpiment, As_2S_3, and realgar, As_2S_2, or of the mixed sulfides, such as mispickel, FeAsS. Orpiment and realgar have been used as pigments since prehistoric times and have been found in some areas in sulfide depilatory creams used for ritual or cosmetic purposes. The sulfides are present in substantial amounts in ores bearing gold, silver, copper, lead, zinc, cobalt, and tin. Arsenic is leached from the minerals and is found in small amounts in water, soil, vegetation, and animal life. It may be concentrated by some marine organisms (Chapman, 1926) and is thus present in appreciable amounts in some sedimentary rocks and in a more soluble form than the sulfides of the older rocks. Ground water collecting in such sedimentary strata may contain sufficient arsenic to be a health hazard if used continually for domestic purposes.

When ores are roasted, arsenic sublimes at 193° C. and may be recovered as arsenic trioxide ("white arsenic") by precipitation from the fumes. Incompletely treated fumes caused widespread arsenism at Reichenstein (Geyer, 1898), in Ohio (Birmingham et al., 1965), and in Peru (Obermayer, 1965). Crude arsenic trioxide may be purified and converted into inorganic or organic compounds. There is disagreement about the carcinogenic hazard to workers in smelting and chemical works (Perry et al., 1948; Holmqvist, 1951; Pinto and Bennett, 1963). The workers in all factories showed increased excretion of arsenic, and those in some showed dermatitis. The absence of carcinogenic effects in the Swedish and American workers is hard to explain in the light of present knowledge. It may be related to the length of follow-up and whether or not reliance is placed on death and other certificates. The latest data (Lee and Fraumeni, 1969) suggest that inhaled arsenical dusts are carcinogenic to the respiratory tract.

Industrial and Argicultural Uses

Arsenic is used in some alloys, in glass manufacturing, and in making enamels. It is a constituent of some paint pigments and dyestuffs. Inorganic arsenicals, such as sodium arsenite and lead arsenate, have been used as insecticides, fungicides, herbicides, defoliants, vermicides, and wood preservatives; they have been sprayed in orchards, vineyards, and cotton, corn, soya bean, and potato fields (Hueper, 1955). A considerable number of workers has thus been exposed to the hazards of arsenic, often with inadequate warning. More recently organic arsenicals, as food additives, have been found to improve the health and feed efficiency of livestock (Frost, 1967), but like the organic preparations used in medical treatment the compounds are probably not carcinogenic.

Chronic Arsenism Due to Occupational Exposure

It is much more difficult to gather data on carcinogenic effects which take two or three decades to appear than on more immediate effects, such as arsenic pigmentation or dermatitis. It has been, for instance, the writer's impression that Bowen's disease of the covered skin was commoner than would be expected in Australian sheep farmers who used arsenical sheep dip, but an epidemiologic survey would be needed to substantiate this impression. There is, however, solid evidence from vine growing areas in France and Germany (Roth, 1956; Thiers et al., 1967; Denk et al., 1969). Arsenate of lead sprays were used on the vines in the Moselle for over 15 years, and the workers were exposed not only to the spray but also to the arsenic residue on the skins which were used to ferment a "house wine" for the employees. Roth calculated that a worker could have taken more than 50 g. of arsenic in 12 years. The incidence of skin and visceral malignancy, particularly of lung cancer, was much increased in the workers. In Beaujolais, arsenate of lead was substituted for copper fungicide sprays between 1939 and 1943. Most of the workmen and some of their wives suffered direct toxic effects, such as polyneuritis, hepatitis, laryngitis, or bronchitis, and most had melanoderma. Palmo-plantar keratoses developed, to be followed by skin cancers with a latent period of 16 to 23 years. This epidemic is important because the relatively short period of exposure allows the sequence of events to be dated more precisely than is possible in some other studies. The true incidence of changes, especially visceral malignancy, may not be known for some years yet.

The difficulty in following up those with occupational exposure to arsenic and the inadequacy of anything less than periodic examination by someone experienced in assessing the skin manifestations make most of the other reported studies of little value. In particular, those which rely on certification and those in which the investigators are employed by a firm deriving benefit from commerce in arsenicals, must be viewed with suspicion.

Arsenic Treatment

The study of Fierz (1966) of the patients of a country doctor who had been using arsenic for up to 26 years shows a dose-response relationship between the amount of arsenic and percentage of patients with keratoses and, at a higher level, with carcinomas. He found, however, no basis for a nontoxic threshold dose and cited a patient who developed skin carcinoma after a total dose of 70 ml. of Fowler's solution, i.e., 0.7 g. of arsenic trioxide. The average latent period of skin cancer was 14 years, and variations in the latent period did not influence the type of carcinoma. This study is of more value than a survey of the reported cases because of the uniformity of assessment and because the dosage was recorded accurately. The general conclusions are being confirmed by examination of a rather similar group of patients in the north of England (Evans, personal communication, 1970).

Chronic Arsenism From Drinking Water

The older epidemics of Reichenstein (Geyer, 1898) and Córdoba province (Arguello et al., 1938) provide good evidence of the noxious effects of arsenic but lack the comprehensive epidemiological character of the Taiwan investigation (Tseng et al., 1968; Yeh et al., 1968). One can perhaps criticize the latter for the decision to separate sharply keratoses from Bowen's disease and to classify the first as benign and the second as carcinoma. Widening the definition of carcinoma to include intraepidermal carcinoma makes comparison with other series difficult and tends, perhaps, to inflate the hazards of arsenic.

In one area of Taiwan the artesian water supply was contaminated with arsenic for 45 years. A complete survey of the population of 37 villages whose water supplies contained differing amounts of arsenic showed a prevalence of skin cancer, which increased with age to a figure of more than 10 percent in people over the age of 59, and a proportional increase in prevalence with increasing contamination of water. There was a consistently higher rate in males than females of the same age and from the same village, which might be attributed to injury, such as cutting away the keratoses with infected knives. The youngest patient with melanosis was 3, with keratoses 4, and with skin cancer 24. A control population whose wells were not contaminated showed no melanosis, keratoses, or skin cancers. The clinical and microscopic features of the lesions and a five-year follow-up study will be referred to in later sections of this chapter.

A rather bizarre epidemic occurred in Iran (Pettit, personal communication). Wells supplying water to a segment of a village were contaminated, and the people living there suffered from chronic arsenism because arsenic was present in the sulfide preparation used for ritual depilation. The drain from the mosque ran through the center of the affected segment, and arsenic escaped into the shallow wells. The severity of the keratoses was directly related to the closeness of the patient's house to the drain.

Arsenic Eaters

The arsenic eaters of Styria caught the popular imagination in England in the nineteenth century and remained notorious long after the custom disappeared. The peasants living in Steiermark, Austria, were accustomed to feeding arsenic to their horses to make them strong and able to work at high altitudes. It also made them look sleek, a trick well known to horse dealers. It has been suggested (Riehl, personal communication) that the men then reasoned they would need to take arsenic to be strong enough to control their horses. There is no local memory of late skin changes in those who indulged in the habit, although a contemporary account (MacLagan, 1864) leaves no doubt the men both ate, and excreted in their urine, excessive amounts of arsenic. The suggestion that the arsenic was harmless because it was taken as the crystalline form of the insoluble sulfide, orpiment (Franseen and Taylor, 1934), is at variance with the report (Poisoned Bath buns, 1860) of acute arsenic poisoning when orpiment was used to color Bath buns in mistake for chrome yellow, which the baker habitually substituted for eggs.

Individual Variation in the Response to Arsenic

The reports of series of cases in which arsenic was given medicinally and the total dose could be estimated show that a small proportion of individuals are much more sensitive to the carcinogenic effect than the majority. At the other end of the curve of biologic variation, some persons exposed to arsenic for a long period suffer no adverse effects. The fundamental cause for this variation in response is unknown. The type of tumors which develop may also vary. Although most patients show keratoses and Bowen's disease, a minority (about 15 percent in the writer's series) have only multiple basal cell carcinoma. It seems likely that the type of response is determined by constitutional factors rather than by the effect of different dose schedules. Patients with basal cell carcinoma caused by arsenic have a much greater chance of developing lung cancer than do those whose basal cell carcinoma is not so caused (Russell, personal communication).

Experiments With Arsenic As a Carcinogen

Only one report of tumors developing in experimental animals following the administration of arsenic has been published (Knoth, 1966). Mice, and their offspring born during the experiment, developed neoplasms of the lung and lymph nodes, while control animals did not. The experimental details in the report are rather inadequate, and the record of the further experiments, which the author promised, does not seem to have been published yet. Other experiments (Hartwell, 1951) have been unsuccessful, and indeed several workers have noticed inhibition of spontaneous lung adenomas and papillomas in mice given arsenic (Kanisawa and Schroeder, 1967), although no such effect has been shown in dogs or rats (Byron, et al., 1967; Kanisawa and Schroeder, 1969). Experiments in which arsenic has been applied to the skin can be disregarded as bearing no relationship to the human situation (Leitch and Kennaway, 1922; Raposo, 1928; Friedewald, and Rous, 1944). Experiments have been designed to test the co-carcinogenic potential of arsenic by mouth combined with either initiating or promoting agents applied to the skin (Baroni et al., 1963), but they have failed to show an effect.

The writer carried out a similar series of experiments, briefly reported (Sanderson, 1961), in which an increasing number of papillomas were found in animals given arsenic in their drinking water, especially when it was combined with croton oil painting. Microscopic examination showed focal sebaceous hyperplasia with progressive loss of the capacity to mature as the lesions progressed. Several lesions ended as circumscribed sebaceous neoplasms (Figs. 19–1 and 19–2). A further series designed to eliminate the influence of infestation by Mycoptes produced no papillomas.

In the absence of an experimental model of human arsenic cancer, theories about the relationship of carcinogenicity to the chemical structure of the arsenicals, and in particular to the valency of arsenic in various compounds, cannot be tested in a rigorous manner. Balance studies in mice have shown that much of the inorganic arsenic ingested is converted in the tissues to forms not recoverable by usual chemical assay methods (Clements et al., 1951). Whether arsenic acts by substituting for phosphorus in the nucleic acid molecules, as an enzyme inhibitor, or in some less direct manner is not certain at the moment. There is evidence that phytohemagglutinin-stimulated lymphocytes have disturbed nuclear division after brief in vitro exposure to dilutions of arsenic in the culture medium, and that the higher concentrations cause 80 to 100 percent of entire metaphase plates to be pulverized. Under the same conditions tritiated thymidine labeling was diminished (Petres and Berger, 1972). These authors believe that arsenic competitively inhibits insertion of phosphorus into the nucleotide chain, as well as inhibiting enzymes containing SH-groups and the "dark repair" mechanism for DNA, as has been shown for human epidermis in vitro (Jung and Trachsel, 1970). It is possible, in view of some of its reputed therapeutic effects, that its action is partly as an immunosuppressant. Experiments to test this hypothesis have not, to the writer's knowledge, been carried out.

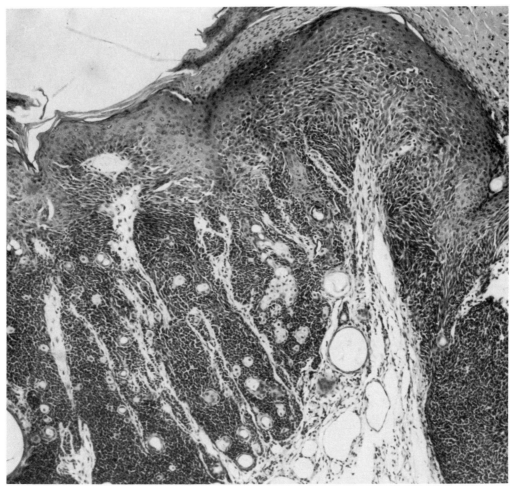

Figure 19–1 Sebaceous neoplasm in mouse fed arsenic and painted with croton oil. Scattered sebaceous cells in columns of immature and undifferentiated cells. *H & E, × 100.*

CLINICAL FEATURES

The individual skin cancers of patients who have been given arsenic do not possess any unique features and hence do not require detailed description here. Dermatologists suspect arsenic as the carcinogen when there are multiple tumors of a particular distribution and type starting before the fifth decade and when there are certain associated phenomena. A positive history of arsenic ingestion is very helpful but is elicited in only a minority of patients at the first interview and must be enquired about directly (Arhelger and Kremen, 1951).

Keratoses

The most distinctive physical sign is the presence of punctate keratoses on the palms and soles (Fig. 19–3). It was this feature which led Hutchinson to link arsenic with cancer, and the older writers (White, 1885; Hutchinson, 1888; Dubreuilh, 1910) have described the keratoses very accurately. Erythema and hyperhidrosis may precede their appearance. Beginning as pinpoint-sized areas of hyperkeratosis, which are usually not noticed by the patient, they may vary in size up to 5 to 10 mm. in diameter. Small keratoses are slightly raised and may be detected more easily by palpation. They can be seen more clearly if the skin is moistened or anointed with Vaseline. The hyperkeratosis is hard, adherent, and not penetrated by vascular papillae, but it may be situated on an erythematous base. The intervening skin may be abnormally rough and dry, and the normal creases may be exaggerated of fissured in severe cases. Al-

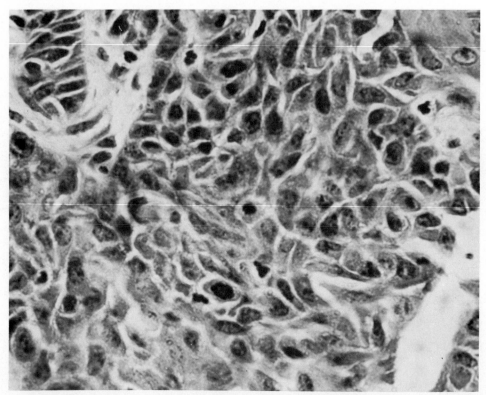

Figure 19–2   Higher magnification of Figure 19–1 to show the undifferentiated cells with frequent mitoses. *H & E,* × 1000.

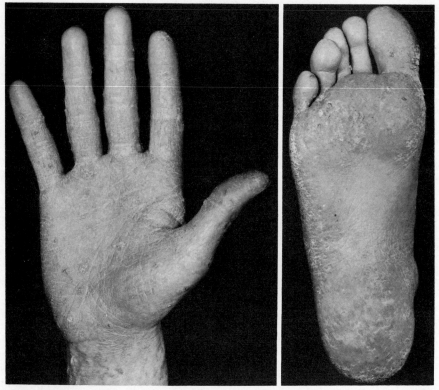

Figure 19–3   The palm and sole of a patient treated with liquor arsenicalis for psoriasis. Cornlike keratoses of different sizes and diffuse hyperkeratosis can be seen. (Case 1, from Sanderson: Trans. St. John's Hosp. Dermatol. Soc., 49:115, 1963.)

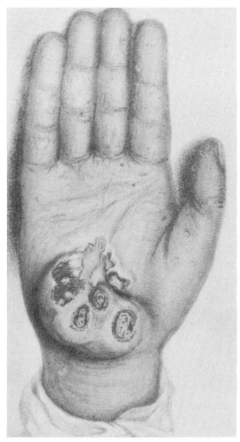

Figure 19-4　The palm of the hand of the physician from Boston described by White and Hutchinson. (Copied from Hutchinson, 1888.) (See also Color Plate I-A.)

most always multiple and symmetrical, the keratoses may occur in great profusion or in quite small numbers and are often more numerous on the soles than on the palms. The favored sites are the thenar eminence and lateral borders of the palms, the roots and lateral surfaces of the fingers, and the soles, heels, and toes (Yeh et al., 1968). They tend to reach a limiting size and then remain stationary, but they can disappear if the arsenic is stopped soon enough (Dubreuilh, 1910; Montgomery, 1935). Although the palmo-plantar keratoses are relatively benign, illustrations from Hutchinson's original paper (Fig. 19-4) show that malignancy is a possibility, and the chance of such change in a patient with them has been put at 20 percent (Montgomery, 1935).

Palmo-plantar keratoses are often associated with keratotic lesions on the dorsa of the extremities (Fig. 19-5), on the limbs, especially over the extensor aspect of joints, and elsewhere. An underlying hyperemia is seen in most of these lesions, and there may be focal telangiectasia as well. The lesions are circumscribed, and the degree of hyperkeratosis is variable. Arsenical keratoses probably occur in about 90 percent of cases of arsenic cancer (Neubauer, 1947).

Bowen's Disease

In any discussion of this disorder it is desirable to use the term only for those lesions which have the classical clinical features and not to include actinic or arsenical keratoses with a Bowenoid histology. In most cases a clinical distinction can be made between arsenical keratoses, which tend to persist more or less unchanging for years, and Bowen's disease, which tends to enlarge progressively. Arsenical Bowen's disease is usually multiple and distributed much more at random over the skin surface, with a smaller number of lesions but more of them on the trunk than is the case with keratoses. In many patients the lower part of the body may be rather more affected than the upper part. Recurrent minor trauma may determine the sites of appearance of Bowen's disease and keratoses (Sommers and McManus, 1953). The individual areas are red, scaly or slightly crusted, and irregular in outline, and they may vary in size from 1 mm. to 10 cm. or more in advanced lesions. There may be pigmentation. Where Bowen's disease is exposed to frequent external stresses, in flexor creases of the fingers or elsewhere on the palm, for instance, it may present as a superficial and intractible ulceration of fixed and somewhat irregular limits. The scale in Bowen's disease is much less adherent than are keratotic protrusions and, when removed, leaves a slightly moist or bleeding surface. A complete description of Bowen's disease is given on p. 487.

Squamous Cell Carcinoma

Keratoses and the lesions of Bowen's disease are both potentially invasive, but only a minority of them become squamous

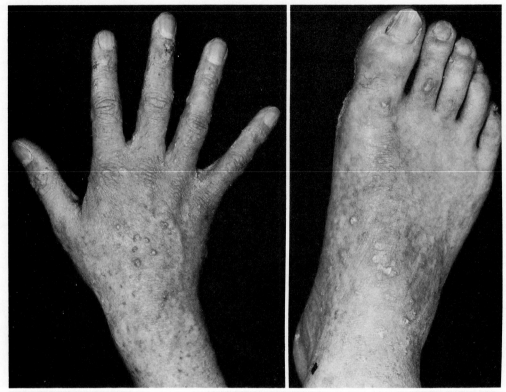

Figure 19–5   Dorsa of hand and foot of the same patient pictured in Figure 19–3, showing numerous scattered keratoses.

cell carcinoma and usually only after many years. The latent interval is 14 years, on the average, from the taking of arsenic medicinally to the evidence of malignancy and does not seem to be shortened by large dosage (Fierz, 1966). Invasion is more likely to occur in Bowen's disease than in keratoses, but, because of the greater total number of keratoses, squamous cell carcinoma is commoner on the extremities than elsewhere (Yeh et al., 1968). Persistent fissuring, erosion, ulceration, and induration are the main signs, and when they occur biopsy is mandatory. Squamous cell carcinoma is described on p. 488.

Basal Cell Carcinoma

In contrast with the detailed precise descriptions of keratoses in the literature, basal cell carcinoma has been given less emphasis than it deserves. This is partly because of the similarity of the lesions on the trunk to those of Bowen's disease clinically, partly because of the use of "benign superficial epitheliomatosis" as a collective diagnosis for both, and perhaps because of some difficulty in the microscopic diagnosis. Quite a number of arsenical basal cell carcinomas are unaccompanied by any of the other stigmata of chronic arsenism, and the prime cause is more likely to be overlooked than in the case of Bowen's disease and squamous cell carcinoma.

In Caucasians arsenic causes lesions of two types in particular: a superficial, spreading (Pagetoid) tumor with an atrophic, erythematous, or scaly center and threadlike margin (Fig. 19–6), or a small and indolent nodular type. Lesions are almost invariably multiple and more likely to be on the trunk than the face, scalp, or extremities. Tumors of the trunk deserve their reputation for indolence and benignity. On the face, their behavior may be more aggressive and in keeping with basal cell carcinoma due to other causes. A higher proportion of deep tumors was found in the Taiwan population than is seen in clinics in the United States or Europe. Basal cell carcinoma is described on p. 485.

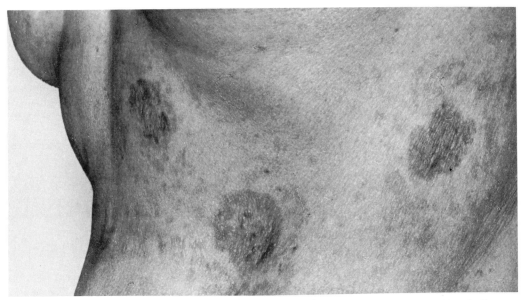

Figure 19–6 Superficial basal cell carcinoma on the trunk following liquor arsenicalis in childhood. The areas are red, scaly, and atrophic, with scattered small-tumor nodules centrally and an irregular threadlike margin.

Associated Phenomena

Pigmentation is frequently present in people who have been taking arsenic for a long time. It is commoner in the dark-complexioned than in the fair-skinned and affects particularly those areas, such as the nipples, linea nigra, axillae, and genital area, which are normally darker than the general skin. On the chest and abdomen there may be "rain-drop" hyperpigmentation where the diffuse brown color is splattered with paler spots. The mucosal surfaces are usually spared. Telangiectasia may be seen at times and, like the pigmentation, may persist long after arsenic has been given up.

In Taiwan peripheral vascular insufficiency ending with gangrene ("black-foot") is a common happening in elderly subjects, and in vintners cirrhosis of the liver is frequent. Evidence has been accumulating over the years of an increased incidence of internal malignant tumors in patients with arsenical skin cancer described, though not explained, by the term "general tumor predisposition" (Büngeler, 1930). These disorders all influence the prognosis but are late events and appear when other features have already suggested arsenic as the cause.

PATHOLOGY

Classification

The most complete description of the microscopic features of arsenic cancer (Yeh et al., 1968) is based on a rather unwieldy classification. The basic classes are: keratoses of two types (one being considered benign), Bowen's disease, intraepidermal epithelioma of Jadassohn, and squamous cell and basal cell carcinomas. Some lesions are made up of combinations of these types, and there are further subdivisions based on macroscopic and other changes. This may be a useful classification for epidemiologic purposes, but it does not assist the understanding of the pathologic processes. Indeed, it causes confusion in at least two ways: by grouping intraepidermal lesions with invasive carcinoma, and by describing combined forms of basal cell and squamous cell carcinoma.

A number of studies have confirmed the fundamental difference between basal cell carcinoma and the other epidermal changes listed above, and this should be the primary division in a classification of arsenic cancer. The other lesions result from two processes. The first is dysplasia, which is slight and orderly in some of the keratoses, especially on the palms and soles, and is severe and disorderly in Bowen's disease. It is convenient to separate the range of changes into three broad categories: keratosis, bowenoid keratosis, and Bowen's disease. The microscopic appearance may be modified by an irregular distribution of dysplastic cells in Bowen's disease, giving nests and squamous eddies of "Jadassohn" type. The second process, which affects the appearance is an inhibition of maturation. This may produce acanthotic thickening of the area, often with an accumulation of basaloid cells in the lower epidermis (Fig. 19–7). This change has caused confusion by being mistaken for basal cell carcinoma, and the similarity may be increased by hyperpigmentation due to increased melanin transfer to the immature cells. Some keratoses may, on the other hand, arise from atrophic epidermis.

It is unnecessary to arrange separate categories to accommodate the various changes described above, and it may be misleading to liken them to other lesions, such as seborrheic keratoses. Retarded maturation, dysplasia, dyskeratosis, and other gross cytologic abnormalities occur to different degrees in different lesions. Insofar as prognosis is possible, it should be based on the severity of the dysplastic changes. Squamous cell carcinoma can arise from keratoses and from Bowen's disease, and glandular or visceral metastases usually preserve the cytologic character of the original lesions.

In a multifocal process like arsenic cancer it is possible to have separate foci of two different types of neoplasia beginning adjacent to each other and eventually colliding and blending together. This may be a cause of compound basal and squamous changes, as Yeh et al. (1968) have suggested. The writer has observed a superficial basal cell carcinoma expand into and invade a seborrheic keratosis. It is, however, likely to be a less common event than might be assumed from reported examples of mixed basal cell and squamous cell carcinoma.

The use of the term "benign superficial

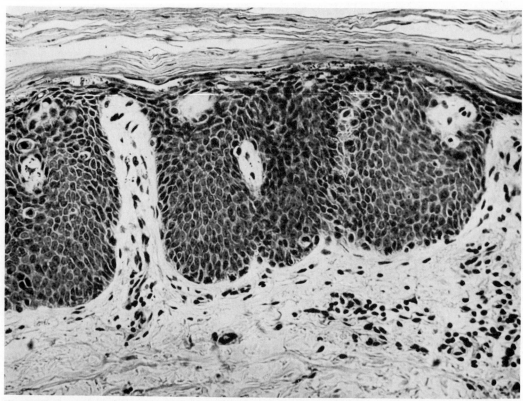

Figure 19–7   Arsenical keratosis with retarded maturation as the main change and with only a minor degree of cellular atypia. *H & E, ×250.*

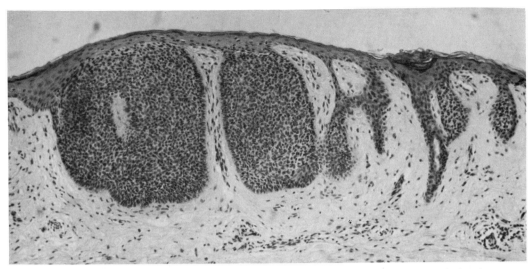

Figure 19–8 Margin of a superficial basal cell carcinoma. The apparent multifocal pattern is due, in part, to spread along interpapillary ridges. The larger nodules produce the threadlike clinical appearance. *H & E,* × *125.*

epitheliomatosis" (Montgomery, 1929 and 1935; Montgomery and Waisman, 1941) seems now to have been largely abandoned. It is a diagnosis which lacks pathologic precision and is best forgotten.

Basal Cell Carcinoma. In the series of

Yeh et al. (1968) 15 percent of arsenical skin cancers were basal cell carcinomas. There were multiple lesions in almost all cases, and more than half the lesions were of the deep type, in contrast to experience elsewhere. It may have been that a higher

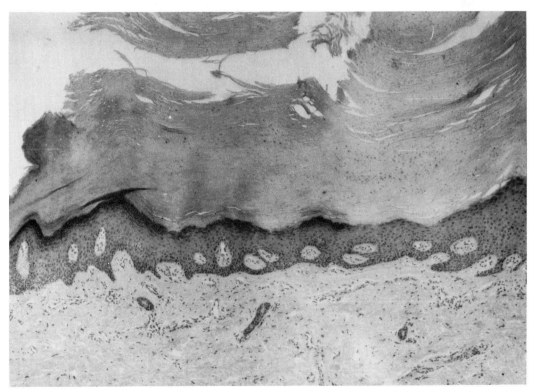

Figure 19–9 Arsenical keratosis showing orderly maturation with acanthosis but little deviation of the malpighian cells from normal, variable diminution of the granular layer, hyperkeratosis, and parakeratosis. *H & E,* × *100.*

proportion of lesions were neglected in Taiwan than in other places. There was also a greater variability of the histologic picture, resembling that of basal cell carcinoma of other causation, except for the relative frequency of cells with bizarre or multiple nuclei. Other reports suggest that the characteristic arsenic-caused basal cell carcinoma is superficial (Fig. 19–8) and neither invades deeply nor ulcerates in the earlier stages of its evolution. In other respects the tumors resemble ordinary basal cell carcinomas (p. 482).

Keratoses. The keratosis which is found on the extremities and which usually behaves in a benign fashion may

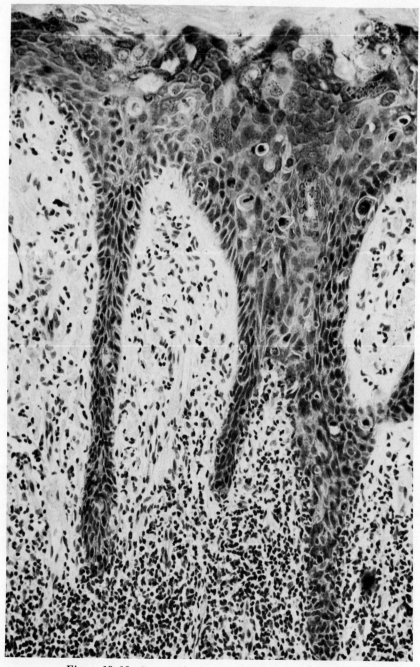

Figure 19–10   Bowenoid arsenical keratosis. *H & E, × 200.*

show little deviation from normal in the malpighian cells. Maturation takes place in an orderly fashion, a granular layer is usually present, and mitoses are normal and not excessively frequent. The main evidence of dysplasia is seen in the stratum corneum, which is hyperkeratotic and perhaps parakeratotic (Fig. 19–9). In some instances there may be acanthosis and papillomatosis; in others the epidermis beneath the hyperkeratosis may be atrophic. There is little inflammatory reaction beneath these keratoses, and the microscopic appearance mirrors their benign behavior.

Bowenoid Keratosis. There are no sharp boundaries between this type and Bowen's disease, on the one hand, and a simple dysplastic keratosis on the other. The epidermal maturation in these lesions is sufficiently orderly to produce a thick, adherent, hyperkeratotic cap, but there are numbers of atypical cells in the epidermis (Fig. 19–10). The cells are atypical in their tendency to premature and individual keratinization and in their large, hyperchromatic or multiple nuclei, and

there are more frequent and abnormal mitoses. The background against which the atypical cells are set is composed of rather large, acidophilic malpighian cells which are present in sufficient numbers to distinguish the lesion from Bowen's disease. Vacuolar degeneration may be seen, although it cannot be regarded as pathognomonic of arsenical lesions. A more intense lymphocytic infiltrate occupies the papillary dermis beneath the lesion.

Bowen's Disease. The epidermis may be thickened with papillomatosis, or it may be atrophic (Fig. 19–11). The loss of polarity is such that the normal malpighian cells are replaced by a disorderly "windblown" array of atypical cells, some undergoing premature keratinization and others showing arrest of maturation. Giant and multinucleate cells, hyperchromatic "freckled" nuclei, abnormal mitoses, and cellular vacuolation are frequent, but there are usually sufficient cells with a normal potential to form granulocytes in the upper epidermis. There is always a chronic inflammatory reaction, usually quite in-

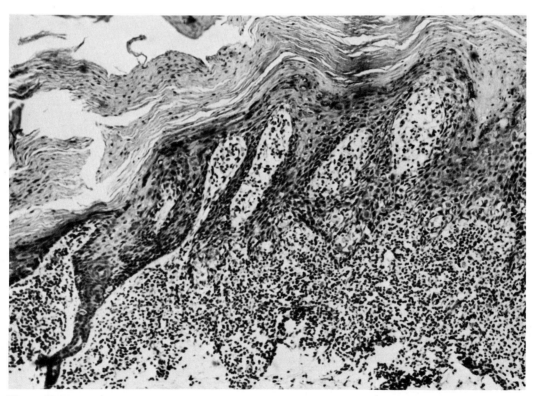

Figure 19–11 Bowen's disease with psoriasiform architecture of epidermis and marked lymphocytic reaction. *H & E, × 100.*

tense. The appendage ducts are not usually replaced by the changes, but the dysplastic cells tend to grow down around them like a sleeve and to straighten and attenuate them as they pass through the epidermis.

Squamous Cell Carcinoma. The criteria for deciding when invasion occurs are discussed on pages 481 and 482. There are two particular problems with arsenical tumors. The tendency to grow down and, to some extent, to strangulate and displace appendage ducts may cause practical problems with Bowen's disease, especially in lesions which have received superficial treatment and been covered by a normal epidermis (Pinkus and Mehregan, 1969). Occasionally a simple dysplastic keratosis may become invasive, and the apparently harmless cytologic appearance may be misleading (as it is with some actinic keratoses). Such lesions may invade locally but are usually late in metastasizing. There is a considerable risk, given by Graham and Helwig (1966) as 37 percent, of metastasis from invasive Bowen's disease in general. The general pathology of squamous cell carcinoma is presented on page 482.

Other Cutaneous Tumors. There are isolated reports of sebaceous and sweat gland tumors (Sommers and McManus, 1953) but not of malignant melanoma, as far as the writer is aware.

DIFFERENTIAL DIAGNOSIS

Two different practical problems arise in arsenical cancer. The more important one is the recognition of arsenic as the etiologic agent in premalignant or malignant lesions when the pathologic diagnosis has been established. The other one is the differentiation of Bowen's disease and keratoses from other dermatoses, such as psoriasis, for which arsenic may have been given.

As mentioned before, a history of arsenic medication or occupational exposure is only obtained in a minority of cases in the first interview and is almost never volunteered by the patient. Repeated questioning aimed at the patient's past medical history and occupations will, in the writer's experience, often reveal either a forgotten exposure or the background that makes exposure possible.

The distinguishing features of arsenic-induced lesions are their multiplicity and distribution. Most other skin carcinogens act from outside, and the effect is limited to areas of exposure. Actinic lesions are concentrated on the head, neck, hands, and forearms, even in these days of maximal exposure in sunbathing. They are accompanied by elastotic degeneration of the skin and are more severe in fair-complexioned people. Lesions due to tar, oil, and other products of fossil fuels affect principally the hands, forearms, and scrotum. Radiation-induced cancer is even more limited and often occurs in skin showing atrophy. By contrast, the arsenic lesions are scattered almost at random. Basal cell carcinoma is usually most profuse on the trunk, although it may have the more usual concentration on the face in fair-skinned people who have also been in the sun a lot. The family history, dental cysts, and skeletal and other abnormalities readily distinguish the basal cell nevus syndrome. The palmo-plantar keratoses are peculiar to arsenical malignancy and do not follow exposure to fossil fuels or radiant energy. Bowen's disease of the classic type is not a consequence of any other known carcinogens, although whether arsenic is the only or major cause is still an open question. Although there may be microscopic evidence of collagen degeneration (Yeh et al., 1968) this produces no gross clinical changes. In the full-blown clinical picture, therefore, there can be little difficulty in making the correct etiologic diagnosis, even with no history of exposure to arsenic.

If the presenting lesion is a solitary basal cell carcinoma or patch of Bowen's disease, objective evidence elsewhere must be sought, particularly on the soles and palms. Arsenic keratoses should be looked for with the skin moistened to accentuate irregular reflections, as well as in the dry state. The initial identification is often more easily made by palpation. The lesions resemble corns in their hard, coherent keratin and are distinguished from viral warts by the absence of a papillary structure. The palmar pits of basal cell nevus syndrome are defects rather than accretions of keratin. Darier's disease causes lesions of a rather similar type but can be distinguished by the changes elsewhere and the previous and family history. Likewise, punctate keratoderma is a disorder present from early in life.

Perhaps the most difficult clinical problem is to distinguish Bowen's disease from superficial basal cell carcinoma or from psoriasis in patients whose arsenic was administered to treat that disease. An atrophic patch of Bowen's disease often appears to have a slightly elevated margin when stretched, and in some cases biopsy is needed to make the distinction. The irregular border, the quality of the scaling, and the long history make the established lesion of either type distinct from psoriasis, but small and early patches may look very psoriasiform. An intelligent patient can often tell the difference from the cutaneous sensation.

PROGNOSIS

From the point of view of the skin tumors, the prognosis depends upon the behavior of the areas of Bowen's disease and bowenoid keratoses. The likelihood that any patch of Bowen's disease will become invasive is probably quite small and has been put at 5 percent (Graham and Helwig, 1966). The probability increases with the total area of the altered skin and the duration of the lesion. The same applies to keratoses, although it is more difficult to assess the probability of invasion from an individual lesion. Montgomery (1935) found epitheliomas in 20 percent of patients with arsenic keratoses, but this would be a gross overestimate in most series. Basal cell carcinoma is rarely life-threatening, and lesions on the trunk behave in a benign fashion.

The ultimate prognosis depends upon the likelihood of visceral tumors. There are no adequate epidemiologic data on which to base a reliable estimate of the probability of visceral malignancy, but individual experience and case reports indicate that it is a very real danger. There is some evidence that epithelia, such as respiratory or genitourinary, liable to squamous metaplasia are more likely to become neoplastic than others, such as the gastrointestinal epithelium (Sommers and McManus, 1953; Denk et al., 1969). Carcinoma of the lung is more likely to be peripheral than is the case with tumors due to smoking. Racial and genetic factors and other environmental carcinogens probably cause considerable variation in the type of internal cancer in different populations.

The cases in Taiwan have been followed up at five years (Yeh, 1973) and the causes of death analyzed for the patients with skin cancer and blackfoot and for the general population of the endemic area and compared with those for the whole population of Taiwan. The percentage mortality for all three groups from the endemic area is higher than for the whole population. Standard mortality ratios showed a much higher mortality rate in patients less than 49 years of age. Bladder, lung, and liver were the most frequent internal organs reported as being involved by neoplasms. In the skin cancer group there was a much greater percentage mortality from cancer than in the two other groups from the endemic area, and the increase was almost entirely due to mortality from the skin cancer itself.

TREATMENT

The details of the treatment of Bowen's disease, bowenoid keratoses, squamous cell carcinoma, and rodent ulcers do not alter because arsenic is the cause and are given elsewhere. If premalignant lesions are numerous, radiotherapy is undesirable because of the extensive scarring that results, and surgery may be difficult. For many patients, therefore, local destructive measures may be the treatment of choice. Many physicians prefer physical destruction, either with diathermy current or galvanocautery combined with curettage. An alternative method is the topical application of cytotoxic substances, such as 5-fluorouracil, methotrexate, or colchicine analogues. Early and superficial lesions usually respond satisfactorily, but well-established Bowen's disease may require prolonged treatment, and relapse rather frequently occurs (Klein et al., 1970). The treatment of such lesions and of superficial basal cell carcinoma by the production of an artificial contact sensitivity dermatitis to dinitrochlorobenzene (DNCB) seems to be a more satisfactory method as judged by the short-term results.

The palmo-plantar keratoses have been reported to respond to 5-fluorouracil cream (Klein et al., 1970).

REFERENCES

Anderson, N. P.: Bowen's precancerous dermatosis and multiple benign superficial epitheliomas; evidence of arsenic as an etiological agent. Arch. Dermatol. Syph., 26:1052, 1932.

Anderson, N. P.: Arsenical keratosis of the palms and soles, prickle cell epithelioma of a finger, multicentric benign superficial epithelioma. Arch. Dermatol. Syph., 35:323, 1937.

Arguello, R. A., Cenget, D. D., and Tello, E. E.: Cancer y arsenicismo regional endémico en Córdoba. Rev. Argent. Dermatosif., 22:461, 1938.

Arhelger, S. W., and Kremen, A. J.: Arsenical epitheliomas of medicinal origin. Surgery, 30:977, 1951.

Baroni, C., Esch, G. J. van, and Saffiotti, U.: Carcinogenesis tests of two inorganic arsenicals. Arch. Environ. Health, 7:668, 1963.

Bean, S. F., Foxley, E. G., and Fusaro, R. M.: Palmar keratoses and internal malignancy. A negative study. Arch. Dermatol., 97:528, 1968.

Berlin, C., and Tager, A.: Psoriasis complicated by cutaneous and visceral carcinomatosis due to ingestion of arsenic. Acta. Dermatol. Venereol. (Stockh.), 42:252, 1962.

Birmingham, D. J., Key, M. M., Holaday, D. A., and Perone, V. B.: An outbreak of arsenical dermatoses in a mining community. Arch. Dermatol., 91:457, 1965.

Bleiberg, J.: Soluble inorganic arsenicals. J. Allerg., 41:236, 1968.

Bloomfield, J. J., Trasko, V. M., Sayers, R. R., Page, R. T., and Peyton, M. F.: A preliminary survey of the industrial hygiene problem in the United States. Public Health Bull., 259:132, 1940.

Büngeler, W.: Tierexperimentelle und zellphysiologische Untersuchungen zur Frage der allgemeinen. Geschwulstdisposition. Frankfurt. Z. Pathol., 39:314, 1930.

Byron, W. B., Bierbower, G. W., Brouwer, J. B., and Hansen, W. H.: Pathologic changes in rats and dogs from 2 year feeding of sodium arsenite or sodium arsenate. Toxicol. Appl. Pharmacol., 10:132, 1967.

Chapman, A. C.: On the presence of compounds of arsenic in marine crustaceans and shell fish. Analyst, 51:548, 1926.

Chapple, R. A.: Treatment of intermittent fevers by large doses of arsenic. Med. Times Gazette, 1:218, 1861.

Clements, R., Tree, H. G., Ewing, P. L., and Emerson, G. A.: Conversion by tissues of inorganic arsenicals to forms not recoverable by the usual assay methods. Texas Rep. Biol. Med., 9:27, 1951.

Denk, R., Holzmann, H., Lange, H. J., and Greve, D.: Über Arsenspätschäden bei obduzierten Moselwinzern. Med. Welt, 11:557, 1969.

Dewar, W. A., and Lenihan, J. M. A.: A case of chronic arsenical poisoning: examination of tissue samples by activation analysis. Scott. Med. J., 1:236, 1956.

Dobson, R. L., and Pinto, J. S.: Arsenical carcinogenesis. In Montagna, W., and Dobson, R. L. (Eds.): Advances in Biology of Skin. Vol. VII. Carcinogenesis. Oxford, Pergamon Press, 1966.

Dobson, R. L., Young, M. R., and Pinto, J. S.: Palmar keratosis and cancer. Arch. Dermatol., 92:553, 1965.

Domonkos, A. N.: Neutron activation analysis of arsenic in normal skin, keratoses and epitheliomas. Arch. Dermatol., 80:672, 1959.

Dubreuilh, W.: Kératose arsénicale et cancer arsénical. Ann. Dermatol. Syphiligr. (Paris), 5th series, 1:65, 1910.

Epstein, E.: Association of mucocutaneous and ceral cancers. Arch. Dermatol. Syph., 69:58, 1954.

Ferguson, A. G., Dewar, W. A., and Smith, H.: Arsenic values in various skin diseases. Arch. Dermatol., 81:931, 1960.

Fierz, U.: Katamnesische Untersuchungen über die Nebenwirkung der Therapie von Hautkrankheiten mit anorganischem Arsen. Arch. Klin. Exp. Dermatol., 227:286, 1966.

Fowler, T.: Medical Reports on the Effect of Arsenic in the Cure of Agues, Remitting Fever and Periodic Headaches. London, J. Johnson, 1786.

Franseen, L. C., and Taylor, G. W.: Arsenical keratoses and carcinomas. Am. J. Cancer, 22:287, 1934.

Friedewald, W. F., and Rous, P.: Determining influence of tar, benzpyrene, and methylcholanthrene on character of benign tumors induced therewith in rabbit skin. J. Exp. Med., 80:127, 1944.

Frost, D. V.: Arsenicals in biology: retrospect and prospect. (review) Fed. Proc., 26:194, 1967.

Geyer, L.: Ueber die chronischen Hautveränderungen beim Arsenicismus und Betrachtungen über die Massenerkrankungen in Reichenstein in Schlesien. Arch. Derm. Syph. (Wein), 43:221, 1898.

Graham, J. H., and Helwig, E. B.: Bowen's disease and its relation to systemic cancer. Arch. Dermatol., 80:133, 1959.

Graham, J. H., and Helwig, E. B.: Bowen's disease and its relationship to systemic cancer. Arch. Dermatol., 83:738, 1961.

Graham, J. H., and Helwig, E. B.: Cutaneous premalignant lesions. In Montagna, W., and Dobson, R. L. (Eds.): Advances in Biology of Skin. Vol. VII. Carcinogenesis. Oxford, Pergamon Press, 1966.

Graham, J. H., Mazzonti, G. R., and Helwig, E. B.: Chemistry of Bowen's disease: relationship to arsenic. J. Invest. Dermatol., 37:317, 1961.

Harter, J. G., and Novitch, A. M.: An evaluation of Gay's solution in the treatment of asthma. J. Allerg., 40:327, 1967.

Hartwell, J. L.: Survey of Compounds Which Have Been Tested for Carcinogenic Activity. Ed. 2. Public Health Service Publication No. 149, 1951.

Hebra, F.: Diseases of the Skin. (Translation by C. H. Fagge and P. H. Pye-Smith.) London, New Sydenham Society, 1868.

Hill, A. B., and Fanning, E. L.: Studies in the incidence of cancer in a factory handling inorganic compounds of arsenic. 1. Mortality experience in the factory. Br. J. Ind. Med., 5:2, 1948.

Holmqvist, I.: Occupational arsenical dermatitis; study among employees at copper ore smelting work including investigations of skin reactions to contact with arsenic compounds. Acta. Dermatol. Venereol. (Stockh.), Suppl. 26, 31:1, 1951.

Hueper, W. C.: A quest into the environmental causes of cancer of the lung. Public Health Monograph No. 36, 27, 1955.

Hueper, W. C.: Cancer hazards from natural and artificial water pollutants. In Proc. Conf. Physiological Aspects of Water Quality, Washington, D. C. Sept 809, 1960. Cited Tseng, 1968.

Hunt, T.: Practical observations on the pathology and

treatment of certain diseases of the skin. London, J. A. Churchill, 1847.

Hutchinson, J.: On some examples of arsenic-keratosis of the skin and of arsenic-cancer. Trans. Pathol. Soc. Lond., 39:352, 1888.

Jung, E. G., and Trachsel, B.: Molekularbiologische Untersuchung zur Arsencarcinogenesis. Arch. Klin. Exp. Dermatol., 237:819, 1970.

Kanisawa, M., and Schroeder, H. A.: Life term studies on the effects of arsenic, germanium, tin and vanadium on spontaneous tumors in mice. Cancer Res., 27:1192, 1967.

Kanisawa, M., and Schroeder, H. A.: Life term studies on the effect of trace elements on spontaneous tumors in mice and rats. Cancer Res., 29:892, 1969.

Kennaway, E. L.: A contribution to the mythology of cancer research. Lancet, 2:769, 1942.

Klein, E. Stoll, H. L., Miller, E., Milgrom, H., Helm, F., and Burgess, G.: The effects of 5-fluorouracil (5-FU) ointment in the treatment of neoplastic dermatoses. Dermatologica, Suppl. 1, 140:21, 1970.

Knoth, W.: Psoriasis vulgaris. Arsenbehandlung. Arch. Klin. Exp. Dermatol., 227:228, 1966.

Lee, A. M., and Fraumeni, J. F., Jr.: Arsenic and respiratory cancer in man: an occupational study. J. Natl. Cancer Inst., 42:1045, 1969.

Leitch, A., and Kennaway, E. L.: Experimental production of cancer by arsenic. Br. Med. J., 2:1107, 1922.

MacLagan, C.: On the arsenic eaters of Styria. Edin. Med. J., 10:200, 1864.

Milner, J. E.: The effect of ingested arsenic on methylcholanthrene-induced tumors in mice. Arch. Environ. Health, 18:7, 1969.

Minkowitz, S.: Multiple carcinomata following the ingestion of medicinal arsenic. Ann. Intern. Med., 61:296, 1964.

Montgomery, H.: Superficial epitheliomatosis. Arch. Dermatol. Syph., 20:339, 1929.

Montgomery, H.: Arsenic as an etiological agent in certain types of epithelioma. Arch. Dermatol. Syph., 32:218, 1935.

Montgomery, H., and Waisman, M.: Epithelioma attributable to arsenic. J. Invest. Dermatol., 4:365, 1941.

Neubauer, O.: Arsenical cancer: a review. Br. J. Cancer, 1:192, 1947.

Obermayer, M. E.: Discussion of Birmingham (1965). Arch. Dermatol., 91:463, 1965.

Osborne, E. D.: Microchemical studies of arsenic in arsenical pigmentations and keratoses. Arch. Dermatol. Syph., 12:773, 1925.

Osborne, E. D.: Microchemical studies of arsenic in arsenical dermatitis. Arch. Dermatol. Syph., 18:37, 1928.

Paris, J. A.: Pharmacologia. Ed. 3. London, W. Phillips, 1820, p. 133.

Pascher, F., and Wolf, J.: Cutaneous sequelae following treatment of bronchial asthma with inorganic arsenic: report of two cases. J.A.M.A., 148:734, 1952.

Perry, K., Bowler, R. G., Bucknell, H. M., Druett, H. A., and Schilling, R. S. F.: Studies in the incidence of cancer in a factory handling inorganic compounds of arsenic. II. Clinical and environmental investigations. Br. J. Ind. Med., 5:6, 1948.

Peterka, E. S., Lynch, F. W., and Goltz, R. W.: An association between Bowen's disease and internal cancer. Arch. Dermatol., 84:623, 1961.

Petres, J., and Berger, A.: Zum Einfluss anorganischen Arsens auf die DNS-Synthese menschlicher lymphocyten in vitro. Arch. Dermatol. Forsch., 242:343, 1972.

Pinkus, H., and Mehregan, A. H.: A Guide to Dermatohistopathology. London, Butterworth & Company, Ltd., 1969.

Pinto, S. S., and Bennett, B. M.: Effect of arsenic trioxide exposure on mortality. Arch. Environ. Health, 7:583, 1963.

Poisoned Bath buns. Pharmacol. J., 2nd series, 1:389, 1860.

Raposo, L. S., cited by Hartwell, J. L.: Survey of Compounds Which Have Been Tested for Carcinogenic Activity. Ed. Public Health Service Publication No. 149, 1951.

Rhodes, E . L.: Pulmar-plantar seed keratoses and internal malignancy. Br. J. Dermatol., 82:361, 1970.

Roth, F.: Uber die chroniche Arsenvergiftung der Moselwinzer unter besonderer Berüsichtigung des Arsenkrebses. Z. Krebsforsch, 61:287, 1956.

Roth, F.: The sequelae of chronic arsenic poisoning in Moselle vintners. Ger. Med. Mon., 2:172, 1957.

Sanderson, K. V.: Arsenic as a co-carcinogen in mice. Rep. Br. Emp. Cancer Campaign, 39:628, 1961.

Sanderson, K. V.: Arsenic and skin cancer. Trans. St. John's Hosp. Dermatol. Soc., 49:115, 1963.

Scott, A.: The retention of arsenic in the late cutaneous complications of its administration. Br. J. Dermatol., 70:195, 1958.

Silver, A. S., and Wainman, P. L.: Chronic poisoning following use of an asthma remedy. J.A.M.A., 150:584, 1952.

Smales, A. A., and Pate, B. D.: The determination of sub-microgram quantities of arsenic by radioactivation. III. The determination of arsenic in biological material. Analyst, 77:196, 1952.

Smith, H.: Estimation of arsenic in biological tissue by activation analyses. Anal. Chem., 31:1361, 1959.

Snegireff, L., and Lombard, O.: Arsenic and cancer. Arch. Ind. Hyg., 4:199, 1951.

Sommers, S. C., and McManus, R. G.: Multiple arsenical cancers of skin and internal organs (review). Cancer, 6:347, 1953.

Stolman, L. P.: Are palmar keratoses a sign of internal malignancy? Arch. Dermatol., 101:52, 1970.

Taub, S. J.: The role of arsenic in chronic asthma and cancer. Eye, Ear, Nose Throat Mon., 49:80, 1970.

Thiers, H., Colomb, D., Moulin, G., and Cohn, L.: Le cancer cutané arsénical des viticulteurs du Beaujolais. Ann. Dermatol. Syphiligr. (Paris), 94:133, 1967.

Tseng, W. P., Chu, H. M., How, S. W., Fong, J. M., Lin, C. S., and Yeh, S.: Prevalence of skin cancer in an endemic area of chronic arsenicism in Taiwan. J. Natl. Cancer Inst., 40:453, 1968.

White, J. C.: Psoriasis, verruca, epithelioma: a sequence. Am. J. Med. Sci., 89:163, 1885.

Wilson, W. E. J.: Melasma arsenicale. J. Cutan. Med. (Lond.), 1:355, 1868.

Wilson, W. E. J.: Lectures on Dermatology. Vol. 2 London, J. A. Churchill, 1873, p. 151.

Woodside, J. R., and Dobson, R. L.: Histopathology of palmar keratoses associated with cancer. Arch. Dermatol., 98:648, 1968.

Yeh, S.: Skin cancer in chronic arsenicism. Hum. Pathol., 4:469, 1973.

Yeh, S., How, S. W., and Lin, C. S.: Arsenical cancer of the skin: histological study with special reference to Bowen's disease. (review) Cancer, 21:312, 1968.

20

Tar Keratosis

Hans Götz, M.D.

SYNONYMS, DEFINITION, HISTORY

Tar keratosis is a collective term for all types of keratosis developing on the skin of persons in prolonged contact with tar, pitch, or coal, or with their products, such as briquettes, or soot and mineral oil products, especially crude paraffin. In the stricter sense of the term, tar keratosis means tar wart, which is identical to what is called verruca picea, soot wart, *poireau de suie*, pitch wart, or briquette wart. These are always small, mostly gray, more rarely brownish, relatively flat, round structures, up to 3 mm. in diameter on the average, and they can be easily scraped off with the fingernail without bleeding, as described by Götz and Zambal (1965).

Tar keratosis can develop into cancer. It is not surprising that the resulting cancer was what first attracted attention as an uncommon finding on the scrotum of chimney sweeps. Only the early date of its first description is historically remarkable. Percival Pott in England described chimney sweep's cancer as an occupational disease in 1775. In Germany it was Volkmann (1875) who not only described tar cancer in brown coal and paraffin workers as an occupational disease and identified it with Pott's scrotal cancer but also observed the early stages of the disease. The frequent irritation and characteristic changes of tar skin were termed "tar itch" by the workers themselves. Volkmann also noticed the verrucous structures which formed under the influence of a certain noxa of coal products or paraffin and eventually led to cancer. Decades later Ehrmann (1909) mentioned skin changes in workers caused by pitch: (1) pitch browning of the skin and yellow discoloration of the sclera; (2) comedones (more rarely folliculitis); and (3) hyperkeratotic structures, such as papillomas, verrucas, or verrucous hyperplasia of the palm of the hand (palmar keratosis). He compared the brown coloration with the appearance of the "skin of a red Indian."

Attempts to produce cancer with tar in animal experiments were of great importance to the understanding of tar skin and tar keratosis. Primary credit is due to the Japanese research workers Yamagiva and Itchikawa (1918), who were the first to produce skin cancer by continual painting with tar. It was proved later that tar-induced skin changes seen in man could also be produced in various animals: after rabbits' ears were painted with tar, skin cornification and transformation into cancer were observed (Itchikawa, 1923). In mice, pigment changes in the form of superficial

492

or deeper melanosis were pointed out (Lipschütz, 1923), and a tendency toward circumscribed hyperkeratosis of the epidermis was observed. There is an interesting parallel reported by Veiel (1924), who for years had treated a man aged 68 for a scrotal eczema of 23 years' standing by painting it with a liquid tar and spirit mixture (1:2), because this treatment seemed the most effective. Warty structures gradually developed which degenerated into cancer. Teutschlaender (1929) reported that he saw such tar warts in briquette workers in Baden, Germany, and South Wales, Britain.

Among the keratotic changes developing in tar skin is the keratoacanthoma. We have seen this only rarely, in contrast to Fabry (1967). Since a separate chapter in this book is dedicated to keratoacanthoma, we do not propose to discuss it in detail at this point. The same applies to the cornu cutaneum.

EPIDEMIOLOGY AND INCIDENCE

All workers employed in plants in which coal products are used are at risk of developing tar skin, with the formation of tar warts and their cancerous sequelae. In 1959 Bönig and Holz listed types of occupations in which long-continued contact with coal products leads to skin lesions:

Tar	Coking plants	Roofing felt manufacture
	Gasworks	Fisheries
	Tar refineries	Rope making
	Road building	
Pitch	Tar refineries	Cable works
	Coal briquette makers	Caulking materials makers
	Cork brick works	Makers of additives to
	Varnish industry	molded plastics
		Shoemakers
Soot	Chimney sweeps	Ship and railway engine
	Carbon black makers	stokers
		Rubber industry
Crude paraffin	Naphthalene industry	Paper industry
	Oil refineries	Munitions industry
	Charcoal burners	Match factories
Asphalt	Roofing felt manufacturers	Insulating tape makers
	Road builders	Protective steel and pipe
	Building industry	paints
	(insulating material)	Linoleum works
	Cable works	Brake and clutch linings
	Electrical industry	
	(sealing compound)	

There are other possibilities, connected mainly with mineral oil products. Contact with mineral, slate, and spindle oils in cotton spinning may lead to changes very similar to those seen in tar skin. It is interesting that, according to Heller (1930), skin lesions—above all, cancer—were found much more rarely in the United States, probably because the machine oils used in spinning are less carcinogenic. In place of coal tar, Americans use the less irritating oil tar in briquette manufacture. Skin cancer in these undertakings is therefore also less common.

In France tar cancer as an occupational disease in miners is extremely rare (Tourraine, 1957); (Huriez in 1954 found only one carcinoma in 80,000 miners.) The question arises, of course, whether these might have all been miners who had hardly any contact with tar products. In German miners who dealt only with natural coal, we have not found any changes which could be interpreted as tar skin. The particular substance to which the skin is exposed is of decisive importance. Other examples of the carcinogenic effects of tar products in different countries are given by Tourraine.

In the optical industry, comedones and excess pigmentation on the face and arms have been described where pitch dust was regularly thrown onto the skin of workers during the grinding of lenses fixed to an adhesive material containing pitch (Koch, 1956; Schröder, 1961). Together with Bill, we have analyzed 111 cases of tar skin at the Skin Clinic, Essen, mainly in workers who have had to be examined because of suspected tar skin or who had left their work after tar skin was diagnosed and presented themselves for follow-up examination. Twenty-seven of the 111 were briquette workers; 21 were pitch loaders, unloaders, carriers, drainers, or squeezer men; 15 were pitch hackers and dischargers; and 22 were weighters-out in pitch or tar plants, as well as other workers in tar or pitch refineries. It was surprising to find nine fitters in pitch plants and four fitters in tar plants. Finally there were one chemical laboratory assistant and 12 distillers in pitch and tar plants. Generally pitch seems to be more aggressive than tar (Barnewitz, 1928). The length of exposure before the formation of tar skin, tar warts, and eventually tar cancer depends on various factors which are discussed in the following section.

ETIOLOGY

When coal tar is distilled in dry heat, fractions are produced that are variously keratogenic and carcinogenic, according to the degree of heat. Compounds that boil below 180° C. form light oil, those boiling from 180 to 230° C. form medium oil (carbolic oil), from 230 to 270° C. heavy oil, and from 270 to 400° C. anthracene oil. Fractions that boil between 400 and 600° C. are called carbonization tar. The retort residue is called pitch.

The substances contained in the various tar fractions as noxae are mainly aromatic hydrocarbons. One particular group capable of producing cancer is derived from benzene, naphthalene, and anthracene, compounds that consist only of carbon and hydrogen and contain no nitrogen. Benzene rings are present, and the compounds are therefore referred to as polycyclic hydrocarbons. Bauer (1963) stressed that, of all the compounds present in tar, 3,4-benzpyrene has the strongest carcinogenic effect. It is fat-soluble, a fact of great importance for the development of tar warts and even cancer. Since keratogenic and carcinogenic substances are discussed in detail elsewhere, it will be mentioned here only that the benzpyrene contents of different tars vary from 0.7 to 4.7 percent. This explains the variable findings in animal experiments, as well as in workers in different countries, especially in the tar industry. Bauer compiled a table of carcinogenic tars of industrial importance: coal tar, lignite tar, tobacco tar, wood tar, terpentine tar, slate tar, gasworks tar, charcoal tar, blast furnace tar, pine tar, coffee tar, and tar pitch from water pipes. Oil tar and peat tar should be added. As stressed by Linser (1962), the "carcinogenic" or, in the wider sense, "skin-damaging hydrocarbons are so for all animals and organs in experiments, but the reactivity of the species varies." No doubt this statement also applies to individual workers in the tar industry.

It is for this reason that various authors have reported widely different results in the induction of skin injuries by tar fractions. For example, Bloch (1922) first provoked wart formation, partly cornua cutanea, and later epitheliomas in mice in 100 percent of his cases. On the other hand, Cookson (1924) described the case of a worker aged 66 who had handled creosol for 33 years and whose skin showed numerous tar warts, only one of which developed into a squamous cell carcinoma. It is by no means mandatory for tar warts to develop into cancer. According to our observations it is even more uncommon than is generally assumed, as will be shown.

The development of cancer after prolonged contact with tar derivatives is always preceded by skin changes which at first look quite harmless. Keratosis or tar warts form on skin which is both susceptible to them and damaged by tar. But *all* irritations leading to cancer formation promote skin changes in the same way. Such accidental irritants may be of various types, such as mechanical (trauma), chemical (arsenic, silver), physical (heat, light, x-rays, radium), biologic (scars, hyperplasia, dyskeratosis), and infectious (tuberculosis, syphilis). Therefore, if cancer develops by way of tar skin or tar warts, it is probably always a combined injury, even if we cannot discover the nature of the combined action of the different factors. A convincing example of such a combined injury (tar plus heat) was reported by Sträuli (1957), who pointed out similar cases described by Bang, Huguenin, Gunsett, and others. A common provoking factor in the formation of tar warts on the scrotum is the rubbing of tight trousers over coal particles, which causes tiny scratches to develop.

According to our observations ultraviolet rays are also of great significance in the formation of tar skin and tar keratosis, and especially in the transition to carcinoma. Teutschlaender (1930) denied any photodynamic effect of light, because tar injuries manifest themselves especially on the scrotum, which is screened from light. But Coulon had shown as early as 1924 that only 1.6 percent of white mice painted with tar and kept in dark cages developed cancer, whereas 9 percent of those exposed to light developed it. There can be no doubt about the injurious effect of ultraviolet rays on the skin. To quote one example, there is the report of Batschwaroff and coworkers (1962) on the incidence of skin cancer in Bulgaria, which is a sunny country. Of 1796 skin cancer patients seen between 1953 and 1959, 75 percent were peasants and 25 percent townspeople. The regions chiefly affected were those exposed to light, such as the nose, lips, ears, and other parts of the face (94 percent), and the neck and upper extremities (2.6 percent).

That light has a decisive effect in the development of tar skin is shown by our own observations. It has been known for a long time that, even many years after leaving the original place of work in the tar industry, former workers may continue to develop tar warts and skin cancer. We asked ourselves, therefore, whether there are any indications in the functional activity of the integument as to why permanent damage to the skin apparently can occur that is due to prolonged contact with tar. Is the skin in a state of increased irritability even after the person leaves the tar industry?

We investigated this question by determining the threshold value for erythema in our 111 patients with tar skin. With the aid of a masking device, eight sections of the skin of the back are exposed to an ordinary ultraviolet lamp for 11.5 to 42 seconds under constant conditions ("light steps" of Wucherpfennig). The amount of radiation increases in geometric progression by 20 percent for each section of skin. The erythema threshold is the number of seconds of irradiation sufficient to cause barely visible reddening 7 hours later.

The determination of the threshold erythema dose in 111 tar workers showed that the majority of older people apparently have a reduced erythema threshold, although it is known that actinic sensitivity usually decreases with age, and in fact our control examinations of men of the same age but with no occupational contact with tar did not reveal any increased light sensitivity. When we arranged the results of the experiment according to the duration of work in the tar industry, it was clearly seen that the tendency to ultraviolet light sensitization increased with increasing length of exposure to tar. At the time of the erythema threshold determination, the 111 former tar workers had not been exposed to the injurious tar for an average of 8.8 years, but 82 percent still showed an increased ultraviolet light sensitivity. Moreover, the group of workers who at some time had had cancer showed a much higher percentage of persistent photosensitization (58 percent) than the group that had not had cancer (33 percent). Persistent ultraviolet light sensitization therefore constitutes another conditional reason why tar warts continue to form and cancer continues to develop even after contact with tar products ceases.

The damage to skin that is done by tar and its derivatives is due in part to the photosensitizing property of certain chemicals, such as anthracene, acridine, methylanthracene, pyrene, fluoranthene, and benzpyrene. The effects of handling tar products are therefore enhanced if certain uncovered parts of the body are subjected to the additional irritation of ultraviolet rays, such as from sunlight.

Another factor, not without importance in our view, is age. According to Vilanova (1958), the skin begins to show signs of aging even from the age of 25. Between 35 and 40 at the latest, age changes are unmistakably present in our northern latitudes. With increasing age the skin tends to dryness, scaling, and keratosis formation. The tendency toward such changes, therefore, must undoubtedly potentiate any similar signs already provoked by tar noxae and ultraviolet light.

Among our 111 tar workers who had left the industry, there were eight men under 40 with tar skin and tar warts. With increasing age up to 60 to 65, the number of cases rose. Parallel with that, of course, went the length of exposure to tar products and to sunlight on the light-exposed parts of the body (nearly all our tar workers worked mainly in the open air). Besides simple senile and atrophic processes, there are additional degenerative changes in the elastic and collagen tissue in the sense of senile elastosis (Götz and Schuppener, 1969). There is a striking clinical and histologic similarity between tar skin, with its tendency towards keratosis and even epithelioma, and aging skin.

So we have a sum of etiologic factors in tar workers which sooner or later leads to tar skin, tar warts, and eventually cancer, and in addition—as already mentioned briefly—there is the individual disposition, which is so difficult to assess.

PATHOGENESIS

Nothing has promoted our knowledge of the pathogenetic processes in the formation of tar warts and tar cancer as much as animal experiments with tar noxae. Itchikawa and Baum (1924) observed the action of tar on rabbit skin (mostly the skin of the ear). First they found signs of inflammation. The epithelium developed a tendency toward hyperplasia and hypertrophy. This was followed by the formation of benign papillomas, which finally merged into the third stage of malignant degeneration of the epithelium.

According to Lipschütz (1923), precancerous warts form the points of origin of invasively growing tumors. A study of the literature, however, shows that cancer apparently develops from tar warts much more frequently in mice than in men. Teutschlaender wrote in 1933 that tumor formation could be produced experimentally in 100 percent of cases by painting mice with tar; it should be mentioned that, of all experimental animals, mice have the greatest tendency toward developing tumors spontaneously.

When prolonged tar painting is discontinued in animal experiments, cell mutation in the epidermis usually goes on and leads to further formation of keratosis and even to cancer. There are always inflammatory changes, followed by degenerative proliferative lesions (warts, papillomas). More recently Linser (1962) stressed the role of the stroma: under the influence of tar noxae the connective tissue is supposed to become "defenseless," allowing the degenerated epidermis cell to penetrate deeply.

On the basis of experiments in rabbits, Babes and Serbanesco (1928) were of the opinion that cancer could develop independently of tar warts, which agrees with our eight years of clinical observations. Although we do not agree with Borst's opinion that the carcinomatous nature of many experimental animal cancers is doubtful, he is right in saying that on the one hand cancer development is not necessarily roundabout via precancerous stages, but on the other hand most so-called precancerous stages do not lead to cancer.

On uncovered parts of the body, carcinogenic tar products can damage the skin just as ultraviolet light rays can do over the course of decades. These carcinogenic substances are lipid-soluble. The fattier the skin surface, the better are the injurious tar products dissolved and able to penetrate into the deeper layers and underlying connective tissue. At the same time the skin becomes more susceptible by exposure to the sun. Much of the sun's infrared light is absorbed in the upper corium layers, where it may cause biologic damage. But the ultraviolet light is only partly absorbed in the horny layers, mainly penetrating to the basal cell layer. Benzpyrene collects preferentially in the cytoplasm of the cells of the germinative layer (Bauer, 1963). Considering that many tar noxae — benzpyrene, for one — also have a light-sensitizing effect, it is understandable that damage to the skin from the combined effect of these factors is enormous.

These facts make it clear why in our 111 tar workers tar warts appeared on sites exposed to light (the face, the dorsum of the hand) in 71 percent of cases — caused by tar noxae plus light — and why the next most frequent site was the scrotum (8 percent of cases) — tar noxae plus high lipid content of the skin. In the case of the scrotum, another factor is the relatively constant temperature of 36.6 to 36.8° C. in the area between the opposed scrotal wall and the inner surface of the thigh. Moreover, the thickness of the epidermis on the inner surface of the thigh is 50 to 60 microns (Southwood, 1955), whereas that of the scrotal skin in our investigations is only about half that figure. Aging processes must be considered too, as the epidermis thins out with increasing age (Cramer, 1968). Components of tar reaching the area between the scrotum and the thigh would be expected to cause damage owing to the high lipid content of the scrotal skin, the constant heat, and the thin epidermis. We have not seen any tar warts on the inner surface of the thigh in any of our 111 patients, although heat and sweat are supposed to provoke tar skin lesions.

The deeper the penetration of fat-soluble carcinogenic tar noxae and the longer it continues, the more damaging must be the effect on connective tissue and epithelium. In body sites that produce little lipids, are not particularly exposed to light, and have a thicker epidermis, such as the dorsum of the foot and the ankle, carcinogenic substances are to a large extent retained in the upper epidermis. During years of work in the pitch and tar industry, traces of noxae fall into a worker's shoes every day and collect on the dorsum of the foot and around the ankle. But here—even with poor hygiene and perhaps only weekly washing of the feet—the mechanical and chemical irritation eventually stimulates the skin to form a warty keratosis, hardly carcinoma. In the history and during our eight years of observation of 111 tar workers, there was only one case of a squamous cell carcinoma on the foot. Tar warts on the dorsum of the foot and around the ankle were the first such lesions to appear primarily in only about 10 percent of our patients, but after years of exposure and even after the men had left the industry warts were present in 57 percent on the dorsum of the foot and in 72 percent on the inner side of the ankle.

It now appears that the effect of these carcinogenic noxae is to induce in the cells of the germinative layer a mutation which is of varying intensity according to the duration of the injury. Ullmann (1933) used the term "engramme," coined by Semon-Teutschlaender, for a stage of preparatory latency. If the injury is of brief duration, the "engrammes" gradually fade. After a number of years, therefore, during which there is no contact with tar products, the tendency toward tar wart formation gradually decreases.

O'Donovan (1929) pointed out the long latent period between tar wart formation and the development of skin cancer in tar workers. The latent period before tumor formation (not necessarily carcinoma), he thought, was between 3 months and 4 years. The longest period before cancer development was 35 years. A railway worker, aged 48, whose job was concerned with the impregnation of wooden ties with tar, after five years developed verrucous structures on the dorsum of the hand and the face, as in experimental tar cancer (Pisani and Izzo, 1961). Fifteen years later these warts developed into cancers. Matras (1960) reported a latent period before malignant degeneration of 3 to 17½ years.

An analysis of our 111 patients shows that the first appearance of tar warts is subject to considerable variation. The workers studied were employed in the tar industry for 15 years on the average before the formation of the first tar warts. The latent period before development to cancer also varied, as did that before the first appearance of carcinoma. We worked out an average of 20 years of work before the first development of tar cancer.

What Mertens (1924) said about tar cancer arising not only from warts and what Oliver (1930) reported about warts in tar workers which *sometimes* go on to form epitheliomas agrees with our experience in Essen. In five years we saw hundreds of typical tar warts in 111 workers, but only in two patients did carcinoma very probably develop from a tar wart. This may have some connection with the fact that in most of our cases the workers were no longer employed in the tar industry.

CLINICAL FEATURES

Many workers with prolonged exposure to tar or pitch products look prematurely old (Fig. 20–1). Upon close examination, the clinical picture is found to consist of two periods. The first change on the face is an inflammatory reddening, especially of exposed parts, accompanied by a burning sensation and sometimes edema and infiltration. After some time conjunctivitis develops, with slight yellow-brown discoloration of the sclera in some cases. Folliculitis and comedones follow. Subjectively, more or less intense itching is noticed (Table 20–1). In many cases, especially after the patients leave the industry, the inflammatory symptoms regress.

It is interesting how frequent itching is; it was not without reason that briquette workers of the last century called their skin condition "tar itch" (Volkmann, 1875). Conjunctivitis was found in 60 percent of cases, primarily owing to the invasion of fine pitch and tar particles which dissolve in the conjunctival space. However, photosensitization also plays an important part. Lacrimation with increased sensitivity to wind and weather was present occasionally. The comedone and hair follicle plugs consist mainly of keratin. Combination with tar

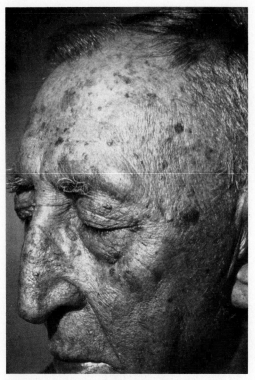

Figure 20–1 A tar worker aged 63 with typical tar skin after 30 years' exposure to pitch and tar products.

TABLE 20–1 SKIN CHANGES ON THE FACE (EXCLUDING TAR WARTS AND CANCER)*

Symptom	Number	Percent
Periocular fibroma	88	80
Brown discoloration	76	68
Conjunctivitis	65	60
Comedones	64	58
Hair follicle plugs	63	57
Itching	46	41
Slate-gray discoloration	31	28
Hyperkeratoses	14	12
Inflammation	6	5
Folliculitis	6	5
Scaling	5	5

*The tables in this section all refer to 111 former workers in the tar industry, with an average exposure to tar products lasting 18½ years.

Among these is atrophy of the skin (to be described under Histology), affecting both epidermis and corium. Others include persistent pigmentation and pigment displacement, as well as occasional telangiectases. According to Table 20–1, nearly all tar workers showed persistent pigmentation of the face, which becomes darker (slate-gray discoloration) with longer exposure to tar products. Table 20–2 shows that, as expected, pigmentation was present only in exposed parts, not on the trunk and legs, despite many years' exposure to tar. Only the scrotum, richer in pigment by nature, showed an intensification of melanin formation after exposure to injurious tar products.

The proliferative changes in the second stage of tar skin development deserve more attention. In Tables 20–1 and 20–2 we have already listed fibroma, hyperkeratosis, and scaling (Figs. 20–2 and 20–3). It is surprising how little attention has been

products makes them appear dark and even black.

By comparison, on the rest of the body we found hardly any signs of inflammation, which is probably explained by the absence of continued action of irritants (Table 20–2).

The first clinical signs of tar skin formation are followed after a variable latent period by the second stage, characterized by degenerative and proliferative changes.

TABLE 20–2 SKIN CHANGES ON THE REST OF THE BODY (EXCLUDING TAR WARTS AND CANCER)

Location	Itching	Pigmentation	Comedones	Inflammation	Hyperkeratosis	Scaling	Fibroma
Neck	23	99	33	4	10	5	27
Dorsum of hand and forearm	33	105	0	3	39	28	2
Trunk	33	0	0	0	11	4	3
Scrotum	9	38	0	1	1	0	3
Legs	10	0	0	1	3	63	2
Inside of ankle	2	0	0	0	7	78	0
Dorsum of foot	5	0	0	0	6	80	0

paid in the literature to fibroma in tar workers, probably because of its benign character. We found fibromas in the region of the eyes in 80 percent of our former tar workers (Table 20–1). They were less common on the neck, dorsum of the hand, forearm, trunk, scrotum, and legs, for a total of 37 fibromas (Table 20–2). The fibromas were nearly always pedunculated, but in three cases we saw broad-based papillomas which we described as a separate type of wart.

Among the proliferative changes we have also included hyperkeratosis and scaling, because they are usually associated with increased acanthosis and thickening of the horny layer. By hyperkeratosis we mean a rather flat, rough thickening observed mostly on the dorsum of the hand, but occasionally also on the palm, and on the forearm (Table 20–2). Scaling was most intense on the legs and feet and affected elderly people more. There is probably a combined effect of age and tar noxae – pigment displacement, circumscribed skin atrophy, scaling, circumscribed keratosis, telangiectasis. In some cases the formation of tar warts, which in

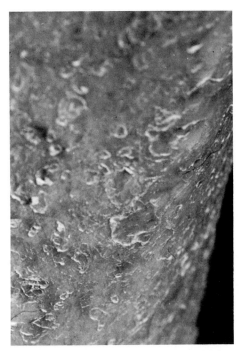

Figure 20–3 Coarse-lamellar scaling on the leg of a tar worker aged 56 with 30 years' tar exposure.

our opinion may be described as an "occupation stigma," allowed us to diagnose tar skin, taking the history into account, of course. We saw only one case of keratoacanthoma and one of cutaneous horn, which developed only after the men had left the tar industry.

We have already emphasized that the period from the start of exposure to the development of the first tar skin symptoms shows considerable individual variation. Months or years after entering the tar industry a worker may develop a clinical picture greatly resembling that of toxic melanodermatitis. Table 20–3 shows the

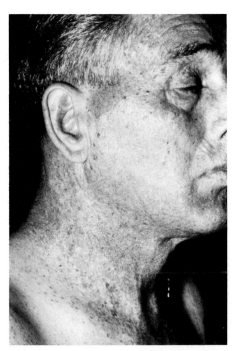

Figure 20–2 Tar skin of the face and neck (light-exposed parts) of a worker aged 42, with pigmentation, wart formation, and periocular fibromas.

TABLE 20–3 LENGTH OF EXPOSURE TO TAR AND PITCH BEFORE THE FIRST SIGNS OF TAR SKIN BEGAN (INCLUDING TAR WARTS AND CANCER)

Less than 5 years	18 workers
5 to 10 years	23
10 to 15 years	10
15 to 20 years	18
20 to 25 years	10
25 to 30 years	10
30 to 35 years	11
35 to 40 years	9
More than 40 years	2
	111

41 } 69

length of tar exposure and the time when skin changes developed.

The shortest exposure before the appearance of pitch skin was only 1½ years. In over one-third of the tar workers (41), early skin changes appeared after an exposure of less than 10 years, whereas another third (42) tolerated exposure to tar and pitch products for more than 20 years without definite signs of disease and developed the typical changes only later. Most cases (51) occurred between the sixth and twentieth years of work, the incidence declining with increasing age. The explanation may be that in the first two decades there is a kind of individual self-selection. Only those workers remain in the tar industry who have not developed skin changes sufficient to disable them within the terms of the Occupational Diseases Regulations. According to Downing (1932) an exposure of 10 to 20 years caused the majority of cases, but he, too, reported a reduction in incidence with longer exposure.

One of the most important clues to the diagnosis of "tar skin" is the formation of tar warts.

Data from our histories show occupational contact with tar or pitch for an average of 18½ years before the worker was removed from his place of work. An average of 15 years passed before tar warts developed, but the length of exposure varied considerably in the individual case. The shortest contact was only 2½ years, the longest 43 years. As seen in Table 20–4, we found primary formation of warts most often on the face (52 percent) and the dorsum of the hand (19 percent).

We have already explained why exposed parts of the body are more affected; cov-

TABLE 20–4 LOCATION OF THE FIRST TAR WARTS TO APPEAR (111 WORKERS)

Face	58 (52 percent)
Neck	10
Arm	2
Forearm	7
Dorsum of the hand	21 (19 percent)
Trunk	3
Scrotum	9 (8 percent)
Leg	4
Dorsum of the foot	6
Inside of ankle	6

TABLE 20–5 LOCATION OF TAR WARTS DURING 5 YEARS OF OBSERVATION (111 WORKERS)

Face	43 (39 percent)
Neck	5
Forearm	21 (19 percent)
Dorsum of the hand	51 (46 percent)
Trunk	6
Scrotum	10 (9 percent)
Penis	1
Leg	11
Dorsum of the foot	64 (57 percent)
Inside of ankle	80 (72 percent)

ered parts offer a less suitable base for the development of tar warts. The picture changes only after many years of contact with tar and pitch products, as seen in Table 20–5. This table takes no account of the history given by the patients but is based solely on our own observations of workers referred to the clinic for initial and follow-up examinations during a period of 5 years.

Here we have a more varied picture with regard to localization. We have to take into consideration the fact that, even after removal of the tar worker from his place of work, the tendency toward formation of tar warts and even carcinoma persists. Among 111 workers with tar skin we diagnosed tar warts in 94 (85 percent). As we saw these small tumors on several parts of the body in some workers, the total number seen is higher than the total number of workers.

It is very remarkable and not mentioned anywhere in the literature except in the first report by Götz and Zambal (1965) and a later one by Fabry (1967) that, with prolonged duration of tar skin disease, the most common location of tar warts is not the face but the dorsum of the foot (Fig. 20–4) and the ankle region (Fig. 20–5). Even if the workers have been out of the industry for many years, the ankle region is the chief location of tar wart recurrences (see under Pathogenesis).

Is there any relation between the formation of tar warts and carcinoma? In Table 20–6 the incidence of tar warts in our 111 tar workers is compared with that of the carcinomas recorded by us. According to the histories and our observations during a 5-year observation period, cancerous degeneration of the skin was found in 46

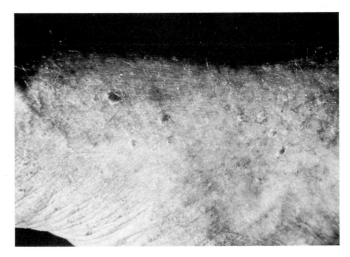

Figure 20–4 Typical tar wart formation on the dorsum of the foot, in addition to diffuse fine-lamellar scaling and moderate flat hyperkeratosis.

workers or about 41 percent of our 111 analyzed cases. A tar wart may certainly represent the precursor of a malignant tumor, as was pointed out under Pathogenesis, but this does not happen very frequently. Table 20–6 shows the tendency toward tar wart formation in the 111 subjects to be much more marked than the tendency toward cancer development. Only the scrotum seems to occupy a special position. Whereas we found 10 tar warts in this region, cancer developed 12 times, not necessarily from tar warts (see Pathogenesis). The most common site of cancer is the light-exposed face, followed by the

scrotum. This agrees in principle with earlier reports by Heller (1930), Henry (1946), and Tourraine (1957), among others.

Since both tar skin alone and its proliferative changes, particularly tar warts, must be regarded as the basis for cancer development, we must here include the incidence of carcinoma in our 111 tar workers. According to Table 20–7, 33 carcinomas were seen in 80 subjects between the ages of 50 and 65. This is 72 percent of the total of 46 recorded carcinomas in 111 workers. In other words, three quarters of all tar cancers developed in the age group most disposed to cancer. An analysis of the 80 workers between 50 and 65 shows that increasing length of tar exposure does not reduce the cancer rate, as might happen by adaptation. The group with 10 years' exposure includes 23 workers, of whom 5 developed cancer. The group with 10 to 20 years of exposure includes 20 workers, of

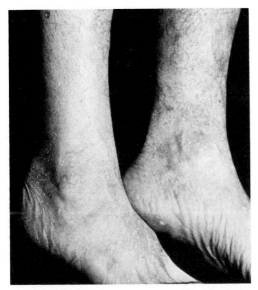

Figure 20–5 Tar wart formation on the lower third of the leg, especially the ankle region, spreading to the dorsum of the foot, in a tar worker aged 44.

TABLE 20–6 TAR WARTS AND TAR CANCER

Location	Incidence of Tar Warts	Incidence of Tar Cancer
Face	43	23
Neck	5	2
Arm	21	3
Dorsum of the hand	51	5
Trunk	6	3
Scrotum	10	12
Penis	1	–
Leg	11	–
Dorsum of the foot	64	1
Inside of ankle	80	–

TABLE 20–7   RELATIONSHIP OF THE AGE OF THE PATIENTS AND THEIR LENGTH OF EXPOSURE TO TAR IN 46 CASES OF CARCINOMA (111 WORKERS)

Length of Exposure To Tar or Pitch (years)	Age							
	Under 40	40 to 45	45 to 50	50 to 55	55 to 60	60 to 65	65 to 70	Over 70
					2			
40				1(1)	4(2)	4(2)		
35				2(2)	2(1)	6(3)	1	
30		1		1(1)	1	4(2)	3(1)	
25				3(1)	5(2)	2(1)		
20	8	1	3(2)	4(3)	7(3)	1(1)	1(1)	1(1)
15				2(1)	5(2)	1	1(1)	1(1)
10	4(2)	1(1)	2	5(1)	5(1)	4(2)	2(1)	
5	4	3(2)		3	5(1)	1	2	
	8	6	5	21	36	23	10	2

Age and number of workers at time of leaving the tar industry; (in brackets) the number of carcinomas during the course of tar skin disease.

whom 10 developed cancer. The group with 20 to 30 years of exposure includes 16 workers, of whom 7 developed cancer, and the group with 30 to 40 years' tar exposure includes 19 workers, of whom 11 developed cancer. With rising age and exposure there is no habituation; on the contrary, the chance of carcinoma development increases distinctly. The clinical signs are always influenced in their intensity and place of appearance by the type of occupation and the properties of the noxae.

HISTOLOGY

Our histologic findings are based on 193 biopsies from tar workers referred to us for assessment in the course of 8 years; in some cases more than one excision was performed. The largest contingent was the group of 111 tar workers from the period 1963 to 1967 analyzed in the preceding sections. Although the number of tar injuries has undoubtedly gone down as a consequence of legislative measures in the Ruhr district, we are still seeing three or four new cases every year. However, it is not only tar warts and carcinomas that are included in the assessment of tar injury, but also, as stressed before, the changes called "tar skin" as the basis from which they originate.

Tar Skin

What is remarkable in tar skin is the finding of *atrophic changes of the malpighian layer in combination with marked hyperkeratosis*. In Figure 20–6 the epidermal cells capable of division show occasional small cell strings or buds in the upper corium. In Figure 20–7 these are more prominent, whereas in Figure 20–8 the papillary body is greatly flattened and shows round cell infiltration while the malpighian layer is better preserved. However, in all these cases the thick, partly lamellar horny layer dominates the picture. On the other hand, we also see flattening of the malpighian layer without significant hyperkeratosis (Fig. 20–9, which also shows deep-sited, tubelike strings of epithelium). The pigmentation in tar skin is due to not only increased melanin accumulation in the clear cells of the basal layer, but in some cases, also to increased accumulation of

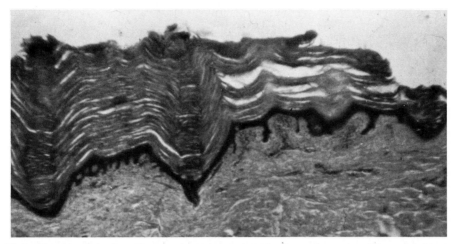

Figure 20-6 Tar skin of the face. Vigorous hyperkeratosis with advanced atrophy of the malpighian layer. No inflammatory reaction in the corium, which after special staining shows senile elastosis (20 years' exposure, worker aged 45).

melanophages and deposition of melanin particles in the upper corium (Fig. 20–10). This was observed by Bettazzi (1932). Occasional findings of newly formed telangiectases in our cases could also be demonstrated histologically (Fig. 20–11).

Another peculiarity of tar skin is the fact—in contrast to Figures 20-7 to 20–11—that in other workers *marked acanthosis was found without corresponding hyperkeratosis* (Fig. 20–12). These lesions, mainly on the face and the neck, with the clinical appearance of comedones, represent keratin plugs in dilated hair follicles (Fig. 20–13).

In some cases these large horn accumulations in the hair follicle ostium set off inflammation (Fig. 20–14). Often mentioned in the past in connection with experimental tar cancer production, but less noticeable in man, is proliferation of the epithelium starting directly from the hair follicle. Figure 20–15 is an example of such an early change demonstrated on the nose of a worker aged 57 after 24 years of contact with tar products. There is a striking absence of sebaceous glands, which are probably atrophied. Tar skin generally is distinguished by unusual dryness.

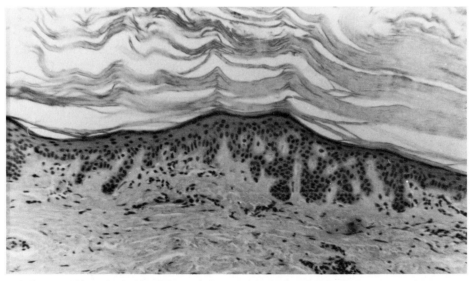

Figure 20-7 Tar skin on the inside of the ankle in a worker aged 61. Vigorous hyperkeratosis with thinning of of the malpighian layer. There is a tendency toward increased epithelium budding, and senile elastosis.

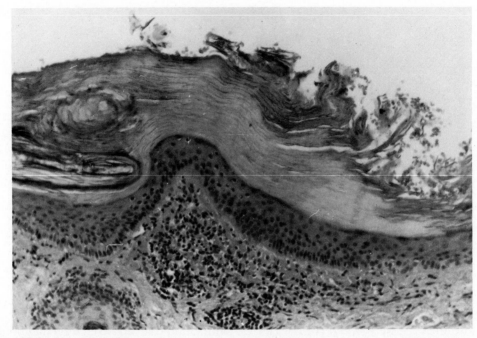

Figure 20–8 Circumscribed keratosis in tar skin of the right wrist. Atrophy of the malpighian layer is less advanced than in the cases shown in Figures 20–6 and 20–7, but there is flattening of the papillary body and an inflammatory reaction in the upper corium.

To summarize the histopathologic findings, as a consequence of chronic tar and pitch action on the skin there is an atrophic effect, especially on the malpighian layer, while on the other hand the keratoplastic action promotes hyperkeratosis. In other cases acanthosis is more prominent, and hyperkeratosis is less marked. Pigmentation or pigment displacements are to be regarded as an expression of a combined injury (tar noxae plus light).

Tar Warts

The acanthogenic and keratoplastic effect becomes much more obvious in the formation of warts, particularly the so-

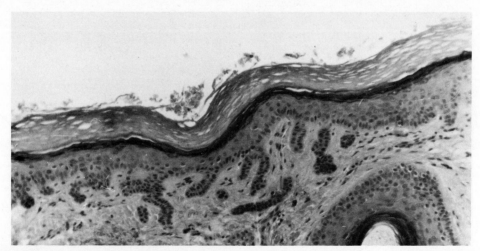

Figure 20–9 Tar skin of the wrist of a worker aged 60. Tubelike, thin, epithelial tracks are seen in the upper corium, but there is no hyperkeratosis.

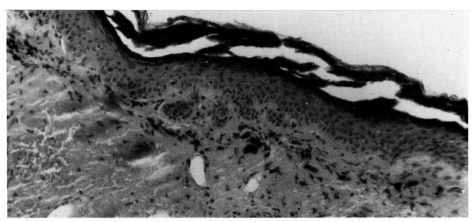

Figure 20–10   Tar skin of the face of a worker aged 57. Note an accumulation of melanophages in the upper corium in addition to numerous fine melanin particles.

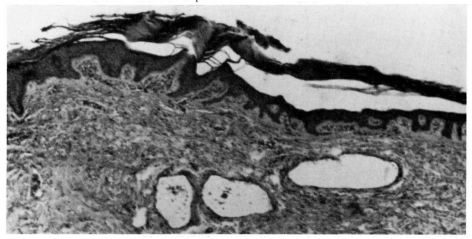

Figure 20–11   Tar skin of the ankle region of a worker aged 51 with new formation of telangiectases. The epidermis and papillary body are well preserved.

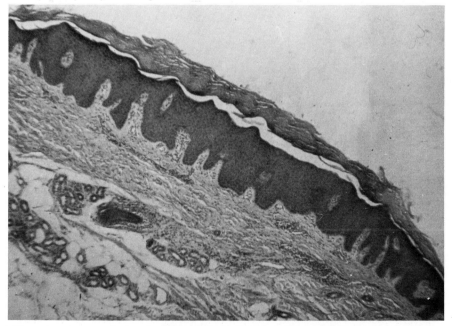

Figure 20–12   Tar skin of a worker aged 48 (neck region). Histologic features are a uniform hyperplasia of the malpighian layer, but a relatively narrow horny layer.

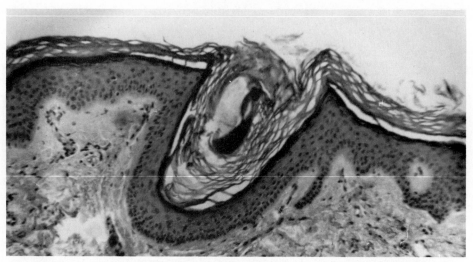

Figure 20–13   Hair follicle keratosis presenting as a comedo in tar skin of the face.

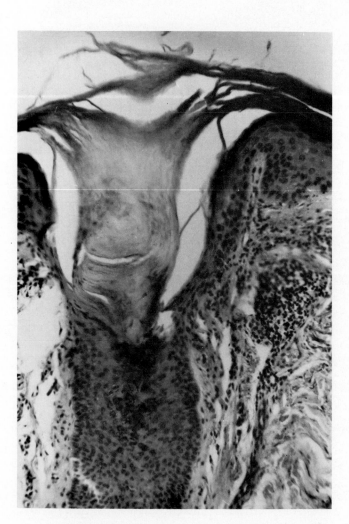

Figure 20–14   Hair follicle keratosis in tar skin of the neck with inflammatory reaction.

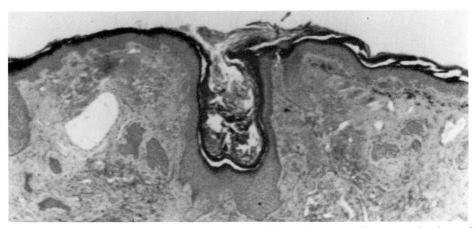

Figure 20–15 Beginning of hyperplasia of hair follicle epithelium into surrounding connective tissue after 24 years' contact with tar products.

called tar warts. On the basis of our latest investigations we delineate three types.

Type I. Owing to its frequency this is the characteristic wart resulting from tar injury to the skin. There is moderate acanthosis, forming contiguous, strikingly pointed, steeplelike cones. Above this, similarly arranged, is a greatly thickened horny layer. The keratin is nearly always free from nuclear debris and more or less loosely layered (Figs. 20–16 and 20–17). The cells of the malpighian layer show nothing atypical and no mitosis. The granular layer may show 12 to 15 layers of keratohyalin as in lichen ruber, though only in circumscribed places (Fig. 20–18).

In other cases the granular layer is less clearly developed (Fig. 20–19).

In this broad tar wart the corium is damaged. Senile elastosis and split-up collagen fibers characterize the changes. The corium as a whole is thinned but shows no inflammatory reaction. In some sections the "steeple tops" are flattened (Fig. 20–20). In these cases there is a suggestion of papillomatosis, by which we mean narrow, markedly elongated but not intertwined, individual papillae. In Figure 20–21 we have a larger wart of this type, but here there is a peculiar vacuolation in the malpighian layer at the left periphery of the picture. In Figure 20–22 this region is seen en-

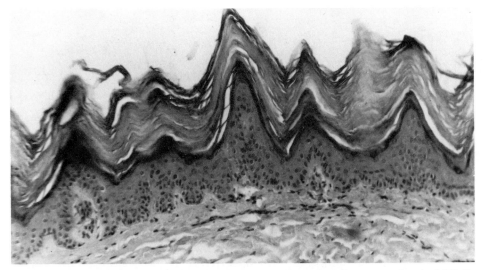

Figure 20–16 Characteristic appearance of tar wart, type I, in the ankle region (tar worker aged 61). Note the "steeple" shape.

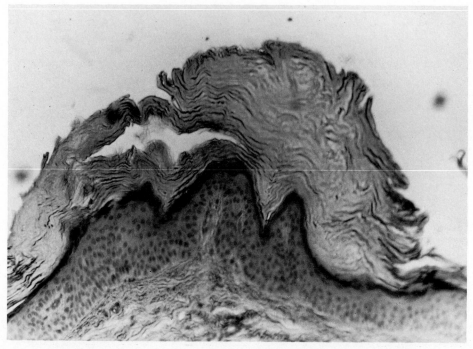

Figure 20–17 Small tar wart, type I, on the leg, with vigorous hyperkeratosis.

larged 400 times; the vacuolation resembles that of arsenical keratosis. Since quite a few tar products contain arsenic, the question arises whether the vacuolation is a result of toxic arsenic action. There was even a time when tar injuries were attributed mainly to the arsenic content (Bayet, 1923). We observed this vacuolation in six of our numerous biopsies.

Type II (Papillomatosis). This type is really more a papilloma, although one that is sometimes not immediately recognizable clinically (Fig. 20–23). It has a broad base and histologically represents papillomatosis. It is characterized by greater ramification and proliferation of the papillae and less hyperkeratosis than type I, and in contrast to type I, cannot be scraped off

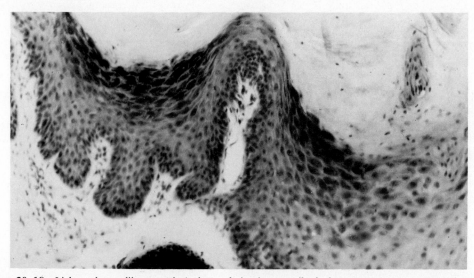

Figure 20–18 Lichen planus–like granulosis, but only in circumscribed places (tar wart, type I, on the neck).

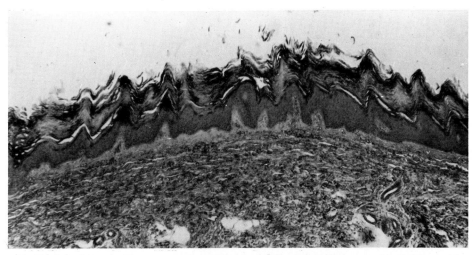

Figure 20–19 Broad-based tar wart, type I (steeple type). The corium is narrowed and damaged by senile elastosis and splitting of collagen fibers (dorsum of the foot of a tar worker aged 53).

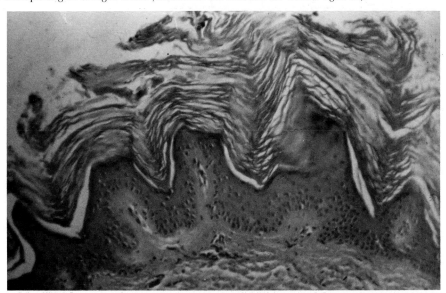

Figure 20–20 Tar wart, type I, but with plateau-like flattening of acanthotic spikes (forearm).

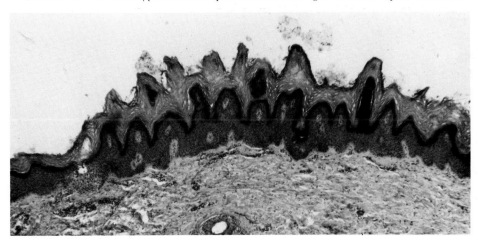

Figure 20–21 Larger tar wart, type I, but with less papillomatosis. At the left border there is marked vacuolation of the malpighian layer (ankle region).

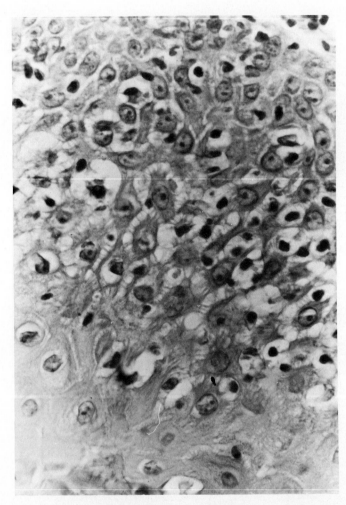

Figure 20–22 Vacuolation in the malpighian layer of the same wart seen in Figure 20–21. Intercellular bridges are partly disturbed. Note the invasion of round cells (?toxic arsenic effect). × *400.*

with the fingernail without causing bleeding. In the course of 8 years we found type II warts on only five occasions.

Pedunculated fibromas, small connective tissue growths mainly in the periorbital region, are frequently seen and are entirely harmless. They do show that tar products are capable of stimulating hyperplasia in connective tissue at some locations (Fig. 20–24).

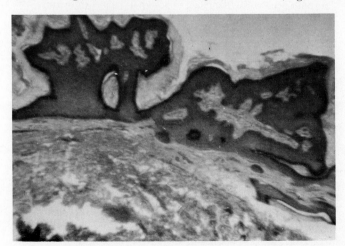

Figure 20–23 Tar wart, type II, on the elbow of a worker aged 61. The characteristic papillomatosis is seen clearly only microscopically.

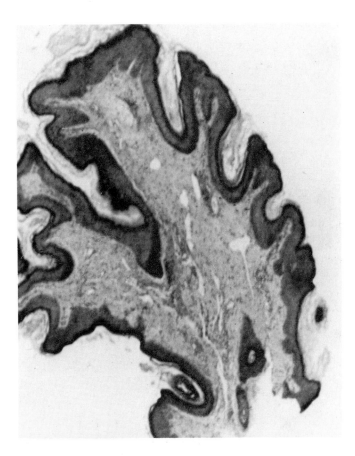

Figure 20–24 Pedunculated fibroma of tar skin in the periorbital region. No hyperplasia of the epidermis (tar worker aged 49).

Type III. Whereas in type I warts we find vigorous proliferation of the malpighian layer toward the periphery, it may be said that in type III it grows in the opposite direction. Here, too, there is hyperplasia of the prickle cell layer, but the cells proliferate in broad or more commonly finger-like branches toward the inside into the upper corium. Figure 20–25 shows an excellent example. It is a biopsy from the dorsum of the hand of a tar worker aged 57. Below an enormous hyperkeratosis there is an unsettled malpighian layer. This is shown more clearly at higher magnification in Figure 20–26. One would be inclined to suspect basal cell epithelioma,

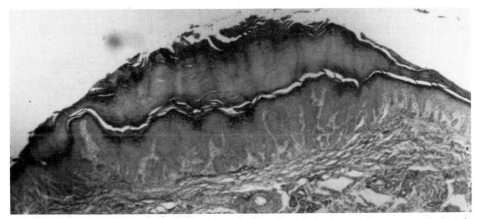

Figure 20–25 Tar wart, type III, on the dorsum of the hand. There is vigorous hyperkeratosis, but also proliferation of the malpighian layer is directed toward the corium (i.e., no "steeples").

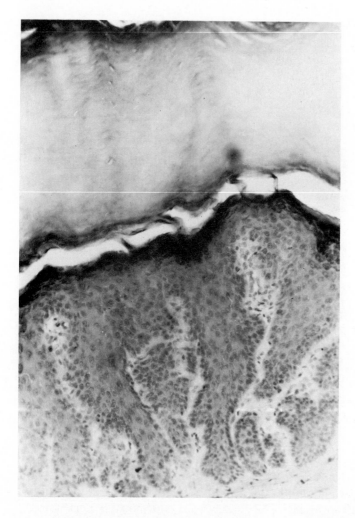

Figure 20–26 Section of Figure 20–25. The fingerlike epithelial tracks proliferating into the corium are reminiscent of those of basal cell epithelioma.

but there are no atypical cells (a kind of pseudoepitheliomatous hyperplasia).

Another example with a more lamellar hyperkeratosis is seen in Figure 20–27. Here, too, the epidermis proliferates downward. In Figure 20–28 the epithelial cones directed toward the corium are plumper and not quite so marked as in Figures 20–25 and 20–27. The lamellar horny layer with circumscribed thickening lies on it almost flat. In these cases a fingernail would be able to remove the wartlike horny layer without causing bleeding.

In the sections shown so far there has been no inflammatory reaction in the corium. There is, however, a very marked one in Figure 20–29 (section of another tar wart, type III), with almost exclusively small lymphocytes and occasional plasma cells. On closer scrutiny of the cells in the epithelial cone a certain atypism (hy-

pochromasia, size differences, clear zones around the nuclei) cannot be excluded. The orthokeratotic horn aggregations should be noted.

Transition to Precancerosis or Carcinoma. The highest degree of tar damage to the skin, which is epithelioma, need not originate from a tar wart. In Figure 20–30 we see a section of tar skin of the face which shows considerable cellular activity in the malpighian layer. There are also atypical cells and proliferation of some epithelial strings downward. If there were a thick parakeratotic horny layer, we should not hesitate to call this a senile keratosis with beginning transformation into a squamous cell carcinoma. However, the horny layer is unusually thin. This is, in fact, a precancerous process developing from tar skin.

The section in Figure 20–31 we also

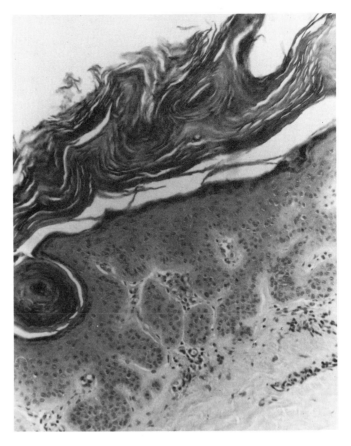

Figure 20–27 Tar wart, type III, of the leg. Above the (downward) hyperplasia of the prickle cell layer lies a thick-lamellar horny layer. At the left border there is a follicular horn plug.

regard as precancerosis with strong inflammatory stroma reaction. It is a biopsy from the scrotal skin of a tar worker with slight circumscribed thickening clinically. Proliferation, apparently of an early invasive type, cell activity, and atypism, as well as vacuolation—shown magnified 400 times in Figure 20–32—suggest that the histopathologic changes indicate early malignancy. Here again the question arises of possible (?additional) arsenical damage.

Figure 20–33 shows a greatly enlarged

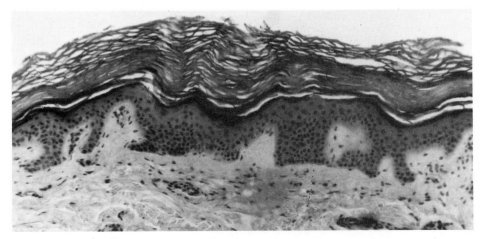

Figure 20–28 Tar wart, type III, of the dorsum of the foot. There are no acanthotic steeples, but broad epithelial rete ridges are seen proliferating into connective tissue. Here, too, a thick horny layer lies almost flat on them.

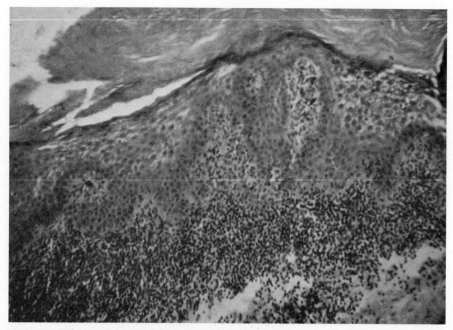

Figure 20–29 Section from a tar wart, type III, of the face. Below an enormous horny layer there is epithelial proliferation toward the corium, causing intense inflammatory cell infiltration (lymphocytes, isolated plasma cells).

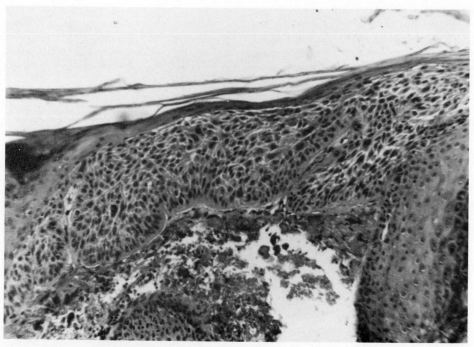

Figure 20–30 Section of tar skin (face). Early precancerosis.

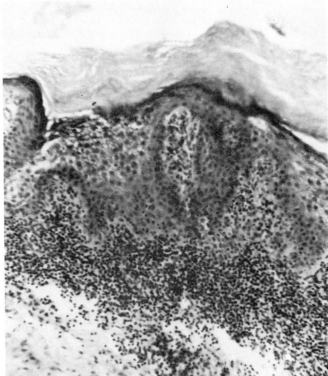

Figure 20–31 Precancerosis of scrotal skin with atypical cells and early intensive growth with intense inflammatory stroma reaction. There is striking vacuole formation in the epithelium on the left side of the picture.

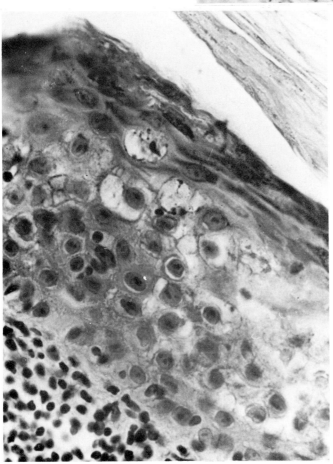

Figure 20–32 Magnification ×500 of the vacuolation in Figure 20–31. The cells show obvious atypism, and there is intraepithelial edema (?arsenic intoxication).

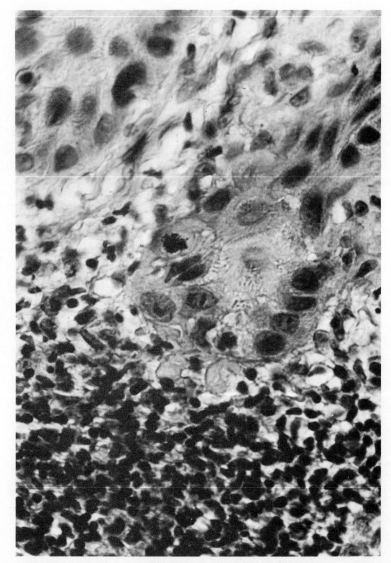

Figure 20–33   Beginning malignant transformation of tar keratosis of the dorsum of the hand. × *500.*

section from the lower edge of a tar keratosis of the dorsum of the hand. Hyperchromasia of the nuclei, varying size, hypochromasia, and mitoses, in addition to a strong inflammatory reaction in the corium, make it certain that malignancy has set in. In a tar worker aged 55 a basal cell epithelioma developed on the outer ear with a slightly horny surface (Fig. 20–34). The infiltrating strings of basal cells led to the formation of horn pearls in one place. The inflammatory changes are regarded as a defense reaction.

In Figure 20–35 we finally demonstrate an example of how a squamous cell carci-

noma can develop from a tar wart. At the left edge of the picture two steeplelike points are still recognizable. Apparently this was originally a tar wart, type I. The biopsy was taken from the nose of a tar worker aged 59. We want to stress again that in our experience the transformation of a tar wart into an epithelioma is rarer today than is supposed in some quarters. Figure 20–36, on the other hand, shows a squamous cell carcinoma that developed in flat tar skin. The tar worker — employed in the industry for 15 years — had the typical symptoms of tar skin but no warts. During a medical examination a small erosion was

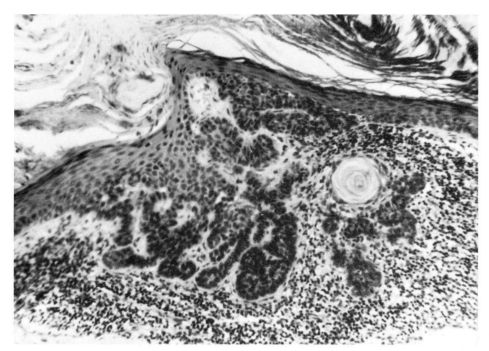

Figure 20–34 Early basal cell epithelioma of the external ear of a tar worker aged 55.

found on the cheek. Histopathologic examination disclosed a squamous cell carcinoma.

As can be gathered from this description, tar skin as well as tar warts may provide the basis for the development of precanceroses and epitheliomas. The tar products act with varying intensity, sometimes causing atrophy of the epidermis and the dermal papillae, and sometimes

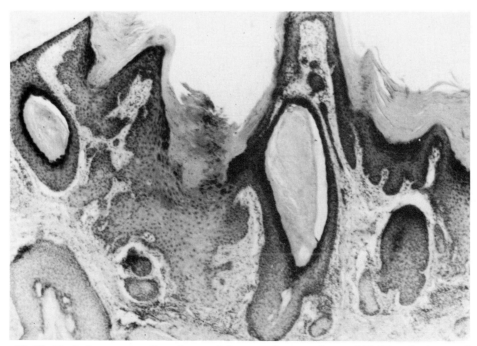

Figure 20–35 Typical squamous cell carcinoma of the nose of a tar worker aged 59. There has been malignant transformation apparently from a tar wart, type I, as steeple formation is still visible at the left border of the picture.

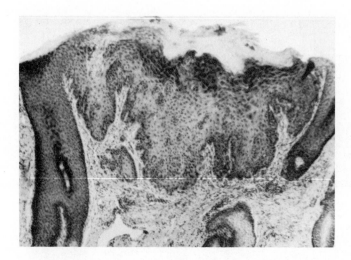

Figure 20–36 Squamous cell carcinoma developing in flat tar skin of a worker aged 40 after 15 years' contact with tar products.

causing proliferation in the form of hyperkeratotic tar warts, papillomas, and fibromas. Why there is an inflammatory reaction in some cases cannot be decided; possibly external irritants play a part. However, in our entire biopsy material, inflammatory changes in the corium were relatively rare, conceivably because the

great majority of our patients were elderly workers who had been in the tar industry for a long time. Acute inflammatory changes were probably present originally, but regressed later. Vacuolation of the cells in the malpighian layer, found on occasion histologically, has been described by Scolari (1938) in tar melanosis.

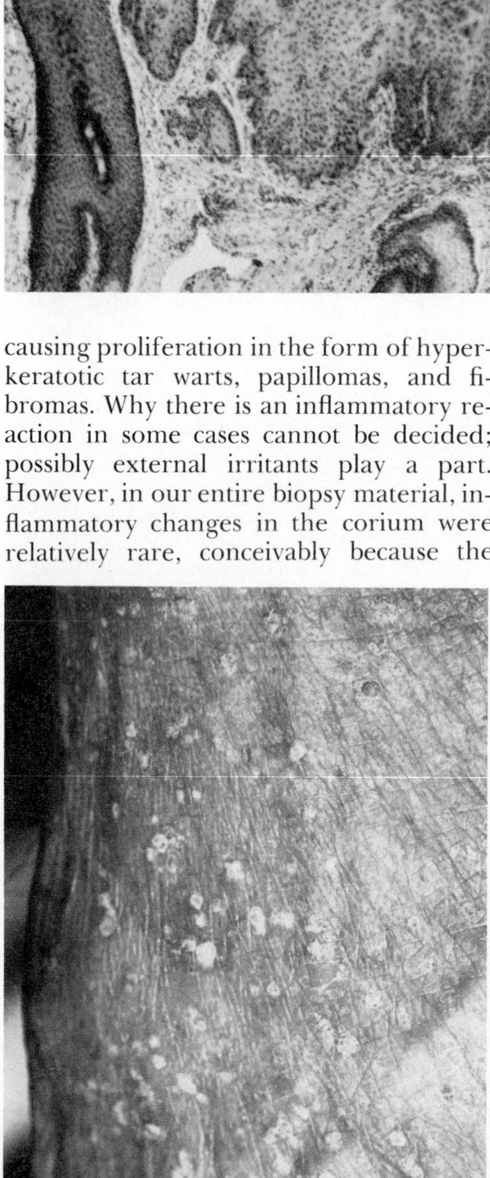

Another interesting point is the behavior of pigment in tar warts. Most of the warts examined by us histologically were without pigment and therefore of a gray-white hue (Fig. 20–37). On the other hand, the melanin content in pure tar skin was high. Melanophages were found more rarely. The pigment lay mainly in the region of the basal cell layer. Finally, although we can state that increased cellular activity in the malpighian layer and the inflammatory stroma reaction call for caution with regard to precancerosis, a reliable histologic criterion of early malignancy could not be found.

DIFFERENTIAL DIAGNOSIS

Differential diagnostic considerations in assessing "tar skin" must first take into account age-induced senile degenerative atrophy of exposed parts of the body. During the aging process the skin of the face and the dorsum of the hand shows hyperpigmentation or depigmentation. It becomes thinner, telangiectases develop, and in places it tends to hyperkeratosis, scaling, and the formation of circumscribed nodules (senile keratosis). Signs of inflammation may supervene. As in "tar skin" due to

Figure 20–37 Typical, almost pigmentless tar warts, type I, on the dorsum of the foot of a tar worker aged 45. Note the strong pigmentation in the vicinity of the warts.

various tar noxae, we find an association of degenerative atrophic and proliferative processes. The connective tissue also shows basophilic degeneration of the elastic layer, atrophy of sebaceous glands, and damage to collagenous tissue.

The toxic melanodermatitis which used to occur after the application of nonpurified petroleum jelly led to similar changes, although inflammation was more prominent. We saw this picture quite frequently even after World War II. Today nonpurified petroleum jelly (a mineral oil product) is no longer used for therapeutic purposes, and the pharmaceutical industry has developed ointment bases (polyethyleneglycol emulsions) which are extremely well tolerated.

Occupational injury due to arsenic must be considered in the differential diagnosis of tar skin. Inorganic arsenic also can produce a pigmentation of the skin, which may become blackish and which more often affects the trunk. This was hardly ever the case in our tar skin patients. Hyperkeratoses develop, particularly in regions rich in sweat glands (palm of the hand, sole of the foot), and in some patients these later develop into carcinomas.

Ore dust containing arsenic of course settles profusely on the head and shoulders of certain workers, and there may be direct resorption of arsenic. Beside pigmentation there is precancerous and epithelial proliferation, as in tar skin, and just as in tar keratosis there is in places histopathologic evidence of thickening of the granular layer, vacuolation of the upper layers of the malpighian layer, and, more commonly, acanthosis with marginal inflammation. Dyskeratotic cells are reminiscent of those seen in Bowen's disease.

In skin damaged by arsenic there are also papillomas, but in our opinion it is of decisive importance that multiple warts, turning into basal cell epithelioma, appear mainly on the trunk and only rarely on the scrotum. In tar skin the typical efflorescences prefer the locations already described; carcinomas occurred only in isolated cases in our tar workers, but sometimes several developed in the same patient at intervals. An impressive example of arsenical skin damage is seen in people with psoriasis of long standing, with the continu-

al formation of new basal cell epithelioma on the trunk and extremities going on for decades. True, prolonged ingestion of inorganic arsenic, a cumulative poison, must be taken into account in these cases.

In the older literature there is an occasional mention of "acute" cancers in tar skin. In our opinion this is a misinterpretation in the majority of cases, and actually these formations were probably keratoacanthomas. We consider the case of Blum and Bralez (1930) to be an example. They described the precipitate development of a nodule within a month and said that it grew to a diameter of 2 cm. in another three weeks. Histologically it was thought to be squamous cell carcinoma. The patient was a stoker who worked daily in hot surroundings full of coal dust. In the present view coal dust by itself is not considered to have any carcinogenic action. The special characteristics of that "acute" cancer were not known at the time. MacCormac and Scarff (1936) described it as "molluscum sebaceum," and later Rook and Whimster (1950) more aptly called it "keratoacanthoma." It can easily be mistaken histologically for a true squamous cell carcinoma. On the other hand, there are cases of actual transition to true carcinomas. In our experience this is not common in tar skin (but see Braun and Enayat, 1960), as we have seen only one keratoacanthoma in the course of eight years. Perhaps that is due to the fact that most of our patients were no longer employed in the tar industry.

Occasionally a cutaneous horn develops in tar-damaged skin. The lesion for which we made this diagnosis is shown in Figure 20–38. To what extent transition from this precancerosis to a squamous cell carcinoma has already occurred can only be decided histologically. The clinical picture presents no diagnostic difficulties, for tar warts never reach this size.

Considerably more diagnostic effort is sometimes required in deciding whether a wart in a worker who left the tar industry some time ago should be described as a "tar wart" or not. Most commonly the senile wart must be excluded. On examining very early keratosis seborrheica one may sometimes encounter a suggestion of the steeplelike epidermis cone which is so char-

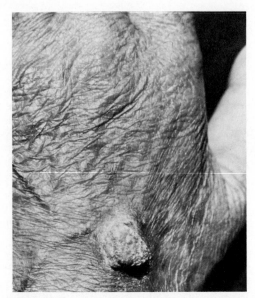

Figure 20–38   Cutaneous horn on the dorsum of the hand of a tar worker aged 63 whose skin is completely atrophic.

acteristic of the tar wart, type I. Sachs et al. (1949) were the first to point out these elongations of the epithelial rete ridges and to describe the lesion as "keratosis seborrheica." Clinically these lesions are distinguished by their brownish pigmentation and fatty consistency. Scratching with the fingernail can remove this *early* type without bleeding, just like a tar wart. The hyperkeratosis of a tar wart, however, never has a fatty character. Histologically there is a thin epidermis with a lamellate horny layer and a granular layer which, though present, is never thickened. Keratosis seborrheica is obviously an immature senile wart. The authors themselves pointed out this transitional stage.

Another affection histologically resembling the typical picture of tar wart, type I, is Hopf's acrokeratosis verruciformis. Apart from the different clinical aspect, the most important differential feature is the history. Hopf's dermatosis is one of the nevoid affections (unless it is a variant of Darier's disease, as has been suggested recently), and it has therefore most often been present since childhood or puberty. Next, epidermodysplasia verruciformis (Lewandowsky-Lutz) should be mentioned, but histologically this is more like verruca vulgaris and shows a typical intracellular edema in the granular layer. We

have never observed similar changes in tar warts.

Tar warts, type III (Fig. 20–27), may possibly be mistaken for verruca plana, but the demonstration of vacuolated cells in the granular layer of the latter should prevent this. Keratosis senilis is characterized histopathologically by parakeratotic columns in the horny layer. Atypical epithelial proliferation in the form of buds and tubes is found in tar warts, type III, as well as in keratosis senilis, but the latter occasionally shows mitoses at the base. Verruca vulgaris cannot be mistaken for tar warts either clinically or histologically. It is characterized by vacuolation of cells of the granular layer and centrally arranged epithelial marginal ledges with vigorous papillomatosis.

In 1958 the Australian dermatologists Kocsard and coworkers reported 24 cases of wart formation on the extremities of 250 elderly men. They described these structures as "stucco keratosis." In a later study Kocsard and Ofner (1966) reported the results of examinations of 388 patients aged 46 to 91 and said that they had discovered "stucco keratosis" in 7 percent of these. Because a senile elastosis generally becomes noticeable with increasing age and therefore is present simultaneously with the wart, which is made conspicuous by the hypertrophy of the epidermis, the authors used the term "keratoelastoidosis verrucosa" of the extremities to describe this lesion. Examination of Figures 2 and 4 in Kocsard and Ofner's publication (1966), showing stucco keratosis on the dorsum of the foot and its histology, will demonstrate that this lesion is identical to the tar wart, type I, described by us in 1965 and in this study, from both clinical and histologic aspects. We therefore agree with the view of Kocsard et al. (1968) that stucco keratosis is identical with the tar warts described by us.

It is perhaps no accident that Kocsard's observations come from sunny Australia. Tar products have a photosensitizing effect on the whole skin, which often persists for many years. Other carcinogenic substances also have a photodynamic effect, and the carcinogens attacking man in the course of his life are extremely numerous as we now know (toxins, minerals, metals, aniline derivatives, tar products, benzol derivatives, body substances, synthetic products, mechanical trauma, thermal injuries, ultraviolet and ionizing rays). To all of these the skin reacts in a definite and constant manner, leading to eventual cancer formation, though with variations in degree. In our opinion the tar wart represents just *one* form of possible malignant transformation, even if it is benign at first. The age-induced stroma change alone promotes the proliferation process, as explained under Etiology and Pathogenesis. This also explains why the tendency toward wart formation persists for years after removal of the carcinogenic irritants, especially as the latent period has to be considered and may extend to decades.

TREATMENT

Therapeutic measures are simple. An emulsion that screens out light should be used by all workers at risk as a matter of course. Since age and length of contact with tar noxae are important, all proliferative skin changes must be surgically removed—the more promptly the older the worker and the longer the exposure. All warts must be excised and histologically examined, for their removal may prevent the development of cancer. The same procedure should be followed in suspected or clinically diagnosable precanceroses. This includes, above all, the circumscribed inflammatory lesions of Bowen's disease. Finally, all carcinomas must be diagnosed as early as possible and excised or treated with x-rays. Personally we prefer surgery because through electrocoagulation we lose the chance of histologic identification. However, one could first take a biopsy and then decide on the type of treatment. Keratoacanthomas and cutaneous horns should be removed in the same way. The worker must leave the tar industry and be kept under regular medical surveillance.

PROPHYLAXIS

Having studied certain etiologic factors, the course of the pathologic processes in the skin, and their respective clinical pictures, we have to consider as necessary preventive measures (1) a change of working conditions, (2) personal precautions, and (3) instruction from outside sources and continuous control of the worker's state of health.

1. In certain processes of work, tar products are whirled up as dust (especially pitch dust) and settle on the skin. In others tar and its products or crude oil and its products are smeared on the skin; in still others heat and steam are present, causing intensive sweating and thus promoting the solution of certain carcinogenic substances. For work done in the open air, a protective roof would reduce the action of the dangerous ultraviolet rays of sunlight. On the other hand, there is deficient ventilation in many workrooms. It follows that it is the task of management to mechanize production processes in order to allow only a minimum of carcinogenic substances to act on the worker's skin.

2. In guarding against any occupational disease, the will to protect oneself is of prime importance. Thorough daily cleansing of the whole body, particularly the genital region, legs, and feet, is decisive. Management must provide suitable protective clothing—plastic safety helmets, respirators, goggles, clean overalls of a material not absorbing tar products—and these should be properly used and frequently changed. In some cases a scarf protects exposed parts. Gloves should be made of synthetic but "breathing" material or of leather, should extend up over the forearm, and should not be too tight to prevent an exchange of sweat-containing air with fresh air. Boots should reach up to the calves and be covered by trousers down to the ankles. The settling of carcinogenic particles on the dorsum of the foot could thus be prevented. Since many tar products are fat-soluble, a fatty skin cream would not be protective. It may be necessary for the pharmaceutical industry to develop new types of barrier lotions. Emulsions protecting against ultraviolet rays are already available.

3. The worker will be all the more willing to wear the issued protective clothing the more thoroughly he is enlightened on the dangers resulting from continuous contact with tar and pitch and allied car-

cinogenic products. Large posters should therefore be displayed in all hazardous workshops, pointing out the disease symptoms and their prevention. Wherever possible, carcinogenic substances should be replaced by less injurious agents in certain processes. Our investigations have shown that, with increasing length of exposure and age, the danger of the development of tar skin and its consequences grows. Teutschlaender therefore suggested once that the length of exposure be limited to a maximum of five years. He also recommended a more frequent change of workplace. Youths are generally less susceptible than older people. In this country, existing mining regulations provide satisfactory controls in workshops in which coal and its derivatives are handled. Specialist examinations at regular intervals are obligatory.

Alkali resistance determinations in our 111 workers have not shown any influence on neutralization time even after many years' contact with tar noxae. Neutralization time did increase in older workers, but this result could not be attributed to long tar exposure but rather to the physiologic aging process which always causes a prolongation of the alkali neutralization time after the age of 50. Extensive pH estimations on different body sites showed no deviation from the norm even after decades of exposure. With regard to prophylaxis these studies provided no means of practical application.

PROGNOSIS

Undoubtedly tar skin and tar warts provide the basis for the development of cancer. According to our observations, however, it seems that the chemical tar noxae must act on the skin *constantly* in order to foster the development of a carcinoma. We have to bear in mind that, even after a period of avoiding tar noxae, the proliferative stimuli of an epidermis cell damaged over the years still persist. Thus Teutschlaender (1933) described all tar skin changes with proliferative growth, particularly tar warts, as "precancerous," even though, as indicated above, cancer formation from a tar wart is not the rule. During an observation period of eight years after the cessation of tar contact, we diagnosed only five definite carcinomas. Richter's remark (1930) that "the so-called chimney-sweep's cancer—essentially a tar cancer—will soon be a thing of the past" was too optimistic. Even after patients leave the industry, carcinogenic factors continue to play their part (increasing age with its disposition to malignancy, sunlight with its ultraviolet rays). Years of contact with tar products cause (at least in some workers) a mutation of cells of the malpighian layer, which explains the formation of tar warts many years after leaving the industry. The persistent light sensitization of the skin detected by us in most tar workers may support the thesis that this mutation causes a persistent alteration of the physiologic chemistry of the epidermis cell in particular. Finally we must not forget that later in the worker's life still other skin-damaging or carcinogenic agents are at work which we do not even know about but which eventually produce malignant degeneration in the previously prepared cells. This explains the long latent period of up to four decades in some cases. It is true that the examining physician has to consider in this kind of carcinoma whether suficient bridging symptoms are present from the time the tar worker left his occupation to justify the assessment of this "late cancer" as occupational tar cancer.

The prognosis is favorable in warts diagnosed early, and in precanceroses and skin carcinoma if the lesions are removed promptly.

REFERENCES

Babes, A., and Serbanesco: Cancer du goudron et verrue du goudron chez le lapin. C. R. Soc. Biol., 98:1642, 1928.

Barnewitz, J.: Die künstliche Erzeugung von Krebs bei Mäusen durch die Einwirkung von Steinkohlenpech. Dtsch. Med. Wochenschr., 54:1162, 1928.

Batschwaroff, B. Profiroff, D., and Toleff, I.: Der Hautkrebs als Berufserkrankung der Landarbeiter im Gebiete von Plovdiv. Symposium dermatologorum, Prague, October 12 to 15, 1960. Prague, Universitas Carolina, 1962, Vol. 1, p. 39.

Bauer, K. H.: Das Krebsproblem. Ed. 2. Berlin, Springer-Verlag, 1963, p. 354.

Bayet, A.: Cancer du goudron et cancer arsenical. Le Cancer, 1:5, 1923.

Bettazzi, G.: Dermatite e processi praecancerosi da catrame nell'uome. Arch. Ital. Chir., 31:69, 1932.

Bloch, B.: Experimentell erzeugte Carcinome bei Mäusen. Vereing. Südwestdeutscher Dermatologen, Frankfurt, October 8 and 9, 1921. Cited in Z. Haut. Geschlechtskr. 3:133, 1922.

Blum, P., and Bralez, J.: L'épithéliome du goudron. Etude clinique et expérimentale. Arch. Derm.-Syph. (Paris), 2:496, 1930.

Bönig and Holz, cited by Bauer.

Borst, M.: Über Teercarcinoide. Z. Krebsforsch., 21:341, 1924.

Braun, W., and Enayat, M.: Molluscum pseudocarcinomatosum (Kerato-Akanthom) und Beruf. Berufsdermatosen, 8:61, 1960.

Cookson, E.: Epithelioma of the skin after prolonged exposure to creosote. Br. Med. J., 1:368, 1924.

Coulon, A.: Action des différentes radiations du spectre visible sur les tumeurs greffées de la souris et sur les tumeurs de goudron. Arch. Physique. Biol., 3:223, 1924.

Cramer, H. J.: Die Altersveränderungen der Haut. *In* Marchionini, A., et al. (Eds.): Normale und pathologische Anatomie der Haut. Handbuch der Haut- und Geschlechtskrankheiten. Berlin, Springer-Verlag, 1968, Vol. 1, part 1, p. 683.

Downing, C. C. R.: Cutaneous papillomas among patent fuel workers in relation to malignant disease. J. Ind. Hyg., 14:255, 1932.

Ehrmann, O.: Die "Pechhaut," eine Gewerbedermatose. Monatshefte Prakt. Dermat., 48:18, 1909.

Fabry, H.: Sogenannte Pechhaut nach Einwirkung von Verbrennungs- und Destillationsprodukten der Kohle. Berufsdermatosen, 15:198, 1967.

Götz, H., and Zambal, Z.: Histologische Untersuchungen bei Pechhautleiden, insbesondere von Verrucae piceae. Arch. Klin. Exp. Dermatol., 222:613, 1965.

Götz, H., and Schuppener, H. J.: Atrophien der Haut. *In* Marchionini, A., et al., (Eds.): Handbuch der Haut- und Geschlechtskrankheiten. Berlin, Springer-Verlag, 1969, Vol. 3, part 2, p. 454.

Heller, I.: Occupational cancers. J. Ind. Hyg., 12:169, 1930.

Henry, S.: Cancer of the scrotum in relation to occupation. London, Oxford University Press, 1946.

Itchikawa, K.: Sur la production expérimentale du cancer. J. Radiol. Électrol., 7:415, 1923.

Itchikawa, K., and Baum, S.: Etude expérimentale et comparée du cancer. III. Réaction locale et histogénèse du cancer expérimental chez le lapin. Bull. Assoc. Fr. Étude Cancer, 8:107, 1924.

Koch, R.: Uber das Vorkommen von Pechschäden in der optischen Industrie. Berufsdermatosen, 4:276, 1956.

Kocsard, E., Ofner, F., Coles, J. L., and Turner, B.: Senile changes in the skin and visible mucous membranes of the Australian male. Aust. J. Dermatol., 4:216, 1958.

Kocsard, E., and Ofner, F.: Keratoelastoidosis verrucosa of the extremities (Stucco keratoses of the extremities). Dermatologica, 133:225, 1966.

Kocsard, E., Baer, C. L., and Constance, T. J.: Hyperkeratosis lenticularis perstans Flegel. Dermatologica, 136:35, 1968.

Linser, K.: Kritisches zum berufsbedingten Krebs der Haut. Symposium dermatologorum, Prague, October 12 to 15, 1960. Prague, Universitas Carolina, 1962, Vol. 1, p. 7.

Lipschütz, O.: Das experimentelle Teercarcinom der Maus. Wien. Klin. Wochenschr., 36:409, 1923.

MacCormac, H., and Scarff, R. W.: Molluscum sebaceum. Br. J. Dermatol., 48:624, 1936.

Matras, A.: Karzinom auf Teerhaut, ein Beitrag zur berufsmässig bedingten Krebsentstehung. Wien. Klin. Wochenschr., 72:416, 1960.

Mertens, V. E.: Beobachtungen über die Entstehung von Teerkrebs an Mäusen. Z. Krebsforsch., 21:494, 1924.

O'Donovan, W. J.: Cancer of the skin due to occupation. Tar carcinoma. Arch. Dermatol. Syph. (Chicago), 19:595, 1929.

Oliver, T.: Coke-men and by-products workers: Their complaints and maladies. Br. Med. J., 1:992, 1930.

Pisani, M., and Izzo, L.: Su un caso di cancro de catrame. Dermatologia (Napoli), 12:259, 1961.

Pott, P.: Chirurgical observations relative to cancer of the scrotum, London, 1775.

Richter, L. E.: Der ausgestorbene Schornsteinfegerkrebs. Z. Krebsforsch., 31:565, 1930.

Rook, A., and Whimster, J.: Le Kératho-acanthome Arch. Belges Dermatol., 6:137, 1950.

Sachs, W., Mackee, G. M., and Sachs, P. M.: Keratosis (seborrheic and senile). Arch. Dermatol. Syph. (Chicago), 59:179, 1949.

Schröder, R.: Über Pechschäden in der optischen Industrie. Z. Haut. Geschlechtskr., 10:61, 1961.

Scolari, E.: Melanodermia da pece con epiteliomi disserminati della faccia. G. Ital. Dermatol., 79:307, 1938.

Southwood, W. F. W.: The thickness of the skin. Plast. Reconstr. Surg., 15:423, 1955.

Sträuli, P.: Das akute Teerverbrennungskarzinom. Oncologica (Basel), 10:72, 1957.

Tentschlaender, O.: Über den Pechkrebs der Brikettarbeiter auf Grund von Fabrikbesuchen in Baden und Südwales. Z. Krebsforsch., 28:283, 1929.

Teutschlaender, O.: Neuere Untersuchungen über die Wirkungsweise von Teer und Pech bei der Entstehung beruflicher Hautkrebse. Z. Krebsforsch., 30:573, 1930.

Teutschlaender, O.: Arbeit und Geschwulstbildung. Monatsschr. Krebsbekämpfung, 1:30; 72; 105; 167; 212; 267, 300, 1933.

Tourraine, A.: Beruflich verursachte Krebse der Haut. Berufsdermatosen, 5:49, 1957.

Ullmann, K.: Krebsbildung in der Gewerbemedizin und ihre Beziehungen zur experimentellen Geschwulstforschung. *In* Jadassohn, J. (Ed.): Handbuch der Haut-und Geschlechtskrankheiten. Berlin, Springer-Verlag, 1933, Vol. 2, p. 642.

Veiel, F.: Teerkrebs beim Menschen. Arch. Dermatol. (Berl.), 148:142, 1924.

Vilanova, X.: La piel senil (Generalidades). Act. dermo-sifiliogr. (Madr.), 49:65, 1958.

Volkmann, R.: Über Teer-, Paraffin- und Rubkrebs (Schornsteinfegerkrebs). *In* Beiträge zur Chirurgie, Leipzig, 1875, p. 370.

Yamagiva, K., and Itchikawa, K.: Experimental study of the pathogenesis of carcinoma. J. Cancer Res., 3:1, 1918.

21

Leukoplakia

Otto P. Hornstein, M.D.

LEUKOPLAKIC AND LEUKOKERATOTIC LESIONS OF THE ORAL CAVITY

Leukoplakia (Schwimmer, 1877) has been described as a disorder of the oral mucosa or the vermilion of the lip which is characterized by thickening and anomalous keratinization of the epithelium, slight inflammation, chronic progress, and no tendency to disappear (Waldron and Shafer, 1960; Shafer and Waldron, 1961; Sprague, 1963; Schuermann et al., 1966; Silverman and Rozen, 1968; Waldron, 1970). Since many authors use the term "leukoplakia" only in this general sense, whereas others include distinct histopathologic criteria of different significance (such as dyskeratosis or nuclear atypia), there is some confusion about the essence and interpretation of this ambiguous term (Sprague, 1963). At a W.H.O. meeting of oral pathologists in Copenhagen in 1967, there was agreement to define leukoplakia as a white spot or plaque which cannot be removed by rubbing and cannot be ascribed to any other definable disorder (cited by Pindborg, 1956b). At present this minimal definition is being tested by some research centers collaborating with the W.H.O. International Reference Center for oral precancerous conditions.

Reversing the cited definition, it is no longer correct to call white hyperkeratotic lesions of the mucosa "leukoplakia" if they are caused by any other known disease. There are many dermatoses and even systemic disorders which induce leukoplakia—so to speak, as a lesion specific to the mucosa. It may be very difficult to discern "idiopathic" leukoplakias from "symptomatic" ones, i.e., leukoplakias associated with nosologically defined diseases (Hirayama, 1966; Schuermann et al., 1966), since the first type of leukoplakia may vary considerably in clinical appearance and may resemble benign as well as premalignant lesions. However, clinical differentiation of each leukoplakic lesion as precisely as possible is very important for exact therapy and clear prognostic evaluation. For this reason, stomatologists and dermatologists should cooperate closely in this clinical field.

In accordance with Greither (1965) and Schuermann et al. (1966) we identify four categories of leukoplakic lesions of the oral cavity:

1. "Idiopathic" leukoplakias.
2. "Symptomatic" leukoplakias (associated with well-defined diseases).

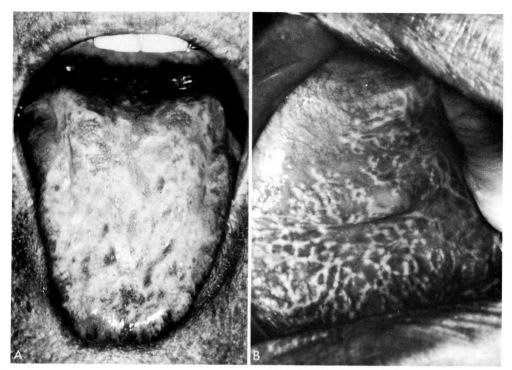

Figure 21–1 *A,* "Symptomatic" leukoplakia of the tongue in a 63 year old patient with lichen planus. The lingual surface is coated with a milky leukoplakia which forms whitish confluent patches and rings, including small areas with remainders of fungiform papillae.

B, Lichen planus of the oral mucosa, forming "cobweb leukoplakia" by a delicate pattern of confluent white strips of keratinized epithelium.

3. "Traumatic" leukoplakias (due to determinable local irritants).

4. Definite precancerous leukoplakias.

Some disorders with relation to the above mentioned types of leukoplakia are listed in Table 21–1.

Many of the enumerated leukoplakic conditions remain in a benign stage throughout life or disappear after removal of the causative factors (such as an ill-fitting denture). Some leukoplakias, on the other hand, may change *facultatively* into

Figure 21–2 "Irritative" leukoplakia like "oral callosity" in a 52 year old man. The postcommissural mucosa presents an opaline, bluish-white, finely fissured area fading into the adjacent buccal mucosa.

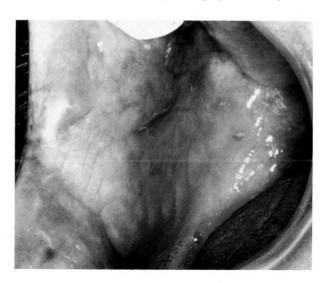

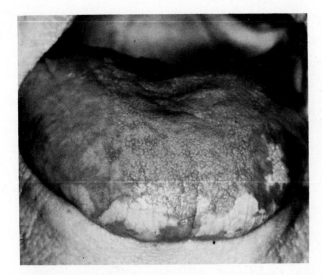

Figure 21–3 Precancerous leukoplakia of the tongue resembling a "sugar coating" in a 78 year old woman. Abrupt, irregular borders of white leukoplakic spots localized in an atrophic epithelium.

Figure 21–4 Normal epithelium of the buccal mucosa with just slight keratinization of the superficial squamous cells.

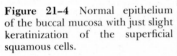
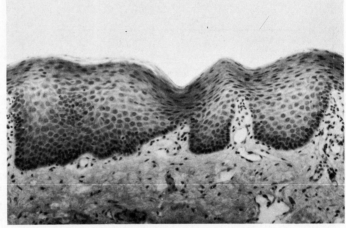

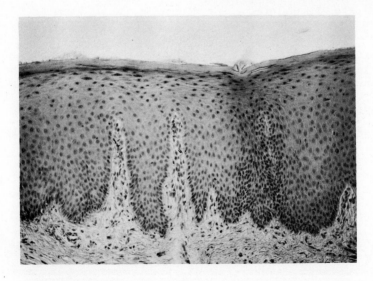

Figure 21–5 "Irritative" leukoplakia of the postcommissural mucosa, showing benign acanthosis of the epithelium and epidermis-like keratinization at the surface.

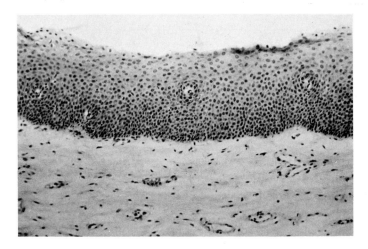

Figure 21-6 Focal dysplasia in a precancerous leukoplakia of the oral mucosa. In the lower strata of the epithelium, small atypical cells are very closely and irregularly arranged.

premalignant lesions if the conditioning irritations continue for a long time (such as inflammation in syphilitic glossitis, or in pemphigoid variety of lichen ruber). Whether a "primary" leukoplakia is a harmless anomaly or a premalignant lesion in many cases cannot be decided clinically with certainty but only by histologic examination of a biopsy specimen.

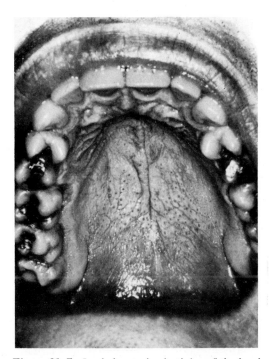

Figure 21-7 Leukokeratosis nicotinica of the hard palate in a habitual pipe smoker. In the adjacent area of the soft palate, the disorder fades gradually.

Clinical and Epidemiologic Features

Leukoplakic lesions may occur at all sites of the oral cavity but most commonly are localized on the buccal mucosa bilaterally behind the commissure of the lips. The pattern of leukoplakia is similar to an angle opening up toward the lips, and tends to continue along the dental contact area of the buccal epithelium. Next to this area, in descending order, the edentulous alveolar ridge of the maxilla, the tongue, lips, palate, floor of the mouth, and gingiva may be involved (Renstrup, 1958; Pindborg, 1968). Shafer and Waldron (1960, 1961), by contrast, found most leukoplakic areas, after the buccal fold, opposite the interdental occlusion level, on the mandibular alveolar ridge and the gingiva. This varying prevalence of location may be due to some racial variations, personal habits, factors of oral hygiene, and so forth.

Although oral leukoplakias may be observed in many people, little is known about their worldwide incidence. In a large series of patients with oral disorders, McCarthy and McCarthy (1954) found leukoplakic lesions in about 15 percent. In particular, oral leukoplakias are a frequent finding among Indians, Malays, Indonesians, and New Guineans (Clinical Oncology, 1973; Forlen et al., 1965; Mehta et al., 1969a and 1969b; Muir and Kirk, 1960; Pindborg, 1963; Pindborg et al., 1967a; Singh and von Essen, 1966; Tenne-

TABLE 21-1

"Idiopathic" leukoplakias

"White spongy naevus of the mucosa" (Cannon)
(identical to the "white folded gingivostomatosis"
of Everett-Noyes or to the "oral epithelial naevus"
"Leukedema"
Focal epithelial hyperplasia
(Heck's disease)

"Symptomatic" leukoplakias

associated with:
Syphilitic glossitis interstitialis
"Glossitis granulomatosa" (peculiar manifestation
of Melkersson-Rosenthal syndrome)
Tuberculosis (e.g., incipient stage of tuberculosis
luposa)
Chronic candidiasis (and other mycotic infections)
Lichen planus
Lupus erythematosus
Abrikosov's tumor ("myoblastoma")
Dyskeratosis follicularis Darier
Some congenital ichthyotic disorders
Dystrophic type of epidermolysis bullosa here-
ditaria (Siemens-Hallopeau)
Deficiency of vitamin A

"Traumatic" (irritative)
leukoplakias

Postcommissural leukoplakia ("oral callosity")
Leukokeratosis nicotinica palati
("smoker's gum," "nicotine stomatitis")
Leukokeratosis caused by chewing tobacco or
betel, or by snuff dipping
Leukoplakia caused by ill-fitting dentures
Leukoplakia caused by carious teeth and similar
disorders (including "electrogalvanic stomatitis")
Habitual cheek biting (Schuermann's "morsicatio
buccarum")
Leukoplakia associated with:
Chronic cheilitic conditions
"Glossitis rhombica mediana" (lingua Brocq-
Pautrier)
Oral submucous fibrosis (Pindborg)

Definite precancerous leukoplakias

"Speckled" leukoplakia (Pindborg)
Bowen's disease of the mucosa
"Oral florid papillomatosis" (Rock-Fisher) (?)
Some varieties of hereditary polykeratoses
(Touraine)

koon and Bartlett, 1969; Wahi et al.,
1965). In epidemiologic studies comprising 30,000 individuals in Indian communities, Pindborg et al. (1966) noted an incidence of leukoplakic lesions varying
between 1.6 and 3.3 percent.

In another ethnographic and histologic study
carried out by Forlen et al. (1965) on the "betel

leukoplakia" of Papuans in New Guinea where
excessive betel chewing and tobacco smoking
are very popular, leukoplakia predominantly
localized on the buccal mucosa was found in a
range from 10 to over 20 percent of the examined males and females, in relation to
the degree of addiction to chewing betel in
different tribes. As will be discussed later in
the section about the etiology of leukoplakic
conditions, the varying frequency of oral leukoplakias in different populations depends on
special customs of smoking, chewing tobacco and
betel blended with various ingredients, and other personal habits (Forlen et al., 1965; Mehta et
al., 1969a and 1969b; Pindborg, 1963, 1965a
and 1965b; Pindborg et al., 1965, 1966, and
1967a). In some southeastern regions of Asia
the male:female ratio of incidence is only
slightly in favor of men (Forlen et al., 1965;
Mehta et al., 1969a; Pindborg et al., 1968a).
About 70 percent of all leukoplakic lesions are
found in persons aged 40 to 70 years; white
people under 30 are rarely affected (Schuermann et al., 1966; Shafer and Waldron, 1961;
Shklar, 1965; Waldron, 1970; Waldron and
Shafer, 1960).

The clinical aspect of leukoplakia may
vary considerably, ranging from a little
spot to vast areas covering almost all of the
oral cavity. In the beginning only a slight
opaline tarnish is to be seen, similar to the
delicate scab after cauterization by silver
nitrate. Later the color of the mucosa
changes to bluish white and becomes more
intensive or pearly, while the primarily
smooth surface shrivels or assumes the appearance of a polygonal mosaic irregularly
furrowed by fine fissures. Some of the
leukoplakic lesions are sharply, almost
jaggedly bordered; others fade gradually
into the normal-appearing adjacent mucosa. In leukoplakic areas of the dorsal
surface of the tongue, most papillae undergo involution, and the tongue looks
glossy, etched, or coated with a frost. Irregularly shaped warty projections arising
from a flat leukoplakic base may lead to a
suspicion of premalignant or even early
malignant transformation. On the lower
lip the entire mucosa or the vermilion
region may be involved, the latter with a
dry, whitish blotched surface and a
blurred outline toward the outer lip. On
palpation, as a rule the lesion is only
slightly firmer than normal mucosa. Symptoms of inflammation are not to be seen. In
some cases pearly-white, jaggedly bor-

dered hyperkeratoses arise from the surface spontaneously or by "nibbling," while the basal leukoplakia, which is firmly adherent to the underlying tissue, cannot be rubbed off. When the palate is affected, leukoplakia usually appears like small polygonal white papules, in some of which a central red dot may be seen.

Even if a leukoplakic lesion arouses little suspicion of premalignancy, a biopsy should be performed. *In case of a nonuniform leukoplakia, it is better to take biopsy specimens from several areas than from just one, since the histologic findings may be different.* Benign leukoplakia reveals a rather regular, well-ordered acanthosis of the epithelium with keratinization and thickening of the superficial layers and with almost complete loss of nuclear remainders like an "epidermization" of the surface. There are well-differentiated cell structures of the enlarged stratum spinosum, as well as regularly polarized nuclei in the basal cell layer. In the underlying tunica propria no, or only faint, symptoms of inflammation are present. This benign type of leukoplakia clinically appears rather uniform and is localized most commonly in the postcommissural area of the buccal mucosa.

In the group of significantly premalignant leukoplakias, different patterns of cellular atypia become evident which imply dyskeratosis of single cells, as well as nuclear hyperploidism and polymorphism (dyskaryosis), degradation of regular cell structure, changing of the nucleus:cytoplasm ratio, or increased mitotic activity. In the early stages of premalignancy, these alterations predominantly are confined to the lower epithelial layers, whereas in advanced stages, the entire epithelium is "replaced" by atypical cells undergoing marked disarray. The rete ridges are deformed into plump pegs, showing an increased number of mitoses, as well as closely arranged basal epithelial cells of irregular shape and size, while the underlying connective tissue is infiltrated by leukocytes and mononuclear cells with increased vascularity and edema.

This condition of highly premalignant epithelium is called either *precancerous dysplasia* or *carcinoma in situ.* According to Sprague (1963), minimal, moderate, and severe forms of precancerous dysplasia may be differentiated. It should be emphasized, however, that various stages of the premalignant evolution may exist at different points of the same leukoplakic area. For this reason some authors attempt exfoliative cytodiagnosis by smears taken from distant places of the leukoplakic lesion (Gardner, 1964 and 1965; Sandler, 1962). This screening method, however, can only supplant, not replace, the histologic examination of a biopsy specimen.

Differential Diagnosis

Since the certainty of the histologic finding depends on the physician's accuracy in taking the biopsy, some notes should be added to facilitate clinical differentiation between benign and premalignant leukoplakias. A benign leukoplakia may be presumed if, in the postcommissural or buccal area of both sides, a rather uniform white patch of epithelium is to be seen, usually exhibiting a smooth, or only finely furrowed, surface without any symptoms of inflammation. Shafer and Waldron (1961) noted this benign type in 82 percent of leukoplakic lesions. If local irritation or a well-defined disease can be proved, the leukoplakia should be classified as a "symptomatic" one, a determination which may facilitate the prognostic evaluation of the lesion, whether it is a harmless or a facultatively premalignant one. On the other hand, if irregular thickening and infiltration of the leukoplakia is present, a precancerous lesion has to be suspected. To be greatly suspected in this respect is the "speckled" type of leukoplakia (Pindborg et al., 1963), which changes into malignancy in a high percentage of cases. *Marked induration or localized ulceration within a leukoplakic area is pathognomonic of cancer formation.* Since the risk of inducing metastatic spread to lymph nodes may be increased in this stage by minor biopsies, wide excision of the entire lesion should be carried out on first admission.

Pipe smokers, and more rarely other tobacco consumers, may undergo a peculiar form of benign leukoplakia designated *leukokeratosis nicotinica* (Krainz and Kumer, 1933; Kren, 1934; Schuermann et al., 1966; Tappeiner, 1941). Most commonly the hard palate is affected less frequently than the soft palate or the alveolar ridge of the maxilla. The gum is coated with diffuse whitish hyperkeratosis interspersed with many little red dots, corresponding to the ductal orifices of the small mucous glands. This type of leukokeratosis being known likewise as "smoker's gum" or "stomatitis nicotinica" (Capman and Redish, 1960; Lewis, 1955; Saunders, 1958; Schwartz, 1965), occurs only in heavy smokers, predominantly elderly men. It almost never turns into a precancerous or cancerous condition. Even after decades of tobacco use, the keratotic disorder may disappear if smoking is stopped. The clinical appearance is such a characteristic one that biopsy is not required in most cases.

The term *leukedema* was used by Sandstead and Lowe (1953) to describe a delicate, filmy opalescence of the mucosa which can be wiped off but tends to recur. Histologically it is characterized by intracellular edema and retention of the superficial parakeratotic cells (Archard et al., 1968). Perhaps more pronounced forms of leukedema represent only a variety of any leukoplakia, whereas minimal forms may pass as a harmless anomaly without pathologic significance (Waldron, 1970). The condition is seen quite often among American Negroes, and it also occurs rather frequently in inhabitants of New Guinea (Pindborg et al., 1968a). In a few of my patients clinically and histologically I also observed a mucosal condition like leukedema. Besides habitual smoking as a possible etiologic factor, I suggest that in younger females a very similar clinical condition periodically occurring on the buccal mucosa may be due to hormonal imbalance during the menstrual cycle.

Other types of idiopathic leukoplakias will not be dealt with, since they remain benign for life, so far as is known.

A peculiar form of leukoplakic disorder designated *oral submucous fibrosis* should be mentioned briefly. Extensive studies carried out by Pindborg et al. (1966, 1967b, 1968) on the nosologic features and epidemiology of this oral disorder revealed an incidence of 0.2 to 0.5 percent in various urban populations of India. Reports to date have been concerned chiefly with Indian people and Indian inhabitants of South Africa (Pindborg and Sirsat, 1966; Pindborg et al., 1967b; Vogler et al., 1962). Women are somewhat more affected than men. Though the question of etiology is open so far, the conditon shows marked symptoms of initial fibrotic degeneration of the submucosal connective tissue associated with atrophic changes of the overlying epithelium.

The condition usually begins with insidious symptoms of a burning sensation and a feeling of stiffness of the tongue and mouth. Blisters, ulcerations, or recurrent stomatitis may precede or accompany the advancing course of the disorder. Fibrous bands develop in the buccal and labial mucosa, in the pterygomandibular raphe, and also in the pharynx. The dorsal surface of the tongue is commonly involved and undergoes loss of papillae. The most striking aspect of the disorder is a blanching of the affected oral mucosa which is firmly attached to the underlying tissue and irregularly interspersed with scarlike and brownish patches. The chief reason why we refer to this peculiar oral condition is its *predisposition to develop leukoplakia*, which may even become a cancer in consequence of the long-standing alteration of the atrophic epithelium.

In this context we want to draw attention to a little known precancerous condition of the oropharynx in patients suffering from so-called *hereditary congenital polykeratoses (Touraine)*. An essential pathologic feature of this group of genodermatoses is systemic hyperplastic proliferation and dyskeratosis of large areas of the skin, as well as of the adjacent mucosa of the mouth, external genitalia, and other orifices, so that leukoplakias, or leukokeratoses, of the oral cavity may be associated with other symptoms of polykeratosis (Schuermann et al., 1966). The mucocutaneous correlation of keratotic dystrophy applies especially to the syndrome of Zinsser-Engman-Cole, inasmuch as the oral leukoplakic lesions which may be observed in this rare hereditary disorder, occasionally, following premalignant dysplasia, undergo malignant transformation. In an unusual case reported by Pindborg (1968), bullous lesions of the buccal and lingual mucosa preceded the leukoplakic hyperkeratoses, but such an exudative stage may be considered as an atypical finding in this peculiar syndrome.

In *epidermolysis hereditaria bullosa dystrophicans (Hallopeau-Siemens)*, another serious genodermatosis confined to the ectodermal tissues, widespread leukoplakic areas in the oral cavity develop as sequelae of recurrent epitheliolytic damage of the dystrophic mucosa (Schuermann et al., 1966). In advanced stages of the disease, scarring synechias and stenosing shrinkage of the vestibular and sublingual mucosa, as well as of the larynx, pharynx, or esophagus, result in impairment of ingestion. Due to the extreme chronicity and seriousness of this hereditary disorder (existing since birth), cancer of the oral or esophageal mucosa may ultimately occur.

Etiology

The etiology of the intraoral and labial leukoplakias, aside from the above-mentioned disorders, comprises some known, but more unknown, factors. With the most important factors ranks *local contact with tobacco,* be it by pipe smoke or by quid (Cooke, 1969; Lewis, 1955; Mehta et al., 1969a; Pindborg et al., 1967a; Schuermann et al., 1966; Shklar, 1965). Snuff as well, applied habitually in the lower sulcus of the buccal mucosa, may give rise to leukoplakia or even carcinoma (Brown et al., 1965; Landy and White, 1961; Pindborg, 1968; Pindborg and Renstrup, 1963; Pindborg et al., 1965; Rosenfeld and Callaway, 1963; Stecker et al., 1964). With strange customs of smoking (such as smoking with the glowing end of the cigarette or cigar inside the mouth as is popular in the Philippines, the Dutch Antilles, and India), leukoplakia arises from chronic stomatitis, primarily at the hard palate, where the local effect of smoke and heat is focused (Quigley et al., 1964; Reddy and Rao, 1957; Sandler, 1962; Schoenfeld and Holzberger, 1964; Tiecke and Bernier, 1954). Apparently local heat intensifies the carcinogenic potency of tobacco, so that the incidence of carcinoma may be increased by smoking (Pindborg, 1968; Quigley et al., 1964; Reddy and Rao, 1957; Schoenfeld and Holzberger, 1964).

A peculiar variety of irritative leukoplakia which chiefly involves the buccal mucosa is due to habitual chewing of betel nut, especially in combination with other ingredients of betel morsel. This *betel leukoplakia* predominantly occurs in Indian people, in the Papuans of New Guinea, and in some other races of southeastern Asia (Forlen et al., 1965; Mehta et al., 1969a and 1969b; Muir and Kirk, 1960; Pindborg et al., 1965, 1966, and 1967a; Singh and von Essen, 1966; Tennekoon and Bartlett, 1969; Wahi et al., 1965). Forlen et al. (1965) noted typical leukoplakias in 17.5 percent of

the Papuans chewing betel as well as smoking tobacco, whereas only 4 percent of those who only smoked presented similar lesions. Changing of betel leukoplakia into carcinoma chiefly depends on whether the morsel is blended with tobacco leaves containing carcinogenic substances (Hirayama, 1966; Mehta et al., 1969a; Muir and Kirk, 1960; Pindborg et al., 1967a).

Traumatic, commonly harmless, causes of leukoplakia are ill-fitting dentures, teeth in an irregular position, and carious dental stumps which may give rise to oral callosity by chronic irritation of the opposite mucosa. Furthermore, inlays of different metals in adjacent teeth may evoke an electrogalvanic leukoplakia, or even ulcerous stomatitis, of the contacting mucosa (Schuermann et al., 1966). Some authors also suppose that leukoplakias develop in long-standing malnutrition with anemia and protein deficiency as well as vitamin A or B deficiency (Ahlbom, 1936; Jacobsson, 1948; Keller, 1963 and 1967; Trieger et al., 1958 and 1959; Wynder and Fryer, 1958). Some leukoplakias localized at the posterior palate also may be induced by neurodystrophic disturbances of the glossopharyngeal nerve (Seifert, 1966).

On the lower lip the most important cause of leukoplakia is undoubtedly chronic exposure to sunlight, especially its ultraviolet radiation. This *actinic leukoplakia* as well as some other cheilopathies of premalignant significance will be discussed further below.

To better understand the histopathologic features of oral leukoplakia, some basic properties of the metabolism of epithelial cells with regard to their glycogen content, as well as the distribution of the mitochondria in the different epithelial strata, should be called to mind. The normal epithelium of the mucosa consists of a glycogen-free basal cell layer which contains mitochondria to a large extent, whereas in the overlying stratum spinosum, glycogen and an increasing number of tonofibrils are visible in contrast to few mitochondria. In the superficial layers, on the other hand, loss of the glycogen content and incipient keratinization occur. Apparently in the lower epithelial layers cellular metabolism involves primarily an oxidative pathway, whereas in the glycogen-containing higher strata of the epithelium, a nonoxidative glycolytic pathway of metabolism is predominant (Fasske and Themann, 1959; Fasske and Morgenroth, 1964). When leukoplakia develops, the functional structure of the basal epithelium is disordered, inasmuch as the content of mitochondria as well as of some reticular cytoplasmic substructures increases, contrasting with a marked decrease of the glycogen. These changes result in a distinct keratinization of the superficial epithelial cells (Fasske and Morgenroth, 1964; Fasske et al., 1959).

Therapy and Prognosis

In many cases of harmless leukoplakia the lesions may disappear completely with careful oral hygiene, avoidance of mucosal irritants (tobacco, hot spices, alcohol), removal of offending tooth stumps, or correction of jutting dental crowns and other irritating prosthetic material. Chronic trauma to the mucosa by habitual cheek biting is also reversible, if the neurotic habit is given up. In cases of symptomatic leukoplakias the basic disease has to be treated. If there is minimal suspicion of malignant transformation, a positive histologic diagnosis must be made. The dentist or physician is not allowed to wait until distinct symptoms of incipient carcinoma arise, but has to carry out one or more biopsies in search of an exact diagnosis. Cauterization by diathermy, or application of x-rays even in minimal dosage, may be dangerous because it increases local irritation. Every clear-cut precancerous leukoplakia should be removed by wide surgical excision (followed by plastic replacement of the mucosa, if necessary), which we prefer to irradiation. All patients who are affected by oral leukoplakia ought to be reexamined at regular intervals.

It is not surprising that there are divergent opinions about prognosis in the literature. In an extensive long-term study of oral leukoplakia in a Swedish population, Einhorn and Wersäll (1967) stated that only 2.4 percent of patients after 10 years, and 4 percent after 20 years, had developed carcinoma. In a series of 248 Danish patients under control for 3.7 years on the average, Pindborg et al. (1968) noted a 4.4 percent incidence of malignant transformation. In the follow-up study of Silverman and Rozen (1968), the rate of cancer development in American patients was 6 percent.

In every case of clinically suspected premalignant or malignant growth, it is important to repeat the biopsy if the first specimen does not confirm the diagnosis. There often exists a clear-cut histologic borderline between apparently benign and malignant areas, so that a biopsy taken from the area close to but outside the malignant proliferation may be inconclusive. Shafer and Waldron (1961) as well as Silverman and Rozen (1968) detected clinically unsuspected stages of early cancer in 10 percent of their biopsy specimens of leukoplakic lesions.

BOWEN'S DISEASE AND CARCINOMA IN SITU OF THE ORAL CAVITY

Bowen's disease arises not only from the skin but also from the oral mucosa, where it has been considered a distinct type of oral precancerosis which predominantly occurs in males in their middle or later decades of life (Gorlin, 1950; Hornstein

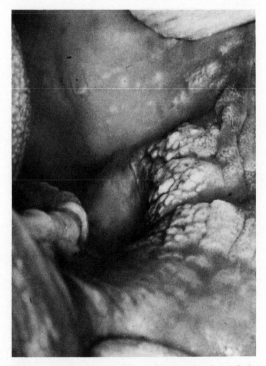

Figure 21–8 Bowenoid carcinoma in situ of the buccal mucosa in a 69 year old man. White warty protuberances arising from a "speckled" leukoplakic area.

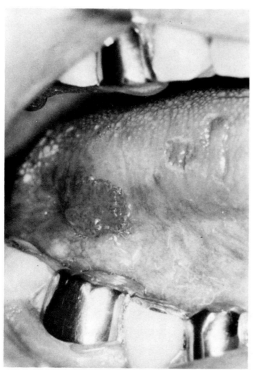

Figure 21–9 "Erythroplakic" type of incipient carcinoma arising from the lateral tongue in a 45 year old man. (Near the coarsely protruding tumor are some delicate patches of exfoliation.)

and Pape, 1965; Moulonguet, 1936; Reich, 1954; Schuermann et al., 1966; Touraine and Solente, 1935). The chief reason why only a few papers on the disease have been published up to now, in my opinion, may be some difficulty in clinically differentiating the lesion from other premalignant ones. All regions of the oropharynx may be affected, particularly the retroangular and buccal areas, less frequently the lips, tongue, or throat.

As to the clinical and histologic findings of Bowen's precancer of the oral mucosa, some authors make a distinction between a dysplastic and a hyperplastic type of the disease. The former shows localized or widespread leukoplakic areas varying in color, size, and surface pattern, and being interspersed with variably shaped erythroplakic lesions with a dark red, slightly granular surface. Faintly opalescent, flat plaques, whitish hyperkeratoses with an irregularly wrinkled surface, and papillary projections may be closely aggregated. In early stages, the firmness of the lesions, as a rule, is only moderately increased. It should be emphasized, however, that in some cases of Bowen's disease a clear-cut clinical distinction from the "speckled" type of leukoplakia (Pindborg, 1968; Pindborg et al., 1963) is impossible. On the other hand, the close aggregation of leukoplakic lesions, differing from each other in aspect and being combined with erythroplakic (pseudoerosive) patches, is rather typical of oral Bowen's disease. Since the ulcerative pattern does not belong to the typical premalignant condition of Bowen's disease, beginning ulceration is indicative of transformation into invasive carcinoma.

The hyperplastic type of oral Bowen's disease (Hudelo and Cailliau, 1933; Lacronique and Dechaume, 1932; Moulonguet, 1936; Reich, 1954; Reich and Bonse, 1955) is characterized by marked exophytic outgrowths with a papillary, whitish, sparkling surface arising from leukoplakic bases. The polypous, papillomatous, or pectinate masses may look like boiled cauliflower. In the old French literature, these fungating oral lesions were designated *hyperplasie pure* of Bowen's disease (Lacronique and Dechaume, 1932; Hudelo and Cailliau, 1933; Touraine and Golé, 1936). In the paragraph about the clinical problem of an allegedly "new" disorder termed "oral florid papillomatosis" (Rock and Fisher, 1960; Samitz and Weinberg, 1963) in its nosologic relation to "verrucous carcinoma" (Ackerman, 1948; Ackerman and Johnson, 1954; Ackerman and McGavran, 1958; Fonts et al., 1969; Goethals et al., 1963), I shall discuss the question of whether this *hyperplasie pure* may be postulated as a distinct variety of Bowen's disease or should better be integrated into another clinicopathologic entity.

Histologically, in the dysplastic type of Bowen's disease one finds considerable structural disorganization, cellular polymorphism, and dyskaryosis of the epithelial cells which involves all layers of the epithelium, while the superficial squamous cells may undergo incomplete keratinization. In many epithelial cells heavily deformed, hyperchromatic, and gigantic nuclei or atypical mitoses are present. The cells in the deeper layers of the dysplastic epithelium are closely and irregularly arranged. The basement membrane usually remains intact, while the underlying connective tissue is infiltrated by mono-nuclear cells or leukocytes.

The histologic picture of *hyperplasie pure* (Hornstein and Pape, 1965; Hudelo and Cailliau, 1933; Lacronique and Dechaume, 1932; Reich, 1954) differs from the above findings insofar as the structure of the epithelial cells appears to be almost regular; on the other hand, there are seen bulky, "blown-out" rete ridges with endophytic as well as exophytic papillomatous projections. As the epithelial proliferation as a whole and its basal cell layers present only minor disorder or polymorphism in spite of an accompanying inflammatory stroma reaction, the deceptive impression of a benign hyperplasia may result.

In the clinicopathologic literature there are divergent opinions with regard to the classification of Bowen's disease of the oral cavity. Since the first report by Lacronique and Dechaume in 1932, several French, German, Italian, British, and American authors have published analogous cases of Bowen's disease with oral, laryngeal, or endonasal localization (see Hornstein and Pape, 1965). On the other hand, many oral pathologists tend to identify Bowen's disease of the different mucosal tissues with the so-called "carcinoma in situ"—that is, a noninvasive stage of early carcinoma (especially of the uterine cervix). Indeed, no stringent histopathologic differences between the dysplastic type of Bowen's disease and carcinoma in situ can be postulated as far as the oral cavity is concerned, because both are characterized by an epithelium with distinct cellular criteria of malignancy, without any invasion of the underlying connective tissue. Furthermore, contrary to focal precancerous leukoplakia, the finding of disorganizing dysplasia involving all cell layers of the epithelium is applicable to both disorders. Since the concept of the uterine carcinoma in situ has been accepted by most clinicians and pathologists, the majority of pathologists apply this term as well in cases of "intraepithelial" or noninvasive neoplasia of the mouth, larynx, esophagus, bronchi, and other mucosal tissues.

The question whether Bowen's disease of the oral mucosa is a nosologic entity or not is made still more complex by some difficulties in classifying the peculiar hyperplastic type. While some European au-thors, for reasons of historic priority, continued to use the ancient French term *hyperplasie pure* (Greither, 1965; Hornstein and Pape, 1965; Reich, 1954; Reich and Bonse, 1955; Schuermann et al., 1966), in 1960 Rock and Fisher described "oral florid papillomatosis," supposedly a new disease of possibly viral origin interpreted as an excessive form of benign epithelial hyperplasia. In the recent edition of Thoma's *Oral Pathology*, Waldron (1970), on the other hand, discards the terms "oral florid papillomatosis" and *hyperplasie pure* of Bowen's disease and, in their place, ranks analogous cases with a peculiar type of noninvasive cancer of low-grade malignancy which had been described, in 1948, by Ackerman as "verrucous carcinoma." There are, indeed, some clinical as well as histologic features of oral verrucous carcinoma remarkably similar to the previously outlined disorders, so the possibility that these conditions are identical has to be discussed more extensively.

Trying in this context to apply the above-mentioned unitary view of the pathologists to the varying clinical appearances and the progress of these lesions, the clinician is tempted to suspect that the different terms in reality are only synonyms of *two different types of intraoral transformation to cancer.* There is an incipiently noninvasive intraepithelial carcinoma in situ (identical with the dysplastic type of Bowen's disease) and, on the other hand, a likewise noninvasive but excessively hyperplastic, pseudobenign initial stage of carcinoma (identical with *hyperplasie pure* of Bowen's disease as well as with the "oral florid papillomatosis" of Rock and Fisher). Apparently both kinds of transformation differ as to the predominant direction of malignant growth, in that the normal epithelium, in the case of carcinoma in situ, is replaced by superficially expanding dysplastic epithelium, whereas in the case of papillomatous hyperplasia, the epithelium tends to proliferate vertically to the surface but not to destroy the underlying connective tissue at this preinvasive stage.

Carcinoma in situ clinically may appear as "speckled" leukoplakia as well as erythroplakia with a red, delicately granular, or velvetlike surface. We doubt whether there exists in the mouth a distinctive nosologic entity of erythroplakia (Mathis and Herrmann, 1963; Pindborg, 1968; Williamson, 1964) (nor "erythroplasia Queyrat" of the penis), and this term is more a clinical description than a histologic entity. Histologically, there is no difference between the erythroplakic and the leukoplakic variants of oral carcinoma in situ. In both the danger of invasive cancer followed by metastatic spread is imminent.

In my opinion carcinoma in situ may be regarded as an *integrating term*, and the variability of clinical appearance should be expressed by additional notes (such as carcinoma in situ of erythroplakic, bowenoid, or speckled type). The wide, multilocular, and discontinuous spread in the oral cavity seems to be a criterion which these three types have in common. The prognosis of oral carcinoma in situ can be considered good only if the diagnosis is made at an early stage and is immediately followed by adequate treatment. Radical surgical excision of all lesions is the therapy of choice. Due to the tendency of the oral carcinoma in situ to grow multicentrically and discontinuously, its recurrence rate is high. Therefore every patient should be kept under careful supervision for at least five years and should be motivated to avoid all well-known etiologic factors, especially tobacco in every form.

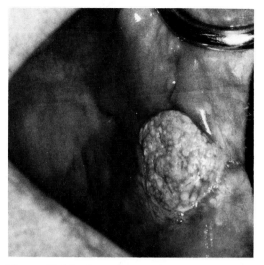

Figure 21–10 Verrucous carcinoma of the postcommissural mucosa in a 52 year old man. There is only slight leukoplakic change of the surrounding mucosal epithelium.

VERRUCOUS CARCINOMA OF THE ORAL CAVITY AND ORAL FLORID PAPILLOMATOSIS

American oral pathologists regard verrucous carcinoma as a distinctive clinicopathologic type of low-grade epidermoid carcinoma, which differs from other oral carcinomas by some clinical, histologic, and prognostic features (Ackerman, 1948;

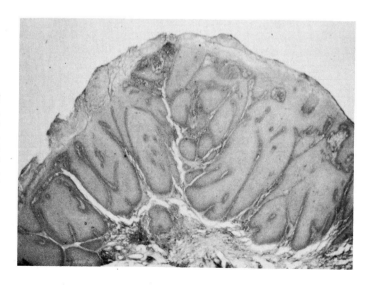

Figure 21–11 Histoligic view of early verrucous carcinoma. × 9. Bulky, ballooned-out rete pegs push into the connective tissue; the pegs are separated from each other by fine, elongated papillae of the connective tissue and coated with a broad hyperkeratosis at the surface.

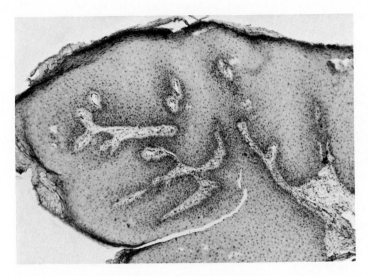

Figure 21–12 Verrucous carcinoma: part of the tumor at low magnification. Vegetating hyperacanthosis of the epithelium resembling a benign papilloma.

Ackerman and Johnson, 1954; Ackerman and McGavran, 1958; Duckworth, 1961; Fonts et al., 1969; Goethals et al., 1963; Sharp et al., 1956; Shatkins, 1963; Waldron, 1970). The frequency of occurrence of verrucous carcinoma compared with other types of oral cancer is uncertain, since the tumor apparently is designated by various names. Of 1217 oral carcinomas diagnosed at the Mayo Clinic, 55 (4.5 percent) met the histologic criteria for verrucous carcinoma (Goethals et al., 1963). According to Duckworth (1961), this cancer represents less than 2 percent of the total of oral carcinomas. It usually occurs in elderly people.

The clinical appearance of verrucous carcinoma is characterized by large, whitish, cauliflower-like masses resembling polypous condyloma acuminatum on a leukoplakic base. These fungating tumors may involve wide areas of the oral cavity but are found most commonly in the mandibular buccal sulcus, adjacent buccal mucosa, and alveolar mucosa of the mandibular ridge. Occasionally the carcinoma involves the margin of the tongue, the maxillary alveolar mucosa, or the lips. The luxuriant tumor masses may grow to a very large size, impeding mastication. The gray-white to white sparkling color depends on the thickness of the surface keratinization. The lesion is rather soft, not having the induration of typical squamous cell carcinomas. When spreading onto the vermilion border, the tumors look like cu-

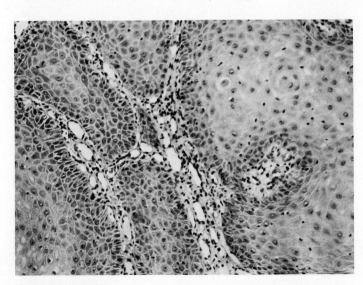

Figure 21–13 Verrucous carcinoma at higher magnification. Well-differentiated epithelium with only moderate atypia and disorientation of the basal cells.

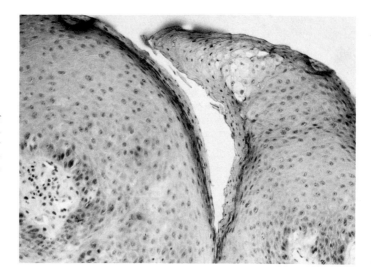

Figure 21-14 Superficial part of verrucous carcinoma showing filiform hyperkeratosis with nuclear remainders in the partly water-clear, partly lamellar squamous cells.

taneous horns superimposed on leukoplakic areas. Intraorally they are composed of multiple papillary vegetations with deep fissures between them. Extended ulceration rarely is found, but small ulcers may occur on the tips or sides of the papillary excrescences.

Verrucous carcinoma, at least in its early stage, grows outward rather than deeply into surrounding tissue. When becoming invasive, however, it penetrates the cheek and may extend to the skin surface as a funguslike protruding mass. The tumor also may destroy the bone of the mandible or maxilla. On the other hand, spread to regional lymph nodes is uncommon, and metastasis in the blood has been only exceptionally observed. Only 3 of 38 patients reported by Ackerman and Johnson (1954) showed metastases, which subsequently developed in two patients during local recurrence of the tumor following treatment.

Histologically, the tumor looks like an exorbitant papillary hyperplasia of the squamous epithelium projecting multiple folds to the surface and swollen blunted pegs at the deep margin. These tend to be bulky, bulbous forms, compressing the papillary ridges of corium interspersed between them. The excessively hyperplastic epithelium as well as its individual cells seems to be in a well-differentiated stage, and distinct nuclear atypia or polymorphism is only rarely found. In most tumor sections the basal cell layer appears to be regularly arranged, showing no break

through the basement membrane. The underlying stroma is infiltrated with lymphocytes and other mononuclear cells in addition to showing increased vascularity. In advanced or recurring stages, however, the histologic features of malignancy may become more prominent, and in repeated biopsies progression may be observed from pseudobenign hyperplasia with dyskeratosis to typical cancer with invading growth.

The misleading "benign" microscopic features of the tumor may explain why many pathologists, particularly if they are not familiar with this peculiar type of oral carcinoma, give an incorrect diagnosis of benign papilloma. Waldron (1970) emphasizes the diagnostic problem of cytology, too, inasmuch as smears taken from clinically and histologically proved verrucous carcinomas, at initial stages, erroneously may be interpreted as class I or II.

Verrucous carcinoma has a relatively high recurrence rate, which seems to be due to the multicentric formation of new lesions of the oral mucosa conditioned by leukoplakia. In the Mayo Clinic series (Goethals et al., 1963), 31 percent of the patients developed new oral carcinomas, some of them of higher grade malignancy. Nevertheless, the survival rate for patients with oral verrucous carcinoma is regarded to be better than that for patients with most other types of oral cancer. Goethals et al. (1963) reported five-year survival in 75 percent of patients treated by diathermy excision. Death usually is due to local complications of the tumor growth and treatment, or to intercurrent disease in elderly patients.

As to etiology, most authors stress the significance of habitual chewing of tobacco or snuff over many years (Ackerman, 1948; Ackerman and Johnson, 1954; Ackerman and McGavran, 1958; Brown and Suh, 1965; Cooke, 1969; Fonts et al., 1969; Landy and White, 1961; Rosenfeld and Callaway, 1963; Stecker et al., 1964). There are some differences in the geographic distribution of the tumor incidence according to local customs of consuming tobacco. For this reason the male:female sex ratio of oral verrucous cancer varies in different populations. The series of the Mayo Clinic (Goethals et al., 1963) included only a few men who admitted tobacco chewing. In some southeastern regions of the United States, on the other hand, verrucous carcinoma may be observed not rarely in elderly, particularly rural, women who have taken snuff for many years. In these regions verrucous carcinoma commonly is referred to as "snuff dippers' cancer" (Brown et al., 1965). Among 300 patients with oral cancer in Nashville, reported by Rosenfeld and Callaway (1963), there were only 125 men, a male:female ratio of 2:3, which differs markedly from the well-known predominance of men with oral cancer in most countries. In 25 female cases of Landy and White (1961), exposure to snuff ranged from 20 to more than 50 years.

It should be mentioned that many oral carcinomas occurring in Indian as well as other populations of southeastern Asia, who are addicted to the habit of chewing a mixture of betel nuts, tobacco, and slaked lime, have the clinical and histologic features of typical verrucous carcinoma (Cooke, 1969). In some patients, nevertheless, especially from northern regions of America or from Europe, the same type of carcinoma may develop with an unknown etiology.

Treatment consists of surgical removal of all lesions as widely as possible. Diathermy excision or curettage may be sufficient in cases of very widespread tumor but usually does not prevent new lesions from recurring within a short time. Radiotherapy should be omitted, since there are reports of such unfavorable clinical courses as extended radionecrosis and rapid progress to a final stage beyond help (Perez et al., 1966). Kanee (1969), in the case of a 79 year old woman treated by methotrexate, achieved marked clinical improvement with at least temporary remissions of the malignant growth. To date the combination of surgical excision and chemotherapy may be regarded as the best method of therapy.

Oral Florid Papillomatosis

In 1960, Rock and Fisher reported on three cases of an unusual papillomatous lesion of the oral cavity and the larynx which they designated "florid papillomatosis," missing earlier reports on the "pure hyperplastic type" of oral Bowen's disease in the French and German literature (Lacronique and Dechaume, 1932; Hudelo and Cailliau, 1933; Moulonguet, 1936; Reich, 1954; Reich and Bonse, 1955; Hornstein and Pape, 1965; Schuermann et al., 1966). The clinical appearance of the lesions as well as their resistance to radiotherapy and other treatment, in association with a marked recurrence rate, pointed to carcinoma, whereas the clinical course with an absence of metastases and some electron microscopic findings of rather normal-appearing epithelial cells seemed to prove the benign character of the tumors. Furthermore, the authors called for conservatism in therapy, especially with x-rays, as they observed tissue necrosis and radionecrosis of bone with superimposed infection following irradiation.

In subsequent years, some dermatologists presented similar cases which seemed to substantiate the relatively benign nature of oral florid papillomatosis (Wechsler and Fisher, 1962; Samitz and Weinberg, 1963; Knossew, 1966; Tappeiner and Wolff, 1969) or "oral florid verrucosis" (Barnett and Hyman, 1968). On the other hand, there are some recent reports of squamous cell carcinomas developing from such lesions on long-term observation (Kaminsky et al., 1966; Samitz et al., 1967; Kanee, 1969). In the cases of Samitz et al. (1967), Knossew (1966), and Kanee (1969), treatment by aminopterin, mercaptopurine (Purinethol), or methotrexate did not succeed in preventing a change for the worse in spite of temporary improvement. Thus *the original concept of the condition as a pseudomalignant one has to be revised,* particularly since all authors describing oral florid papillomatosis have failed to notice the reports on verrucous carcinoma referred to above. This condition has been listed in the standard tumor classification of oral pathology since the first paper by Ackerman in 1948. When Ackerman's diagnostic criteria for verrucous carcinoma are compared with those of "florid papillomatosis," the latter condition obviously meets some striking histologic standards of the former, such as verrucous papillary lesions and blunted pseudoepitheliomatous hyperplasia. Histologic symptoms of higher-grade malignancy, such as cellular dysplasia as in carcinoma in situ, or invasive foci, may also appear in advanced stages (Kanee, 1969; Samitz et al., 1967). Furthermore, the considerable recurrence rate of the lesions and their marked resistance to therapeutic irradiation are important properties common to both affections. In summary, there remains little proof of a "new" clinicopathologic entity.

Attention of dermatologists and pathologists should nevertheless be drawn to reports on hyperplastic Bowen's disease in the oral cavity by French authors as far back as the early 1930's (Lacronique and Dechaume, 1932; Hudelo and Cailliau, 1933). Not only the clinical and histologic features of the lesions but also their resistance to radiotherapy (Reich, 1954; Reich and Bonse, 1955; Schuermann et al., 1966), as well as the dubious clinical course of the disease, are very similar, if not identical, to the "oral florid papillomatosis" above-mentioned. In 1965, Hornstein and Pape reported on another four cases of oral Bowen's disease with regard to the peculiar type of *hyperplasie pure* described long ago. Tappeiner and Wolff (1969), on the other hand, gave Scheicher-Gottron the recognition of having first described the condition of "oral florid papillomatosis" under the name of "papillomatosis mucosae carcinoides" in an analogous case in 1958.

Reviewing the scattered papers on this topic and also paying attention to some older publications on it, a feeling of some confusion in nomenclature arises from obviously insufficient information about an important problem of oral pathology running under various terminologic flags. From an historic viewpoint, there is little doubt that Lacronique and Dechaume (1932) were the first to describe the condition as a particular type of oral Bowen's disease and to use the term *hyperplasie pure.* This interpretation has been endorsed by some German authors (Reich, 1954; Reich and Bonse, 1955; Schuermann et al., 1966; Hornstein and Pape, 1965), who have contributed additional cases since 1954. It should be mentioned that, in Ackerman's concept of oral verrucous carcinoma, the prior reports of French authors, which used another term, were not taken into consideration. Nevertheless, regarding the imposing number of case reports on oral verrucous carcinoma, chiefly by American authors within the past 25 years and comparing these to the divergent nomenclature for an obviously analogous condition in the dermatologic literature, it seems to me best to come to an agreement about a joint designation of a distinct tumor condition erroneously being divided into fictitious entities. It may be regarded as a question of oncologic definition (and of judging the priority of historic data or of prevailing usage of terms) whether the condition being discussed should be designated "hyperplastic type of Bowen's disease" or "verrucous carcinoma" as defined above. I suggest aggreement on the latter term, as it is difficult, in fact, to reduce the histologic features of a markedly "dysplastic" and of a predominantly "hyperplastic" epithelial proliferation to the same nosologic denominator of Bowen's disease, though in both conditions the initially malignant, or at least highly premalignant, properties of growth are proved. (For further information see Chapter 33.)

CARCINOMA AND PRECANCEROUS CONDITIONS OF THE LIP

Cancer of the lip accounts for 25 to 30 percent of all oral cancers (Ackerman and

Del Regato, 1962; Clinical Oncology, 1973; Schuermann et al., 1966; Pindborg, 1968; Sharp et al., 1956; Waldron, 1970). The lower lip is estimated to be affected at least 10 times (Clinical Oncology, 1973), more probably 20 times (Schuermann et al., 1966), or even 60 times (Pindborg, 1968) more frequently than the upper one. Lip cancer predominantly occurs among white men, with a sex ratio varying from 50:1 to 10:1, according to location. In the United States the male:female ratio is about 14:1 (Waldron, 1970). In Australia (Belisario, 1959), as well as in the southern states of the United States, lip carcinomas are rather often seen, whereas in India, for instance, the lip is an uncommon site of cancer, contrasting with the extraordinarily high incidence of cancer inside the oral cavity (Mehta et al., 1969b; Pindborg, 1963 and 1965a; Pindborg et al., 1967a; Singh and von Essen, 1966; Wahi et al., 1965). Furthermore, in the Negro race, labial carcinoma rarely occurs (Leffall and White, 1965). Of 827 patients with lip carcinoma reviewed by Bernier and Clark (1951) in an extensive study dealing primarily with American soldiers during World War II, only four were Negroes. The enormous geographic as well as racial variations of the incidence rate of labial carcinoma may indicate the influence, above all, of racial factors in its etiology. There is also a wide range of age incidence, from under 40 years to very old people with a peak in the fifth to seventh decades (Ashley et al., 1965; Belisario, 1959; Clinical Oncology, 1973; Cross et al., 1948; Judd and Beahrs, 1949; Keller, 1963; Schuermann et al., 1966; Sharp et al., 1956).

Carcinoma of the lower lip usually develops on the vermilion region outside the borderline of contact with the upper lip. In most cases it arises from the lateral part of the lip about halfway between the midline and the commissure. In the large series of Bernier and Clark (1951), a midline location accounted for only 15 percent. In almost all cases of carcinoma the vermilion shows a dry, atrophic, or widely leukoplakic condition which has developed over years. This labial alteration, which may become fissurated, sore, and covered by adherent crusts or hyperkeratotic scales, has to be regarded as a precancerous con-

dition of low grade (Schuermann et al., 1966).

Etiologically, in the majority of cases, an association with a fair or ruddy complexion is striking, particularly in persons engaged in outdoor occupations with prolonged exposure to sun, wind, and frost. Farmers and sailors used to be affected by lip cancer at a considerably higher rate than other groups. In the past decades, obviously owing to changing economic, and social conditions in western countries, the prevalent occurrence of lip carcinoma in men with rural occupations has become more and more vague. Next, racial as well as complexion factors, and increased exposure to the sun and other environmental influences, are of importance in the etiology of lip carcinoma. Furthermore, the rare involvement of the upper lip can be explained primarily by the small exposure of this region to actinic radiation. Habitual pipe smoking or chewing tobacco is another, probably less important, etiologic factor.

Arising from its precancerous basis the incipient carcinoma usually presents as a localized, whitish, slightly indurated plaque or nodule that may be covered by a brownish adherent scale or crust. Until the patients seek the doctor's attention, and the lesion is diagnosed as precancer or carcinoma, on the average more than a year has passed (Schuermann et al., 1966). Unfortunately, in many cases rather a long time is spent in treatment with a corticoid-containing ointment. It should be emphasized that, *in every suspicious labial lesion that persists rather than heals, a biopsy has to be performed.* Another clinical examination that is simple and helpful for diagnosis of precancerous or cancerous lesions is staining of the lip by toluidine blue dye (Shedd et al., 1967; Wang et al., 1973). In contrast to the normal surrounding epithelium, and to benign hyperplasia, a precancerous lesion or carcinoma remains markedly stained after removal of the dye with water.

Clinically, there are two main types of lip carcinoma: an *exophytic, hyperkeratotic tumor* and an *infiltrating ulcer.* A third papillary pattern like verrucous carcinoma only rarely occurs on the lip. The exophytic type apparently is the most common. It appears as a slow-growing warty or nodular

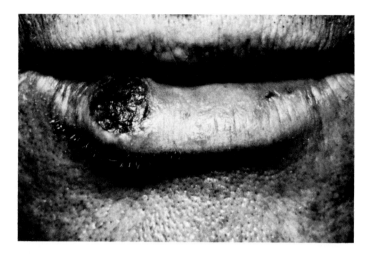

Figure 21–15 Ulcerative type of lip carcinoma in a 60 year old man.

lesion with closely adherent grayish brown horn prickles on its surface. In a very hyperkeratotic outgrowth the lesion may resemble a wide-based cutaneous horn. Lamellar scaling surrounding or covering the tumor is often observed. As the cancer enlarges, its clinical appearance may change into a flat ulcerative or extended erosive lesion with hemorrhagic crusts on a coarsely vegetating ground. This type of labial carcinoma has a lower grade of malignancy than the primarily ulcerative one, with less of a tendency to deep invasion or lymphatic spread.

The second type of lip cancer assumes an ulcerous form from the outset and tends to infiltrate the borders and the underlying tissues more rapidly than the exophytic type does. The tumor may invade the adjacent structures more extensively than the surface ulceration indicates. The margins of the ulcer are firm and sometimes raised in an irregularly thickened rim, whereas the base is covered by a greasy yellowish brown exudate interspersed with necrotizing cell detritus. Carcinomas of this type of growth usually present a higher grade of malignancy than the exophytic type.

Pathologically, most lip carcinomas show a rather well-differentiated epidermoid pattern, whereas the more anaplastic type accounts for only a minority. In the large series reported by Judd and Beahrs (1949), Ward and Hendrick (1950), and Bernier and Clark (1951), lip carcinomas of higher histologic grades of malignancy comprise only about 15 percent of all

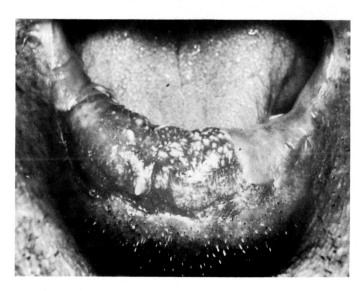

Figure 21–16 Widespread lip carcinoma with "speckled" leukoplakia within a flat ulcerative area. Enlargement of the lower lip by invasion of the deeper tissues.

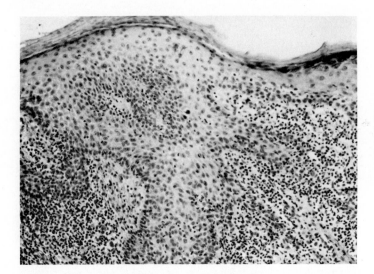

Figure 21-17 Incipient lip carcinoma with irregular rete ridges invading the adjacent connective tissue, which shows marked cellular infiltration.

cases. Long-standing carcinomas, however they may be differentiated, tend to spread to the lymph nodes of the ipsilateral submandibular (less frequently submental) region and may also invade the mandibular bone and surrounding structures. In rare cases, spread along the perineural lymph

sheaths with extension through the mental foramen into the mandible has been observed to be a sign of an unfavorable prognosis (Balantyne et al., 1963).

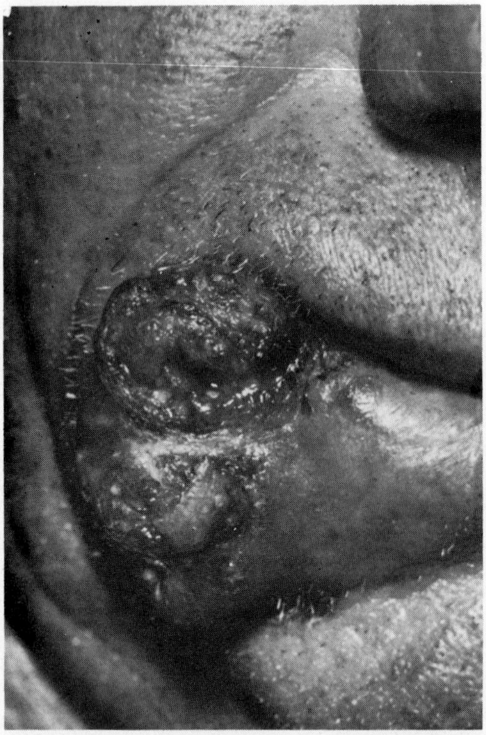

The extent of *metastasis* to regional lymph nodes depends on the time of admission for therapy. In the series of Krantz et al. (1957), 18 percent of all patients showed metastases at the first clinical examination. Apparently, the higher the histologic grade of malignancy, the greater the occurrence of local metastases. This opinion is well supported by the study of Cross et al. (1948), who observed in a large clinicopathologic series metastatic growth in about one-third of the patients with anaplastic carcinomas but in only 7 percent of those with well-differentiated carcinomas. Furthermore, it should be noted that carcinomas arising from the labial commissures are more likely to spread by the lymphatics than those confined to the other parts of vermilion. Blood-borne metastases occur only in very rare cases of lip cancer (Ackerman and Del Regato, 1962; Schuermann et al., 1966; Sharp et al., 1956; Waldron, 1970).

Some years ago Greene and Bernier (1959) drew attention again to a rare, peculiar variant of lip carcinoma that was designated "spindle cell epidermoid carcinoma" by Martin and Stewart as far back as 1935. Histologically, this tumor differs distinctly from the usual anaplastic type of carcinoma, as it is composed of uniformly spindle-shaped cells which tend to infiltrate the adjacent tissues without forming compact clusters or ramifications. This histologic feature may resemble spindle cell sar-

Figure 21-18 Advanced stage of squamous carcinoma at the lip commissure. Wide infiltration of the lateral area of lower lip being secondarily ulcerated.

coma, but the tumor's true origin from epithelium was proved in serial sections by Greene and Bernier (1959).

As stated above squamous cell carcinoma of the *upper lip* is very uncommon. Tumors of this region chiefly comprise genuine basaliomas of varying clinical as well as histologic pattern, as well as adenocarcinomas of small mucosal or minor salivary glands, malignant melanomas, cystic adenopapillomas of benign nature, and mucoepidermoid carcinomas (exceptionally arising from the lip). The same variety of malignant or semimalignant tumors, of course, may be observed on the lower lip (Keen and Elzay, 1964; Lucas, 1964) but usually involve more its dermal or mucosal portion than its vermilion border (Schuermann et al., 1966). In a series of squamous cell carcinomas of both lips, Martin et al. (1941) found a lower five-year survival rate (41 percent) for patients with upper lip carcinoma than for those with lower lip involvement (better than 70 percent).

The choice of treatment in each case depends on the tumor stage, both for the primary lesion and the lymph nodes. While most German and Swiss dermatologists and oncologists preferred radiotherapy by Chaoul's method of application from the 1930's until the 1960's, in recent years they have again turned to surgical treatment. Radiotherapy, however, gives equally good results if the primary tumor is in an early, or strictly superficial or exophytic, stage, not exceeding 2 cm. in its largest diameter. When the carcinoma advances to a larger size, or presents primarily as the ulcerative type, preference should be given to surgery with V-shaped wide excision. Furthermore, when deeper structures of the lip appear to be involved, an oral surgeon should be charged with therapy. Block dissection of submandibular and submental lymph nodes is imperative if enlarged or indurated nodes might contain metastases. Prophylactic irradiation of regional nodes when the tumor is clearly of stage I is not indicated. Palliative radiotherapy may be attempted in cases beyond surgical help.

General *prognosis* of epidermoid carcinomas of the lower lip, though better than for most other types of intraoral cancer, does not equal the high cure rate of most skin cancers. However, a five-year cure rate of 90 percent was reported by Ashley et al. in 1965. There is, of course, a marked change for the worse when metastatic nodes are present just before initial treatment or following it. In such cases, the cure rate may fall from more than 90 percent in tumor stage I to about 50 percent (Krantz et al., 1957). Nevertheless, the five-year cure rate of all lip carcinomas is still better than that of the total of human cancers, which has been regarded as about 18 percent (Schuermann et al., 1966). It should be mentioned, on the other hand, that in a few cases of "spindle cell epidermoid carcinoma" a very poor prognosis has been reported (Goldman and Grady, 1945; Martin and Stewart, 1935).

Chronic Cheilitis Predisposing to Lip Carcinoma

As opposed to the well-defined premalignant lesions occurring on the lips, such as cutaneous horn or precancerous leukoplakia, less attention is usually paid to the sequelae of long-standing inflammatory alterations of the lower lip. Certain forms of chronic, noneczematous cheilitis are known to precede distinct premalignant as well as malignant lesions. There are three chief patterns: cheilitis glandularis of a simple as well as a purulent type, cheilitis actinica (exfoliativa), and Manganotti's "abrasive precancerous cheilitis."

The simple type of *cheilitis glandularis* that was described by Puente and Acevedo in 1927 primarily affects the lower lip in younger or middle-aged persons, mainly males. In spite of some reports implicating a southern climate or chronic irritation of the labial mucosa by poor dental care, the real etiologic factors remain unknown (Ambrosetti, 1953; Schuermann et al., 1966; Seifert, 1966; Touraine and Solente, 1935; Wendlberger, 1938; Wise, 1931).

Most cases of cheilitis glandularis simplex are regarded by physicians as minor, especially because patients usually do not complain of it. On the mucosal surface of the lower lip and extending to its vermilion border, some tiny red-dotted granular lesions are visible. Each consists of a minute

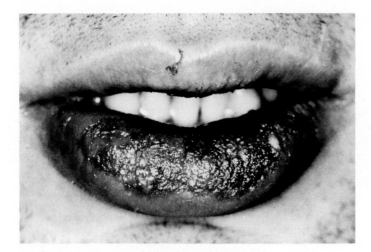

Figure 21-19 "Cheilitis glandularis apostematosa" in a 27 year old man. Diffuse erosion of the vermilion of the lower lip, covered with crusts and scales.

inflammatory spot around the opening of a small mucous or heterotopic salivary gland. On palpation, the lip is found to include small nodules which, on pressure, excrete a minute droplet of water-clear saliva. The entire lip may be somewhat swollen and everted. Leukoplakia may sur-

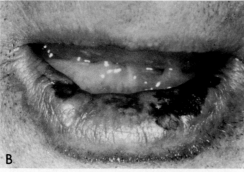

Figure 21-20 *A,* "Cheilitis abrasiva praecancerosa" (Manganotti) in a 56 year old man.

B, Cheilitis of the same patient after staining by toluidine blue. The precancerous lesions remain markedly stained when the dye is washed off with water.

round the small red spots if the condition is chronic.

Histologically, the small mucosal glands are found to be hyperplastic without remarkable surrounding inflammation, while the excretory ducts are dilated. Some connective tissue may accumulate around the enlarged glandular lobules. Changing of the ductal epithelium to squamous cell metaplasia has to be regarded as the beginning of a precancerous stage.

About 100 years ago, Volkmann described a peculiar type of chronic cheilitis called "cheilitis glandularis apostematosa." This is apparently a variety of cheilitis glandularis with a more inflammatory, at times purulent, stage (Everett and Holder, 1955; Schuermann et al., 1966). Inflammation occupies the entire surface of the lower lip, which becomes painful with a burning sensation, especially when touched and during eating and speaking. The lip is edematous and its surface becomes irregularly erosive, with small superficial ulcers being coverved with a scabbed or yellowish brown greasy coat. The regional lymph nodes only rarely are enlarged, and the patients usually remain in good general condition. The purulent stage of cheilitis may subside and be followed by leukoplakia, which also occurs on the buccal mucosa extending from the labial commissures.

Biopsy specimens from the lip show a marked cellular stroma reaction around the enlarged mucosal glands, which contain masses of leukocytes, scaled-off epithelial cells, and bacteria, particularly in the intralobular ductal

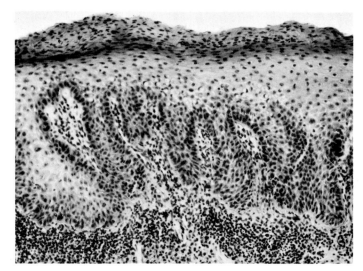

Figure 21–21 Histologic view of "cheilitis abrasiva praecancerosa," showing atypical rete ridges of the epithelium with cellular infiltration of the underlying tunica propria.

segments. Some acinous lobules as well as small ductal cysts with congested mucous and cell detritus may be destroyed. The surface erosions and flat ulcers are coated by an exudate and surrounded by acanthotic epithelium. In more chronic stages mononuclear cells, primarily lymphocytes and plasma cells, predominate in

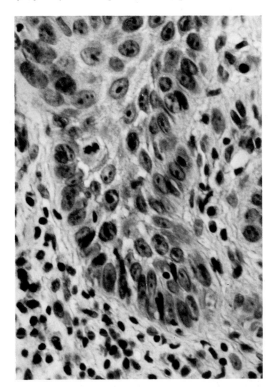

Figure 21–22 Atypical structure of small epithelial ridge in a patient with precancerous "cheilitis." × *360*. The basal layer of the epithelium shows closely packed and irregularly ordered cells with enlarged or polymorphous nuclei or both.

the infiltration of the periglandular connective tissue.

"Cheilitis actinica (exfoliativa)" is another chronic inflammatory condition of the lower lip which has been observed mainly among inhabitants of the eastern Mediterranean countries (Katzenellenbogen, 1939; Marchionini and Tor, 1939), southeastern Europe (Nicolau and Balus, 1964), and California (Ayres, 1923). Marchionini and Tor (1939), describing the condition as "Anatolian summer cheilitis," emphasized the complexity of etiologic factors, such as outdoor occupation under prolonged sunshine in a very dry, dusty, and warm climate. Apparently the etiology also may be influenced by racial and other endogenous conditions. Furthermore, local reaction to photosensitizing food ingredients or drugs may be of importance in some cases. There is a question whether a deficiency of the B-group vitamins plays an etiologic role. It should be noted that pellagra, as a well-defined nosologic entity caused by a diet lacking amino-nicotinic acid, presents other dermal as well as general symptoms.

Manganotti's "abrasive cheilitis" (Manganotti, 1934; Schuermann et al., 1966) is a peculiar type of cheilopathy which shows more distinct clinical as well as histologic features of a premalignant condition than both types of cheilitis mentioned previously. Apparently the disease has a higher incidence rate in Mediterranean than in other European countries. In my dermatologic practice in recent years, I observed it in only about 1 in 2000 patients. Males in their middle or senior years are most commonly affected.

Clinically, irregular erosions and small flat ulcers alternate with fissures, cicatrizing or atrophic spots, and leukoplakic areas on the vermilion of the lower lip, usually originating from the midline area and spreading laterally. The erosive or "abrasive" condition may persist for years and tends to become resistant to almost all topical treatment by anti-inflammatory ointments. On palpation, the surface of the lip is only slightly infiltrated and the deeper structures are of normal consistency. Nevertheless, from its beginning the lesion is a *real precancerosis* which may change into carcinoma after years or only months. Progress to extensive ulceration is a striking clinical indication of initial malignant transformation.

The histologic features of Manganotti's abrasive precancerous cheilitis are characterized by marked parakeratosis and hyperkeratosis with irregular proliferation of the epithelial rete ridges forming pegs of varying shapes. In the early stage the epithelial cells remain well differentiated, whereas in more advanced stages, the lower strata of the epithelium are replaced by irregularly and closely arranged cells showing atypia with dyskaryosis, changes in cellular orientation, increased nuclear:cytoplasmic ratio, and some abnormal mitoses. The underlying connective tissue is infiltrated by leukocytes and mononuclear cells with increased vascularity.

Clinical diagnosis of Manganotti's precancerous lesion can be supported by in vivo staining with toluidine blue according to Wang et al. (1973). By this simple method the premalignant areas can be demonstrated as clear-cut dark blue plaques which attract the dye much more than the benign epithelium. The staining may facilitate recognition of precancerous areas during surgical removal.

For treatment, careful excision of all precancerous areas in a wedge-shaped form gives good results from an esthetic as well as a functional viewpoint. Nevertheless, relapses occur after incomplete removal, or if the etiologic conditions continue. Such factors may be broad exposure to sun without light protection, and habitual smoking of a pipe or cigarettes with repeated pulling away of the cigarette paper from the lip area where it sticks. Radiotherapy in any form is contraindicated, as it may produce another long-acting alteration of the lip afterward. All patients have to be urged to protect their lips from drying and peeling by fatty pomades containing ultraviolet-absorbing substahces.

Prognosis of all chronic noneczematous conditions of the lower lip has to be cautious. There is only poor information about the incidence of malignant transformation. In the series of cheilitis glandularis reported by Touraine et al. (1935 and 1936), 5 out of 40 patients subsequently developed lip carcinomas. In Argentina and other South American countries the rate of malignant transformation of this type of chronic cheilitis is regarded to be higher than in European countries, exceeding 30 per cent of cases (Ambrosetti, 1953; Schuermann et al., 1966).

In seasonally occurring actinic cheilitis, as in the Anatolian variety, there is a lesser potential for carcinoma. Manganotti's type of cheilitis presents suspicious histologic criteria of premalignancy and frequently changes into carcinoma later on. (See also Chapter 25.)

CARCINOMA OF THE TONGUE

Next to the lower lip the tongue is the most common site of oral cancer, exceeding or closely approximating the total incidence of all other intraoral primary sites combined (Tiecke and Bernier, 1954). In contrast to lip carcinoma the prognosis for cancer of the tongue, including all stages, is rather poor. Early diagnosis is imperative for amelioration of the overall five-year cure rate, which is only about 30 percent (Clinical Staging System, 1967; Clinical Oncology, 1973; Dargent et al., 1959; Flamant et al., 1964; Frazell and Lucas, 1962; Montana et al., 1969; Sharp, 1948; Sharp et al., 1956; U.S. Public Health Service, 1964; Waldron, 1970).

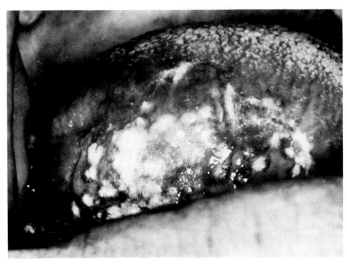

Figure 21-23 Carcinoma of the tongue, resembling "speckled" leukoplakia interspersed among small, flat ulcers with coarse ground. Contrary to the clinical appearance of precancerosis, on palpation the deeper structures of the tongue feel widely infiltrated by invading cancer.

In most countries tongue cancer occurs predominantly in men, with a male:female ratio of more than 10:1. According to Waldron (1970), in the United States the sex ratio is only 4:1 at present, and in the Scandinavian countries there is also a trend toward some lowering of this ratio, probably caused by the higher prevalence of Plummer-Vinson's syndrome in these regions (Pindborg, 1968). In a larger series of tongue cancer reported by Martin et al. in 1940, 87 percent of the patients were males. After 22 years, in a renewed extensive series of 1554 cases from the same institution, the percentage of males had changed to 78 (Frazell and Lucas, 1962). The authors speculate that the clear, though moderate, increase in tongue cancer in women may be due to their increased use of tobacco and alcohol. Such variations according to country, however, only modify the striking predominance in men, which is, however, contrary to the physician's experience that it is chiefly women who seek attention for harmless lesions of the tongue and are anxious about cancer. Most patients with real carcinoma, indeed, ignore the early symptoms and often delay in consulting the doctor.

Carcinoma of the tongue occurs mainly in late middle-aged and elderly persons (Flamant et al., 1964; Sharp, 1948; U.S. Public Health Service, 1964; Waldron, 1970). In the extended series of Frazell and Lucas (1962), four-fifths of the patients were in the sixth to eighth decades. Young persons are rarely affected by tongue cancer.

In about 75 percent of cases the car-

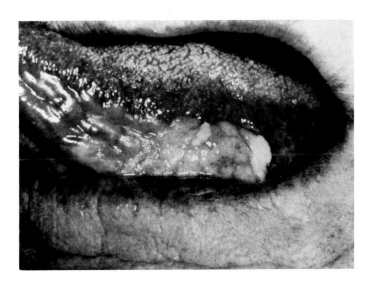

Figure 21-24 Carcinoma of the tongue which had developed from Bowen's disease in a 69 year old woman. Cauliflower-like appearance of the tumor surface. The adjacent ventrolateral mucosa of the tongue shows atrophic epithelium and patchy leukoplakia.

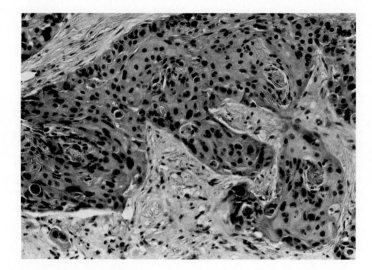

Figure 21–25 Bowen's carcinoma with pronounced dysplasia of the tumor cells, showing dyskeratosis, hyperchromatic and polymorphous nuclei, and loss of polarization of the basal cell layers.

cinoma arises from the anterior two-thirds of the tongue. The primary sites of origin most commonly are the lateral borders, whereas the dorsal surface, tip, and ventral areas are involved less frequently. In the remainder of cases the carcinoma develops from the posterior third of the tongue, which is, on the other hand, the prevailing site of sarcoma or malignant lymphoma (Schuermann et al., 1966; Sharp et al., 1956; Waldron, 1970). Squamous cell carcinoma accounts for at least 90 to 95 percent of all lingual malignant lesions and for 97 percent in the recent report of the International Union Against Cancer (Clinical Oncology, 1973).

The early appearance of tongue cancer may be as a hard nodule, ulcer, deep fissure, papillary or verrucous outgrowth, indurated patch, or leukoplakia. At this initial stage, patients only rarely complain of local ache or discomfort. Dysphagia or pain, often simulating sore throat, is the most important subjective symptom of a growing tumor, particularly when the basal region of the tongue is involved or the lingual or glossopharyngeal nerve becomes affected. *The minimal trouble caused by incipient lingual carcinoma and the lack of prominent clinical symptoms stresses the importance of careful inspection and palpation in each examination of the tongue.*

Further evolution of lingual cancer is characterized by an infiltrating or exophytic pattern of growth. In advanced stages of invasive carcinoma the tongue becomes

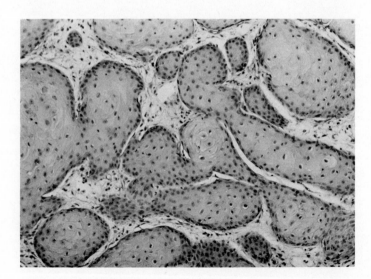

Figure 21–26 Squamous cell carcinoma of low-grade malignancy, showing clusters of rather well-differentiated epithelial cells infiltrating the edematous stroma.

difficult to move because of involvement of its musculature as well as fixation to the surrounding structures. This complication especially applies to carcinomas originating from the posterior lingual region.

There is a *high incidence of spread to regional lymph nodes* in all carcinomas of the tongue. Some patients complain of a feeling of a lump at the side of the neck or in the throat as the first symptom. In the series of Frazell and Lucas (1962), 40 percent of patients presented lymph node involvement on admission, and in about one-fifth of this group bilateral nodes were involved. Nevertheless, the absence of palpable adenopathy does not preclude the possibility of metastases that may have already developed in another region, such as the lung by spread along the bronchial tree (Schuermann et al., 1966). As a rule, however, carcinomas of the anterior two-thirds of the tongue metastasize into the deep middle and upper cervical node groups. The submandibular or submental lymph nodes less frequently become involved. As the lymphatics of the posterior third of the tongue drain into the upper deep cervical nodes and commonly cross into the opposite side as well, metastases of carcinomas localized at the posterior lingual region usually spread by this route. Unfortunately, tumors of the poorly visible base of the tongue only rarely are detected in an early stage. Distant blood-borne metastases are unusual.

The prognosis of lingual carcinoma has to be considered as serious. In the recent report of the U.I.C.C. (Clinical Oncology, 1973), the absolute rate of five-year survival was 26.9 percent, whereas in stage I or II, this rate improves to 53 percent. In the United States Public Health Service Report on the end results in cancer published in 1964, the five-year survival rate in 837 patients with lingual carcinoma of all stages was 30 percent in men and 44 percent in women subjected to treatment between 1950 and 1954.

Factors of importance in prognosis are the site of origin of the tumor (anterior is better than posterior), the size as well as the stage of the primary lesion, and the degree of metastasis. Of 904 cases reviewed by Flamant et al. (1964), late survival ranged from 57 percent in patients with cancer less than 2 cm. in diameter at the tip of the tongue to 3 percent in patients with fixed tumors at the base. In the series of Frazell and Lucas (1962), 45.8 percent of patients with carcinomas of the anterior third of the tongue survived five years, whereas of those with malignant lesions on the posterior third, only 20.7 percent did so. The presence or absence of metastases apparently is of greater prognostic significance than the histologic degree of malignancy (Waldron, 1970).

A particular set of nosologic conditions bearing on the etiology of lingual cancer are the chronic and cicatrizing forms of glossitis, primarily the chronic interstitial glossitis which mainly affects men during the third stage of syphilis. A positive complement-binding serum reaction in some cases of lingual cancer may be due to prolonged syphilis with insidious interstitial glossitis causing malignant epidermoid transformation. Of 108 patients with carcinoma of the tongue recorded by Wynder et al. (1957), 18.5 percent had positive serologic tests for syphilis. Vogler et al. (1962) and Keller (1963), on the other hand, tend to discount the prevailing significance of syphilis in the etiology of lingual cancer.

In rare cases of chronic erosive lichen ruber of the buccal and lingual mucosa and of other long-standing pemphigoid lesions or hereditary epitheliolytic conditions of the oral cavity, such as epidermolysis bullosa dystrophicans (of Hallopeau-Siemens), prolonged inflammatory irritation of the lingual epithelium may dispose to its cancerous transformation (Koberg et al., 1965; Schuermann et al., 1966). In a peculiar case of "glossitis granulomatosa" as a variety of Melkersson-Rosenthal syndrome, I observed the development of cancer in the anterior lateral part of the tongue after persistence of an inflammatory macroglossia for more than 20 years (Hornstein, 1965).

Wynder et al. (1957) noted liver cirrhosis as a pathologic condition associated with lingual carcinoma in 44.4 percent of their cases, mostly heavy drinkers or smokers. Trieger et al. (1958 and 1959) drew attention to a remarkably poorer survival rate in cancer of the tongue in patients suffering from liver cirrhosis than in those without evidence of hepatopathy. Alcoholism or deficiency of iron or vitamins may appear to be intrinsic factors in lingual as well as other oral cancers (Ahlbom, 1936; Jacobsson, 1948; Keller, 1967; Wynder et al., 1957; Wynder and Fryer, 1958). Occasionally traumatic irritation from carious teeth or sharp-edged stumps may also play a part in inducing cancer at the lateral lingual border. Habitual consumption of tobacco by pipe smoking or quid chewing has to be regarded as an etiologic factor of importance (Clinical Oncology, 1973; Frazell and Lucas, 1962; Gibbel et al., 1949; Moore, 1964; Sharp et al., 1956; Trieger et al., 1958; U.S. Public Health Service, 1964; Waldron, 1970).

The choice of treatment depends on the factors mentioned above with regard to prognosis. If possible, wide excision of the primary malignant lesion with surrounding tissue is mandatory. In advanced stages, most of the tongue has to be resected. In each case of obvious, or even suspected, involvement of the lymph nodes, radical unilateral or bilateral block dissection is necessary.

Radiotherapy by high-energy external irradiation or by local application of radium needles should be restricted to cases beyond surgical help, or in general most tumors of the posterior third of the tongue. As carcinomas of this region usually are in a more anaplastic histologic grade than those of other lingual areas, their immediate response to radiotherapy may be good (Jacobsson, 1948). Unfortunately, very often they recur and become resistant to radiation therapy.

CARCINOMAS OF OTHER SITES OF THE ORAL CAVITY

Cancer of the floor of the mouth comes next in frequency after lingual cancer. It also occurs mainly in males with an incidence peak in the sixth and seventh decades. As Leffall and White reported (1965), the floor of the mouth is the most common intraoral site of carcinoma in Negroes.

The early clinical symptoms of cancer are usually minimal, and the primary picture of the tumor may be that of a harmless leukoplakic or erythroplakic condition without discomfort or pain. As the lesion may be felt by the tip of the tongue it will not pass unnoticed for long. Subsequently an ulceration with irregularly shaped margins and marked induration arises. Since the ulcerated tumor also infiltrates the deeper structures of the floor of the mouth, it often becomes painful and infected. In this stage it may be difficult to differentiate clinically an inflammatory enlargement of the submandibular lymph nodes from involvement by tumor metastases. Since the majority of carcinomas originate from the anterior area of the floor of the mouth near the midline, bilateral metastasis occurs in many cases (Montana et al., 1969). Though the spread to the regional nodes is somewhat delayed in comparison to the early metastatic spread of lingual cancer (Waldron, 1970), in about 25 to 40 percent of cases tumor involvement of nodes is present on examination (Erich and Kragh, 1959b).

In differential diagnosis, cystic enlargement of the duct of the sublingual salivary gland following calculus obstruction (so-called "ranula") and sublingual sialadenitis should be excluded. Tumors of the major or minor submandibular (submucosal) gland may also resemble advanced stages of carcinoma when they secondarily destroy the adjacent mucosa.

In early cancer of the floor of the mouth, irradiation may be as successful as surgical excision. In advanced stages, on the other hand, or when the regional lymph nodes undoubtedly are involved by metastases, radical excision with hemimandibulectomy and block dissection of the neck nodes yields the best results (Clinical Oncology, 1973; Erich and Kragh, 1959b). The five-year survival rate of about 70 percent of perfectly treated early carcinomas without lymph node involvement decreases to about 35 percent in advanced stages with metastases (Clinical Oncology, 1973).

Cancer of the alveolar mucosa occurs less commonly than that of the lower lip, tongue, or floor of the mouth. Nevertheless, its early recognition by dentists or stomatologists is extremely important because of the high risk of diagnostic confusion with other benign inflammatory or hyperplastic lesions occurring so frequently in the gingiva and alveolar ridge

(Duckworth, 1961; Erich and Kragh, 1959a; Schreiber and Waldron, 1958). Elderly male patients are most often affected, but the marked prevalence of males in most western countries changes to an approximately even sex ratio in some southern regions of the United States (Brown et al., 1965; Rosenfeld and Callaway, 1963).

As a rule, the tumor arises more often from the mandibular alveolar mucosa than from the maxillary (Cady and Catlin, 1969). Furthermore, carcinomas mainly occur in edentulous areas, while those developing from the gingiva account for only a minority of cases (Erich and Kragh, 1959a). The early lesion may show clinical features similar to those of other intraoral cancers. When the carcinoma arises like a verrucous or nodular outgrowth, it may be misdiagnosed as virus papilloma or common fissurated epulis. When it develops in close contact with an ill-fitting denture, it may be mistaken for a harmless traumatic leukoplakia or ulcer. It should be emphasized once more that, in each case of poorly healing ulcer or papillary lesion of the mucosa, particularly when it appears in a leukoplakic area, a biopsy for histologic evaluation of the lesion is mandatory. Cytologic screening (Sandler, 1962) or in vivo staining of the suspicious area by toluidine blue (Shedd et al., 1967) may be helpful in detecting early cancer but does not equal the diagnostic accuracy of histologic examination.

Invasion of adjacent bone is typical of many alveolar carcinomas and may be found in about 50 percent of all cases. In the literature there are some differences in the incidence rate of metastasis to lymph nodes, ranging from 9 to 30 percent (Erich and Kragh, 1959a). This variation may be due to some degree to a high error rate when the clinical estimation of metastatic node involvement is not verified by histology.

For the therapy of cancer of the alveolar mucosa, readers are referred to textbooks of dentistry and oral surgery.

Cancer of the buccal mucosa shows considerable variation in incidence in different regions of the world. Carcinomas of the mucosal surface of the cheek (including postcommissural lesions) in Southeast Asia

account for more than 20 percent of all oral cancers (in southern India, as high as 50 percent: Clinical Oncology, 1973; Singh and von Essen, 1966), whereas in most western countries the incidence fluctuates around 10 percent or less (Bhansali, 1961). Men beyond their fifties are usually affected (Muir and Kirk, 1960; Pindborg, 1963 and 1965a; Singh and von Essen, 1966), but in India and in some parts of the United States (Brown, et al., 1965), buccal carcinomas are as often observed in women as in men. This striking change of the usual predominance of males may be due to the popularity of taking snuff by mouth among rural women of some southeastern regions of the United States, on the one hand, and by habitual chewing of betel in the Indian population (Pindborg, 1963 and 1965a; Pindborg et al., 1965, 1966, and 1967a; Singh and von Essen, 1966; Wahi et al., 1965). It should be mentioned that these customs coincide with those noted as important for the development of oral verrucous carcinoma. Apparently the composition of snuff as well as of betel quid varies from region to region. In extensive ethnographic and epidemiologic studies of the Indian population (Hirayama, 1966; Pindborg et al., 1965, 1966 and 1967a; Wahi et al., 1965), it was clearly demonstrated that chewing pure betel nut or leaves is not enough to stimulate malignant growth of the buccal mucosa. Only when the quid is habitually blended with tobacco and other irritating ingredients may the epithelium undergo malignant transformation. It has also been shown that the habitual placement of the quid influences the location of the consequent carcinoma. As Indian people prefer to keep the quid in the lower buccal sulcus, in many cases even while they sleep, the risk of cancer of the chronically irritated epithelium is very high compared with the relatively rare incidence of cancer of the floor of the mouth in India (Hirayama, 1966). It should be noted that chronic submucous fibrosis (Pindborg, 1965b; Pindborg and Sirsat, 1966; Pindborg et al., 1967b) very often precedes malignant transformation of the adjacent superficial epithelium.

The clinical evolution of carcinoma of the buccal mucosa may show some patterns of growth. In many cases the primary lesion resembles the speckled type of leukoplakia (Pindborg et al., 1963) interspersed with erythroplakic patches or enlarged leukoplakic areas, which may vary as to the thickness of keratinization (demonstrated by the intensity of the whitish color) and the surface pattern. In other cases an extending ulceration with invasion of the surrounding tissue is the predominant clinical feature, whereas the type of exophytic verrucous growth which is also known as "Ackerman's carcinoma" or verrucous carcinoma occurs less frequently (Bhansali, 1961; O'Brien and Catlin, 1965; Shedd et al., 1968).

Therapy depends on the clinicopathologic assessment, as well as on the actual stage of the tumor. Early carcinomas should be widely removed by excision, whereas radiotherapy, if a clear-cut indication is given, achieves results approximately as good as those of surgical treatment. However, in carcinomas of the Ackerman type irradiation has to be omitted, as it may produce local complications leading to an unfavorable clinical course, including stimulation of metastatic spread when the tumor recurs (Perez et al., 1966).

Cancer of the palate most often arises from the posterior part. In the hard palate, tumors of the small mucous glands are predominant. Nevertheless, in some parts of the world, particularly in southern India, the Philippines, and some islands or countries around the Caribbean Sea, epidermoid cancer arising from the hard palate is well known and is in contrast to the relative rarity of squamous cell cancer of this site elsewhere. The reason is the habit of "reverse smoking" cigars or cigarettes with the burning end inside the mouth (Pindborg, 1968; Quigley et al., 1964; Reddy and Rao, 1957; Schoenfeld and Holzberger, 1964). In an Indian district where this strange practice is very popular (Reddy and Rao, 1957), palatal cancer comprised 45 percent of all oral cancers.

The clinical picture and evolution of palatal carcinomas depend on the primary site of origin. Cancers arising from the hard palate may destroy the underlying bone and penetrate into the maxillary sinuses or perforate the nasal floor (Sharp et al., 1956; Waldron, 1970). In the early

stages of cancer, however, difficulty in wearing a denture may be the first symptom prior to local pain, leading to the false assumption of a decubital ulcer. Carcinomas arising from the soft palate usually invade the anterior faucial pillars and the pterygoid fossa, so that disturbances of swallowing, severe pharyngeal pain, and trismus become clinically prominent. Regional metastasis involves the upper deep cervical or submandibular lymph nodes, rarely the retropharyngeal nodes (Clinical Oncology, 1973; Tiecke and Bernier, 1954; Waldron, 1970).

Radical excision combined with surgical or prosthetic reconstruction of the palate, if necessary, is regarded by most authorities as giving better results than irradiation (Clinical Oncology, 1973). The late prognosis of the tumor is influenced not only by its anatomic location and clinical stage but also by its histogenesis and histologic grade of malignancy. Adenocarcinomas originating from the small palatal mucous glands have a somewhat better survival rate than epidermoid carcinomas of the mucosal epithelium (Brown et al., 1965; Clinical Oncology, 1973).

Concluding this chapter as a whole, I want to stress the responsibility of every physician, be he a stomatologist, dermatologist, or general practitioner, to make an effort at correct diagnosis of every leukoplakic disorder of the oral cavity, and to leave nothing undone to obtain full information on it by experts in oral pathology, for in the incipient stages of malignant lesions their true nature may be disguised by a harmless-appearing leukoplakic condition. The earlier an exact diagnosis is obtained, the more can be expected in improvement of the end results. It may justify the challenge of the above postulate

TABLE 21–2

Anatomic Site	Absolute Five-Year Survival	Stage I or II Five-Year Survival
Lip	67.7%	85.2%
Tongue	26.9%	53.0%
Floor of mouth	33.7%	59.5%
Buccal mucosa	37.0%	60.6%
Gingiva	33.9%	62.7%
Palate	26.7%	46.6%

to point to the most recent study of the U.I.C.C., which comprises worldwide inquires on the prognosis of malignant tumors in terms of five-year survival according to the anatomic sites. The data from this report are cited in Table 21–2.

REFERENCES

Ackerman, L. V.: Verrucous carcinoma of the oral cavity. Surgery, 23:670, 1948.

Ackerman, L. V., and Johnson, R.: Present day concepts of intraoral histopathology. *In* Proceedings of the Second National Cancer. New York, American Cancer Society, Inc., 1954, pp. 403–414.

Ackerman, L. V., and McGavran, M. H.: Proliferating benign and malignant epithelial lesions of the oral cavity. J. Oral Surg., 16:400, 1958.

Ackerman, L. V., and Del Regato, J. A.: Cancer: Diagnosis, Treatment and Prognosis. Ed. 3, St. Louis, C. V. Mosby Company, 1962, pp. 82, 260, 314.

Ahlbom, H. E.: Simple achlorhydric anemia, Plummer-Vinson syndrome and carcinoma of the mouth, pharynx and esophagus in women. Br. Med. J., 2:331, 1936.

Altmann, F., Basek, M., and Stout, A. P.: Papilloma of the larynx with intraepithelial anaplastic changes. Arch. Otolaryngol. (Chicago), 62:478, 1955.

Ambrosetti, F. E.: Queilitis glandular simple. Enfermedad de Puente y Acevedo. Arch. Argent. Dermatol., 3:543, 1953.

Anderson, D. L.: Significance of surface size of intraoral carcinoma. J. Can. Dent. Assoc., 32:212, 1966.

Archard, H. O., et al.: Leukoedema of the human mucosa. Oral Surg., 25:717, 1968.

Ash, C. L.: Oral cancer, a twenty-five year study. Am. J. Roentgenol., 87:417, 1962.

Ashley, F. L., et al.: Carcinoma of the lip: A comparison of five-year results after irradiation and surgical therapy. Am. J. Surg., 110:549, 1965.

Ayres, S.: Chronic actinic cheilitis. J.A.M.A., 81:1183, 1923.

Balantyne, A. J., et al.: The extension of cancer of the head and neck through peripheral nerves. Am. J. Surg., 106:651, 1963.

Barnett, J. G., and Hyman, A. B.: Oral florid verrucosis. Arch. Dermatol., 97:479, 1968.

Belisario, J. C.: Cancer of the Skin. London, Butterworth's, 1959.

Bernier, J. L., and Clark, M. L.: Squamous cell carcinomas of the lip. Milit. Surg., 109:379, 1951.

Bhansali, S. K.: Malignant tumours of the buccal cavity: A clinical analysis of 970 cases. Clin. Radiol., 12:299, 1961.

Broders, A. C.: Carcinomas of the mouth: Types and degrees of malignancy. Am. J. Roentgenol., 17:90, 1927.

Brown, R. L., Suh, J. M., Scarborough, J. E., Wilkins, S. A., and Smith, R. R.: Snuff dipper's intraoral cancer: Clinical characteristics and response to therapy. Cancer, 18:2, 1965.

Cady, B., and Catlin, D.: Epidermoid carcinoma of the gum. Cancer, 23:551, 1969.

Capman, I., and Redish, C. H.: Tobacco-induced epithelial proliferation in human subject. Arch. Pathol., 70:133, 1960.

Clinical Oncology. Ed. by Committee on Professional Education of U.I.C.C. (International Union Against Cancer). Berlin, Springer-Verlag, 1973.

Clinical Staging System for Carcinoma of the Oral Cavity. American Joint Committee for Cancer Staging and End Results Reporting, Chicago, 1967.

Cooke, B. E. D.: Leukoplakia buccalis and oral epithelial naevi. A clinical and histological study. Br. J. Dermatol., 68:151, 1956.

Cooke, B. E. D., and Morgan, J.: Oral epithelial naevi. Br. J. Dermatol., 71:134, 1959.

Cooke, R. A.: Verrucous carcinoma of the oral mucosa in Papua-New Guinea. Cancer, 24:397, 1969.

Cross, J. A., et al.: Carcinoma of the lip. Surg. Gynecol. Obstet., 87:153, 1948.

Dargent, M., Mayer, M., and Bertoin, P.: Le cancer de la langue. Étude d'ensemble. Principes thérapeutiques. Ann. Chir., 13:135, 1959.

Darling, A. I., and Fletcher, J. P.: Familial white folded gingivostomatosis. Oral Surg., 11:296, 1958.

Duckworth, R.: Verrucous carcinoma presenting as mandibular osteomyelitis. Br. J. Surg., 49:332, 1961.

Einhorn, J., and Wersäll, J.: Incidence of oral carcinoma in patients with leukoplakia of the oral mucosa. Cancer, 20:2189, 1967.

Erich, J. B., and Kragh, L. V.: Results of treatment of squamous cell carcinoma arising in mandibular gingiva. Arch. Surg. (Chicago), 79:100, 1959a.

Erich, J. B., and Kragh, L. V.: Treatment of squamous cell carcinoma of the floor of the mouth. Arch. Surg. (Chicago), 79:94, 1959b.

Everett, F. G., and Holder, T. D.: Cheilitis glandularis apostematosa. Oral Surg., 8:405, 1955.

Fasske, E., and Themann, H.: Über das Deckepithel der menschlichen Mundschleimhaut. Licht- und elektronenmikroskopische Untersuchungen. Z. Zellforsch., 49:447, 1959.

Fasske, E., and Morgenroth, K.: Pathologische Histologie der Mundhöhle. Hirzel, Leipzig, 1964.

Fasske, E., Hahn, W., Morgenroth, K., and Themann, H.: Die formale und kausale Genese der Leukoplakia oris. Z. Haut. Geschlechtskr. 26:339, 1959.

Flamant, R., Hayem, M., Lazar, P., and Denoix, P.: Cancer of the tongue. A study of 904 cases. Cancer, 17:377, 1964.

Fonts, E., et al.: Verrucous squamous cell carcinoma of the oral cavity. Cancer, 23:152, 1969.

Forlen, H. F., Hornstein, O. P., and Stüttgen, G.: Betelkauen und Leukoplakie. Arch. Klin. Exp. Dermatol., 221:463, 1965.

Frazell, E. L., and Lucas, J. C., Jr.: Cancer of the tongue. Cancer, 15:1085, 1962.

Gardner, A. F.: The cytologic diagnosis of oral carcinoma: A review of the literature. J. Calif. Dent. Assoc., 40:9, 1964.

Gardner, A. F.: An investigation of 890 instances of oral malignancies: Incidence, etiology, prognosis and relationship to oral exfoliative cytology. Acta Cytol. (Baltimore), 9:273, 1965.

Gardner, A. F.: Pathology in Dentistry. Oral Manifestations of Systemic Diseases. Springfield, Ill., Charles C Thomas, Publisher, 1968, pp. 176–183.

Gibbel, M. J., Cross, H. M., and Ariel, J. M.: Cancer

of the tongue. A review of 330 cases. Cancer, 2:411, 1949.

Goethals, P. L., et al.: Verrucous squamous carcinoma of the oral cavity. Am. J. Surg., 106:845, 1963.

Goldman, H. M., and Grady, H. G.: Case reports from the Army Institute of Pathology. Am. J. Orthod. Oral Surg., 31:189, 1945.

Gorlin, R. J.: Bowen's disease of mucous membrane of the mouth: Review of literature and presentation of cases. Oral Surg., 3:43, 1950.

Gorlin, R. J., and Pindborg, J. J.: Syndromes of the Head and Neck. New York, McGraw-Hill Book Co., 1964.

Greene, G. V., Jr., and Bernier, J. L.: Spindle cell squamous carcinoma of the lip. Oral Surg., 12:1008, 1959.

Greither, A.: Keratotische Zustände und Krankheiten der Mundschleimhaut. Fortschr. Prakt. Dermat. Vener., 5:71, 1965.

Hirayama, T.: An epidemiological study of oral and pharyngeal cancer in Central and South-East Asia. Bull. W.H.O., 34:41, 1966.

Hornstein, O. P.: Plattenepithelkrebs auf Glossitis granulomatosa. Ein Beitrag zu deren Spätprognose. Hautarzt, 16:90, 1965.

Hornstein, O. P., and Pape, H.-D.: Morbus Bowen der Mundschleimhaut. Dermatologica, 131:325, 1965.

Hudelo, L., and Cailliau: La maladie de Bowen des muqueuses envisagée comme cancer d'emblée. Ann. Dermatol. Syphiligr. (Paris), 7:813, 1933.

Jacobsson, F.: Carcinoma of the tongue: Clinical study of 277 cases treated at Radiumhemmet, 1931–1942. Acta Radiol. (Stockh.), 68 (Suppl.): 1, 1948.

Judd, E. S., and Beahrs, O. H.: Epithelioma of the lower lip. Arch. Surg. (Chicago), 59:422, 1949.

Kaminsky, A. R., Kaminsky, C. A., Abulafia, J., and Kaminsky, A.: Papilomatosis florida oral: Su Tratamiento con Methotrexate. G. Ital. Dermatol., 107:821, 1966.

Kanee, B.: Oral florid papillomatosis complicated by verrucous squamous carcinoma. Arch. Dermatol., 99:196, 1969.

Katzenellenbogen, J.: Cheilitis exfoliativa actinica. Acta Derm. Venereol. (Stockh.), 18:319, 1939.

Keen, R. R., and Elzay, R. P.: Basal cell carcinoma from mucosal surface of lower lip: Report of case. J. Oral Surg., 22:453, 1964.

Keller, A. Z.: Epidemiology of lip, oral and pharyngeal cancer and association with selected systemic diseases. Am. J. Public Health, 53:1214, 1963.

Keller, A. Z.: Cirrhosis of the liver, alcoholism and heavy smoking associated with cancer of the mouth and pharynx. Cancer, 20:1015, 1967.

Knossew, L. S.: Papillomatous granulomatosis (florid oral papillomatosis). Aust. J. Dermatol., 8:173, 1966.

Koberg, W., Schettler, D., and Selle, G.: Zur Frage der Karzinomentstehung auf dem Boden eines Lichen ruber planus der Mundschleimhaut. Münch. Med. Wochenschr., 107:463, 1965.

Krainz, W., and Kumer, L.: Über eine Raucherleukokeratose des Gaumens. Arch. Dermatol., Syph. (Berl.), 168:224, 1933.

Krantz, S., et al.: Results of treatment of carcinoma of lower lip. Am. J. Roentgenol., 78:780, 1957.

Kraus, F. T., and Perez-Mesa, C.: Verrucous carcinoma. Cancer, 19:26, 1966.

Kren, O.: Mundschleimhautaffektionen. Z. Haut. Geschlechtskr., 3:111, 1934.

Lacronique, G., and Dechaume: Maladie de Bowen de la muqueuse buccale. Rev. Stomatol., 34:95, 1932.

Landy, J. J., and White, H. J.: Buccogingival carcinoma in snuff dippers. Am. Surg., 27:442, 1961.

Leffall, L. D., and White, J. E.: Cancer of the oral cavity in Negroes. Surg. Gynecol. Obstet., 120:70, 1965.

Lewis, A. B.: Effects of smoking on the oral mucosa. Oral Surg., 8:1026, 1955.

Lucas, C. M.: Pathology of Tumors of the Oral Tissues. Boston, Little, Brown and Company, 1964, p. 118.

Manganotti, G.: Cheilitis abrasiva praecancerosa. Atti 3. Conv. nat. per la Lotta contro ie Cancro, Roma, 1934, p. 536.

Marchionini, A., and Tor, S.: Zur Klimatophysiologie und -pathologie der Haut. I. Die Sommercheilitis in Zentralanatolien. Arch. Dermatol. Syph. (Berl.), 179:421, 1939.

Martin, H. E., and Stewart, F. W.: Spindle-cell epidermoid carcinoma. Am. J. Cancer, 24:273, 1935.

Martin, H. E., and Sugarbaker, E. L.: Cancer of the floor of the mouth. Surg. Gynecol. Obstet., 71:347, 1940.

Martin, H. E., Munster, H., and Sugarbaker, E.: Cancer of the tongue Arch. Surg. (Chicago), 41:888, 1940.

Martin, H. E., et al.: Cancer of the lip. Ann. Surg., 114:226, 341, 1941.

Mathis, H., and Herrmann, D.: Erythroplasie de Queyrat an der Mundschleimhaut. Osterr. Z. Stomatol., 60:170, 1963.

McCarthy, F. P., and McCarthy, P. L.: Diseases of the mouth. New Engl. J. Med., 250:493, 1954.

Mehta, F. S., et al.: Clinical and histologic study of oral leukoplakia in relation to habits. Oral Surg., 28:372, 1969a.

Mehta, F. S., et al.: Epidemiologic and histologic study of oral cancer and leukoplakia among 50,915 villagers in India. Cancer, 24:832, 1969b.

Moertel, C. G., and Foss, E. L.: Multicentric carcinomas of the oral cavity. Surg. Gynecol. Obstet., 106:652, 1958.

Montana, G. S., et al.: Carcinoma of the tongue and floor of the mouth. Cancer, 22:1284, 1969.

Moore, C.: Smoking and mouth-throat cancer. Am. J. Surg., 108:565, 1964.

Moulonguet, A.: Un cas de maladie de Bowen de la bouche. Ann. Otolaryngol. (Paris), pp. 714–717, 1936.

Muir, C., and Kirk, R.: Betel tobacco and cancer of the mouth. Br. J. Cancer, 14:597, 1960.

Nicolau, S. G., and Balus, L.: Chronic actinic cheilitis and cancer of the lower lip. Br. J. Dermatol., 76:278, 1964.

Niver, F. D., Strong, S., and Goodman, M. L.: Mucoepidermoid carcinoma of buccal mucosa: Report of a case. Oral Surg., 27:1, 1969.

O'Brien, P. H., and Catlin, D.: Cancer of the cheek (mucosa). Cancer, 18:1392, 1965.

Perez, C. A., et al.: Anaplastic transformation in verrucous carcinoma of the oral cavity after radiation therapy. Radiology, 86:108, 1966.

Pindborg, J. J.: Ethnic and environmental aspects of oral cancer. Dent. Progr., 3:70, 1963.

Pindborg, J. J.: Oral cancer from an international point of view. J. Can. Dent. Assoc., 31:219, 1965a.

Pindborg, J. J.: Oral precancerous conditions in South East Asia. Int. Dent., 15:190, 1965b.

Pindborg, J. J.: Atlas of Diseases of the Oral Mucosa. Copenhagen, Munksgaard, 1968.

Pindborg, J. J., and Renstrup, G.: Studies in oral leukoplakias. II. Effect of snuff on oral epithelium. Acta Derm. Venereol. (Stockh.), 43:271, 1963.

Pindborg, J. J., and Sirsat, S. M.: Oral submucous fibrosis. Oral Surg., 22:764, 1966.

Pindborg, J. J., Renstrup, G., Poulsen, H. E., and Silverman, S., Jr.: Studies in oral leukoplakias. V. Clinical and histologic signs of malignancy. Acta Odontol. Scand., 21:407, 1963.

Pindborg, J. J., et al.: Frequency of oral leukoplakia and related conditions among 10,000 Bombayites. J. All-India Dent. Assoc., 37:228, 1965.

Pindborg, J. J., Bhat, M., Devanath, K. R., Narayana, H. R., and Ramachandra, S.: Frequency of oral white lesions among 10,000 individuals in Bangalore, South India. Indian J. Med. Sci., 20:349, 1966.

Pindborg, J. J., Klaer, J., Gupta, P. C., and Chawla, T. N.: Prevalence of leukoplakia among 10,000 persons in Lucknow, India, with special reference to tobacco and betel nut usage. Bull. W.H.O., 37:109, 1967a.

Pindborg, J. J., Poulsen, H. E., and Zachariah, J.: Oral epithelial changes in thirty Indians with oral cancer and submucous fibrosis. Cancer, 20:1141, 1967b.

Pindborg, J. J., et al.: Epidemiology and histology of oral leukoplakia and leukoedema among Papuans and New Guineans. Cancer, 22:379, 1968a.

Pindborg, J. J., Jølst, O., Renstrup, G., and Roed-Petersen, B.: Studies in oral leukoplakia. XII. A preliminary report on the period prevalence of malignant transformation in leukoplakia based on a follow-up study of 248 patients. J. Am. Dent. Assoc., 76:767, 1968b.

Puente, J. J., and Acevedo, A.: Queilitis glandular. Rev. Med. Lat. Am. (Buenos Aires), 12:671, 1927.

Quigley, L. F., Cobb, C. M., Schoenfeld, S., Hunt, E. E., and Williams, P.: Reverse smoking and its oral consequences in Caribbean and South American peoples. J. Am. Dent. Assoc., 69:427, 1964.

Reddy, D. G., and Rao, V. K.: Cancer of the palate in coastal Andhra due to smoking cigars with the burning end inside the mouth. Indian J. Med. Sci., 11:791, 1957.

Reich, H.: Zur Bowenschen Krankheit der Mundschleimhaut. Arch. Dermatol. Syph. (Berl.), 197:145, 1954.

Reich, H., and Bonse, G.: Die Bowensche Krankheit der Mundschleimhaut. Strahlentherapie, 96:415, 1955.

Renstrup, G.: Leukoplakia of the oral cavity. Acta Odontol. Scand., 16:99, 1958.

Renstrup, G.: Studies in oral leukoplakias. IV. Mitotic activity in oral leukoplakias. Acta Odontol. Scand., 21:333, 1963.

Robinson, H. B. G.: Neoplasms and "precancerous" lesions of the oral regions. Dent. Clin. N. Amer., 3:621, 1957.

Rock, J. A., and Fisher, E. R.: Florid papillomatosis of the oral cavity and larynx. Arch. Otolaryngol. (Chicago), 72:593, 1960.

Rosenfeld, L., and Callaway, J.: Snuff dipper's cancer. Am. J. Surg., 106:840, 1963.

Samitz, M. H., and Weinberg, R. A.: Oral florid papillomatosis. Arch. Dermatol., 87:478, 1963.

Samitz, M. H., Ackerman, B. A., and Lantis, L. R.: Squamous cell carcinoma arising at the site of oral florid papillomatosis. Arch. Dermatol., 96:286, 1967.

Sandler, H. C.: Cytological screening for early mouth cancer (Interim report of the Veterans Administration Cooperative Study of oral exfoliative cytology). Cancer, 15:1119, 1962.

Sandstead, H. R., and Lowe, J. W.: Leukoedema and keratosis in relation to leukoplakia of the buccal mucosa in man. J. Natl. Cancer Inst., 14:423, 1953.

Saunders, W. H.: Nicotine stomatitis of the palate. Ann. Otolaryngol. (Paris), 67:618–627, 1958.

Scheicher-Gottron, E.: Papillomatosis mucosae carcinoides der Mundschleimhaut bei gleichzeitigem Vorhandensein eines Lichen ruber der Haut. Z. Haut. Geschlechtskr., 24:99, 1958.

Schoenfeld, S., and Holzberger, P. C.: Palatal leukokeratosis secondary to candela pa Den. A geographic-medical note. Arch. Dermatol., 90:89, 1964.

Schreiber, H. R., and Waldron, C. A.: Carcinoma of the gingiva simulating gingival hyperplasia. J. Periodontol., 29:196, 1958.

Schuermann, H., Greither, A., and Hornstein, O.: Krankheiten der Mundschleimhaut und der Lippen. Ed. 3., München, Urban & Schwarzenberg, 1966, pp. 285–290, 409–416, 435–440, 450–456.

Schwartz, D. L.: Stomatitis nicotina of the palate. Oral Surg., 20:306, 1965.

Schwimmer, E.: Die idiopathischen Schleimhautplaques der Mundhöhle; Leukoplakia buccalis. Vjschr. Dermatol. (Berlin), 9:511, 1877.

Seifert, G.: Die Mundspeicheldrüsen. In Doerr, W., and Ühlinger, E. (eds.): Spez. Pathol. Anat., Vol. I. Berlin, Springer-Verlag, 1966, p. 161.

Shafer, W. G., and Waldron, C. A.: A clinical and histopathologic study of oral leukoplakia. Surg. Gynecol. Obstet., 112:411, 1961.

Sharp, G. S.: Cancer of the oral cavity. Oral Surg., 1:614, 1948.

Shatkins, S.: Verrucous squamous carcinoma of palate. New York Dent. J., 29:106, 1963.

Shear, M., Lemmer, J., and Dockrat, I.: Oral submucous fibrosis in South African Indians. S. Afr. J. Med. Sci., 32:41, 1967.

Shedd, D. P., et al.: In vivo staining property of oral cancer. Arch. Surg. (Chicago), 95:16, 1967.

Shedd, D. P., et al.: Cancer of the buccal mucosa, palate and gingiva in Connecticut. Cancer, 21:440, 1968.

Shklar, G.: The precancerous oral lesion. Oral Surg., 20:58, 1965.

Silverman, S., Jr., and Rozen, R.: Observations on the clinical characteristics and natural history of oral leukoplakia. J. Am. Dent. Assoc., 76:772, 1968.

Singh, A. D., and von Essen, C. F.: Buccal mucosal cancer in South India: Etiologic and clinical aspects. J. Am. Roentgenol., 96:6, 1966.

Sprague, W. G.: A survey of the use of the term "leukoplakia" by oral pathologists. Oral Surg., 16:1067, 1963.

Stecker, R. H., et al.: Verrucous snuff dipper's carcinoma of the oral cavity. J.A.M.A., 189:838, 1964.

Tappeiner, J., and Wolff, K.: Papillomatosis mucosae carcinoides ("oral florid papillomatosis"). Hautarzt, 20:102, 1969.

Tappeiner, S.: Über tabakbedingte Leukokeratosen des Gaumens. Arch. Dermatol. Syph. (Berl.), 181:173, 1941.

Tennekoon, G. E., and Bartlett, G. C.: Effect of betel chewing on the oral mucosa. Br. J. Cancer, 23:39, 1969.

Tiecke, R. W., and Bernier, J. L.: Statistical and morphological analysis of four hundred and one cases of intraoral squamous cell carcinoma. J. Am. Dent. Assoc., 49:684, 1954.

Touraine, A., and Golé, L.: Maladie de Bowen à type leucoplasiforme de la muqueuse jugale, associée à un cancer de la lèvre sur cheilite glandulaire. Bull. Soc. Fr. Dermatol. Syphiligr., 43:740, 1936.

Touraine, A., and Solente, G.: La chéilite glandulaire: sa fréquence, son ancienneté. (Une observation du XVIIe siècle.) Bull. Soc. Fr. Dermatol. Syphiligr., 42:777, 1935.

Trieger, N., et al.: Cirrhosis and other predisposing factors in carcinoma of the tongue. Cancer, 11:357, 1958.

Trieger, N., et al.: Significance of liver dysfunction in mouth cancer. Surg. Gynecol. Obstet., 108:230, 1959.

United States Public Health Service: End Results in Cancer (Report No. 2). Publication No. 1149, 1964.

Vogler, W. R., et al.: A retrospective study of etiological factors in cancer of the mouth, pharynx and larynx. Cancer, 15:246, 1962.

Wahi, P. N., Kehar, U., and Lahiri, B.: Factors influencing oral and oropharyngeal cancers in India. Br. J. Cancer, 19:642, 1965.

Waldron, C. A., and Shafer, W. G.: Current concepts of leukoplakia. Int. Dent. J., 10:350, 1960.

Waldron, C. H.: Oral epithelial tumors. In Gorlin, R. J., and Goldman, H. M. (Eds.): Thoma's Oral Pathology. Ed. 6. St. Louis, C. V. Mosby, Vol. II, pp. 801–860, 1970.

Wang, P., Wang, I., and Hornstein, O. P.: Vitalfärbung mit Toluidinblau als klinische Methode zur Früherkennung von Praecancerosen und Carcinomen der Lippen. Therapiewoche, 23:7647, 1973.

Ward, G. E., and Hendrick, J. W.: Results of treatment of carcinoma of the lip. Surgery, 27:321, 1950.

Wechsler, H. R., and Fisher, E. R.: Oral florid papillomatosis. Clinical, pathological and electron microscopic observations. Arch. Dermatol., 86:480, 1962.

Wendlberger, J.: Die Cheilitis glandularis simplex und ihre Rolle als Vorläufer maligner Entartung. Arch. Dermatol. Syph. (Berl.), 176:76, 1938.

Williamson, J. J.: Erythroplasia of Queyrat of the buccal mucous membrane. Oral Surg., 17:308, 1964.

Wise, F.: Cheilitis glandularis apostematosa. Arch. Dermatol., 23:816, 1931.

Wookey, H., et al.: Treatment of oral cancer by combination of radiotherapy and surgery. Ann. Surg., 134:529, 1951.

Wynder, E. L., Bross, I. J., and Feldman, R. M.: A study of the etiological factors in cancer of the mouth. Cancer, 10:1300, 1957.

Wynder, E. L., and Fryer, J. H.: Etiologic consideration of the Plummer-Vinson (Paterson-Kelly) syndrome. Ann. Intern. Med., 49:1106, 1958.

22

Cutaneous Horns

Robert S. Bart, M.D.

INTRODUCTION

At the outset, it must be stressed that "cutaneous horn" is a clinical description like "papule" or "nodule"; it is the microscopic picture of what is at the base which is most important. However, as with a papule or nodule a correct estimate of the histologic picture can frequently be made on the basis of a careful clinical inspection of the lesion and the patient as a whole.

DEFINITION

The term "cutaneous horn" (cornu cutaneum) has been used to describe those markedly hyperkeratotic growths arising from the skin which in shape and hardness resemble the horns of animals (Moncorps, 1931). Until recent years this designation was most often applied to very large, sometimes astounding, horny excrescences. Such types have been illustrated by several authors (Gould and Pyle, 1896; Charache, 1935; Smialowski and Currie, 1960; Batschwarov and Profirov, 1964; Semins and Null, 1969). Today the tendency is to apply the name "cutaneous horn" in a less restrictive way (Lennox and Sayed, 1964; Mehregan, 1965; Bart et al., 1968a), to describe a *markedly hyperkeratotic growth, re-gardless of size, in which the bulk or major part of the growth is made up of more or less compact keratinous material, approximately conical or cylindrical in form* (Fig. 22–1).

Definitions which stress the criterion of resemblance to animal horns are verbally and imaginatively attractive, but they are too restrictive clinically and tend to limit the diagnosis to the rare, large lesions. Extreme "horns" are not often encountered in practice, especially not in areas of the world where medical attention is sought early. This chapter concerns itself with

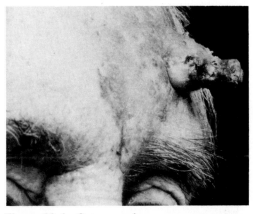

Figure 22–1 Cutaneous horn upon a squamous cell carcinoma. Note evidence of actinic damage in the surrounding skin. The patient was 68 years old and had blue eyes. (Courtesy of Skin and Cancer Unit, New York University.)

TABLE 22–1 CUTANEOUS HORNS: LOCATIONS AND HISTOPATHOLOGY*

Location	Number (37)	Seborrheic Keratosis† (14)	Benign Hyperplastic Epithelium (6)	Angioma (1)	Actinic Keratosis (8) and Early Squamous Cell Carcinoma (6) (14)	Frank Squamous Cell Carcinoma (2)
Scalp	1					1
Face	14	9	2		3	
Ear lobe	2	2				
Aural pinna, cartilaginous	5				5	
Nostril	1		1			
Neck	3	1	1		1	
Chest	1		1			
Hand, dorsum	3				2	1
Forearm	1				1	
Thigh	1	1				
Popliteal space	1	1				
Leg	4		1	1	2	

*From Bart et al.: Acta Derm. Venereol. (Stockh.), 48:507, 1968.
†Includes basosquamous papilloma and inverted follicular keratosis.

growths meeting the definition given above, so that most lesions fall somewhere between the rare astonishing lesions and those excrescences which may be designated as merely hyperkeratotic. It seems appropriate, especially in view of the purposes of this book, to exclude viral verrucae, as well as those hornlike lesions which sometimes arise on a more or less widespread dermatosis, such as verrucous nevus or ichthyosis, even though in the strictest sense these excrescences might meet the morphologic definition of cutaneous horns.

PATHOLOGY

In a study published by us a few years ago (Bart et al., 1968a) we found that more than half the number of cutaneous horns we studied were benign. This had been reported previously by others (Lennox and Sayed, 1964; Cramer and Kahlert, 1964). Table 22–1 shows the locations and histopathologic findings of the cutaneous horns in our study. Table 22–2, compiled from numerous sources, summarizes the various histologic pictures found in the bases of cutaneous horns, the estimated

TABLE 22–2 CUTANEOUS HORNS: HISTOLOGIC TYPES, RELATIVE INCIDENCE, AND MALIGNANT POTENTIAL

Histology	Relative Incidence	Malignant Potential
Seborrheic keratosis, basosquamous papilloma, and inverted follicular keratosis	common	benign
Benign hyperplastic epithelium	common	benign
Actinic keratosis with or without early squamous cell carcinoma	common	premalignant or malignant
Frank squamous cell carcinoma	uncommon	malignant
Keratoacanthoma	rare	benign
Bowen's disease	rare	carcinoma in situ
Histiocytoma	rare	benign
Basal cell epithelioma	rare	malignant
Angioma	rare	benign
Kaposi's sarcoma	rare	malignant
"Penile horn"	uncommon	benign to malignant
Keratotic and micaceous pseudoepitheliomatous balanitis	uncommon	presumably benign
Sebaceous adenomatous proliferation	rare	benign
Acquired digital (acral) fibrokeratoma	uncommon	benign

TABLE 22–3 TERMINOLOGY: SYNONYMS AND VARIANTS

Seborrheic Keratosis
  Seborrheic verruca
  Verruca senilis
  Senile wart
  Basosquamous papilloma
  Inverted follicular keratosis
Benign Hyperplastic Epithelium
  "Open epithelial cyst"
  "Molluscum-like" horns
  Pseudoepitheliomatous hyperplasia
  "Keratoacanthoma"
  Hyperkeratotic papilloma
Actinic Keratosis
  Solar keratosis
  Senile keratosis
  Keratosis senilis
  Squamous keratosis (Lennox and Sayed, 1964)
  Bowenoid actinic keratosis
  "Bowen's disease"
Squamous Cell Carcinoma
  Prickle cell epithelioma
  Epidermoid carcinoma

relative incidence of types, and their respective malignant potentials.

The horns themselves are composed of compact keratin, sometimes with para-keratotic elements. The histologic pictures at the bases of the horns vary from completely innocuous to unquestionably malignant, e.g., from seborrheic keratosis to infiltrating squamous cell carcinoma. Fortunately, infiltrating squamous cell carcinomas are found only rarely under cutaneous horns, probably because the differentiation necessary to make large amounts of adherent keratin is usually lost in the carcinomatous transformation of the keratinocytes. Table 22–3 lists those histologic diagnoses most often applied in describing the bases of cutaneous horns. I have grouped them under four headings: *seborrheic keratosis, benign hyperplastic epithelium, actinic keratosis,* and *squamous cell carcinoma.* The other titles, used by other authors, are either synonyms for these four or represent probable histologic variants. Although cutaneous horns may rarely occur over true keratoacanthomas, open epithelial cysts, or Bowen's disease, it is likely that many of the lesions reported by others as examples of these entities really are examples of benign hyperplastic epi-

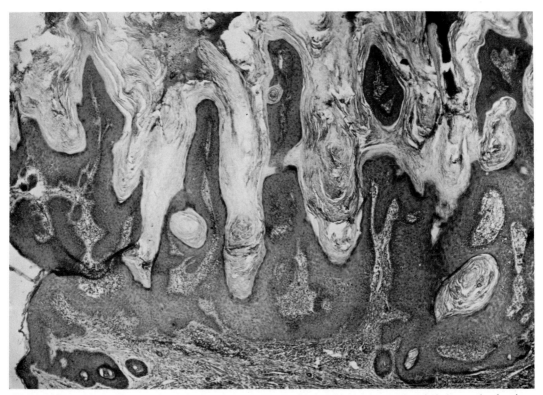

Figure 22–2 Photomicrograph of the base of a cutaneous horn arising from a seborrheic keratosis, showing papillomatosis and pseudohorn cysts. *H & E, ×46.* (Courtesy of Skin and Cancer Unit, New York University.)

thelium or bowenoid actinic keratoses. Such diagnoses may have been based on purely histologic grounds rather than on the more revealing method of correlating histologic picture and clinical behavior.

Cutaneous Horns Over Seborrheic Keratoses and Variants

The typical histologic picture of seborrheic keratosis may be seen, in which there is an irregular epithelial proliferation with invagination of the keratin into the epidermal folds, pseudohorn cysts, and papillomatosis (Fig. 22–2). The proliferation is formed by small keratinocytes, which may dispose themselves in a disorderly pattern. Such cells have well-formed intercellular bridges (Andrade and Steigleder, 1959) and may contain melanin. Sometimes melanocytes are interspersed between the keratinocytes. Variations in the histologic features occur. Groups of larger, polygonal cells with more obvious intercellular bridges and with paler, more abundant cytoplasm are sometimes seen. The presence of those cells in a seborrheic keratosis results in the picture of so-called ba-

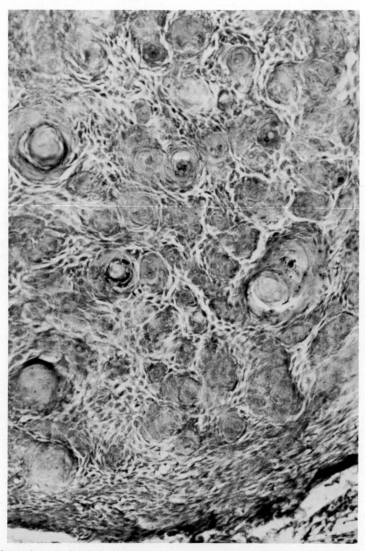

Figure 22–3 Photomicrograph of the base of a cutaneous horn showing histology of inverted follicular keratosis. Note prominence of whorls (squamous eddies). Features of malignancy are absent. *H & E, ×183.* (From Bart et al.: Acta Derm. Venereol. (Stockh.), 48:507, 1968.)

sosquamous papilloma (Civatte, 1957). When the predominant feature consists of groups of these paler cells in whorls (Fig. 22–3), the appearance is that of inverted follicular keratosis, described by Helwig (1955).

Cutaneous Horns Over Benign Hyperplastic Epithelium

In such lesions microscopy reveals varying degrees of irregular acanthosis topped by horn (Fig. 22–4). The rete ridges in some lesions are short and broad, in others elongated and tortuous. The individual epidermal cells are ordinary in appearance. When the epithelium is disposed in a cuplike manner, and when the acanthosis is not very marked or irregular, the histology may suggest that the horns have arisen from the acanthotic walls of epithelial cysts which have opened to the surface (Fig. 22–5); if the acanthosis is somewhat greater, the lesions look like the "molluscum-like lesions" described by Lennox and Sayed (1964). At times the acanthosis

is so marked and so irregular that it borders on pseudoepitheliomatous hyperplasia. Such changes, when disposed in a cup shape, result in an appearance suggestive of keratoacanthoma. Many of the cutaneous horns occurring over benign bases have sufficient papillomatosis to qualify as examples of what Cramer and Kahlert (1964) have termed "hyperkeratotic papillomas."

Cutaneous Horns Over Actinic Keratoses and Early Squamous Cell Carcinomas

These two types are considered together because of their clinical and histologic similarities. In actinic keratoses, there is moderate to marked irregular acanthosis with elongated rete ridges and epithelial buds (Fig. 22–6A). The epidermal cells are arranged in disorderly fashion, are relatively light-staining, and differ in size and shape. Hyperchromatic nuclei, mitotic figures, bi- and multinucleated cells, and isolated prematurely keratinized cells are

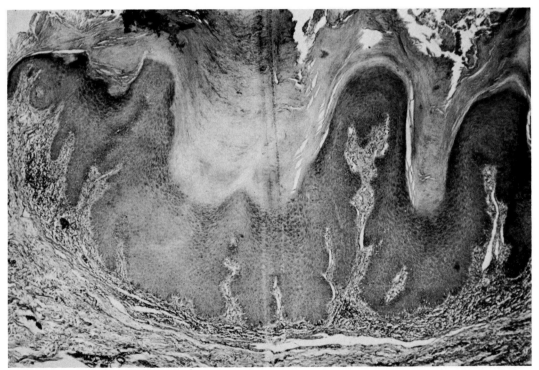

Figure 22–4 Photomicrograph showing benign hyperplastic epithelium. *H & E, ×46.* (Courtesy of Skin and Cancer Unit, New York University.)

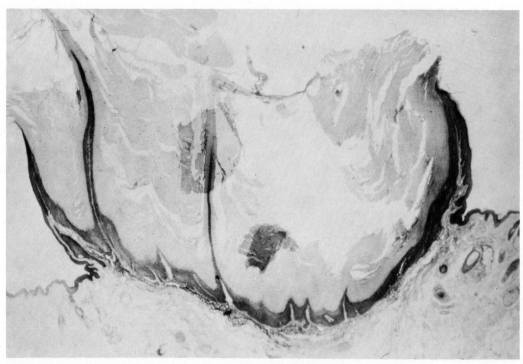

Figure 22–5 Photomicrograph of a cutaneous horn arising upon benign hyperplastic epithelium which resembles the acanthotic wall of an open cyst. *H & E, ×18.* (From Bart et al.: Acta Derm. Venereol. (Stockh.), 48:507, 1968.)

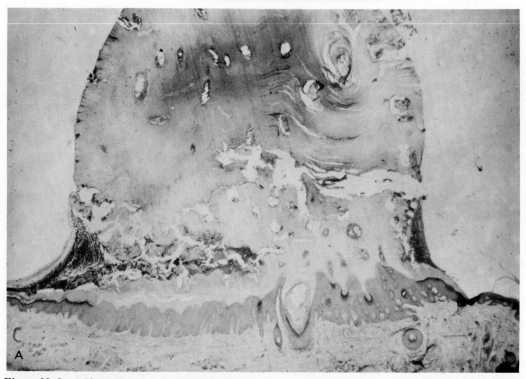

Figure 22–6 *A*, Photomicrograph of a cutaneous horn arising from an actinic keratosis. *H & E, ×18.* (Courtesy of Skin and Cancer Unit, New York University.)

Illustration continued on opposite page.

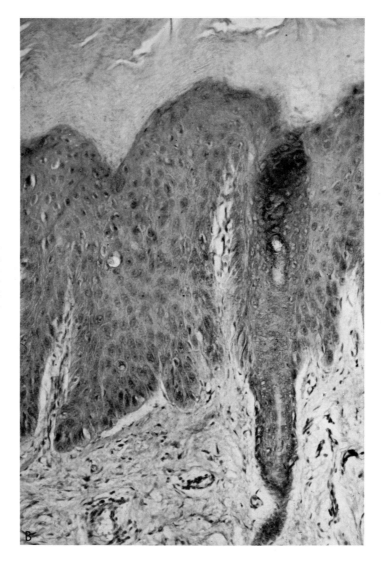

Figure 22–6 *(Continued) B,* Higher power photomicrograph of actinic keratosis shown in *A.* The sweat duct remains uninvolved. *H & E. ×183.* (From Bart et al.: Acta Derm. Venereol. (Stockh.), 48:507, 1968.)

sometimes seen. In some areas, the granular layer is absent and there is overlying parakeratosis. An abrupt transition may be seen between the normal epidermis of the unaffected surrounding skin and the abnormal areas under the horn. Frequently the adnexal intraepidermal epithelium is spared (Fig. 22–6B). In some of the actinic keratoses, areas with bowenoid features are found; occasionally poikilokarynosis is so marked that the histology of a lesion is essentially indistinguishable from that of Bowen's disease. However, the adnexal epithelium may be spared. Early squamous cell carcinomas present essentially the same features as the actinic keratoses, but the rete ridges grow downward into the

dermis further, and some buds of epithelium appear to be separated from the anaplastic epidermis above (Fig. 22–7). Unaffected intraepidermal adnexal epithelium is less often found.

Cutaneous Horns Over Frank, Invasive Squamous Cell Carcinomas

Microscopically these lesions show invasive, but well-differentiated squamous cell carcinomas (Figs. 22–8 and 22–9). Horn pearls may be present in large numbers. There may be histologic evidence that the tumors have arisen from actinic keratoses.

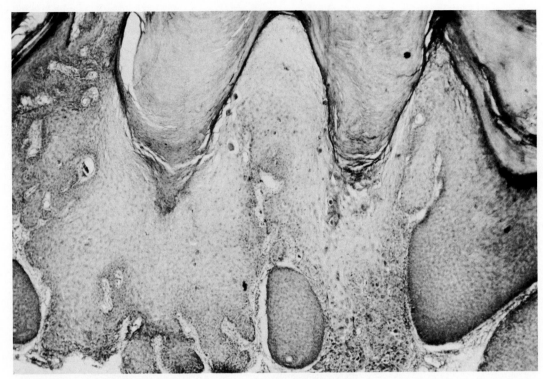

Figure 22-7 Photomicrograph of the base of a cutaneous horn, showing early squamous cell carcinoma developing in an actinic keratosis. *H & E, ×46.* (Courtesy of Skin and Cancer Unit, New York University.)

CLINICAL DESCRIPTIONS

By definition, all cutaneous horns, regardless of cause, are approximately conical or cylindrical in form and composed mostly of keratin. The important question is whether or not there are further clinical features of a particular lesion or of the patient bearing it which may serve as worthwhile clues to the histologic pattern at the base. In many instances careful examination of the horn and the patient will lead the physician to correctly anticipate the histologic diagnosis. The clinical pictures of the most common types of cutaneous horns are described below.

Cutaneous Horns Over Seborrheic Keratoses

Although there are considerable variations in the appearances of these lesions, some of these horns bear enough resemblance to ordinary seborrheic keratoses for the true diagnosis to be made clinically. In those cases, the horn tends to be dark brown with a greasy verrucoid surface

(Fig. 22–10), and it can sometimes be crumbled by firm digital pressure. The inverted follicular keratosis, which may be considered as a variety of seborrheic keratosis (Andrade, 1971), may present as a light-colored horn arising from a firm, pinkish, nodular base (Fig. 22–11). Such a lesion usually requires histologic resolution.

Cutaneous Horns Over Benign Hyperplastic Epithelium

Cutaneous horns upon benign hyperplastic epithelium are variable in their clinical appearance. The horn itself is frequently light in color; it may arise directly from the level of the skin or from a sessile, bulging, sometimes erythematous base (Fig. 22–12).

Cutaneous Horns Over Actinic Keratoses and Early Squamous Cell Carcinomas

The horny material over actinic keratoses and early squamous cell carcinomas

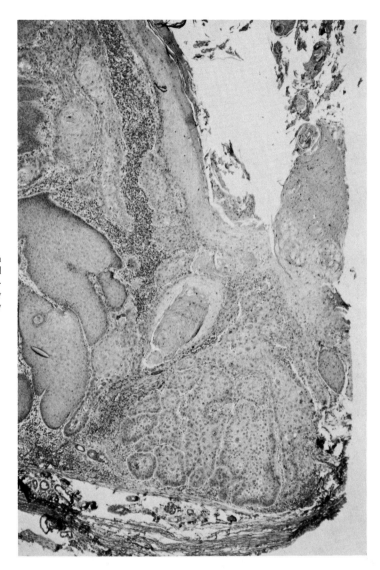

Figure 22–8 Photomicrograph of a frank, invasive squamous cell carcinoma at the base of a cutaneous horn. *H & E, ×46.* (Courtesy of Skin and Cancer Unit, New York University.)

tends to be hard and yellowish brown, and frequently seems to arise directly from the surface of the skin (Figs. 22–13 and 22–14). Sometimes there is an erythematous, nodular base, but the presence of such a nodular base does not necessarily mean that there will be histologic evidence of early carcinomatous changes. There is frequently marked actinic damage of the skin surrounding the cutaneous horn.

Cutaneous Horns Over Frank, Invasive Squamous Cell Carcinomas

In the cutaneous horns over frank squamous cell carcinomas, the horn may arise directly from the skin surface (Fig. 22–15) or from an erythematous nodular base (Fig. 22–16) (Bart et al., 1968a). The bases of such horns tend to be large, perhaps 2 cm. or more in diameter, and to arise from actinically damaged skin.

PATHOGENESIS

The causes of cutaneous horns are those of the various entities found at their bases (Table 22–2). For most of these lesions, the pathogenesis is poorly understood and will not be discussed here, except to say that their incidence increases with age. More is known about actinic keratoses and the squamous cell carcinomas which develop

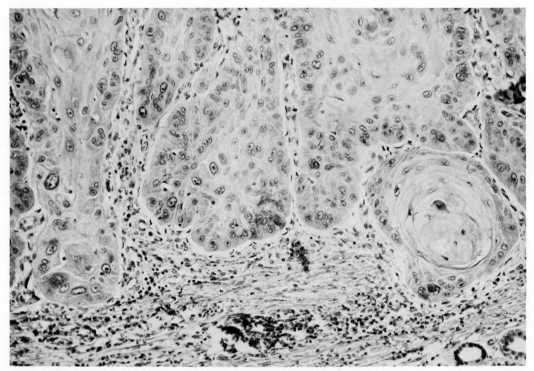

Figure 22–9 Higher power photomicrograph of carcinoma shown in Figure 22–8. A different field is represented. Note variations in sizes and staining qualities of nuclei and cells, and their disorderly arrangement. The horn pearl characterizes the tumor as a well-differentiated squamous cell carcinoma. *H & E, ×457.* (From Bart et al.: Acta Derm. Venereol. (Stockh.), 48:507, 1968.)

from them; although the subject of "actinic skin" is discussed in depth elsewhere in this book, it is appropriate to mention it here because it is so intimately related to the occurrence of cutaneous horns over actinic keratoses and squamous cell carcinomas. The degree of actinic damage to the skin is directly related to the intensity

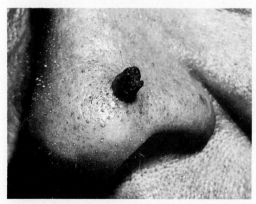

Figure 22–10 Cutaneous horn upon a seborrheic keratosis. Note the dark color and the "stuck-on" appearance. (From Bart et al.: Acta Derm. Venereol. (Stockh.), 48:507, 1968.)

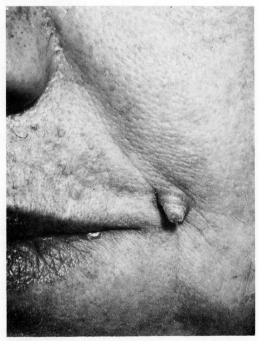

Figure 22–11 Cutaneous horn arising from an inverted follicular keratosis. Note the nodular base. (Courtesy of Skin and Cancer Unit, New York University.)

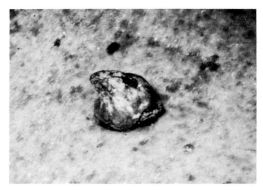

Figure 22–12 Cutaneous horn upon benign hyperplastic epithelium. (Courtesy of Dr. Rudolf L. Baer.)

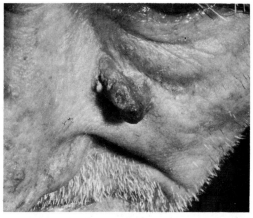

Figure 22–13 Cutaneous horn upon bowenoid actinic keratosis. (Courtesy of Skin and Cancer Unit, New York University.)

and duration of sun exposure and inversely to the protection afforded by the degree of melanization of the skin. Thus in our study (Bart et al., 1968a) we found that, whereas entirely benign cutaneous horns occurred with equal frequency in persons with light or dark eyes, those arising upon actinic keratoses and squamous cell carcinomas occurred much more frequently in light-eyed individuals, that is, in those who—by virtue of associated fair skin—were more likely to incur actinic damage. Similarly it was much more common to find associated premalignant and malignant skin lesions—actinic keratoses, basal cell epitheliomas, and squamous cell carcinomas—other than the cutaneous horns themselves, when the horns were upon actinic keratoses and squamous cell carcinomas than when they were upon benign bases.

In most studies (Cramer and Kahlert, 1964; Mehregan, 1965; Bart et al., 1968a) cutaneous horns were found to be unusual before the sixth decade, and somewhat more common in men (Mehregan, 1965; Bart et al., 1968a). Cutaneous horns upon both benign and malignant underlying lesions occur most frequently on the exposed areas, especially the face (Marcuse, 1902; Moncorps, 1931; Cramer and Kahlert, 1964; Mehregan, 1965; Bart et al., 1968a). In our study (Bart et al., 1968a) all lesions on the cartilaginous portions of the aural pinnae and on the dorsa of the hands were malignant or premalignant (Table 22–1). Location on these sites would seem to be a helpful clinical clue.

DIFFERENTIAL DIAGNOSIS

The differential diagnosis concerns the various entities which are found at the bases of cutaneous horns. As stated above, there are clinical clues which may help the

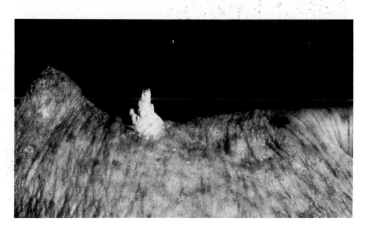

Figure 22–14 Cutaneous horn upon an early squamous cell carcinoma. It seems to arise directly from skin showing marked actinic damage. (Courtesy of Skin and Cancer Unit, New York University.)

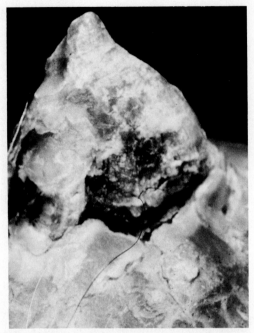

Figure 22–15 Cutaneous horn upon a frank, invasive squamous cell carcinoma. It appears to arise directly from the actinically damaged bald pate of this elderly man. (Courtesy of Dr. Alfred W. Kopf.)

and (3) location on the dorsum of a hand or over the cartilaginous portion of the pinna of an ear. The acquired digital or acral fibrokeratoma (see below) is a distinct clinical entity and should pose little problem in diagnosis to those who are familiar with it. We have not found that the occurrence of erythema, nodularity of the base, or symptoms, with the possible exception of bleeding, help to differentiate benign from premalignant or malignant lesions. Final diagnosis, of course, depends on histologic examination. However, even upon histologic examination, error may be made. Sometimes inverted follicular keratoses, and occasionally even ordinary seborrheic keratoses, are misdiagnosed microscopically as squamous cell carcinomas. About one-third of the seborrheic keratoses in our series (Bart et al., 1968a) had originally been "overdiagnosed" in this way. Rowe (1957) pointed out the histologic resemblance between certain seborrheic keratoses and squamous cell carcinomas.

clinician to make a correct guess as to the histologic picture of the base (Bart et al., 1968a). Those clinical features which favor premalignancy or malignancy are (1) absence of resemblance to seborrheic keratosis; (2) occurrence in a person with light eyes, especially if there is other evidence of cutaneous premalignancy or malignancy;

TREATMENT

The "shave biopsy" which is often useful in substantiating the diagnosis of basal cell epithelioma is much less frequently a useful approach to cutaneous horns, when it may be important to see the depth of the pathology in order to rule out squamous

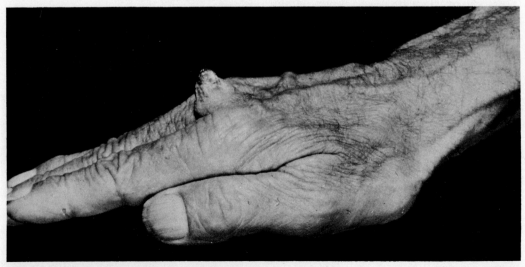

Figure 22–16 Cutaneous horn upon a frank, invasive squamous cell carcinoma. Note the nodular base. (From Bart et al.: Acta Derm. Venereol. (Stockh.), 48:507, 1968.)

cell carcinoma. However, some find a "saucerization" biopsy, which goes deeper, useful at times (Popkin, 1971). This can be followed by further treatment, if indicated. Fusiform excision with histologic examination of the specimen is often indicated. Since the histologic diagnosis may not justify an extensive procedure, initial excision should be conservative, with rarely more than a 3- to 5-mm. border of normal-appearing skin included in the short diameter of the specimen. Wider excision can be carried out subsequently if the histologic picture warrants. This will rarely be indicated, since frank squamous cell carcinoma is uncommon at the base of a cutaneous horn. Obviously, if the skin is very lax around a lesion suspected of being malignant, it may be desirable to take a wider border initially. X-ray therapy may also be used in selected cases for squamous cell carcinomas found at the bases of cutaneous horns. However, such therapy should be used with caution for lesions other than those on the head or neck and in persons under 40 years of age (Bart et al., 1970; and refer to chapter on "Radiotherapy," this book).

PROGNOSIS

Although adequate follow-up statistics for a large series of cutaneous horns are not available, recurrence is apparently unusual after adequate conservative removal. Shapiro (1971) saw a man with a hornlike squamous cell carcinoma of a popliteal fossa metastatic to an inguinal node, but metastatic disease must be rare, and I have not seen it. Since those squamous cell carcinomas found at the bases of cutaneous horns usually arise from actinic keratoses, the findings of Graham and Helwig (1966) and of Bendl and Graham (1970) seem pertinent in this regard. They reported that metastases from squamous cell carcinomas arising from actinic kerastoses rarely, if ever, occur.

MISCELLANEOUS ENTITIES

It is evident from the foregoing that the majority of cutaneous horns occur on the basis of four lesions: (1) actinic keratoses; (2) such squamous cell carcinomas as derive from them; (3) seborrheic keratoses and variants; and (4) a number of histologic patterns all of which may be regarded as varieties of "benign hyperplastic epithelium." In addition, cutaneous horns occur less commonly over a miscellaneous assortment of benign and malignant conditions, most of which are discussed briefly below.

Many of the horns said to have arisen upon keratoacanthomas very likely represent examples of benign hyperplastic epithelium in cup-shaped pattern rather

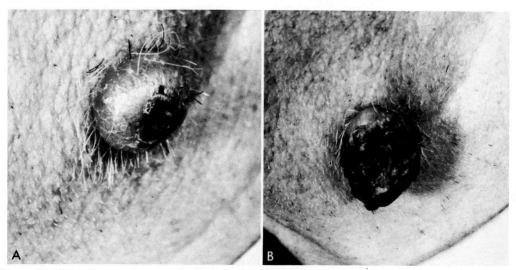

Figure 22–17 *A*, Keratoacanthoma of about six weeks' duration. *B*, The same lesion four months later presenting as a cutaneous horn. Over the next three months, it involuted completely without treatment. (Courtesy of Skin and Cancer Unit, New York University.)

than true keratoacanthomas. On the other hand, occasionally a true keratoacanthoma may be capped by a cutaneous horn. We have seen such a lesion (Fig. 22–17) which spontaneously resolved over several months. A similar growth was illustrated by Stevanović (1965).

It is likely that cutaneous horns occasionally arise upon true Bowen's disease; however, many reported lesions could have been bowenoid actinic keratoses. In the Oncology Section of the Skin and Cancer Unit we have not encountered any cutaneous horns over indubitable lesions of Bowen's disease.

Cutaneous horns upon histiocytomas have been reported (Mehregan, 1965; Shapiro, 1971), but are very unusual.

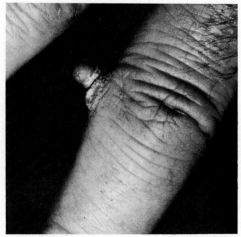

Figure 22–18 Acquired digital fibrokeratoma. (From Bart et al.: Arch. Dermatol., 97:120, 1968.)

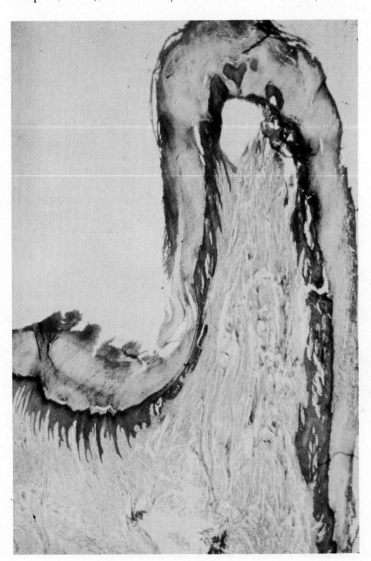

Figure 22–19 Photomicrograph of fibrokeratoma shown in Figure 22–18. There is a normal-appearing core of connective tissue covered with a hyperkeratotic, acanthotic epidermis. *H & E, ×18.* (From Bart et al.: Arch. Dermatol., 97:120, 1968.)

Although I have not seen such lesions, cutaneous horns over basal cell epitheliomas have been reported (Cramer and Kahlert, 1964). I wonder how such characteristically soft proliferations can support such hard superstructures.

Benign angiomas may be found in the bases of cutaneous horns (Bart et al., 1968a). In the case of Kaposi's sarcoma reported by Gibbs and Hyman (1968), no lesions of Kaposi's sarcoma other than those under dense hyperkeratosis were to be found, so that the microscopic diagnosis came as a surprise.

Several instances of cutaneous horns occurring on the penis, usually on the glans, have been reported (Goldstein, 1933; Van der Velde, 1936; Winterhoff and Sparks, 1951; Lillie, 1961). Malignancy and metastases have been reported (Goldstein, 1933). Some of the penile horns may have occurred upon keratotic and micaceous pseudoepitheliomatous balanitis (Lortat-Jacob and Civatte, 1966); as the name implies, they are thought to represent instances of pseudocancer. However, more observations are probably in order before we accept these lesions as entirely benign. Long-standing phimosis frequently precedes horn formation.

Sebaceous adenomatous proliferation has been found at the base of a cutaneous horn (Ritchie and Mullins, 1968).

Acquired digital or acral fibrokeratomas do not meet the definition of cutaneous horns, since they are composed primarily of connective tissue. I have included them in this chapter because their overall configurations are similar to cutaneous horns and because they may be misdiagnosed as such, especially when they are very hyperkeratotic. Acquired fibrokeratomas are benign, solitary, firm, more or less hyperkeratotic projections—often arising out of collarettes of slightly raised skin—that occur most frequently on the digits of the hands (Fig. 22–18) (Bart et al., 1968b; Hare and Smith, 1969). They have also been reported on the toes, palm, dorsum of hand, sole, prepatellar area, and ankle (Verallo, 1968). Acquired fibrokeratomas most commonly occur in males of middle years. None has ever been known to become malignant. Microscopically a fibrokeratoma is composed of a core of normal-appearing connective tissue covered with an acanthotic epidermis which produces a dense enveloping hyperkeratosis (Fig. 22–19). The treatment for acquired fibrokeratomas is conservative surgical excision or "shave" removal with a scalpel and electrodesiccation of the base. Recurrence has not been reported.

REFERENCES

Andrade, R.: Personal communication, 1971.

Andrade, R., and Steigleder, G. K.: Contribution á l'étude histologique et histochimique de la verrue séborrhéique (papillome basocellulaire). Ann. Dermatol. Syphiligr. (Paris), 86:495, 1959.

Bart, R. S., Andrade, R., and Kopf, A. W.: Cutaneous horns: a clinical and histopathologic study. Acta Derm. Venereol. (Stockh.), 48:507, 1968a.

Bart, R. S., Andrade, R., Kopf, A. W., and Leider, M.: Acquired digital fibrokeratomas. Arch. Dermatol., 97:120, 1968b.

Bart, R. S., Kopf, A. W., and Petratos, M. D.: X-ray therapy of skin cancer: evaluation of a "standardized" method for treating basal-cell epitheliomas. *In* Proceedings Sixth National Cancer Conference. Philadelphia, J. B. Lippincott, 1970.

Batschwarov, B., and Profirov, D.: Kasuistik in Bildern. Dermatol. Wochenschr., 150:91, 1964.

Bendl, B. J., and Graham, J. H.: New concepts on the origin of squamous-cell carcinomas of the skin: solar (senile) keratosis with squamous-cell carcinoma—a clinicopathologic and histochemical study. *In* Proceedings Sixth National Cancer Conference. Philadelphia, J. B. Lippincott, 1970.

Charache, H.: Cutaneous horn of the scalp. Am. J. Surg., 29:297, 1935.

Civatte, A.: Atlas d'histopathologie cutanée. Paris, Masson, 1957.

Cramer, H. J., and Kahlert, G.: Das Cornu cutaneum: Selbständiges Krankheitsbild oder Klinishches Symptom? Dermatol. Wochenschr., 150:41, 1964.

Gibbs, R. C., and Hyman, A. B.: Kaposi's sarcoma at the base of the cutaneous horn. Arch. Dermatol., 98:37, 1968.

Goldstein, H. H.: Cutaneous horns of the penis. J. Urol., 30:367, 1933.

Gould, G. M., and Pyle, W. L.: Anomalies and curiosities of medicine. Philadelphia, W. B. Saunders Company, 1896.

Graham, J. H., and Helwig, E. B.: Cutaneous premalignant lesions. *In* Montagna, W., and Dobson, R. L. (eds.): Advances in Biology of Skin Carcinogenesis. Oxford, Pergamon Press, 1966, pp. 296–305.

Hare, P. J., and Smith, P. A. J.: Acquired (digital) fibrokeratoma. Br. J. Dermatol., 81:667, 1969.

Helwig, E. G.: Inverted follicular keratosis. *In* Seminar on the Skin: Neoplasms and Dermatoses. American Society of Clinical Pathologists, International Congress of Clinical Pathology, Washington, D.C., September, 1954. Published by American Society of Clinical Pathology, 1955.

Lennox, B., and Sayed, B. R.: Cutaneous horns. J. Pathol. Bacteriol., 88:575, 1964.

Lillie, G. V.: Penile horn. Arch. Dermatol., 84:322, 1961.

Lortat-Jacob, E., and Civatte, J.: Balanite pseudo-épithéliomateuse kératosique et micacée (balanite synéchiante à évolution kératosique). Bull. Soc. Fr. Dermatol. Syphiligr., 73:931, 1966.

Marcuse, M.: Zur Kenntniss der Hauthorner. Arch. Dermatol. Syph. (Berl.), 60:197, 1902.

Mehregan, A. H.: Cutaneous horn: a clinicopathologic study. Dermatol. Digest, 4:45, 1965.

Moncorps, C.: Cornu cutaneum, Hauthorn. *In* Jadassohn, J. (ed.): Handbuch der Haut- und Geschlechtskrankheiten. VIII, 2, Berlin, Springer-Verlag, 1931.

Popkin, G.: Personal communication, 1971.

Ritchie, E. B., and Mullins, J. F.: Sebaceous adenomatous proliferation at the base of a cornu cutaneum. Arch. Dermatol., 98:392, 1968.

Rowe, L.: Seborrheic keratoses: "pseudoepitheliomatous hyperplasia" (Weidman). J. Invest. Dermatol., 29:165, 1957.

Semins, H., and Null, H. M.: Giant cutaneous horn. J.A.M.A., 210:2285, 1969.

Shapiro, L.: Personal communication, 1971.

Smialowski, A., and Currie, D. J.: Photography in Medicine. Springfield, Ill., Charles C Thomas, Publisher, 1960, p. 159.

Stevanović, D. V.: A comparative morphological and dynamic study of the pseudocarcinomatous process of man and hairless mouse. Dermatologica, 131:367, 1965.

Van der Velde, O.: Cornification of the glans penis: review of the literature: case report. J. Mich. Med. Soc., 35:317, 1936.

Verallo, V. V. M.: Acquired digital fibrokeratomas. Br. J. Dermatol., 80:730, 1968.

Winterhoff, E., and Sparks, A. J.: Penile horn. J. Urol., 66:704, 1951.

23

Xeroderma Pigmentosum

José M. Mascaró, M.D.

The name *xeroderma pigmentosum* is no more appropriate than the majority of the synonyms that have been proposed. As Civatte (1936) correctly observed, the designation places excessive emphasis on two characteristics which exist in other dermatoses, the dryness and the pigmentation, and furthermore does not suggest the preneoplastic quality of the disorder. Nevertheless the term has been universally accepted, and it would be illogical now, a century after the original description, to look for a more appropriate designation.

SYNONYMS

Some of the synonyms recorded are senilitas cutis praecox (Kaposi), atrophoderma pigmentosum (Crocker), melanosis lenticularis progressiva (Pick), lioderma essentiale cum melanosi et telangiectasi, angioma pigmentosum et atrophicum (Taylor), malignant juvenile lentigo, lentigo mélanique, maladie pigmentaire épithéliomateuse or lentigo épithéliomateux (Quinquaud), epithéliomatose pigmentaire (Besnier), multiple hereditary carcinomatosis (Siemens), actinic epitheliomatous atrophy, Kaposi's dermatosis (Vidal), Lichtschrumpfhaut (Hofman),

parchment skin, mesodermal dysplasia (Montgomery), and blastomatogenous heliodermatrophy.

DEFINITION

Xeroderma pigmentosum is a complex genodermatosis characterized by the appearance of atrophy, dryness, and pigmentation of the skin, which gives way to the early appearance of keratoses and carcinomas, especially on skin exposed to actinic radiation. Frequently it is accompanied by neuroendocrine manifestations.

HISTORY

In 1870 Moritz Kohn (Kaposi), in the *Treatise on Diseases of the Skin* by Ferdinand von Hebra, described a hitherto unknown cutaneous process. In the chapter on xeroderma ("parchment skin," a term which had been created by Erasmus Wilson to group diseases which were characterized by "a dry and parched skin"), he described a peculiar type of cutaneous alteration in two patients he had studied since 1863. The disease was characterized by parchment-like dryness of the skin

573

with pigmentation and a tendency toward the precocious development of tumors. A few years later, in 1882, Kaposi enlarged upon the description of this new process in a complete work which added four more cases to the two original ones. The author gave a minutely detailed description of the disease, which he said was characterized by "dark spots between which depressions existed which were similar to the scars of smallpox and were a brilliant white in color, and found on the face, ears, the neck and the nape of the neck, the back, the chest as far as the third rib, the arms, the back of the hands, and sometimes the legs and the dorsum of the feet, with punctiform vascular dilatations."

Kaposi s description was soon confirmed by various authors, and over the years additional studies appeared and enlarged understanding of the disease. Although Kaposi himself had mentioned photophobia, the ocular manifestations of xeroderma pigmentosum were studied for the first time by Archambault in 1890. The neuropsychologic alterations, also perceived by the original author, were better studied by Neisser (1883), Audry (1907), Leredde (cited by Hadida et al., 1963), and Siemens and Kohn (1925). In 1933 De Sanctis and Cacchione completed the study of these alterations by describing the complex syndrome of xerodermic idiocy, which is associated with the cutaneous process, mental retardation, and neurologic and endocrine disorders (testicular aplasia and delayed growth). In fact, a year earlier Ajello and Follman (1932; cited by Hadida) had observed the existence of endocrine lesions (in the hypophysis, thyroid, ovary, and adrenal glands) in autopsies of patients affected with xeroderma pigmentosum.

The first histologic description, as Kaposi indicates, was given by Geber. Kaposi (1883), Neisser (1883), and Vidal and Leloir (1883) soon afterward presented these data in a more precise manner, and they were to be subsequently amplified in successive publications.

In regard to the pathogenesis, since Archambault (1890), one of the first to discuss it, there have been experiments on the action of different radiations on the skin of these patients reported by Low (1906), Hahn and Weik (1907), Rothman (1923), Lynch (1934), Anderson and Begg (1950), and Berlin (1958) and studies on the genetics of the disease by Cockayne (1933), Haldane (1936), and Macklin (1936, 1944, and 1945), all of which have contributed to defining it more precisely.

It would be impossible to mention all the important work which has been done on xeroderma pigmentosum. Historically, however, we cannot overlook the recent and exhaustive etiologic and histopathologic studies of Hadida et al. (1963), or the fundamental investigations on the genetics, biochemistry, and clinical oculocutaneous and neuropsychic manifestations by El-Hefnawi and his collaborators (1962–1965). Likewise the investigations of Cleaver (1968) and Bootsma (cited by Veldhuisen and Poowels, 1970) on the replication of DNA in cell cultures of fibroblasts from patients with xeroderma pigmentosum constitute an important landmark in our knowledge of this complex process. Rasheed et al. (1969) made a very interesting study on the ultrastructure of the skin lesions of xeroderma pigmentosum.

EPIDEMIOLOGY AND INCIDENCE

Frequency

This process has been known for a century and some hundreds of cases of xeroderma pigmentosum have been published. In his extremely thorough work, Siemens and Kohn (1925) already collected 333 cases from 222 families. The frequency among the general population varies between 1:65,000 and 1:100,000, according to Dorn (1959). This is an indication that, although we are not confronted with a frequent genodermatosis, we are not dealing with an exceptionally rare disease.

Cases have been described in Europe, North and South America, North Africa—where it appears to be very frequent—and Asia. The greater incidence of the disease in certain regions, such as the south coast of the Mediterranean, seems to be dependent on two factors: the frequency of consanguineous marriages, which facilitates the expansion of the genodermatosis and determines the appearance of severe cases, and the intensity of solar irradiation, which results in the forms of medium intensity presenting a richer symptomatology in these regions than they would in more temperate zones.

Race

Patients with xeroderma pigmentosum frequently have fair skin and blond hair, but the disease is not rare in individuals who are heavily pigmented (Lowenthal and Trowel, 1938; Hadida et al., 1963). Even though this process is observed principally in people with white skin, it can be seen in all races and ethnic groups. Xeroderma pigmentosum is rarely found in Negroes (Carney, 1954), but some cases have been described (Hopkins and Van Studdiford, 1934; Lowenthal and Trowel, 1938; King, 1940; Kesten and Slatkin, 1952). Among people of yellow skin, if one is to judge from published works, xeroderma pigmentosum would appear to be much more frequent in Japan than in China (Canright, 1934). Different authors have emphasized the particular frequency of xeroderma pigmentosum among Jews, among whom the incidence is greatest in those of Asiatic descent (Czerniak, 1954). However, the percentage of cases described among Jews is variable, ranging from 7 percent (Siemens and Kohn, 1925) to 24 percent (Elsenber, 1890) and even to 70 percent (Hoede, 1940); this is so because the result depends on the region or country in which the compilation was done. The disease is also frequent among Arabs (Hadida et al., 1963). The greater incidence among Jews and Arabs is undoubtedly due to the frequency of consanguineous marriages in both groups.

Age

Normally the symptoms begin to occur toward the end of the first year of life or at the beginning of the second. Siemens and Kohn (1925) pointed out that 80 per-

cent of cases begin within the first three years. Nevertheless, as we shall shortly see, cases exist in which the onset of the disease occurs much later.

Sex

In general, the disease affects both sexes in equal proportion. In 1925, Siemens and Kohn found that out of 333 patients 149 were male and 152 female. But not all authors find an equal incidence in both sexes. Lowenbach (cited by Ballarini, 1938) pointed out that even among siblings it is not uncommon to find only those of the same sex affected. And in Algeria, Hadida also noted a greater frequency in males, who represent about two-thirds of the 80 cases he gathered. This does not constitute a sufficient argument in support of Cockayne (1933) and Macklin (1945), who asserted that transmission is recessive and partially sex-linked.

Other Factors

The existence of consanguinity in the patients' forebears is very frequent (Siemens and Kohn, 1925) and is found in proportions which vary according to different authors (14.7 percent by Rouvière, 1910; 21.2 percent by Macklin, 1936; and 58.6 percent by Cockayne, 1933). It is precisely the greater frequency of consanguineous marriages which determines the greater incidence of xeroderma pigmentosum in certain ethnic groups. In fact, consanguineous marriages are frequent among Jews, as a result of the isolation in which they find themselves, and among Arabs because of economic reasons (Reed et al., 1965).

ETIOLOGY AND PATHOGENESIS

Inheritance

It is universally acknowledged that xeroderma pigmentosum is a familial hereditary disease, both in the pure cutaneous forms and in the complex cutaneo-neuroendocrine forms. From the numerous studies on the genetics of the process, we can deduce that it is transmitted by means of an incompletely recessive autosomal gene (Dorn, 1959; Koller, 1948), which in some pedigrees appears to show a partial sex linkage. However, not all the authors reach identical conclusions, since recent studies (El-Hefnawi and Smith, 1965) tend to demonstrate a linkage between the locus of xeroderma pigmentosum and the ABO blood group, with an association of the disease and blood group O in 80.4 percent of the patients, and complete absence of AB. This supports the idea of transmission by a recessive autosomal gene without partial sex linkage.

Korn-Heydt (1966), in his chapter on aplasias, hyperplasias, and hereditary tumors in the Jadassohn *Handbuch* edited by Gottron and Schnyder, distinguished a recessive autosomal form, which would be the most frequent, and a rare autosomal dominant form, illustrated by the cases of Vilanova (1932) and Anderson and Begg (1950). Perhaps these two hypotheses are not completely incompatible, and in the recessive cases there exists a partial sex linkage. Heavily freckled relatives of the patients may then represent the heterozygous forms of the process, whose expression would depend on the individual phenotype (Anderson and Begg, 1950).

Raphael, Martin, Inwood, and Fimlt (1961) did not find chromosomal abnormalities in one case, and neither did Goldman and Owens (1964) in two more. Esteller and coworkers (1964) found a normal trisomy G mosaicism in one patient and a normal karyotype in another. The dermatoglyphic examination of the mosaic case showed a high axial triradium. Later these same authors examined two other cases (1966) and found normal karyotypes. Kamimura and Sato (1963) examined a Japanese family with a high incidence of xeroderma pigmentosum and likewise found no chromosomal alterations.

Variations in the clinical picture from single cutaneous manifestations to the complex picture of xerodermic idiocy can be attributed to the variable degree of penetration of the gene, as Gawad and El-Hefnawi (1968) indicate.

Sensitivity to Light

In general, the cutaneous and ocular manifestations of xeroderma pigmentosum are due to hypersensitivity to actinic light and especially to the ultraviolet rays of the solar spectrum. However, the nature and mechanism of this hypersensitivity are still not clarified. On the other hand, there does not seem to be any obvious relation between the degree of light sensitivity and the severity of clinical symptoms (Berlin and Tager, 1958). There are also patients without any manifest hypersensitivity to light (Goldman, 1961), and in photobiologic studies, alongside patients with increased sensitivity to wavelengths between 280 and 310 nm. (Luger, 1962; Lynch, 1934), there are others in whom the response to light is completely normal (Kesten and Slatkin, 1952). Notable variations can be observed in the same individual: hypersensitivity demonstrated early in the course of the disease can subsequently disappear without our being able to consider the patient's pigmentation a sufficient sunscreen to justify such a change in the reaction to light.

Different experiments performed on sensitivity to light in xeroderma pigmentosum are difficult to compare, because the authors have worked under different conditions and with nonstandardized light sources. Those of Berlin and Tager (1958) are worth citing: after they exposed skin to rays from a quartz light, they observed a marked and persistent abnormal erythematous reaction, which was followed by a lasting pigmentation. These abnormally intense reactions can be avoided with the use of protective sunscreen creams. X-rays (100 to 200 R. with or without filter) (Berlin and Tager, 1958) and grenz rays (100 R.) (Bachrach, 1958, cited by Berlin) likewise have a pigmentogenic effect.

These experiments are confirmed by clinical observations that the disease gets worse during exposure to the sun and progresses more slowly when patients are protected from such exposure. Moreover, in two cases Hadida et al. (1963) have seeen pigmented lesions in autografts from covered areas after these have been used to replace skin lost through extirpation of tumors in light-exposed areas. With the monochromator Cripps (1970) has been able to determine the type of radiation that affects the skin of xeroderma pigmentosum patients. Radiation at 340 nm. produces maximal erythema within 72 hours, which persists for more than 10 days.

Metabolic and Endocrine Disorders

Recent investigations have been able to demonstrate the existence of metabolic and endocrine disorders; knowledge of this can contribute to the clarification of the pathogenic mechanisms of xeroderma pigmentosum. Many of these disorders appear in sequential order.

El-Hefnawi et al. (1962c) found an increase in serum copper in patients with xeroderma pigmentosum, accompanied by a parallel decrease in glutathione. Likewise an increase in α_2-globulin exists (El-Hefnawi et al., 1962b), perhaps at the expense of ceruloplasmin, since in human plasma copper is combined with this, which is an α-globulin (Holmberg and Laurell, 1948). Melanin formation would be altered in these patients because of the disequilibrium between tyrosinase activity and the proportion of sulfhydrilic compounds, such as serum glutathione. Nevertheless, as Perry and coworkers (1970) pointed out, the increase in serum copper is not necessarily related to the pathogenesis, since it is also increased in certain viral and microbial infections, and also in neoplasias, and therefore could be only a secondary phenomenon.

Another interesting finding is the increased level of amino acid excretion observed in the urine of these patients (El-Hefnawi and El-Hawary, 1963a), which is mainly represented by cysteine, cystine, histidine, lysine, arginine, aspartic and glutamic acids, serine, and alanine, with less of an increase in the remaining amino acids, with the exception of tryptophan and valine, which are absent. Normal blood levels of the amino acids and normal urea clearance support the idea that the aminoaciduria is caused by a lack of tubular reabsorption, as exists for example in cystinuria and glycinuria, and in the syndromes of Fanconi, Lowe, and Hartnup. According to El-Hefnawi the loss of cysteine (which is a sulfhydrilic amino acid) could explain the decreased protection against actinic radiation, since the cysteine plays a preponderant role in the defense against radiation and also is a very important factor in the formation of glutathione, which is diminished in xeroderma pigmentosum.

As Ashurst pointed out (1969), it is interesting that in different photodermatoses (xeroderma pigmentosum, Hartnup's disease, and vacciniform hydroa) in which aminoaciduria has been noted, the common denominator is excessive excretion of alanine and glutamine.

Finally, within this same group of sequential findings investigated by El-Hefnawi et al. (1963), there was a decrease in the urinary elimination of the 17-ketosteroids and the 17-hydroxycorticosteroids which could not be offset by corticotropin stimulation. Serum electrolytes were completely normal. These conclusions appear to agree with those previously cited, since the level of serum copper decreases in proportion to the administration of adrenal corticosteroids, according to Lipkin et al. (1962), and in animal experiments adrenalectomy raises the level of serum copper (El-Mofty et al., 1961). Melanocyte-stimulating hormone controls pigmentation in mammals by regulating serum copper, which in turn activates cutaneous tyrosine (Lorincz, 1954).

El-Hefnawi deduced from this sequence of changes that a secondary adrenal hypofunction exists through deprivation of proteins or amino acids from the anterior pituitary. If pituitary hypofunction were secondary to adrenal disease, the secretion of aldosterone would be normal (Nabarro, 1960). One cannot, however, exclude the possibility of a hereditary corticotropin defect as part of a multiple disorder.

Photosensitizing substances do not exist in the urine of xeroderma pigmentosum patients. Passive transfer to an animal of hypersensitivity to light cannot be accomplished through an injection of the blood of these patients (Rothman, 1923).

Other Findings

Among more recent investigations, those with the most interesting findings are those of Cleaver (1968) to the effect that cultured fibroblasts from patients with xeroderma pigmentosum cannot carry out repair replication of DNA. Repair replication is a form of DNA replication which occurs in PPLO, bacteria, normal mammalian cells, and even certain cancerous cells, such as HeLa cells. It consists of replacement of altered bases in the molecule of the DNA, with elimination of damaged ones and insertion of new ones. The fibroblasts of patients with xeroderma pigmentosum exposed to and damaged by ultraviolet rays do not undergo repair replication, whereas the fibroblasts of healthy subjects do so. According to Cleaver, with the persistence of the alterations produced in DNA by ultraviolet rays or solar light, its functions can become modified and the surviving cells can be converted into malignant ones. In part and as a way of compensation, the surviving cells may proliferate to replace the destroyed ones; in this way they would be able to form the cutaneous tumors of xeroderma pigmentosum.

The fibroblasts' inability to undergo repair replication could be the result of the enzymatic defect thought by many workers to exist in xeroderma pigmentosum. Nevertheless, the relationship between repair replication of DNA and carcinogenesis is neither simple nor obvious, and these experiments need confirmation and more profound study.

Bootsma (cited in Veldhuisen and Poowels, 1970) has demonstrated that an inversely proportional relation exists between the capacity for repair replication and the severity of the clinical symptoms of xeroderma pigmentosum. An interesting observation by Burk et al. (1970) is that DNA in lymphocytes from patients with xeroderma pigmentosum incorporates tritiated thymidine more slowly but for a longer time than does DNA from normal subjects.

Conclusions on Pathogenesis

The findings of the investigators and the reflections of the authors who have occupied themselves with this problem certainly open up new perspectives and point toward comprehension of the complex pathogenesis of xeroderma pigmentosum, but we are very far from knowing the secret of this process.

The pigmentary disorders of xeroderma pigmentosum can be caused by the cited increase of serum copper, since equal hypercupremia has been observed in other cutaneous processes which evolve into hypermelanogenesis (Riehl's melanosis, bronzed diabetes, pregnancy pigmentation) (El-Hefnawi et al., 1962c). In its turn the serum copper, transported by the ceruloplasmin, increases with the decrease in circulating adrenocortical hormones, and these can be diminished by an adrenal hypofunction of pituitary origin. This is the pathogenetic sequence which El-Hefnawi deduces as the result of his investigations and the associated protein deficiency which leads one to imagine the existence of a nephrotubulopathy, which is probably congenital. Thus xeroderma pigmentosum appears today as a complex hereditary process which manifests itself solely through cutaneous symptomatology or shows itself as a complex cutaneo-neuroendocrine-somatic expression; it is probably the result of a complex metabolic error, in which the fundamental defect is a lack of one or a number of enzymes. Through an alteration in sulfur metabolism, xeroderma pigmentosum would be characterized in skin by either a hypersensitivity or a nonsensitivity to ultraviolet radiation. There would be a tubulopathy in the kidney with a congenital reabsorption defect. And to these enzymopathies many others poorly known would be added, which would be responsible for the neuroendocrine-somatic features. Probably there are also defects in the enzymes in charge of DNA replication.

CLINICAL DESCRIPTION

Natural History

Parents normally do not reveal any abnormality, with the exception of profuse freckles in certain cases (Cockayne, 1933), and at birth the infant has a completely normal skin. In 75 percent of cases, the first symptoms appear between six months and three years of age. Cutaneous manifestations normally appear after exposure to sunlight; but cases following both vaccination for smallpox and acute infection such as measles have been described (Shuermann, 1938; Alajmo, 1933; Berlin, 1939; Nödl, 1955a and 1955b; Ballarini, 1938).

The first signs generally consist of a transitory sunburn of the exposed areas of skin, which can be accompanied by edema and exuding vesiculobullous lesions and which is followed by desquamation. Frequently the lesions impetiginize. In exceptional cases a brief exposure to

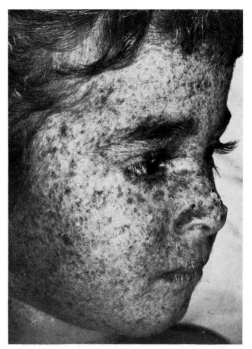

Figure 23–2 Typical appearance of xeroderma pigmentosum. (Patient of Professor Duperrat, Paris.)

sunlight can produce a picture similar to a burn with formation of large blisters (Delacrétaz, 1959). This is followed by an increased dryness of the skin in the exposed areas.

Finally lentiginosis of the exposed cutaneous areas appears: on the face, the back of the hands, the neck, the arms and forearms, the lower part of the legs, and sometimes the lips and the conjunctiva. At first these lentigines are transitory and disappear in the winter months, but then they return permanently, are not influenced by the seasons, and progressively increase in number and intensity.

Rarely, in a few cases, the pigmentations appear without an inflammatory erythematous phase preceding them (Bering, 1932, cited by Delacrétaz, 1959), although it is probable that there has been a discrete erythematous phase which has passed unnoticed. Likewise cases exist in which the covered areas are equally affected by the lentigines, as for instance the trunk, and they can even appear on the covered parts first (Lesser, 1898; Pick and Amicis, cited by Civatte, 1936).

Another element of the disorder develops after the lentigines: capillary dilata-

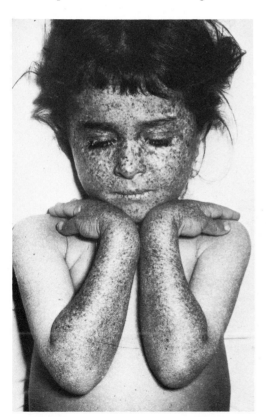

Figure 23–1 Mottled lesions in sun-exposed areas. (Patient of Professor Duperrat, Paris.)

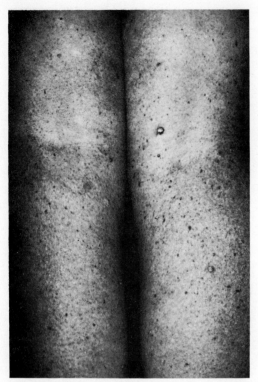

Figure 23-3 Poikilodermic lesions of the legs, with pigmented spots, atrophic plaques, and very abundant telangiectases and small vascular tumors.

tions (telangiectases and angiomas) which, though predominantly affecting parts of the body exposed to light, can be found on the skin of the covered areas and in the buccal and lingual mucosa (Goldman, 1961).

Finally the third element comes to be added to the picture: small, irregular or round, atrophic white spots, which can either follow the vesiculobullous lesions or appear earlier.

The affected skin becomes progressively thinner, dried, and covered with scales (Figs. 23–1 to 23–4). It cracks and can form ulcerations. These are slow to heal and produce retractile scars, which in some locations can produce considerable functional alterations; ectropion may occur in the eyelids and atresia in the mouth and the nasal orifices.

Numerous keratoses and also benign and malignant tumors develop on this dry, atrophic, and mottled skin. Occasionally this can begin from the first year of life (Berlin, 1939; Gay Prieto and Lopez, 1939), but generally the onset is between three and four years of age.

The evolution of xeroderma pigmentosum is not predictable. In general, it is found that cases which begin in early childhood reach the tumoral phase before the 20th year, and those which begin later evolve more slowly. However, there is no constant relation between the more or less rapid and malignant evolution, and the age of onset of the disease.

The malignant tumors can be basal cell carcinomas, which will give way to penetrating ulcerations; cutaneous or conjunctival squamous cell carcinomas (Fig. 23–5), which produce lymph node metastases; or malignant melanomas. These are not rare and may be numerous (Van Patten and Drummond, 1953); they can lead to early

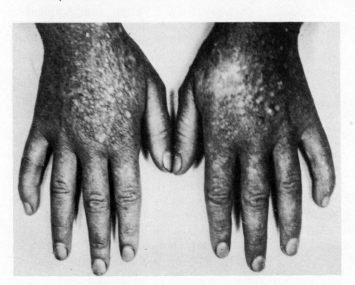

Figure 23-4 Lesions on the back of the hands. On the left hand there is a scar created by electrocoagulation of an epithelioma. (Patient of Professor Duperrat, Paris.)

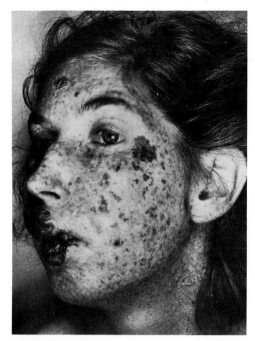

Figure 23–5 Appearance of various squamous cell epitheliomas in xeroderma pigmentosum. (Patient of Professor Duperrat, Paris.)

death from widespread metastases or present a slow and benign evolution, which is in contrast to their obvious malignancy (Ronchese, 1953).

Where they exist, ocular manifestations arise slowly. Mental debility is revealed through progressive deterioration. Spastic paralysis appears, and with the growth of the child, endocrine alterations become apparent and are manifested as gonadal underdevelopment and dwarfism.

Frequently xeroderma pigmentosum is fatal within 10 years, and two-thirds of the patients die before they are 20 years old. However, instances of survival until age 70 have been reported (Herxheimer, 1908). The causes of death normally are neoplastic cachexia through multiple metastases of a squamous cell carcinoma or a malignant melanoma, hemorrhages, secondary meningitis due to a neoplastic invasion (Hadida et al., 1963), and intercurrent diseases like tuberculosis (Hoede, 1960). If the patient is watched regularly, however, early treatment of tumors and protection from sunlight can contribute to a considerable extension of survival.

Within the same family, notable varia-tions have been described in the survival of those affected (Lemaire and Gaumond, 1965).

Cutaneous Symptomatology

In speaking about the natural history of the process, we have mentioned the phases through which the lesions pass in their evolution, which can be characterized as follows:

The first phase is characterized by the appearance of blotches of spring or summer erythema after exposure to the sun. The erythema can be accompanied by edema (which can be pseudoerysipelatous) and by vesiculobullous eruptions which exude liquid and impetiginize; moreover, there can be congestive conjunctivitis with photophobia of the eyes. Already at this stage, which is reversible, the paradoxical intensity of the symptomatology is very evident when compared with the short period of exposure to the sun.

After the inflammatory phase the freckles develop: these can be round, oval, or irregular and either yellowish, brown, or black. If there is no further exposure to sunlight, they can disappear, but soon they become persistent and definitive, and they tend to darken. We have mentioned that they can also appear in areas which are not exposed, and they can even be seen in the perianal region (Marill, 1970). Each time more intense, the pigmentations can slowly come together in irregular plaques of greater size. They are not only to be observed on the skin but also can be seen on the lips and mouth and frequently on the conjunctivae.

The second phase includes development of vascular dilatations and angiomas, and atrophic spots. The vascular dilatations are present in the form of telangiectases, vivid red or dark in color, which appear in the areas exposed to the sun, but they can also develop in the covered regions and in the mucosa (buccal, lingual, or conjunctival). According to Goldman (1961), the angiomatous formations can correspond to the senile type of angiomas, bright red or blackish blue in color, or to more voluminous vascular tumors. Hadida et al.

(1965) described tumors on the tongue, near the tip and along the midline, which present as pyriform elevations with a red depapillated surface and a wide base, and which under the microscope reveal a picture reminiscent of telangiectatic granuloma, or benign angioendothelioma with inflammatory reaction.

The atrophic spots can appear on apparently normal skin or can follow the inflammatory elements of the previous phase. They are oval, round, or irregular, of a few millimeters in diameter, and white or occasionally pearl-colored. Their surface can be smooth or scaly, but it is always dry. They may or may not be atrophic.

The conjunction of all these manifestations gives a variegated look to the skin, which appears thinned, atrophic, and senile. This atrophy produces a peculiar facies, with a thinning of the nose; atresia at the mouth and nose, which are found to be surrounded by radiated fissures; and ectropion of the lower eyelid, which secondarily will cause conjunctivitis and keratitis.

There are no alterations in the hair. More or less serious dental malformations may exist.

Hadida et al. (1963) described lesions in the covered areas which are not usually found. They are bandlike lesions which are localized in the lumbar region and are made up of achromic spots which may or may not be atrophic.

In *the third (tumoral) phase* diverse neoplasms develop. One may be dealing with benign epithelial tumors, such as papillomas and acanthomas; with adnexal tumors, such as pilomatrixomas (Lund, 1957); or with junctional nevi (Allen, 1966). Keratoacanthomas are exceptional (Bessiere, 1960; Stevanovic,1961; Marill, 1970). One can also see every type of benign conjunctival tumor: fibromas, xanthomas, angiomas, and neuromas (Nödl, 1955a and 1955b). Lesions of the precancerous type are the most frequent.

The characteristic feature is the appearance of malignant tumors, because of which many publications refer to this phase as the cancerous period. It normally develops a year or two after onset, producing malignant neoplasms in the region of the face, affecting the eyelids,

the nose, and the nasogenian folds. Crusts and verrucous formations develop, which bleed easily on contact, together with vegetating irregular masses which can reach great size (even as much as the volume of a child's head). They are squamous cell carcinomas, which may produce lymph node metastases but which do not normally produce visceral metastases (even though this has been described in one patient by Lade and Handreke, 1960, cited by Hadida et al., 1963). On other occasions ulcerating lesions appear, which can cause widespread and profound destruction on the face; these are the penetrating basal cell carcinomas. Finally, although with less frequency, sarcomas and malignant melanomas can develop, whose evolution, as we have seen, can be either fatal or paradoxically benign.

Ocular Symptomatology

Ocular lesions caused by xeroderma pigmentosum are very important, as much for their frequency as for their gravity. They are present in approximately 80 percent of patients (Labib et al., 1961), and they have been the object of important studies, such as those of Magni (1950), Duke-Elder (1940), and El-Hefnawi and Mortada (1965). Above all, these manifestations affect the structures which are directly exposed to the sunlight. Therefore, they are frequent in the eyelids, the conjunctiva, and the epibulbar region, including the cornea; however, lesions of the iris, the lens, and the retina are exceptional.

Eyelid. In the eyelid the lesions are similar to those on the exposed skin, with modifications due to its structure and function. The pigmentation can be intense, and the atrophy causes either entropion or much more often ectropion, which secondarily produces conjunctivitis and keratitis through a lack of palpebral protection. Ectropion is especially evident in the lower eyelid, which furthermore is the most intensely affected in xeroderma pigmentosum. Normally blepharitis exists, which is accompanied by madarosis or distichia. Alterations in the tarsus can produce serious functional disorders.

The malignant tumors are most often basal cell carcinomas, although squamous cell carcinomas, sarcomas, and melanomas can also develop. These neoplasms are found particularly in the internal or external canthus, from where they progress circumferentially to the neighboring skin, infiltrating the angle of the eye and entering the orbit. Timsit (1954) described an irregular appearance of the ciliary border through coalescence of translucid miliary pearls, which are then transformed into a typical epithelioma. These pearls are frequently observed on the posterior rim of the ciliary border in the transition zone of the epithelium.

Conjunctiva. Here, likewise, lesions similar to those of the skin are observed. A more or less intense hyperemia exists, and phlyctenoid formations appear frequently. The lesions are located mainly in the bulbar conjunctiva, where they are arranged horizontally in the areas most exposed to sunlight and also in the areas of the palpebral conjunctiva uncovered by ectropion. They are accompanied by photophobia, epiphora, and blepharospasm, with a bright color and with mucopurulent secretions. Occasionally the blepharospasm is so intense that in order to examine the eye an anesthetic is necessary. All these manifestations combine in time to produce a symblepharon. The neoplasms are all epidermoid metastasizing epitheliomas, which appear with greater frequency in the region of the sclerocorneal limbus, and which raise up a fold in the conjunctiva which advances in the form of a pseudopterygium (Heine, 1906).

Cornea. Keratitis is frequent and causes ulcerations and opacities with vascularization. More serious are the neoplastic infiltrations which are present in the form of either grayish micronodules surrounded by deposits of pigment (Sulzer, cited by Hadida et al., 1963) or pannus, or leukoma, which can be benign or pseudotrachomatous in appearance, but which is epitheliomatous in fact. Superimposed infection of the corneal lesions is frequent. Malignant tumors that develop in the cornea are epidermoid epitheliomas, which, according to Reese (1951) and El-Hefnawi and Mortada (1965), can arise by invasion of the cornea by neoplasms from the limbus or, more rarely, from the malignant degeneration of a corneal ulcer.

The melanomas of the limbus, of the caruncle, and of the palpebral rim, which appear in the course of xeroderma pigmentosum, normally follow a benign evolution, but they can be malignant and cause metastases. Beside the epidermoid epitheliomas and the melanomas, some cases of sarcoma of the conjunctiva have been described. Likewise lesions of the lacrimal apparatus have been described, as has retraction of the fundus of the conjunctival sac.

One can observe atrophy in the iris, especially in the lower part (Max, 1912), and pigmentation (Alajmo, 1933; Huerkamp, 1951). Likewise, the possibility that a congenital cataract might exist has been mentioned (Dougherty, 1960). Lesions in the retina during the course of xeroderma pigmentosum are exceptional.

In terminal cases atrophy of the ocular globe can occur (Max, 1912). In the same manner secondary glaucoma through neoplastic infiltration can appear following the closing of the angle of filtration.

Neurologic Symptomatology and Other Manifestations

Neurologic manifestations are those which most frequently accompany the oculocutaneous syndrome. When, at the same time, other endocrinologic disorders exist, we have the syndrome of de Sanctis and Cacchione (1932), of which, according to Reed et al. (1965), only 22 complete, published cases exist (Fig. 23–6). The complete syndrome comprises the following:

(1) Oculocutaneous lesions of the type seen in xeroderma pigmentosum, with hypersensitivity to sunlight and early development of malignant tumors (Fig. 23–7).

(2) Microcephalia, with spastic paralysis and mental retardation progressing from deficiency to idiocy. Spastic paralysis is accompanied by alteration of reflexes and coordination, presenting a picture similar to that of Friedreich's ataxia. Also reported are speech abnormalities, deafness, dumbness (Civatte, 1936), choreal movements, facial paralysis with

contractures, and changes in ocular perception (Gawad and El-Hefnawi, 1968).

(3) Gonadal underdevelopment in males manifested objectively by testicular hypoplasia. The 17-ketosteroids in the urine are found to be consistently decreased.

(4) Dwarfism, with delay in bone maturation, together with congenital deformities. In general, the patients are poorly developed physically. Malformations of teeth are not rare.

(5) A history of maternal miscarriages is frequently found.

Incomplete forms exist in which the oculocutaneous picture accompanies only minor neurologic or endocrinologic manifestations, or merely a deficiency in body weight.

Psychologic manifestations are quite frequent in xeroderma pigmentosum, and out of 286 cases which El-Sasser et al. (1950) collected, they found such symptoms in 41. Psychologic manifestations have been studied by Hadida et al. (1963), Orusco et al. (1970), and Gawad and El-Hefnawi (1968). Some children with xeroderma pigmentosum avoid the company of other children, although this may be due to the photophobia which prevents them from playing in the open air. Frequently they are timid and may even on occasion be hostile. They are unstable and intro-

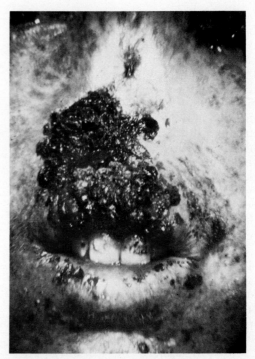

Figure 23–7 Squamous cell epithelioma in De-Sanctis-Cacchione syndrome. (Patient of Professor Nazzaro, Rome.)

verted, and they have a tendency to be melancholy. Many of them are dull and listless. According to El-Hefnawi, some relationship exists between the degree of cutaneous involvement and the importance of the neuropsychic symptoms.

The electroencephalogram (Hadida et al., 1963; Gawad and El-Hefnawi, 1968) shows modifications in the type of dysrhythmia with slow and irregular rhythms, alterations in basic pattern, and, exceptionally, signs of diffuse or irritative cerebral pain in the temporal or occipital regions (Hadida et al., 1963). Pneumoencephalography practiced once by El-Sasser showed a dilatation of the subarachnoid spaces and of the ventricles, but in 10 cases Timsit (1954) did not find any alteration.

Among diverse manifestations reported, the coexistence of xeroderma pigmentosum with the following has been mentioned: serofibrinous pericarditis (El-senber, 1890); anemia; hemoglobinuria (Gagey, 1890, cited by Lowenbach, 1905); painless polyadenopathy (Hahn and Weik, 1907); vascular alterations, such as rigidity of the radial artery in a child of four (Lesser-Bruhns, 1898, cited by Lo-

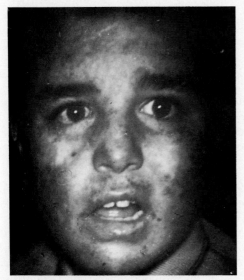

Figure 23–6 De-Sanctis-Cacchione syndrome. (Patient of Professor Cabre, Cádiz.)

wenbach, 1905); generalized amyloidosis with multiple thrombosis, pulmonary embolus, and cardiac hypertrophy seen at autopsy (Froboese, 1951); and tumor at the base of the cranium (Thomas et al., 1947).

From the dermatologic point of view, the association of xeroderma pigmentosum with keratosis suprafollicularis alba et rubra (Baumann, 1953), punctiform congenital leukoderma (Borda et al., 1955), and congenital ichthyosis (Lynch et al., 1967) has been described.

Clinical Forms

According to Hadida et al. (1963), we can distinguish the clinical forms of xeroderma pigmentosum in three ways: from the morphology of the lesions, their topographic distribution, and their mode of evolution.

Morphology. There are hyperchromic and hypochromic varieties. Among the latter, exceptional cases in which the pigmentation is completely absent deserve mention (Audry, 1907). Similarly there are predominantly atrophic forms and others with a large angiomatous component, as in the case of Goldman (1961) (see Figs. 23–3 and 23–11).

Topography. Localized forms either predominantly or exclusively affect a particular area, such as the face, which for a long time may be the only area affected. At the opposite extreme, diffuse or universal forms exist with lesions distributed throughout the whole integument (as in the case of Goldman, 1961). Finally there are inverse forms affecting the covered parts (Rollier, 1957; Hadida et al., 1963), which can be manifest as whitish lumbar lesions, and which may or may not be atrophic; or, as Rollier (1957) pointed out, they may exist in the form of atrophic, keratotic white spots with pigmentation and telangiectasis in the areas where clothes cause friction (sacro and lumbar regions).

Evolution. Acute forms begin in the first months of life and present a galloping evolution producing malignancy in the first year (Berlin, 1939; Gay Prieto and López, 1939); there are also chronic forms with slow evolution and survival for many years. Patients with the chronic form normally have few lesions, which makes the disease compatible with an almost normal life. The late form is found in the adult, sometimes even in old age. Its authenticity is questioned by various authors, since some of them consider it a keratosis with senile or presenile melanosis. It can be considered as xeroderma pigmentosum which appears late only if ocular, neurologic, or associated somatic alterations exist. As Halberstaedter (1946) correctly pointed out, the fundamental difference between these forms of senile or presenile involution of the skin and xeroderma pigmentosum is that, in the latter, the lesions are not dependent on the time or the intensity of exposure to the radiation but rather on the hypersensitivity of the individual to UV rays.

Laboratory Data and Complementary Investigations

Some authors have described a marked or moderate lymphocytosis (Berlin and Tager, 1958; Rothman, 1923) seen only during the phases of photosensitivity. Hadida et al. (1963), however, not only have not observed lymphocytosis but also in 23 or 40 cases found a figure lower than normal.

We have already mentioned El-Hefnawi's findings (1962b) of a hyper α_2-globulinemia without any other alteration of the serum proteins, which is sometimes found along with an increase in ceruloplasmin. However, for Orusco et al. (1970), this increase of the α_2-globulins was associated with an increase in the macroglobulin. Gómez Orbaneja (1971) found normal values of ceruloplasmin in two cases. El-Hefnawi and coworkers (1962c) likewise have shown the existence of abnormally high values of serum copper (the mean value being 227 mg. per 100 ml.), contrasting with abnormally low values of serum glutathione (mean value 20.9 mg. per 100 ml.). The normal values of both are 153 mg. per 100 ml. and 26.8 mg. per 100 ml., respectively, for which the proportion of Cu/Glut in the patients is of the order of 11.3, whereas in the normal subject the mean is 5.8.

In a patient studied by Gianotti (1953), the values for serum vitamin A were found to be very low, but their normalization by administering vitamin A did not lead to any improvement in the patient.

Moss (1965) observed a slight increase in the glucose-6-phosphate dehydrogenase activity in erythrocytes.

In the urine the decrease of the 17-ketosteroids and the 17-hydroxycorticosteroids with abnormal and delayed response to ACTH has already been mentioned in the section on etiology. Porphyrins are not to be found, and the figures from those who have studied them (El-Sasser et al., 1950) fall within normal ranges. Amino acid excretion is very high (El-Hefnawi and El-Hawary, 1963a) manifested as is indicated in Etiology and Pathogenesis, through greatly increased excretion of certain amino acids, less of others, and by the absence of tryptophan and valine.

Other Investigations

The results of electroencephalographic and pneumoencephalographic studies and those on photobiology have already been described in the corresponding sections. With certain authors (El-Sasser et al., 1950) radiography of the skull has regularly shown a small or closed sella turcica, whereas other authors despite systematic research have not encountered such alterations (Hadida et al., 1963). Langhof and Muting (1955) observed quantitative alterations in the content of amino acids in the skin of patients affected with xeroderma pigmentosum.

PATHOLOGY

Cutaneous Alterations

The histologic alterations of the skin in xeroderma pigmentosum are quite characteristic, although as Hadida et al. (1963) have correctly pointed out, a pathognomonic sign of the process does not exist (Figs. 23–8 to 23–11). Microscopic diagnosis can be made only by noting the appearance of various alterations, well studied by Gans (1928), Gans and Steigleder (1957), Montgomery and Reuter (1932), Montgomery (1967), Lynch (1934),

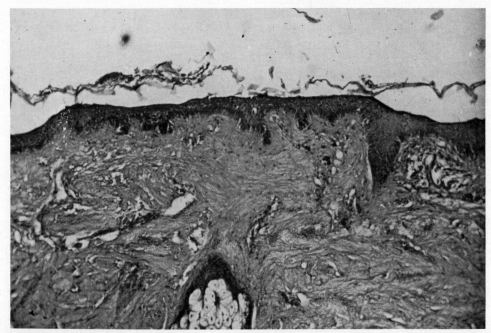

Figure 23–8 Histopathology of xeroderma pigmentosum. Initial lesion with vacuolization of the basal layer and hyperactivity of the melanocytes in the epidermal interpapillary ridges.

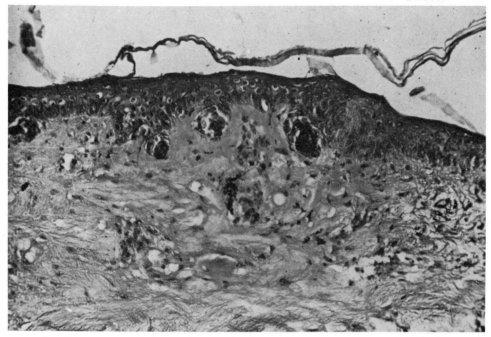

Figure 23–9 The initial appearance is similar to that of precancerous melanosis or the "malignant freckle" of Hutchinson-Dubreuilh. There is hyperplasia and hyperactivity of the melanocytes of the epidermal inter-papillary ridges, involution of the dermis, and lymphocytic reaction.

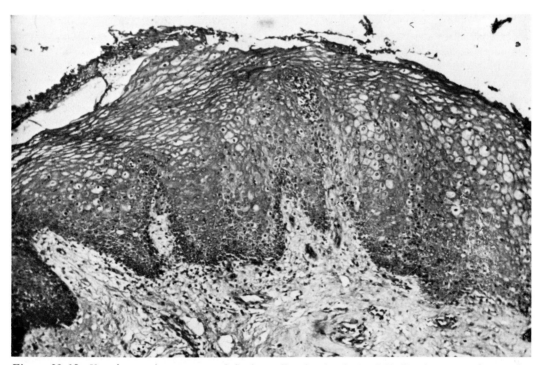

Figure 23–10 Xeroderma pigmentosum of the lower lip, showing leukoplakia-like features and a massive vasocongestive reaction in the dermis.

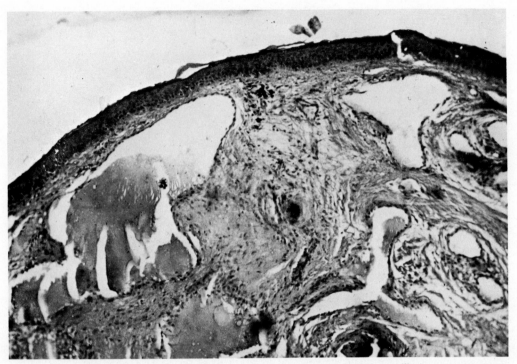

Figure 23–11 Angiomatous lesions with massive ectasia of the capillaries.

Hadida et al. (1963), and Delacrétaz (1959). As do the majority of the authors, we will distinguish three different aspects of the histologic picture which correspond to the successive clinical phases—erythematous, pigmentary, and atrophic. However, the transition between the different phases is progressive and not abrupt, so that in a particular section one can find intermediate pictures between them.

Erythematous Phase. In this phase the epidermal changes are not important unless the postirradiation reaction is intense and erythemato-vesiculobullous, in which case the modifications are similar to those of a burn with vacuolization and rupture of the cells of the germinative layer. There is vasodilation with turgescence of the endothelial cells of the capillaries, which protrude into the vascular lumen. There is edema of the papillary and mid-dermis due to permeability of the capillary walls. However, together with the exudative process, proliferative manifestations soon appear, such as histiolymphocytic infiltrates around the capillaries and the adnexae, disposed in ever denser cuffs. Occasionally the infiltrate is arranged in a thick band and oc-

cupies the papillary dermis, causing exocytosis and dissociation of the basal layer where the inflammatory infiltrate contacts the epithelium. The cells of the basal layer begin slowly to show an overload of melanin through hyperactivity of the melanocytes. Here and there a germinative cell presents cytoplasmic vacuolization and pyknosis. The collagen and the elastic fibers are not altered in this stage.

Hyperpigmentary Phase. Little by little the above modifications are accentuated. The epidermal changes become more notable. The epidermis is progressively thinned in an irregular way, and so the areas in which the epithelium has diminished in thickness alternate with other papillomatous areas in which the interpapillary processes are thin and irregular. The horny layer can be thick and presents areas of parakeratosis. The hyperpigmentation is irregular and extends from the basal layer into the malpighian layer, even reaching the granular layer; melanin granules are found in all epidermal layers.

The interpapillary ridges are sometimes very thin and elongated, and loaded with pigment, and they show the same appearance that can be observed in the senile lentigo. Some cells of the basal and the malpighian layers undergo a pseudovacuolization through intracellular edema, showing a pyknotic and retracted nucleus and occasionally karyorrhexis. The picture is common in various genodermatoses. At worst, there is loss of cellular and nuclear outlines. Edema is considerable in the dermis, which takes on a homogeneous appearance reminiscent of radiodermatitis. The inflammatory infiltrates persist and become accentuated. Phenomena of incontinentia pigmenti exist, with the presence of numerous deposits of pigment in the dermis, which are either intracellular in elongated or rounded melanophages, or extracellular in thick clumps. Likewise, in the dermis changes begin to appear which are characterized by basophilic degeneration and homogenization of the collagen, and in those areas where the inflammatory cellular infiltrate is intense, there is dissociation, thinning, and sometimes rupture of the elastic fibers which lose their habitual stain affinity.

Atrophic Phase. Here there is a regular thinning of the epidermis, which appears atrophic and has no rete ridges. The epithelium shows a tendency to cellular eosinophilia, with pseudovacuolized cytoplasm and marked nuclear pyknosis. Connective tissue changes are found to be situated mainly in the upper two-thirds of the dermis, with homogenization and basophilic fragmentation of the collagen until it acquires a markedly senile appearance. Likewise, involution of the elastic fibers is frequent, and at certain points they can disappear completely. Depending on the age of the lesions, a more or less intense sclerosis can exist, which is poor in cells. The pigment that tatoos the epidermis has disappeared. More or less dense inflammatory infiltrates can persist in the dermis. Capillaries are numerous and dilated in certain areas but absent in other areas. The adnexae may be preserved, but their disappearance is not rare, with the exception of arrector muscles and sometimes sweat glands. All these changes are variable, and there can be a discordance between the degrees of epidermal and dermal involvement.

These three phases, which characterize xeroderma pigmentosum properly speaking, lead to pre-epitheliomatous keratoses which show poikilocytosis, cytoplasmic vacuolization, poikilokaryosis, and nuclear pyknosis. A dense band of lymphocytic infiltrate is present in the dermis, containing some mast cells and on rare occasions plasmocytes. After this a kind of bowenoid carcinoma in situ slowly develops.

Finally the picture is that of a malignant tumor: basal cell carcinoma, squamous cell carcinoma, metatypical epithelioma, sarcoma, or malignant melanoma. In fact some tumors which are classified as fusocellular sarcomas are undifferentiated squamous or basal cell carcinomas.

Nödl (1955a and 1955b) insisted on the importance of the stroma reaction and on the neogenesis of sebaceous cells in xeroderma pigmentosum. In a case described by Froboese (1951), a fusocellular sarcoma which appeared in a patient who had presented numerous epitheliomas may have been an x-ray fibrosarcoma.

Each of the different benign tumors described in the course of xeroderma pigmentosum (fibromas, neuromas, angiomas, keratoacanthomas, and others) has the appropriate histologic structure, although according to Nödl (1955a and 1955b) the senile angiomas in xeroderma pigmentosum are deeper than genuine senile angiomas. Goldman (1961) pointed out a curious aspect of the cellular nuclei in fibrous tumors which gives them a pseudosarcomatous appearance, as can be seen in the connective tissue a few weeks after roentgen irradiation.

Rollier (1957), Hadida et al. (1963), and Mascaró (unpublished data) have studied the histologic structure of the skin of patients with xeroderma pigmentosum in areas which are not exposed to the sun and which are apparently healthy. The microscopic findings are of lesser intensity but similar to those observed in the areas of skin exposed to sunlight. What appears most characteristic is pseudovacuolization by intracellular edema, with pyknosis and retraction of the nuclei of some epithelial cells scattered in the epithelium, a picture which is common in a number of genodermatoses.

Ultrastructural Studies

In a very complete investigative work, Rasheed et al. (1969) found both epidermal and dermal alterations. In the epidermis there is shrinkage of the keratinocytes and widening of the intercellular spaces, degeneration and fragmentation of desmosomes, and subsequent formation of microvillus-like processes on the epidermal cell surfaces. There is also an increase in the number of the melanosomes in melanocytes. In the dermis they found marked changes of the connective fibers (collagen and elastic) similar to those found in the cutaneous elastoses. Ultrastructural differences between clinically affected and nonexposed apparently healthy skin are more quantitative than qualitative. The authors suggest that collagen fibers or their decomposition products have their part in the formation of the elastotic masses; this interpretation is concordant with the opinion of different authors on the genesis of elastic tissue in vitro (Hall, 1963–64; Hall et al., 1952 and 1955), in senile elastosis (Mitchell, 1967), and in other connective tissue diseases, such as Ehlers-Danlos syndrome (Duperrat and coworkers, 1968; Mascaró, 1970).

Ocular Alterations

In the conjunctiva the histologic picture is somewhat similar to that of the skin, with natural variations due to the different anatomic structures of each epithelium. It is of interest to point out the phenomena of cytoplasmic vacuolization (El-Hefnawi and Mortado, 1965) and pyknosis of some epithelial cells. Dilation of the capillaries, edema, and the inflammatory infiltrate (here with numerous plasmocytes) are important. Similarly there are deposits of melanin. The connective tissue presents progressive hyalinization with disappearance of the fibrils and thickening of the collagen bundles. Between the benign tumor formations, phlyctenoid proliferations, pinguecula, and pseudopterygium are to be observed, among which the degenerative changes of the connective tissue stand out. One can observe active junctional nevi with a lymphoplasmocytic infiltrate in the stroma. With regard to the malignant tumors, most of them are nonkeratinizing epidermoid epitheliomas, but malignant melanomas or fusocellular sarcomas can develop.

In the tarsus marked alterations with pseudocystical degeneration have been described (Ischrey, cited by Renard et al., 1955).

Neurologic Alterations

The autopsy of one of the first cases of xerodermic idiocy showed macroscopically an abnormally small brain and histologically a gliosis with loss of neurons of the cortex in the temporal and frontal regions. Yano (1950), who performed the autopsies on two of the cases of this particular syndrome studied and published by Mitsuda (1940), observed pathologic alterations completely similar to those which are found in Friedreich's ataxia.

DIFFERENTIAL DIAGNOSIS

In the complete form of xeroderma pigmentosum, the clinical diagnosis is easy, and there is almost no possibility of confusion. However, in the early phases with incomplete symptoms and in the atypical forms, the diagnosis may not be obvious. The only two clinical pictures that might be confused with xeroderma pigmentosum are profuse freckling—which can lead to confusion with the heterozygous form—and so-called sailor's skin, which can present difficulties in differentiation from the type of xeroderma pigmentosum that appears late in life. We have already mentioned that different authors believe that these late forms are not the same as genuine xeroderma pigmentosum and consider them to be a type of senile or presenile skin degeneration. The same authors accept as xeroderma pigmentosum only those cutaneous lesions accompanied by extracutaneous symptoms.

It is traditional to mention that in a particular case the differential diagnosis will have to be established with the Rothmund-Thomson syndrome, acrogeria, the Peutz-Touraine-Jeghers syndrome, poikiloderma of Petges-Jacobi or of Civatte, the congenital porphyria of Günther, erythropoietic protoporphyria, hydroa vacciniformis, arsenical pigmentation, scleroderma, and even mastocytosis in its urticaria pigmentosa variety. Although the similarity of the cutaneous lesions to those of chronic radiodermatitis should be pointed out, the problem of differential diagnosis in this case never presents itself in practice.

The picture of xerodermic idiocy ought to be distinguished from Friedreich's ataxia, with which at the beginning it is frequently confused because of the spastic gait and the muscular atrophy which these patients present (Reed et al., 1965). Likewise, confusion may arise with ichthyotic idiocy, which combines mental retardation and ichthyosis.

One could confuse the histologic picture with that of chronic radiodermatitis, if one did not possess the clinical data, or with a lentigo in the pigmentary phase. But, in fact, if one has a solid clinical orientation, such an error is not possible. In the early erythematous phase with hypersensitivity to light, there exists the possibility of confusing the histologic picture with that of a polymorphous light eruption, or with the Rothmund syndrome—in the first case because of the lymphoid infiltrate of the dermis, and in the second because of cellular vacuolization with pyknosis of the nuclei, histologic findings which, as we have already mentioned, are common to various genodermatoses.

TREATMENT

No effective treatment exists. The most effective approach is protection of the skin and mucous membranes by avoiding exposure to the sun and other light sources whose spectrum contains ultraviolet rays. Protection from radiation is achieved by the use of clothes which cover the greatest possible area of integument, together with hats and glasses with lenses which filter ultraviolet rays. Sunscreen creams are useful if they contain quinine,

tannin, methyl salicylate, and 25 percent titanium dioxide in vanishing cream (Rook, 1968) and American red Vaseline. We use a solution of 10 percent sulisobenzone in polyethylene glycol with good results.

General treatment, consisting of administration of chloroquine, vitamins A and C, PP (nicotinic acid, nicotinamide), corticoids, resorcin, gonadotropin, urethane, or nitrogen mustard (Johne and Timper, 1950), which have been used by different authors, has not achieved any appreciable results. Perry et al. (1970) tried penicillamine, since this has yielded good results in the hepatolenticular degeneration of Wilson, which presents as hypercupremia; however, one is still not able to judge its effectiveness in xeroderma pigmentosum. The administration of antibiotics is often useful, since the existence of superimposed infection is not rare.

It is very important to supervise the patient regularly, so that one is prepared to excise or destroy malignant tumors or the precancerous lesions. In lesions of the precancerous keratosis type, cryotherapy with carbon dioxide or liquid nitrogen, or electrocoagulation followed by curettage can be used. But these methods have been superseded by the use of 1 or 2 percent 5-fluorouracil in propylene glycol, which gives excellent results (Perry et al., 1970; Carter et al., 1968), and application on wide surfaces manages to destroy subclinical keratoses.

Electrocoagulation, surgical excision, ionizing radiation, or chemosurgery can be used for more extensive lesions. The use of ionizing radiation (radiotherapy, radium therapy, ^{32}P, cobalt therapy) is discouraged by numerous authors, since radiation tends to aggravate the lesions of the dermis and can stimulate the formation of sarcomas. However, in many cases in the treatment of epitheliomas it has been used with success. Mohs' chemosurgery is indicated for penetrating epitheliomas. Beirne and Wheeless (1956) have successfully used skin planing. In multiple epitheliomas with diffuse involvement of the facial skin, monobloc resections of the skin of the face have been practiced (Woolf et al., 1959; Martins, 1964; Grinspan, 1970).

As a prophylactic measure one has to warn the family against consanguineous marriages and point out that the patient should not receive photosensitizing drugs (PAS, Gonacrine, griseofulvin) (Hadida et al., 1963). However, psoralens—8-methoxypsoralen, 10 mg. three times a day (Hopkins, 1959), and trimethylpsoralen, 5 mg. a day for four weeks (Becker, 1960) —have been used, and although in the initial phase they act as photosensitizers and aggravate the condition, they soon show a protective action in developing a pigmentary protective barrier.

In every case the therapeutic method should be chosen in relation to the type and the size of the neoplasm, but also in relation to the age of the patient and the areas affected.

For incipient ocular lesions, local and general steroid therapy is useful and improves the keratoconjunctivitis. In malignant ocular tumors, depending on their location, electrolysis, diathermocoagulation, excision, or ionizing radiations may be indicated. It may be necessary to enucleate the eye in cases of invasive tumors.

PROGNOSIS

The general prognosis of xeroderma pigmentosum is gloomy. When referring to the natural history of the process, we said that death occurs frequently within 10 years and that two-thirds of patients die before they are 20 years old. Nevertheless, death does not always occur; there is a certain relation between the age at which the initial symptoms occur and the gravity and rapidity of the disease's evolution. Patients who show early symptoms will probably die before adulthood. On the other hand, when the symptoms occur late, evolution of the disease is normally slower. Atypical forms with hypersensitivity to light and profuse freckles are compatible with a prolonged and practically normal life (Anderson and Begg, 1950). If prophylactic and therapeutic measures are established and rigorous control is exercised, it is possible to achieve a longer survival than would be the case if the patient were left to his fate.

ACKNOWLEDGMENTS

Thanks are offered to Professors Duperrat (Paris), Hadida (Marseille), Nazzaro (Rome), Offret (Paris), Piñol (Barcelona), Cabré (Cádiz), and Sayag (Marseille) and to Doctors Dhermy (Paris) and Marill (Argel) for their help and material (histologic slides and photographs) which made possible the writing of this chapter.

REFERENCES

Alajmo, B.: Rass. Ital. Ottal., 2:695, 1933, cited by El-Hefnawi and Mortada (1965).

Allen, A. C.: The Skin. A clinico-pathological treatise. New York, Grune & Stratton, 1966, p. 849.

Anderson, T. E., and Begg, M.: Xeroderma pigmentosum of mild type. Br. J. Dermatol., 62:402, 1950.

Andrade, R.: Die praecanceröse und canceröse Wucherung von Epidermis und Anhangsgebilden. *In* Gans, O., and Steigleder, G. K.: Handbuch der Haut- und Geschlechtskrankheiten. Vol. 1, Part 2. Berlin, Springer-Verlag, 1964, p. 344.

Archambault: De la dermatosi de Kaposi (xeroderma pigmentosum). Thèse, Bordeaux, 1890.

Ashurst, P. J.: Hydroa vacciniforme occurring in association with Hartnup disease. Br. J. Dermatol., 81:486, 1969.

Audry, C.: Sur un cas de xeroderma pigmentosum sans pigmentation. Ann. Dermatol. Syphiligr. (Paris), 8:199, 1907.

Ballarini, M.: Considerazioni su due casi di xeroderma pigmentoso famigliare. Arch. Ital. Dermatol. Sif. Venereol., 14:595, 1938.

Baumann, R.: Xeroderma pigmentosum und keratosis suprafollicularis alba et rubra. Hautarzt, 4:338, 1953.

Becker, S. W., Pautrier, L. M., and Woringer, F.: A case of xeroderma pigmentosum. Arch. Dermatol. Syph., 25:915, 1932.

Becker, S. W., in discussion of Rostemberg, A.: Xeroderma pigmentosum. Arch. Dermatol. Syph., 81:631, 1960.

Beirne, G. A., and Wheeless, J.: Xeroderma pigmentosum. Arch. Dermatol. Syph., 74:112, 1956.

Bering, F., and Barnewitz, J.: Xeroderma pigmentosum. *In* Jadassohn, J.: Handbuch der Haut- und Geschlechtskrankheiten. Berlin, Springer-Verlag, 1932, p. 128.

Berlin, C.: Xeroderma pigmentosum. Recherche sur la sensibilité de la peau à l'égard des divers rayons. Rev. Fr. Dermatol. Venereol., 5:213, 1938.

Berlin, C.: Zentralbl. Hautkrankh., 61:61, 1939.

Berlin, C., and Tager, A.: Xeroderma pigmentosum. Report of eight cases of mild to moderate type and course: A study of response to various irradiations. Dermatologica, 116:27, 1958.

Bessière, L.: Kérato-acanthomes et xeroderma pigmentosum. Bull. Soc. Fr. Dermatol. Syphiligr., 67:1012, 1960.

Borda, J. M., Grageb, H., and Abulafia, J.: Xeroderma pigmentosum y leucodermia punteada congénita. Arch. Argent. Dermatol., 5:95, 1955.

Burk, P. G., Lutzner, M. A., and Robbins: Clin. Res., 28:346, 1970.

Canright, C. M.: Xeroderma pigmentosum. Arch. Dermatol. Syph., 29:668, 1934.

Carney, J. W.: Discussion d'une présentation de Obermeyer et Storkan. Arch. Dermatol. Syph., 69:236, 1954.

Carter, V. H., Smith, K. W., and Noojin, R. O.: Xeroderma pigmentosum. Treatment with topically applied FU. Arch. Dermatol. Syph., 98:526, 1968.

Civatte, A.: Xeroderma pigmentosum. Nouv. Prat. Derm., 6:629, 1936.

Cleaver, J. E.: Defective repair replication of DNA in xeroderma pigmentosum. Nature (Lond.), 218:652, 1968.

Cockayne, E. A.: Inherited Abnormalities of the Skin and its Appendages. London, Oxford University Press, 1933.

Cripps, D. J., and Ramsay, C. A.: Xeroderma pigmentosum. Abnormal monochromatic spectrum action and autoradiographic studies. Abstract. 31st annual meeting, Society for Investigative Dermatology, Chicago, 1970.

Czerniak, P.: Xeroderma pigmentosum. Harefuah, 46:260, 1954.

Degos, R.: Dermatologie. Paris, Flammarion, 1953, p. 718b.

Delacrétaz, J.: Les états pré-épitheliomatheux cutanés. Rapports du X Congrès des Dermatologistes et Syph. de Langue Française, Alger, 1959, p. 41.

de Sanctis, C., and Cacchione, A.: L'idioza xerodermica. Riv. Sper, di Frenita, 56:269, 1932.

Dorn, H.: Xeroderma pigmentosum. Acta Genet. Med., 8:395, 1959.

Dougherty, J. W., in discussion Diagnosis: Xeroderma pigmentosum? Arch. Dermatol. Syph., 81:1029, 1960.

Duke-Elder, W. S.: Textbook of Ophthalmology. Vol. 2. London, Kimpton, 1940.

Duperrat, B., Vanbremeersch, F., and Mascaro, J. M.: Le syndrome d'Ehlers-Danlos. XII Congrés des Dermatologistes de Langue Française, Paris, June, 1965. Paris, Masson et cie, 1968, p. 115.

El-Hefnawi, H., and El-Hawary, M. F. S.: Chromatographic studies of amino acids in sera and urine of patients with xeroderma pigmentosum and their normal relatives. Br. J. Dermatol., 75:235, 1963a.

El-Hefnawi, H., and El-Hawary, M. F. S.: Studies of serum transaminases in xeroderma pigmentosum. J. Invest. Dermatol., 41:479, 1963b.

El-Hefnawi, H., and Mortada, A.: Ocular manifestations of xeroderma pigmentosum. Br. J. Dermatol., 77:261, 1965.

El-Hefnawi, H., and Rasheed, A. J. Egypt. Med. Assoc., 45(Suppl.):106, 1962, cited by El-Hefnawi and Mortada (1965).

El-Hefnawi, H., and Smith, S. M.: Xeroderma pigmentosum. A brief report on its genetic linkage with ABO blood groups in the United Arab Republic. Br. J. Dermatol., 77:35, 1965.

El-Hefnawi, H., El-Nabawi, M., and Rasheed, A.: Xeroderma pigmentosum. I. A clinical study of 12 Egyptian cases. Br. J. Dermatol., 74:201, 1962a.

El-Hefnawi, H., El-Nabawi, M., and El-Hawary, M. F. S.: Xeroderma pigmentosum. II. Electrophoretic studies of serum proteins. Br. J. Dermatol., 74:214, 1962b.

El-Hefnawi, H., El-Nabawi, M., and El-Hawary, M. F. S.: Xeroderma pigmentosum. III. Studies of serum copper and blood glutathione. Br. J. Dermatol., 74:218, 1962c.

El-Hefnawi, H., El-Hawary, M. F. S., El-Komy, H. M., and Rasheed, A.: Xeroderma pigmentosum. V. Studies of 17-ketosteroids and total 17-hydroxycorticosteroids. Br. J. Dermatol., 75:484, 1963.

El-Mofty, A. M., El-Hawary, M. F. S., and Farag, F. B.: J. Egypt. Med. Assoc., 44:13, 1961, cited by El-Hefnawi et al. (1962c).

El-Sasser, G., Freusberg, O., and Thieml, F.: Das Xeroderma pigmentosum und die "xerodermische Idiotie." Arch. Dermatol. Syph. (Berl.), 188:651, 1950.

Elsenber, A.: Xeroderma pigmentosum (Kaposi) melanosis lenticularis progressiva (Pick). Arch. Dermatol. Syph., 22:49, 1890.

Esteller, J., Forteza, G., and Sorni, G.: Estudio citogenético de dos casos de xeroderma pigmentosum y uno de queratodermia de Brauer. Act. Dermosifiliogr. (Madr.), 55:520, 1964.

Esteller, J., Forteza, G., and Sorni, G.: Estudios citogenéticos en el xeroderma pigmentosum. Dermatol. Ibero Lat. Am., 8:1953, 1966.

Feuerstein, M., and Langhof, H.: Untersuchungen über die freien Aminosäuren im Harn und den Aminosäurengehalt der Haare bei Xeroderma pigmentosum. Arch. Klin. Exp. Dermatol., 220:486, 1964.

Froboese, C.: Über das Xeroderma pigmentosum blastomatosum malignum. Gaz. Med. Portug., 4:593, 1951.

Gans, O.: Histologie der Hautkrankheiten. Vol. 2. Berlin, Springer-Verlag, 1928.

Gans, O., and Steigleder, G. K.: Histologie der Hautkrankheiten. Ed. 2. Berlin, Springer-Verlag, 1957.

Gawad, M. S. A., and El-Hefnawi, H.: Neuropsychiatric manifestations in xeroderma pigmentosum. XIII Congressus Int. Derm. München, 1967. Vol. I. Berlin, Springer-Verlag, 1968, p. 654.

Gay Prieto, J., and López, B.: Xeroderma pigmentosum con tumoraciones múltiples en un niño de 23 meses de edad. Act. Dermo-sifiliogr. (Madr.), 30:644, 1939.

Gianotti, F.: Esperienza terapeutica con vitamina A e successivamente con ormoni gonadotropici e testosterone in un caso di xeroderma pigmentoso. G. Ital. Dermatol., 94:209, 1953.

Goldman, L.: Features uncommon to xeroderma pigmentosum. Case report with a study of 92 biopsy specimens. Arch. Dermatol. Syph., 83:272, 1961.

Goldman, L., and Owens, P. L.: Chromosome studies in dermatology. Acta Derm. Venereol. (Stockh.), 44:68, 1964.

Gómez Orbaneja, J.: Personal communication, 1971.

Grinspan, D.: Estudios genéticos en varias dermatosis. VI Congreso Ibero Latino Americano Dermat., Barcelona, 1967. Barcelona, Edit. Cientifico Medica, 1970, p. 269.

Hadida, E., Marill, F. G., and Sayag, J.: Xeroderma pigmentosum (A propos de 48 observations personnelles). Ann. Dermatol. Syphiligr. (Paris), 90:467, 1963.

Hadida, E., Marill, F. G., and Sayag, J.: Tumeurs bénignes de la langue au cours du xeroderma pigmentosum. Bull. Soc. Fr. Dermatol. Syphiligr., 72:168, 1965.

Hahn, G., and Weik, H.: Zwei Fälle von Xeroderma pigmentosum, mit experimentellen Untersuchungen über die Einwirkung verschiedener Lichtarten. Arch. Dermatol. Syph. (Berl.), 88:371, 1907.

Halberstaedter, L.: Skin carcinoma of xeroderma pigmentosum, seaman's skin, and x-ray dermatitis. Acta Med. Orient. (Tel-Aviv), 4:279, 1945. Abstracted in Year Book of Dermatology, Chicago, Year Book Medical Publishers, 1946, p. 333.

Haldane, J. B. S.: Ann. Eugen. (Lond.), 7:28, 1936, cited by El-Hefnawi et al. (1962a).

Hall, D. A.: International Review of Connective Tissue Research. Vols. 1 and 2. New York, Academic Press, 1963–64.

Hall, D. A., Reed, R., and Tunbridge, R. E.: Structure of elastic tissue. Nature (Lond.), 170:264, 1952.

Hall, D. A., Keech, M. K., Reed, R., Saxl, H., Tunbridge, R. E., and Wood, M. J.: Collagen and elastin in connective tissue. J. Gerontol., 10:388, 1955.

Heine, L.: Klin. Monatsbl. Augenheilkd., 44:460, 1906.

Herxheimer, H.: Présentation d'un cas de xeroderma pigmentosum à la séance de la Soc. Allemande de Dermatologie. 10 Juillet 1908. Arch. Dermatol. Syph. (Berl.), 91:378, 1908.

Hoede, K.: Hdb. Erbbiol., 3:455, 1940.

Hoede, K.: Erbkrankheiten mit Ausnahme von Ichtyosis und Follikularkeratosen. In Gottron, H. A., and Schönfeld, W. (Eds.): Dermatologie und Venereologie. Stuttgart, Thieme, V. 1960, p. 48.

Holmberg, C. G., and Laurell, C. B.: Acta Chem. Scand., 2:550, 1948.

Hopkins, C. E.: Psoralen prophylaxis against skin cancer: Progress of field trials. J. Invest. Dermatol., 32:383, 1959.

Hopkins, R., and Van Studdiford, M. T.: Multiple epitheliomas and pigmentary dermatosis in a Negro boy. Arch. Dermatol. Syph., 29:408, 1934.

Huerkamp, B.: Irisschwund bei Xeroderma pigmentosum. Klin. Monatsbl. Augenheilkd., 119:286, 1951.

Johne, H. O., and Timper, R.: Über Xeroderma pigmentosum. Z. Haut. Geschlechtskr., 9:89, 1950.

Jonquieres, E. D. L., Mazzini, M. A., and Sanchez Caballero, H. J.: Actinodermatitis papulofigurada eritematoide recidivante. Arch. Argent. Dermatol., 8:105, 1958.

Kamimura and Sato (1963), cited by Piñol-Aguade et al. (1968).

Kaposi, M.: Xeroderma pigmentosum. Wiener Mediz. Jahrbücher, October, 1882. Reprinted in French by Ann. Dermatol. Syphiligr. (Paris), 4:29, 1883.

Kesten, B. M., and Slatkin, M. H.: Xeroderma pig-

mentosum exhibiting skin reactions in the shorter ultraviolet wavelengths. Arch. Dermatol. Syph., 65:248, 1952.

King, H.: Xeroderma pigmentosum in a Negress. Arch. Dermatol. Syph., 42:570, 1940.

Koller, P. C.: Inheritance of xeroderma and its chromosome mechanism. Br. J. Cancer, 2:149, 1948.

Korn-Heydt, G. E.: Erbliche Aplasien, Hyperplasien und Tumoren. In Jadassohn, J. (Ed.): Handbuch der Haut- und Geschlechtskrankheiten. Berlin, Springer-Verlag, 1966, p. 611.

Labib, M. A., Barrada, A., Choukry, I., and El-Komi, M.: Bull. Soc. Ophthalmol. Egypt., 54:51, 1961.

Lack, H.: Xeroderma pigmentosum blastomatosum malignum with lung involvement. Strahlentherapie, 113:264, 1960.

Langhof, H.: Aminosäurebestimmung bei Lichtdermatosen. Arch. Dermatol. Syph. (Berl.), 200:86, 1955.

Langhof, H., and Muting, D.: Über Aminosäurenhaushalt und Therapie der Lichtdermatosen. Hautarzt, 6:27, 1955.

Larmande, A.: A propos de 20 cas de xeroderma pigmentosum. Algérie Méd., 59:557, 1955.

Lee, M. F.: Ocular manifestations in xeroderma pigmentosum with report of three cases. Chinese Med. J., 73:429, 1955.

Lemaire, M., and Gaumond, E.: Xéroderma pigmentosum. Huit cas d'évolution différente dans deux familles. Can. Med. Assoc. J., 92:406, 1965.

Lipkin, G., Hermann, F., and Mandol, L.: Studies on serum copper. II. The copper levels in relation to corticosteroid administration. J. Invest. Dermatol., 39:547, 1962.

Lorincz, A. L.: Pigmentation. In Rothman, S. (Ed.): Physiology and Biochemistry of the Skin. Chicago, University of Chicago Press, 1954.

Loewenthal, L. J. A.: S. Afr. Med. J., 30:984, 1956.

Loewenthal, L. J. A., and Trowel: Xeroderma pigmentosum in African Negroes. Br. J. Dermatol., 50:66, 1938.

Lowenbach, G.: Xeroderma pigmentosum. In Mradcek, Handbuch der Hautkrankheiten, 3:240, 1905.

Luger, A.: Experimental studies on the causal genesis of xeroderma pigmentosum. Arch. Klin. Exp. Dermatol., 214:432, 1962.

Lund, H. Z.: Tumors of the skin. In Atlas of Tumor Pathology. Washington, D.C., Armed Forces Institute of Pathology, 1957, p. 157.

Lynch, F. W.: Xeroderma pigmentosum, a study in sensitivity to light. Arch. Dermatol. Syph., 29:858, 1934.

Lynch, H. T., Anderson, D. E., Krush, A. J., and Mukerjee, D.: Cancer, heredity and genetic counseling. Xeroderma pigmentosum. Cancer, 20:1796, 1967.

Macklin, M. T.: Xeroderma pigmentosum. Arch. Dermatol. Syph., 34:656, 1936.

Macklin, M. T.: Xeroderma pigmentosum. Arch. Dermatol. Syph., 49:157, 1944.

Macklin, M. T.: Xeroderma pigmentosum; additional notes on 6 cases of Dr. Mayrand and Dr. Gaumond. Arch. Dermatol. Syph., 52:176, 1945.

Magni, S.: Le manifestazioni oculari nello xeroderma pigmentoso (Rilievi clinici ed istopatologici). Boll. Oculist., 29:84, 1950.

Marill, F. G.: Personal communication, 1970.

Martins, A. G.: Sobre xerodermia pigmentosa. Acerca dum caso de extirpaçao de pele da face en monobloco. J. Soc. Ciénc. Med. Lisboa, 128:759, 1964.

Mascaró, J. M.: Acción del complejo enzimático elastasa sobre las fibras orceinófilas del tejido conjuntivo. Actas del VI Congreso Ibero Latino Americano de Dermatologia, Barcelona, 1967. Barcelona, Edit. Cientifico-Medica, 1970, p. 209.

Max, W.: Klin. Monatsbl. Augenheilkd., 50:750, 1912.

Mehregan, A. H.: Dermatitis solaris related to xeroderma pigmentosum. Arch. Dermatol. Syph., 87:469, 1963.

Mitchell, R. E.: Chronic solar dermatosis: A light and electron microscopic study of the dermis. J. Invest. Dermatol., 48:203, 1967.

Mitsuda, H.: Xeroderma pigmentosum with disturbances of central nervous system. Psychiatr. Neurol. Jap., 44:7, 1940.

Montgomery, H.: Dermatopathology. Vol. 1. New York, Harper & Row, 1967. p. 123.

Montgomery, H., and Reuter, M. J.: Xeroderma pigmentosum; report of mild case with histopathologic studies. Arch. Dermatol. Syph., 26:256, 1932.

Moss, H. V., Jr.: Xeroderma pigmentosum. Arch. Dermatol. Syph., 92:638, 1965.

Muting, D.: Über die Aminosäurenzusammensetzung gesunder und kranker menschlicher Haut. Klin. Wochenschr., 31:618, 1953.

Nabarro, J. D. N.: *In* McGowan, G. K., and Sandler, M. (Eds.): The Adrenal Cortex. London, Pitman, 1960, cited by El-Hefnawi et al. (1963).

Neisser, A.: Über das Xeroderma pigmentosum (Kaposi). Lioderma essentialis cum melanosis et telangiectasis. Wschr. Dermatol. Syph., 47:1883.

Nödl, F.: Über mesenchymale und epitheliale Neubildungen bei xeroderma pigmentosum. Arch. Dermatol. Syph. (Berl.), 199:287, 1955a.

Nödl, F.: Über echte Neurome bei Xeroderma pigmentosum. Arch. Klin. Exp. Dermatol., 201:277, 1955b.

Orusco, M., Catanzano, and Baumes: Xeroderma pigmentosum. Actas VI Congreso Ibero Latino Americano de Dermatologia, Barcelona, 1967. Barcelona, Edit. Cientifico-Medica, 1970, p. 239.

Perry, H. O., MacCall, J. T., and Goldstein, N. P.: Tratamiento del xeroderma pigmentoso con penicilamina y 5-fluorouracilo. Actas VI Congreso Ibero Latino Americano de Dermatologia, Barcelona, 1967. Barcelona, Edit. Cientifico-Medica, 1970, p. 379.

Piñol-Aguade, J., Esteller, J., Aliaga, A., and Gimferrer, E.: Citogenética en dermatologia. Barcelona, Edit. Cientifico-Medica, 1968.

Raphael, S. A., Martin, J., Inwood, J., and Fimlt, F.: Xeroderma pigmentosum. The Human Chromosome Newsletter, 4:9, 1961.

Rasheed, A., El-Hefnawi, H., Nagy, G., and Wiskemann, A.: Elektronenmikroskopische Untersuchungen bei Xeroderma pigmentosum. Arch. Klin. Exp. Dermatol., 234:321, 1969.

Reed, W. B., May, S. B., and Nickel, W. R.: Xeroderma pigmentosum with neurological complications. The de Sanctis-Cacchione syndrome. Arch. Dermatol. Syph., 91:224, 1965.

Reese, A. B. (1951), cited by El-Hefnawi and Mortada (1965).

Reese, A. B., and Wilbur, I. E.: Am. J. Ophthalmol., 26:901, 1943.

Renard, G., Lelièvre, A., and Bierent, P.: A propos d'un cas de xeroderma pigmentosum. Presse Med., 63:313, 1955.

Rollier, R.: Aspects cliniques et histologiques des régions cutanées non isolées dans le xeroderma pigmentosum. Bull. Soc. Fr. Dermatol. Syphiligr., 3:280, 1957.

Ronchese, F.: Melanomata pathologically malignant, clinically nonmalignant, in a case of xeroderma pigmentosum. Arch. Dermatol. Syph., 68:355, 1953.

Rook, A., and Wells, R. S.: Genetics in dermatology. *In* Rook, A., Wilkinson, D. S., and Ebling, F. J. G. (Eds.): Textbook of Dermatology. Vol. 1. Oxford, Blackwell, 1968.

Rothman, S.: Untersuchungen über Xeroderma pigmentosum. Arch. Dermatol. Syph. (Berl.), 144:440, 1923.

Rouvière, G.: Xeroderma pigmentosum. Thèse, Université de Toulouse, 1910.

Rowe, L.: Essential amino acids and disease processes. Arch. Dermatol. Syph., 81:405, 1960.

Schuermann, H.: Zblt. Hautkrankh., 59:248, 1938.

Siemens, H. W., and Kohn, E.: Studien über Verernung von Hautkrankheiten. IX. Xeroderma pigmentosum (mit mitteibung von 5 neuen Fällen). Z. Indukt. Abstamm. Vererb.-L., 38:1, 1925.

Silberberg, I., abstracted in Year Book of Dermatology, 1970, p. 209.

Stevanovic, D.: Keratoacantome in Xeroderma pigmentosum. Arch. Dermatol. Syph., 84:53, 1961.

Thomas, A., Puech, Naudascher, Rouault de la Vigne: Xeroderma pigmentosum associé à une tumeur de la base du crâne. Rev. Neurol. (Paris), 79:57, 1947.

Timsit, E.: Contribution à l'étude des manifestations oculaires du xeroderma pigmentosum. Thèse, Alger, Decembre, 1954.

Van Patten, H. T., and Drummond, J. A.: Malignant melanoma occurring in xeroderma pigmentosum; report of a case. Cancer, 6:942, 1953.

Veldhuisen, G., and Poowels, P. H.: Transformation of xeroderma pigmentosum cells by SV_{40}. Lancet, 2:529, 1970.

Vidal, E., and Leloir, H.: De la dermatose de Kaposi (xeroderma pigmentosum). Ann. Dermatol. Syphiligr. (Paris), 4:621, 1883.

Vilanova, X.: Xeroderma pigmentosum retardado hereditario. Ecos Esp. Derm., 8:57, 1932.

Woolf, R., Kepes, J., Giorgiade, N., and Pickrell, K.: Xeroderma pigmentosum. Report of a case treated by total resurfacing of the face. Plast. Reconstr. Surg., 24:214, 1959.

Yano, K.: Xeroderma pigmentosum mit Störungen des ZNS. Folia Psychiatr. Neurol. Jap., 4:143, 1950.

24

Epidermodysplasia Verruciformis

A. Poiares Baptista, M.D., and A. Bastos Araújo, M.D.

Lewandowsky and Lutz described epidermodysplasia verruciformis (E.V.) in 1922 as a rare skin disease characterized by wartlike eruptions, often of a familiar character and generally starting in infancy, of which a high percentage develops into cancer.

Initially, it was considered an autonomous etiologic entity, like genodermatosis; today it has been proved to be a virus infection of the verruca vulgaris type ("verrucosis generalisata" – Hoffmann) with clinical and evolutionary characteristics sui generis conditioned by genetic factors.

CLINICAL DESCRIPTION

E.V. is often characterized by papulous, scaly lesions of various sizes, in groups or isolated. The smallest lesions are circular, oval, or polygonal papules measuring 2 to 5 mm. in diameter; they have distinct, well-defined borders limiting a smooth, slightly elevated surface without appreciable infiltration. For the most part, such lesions are covered with

thin, whitish-grey, or somewhat thicker yellowish, fatty scales, depending upon the location. When discarded, the scales leave fine furrows or wrinkles in polygonal facets on the smooth surface. In some places, the confluence of the papules gives rise to plaques, 1 to 3 cm. in diameter, of an irregular polycyclic outline (Figs. 24–1 and 24–2).

The color of the lesions, which varies from light pink to dark red according to location, disappears on vitropressure. According to Ferreira Marques and Vidal (1948), there is intense fluorescence on examination under Wood's light.

The skin between the lesions is normal, but in some cases it is brownish and covered with furfuraceous, pityriasic scales. On other occasions, the skin is slightly thickened and has a lichenified aspect.

Some lesions can take on particular aspects morphologically as well as topographically. Thus, if scales are absent, the papules may resemble those of juvenile verruca plana, especially if they are on the face or the dorsa of the hands. A small central umbilication can simulate lichen planus. In other cases, a verrucous sur-

596

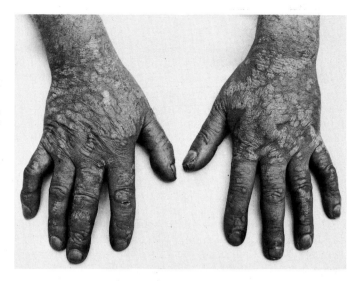

Figure 24–1 Confluent verrucous lesions of dorsa of the hands. There is a reticulated pattern in some areas. (*From* Degos and Baptista: Bull. Soc. Fr. Dermatol. Syphiligr., *64*:279, 1957.)

face can give the papules of E.V. the aspect of verruca vulgaris or senile keratosis (Lewandowsky and Lutz, 1922); the thickness and the abundance of the scales in some lesions suggest psoriasiform lesions. Sometimes, the papules assume a ringlike, netlike, or bandlike appearance, resembling a real Koebner phenomenon

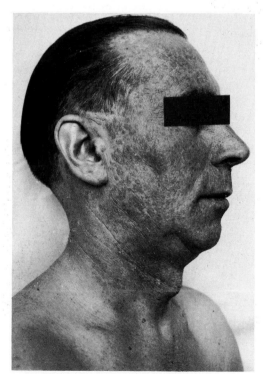

Figure 24–2 Papular and verruciform lesions of the face and neck. (*From* Degos and Baptista: Bull. Soc. Fr. Dermatol. Syphiligr., *64*:279, 1957.)

(Jablonska et al., 1966). Cases have been described resembling pityriasis lichenoides (Midana, 1949; Bizzozero, 1942); pagetoid basal cell epithelioma (Grinspan et al., 1949); xeroderma pigmentosum (Bizzozero, 1942; Midana, 1949); Darier's disease and Pringle's sebaceous adenomas (Chiale, 1942); sebaceous nevus; porokeratosis of Mibelli; pityriasis versicolor; erythema elevatum diutinum (Degos et al., 1953, 1957a, and 1957b); and so forth. On the palms and soles, the lesions appear to be those of verruca vulgaris or can be confused with them. On the scalp yellowish, fatty, adhering scales have been observed, almost never associated with papules.

Not infrequently, typical E.V. lesions are associated with other cutaneous lesions, such as *pigmented macules,* which are pink-brown, well-defined, flat, frecklelike, and usually located in the face (Hamdi and Hulusi, 1933; Ferriera Marques and Vidal, 1948); *pigmented nevi,* which are found in great numbers in variable locations, but principally on the face; *senile keratosis* and *senile skin;* and *palmoplantar keratosis* (two cases with hereditary factors, Teodorescu et al., 1949). The relationship between E.V. and condyloma acuminatum, neurodermatitis, eczema, facial edema, and macrocheilitis is difficult to determine. This polymorphism of the lesions found in the majority of published cases contrasts with the monomorphism of the histology, which has been stressed by Chiale (1942), Midana (1949), and Poiares Baptista (1957).

LOCATION

E.V. is nearly always generalized over the whole cutaneous integument and symmetrically disposed. However, there are sites of predilection, which in some cases are exclusive: (1) the dorsa of the hands and fingers (very common as site of onset) (Fig. 24–1); (2) the extensor surfaces of the forearms; (3) the neck (lateral aspects and nape of the neck in particular); (4) the face (forehead, temples, cheeks, and chin) (Fig. 24–2); (5) the thorax: the dorsal (upper part), pre-sternal, and clavicular areas; and (6) the dorsa of the feet and the extensor surfaces of the legs. Nevertheless, atypical sites are indicated in the literature: abdomen, eyelids, lips, breasts, dorsum of the penis, popliteal areas, thighs, elbows, knees, the perianal area, and so forth.

The mucosae and semimucosae can also be sites of the lesions, although this is rare: reported areas of occurrence include the balanopreputial fold, the lips of the urinary meatus (Louste et al., 1934), the palate, and the tip of the tongue (Midana, 1949). Histologically, such lesions are identical with cutaneous lesions. In general, the skin appendages are unaffected.

CONDITIONS OF ONSET

Usually E.V. occurs before the age of 15 years; less frequently, it is congenital or occurs in the adult.

In some cases the disease follows immediately upon a variety of other diseases, such as measles, whooping cough, pneumonia, diphtheria, furunculosis, brain traumas, sunstroke, and digestive upsets. It is conceivable that these factors act as site or "terrain" modifiers.

The *initial lesions* can, at the very onset, show the appearance already described. However, Wise and Satenstein (1939) described the primary lesions as similar to those of verruca vulgaris, 1 to 2 mm. in diameter, flat or slightly scaly, isolated or in groups, with a histology similar to that of the verruga vulgaris lesion but showing hollow cells in the basal layer of the epidermis. Rechter and Castañe (1945), on the other hand, referred to the primary lesions as "erythematous lentil-shaped macules, which after 10 days become more difficult to distinguish and take on a characteristic appearance." Such lesions can be generalized, appearing as an eruption, or limited to certain areas of the skin (the dorsa of the hands, the forearms, the face, the neck, the dorsa of the feet).

EVOLUTION

Once established, the lesions can become generalized in periods of time ranging from a few days to a number of years, either continuously or intermittently. As a rule, after a certain period of development the lesions become definitely established. Some authors report cases of partial regression with disappearance of the papules, leaving residual pigmented spots. Total regression has also been described, but it is very rare.

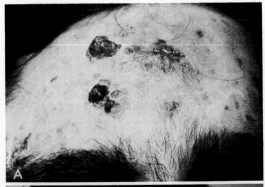

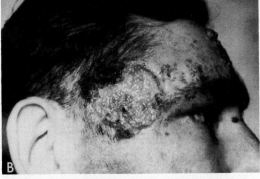

Figure 24–3   *A*, Verrucous, infiltrated lesions of the forehead undergoing malignant transformation. *B*, Squamous cell carcinoma which developed on verruciform lesions.

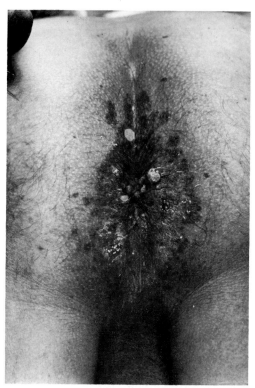

Figure 24-4 Perianal verruciform lesions undergoing transformation into Bowen's disease. *(From* Degos and Baptista: Bull. Soc. Fr. Dermatol. Syphiligr., *64:* 279, 1957.)

MALIGNANT TRANSFORMATION

One of the most important characteristics of E.V. is the frequency with which one or more lesions undergo cancerous transformation. In effect, 22 per cent of E.V. cases result in cancer (Poiares Baptista, 1957). Carcinomas usually develop between 20 and 30 years of age and predominate in regions exposed to light, especially the face (Fig. 24-3); more rarely, they appear on the dorsa of the hands and in the cervical area; exceptionally they are found in the perianal region (Jaeger and Delacretaz, 1953; Degos et al., 1957) (Fig. 24-4). In the majority of cases they are squamous cell carcinomas. Basal cell carcinomas and, more infrequently, Bowen's disease are also found, however (Degos et al., 1957; Wolfowicz, 1959; Jablonska et al., 1970; Baker, 1968; Ruiter, 1969; Ruiter and Mullen, 1970a and 1970b; Grupper et al., 1971). In cases of multiple malignancies, any combination of these cancers can be found (Relias et al., 1967).

The relationship between the verrucous lesions of E.V. and these carcinomas has been confirmed by observation of the cancerous cells, in which there are the same cavity formations as in the verrucous lesions, and of the areas of gradual transition between carcinomas and verrucous lesions. Thus, the name "epidermodysplastic carcinomas," proposed by Ferreira Marques and Vidal (1948), seems justified.

The frequency of malignant transformation and the young age at which it develops as a rule justify E.V. being considered a "precancerous dermatosis."

ETIOLOGY

Initially, E.V. was considered a genodermatosis, based on the following arguments (Poiares Baptista, 1957): (1) consanguinity of the parents in 12 percent of the cases; (2) a familial character in the collaterals or the descendants in 18 percent of the cases; (3) coexistence of neuropsychic or endocrine disorders (idiocy, cretinism, epiloia, hypophyseal disorders, hypothyroidism, ataxia, somatic malformations, and so forth) in 20 percent of the cases; and (4) the stability and resistance of the lesions to treatment. However, the viral etiology, initially defended with clinical arguments by Kogoj (1926), Hoffmann (1926 and 1928), Maschkilleissen (1931), and Tarnabuoni (1929) and later defended experimentally with positive inoculations by Lutz (1946 and 1957) and Jablonska and Milewski (1957), has today been fully demonstrated. Ruiter and Mullen in 1970 showed the presence of an intranuclear virus in E.V. whose morphologic characteristics are identical to the virus of human verrucae.

Electron microscopic studies by Jablonska et al. (1966), Yabe et al. (1969), Schellander and Fritsch (1970), and Tsuji et al. (1970), among others, integrated the virus into the group papova (I), comparing it to or identifying it with the virus of verruca vulgaris (Figs. 24-5 and 24-6). The coexistence of verruca vulgaris, verruca plana, verruca plantaris, and condy-

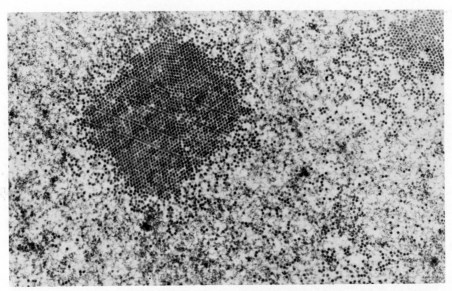

Figure 24-5   Virus in the granular layer. (Courtesy of Dr. Grupper and Dr. Pruniéras.)

loma acuminatum in E.V., observed by Schellander and Fritsch (1970), is in agreement with this concept.

More important, however, are the electron microscopic observations by Jablonska and colleagues (1966), Cornelius and colleagues (1968), Ruiter and Mullen (1970a and 1970b), and Grupper and colleagues (1971), demonstrating the presence of an intranuclear virus with 42 capsomers. In a detailed study of the virus structure, Yabe and colleagues (1969) found that the virus measured 56 millimicrons and possessed 72 capsomers dis-

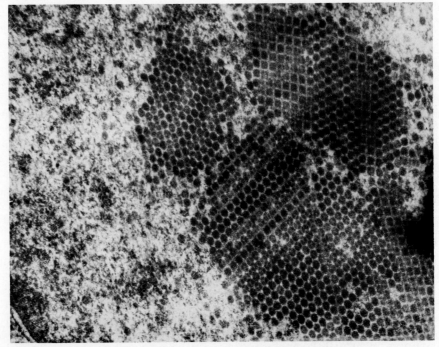

Figure 24-6   Detail of the virus. (Courtesy of Dr. Jablonska.)

posed in a form oriented toward the right, characteristics which evidently coincide with those described by Klug and Finsh in verruca vulgaris. Like the viruses in the papova* group, the E.V. virus is made up of deoxyribonucleic acid forming little ether-resistant particles.

In E.V. the virus occupies an intranuclear position in the vacuolized cytoplasm—demonstrated by Jablonska and colleagues (1966) by autoradiographic methods—and is found following rupture of the nuclear membrane.

The virus has been observed in nearly all layers of the epidermis (horny layer, granular layer, malpighian layer), although it does not seem to occur in the deeper layers, such as the basal layer.

The disappearance of the virus in lesions of arrested development could result in its incorporation into the genetic material of damaged cells (Rubin, 1964; McNulty, 1966; Jablonska et al., 1966).

Rueda and Rodriguez (1972), in their electron microscopic studies, found certain characteristics in the virogenesis which permit the differentiation of E.V. from verruca plana.

The role of the virus in the malignant transformation of E.V. lesions has been much discussed. As stressed by Cornelius and colleagues (1968), the viruses of the papova and the molluscum contagiosum groups are the only ones capable of provoking tumors in man. However, even though the behavior of the virus in malignant degeneration of E.V. is similar to that in Shope's papilloma (the virus ceases to be detectable in the tumor cells), it has still not been possible to demonstrate satisfactorily the cancerous potential of the virus in E.V.

In effect, Caso (1965) proved that the tumor cells do not synthesize viral DNA, and, according to Negroni (1968) the multiplication of the virus does not seem to be important in the malignant transformation of E.V.

Schellander and Fritsch (1970) concluded, on the basis of the sites of degenerated lesions, that in the epitheliomatous transformation the actinic aggression is the decisive factor and the presence of the virus is at most only a precipitating factor.

For the past few years, particular attention has been paid to the behavior of the virus in the various types of malignant transformation in E.V., which has many phases.

From the analysis of studies made, it can be concluded that, once cancerized, the lesions of E.V. cease showing the virus under the electron microscope (Grupper and Arouète, 1969; Ruiter, 1969; Ruiter and Mullen, 1970a and 1970b; Yabe et al., 1969; Jablonska et al., 1966). Such behavior is not constant, however, as the study by Ruiter and Mullen showed; the authors identified the virus in intraepidermal carcinomas as probably being derived from E.V. lesions. On the other hand, they confirmed the absence of viral elements in invasive bowenoid carcinomas and formulated the hypothesis that intraepidermal alterations, transforming E.V. lesions into carcinomas, interfere with the formation of the virus, which then disappears—at least apparently—into more developed forms of carcinoma, perhaps by way of provirus.

Once the viral origin of E.V. lesions is accepted, it must be acknowledged that the clinicoevolutionary characteristics that give the E.V. its particular aspect are different from those of verruca vulgaris. They are conditioned by a *genetic factor*, by a particular "terrain" as shown by the consanguinity of the parents, by a familial character, and by malignant transformation. *Consequently, E.V. is a genodermatosis characterized by a congenital predisposition for infection by the verruca vulgaris virus* (Wolfowicz, 1959).

PATHOLOGY

E.V. Lesions

The histopathology of E.V. reveals a monomorphism contrasting with the clinical polymorphism. Alterations occur exclusively in the epidermis, characterized by a particular transformation of the cells of the malpighian layer and by an accen-

---

*Papova group: virus of verruca vulgaris, virus of rabbit papilloma (Shope papilloma), virus of mouse papilloma, vacuolizing monkey virus.

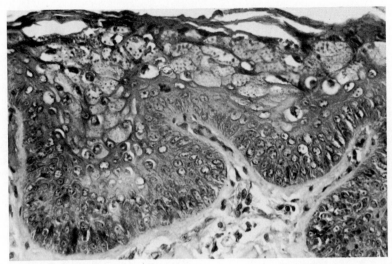

Figure 24–7   Typical histologic aspect of verruciform lesion of dorsa of the hands. Note the pale aspect of the epidermal cells in the upper levels of the malpighian layer.

tuated circumscribed acanthosis, resulting in a verruca vulgaris–like appearance. The lower level is normal and, at times, poor in melanin (Fig. 24–7).

The thickened malpighian layer shows the characteristic lesion: intracellular edema ("dégénération cavitaire"). This affects a group of cells located, for the most part, in the upper half of the malpighian layer (Fig. 24–8) but which can, at times, reach the deeper levels and, more rarely, the basal layer (Figs. 24–7 and 24–9). These malpighian cells are con-

siderably increased in size, with a clear, vacuolated cytoplasm, a deeply stained peripheral or central nucleus, and a relatively well-outlined cellular membrane. These alterations—isolated in fresh lesions or in the majority of the lesions, grouped in relatively well-defined areas, with preservation of cellular cohesion but loss of the intercellular bridges—give the epidermis a very characteristic reticulated aspect.

The granular layer is frequently absent, rarely hypertrophic (Wise and Satenstein,

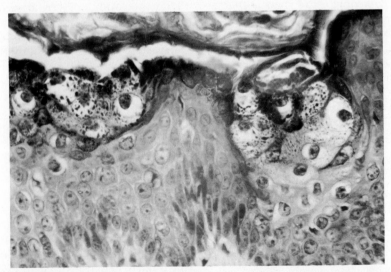

Figure 24–8   Detail of degeneration of the epidermal cells in an initial lesion. Superficial level of the malpighian layer.

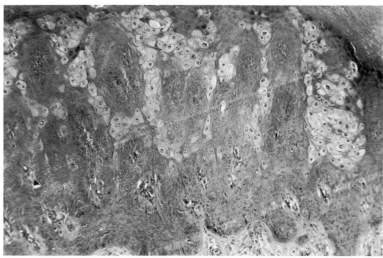

Figure 24–9   Histologic features typical of epidermodysplasia verruciformis (perianal lesions). There are groups of cells with a clear, abundant cytoplasm at various levels of the acanthotic epidermis.

1939). Sometimes the same process of intracellular edema is seen (Lutz, 1946 and 1957; Jablonska et al., 1966). The horny layer is very thick and parakeratotic with rounded nuclei and the reticulated appearance already noted by Lewandowsky and Lutz (1922).

The superficial dermis shows elongated and threadlike papillae and a moderate lymphohistiocytic perivascular infiltrate. The dermis of the light-exposed areas can show an intense actinic elastosis (Ruiter and Mullen, 1970a and 1970b). The appendages are always normal.

The successive stages of the "dégénération cavitaire" (intracellular edema), well studied by Waisman and Montgomery (1942), Bizzozero (1942), Fruhling and Bonjean (1945), and Midana (1949), among others, can be summarized as follows: initially the cytoplasm becomes more voluminous and clear, the perinuclear zone is empty, the nucleus increases in volume, and the cellular membrane thickens; the progression of the perinuclear vacuum, which finally spreads all over the cell, is accompanied by gradual pyknosis of the nucleus, which stays in the center of the cavity or is pushed to the periphery. The cells become oval or polyhedral with a well-defined outline.

Carcinomas

The squamous cell carcinomas, basal cell carcinomas, and Bowen's disease that develop in E.V. do not present any particular characteristics. Nevertheless, numerous authors have noted that, in any of these carcinomas, there are groups of cells with the same cellular alterations as in the malpighian cells of nonmalignant lesions (Figs. 24–10 and 24–11). This discovery and the observation of features of gradual transition from verrucous lesions to carcinomas point to the close relationship between the E.V. lesions and the carcinomas.

The mechanism of malignant transformation of the verrucous lesions through the influence of the virus has recently been analyzed ultrastructurally as well as autoradiographically through the studies of the incorporation of tritiated thymidine (Langner et al., 1968; Grupper et al., 1971). According to the latter authors, "the virus gives rise to a lesion that is essentially lithic, with viral multiplication in the epidermal cells of a normal individual, whereas there would be simultaneously lysis and transformation of the epidermal cells in certain genetically abnormal and therefore different individuals." This behavior is the rule for carcinogenic viruses with DNA, which behave differently in different animals (virus SV40, adenovirus types 2 and 3) or in animals of the same family but of different gender (Shope papilloma). In E.V. the cells with a clear cytoplasm are in the process of lysis

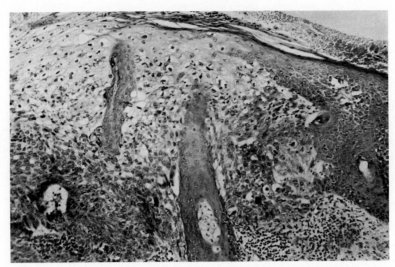

Figure 24-10 Bowenoid epithelioma on epidermodysplasia verruciformis with an intense vacuolation of the cells. The dermis shows foci of inflammatory cells.

and do not incorporate tritiated thymidine — in contrast to the remaining proliferating cells (Grupper et al., 1971). The verruca

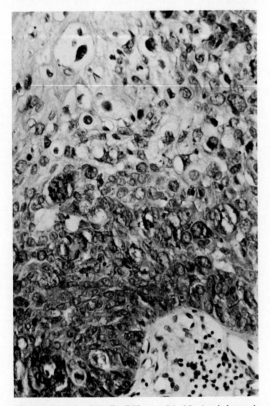

Figure 24-11 Detail of Figure 24-10. At right, epidermal cells in different stages, from the pale aspect of the abundant cytoplasm to the vacuolation and nuclear pyknosis. At left, the poikilokarynosis which is typical of Bowen's disease.

virus would therefore provoke lysis of the majority of the epidermal cells in E.V., while other surviving ones would transform and multiply, giving rise to carcinomas. However, Ruiter and Mullen (1970a and 1970b) admit that, concomitant with the viral degeneration, an autochthonous malignant alteration can exist through the influence of actinic radiation. The reasoning is based on the presence of intense solar elastosis in the dermis underlying the lesions, especially in young patients, and the observation of the virus in the deepest cells of the horny layer, covering incipient intraepidermal carcinomas of the Bowen type which are identical to senile and actinic keratosis.

THERAPY

E.V. is characterized by its extreme resistance to treatment. The general application of *arsenic, bismuth,* and *mercury* does not give any result; the same can be said of topical *keratolytics,* which do, however, at least reduce and remove scabs. Galvanocautery, electrocoagulation, and cryotherapy have restricted uses and are reserved for the treatment of extensive lesions.

The use of *trichloroacetic acid* and *glacial acetic acid* in conjunction with curettage of the lesions, recommended by Lutz (1946 and 1957) resulted in progressive cure over seven years in two patients with E.V. treated by this author. Prolonged treatment using vitamin A in increasing doses, mentioned by Landes et al. and Palitz and Caro, gave contradictory results, and in the case of Lazzaro et al. (1966) the results were negative.

The topical application of antimitotics (5-fluorouracil and Purinethol) does not seem to yield much better results. The use of lysozyme and xenalamine (Montagnani and Izzo, 1962) has produced uncertain or negative results.

REFERENCES

Baker, H.: Epidermodysplasia verruciformis with electron microscopic demonstration of virus. Proc. R. Soc. Med., *61*:589, 1968.

Beurey, J., Jeandidier, P., Rousselot, R., Mougeolle, J. M., Duc, M., and Wolfowicz, G.: Sur deux frères atteints d'epidermodysplasie verruciforme. *In* Epithéliomas et états préépithéliomateux cutanés (Communications). Paris, Masson & Cie, 1961, p. 45.

Bizzozero, E.: Epidermodysplasia verruciformis (Lewandowsky-Lutz). Dermatologica, 85:217, 1942.

Caso, L. V.: The relation of the immune reaction to cancer. *In* Haddow, A., and Weinhouse, S. (Eds.): Advances in Cancer Research. Vol. 9. New York, Academic Press, 1965, pp. 47–191.

Chiale, J.: Epidermodisplasia verruciformis. G. Ital. Dermatol. Sif., 83:303, 1942.

Cornelius, C., Witkowski, J., and Wood, M.: Viral verruca, human papova virus infection. Epidermodysplasia verruciformis, vacuolar degeneration of epidermis. Arch. Dermatol., 98:377, 1968.

Degos, R., Lortat-Jacob, E., and Lefort, P.: Epidermodysplasie verruciforme. Bull. Soc. Fr. Dermatol. Syphiligr., 60:6, 1953.

Degos, R., Delzant, O., and Baptista, A. P.: Epidermodysplasie verruciforme avec transformation bowenienne. Bull. Soc. Fr. Dermatol. Syphiligr., 64:279, 1957a.

Degos, R., Lefort, P., and Baptista, A. P.: Epidermodysplasie verruciforme (Lewandowsky-Lutz). Bull. Soc. Fr. Dermatol. Syphiligr., 64:278, 1957b.

Ferreira Marques, J., and Vidal, Z.: Contribución al estudio de la Epidermodisplasia verruciforme de Lewandowsky-Lutz (discusión de los casos hasta hoy publicados; descripción de un caso típico de epidermodisplasia verruciforme y de un epitelioma que reproduce su citologia: Epitelioma epidermodisplásico). Act. Dermo-sifiliogr. (Madr.), 39:399, 1948.

Fruhling, L., and Bonjean, M.: Contribution à l'étude histopathologique de l'Epidermodysplasie verruciforme de Lewandowsky-Lutz. Dermatologica, 91:281, 1945.

Grinspan, D., Pomposiello, I., and Navarro, J. S.: Epidermodisplasia verruciforme de Lewandowsky-

Lutz. Sesiones Dermatológicas en homenaje al Prof. L. Pierini, 383, 1949.

Grupper, C., and Arouète, J.: Epidermodysplasie verruciforme et épithéliomatose multiple bowenoide. Bull. Soc. Fr. Dermatol. Syphiligr., 76:307, 1969.

Grupper, C., Pruniéras, M., Delescluse, C., Arouète, J., and Garelly, E.: Epidermodysplasie verruciforme: étude ultrastructurale et autoradiographique. Ann. Dermatol. Syphiligr. (Paris), 98:33, 1971.

Hamdi, H., and Hulusi: Epidermodysplasia verruciformis. Virchows Arch. Pathol. Anat., 291:738, 1933.

Hoffmann, E.: Verallgemeinerte Warzenerkrankung — Verrucosis generalisata aut disseminata. Dermatol. Z., 48:241, 1926.

Hoffmann, E.: Verrucosis generalisata. Arch. Dermatol. Syph. (Berl.), 155:318, 1928.

Jablonska, S., and Milewski, B.: Zur Kenntnis der Epidermodysplasia verruciformis Lewandowsky-Lutz. Dermatologica, 115:1, 1957.

Jablonska, S., Fabjanska, L., and Formas, I.: On the viral etiology of epidermodysplasia verruciformis. Dermatologica, 132:369, 1966.

Jablonska, S., Biczysko, W., Jakubowicz, K., and Dabrowski, H.: The ultrastructure of transitional states to Bowen's disease and invasive Bowen's carcinoma in epidermodysplasia verruciformis. Dermatologica, 140:186, 1970.

Jaeger, H., and Delacretaz, J.: Epidermodysplasie verruciforme de Lewandowsky et Lutz et Épithélioma spinocellulaire de la marge anale. Dermatologica, 106:306, 1953.

Kogoj, F.: Die Epidermodysplasia verruciformis. Acta Derm. Venereol. (Stockh.), 7:170, 1926.

Langner, A., Jablonska, S., and Darzynkiewicz, Z.: Autoradiographic study of DNA synthesis by epidermal cells in epidermodysplasia verruciformis. Acta Derm. Venereol. (Stockh.), 48:501, 1968.

Lazzaro, C., Giardina, A., and Randazzo, S.: Sulla Epidermodysplasia verruciformis Lewandowsky-Lutz. Minerva Dermatol., 41:4, 1966.

Lewandowsky, F., and Lutz, W.: Ein Fall einer bisher nicht beschriebenen Hauterkrankung (Epidermodysplasia verruciformis). Arch. Dermatol. Syph. (Berl.), 141:193, 1922.

Louste, Levy-Franckel, A., Cailliau, and Schwartz: Epidermodysplasie verruciforme avec lésions papillomateuses de la muqueuse uréthrale. Bull. Soc. Fr. Dermatol. Syphiligr., 41:270, 1934.

Lutz, W.: Epidermodysplasia verruciformis. Dermatologica, 92:30, 1946.

Lutz, W.: Zur Epidermodysplasia verruciformis. Dermatologica, 115:309, 1957.

McNulty, W. P., Jr.: Tumor viruses. *In* Montagna, W., and Dobson, R. (Eds.): Carcinogenesis. Oxford, Pergamon Press, 1966, pp. 133–151.

Maschkilleissen, N. L.: Ist die Epidermodysplasia verruciformis (Lewandowsky-Lutz); eine selbständige Dermatose? Ihre Beziehungen zur verrucositas. Dermatol. Wochenschr., 92:569, 1931.

Midana, A.: Sulla questione dei rapporti tra Epidermodisplasia verruciformis e Verrucosi generalizzata; osservazioni su 4 casi de l'E.V. a carattere famigliare. Dermatologica, 99:1, 1949.

Montagnani, A., and Izzo, L.: Epidermodysplasia

verruciforme, acrocheratosi, malattia di Darier. Minerva Dermatol., 37:179, 1962.

Negroni, G.: Progress with some tumor viruses of chickens and mammals; the problem of passenger viruses. *In* Haddow, A., and Weinhouse, S. (Eds.): Advances in Cancer Research. New York, Academic Press, 1968, pp. 515–561.

Poiares Baptista, A.: Epidermodysplasie verruciforme de Lewandowsky-Lutz. Mémoire de la Fac. Méd. Paris, 1957.

Rechter, M., and Castañe, A. D.: Epidermodysplasia verruciforme de Lewandowsky-Lutz. Rev. Argent. Dermatosif., 29:49, 1945.

Relias, A., Sakellariou, G., and Tsoitis, G.: Epidermodysplasie verruciforme de Lewandowsky-Lutz à multiples épithéliomas. Ann. Dermatol. Syphiligr. (Paris), 94:501, 1967.

Rubin, H.: Carcinogenic interaction between virus, cell and organism. J.A.M.A., 190:727, 1964.

Rueda, L. A., and Rodriguez, G.: Comparación de la virogenesis en la epidermodisplasia verruciforme y en las verrugas planas. Med. Cutan., 6:451, 1972.

Ruiter, M.: On malignant degeneration of skin lesions in epidermodysplasia verruciformis. Acta Derm. Venereol. (Stockh.), 49:309, 1969.

Ruiter, M., and Mullen, P.: Behavior of virus in malignant degeneration of skin lesion in epidermodysplasia verruciformis. J. Invest. Dermatol., 54:324, 1970a.

Ruiter, M., and Mullen, P.: Further histological investigations on malignant degeneration of cutaneous lesion in epidermodysplasia verruciformis. Acta Derm. Venereol. (Stockh.), 50:205, 1970b.

Schellander, F., and Fritsch, P.: Epidermodysplasia verruciformis. Neue Aspekte zur Symptomatologie und Pathogenese. Dermatologica, 140:251, 1970.

Tarnabuoni, G.: Epidermodysplasia verruciformis. G. Ital. Dermatol. Sif., 70:557, 1929.

Teodorescu, S., Fellner, M., and Conu, A.: Zwei Fälle von Epidermodysplasia verruciformis Lewandowsky-Lutz. Arch. Dermatol. Syph. (Berl.), 188:423, 1949.

Tsuji, T., Abe, Y., and Saito, T.: Generalized verruca plana. Dermatologica, 140:142, 1970.

Waisman, M., and Montgomery, H.: Study of Epidermodysplasia verruciformis in relation to verruca plana and epithelial nevus. Arch. Dermatol. Syph., 45:259, 1942.

Wise, F., and Satenstein, D. L.: Epidermodysplasia verruciformis (Lewandowsky-Lutz). Arch. Dermatol. Syph., 40:742, 1939.

Wolfowicz, G.: L'Epidermodysplasie verruciforme de Lewandowsky-Lutz. Maladie génétique ou virale? Thèse, Faculté de Médecine de Nancy, 1959.

Yabe, Y., Okamoto, T., Ohmori, S., and Tanioku, K.: Virus particles in epidermodysplasia verruciformis with carcinoma. Dermatologica, 139:161, 1969.

25

Cheilitis

I. Katzenellenbogen, M.D., and M. Sandbank, M.D.

INTRODUCTION

Squamous cell carcinoma of the lip is the most common form of cancer of the oral cavity, accounting for approximately 25 to 30 percent of the total (Ackermann and Del Regato, 1962). It occurs on the lower lip in 89 percent of cases, on the upper lip in 3.1 percent and at the angle of the lip in 7.9 percent (Venkei and Sugar, 1965). Development of malignant tumors on the lip is often preceded by tissue changes of the vermilion, hence the importance of cheilitis in case histories of lip cancer. Long-standing exposure to sunshine, wind, and frost (as in farmers, sailors, and others who work outdoors) is by far the most frequent cause of carcinoma of the lower lip (Ackerman and Del Regato, 1962; Ariel, 1958; Atkin et al., 1949; Cockerell et al., 1961; Spatz, 1964; Versluys, 1949). Cheilitis actinica, a counterpart to actinic keratosis (Andrade, 1964; Steigleder, 1962), is a precancerosis in the broader sense. Another form of cheilitis—cheilitis glandularis—is regarded by several authors as a precancerosis (Bejarano, 1933–34; Gay Prieto et al., 1959; Michalowski, 1948; Touraine, 1950), but this assessment has been questioned by others (Bâlus, 1965; Duperrat et al., 1961;

Grinspan et al., 1961). No case of malignancy was reported as a complication of cheilitis granulomatosa, the Melkersson-Rosenthal syndrome, or cheilitis plasmacellularis, by Miescher (1945). A precise determination of the type of cheilitis may help in the prognosis of the case.

NORMAL ANATOMY AND HISTOLOGY OF THE LIP

The upper and lower lips are covered by skin on the outside and mucous membrane on the inside (Fig. 25–1). The skin of the lip ends in a sharp line, to be replaced by the red or vermilion zone of the lips, the transitional zone between the skin and the mucous membrane. This feature was said by Sicher (1952) to be characteristic only of man, but according to Brans (1956) some higher apes also show signs of the vermilion. The skin of the lips has all the characteristics of ordinary skin, containing sweat glands, hairs, and sebaceous glands. The thickness of the skin, especially that of the dermis, shows distinct sexual difference.

According to Sicher (1952), the epithelium of the vermilion is thinner than that of the skin, although Brans (1956) disputed this notion. The epithelium is not

607

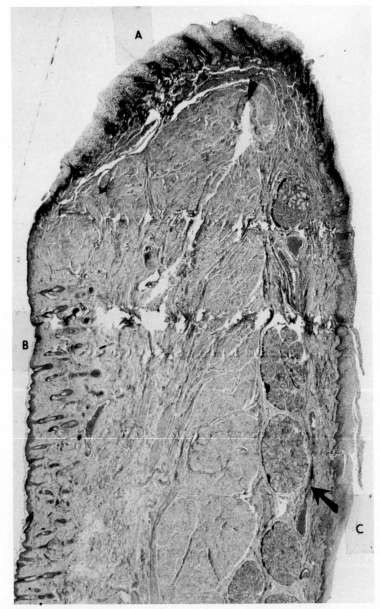

Figure 25–1   Sagittal section through lip of newborn. *H & E, × 15. A,* Vermilion zone of lip: thickened epithelium for sucking. *B,* Skin side: hairs, sebaceous glands, and sweat glands. *C,* Oral mucosa: numerous labial salivary glands.

hornified. Papillae are numerous, densely arranged, slender, and reach far into the epithelium, so that their tips are covered by only a very thin layer of epithelium. Thus the wide and rich capillaries of the papillae are seen through the thin epithelium, creating the red color of this area.

The vermilion does not contain hair or sweat glands. However, in about 50 percent of individuals examined, according to

Sicher, small or larger isolated sebaceous glands can be detected. According to Brans, only 20 percent of men have these glands and only 6 percent of women. No melanin pigment is found in this area.

The mucous membrane is covered by nonhornified, stratified, squamous epithelium. It contains numerous mixed glands of variable size, the largest of which can be felt through the thin mucous membrane.

Sometimes they form an almost continous layer in the upper and lower lip. The submucosa is not sharply separated from the underlying muscle, thus giving high mobility. No pigment is found in the epithelial cells. The submucosa is composed of reticulated loose connective tissue, so that severe edema develops in inflammatory conditions.

Sensory innervation of the upper lip is by the second branch of the trigeminal nerve, and that of the lower lip by the third branch of the trigeminal nerve. Motor innervation is by the facial nerve. Lymph from both lips is drained into the submandibular and superior cervical lymph nodes. The lymphatics immediately below the skin drain into the submental lymph nodes (Brans, 1956). Recent study (Larson et al., 1967) has demonstrated that lymphatic drainage from the upper lip also goes to the submental lymph nodes. The lymphatics have a high incidence of contralateral flow after passing through one or two lymph nodes on the ipsilateral side.

The lips obtain their vascular supply from two branches of the facial artery, the superior and inferior labial arteries. The inferior and superior labial veins drain the lower and upper lips respectively into the anterior facial vein.

Electron microscopy demonstrates these differences between keratinizing human skin and nonkeratinizing oral mucosa:

(1) There is no keratin formation; the tonofilaments are shorter, finer, and fewer in number.

(2) The number of desmosomes seems to be smaller.

(3) Keratohyalin granules are absent.

(4) Stratum lucidum and stratum corneum are absent.

(5) A close relation of the corium and epithelium is observed.

Both layers are separated only by subepithelial membrane of a fibrillar nature.

Irregular projections of basal cells into the corium are seen. An abundance of mitochondria and well developed Golgi apparatus indicate that the cells of the oral mucosa are active metabolically. The electron microscope shows melanocytes with several dendritic processes located at the basal layer, but they were found to be inactive, with no fully formed melanin granules. For further information the reader may consult the papers of Zelikson and Hartman (1962) and Wechsler and Fischer (1962).

CHEILITIS EXFOLIATIVA

Under this heading, devised by Mikulicz and Kümmel (1922) for the *persistent exfoliation of the lips* of Stelwagon (1900), a group of exfoliative conditions of the lips with a polygenic etiology is included. Cheilitis exfoliativa is manifested by chronically inflamed lips, covered with crusts which tend to desquamate, leaving rough-surfaced erosions upon which new crusts tend to form. The lower lip is generally involved (Fig. 25–2). Contact dermatitis (Sulzberger and Goodman, 1938), atopic dermatitis, seborrheic dermatitis (Chalmers and McDonald, 1921), riboflavin deficiency (Decker, 1941), pyorrhea, ill-fitting dental protheses, smoking, and psychogenic factors have been called responsible for this exfoliative condition (Curtis and Rogers, 1952; Savkina, 1962). Because numerous types of cheilitis of

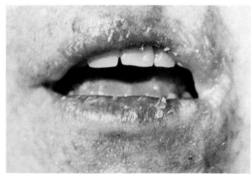
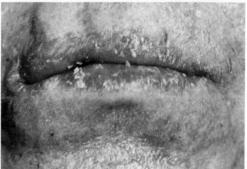

Figure 25–2 Cheilitis exfoliativa; chronic desquamation of lips.

various causes pass through an exfoliative stage, the question arises whether exfoliative cheilitis should be regarded as a nosologic entity (Höfer and Honemann, 1968; Zinsser, 1930).

CHEILITIS ACTINICA

Ayres (1923) described *chronic actinic cheilitis* in five patients from California with a chronic inflammatory disorder of the lower lip, apparently due to sunlight. He regarded this condition as a variety of exfoliative cheilitis. Further cases were reported by Katzenellenbogen (1936 and 1937) from Jerusalem, Grin (as *cheilitis aestivalis*) (1938) and Dojmi (1939) from Yugoslavia, Marchionini and Tor (1939) from Turkey (as *summer cheilitis*), and Nicolau and Bâlus (1964) from Rumania. Single cases have been reported in regions of temperate climate (Bielicky, 1965; Höfer and Honemann, 1968; Michalowski, 1948).

Actinic cheilitis usually occurs during the summer months in places where sunshine is most intense, such as the hot, dry, interior regions of California (Ayres, 1923), highlands and steppes of the Anatolian mountains (Marchionini and Tor, 1939), hills of Jerusalem (Katzenellenbogen, 1936 and 1937), the agricultural regions of Rumania (Nicolau and Bâlus, 1964), and in the high mountains (Canizares, 1964).

Cheilitis actinica occurs most commonly in those people who are habitually exposed to sunlight, such as farmers and outdoor-workers, and accordingly men are far more often affected than women. Fair-skinned people are more prone to the condition than those with darker skin (Ackermann and Del Regato, 1962; Ayres, 1923; Hall, 1950; Katzenellenbogen, 1936; McDonald, 1959; Ratzkowski et al., 1966; van Ziel, 1965). In addition to the sun's rays, exposure to photosensitizing agents, tar, and dust has to be considered (Bielicky, 1965; Gougerot, 1936; Hämäläinen, 1955; Höfer and Honemann, 1968; Marchionini and Tor, 1939; Schuermann et al., 1966).

Acute Form (Fig. 25-3)

There is a rare episodic form of actinic cheilitis following a prolonged exposure to

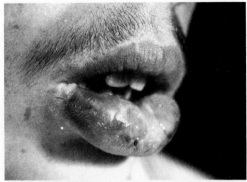
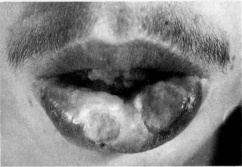

Figure 25–3 Acute actinic cheilitis; swollen lower lip with superficial erosions and crusts.

sunlight ("light trauma") (Katzenellenbogen, 1936). The lower lip is considerably swollen and red. Vesicles appear on the vermilion, become confluent, and burst rapidly, resulting in superficial erosions of various shapes. Persistent serum exudes from the erosions, coagulates, and forms yellowish brown crusts. They often cover the whole vermilion surface, leaving thin strips of intact mucosa. The painful lip impedes eating and speaking. This acute form of cheilitis corresponds to acute sunburn of the skin. If additional exposure to sunlight is avoided, these lesions subside in two or three weeks, and the lip recovers its former size; otherwise the inflammation continues and the cheilitis assumes the chronic form.

Pathologic findings include edema and congestion of the corium with a mild inflammatory infiltrate composed mainly of polymorphonuclear leukocytes. The epidermis shows an intercellular edema which is followed by destruction and shedding of the epithelium. Leukocytes and, according to Bielicky (1965), many eosinophils penetrate the degenerating epithelium. In regions where epithelium is already miss-

ing, a layer of fibrin with embedded leukocytes covers the erosion. The histologic
picture is that of an acute, nonspecific inflammatory reaction.

Chronic Form

The chronic form of actinic cheilitis develops gradually in people exposed to sunlight for years. There is a thickening of the
vermilion of the lower lip in summer and a
mild scaling in winter. The degree of scaling is not uniform, with the middle part
usually more involved. The vermilion be-

comes constantly dry and scaling with occasional fissures. Thin horny layers of whitish gray or brownish color superimposed
one upon another cover the vermilion,
which loses its reddish color and becomes
rigid and callous with a tendency to crack.
A secondary infection of the lip often results in erosions and ulcerations. They
heal, leaving leukoplakia-like scars (Fig.
25–4). The chronic actinic cheilitis may
sometimes assume a pattern of leukoplakia; Nicolau and Bâlus (1964) isolated
small plaques of various shapes with a
milky appearance arising within the general process of cheilitis. In some cases

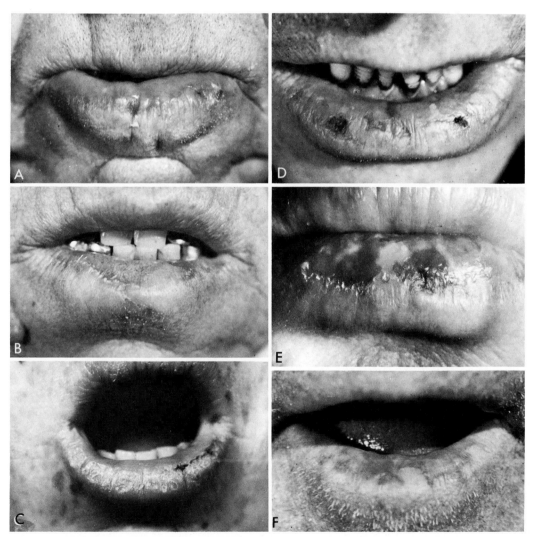

Figure 25–4 Chronic actinic cheilitis; lesions located on the vermilion of lower lip; middle part is more involved. *A* to *D*, Vermilion dry, scaly, with fissures. *E* and *F*, Erosions and ulcerations leaving leukoplakia-like
scars.

there is a tendency to deteriorate with every summer, and the flaking or scaling aspect of the lip remains in winter. In others, the vermilion assumes an exfoliative pattern of slight scaling in summer and winter.

Because of the lack of protection from sunlight (neither keratin nor melanin is present), the vermilion is the principal site of the lesions. The epidermis shows two different types of pathologic changes: it is thin, with loss or flattening of the rete ridges, and the epithelium may be only two to three cells thick (Fig. 25–5*A*), and there is hyperkeratosis with parakeratosis and acanthosis. Cellular or nuclear atypia is absent. Only a few mitotic figures are seen, no more than in normal epidermis (Fig. 25–5*B*). According to Schmitt and Folsom (1968) a large amount of glycogen was found in the epithelium in three of his cases, but the significance of this finding is not understood.

When ulcerations occur they are shallow and essentially start as erosions. Surrounding the ulceration is a heavy inflammatory infiltration composed of polymorphonuclear leukocytes and fibrin. The ulceration is covered by a crust of coagulated fibrin intermingled with leukocytes (Fig. 25–6).

Basophilic degeneration of the upper dermis is observed in all cases (Schmitt and Folsom, 1968). The significance and nature of this type of degeneration is dealt with in another chapter of this book. A heavy band of inflammatory exudate composed of lymphocytes, monocytes, plasma cells, and histiocytes is seen immediately below the epithelium (Höfer and Honemann, 1968; Koten et al., 1967), and also in our own experience a large number of plasma cells are present. Bielicky (1965) and Höfer and Honemann (1968) were impressed by the large number of eosinophils in the exudate. Blood vessels, arterioles, capillaries, and venules show

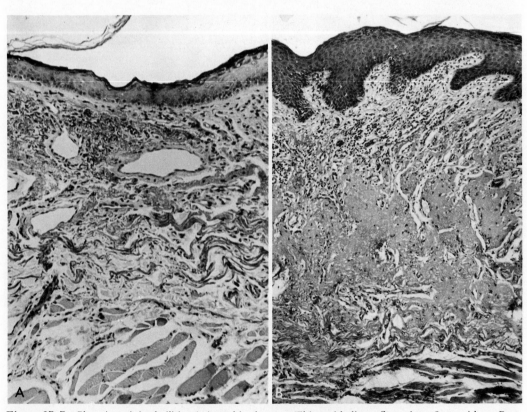

Figure 25–5   Chronic actinic cheilitis. *A*, Atrophic changes. Thin epithelium, flattening of rete ridges. Basophilic degeneration of corium. Dilatation of capillaries. *H & E, 16 × 8. B*, Hypertrophic changes. Acanthotic epithelium with hyper- and parakeratosis. Basophilic degeneration of corium. Dilatation of capillaries. *H & E, 6.3 × 8.*

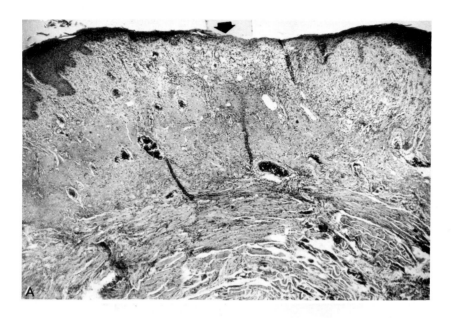

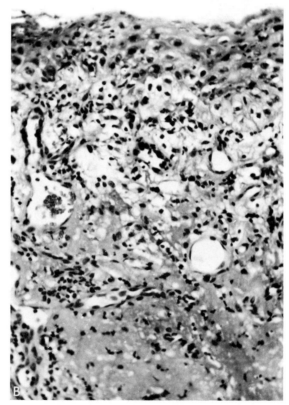

Figure 25–6   Chronic actinic cheilitis. *A,* Shallow ulceration. Basophilic degeneration of upper corium. Dilatation of blood vessels, hypertrophy of endothelial lining. *H & E, 2.5 × 8. B,* Enlargement of *A.* Surrounding the ulceration is an infiltrate composed of polymorphonuclear leukocytes. *H & E, 16 × 8.*

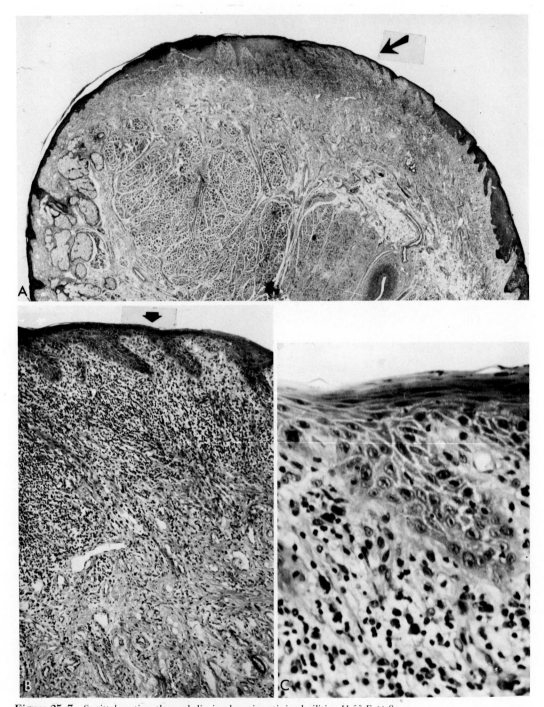

Figure 25–7   Sagittal section through lip in chronic actinic cheilitis. *H & E,* × *8.*
Right, (*A*) vermilion zone; (*B*) skin side; (*C*) oral mucous membrane.
   Left, (*A*) enlargement of figure at right. The lesion is located on the vermilion zone. Band form inflammatory exudate immediately below the epithelium. Arrow indicates (*B*). *H & E,* × *15.*
   (*B*) Enlargement of figure at right. Irregular acanthosis. Inflammation, basophilic degeneration, dilatation of blood vessels in upper corium. Arrow indicates (*C*). *H & E, 6.3* × *8.*
   (*C*) Enlargement of figures at right. Atypical cells in epithelium. Large number of plasma cells in inflammatory infiltrate. *H & E, 25* × *8.*

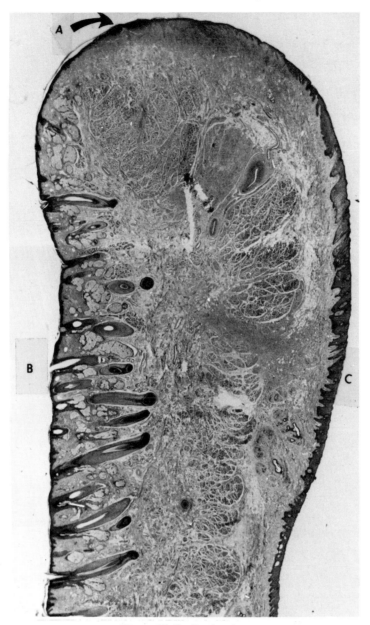

Figure 25–7 *Continued.*

dilatation and hypertrophy of the endothelial lining, manifested by swelling and prominence of the endothelial cells.

Malignant degeneration of actinic cheilitis is clinically suggested by the appearance of small areas of intense hyperkeratosis with slight infiltration on the surface affected by diffuse scaling (Fig. 25–7). The horny prominence develops in the course of time into hard, dry nodules the size of millet seeds or lentils. In other instances limited ulcers develop from linear fissures (Figs. 25–8 to 25–11).

In a survey of cheilitis actinica, 83 of our patients were reexamined 10 years after the onset of the condition: 49 were then free of clinical symptoms of cheilitis. In 10 there were occasional scaling and fissures after exposure to sunlight. In eight cases small leukoplakia-like scars were visible on the vermilion. Squamous cell carcinoma was found in 16 cases, although in four of them all clinical signs of previous cheilitis were no longer present.

In a five year survey made by Shakhova (1964) of 183 patients with cheilitis, 18 were found with incipient forms of cancer. Numerous investigators have noted the relation between cancer of the lower lip and overexposure to sunlight. According to Molesworth (1934), out of 150 patients with cancer of the lower lip, only three had not been exposed to sunlight for a prolonged period. In the larger series of 284 patients with carcinoma of the lower lip studied by Gay Prieto et al. (1959), all were outdoor workers. Richter (1960) reported

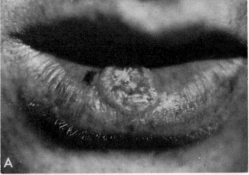

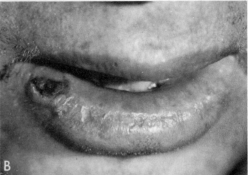

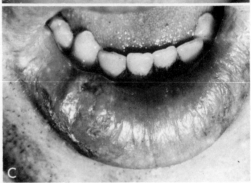

Figure 25–9 Squamous cell carcinoma developing in chronic actinic cheilitis.

A, Verrucous type of squamous cell carcinoma.

B and *C*, Ulcerating type of squamous cell carcinoma.

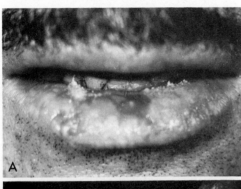

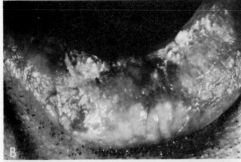

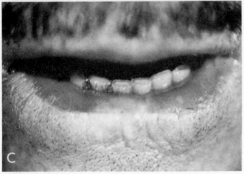

Figure 25–8 Early malignant development in chronic actinic cheilitis (precancerosis).

A and *B*, Early malignant development in chronic actinic cheilitis.

C, Same patient after lip shaving.

103 cases of carcinoma of the lower lip; in those patients the existence of actinic cheilitis was recorded either in the past or at the time of malignancy. Whereas Nicolau and Bâlus (1964), Richter (1960), Grinspan et al. (1961), and Ackermann and Del Regato (1962) regarded cheilitis actinica as a definite precancerous affection, Kuske (1965) stated that only a certain number of the chronic, relapsing forms of actinic cheilitis became precancerous. It is a facultative precancerosis in the broader sense of the term (Andrade, 1964; Steigleder, 1962).

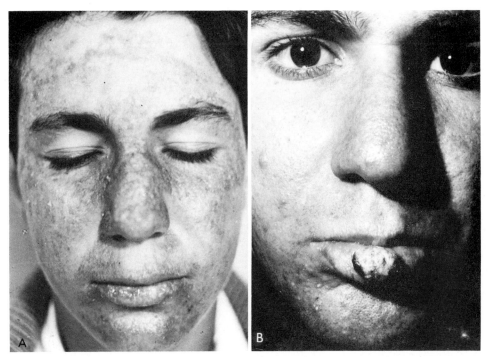

Figure 25–10 *A*, Chronic actinic cheilitis. *B*, Squamous cell carcinoma one year later.

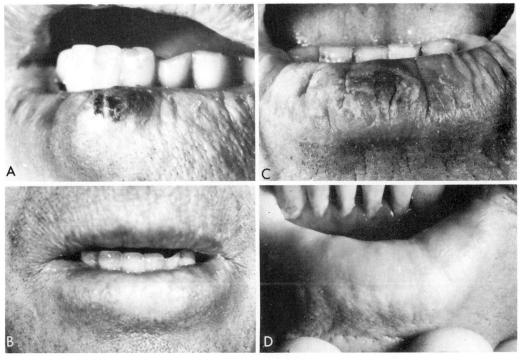

Figure 25–11 Chronic actinic cheilitis and carcinoma (before and after treatment).
A and *B*, Same patient before and after lip shaving.
C and *D*, Same patient before and after lip shaving.

Persons with existing malignancy in the face and concomitant chronic actinic cheilitis are in our experience more prone to cancer of the lip. The histologic criteria for the malignant changes are atypia and loss of polarity of the basal layer cells, hyperchromatism of the nuclei, and an increasing number of mitotic figures. The nuclei becomes larger and irregular in shape, and individual cell keratinization-dyskeratosis is present. This stage of hyperkeratosis and parakeratosis, basal cell atypia with cell keratinization, yet without infiltration, is regarded as precancerosis (Figs. 25–12 and 25–13).

The development of actinic cheilitis into carcinoma is often difficult to detect. Schmitt and Folsom (1968) proposed con-

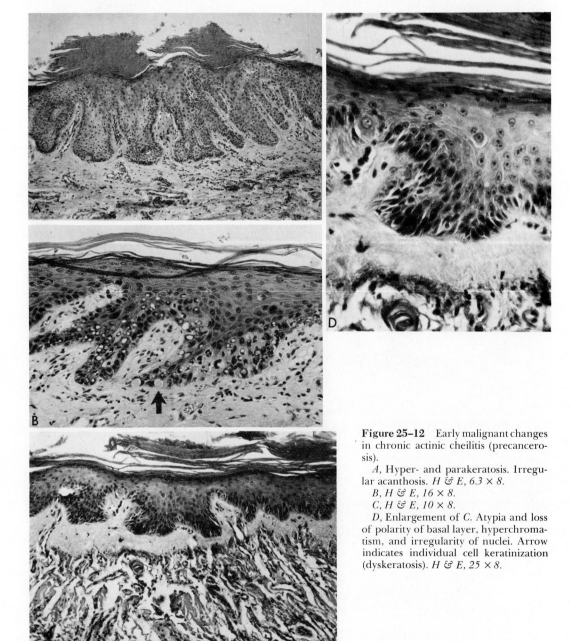

Figure 25–12 Early malignant changes in chronic actinic cheilitis (precancerosis).

A, Hyper- and parakeratosis. Irregular acanthosis. *H & E, 6.3 × 8.*

B, H & E, 16 × 8.

C, H & E, 10 × 8.

D, Enlargement of *C.* Atypia and loss of polarity of basal layer, hyperchromatism, and irregularity of nuclei. Arrow indicates individual cell keratinization (dyskeratosis). *H & E, 25 × 8.*

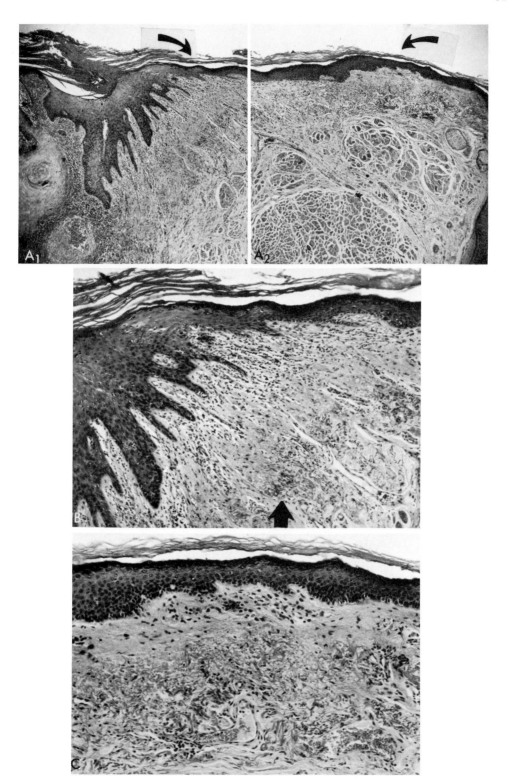

Figure 25–13 *A*, Squamous cell carcinoma developing in chronic actinic cheilitis. Arrow indicates *B* and *C*. *H & E, 2.5 × 8.*

B, Enlargement of *A*. Malignant development in area of basophilic degeneration. Arrow indicates basophilic degeneration. *H & E, 6.3 × 8.*

C, Enlargement of *A*. Changes of chronic actinic cheilitis. Hyper- and parakeratosis, flattening of epithelium; basophilic degeneration of upper corium. *H & E, 10 × 8.*

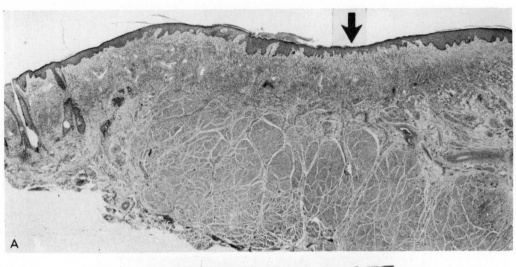

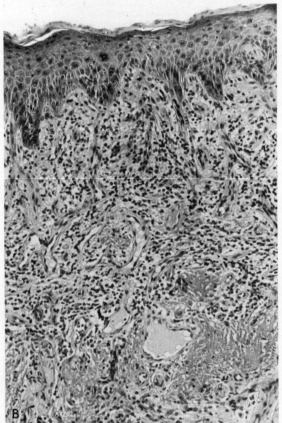

Figure 25–14 *A,* Lip shaving specimen: malignant changes in vermilion, area of clinical normal appearance. Arrow indicates *B. H & E,* × *14.*

B, Enlargement of *A.* Early signs of malignancy in epithelium, inflammation, basophilic degeneration, dilation of blood vessels in upper corium. *H & E, 10* × *8.*

servative treatment of patients with lower lip atrophic degenerative changes for up to six weeks. When the patient failed to respond to such treatment, a horizontal wedge resection of the lower lip was performed, and the surgical specimen was step-sectioned at 1-cm. intervals. Of 13 cases in which this procedure was followed, 12 showed premalignant lesions. Schmitt stressed the multicentric origin of premalignant or malignant lesions of the lower lip. Meyer (1965) supported the notion that dyskeratosis and early carcinoma are frequent findings in regions that clinically appear normal, and he therefore recommended multiple histologic examinations of the specimen removed. This corresponds to our own experience in cases of multiple carcinoma of the lip; histologic examination of material obtained by lip-shaving in cases of carcinoma of the lip revealed considerable deterioration of areas with a clinically normal appearance (Fig. 25–14).

Treatment

Preventive measures are suggested by all authors; the patient should avoid solar radiation by wearing broad-brimmed hats and by application of sun-screening ointments to the lips. The use of anti-malarial drugs (chloroquine, resorcin) to prevent skin cancer of the lip was recommended by Knox (1960), Maskilleison (1967 and 1969), Pashkov (1927), Bielicky (1965), and Höfer and Honemann (1968). Vitamin A ointments are used by Russian authors (Pashkov, 1927, Maskilleison, 1967 and 1969; Savkina, 1962). Corticosteroid ointments and antibiotics were found to be helpful in some cases (Pashkov, 1927; Bielicky, 1965) and harmful in others (Maskilleison, 1967 and 1969).

Grenz rays therapy has been recommended by Pashkov (1927), Savkina (1962), Bezzabotnov and Savkina (1964). In mild cases the recommendation was a single dose of 100 R. and a total of 1000 R.; in more extensive forms of actinic cheilitis, 200 to 500 R. as a single dose and 1700 to 2500 R. as a total dose were suggested. Lip shaving (chelioplasty) is an important procedure in patients with actinic keratosis of the lower lip (Van Ziel, 1965). Electrodesiccation was advised by Cipollaro and Costello (1948), Costello (1948), and Nicolau and Bâlus (1964), and rejected by Maskilleison (1967 and 1969). Solid carbon dioxide treatment has been previously used by us (Katzenellenbogen, 1937); at present lip shaving is practiced in chronic cases (Figs. 25–8, 25–11, and 25–16).

Differential Diagnosis

Cheilitis is an associated symptom of some skin conditions that may precede the skin lesions; actinic cheilitis therefore has to be considered in the differential diagnosis of any exfoliative cheilitis. In lichen planus, adhering whitish scales cover one or both lips. Milky white papules, more commonly aggregations of them, form irregular reticulated or lace-like patterns. Unlike actinic cheilitis, however, the desquamation is mild, and there is no inflammation or crusting of the lips (Fig. 25–15A).

In lupus erythematosus, circumscribed and exceptionally diffuse areas of scaling with tiny deep red borders may cover the lower lip. Thickening of the epithelium, and telangiectases and erosions side by side are combined with bleeding of the vermilion and subsequent hemorrhagic crusts. Concomitant changes on the cheeks or palate contribute to the differential diagnosis.

In pemphigus vulgaris, the lips are painful, covered with hemorrhagic brownish crusts, and bleed readily. Vesicles of a transitory character rupture rapidly, leaving only remnants on the borders. The erosions incline to secondary infection. Pemphigus of the lips and oral cavity, preceding by many months the spreading of the lesions on the skin, was described by Katzenellenbogen and Sandbank in 1959 (Fig. 25–15 C). Primary pemphigus on the vermilion of the lower lip simulating exfoliative cheilitis was more recently reported by Markewich (1967). The pemphigus eruptions of the skin appeared two months later. The occurrence of cheilitis in all the above mentioned conditions is independent of the season.

CHEILITIS ABRASIVA PRECANCEROSA (MANGANOTTI)

This form of cheilitis is regarded by many authors as a late and clinically more serious variant of cheilitis actinica (Grinspan et al., 1961; Andrade, 1964; Maskilleison, 1967 and 1969). Manganotti (1934) described it as a disorder of old age.

The entire breadth of the lower lip, particularly the middle part of the vermilion, is involved. Chronic relapsing erosions and superficial ulcerations alternate with leukoplakia-like scars and lamellar scaling. There is no palpable infiltration, and salivary glands are not affected (Fig. 25–16).

Hyperkeratosis with proliferation of the epithelium and formation of epithelial pegs of varying shapes is an important pathologic finding. The epithelial cells often show hyperchromatism of the nuclei. There is a considerable inflammatory infiltration of the corium with lymphocytes, leukocytes, and plasma cells; a basophilic degeneration of the upper dermis is observed in all cases. First malignant changes are often manifested by atypia and mitoses

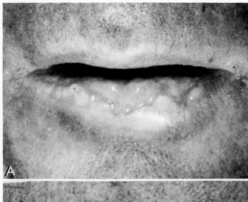
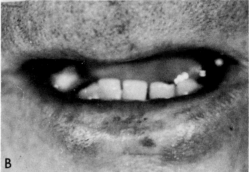

Figure 25–16   Cheilitis abrasiva precancerosa Manganotti.
A, Chronic superficial ulceration in middle part of vermilion.
B, After lip shaving.

of the basal layer cells, which then show further loss of polarity, and their nuclei become larger and irregular in shape. Individual cell keratinization is regarded as an early sign of carcinoma (Schmitt and Folsom, 1968) (Fig. 25–17).

Differential Diagnosis

See discussion of actinic cheilitis.

Treatment

Lip shaving gives the best results (Fig. 25–16).

CHEILITIS GLANDULARIS

Cheilitis glandularis develops in heterotopic hyperplastic salivary glands in the inner part of the mucosa of the lower lip. Clinically three forms of this disorder are distinguished: cheilitis glandularis simplex

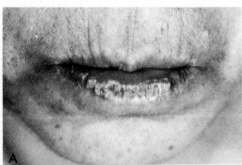
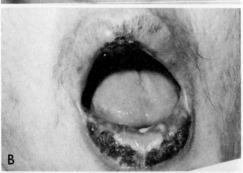
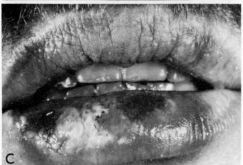

Figure 25–15   Differential diagnosis; involvement of lower lip, in lichen planus (*A*), fixed drug eruption (*B*), and pemphigus vulgaris (*C*).

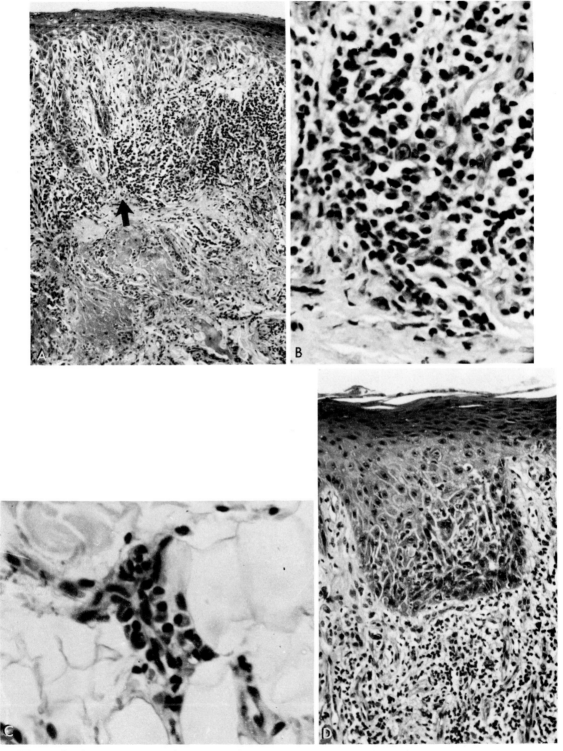

Figure 25–17   Early malignant changes in cheilitis abrasiva precancerosa.

A, Proliferation of epithelium, massive inflammatory infiltrate in upper corium, basophilic degeneration. Arrow indicates *B*. H & E, 10 × 8.

B, Enlargement of *A*. H & E, 40 × 8.

C, Large number of plasma cells in the inflammatory exudate in upper corium and around blood vessels. H & E, 40 × 8.

D, Enlargement of proliferating epithelium. H & E, 40 × 8).

(Puente and Acevedo, 1927); cheilitis glandularis purulenta superficialis (Baelz, 1890); and cheilitis apostematosa (Volkmann, 1870).

Cheilitis Glandularis Simplex

Cheilitis glandularis simplex is regarded as a hereditary anomaly of primordial origin, evidenced by its familial occurrence; males are twice as often involved as females. It has been found in 3 percent of patients in South America (Puente and Acevedo, 1927) and in 0.1 percent in Austria (Wendelberger, 1957). A noncongenital cheilitis glandularis with some dilatation of the gland orifice was recorded by Woodburne and Philpott (1950). It is related to a manifestation of an emotional disturbance.

Cheilitis glandularis simplex is clinically distinguished by red pinhead-sized spots on the mucosa of the lower lip, around the openings of heterotopic salivary glands usually located in the inner part of the mucosa. With pressure upon the glands, water-clear saliva drops appear in the openings of the ducts. In the milder form there is a normal appearance of the lip, while swelling and ectropion mark advanced cases, giving an appearance of macrocheilia (Figs. 25–18 and 25–19). The enlarged mucous glands are palpable through the mucous membrane. Several authors have noted that the facial skin of the patient shows changes of precocious senility (Michalowski, 1962; Puente and Acevedo, 1927; Touraine and Solerrte, 1934; Wendelberger, 1938a and b; Schuermann et al. 1966).

The lesions are localized in the labial glands of the lower lip. The major pathologic manifestation consists of an adenomatous hypertrophy of the glands, which may attain several times their original size. The glands are essentially of the mucous type, although a few serous cells may be observed (Wendelberger, 1938a and b). The mucus-secreting cells are at different phases of secretory activity. Whereas some show maximal activity and the cytoplasm is

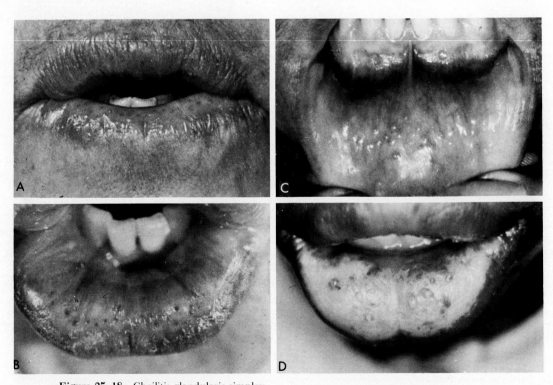

Figure 25–18   Cheilitis glandularis simplex.
A and *B*, Red pinhead-sized spots on the mucosa of lower lip.
C, Hypertrophied heterotopic salivary glands in the inner part of the mucosa of lower lip.
D, Clear saliva drops in the openings of the ducts.

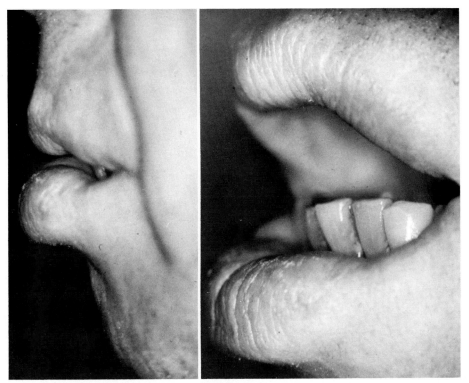

Figure 25-19 Cheilitis glandularis. Macrocheilia and ectropion of lower lip.

filled with mucus, others are small and in their cytoplasm very little mucus can be detected. Thus the hypertrophic labial glands resemble not the submaxillary but the sublingual salivary glands (Puente and Acevedo, 1927). The excretory ducts, both inside and outside the glands, show a marked dilatation and sometimes a cystic appearance of their lumina. The ducts are lined by one or two layers of epithelial cells and contain acidophilic material. Keratotic rings encircle the openings of the ducts (Figs. 25–20 and 25–21C).

In addition to the hypertrophy of the normally located labial glands, groups of heterotopic glands are seen in the transitional zone of the lip extending to the vermilion. These heterotopic glands are equally hypertrophic and show dilatation of their excretory ducts.

Whereas small perivascular inflammatory cells are seen, no inflammatory cells are generally observed within or around the hypertrophic, heterotopic glands (Wendelberger, 1938a and b). According to Wendelberger (1938a and b), senile atrophy of the overlying epithelium is commonly found covering the glandular cheilitis. The underlying corium shows

actinic senile changes manifested by basophilic degeneration.

Differential Diagnosis. The red pinhead-sized spots on the mucosa in mild cases are reminiscent of small angiomas or the Osler syndrome, while cases with macrocheilia may suggest lymphangioma or cheilitis granulomatosa (Miescher, 1945).

Treatment. No treatment is required in mild forms. X-ray treatment was suggested by some authors but rejected by others (Schuermann et al., 1966). Intralesional injections of corticosteroids gave good results (Schweich, 1964). Operative corrections should be considered in all advanced cases (Conway, 1938; Schuermann et al., 1965).

Cheilitis Glandularis Purulenta Superficialis (Baelz)

Unna (1890) reported Baelz's observation of a superficial purulent form of glandular cheilitis which is now regarded as a superficial pyogenic superinfection of the heterotopic salivary glands of the cheilitis glandularis simplex type. A more chronic and severe form was previously

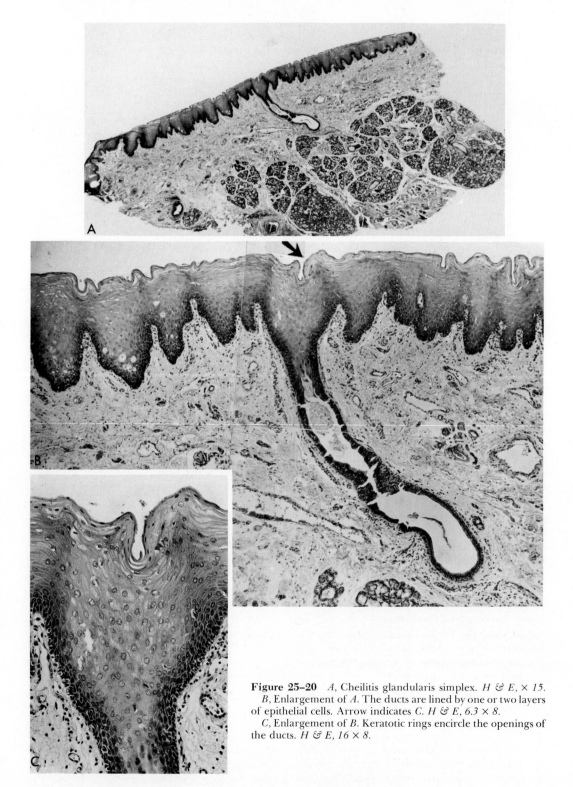

Figure 25–20 *A*, Cheilitis glandularis simplex. *H & E*, × 15.
B, Enlargement of *A*. The ducts are lined by one or two layers of epithelial cells. Arrow indicates *C*. *H & E*, *6.3* × *8*.
C, Enlargement of *B*. Keratotic rings encircle the openings of the ducts. *H & E*, *16* × *8*.

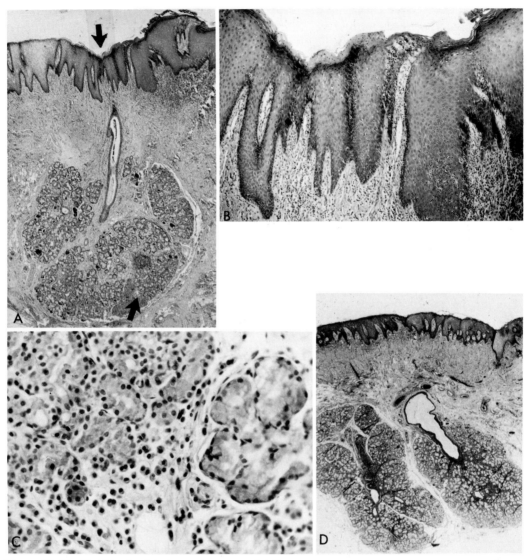

Figure 25–21 Cheilitis glandularis purulenta superficialis.

A, Cheilitis glandularis purulenta superficialis. Arrows indicate *B* and *C. H & E, 1.6 × 8.*

B, Enlargement of *A.* Marked acanthosis of mucosal epithelium. Fibrinous exudate with leukocytes covering erosions. Inflammatory infiltrate in upper corium. *H & E, 16 × 8.*

C, Enlargement of *A.* Numerous plasma cells in inflammatory infiltrate in the gland. *H & E, 25 × 8.*

D, Cystic appearance of excretory ducts. *H & E, 1.25 × 8.*

described by Volkmann (1870) as cheilitis glandularis apostematosa (myxadenitis labialis).

Cheilitis Glandularis Apostematosa

Volkmann (1870) described this conditon of the lower lip due to the association of congenital hyperplasia of heterotopic salivary glands (cheilitis glandularis simplex) with bacterial infection of the glandular acini and ducts. With long duration, the infection proceeds gradually with increasing swelling and greatly reduced mobility of the lip. Everett and Holder (1955) have suggested that infection of the glandular cheilitis is primarily due to chronic chapping, scarring, and subsequent eversion of the lower lip. This ectropion is followed by irritation of the exposed labial mucosa due to drying, actinic influences, and possibly airborne chemicals.

The disorder occurs chiefly on the lower lip, which becomes hard and swollen. The dense swelling may reach the hollow of the chin. The reduced mobility of the lip renders eating and speaking difficult. The mucous glands are palpable through the mucous membrane and give the impression of nodules. With pressure on the affected lip, a mucopurulent secretion can be expressed from the dilated openings of the excretory ducts. The exuded pus forms a gluey film over the lips. Erosions, ulcerations with adherent malodorous crusts, abscesses, and fistulas from the circumglandular fibrous tissue characterize this disorder.

Pathologically, the acini of the heterotopic salivary glands are filled with leukocytes and detritus of desquamated glandular epithelial cells. In the periglandular connective tissue, infiltration of lymphocytes and plasma cells is seen, with an increase of fibroblasts. There is a marked acanthosis of the mucosal epithelium, and a fibrinous exudate with leukocytes covers the erosions and ulcerations (Fig. 25–21).

Differential Diagnosis. The intraacinar and intraductal inflammatory exudate distinguishes glandular cheilitis from granulomatous cheilitis (Miescher, 1945) and the Melkersson-Rosenthal syndrome.

Treatment. Good results with local iodine treatment were obtained by earlier authors (Volkmann, 1870; Unna, 1890; Jordan and Taratuchin, 1935). In one of his cases Sutton (1914) saw improvement following x-ray treatment. Schiavi and Mazzanti (1963) recorded good results with contact roentgen therapy, while Schuermann et al. (1966) saw no benefit from this treatment. Antibiotics and sulfa drugs should be tried (Schuermann et al., 1966), but surgical treatment gives the best results (Doku et al., 1965).

Malignant Development of Glandular Cheilitis

Puente and Acevedo (1927) reported the first case of cheilitis glandularis simplex associated with cancer. Bejarano (1933–34) reiterated the notion of the precancerous origin of cheilitis glandularis simplex, admitting that it would be an error to generalize cheilitis glandularis as a genetic factor in epithelioma of the lip. Touraine (1950), reviewing 132 cases of glandular cheilitis in the literature, emphasized the frequency of cancerous degeneration (36 cases). The periorificial leukoplakic rings encircling the openings of ectopic glands of the lip have been reported to be precancerous, in certain instances giving rise to squamous cell carcinoma. Touraine (1950) and Bejarano (1933–34) stated that many of these epitheliomas developed from the main excretory ducts of aberrant salivary glands. Grinspan et al. (1961) considered cheilitis glandularis as a concomitant symptom but not the starting point of the squamous cancer of the lip. Duperrat et al. (1961), presenting two cases of cheilitis glandularis with carcinoma-like changes seen clinically, found histologically a pseudoepitheliomatous hyperplasia. They maintain that some of the cases reported as malignant degeneration were in fact pseudoepitheliomatous hyperplasias, which often cannot be distinguished from the actual malignancy. Michalowski (1962), reporting six cases of cheilitis glandularis associated with epithelioma of the lower lip, could not trace histologically a relation between the cancer and salivary glands. All his patients were outdoor workers, aged over 40. Exposure of the protruded lip to the sun may have been the cause of malignancy, while the heterotopic glands were a contributory factor. Bâlus (1965), analyzing 97 cases of cancer of the lower lip, found that in 36 cases (37 percent) heterotopic glands and even cheilitis glandularis were close to the tumor but had no part in the origin of the malignancy. Bâlus further claims that in the majority of his cases actinic changes were the precancerous lesions and the glandular cheilitis was a mere coincidence. In two of our cases of cheilitis glandularis simplex, squamous cancer of the lip was detected. No connection of the cancer to the ectopic glands or the leukoplakic rings encircling the openings of the ectopic glands could be traced (Figs. 25–22 and 25–23).

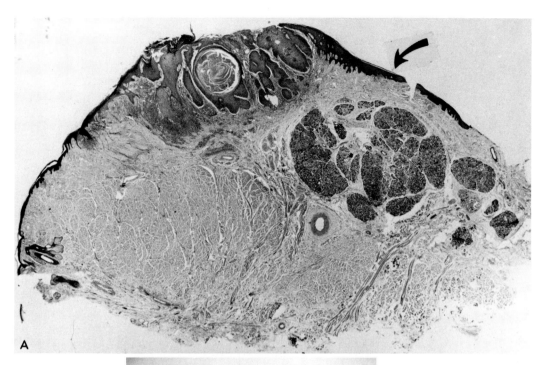

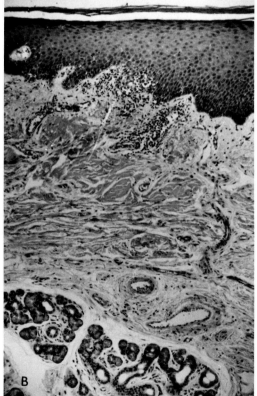

Figure 25–22 Cheilitis glandularis and squamous cell carcinoma.

A, Squamous cell carcinoma developing in area of chronic actinic changes in vermilion. Arrow indicates *B*. *H & E*, × *10.*

B, Enlargement of *A*. Hypertrophic epithelium, basophilic degeneration of corium above the heterotopic glands. *H & E*, *6.3 × 8.*

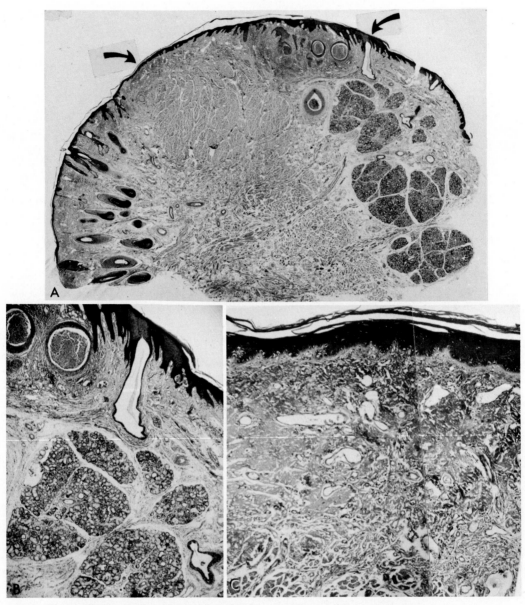

Figure 25–23   Cheilitis glandularis and squamous cell carcinoma.
A, Arrows indicate *B* and *C*. *H & E*, × *10*.
B, Enlargement of *A*. Close neighborhood of ectopic glands and carcinoma. *H & E*, *2 × 8*.
C, Severe actinic changes in area of carcinoma. *H & E*, *6.3 × 8*.

CHEILITIS PLASMA-CELLULARIS

In the last two decades several authors have emphasized the abundance of plasma cells around the natural orifices of the body at the conjunction of skin and mucous membranes (Zoon, 1952 and 1955; Nödl, 1954; Nikolowsky and Wiehl, 1955-56; Woringer and Malhuret, 1959; Hornstein, 1960). Schuermann (1960) named it plasmocytosis circumorificialis.

The lower lip is involved in all cases described so far (Luger, 1968; Molden-hauer, 1966; Peirone, 1968; Zina and Peirone, 1968). Edema and infiltration of the lip, tiny fissures, superficial erosions, and shallow ulcers with leukokeratotic borders mark the changes on the vermilion. Luger (1968) stressed the dark red color with lacquer-like glaze of the lesions, while Zina and Peirone (1968) recorded a granulomatous aspect in one case and keratotic lesions in a second.

The epithelium is atrophic, in places reduced to a few cellular layers, only isolated rete ridges being recognizable. The central part of the lesion may be eroded and the covering epithelium replaced by scales formed by fibrin and leukocytes. The whole corium is filled with massive infiltrate consisting almost exclusively of plasma cells, obliterating the mucosal papillae (Luger, 1968; Zina and Peirone, 1968). An infiltrate-free subepidermal border strip was recorded by Schuermann (1960) and a streaked arrangement of the plasma-cellular infiltrate by Nikolowsky and Wiehl (1955–56).

The vessels of the entire corium, including the capillaries, are dilated and congested. The endothelial cells are in many places arched cushion-like against the tumor (Luger, 1968). Some plasma cells grouped around the blood vessels in a sleeve-like arrangement have large nuclei with irregular chromatin distribution (Zina and Peirone, 1968). In none of the recorded cases was malignancy suspected.

Differential Diagnosis

Luger (1968) considered that the lacquer-like glaze and livid red color of the vermilion helps clinically to differentiate cheilitis plasma-cellularis from cheilitis precancerosa-abrasiva (Manganotti, 1934), and the absence of palpable ectopic glands helps distinguish it from cheilitis glandularis. It is the histologic examination which confirms the diagnosis. The large number of plasma cells present in cases of actinic cheilitis should be taken into account.

SUMMARY

In reviewing the different types of cheilitis and their connection with lip cancer it becomes obvious that sun exposure is the main factor in the development of this malignancy. Sun exposure is implicated as the cause of lip cancer because of the prevalent occurrence of lip cancer of the sun-damaged lower lip in outdoor workers and in light-complexioned persons who have less inherent protection.

Cheilitis actinica belongs to the facultative precanceroses in the broader sense of the term. Persons with existing malignancies in the face and concomitant chronic actinic cheilitis are more prone to cancer of the lip.

Malignant degeneration of actinic cheilitis is clinically expressed by the appearance of horny prominences, ulcers, and deep fissures. However, cancer of the lower lip may occur years after the cheilitis has been clinically cured. The histologic criteria for the malignant changes of actinic cheilitis are manifested by atypia and loss of polarity of the basal layer cells, hyperchromatism of the nuclei, increased number of mitotic figures, and individual cell keratinization. Histologic examination of the entire mucosa of the lip in material obtained by lip shaving of cases of circumscribed carcinoma has disclosed considerable deterioration of the area with a normal clinical appearance. This could explain certain relapses and new malignancies in the mucosa of the lip following radical operation of the cancer and many so-called "denova" cases of cancer of the lip.

Cheilitis abrasiva precancerosa of Manganotti is a late variant of cheilitis actinica and a precancerosis in the strict sense. Many authors are reluctant to accept glandular cheilitis as a precancerosis per se and have a tendency to relate cancer to an actinic cheilitis following upon the glandular cheilitis.

REFERENCES

Ackermann, L. V., and Del Regato, J. A.: Cancer: Diagnosis, Treatment, and Prognosis. Ed. 3. St. Louis, C. V. Mosby, 1962, p. 258.

Andrade, R.: Die präcanceröse und canceröse Wucherung von Epidermis und Anhangsgebilden. *In* Jadassohn, J. J.: Handbuch der Haut- und. Geschlechtskrankheiten. 1,2:344–415, Berlin, Springer-Verlag, 1964.

Ariel, I. M.: Principles in the treatment of lip cancer. *In* Pack, G. F., and Ariel, I. M.: Treatment of Cancer and Allied Diseases. Vol. 3. Ed. 2. New York, Harper & Row, 1958, p. 53.

Atkin, M., Fenning, J., Heady, J. A., Kennaway, E. L., and Kennaway, N. M.: Mortality from cancer of skin and lip in certain occupations. Br. J. Cancer. 3:1, 1949.

Ayres, S., Jr.: Chronic actinic cheilitis. J.A.M.A., 81:1183, 1923.

Baelz, cited by Unna, P. G.: Uber Erkrankungen der Schleimdrusen des Mundes. Monatsschr. Prakt. Dermatol., 11:317, 1890.

Bâlus, L.: Ist die Cheilitis glandularis eine präcanceröse Erkrankung? Hautarzt. Jan. 16, 364, 1965.

Bejarano, J.: Queilitis glandular y epithelioma. Act. Dermo-silfiliogr. (Madr.), 21:504, 1929.

Bejarano, J.: La quelitis glandular como afección cancerígena accidental. Act. Dermo-sifiliogr. (Madr.), 26:535, 1933–34.

Bejarano, J.: Nueva contribución al estudio clinico de la queilitis glandular. Act. Dermo-sifiliogr. (Madr.), 4:405, 1935.

Bezzabotnov, A. S., and Savkina, J. D.: Bucky-rays in the treatment of certain forms of cheilitis. Vestn. Dermatol. Venerol., 38:41, 1964.

Bielicky, T.: Die akute Cheilitis actinica im gemässigten Klima. Hautarzt, Jan. 16, 25, 1965.

Brans, H.: Anatomie des Menschen. Berlin, Springer-Verlag, 1956.

Canizares, O.: Actinic Cheilitis. Arch. Dermatol., 89:286, 1964.

Chalmers, A. J., and McDonald, N.: Some cosmopolitan Sudan skin affections. III. Cheilitis exfoliativa. J. Trop. Med. & Hyg., 24:69, 1921.

Cipollaro, A. C., and Costello, N. J.: Cheilitis exfoliativa. Arch. Dermatol., 57:459, 1948.

Cockerell, E. G., Freeman, R. G., and Knox, J. M.: Changes after prolonged exposure to sunlight. Arch. Dermatol., 84:467, 1961.

Conway, H.: Macrocheilia due to hyperplasia of labial salivary glands, operative correction. Surg. Gynecol. Obstet., 66:1024, 1938.

Costello, M. J.: Cheilitis exfoliativa. Arch. Dermatol., 57:459, 1948.

Costello, M. J., and Délacrétaz, J.: Epithéliomas et états préepithelimateux cutanés. Congrès Dermat. et Syph. de Langue Franc., Alger, 1959, Paris, Masson, 1961.

Covisa, I. S., Bejarano, J., and Gay Prieto, J. G.: Cheilitis glandularis simplex, ses rélations avec les épithéliomes de la lèvre. Ann. Dermat., 1931, p. 111.

Cruickshank, A. H.: Malignant tumors of the lips, tongue, mouth and jaws. In Cancer. Vol. 2. London, Butterworth, 1958, p. 58.

Curtis, G. H., and Rogers, F. J.: Cheilitis exfoliativa. Arch. Dermatol., 66:534, 1952.

Decker, A.: Cheilitis exfoliativa controlled by Riboflavin. Arch. Dermatol. Syphiligr. (Paris), 43:591, 1941.

Dojmi, L.: Ist Cheilitis aestivalis eine Avitaminose? Z. Haut. Geschlechtskr., 61:401, 1939.

Doku, H. C., Shklar, G., and McCarthy, P. L.: Cheilitis glandularis, Oral Surg., 20:563, 1965.

Duperrat, B., and Golé, L.: Chéilite glandulaire à microkystes douloureux. Bull. Soc. Fr. Dermatol., 62:139, 1955.

Duperrat, B., Mascaro, J. M., and Préaux, J. L.: Problèmes diagnostiques, pronostiques et thérapeutiques posés par les chéilites glandulaires. Bull. Soc. Fr. Dermatol. Syphiligr., 68:185, 1961.

Everett, F. G., and Holder, T. D.: Cheilitis glandularis apostematosa. Oral Surg., 8:405, 1955.

Fox, H.: Cheilitis glandularis. J. Cutan. Dis., 31:415, 1913.

Fraenkle, H. L.: Routine management of carcinoma of the skin and lips. N.Y. State J. Med., 49/14, 1949, p. 1659.

Freeman, R. G.: Carcinogenetic effects of solar radiation and preventive measures. In Cancer. London, Butterworth and Company, Ltd., June 21, 1968, p. 1114.

Fritsch, H.: Die Geschwülste der Haut. Stuttgart, G. Thieme, 1957.

Gay Prieto, J., Jaqueti, J., and Alvarez-Cascos, M.: Epitheliomes et états pré-épithéliomateux cutanés. Paris, Masson, 1959.

Gougerot, H.: Chéilites solaires. Lucites solaires labiales et causes sensibilisantes. Bull. Soc. Fr. Dermatol. Syphiligr., 43:1592, 1936.

Grin, F. J.: Cheilitis aestivalis. Lijcnicki Vjesnik (Poseban Otisak), 1:60, 1938.

Grinspan, D., and Abulafia, J.: Carcinoma der Unterlippe nach Leukoplakie. In Cancer. London, Butterworth, 8:1047, 1955.

Grinspan, D., Villapol, L. O., Diaz, J., Israelson, M., Belin, S., and Bongiorno, R.: Etats pré-épithéliomateux de la lèvre. Xe Congrès de Dermat. et Syph. de Langue Franc., Alger, 1959. Paris Masson, 1961.

Hall, A. F.: Relationship of sunlight, complexion and heredity to skin carcinogenesis. Arch. Dermatol. Syph. (Berl.), 61:589, 1950.

Hämäläinen, M. J.: Cancer of the lip with special reference to predisposing influence of sunlight and other climatic factors. Ann. Chir. Gynaecol. Fenn., 44 (Suppl. 175), 1955.

Hissing, A. C.: Cheilitis. Nederland Tijdschr. Geneesk. 1921, II. 65, p. 1399; Ref.; Z. Haut. Geschlechtskr., 3:451, 1922.

Höfer, W., and Honemann, W.: Beitrag zur Problematik der Cheilitis actinica. Hautarzt, 19:175, 1968.

Hornstein, O.: Vulvitis chronica plasmacellularis. Hautarzt, 11:165, 1960.

Johnson, T. B., and Whillis, J.: Gray's Anatomy. Ed. 13. London, Longmans Green Co., 1949.

Jordan, A., and Taratuchin, A.: Über Cheilitis exfoliativa und glandularis. Dermatol. Z., 70:249, 1935.

Katzenellenbogen, I.: Cheilitis exfoliativa actinica. Harefuah, 11:62, 1936.

Katzenellenbogen, I.: Cheilitis exfoliativa actinica. Acta Derm. Venereol. (Stockh.), 18:319, 1937.

Katzenellenbogen, I., and Sandbank, M.: Beitrag zum Pemphigus vulgaris. Hautarzt, 10:363, 1959.

Knox, J. M.: Harmful effects of sunlight. Texas J. Med., 56:653, 1960.

Knox, J. M., Griffin, A. C., and Hakim, R. E.: Protection from ultraviolet carcinogenesis. J. Invest. Dermatol., 34:51, 1960.

Kopf, A. W.: Cheilitis glandularis simplex. In discussion of L. Schweich. Arch. Dermatol., 89:301, 1964.

Koten, J. W., Verhagen, A. R. H. B., and Frank, G. L.: Histopathology of Actinic Cheilitis. Dermatologica, 135/6, 1967, p. 465.

Kuske, H.: Actinic chronic cheilitis. Jadassohn, J.:

Handbuch der Haut- und Geschlechtskrankheiten. Berlin, Springer-Verlag, II, 2, 1965.

Lane, S. L.: Oral cancer. Oral Surg., 6:258, 1953.

Larson. D. L., Coers, C. R., Rodin, A. E., Parcansky, G. M., Corujo, M. R., and Lewiss, S. R.: Lymphatics of the upper and lower lip. A clinical and experimental study. Am. J. Surg., 114:525, 1967.

Luger, A.: Cheilitis plasmacellularis. Hautarzt, 17:244, 1968.

Lynch, G. A.: Cancer of the lip. Ulster Med. J., 36:44, 1967.

McDonald, E. J.: The epidemiology of skin cancer. Invest. Dermatol., 32:379, 1959.

Maisler, A.: Cheilitis glandularis and cancer. Z. Haut. Geschlechtskr., 56:436, 1937.

Manganotti, G.: Cheilitis abrasiva precancerosa. Arch. Ital. Dermatol., 10:25, 1934.

Marchionini, A., and Tor, S.: Zur Klimatophysiologie und Pathologie der Haut. Die Sommercheilitis in Zentralanatolien. Arch. Dermatol. Syph. (Berl.), 179:421, 1939.

Markewich, V. S.: A primary pemphigus focus running a course of exfoliative cheilitis. Vestn. Dermatol. Venerol., 41:82, 1967.

Maskilleison, A. L.: Precancerous cheilitis abrasiva. Klin. Med. Moscow, 45:93, 1967.

Maskilleison, A. L.: Uber die Vorkrebserkrankungen der Lippen, Cheilitis abrasiva, Manganotti, Dermatol. Wochenschr., 155:103, 1969.

Meyer, L.: Comment to van Ziele. W. N. J. Oral Surg., 25:56, 1956.

Michalowski, R.: Chéilite glandulaire suppurée en surface ou maladie de Baelz. Acta Derm. Venereol. (Stockh.), 27:31, 1946.

Michalowski, R.: La chéilite glandulaire et le cancer de la lèvre inférieure. Dermatologica, 96:15, 1948.

Michalowski, R.: La chéilite actinique et héterotopie labiale des glandes salivaires, un syndrome inédit. Dermatologica, 114:373, 1957.

Michalowski, R.: Cheilitis glandularis, heterotopic salivary glands and squamous cell carcinoma of the lip. Br. J. Dermatol., 74:445, 1962.

Miescher, G.: Über essentielle granulomatöse Macrochilie (Cheilitis granulomatosa). Dermatologica, 91:57, 1945.

Mikulicz, J., and Kümmel, W.: Krankheiten des Mundes. G. Fischer Verlag, Jena, IV. Auflage, S. 217, 1922.

Moldenhauer, E.: Cheilitis plasmacellularis, ein Beitrag zur Plasmocytosis circumorificialis. Dermatol. Wochenschr., 152:636, 1966.

Molesworth, E. H.: Die Aetiologie und Zellpathologie des Haut-und Lippenkrebses in Australien.Dermatol. Wochenschr., 99:945, 1934.

Nicolau, S. G., and Bâlus, L.: Chronic actinic cheilitis and cancer of the lower lip. Br. J. Dermatol., 76:278, 1964.

Nikolowski, W., and Wiehl, R.: Pareiitis and Balanitis plasmacellularis. Arch. Klin. Exp. Dermatol., 202:347, 1955–56.

Nödl, F.: Zur Klinik und Histologie der Balanoposthitis chronica circumscripta benigna, plasmacellularis (Zoon). Arch. Dermatol. Syph. (Berl.), 198:557, 1954.

Pashkov, B. M.: Lesions of the oral mucosa and red border of the lips in certain dermatoses. Vestn. Dermatol. Venerol., 43:3, 1927.

Peirone, C. A.: Su due casi di cheilite circumscritte chronica plasmacellulare, Minerva Dermatol., 43:443, 1968.

Pilheu, F. R., and Pradier, R. N.: Cancer del labio, nuestra experiencia de 223 enfermos. Bol. Soc. Argent. Ciruj., 24/22:659, 1963.

Puente, J. J., and Acevedo, A.: Queilitis glandular. Rev. Méd. Lat. Am.. 12:671, 1927.

Purdon, H. S.: Four cases of cheilitis glandularis. Br. J. Dermatol., 70:293, 1954.

Ratzkowski, E., Hochman, A., Buchner, A., and Michman, J.: Cancer of lip. Review of 167 cases. Oncologia, 20:129, 1966.

Richter, R.: Das Hautcarcinom in seinen Formen und seinen Beziehungen zu ethiologischen und klimatologischen Faktoren. Dermatol. Wochenschr., 42:1025, 1960.

Savkina, G. D.: The clinical picture and treatment of exfoliative cheilitis. Vestn. Dermatol. Venerol., 36:43, 1962.

Schiavi, J. F., and Mazzanti, J.: Resultati della radiotherapia nel trattamento de alcune alterazioni precancerose del labbro inferiore (Cheilitis glindolari leucoplassie). Radiobiol. Radioter. Fis. Med., 18:294, 1963.

Schweich, L.: Cheilitis glandularis simplex. Arch. Dermatol., 89:301, 1964.

Schmitt, C. K., and Folsom, T. C.: Histologic evaluation of degenerative changes of the lower lip. J. Oral Surg., 26:51, 1968.

Schuermann, H.: Plasmocytoses circumorificialis. Dtsch. Zahnaerztl. Z., 15:601, 1960.

Schuermann, H., Greither, A., and Hornstein, O.: Krankheiten der Mundschleimhaut und der Lippen. (Ed. 3. München, Urban & Schwarzenberg, 1966.

Shakhova, T. V.: Cheilitis as a precancerous disease. From the book Nauchnaya Sessia postvyaschennaya 100-letin, 1963; cit.: Experta Medica, Section XIII, 18, 1964, p. 720.

Sicher, H.: Oral Anatomy. St. Louis, C. V. Mosby Company, 1952, pp. 178–180.

Spatz, S.: Solar cheilitis with carcinomatous changes of a case. J. Oral Surg., 22:520, 1964.

Steigleder, G. K.: Die Präcancerosen in moderner Sicht. Hautarzt, 14:2, 89, 1962.

Sulzberger, M. B., and Goodman, J.: Acquired specific hypersensibility to simple chemicals: Cheilitis with special reference to sensitivity to lipstick. Arch. Dermatol., 37:597, 1938.

Sutton, R. L.: The symptomatology and treatment of three common diseases of the vermilion border of the lip. Internatl. Clinic, 3:123, 1914.

Touraine, A.: Sept. observations de chéilites glandulaires dont cinq avec cancer. Bull. Dermatol. Syphiligr., 42:1539, 1935.

Touraine, A.: Les chéilites glandulaires et leur cancer. Presse Méd., 58/78:1369, 1950.

Touraine, A., and Lambergeon, S.: Epithelioma spino-cellulaire sur chéilite glandulaire simple, type Puente. Bull. Soc. Fr. Dermatol. Syphiligr., 5:506, 1949.

Touraine, A., and Solente, A.: La chéilite glandulaire: état précancereux de la lèvre inférieure. Presse Méd., 42:191, 1934.

Unna, P. G.: Über Erkrankungen der Schleimdrüsen des Mundes. Monatschr. Prakt. Dermatol., 11:317, 1890.

Venkei, T., and Sugar, J.: Early diagnosis, pathology

and treatment of malignant tumors of the skin. Budapest, Akademiaii Kado (Publishing House of the Hungarian Academy of Science), 1965.

Versluys, J. J.: Cancer and Occupation in the Netherlands. Br. J. Cancer, 3:161, 1949.

Volkmann, R.: Von einigen Fällen von Cheilitis glandularis apostematosa. Virchows Arch. [Pathol. Anat.], 50:142, 1870.

Wechsler, H. L., and Fischer, E. T.: Oral florid papillomatosis. Arch. Dermatol., 86:480, 1962.

Wendelberger, J.: Cheilitis glandularis simplex (Acevado) mit beginnender maligner Degeneration. Osterr. Dermatol. Ges. Ztbl. Haut. Geschl., 57:648, 1938a.

Wendelberger, J.: Die Cheilitis glandularis simplex and ihre Rolle als Vorläufer maligner Entartung. Arch. Dermatol. Syph. (Berl.), 76:176, 1938b.

Wendelberger, J.: Cheilitis glandularis simplex. Familiäres Vorkommen. Klin. Wochenschr., 84:542, 1957.

Woodburne, A. R., and Philpott, O. S.: Cheilitis glandularis: A manifestation of emotional disturbance. Arch. Dermatol., 62:820, 1950.

Woringer, F., and Malhuret, R.: Plasmocytic balanoposthitis. Bull. Soc. Fr. Dermatol. Syphiligr., 5:831, 1959.

Zelikson, A. S., and Hartman, J. F.: An electron microscopic study of normal human non-keratinizing oral mucosa. J. Invest. Dermatol., 38:99, 1962.

Ziel, W. N., van: Early carcinoma of the lip. Diagnosis and treatment. J. Oral Surg., 25:50, 1965.

Zinsser, F.: Handbuch f. Hautkrankheiten und Mundschleimhaut, Jadassohn, Springer-Verlag, Berlin, Bd. 14, I. Teil, 1930.

Zina, G., and Peirone, C. A.: Chéilite circonscrite chronique à plasmocytes (à propos de deux cas). Bull. Soc. Fr. Dermatol. Syphiligr., 75:344, 1968.

Zoon, I. J.: Balanoposthite chronique circonscrite benigne à plasmocytes. Dermatologica, 105:1, 1952.

Zoon, I. J.: Balanitis und vulvitis plasmocellularis. Dermatologica, 111:175, 1955.

26

Lichen Sclerosus et Atrophicus

G. K. Steigleder, M.D., and M. Schlüter, M.D.

DEFINITION

Lichen sclerosus et atrophicus (LSA) is a disease of unknown origin involving the superficial connective tissue of the skin and adjacent mucous membranes. The most important symptom is pruritus (Oberfield, 1961), which, however, is not always present. The most important visible manifestations are ivory-colored papules, which have a tendency to run together in large patches (Chernosky et al., 1957). The center of the patches shows a "cigarette paper" atrophy. The genital area is a favorite location for LSA; often, especially in males, this area alone is involved. Unfortunately LSA in the genital area has been called kraurosis, a term which has caused much confusion and is better avoided (Wilkinson and Sanderson, 1968). Most cases of kraurosis are LSA, but others are just senile genital atrophy combined with inflammatory processes. We believe that primary vulval atrophy is identical to LSA. In all phimoses developing later in life, LSA is to be suspected; histologic examination confirms the diagnosis. The histologic pattern of LSA is diagnostic.

SYNONYMS

Several names have been given to LSA, for example:
Lichen planus sclerosus et atrophicus (Hallopeau)
Lichen planus sclerosus
Lichen albus (von Zumbusch)
Lichen porcelainé
Lichen sclerosus
Lichen atrophicus
Lichen sclerosus et atrophicus
Dermatitis lichenoides chronica atrophicans (Czilak)
Sclerodermia superficialis circumscripta Unna
Unna's cardlike scleroderma
Patchlike scleroderma
Morphaea guttata
White spot disease
Kraurosis vulvae (Breisky)
Atrophic leukoplakic vulvitis (Taussig)
Kraurosis penis
Kraurosis glandis et praeputii penis (Delbanco)
Balanitis xerotica obliterans (Stühmer)
Balanite interstitielle et profonde (Fournier)

635

Scleratrophy of the glans and the preputium

In 1965 Steigleder et al. coined the term "lichenatrophy" in order to have a simple designation, but this name has not yet caught on. The first description of the disease was given in 1887 by Hallopeau; the histologic examination and description by Darier.

CLINICAL FEATURES

The following facts are based on an analysis of the literature from 1910 to 1970 and on personal observation of 136 patients—66 at the Department of Dermatology of the University of Frankfurt, and 70 at the Department of Dermatology of the University of Cologne. The numbers are based on the data concerning 1528 patients in the literature from 1959 to 1970, unless otherwise stated.

INCIDENCE

The incidence of LSA varies according to the ethnic background of the population (Barclay et al., 1966). Apparently Caucasian patients are particularly prone. The incidence varies between 0.15 and 2 per thousand of the patients of a dermatologic department (Findley, 1969; Perry and Homme, 1965). In an army hospital in Vienna, 0.2 percent of the male patients of the department of dermatology had LSA of the penis (Steppert et al., 1970). LSA is said to involve 4.4 times as many females as males, but in Cologne 26 of the patients with LSA were males and 44 were females, the sex ratio being 1 to 1.7. This difference may be due to the fact that most male cases we diagnosed as LSA may be considered as secondary phimoses by others.

CLINICAL APPEARANCE

The primary lesion is a round or polygonal papule, 2 to 4 mm. in diameter (Fig. 26–1). The papules may be reddish blue but more often are white or ivory colored; on the mucous membranes they are

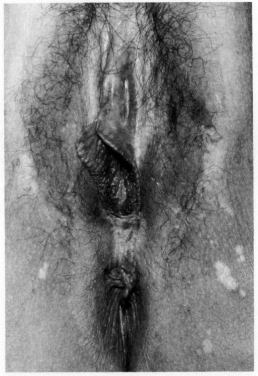

Figure 26–1 Early stage of LSA of the vulva. Small whitish papules are seen on the skin, with more diffuse involvement of the labia and the perineum.

yellowish. The consistency of the papules is variable, sometimes harder and sometimes softer than the surrounding skin. The head of the papule is at first slightly elevated above the surrounding skin; later on, the surface of the papule may be beneath the level of the skin. The papules tend to form large round, oval, polygonal, or bandlike patches. In the center of the patch the skin folds like cigarette paper. The edges of the patches are often hyperpigmented or red. In some cases the edge resembles the lilac ring of localized scleroderma. LSA affects the skin with individual lesions, multiple small papules, large patches which cover entire sections of the skin, or intertriginous, verrucous, bullous, or hemorrhagic lesions (Feldman and Lerner, 1961; Miller, 1957; Montgomery, 1967). Sometimes the appearance is similar to that of vitiligo (Borda, 1961). In the lesions follicular hyperkeratoses are often present. Rubbing the skin feels like rubbing a grater (Nicolau and Balus, 1966).

TABLE 26–1 FIRST LOCALIZATION OF LSA LESIONS ACCORDING TO THE STATEMENTS OF 207 PATIENTS

	♀		♂		
Face	4	+	1	=	5
Neck	15	+	2	=	17
Trunk	4	+	1	=	5
Breast	19	+	2	=	21
Shoulders	10	+	3	=	13
Upper extremities	10	+	3	=	13
Belly	5	+	1	=	6
Hips	5	+	0	=	5
Back	19	+	7	=	26
Lower extremities	8	+	0	=	8
Vulva	24	+	0	=	24
Penis	0	+	64	=	64
					207

Hatched areas of the columns: females; white areas: males.

LOCALIZATION

LSA can in theory occur in any region of the skin, but it favors the genital region, the neck, the upper thorax, and especially the shoulders (Haustein, 1968); it is also found in the submammary area, in the axillae, and on the flexor surfaces of the extremities. Table 26–1, covering 207 patients collected by Schlüter from the literature of 1959 to 1970, shows the location of the lesions of LSA first recognized by the patients. Schlüter also described the localization of lesions in 516 other patients when the diagnosis was first made. Of 943 lesions in those patients, 36.3 percent were in the genital area, 12 percent on the male genitals and 24.3 percent on the female genitals. In 40 cases LSA was generalized. The lips and the scalp were rarely affected. Even the palms and soles may be involved (Purres and Krull, 1971; Wüstner and Gartmann, 1974).

The distribution of LSA-lesions in 539 females and 175 males at the time of diagnosis is shown in Tables 26–2 and 26–3. In this group of patients the only differentiation was between involvement of the anogenital region and the rest of the body.

LSA OF THE FEMALE GENITALS

In females the vulva is chiefly affected (Fig. 26–1). In patients less than 15 years old, the anogenital region is affected twice as often as in adults. The symptoms are pruritus, burning, a stabbing sensation, and pain while urinating and while having intercourse.

The first signs in the female genital area are redness, erythema, and swelling. The physician, however, rarely sees the early stages of LSA. At the time of diagnosis, the vaginal introitus is narrowed, and the labia minora are atrophic. In other words the clinical picture corresponds to what was described as kraurosis vulvae by Breisky in 1885 (Figs. 26–1 and 26–2). Diagnostic for LSA are the already mentioned white papules in the perivulval and perianal areas, especially on the perineum (Fig. 26–1).

Usually LSA begins at the dorsal area of the labia minora (Grimmer, 1970); later LSA surrounds the vulva, the perineum, and the anus like a figure 8 and continues in the shape of an acute angle into the anal rim (Höfs, 1964). LSA also involves the genitocrural folds and the mons pubis. At

TABLE 26–2 DISTRIBUTION OF LSA LESIONS IN 539 FEMALES AT THE TIME OF DIAGNOSIS

	♀		♂		
Vulva alone	8	+	79	=	87
Anogenital region	29	+	157	=	186
Body and anogenital region	11	+	125	=	136
Body alone	12	+	118	=	130
					539

The hatched areas of each column mark the number of patients up to the 15th year of life (left numbers); the white areas mark the number of patients older than 15 years.

TABLE 26–3 DISTRIBUTION OF LSA LESIONS IN 175 MALES AT THE TIME OF DIAGNOSIS

Glans and preputium penis	7 + 130 = 137	
Body and genital area	0 + 22 = 22	
Body alone	1 + 15 = 16	
	175	50 100 150

The hatched areas of each column mark the number of patients up to the 15th year of life (left numbers); the white areas mark the number of patients older than 15 years.

the first stage, the labia minora have disappeared, the vaginal introitus is narrow and sclerotic, the skin is atrophic, and the surface of the skin appears shiny like a tendon or like parchment. We have not found any indication that the hairs of the pudendal area are reduced by LSA.

This typical picture is changed by secondary lesions, by scratching, by microbial infection and vaginal discharge caused especially by *Candida* and *Trichomonas* organisms, and by eczematous reactions caused by hypersensitivity to therapeutic procedures, especially anesthetics. Wetness, warming, rubbing, scratching, sweating, and discharge enhance eczema and pruritus, with the result that LSA as the real disorder is easily overlooked.

Differential Diagnosis

As already mentioned, physiologic involution of the female genitals, combined with eczematous reaction, is to be distinguished from LSA. Lichen planus of the genital area must be considered in the differential diagnosis (Fig. 26–3). The annular lesions and the netlike involvement of the mucous membranes, and the characteristic papules of lichen planus on the areas most affected, may help to make the distinction. Vitiligo never causes atrophy. Localized scleroderma does not cause the same changes in the female genital area. Differentiation between LSA and localized scleroderma in other areas is difficult, even in histologic sections (see Table 26–4).

Differentiation between LSA and leukoplakia is most important, since LSA and leukoplakia are often combined, and leukoplakia may give rise to carcinoma. Leukoplakia is not a disease but a manifestation involving the thickening of the epithelium of the mucous membranes with hyperkeratosis (Montgomery, 1967). Other authors (such as Suurmond, 1964) call this phenomenon leukokeratosis and diagnose leukoplakia only if an atypical proliferation of the epithelium is found. In

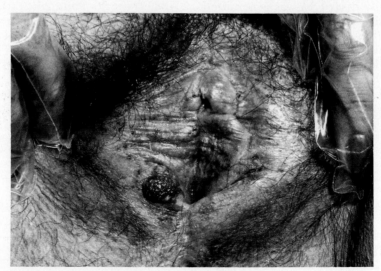

Figure 26–2 Late stage of LSA, or so-called kraurosis vulvae. The labia minora have disappeared, and the introitus vulvae is narrowed; a prickle cell carcinoma is present at the left lower edge.

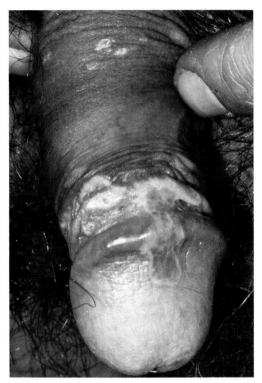

Figure 26-3 Lichen planus of the penis for comparison, showing characteristic annular papules and netlike involvement of the glans.

our opinion, this last lesion should be diagnosed as Bowen's disease of the mucous membranes, which, it is generally accepted, does not have the characteristic pattern of Bowen's disease of the skin. Both leukoplakia and Bowen's disease develop on the LSA of the female genitals. Therefore, LSA of mucous membranes and especially of the female genitals may be considered as a precancerous condition (Banker and Gross, 1962; Steigleder et al., 1965; Suurmond, Wilkinson and Sanderson, 1968).

LSA OF THE MALE GENITALS

In males 90 percent of the LSA lesions are found in the genital area; in nearly 80 percent the genital area alone is affected. The first sign of LSA in this region is a narrowing and sclerosis of the preputial ring (Layman and Freeman, 1944) (Figs. 26-4 and 26-5). In addition, typical papules may be found on the penis, the glans, and especially the preputium. In the early

stages the lips of the external opening of the urethra are swollen, red or white, and surrounded by an erythematous halo (Harkness and Haber, 1960) (Fig. 26-4). Often the opening of the urethra is narrowed. The frenulum and the sulcus coronarius are occasionally affected, but the more distal parts of the urethra, up as far as the fossa navicularis, are only rarely involved. The narrowing of the external opening of the urethra may hamper urination. In contrast to the female genital area, leukoplakia is rarely found on the male genitalia (Tritsch, 1968).

Differential Diagnosis

In the male genital area the diagnosis is easier than in the female genitalia, although LSA is often misdiagnosed as simple phimosis. As far as lichen planus is concerned, the same factors apply as mentioned in the differential diagnosis of LSA of the female genitalia. The characteristic papules of lichen planus, and the annular lesions and netlike lesions of the mucous membranes, are absent in LSA. Dequalinium, a quaternary ammonium antibacterial agent, may cause deep, sharply edged ulcers covered with a "dead-white slough" (Wilkinson and Sanderson, 1968).

HISTOLOGY

Biopsy is highly important in LSA, since the diagnosis can often be easily confirmed by histologic examination. Typical findings in LSA are superficial infiltrations which surround a shell-like edema beneath the epidermis. This edematous connective tissue gives the impression of sclerosis, but only in sections stained with hematoxylin and eosin (Fig. 26-6). Examination in polarized light or by x-ray diffraction reveals that there are less collagen bundles present than in normal skin or, especially, in scleroderma (Steigleder and Raab, 1961) (Fig. 26-7). At first the elastic fibers are pushed aside by edema, but later they are destroyed (Miller, 1957) (Fig. 26-8), as are the reticulum fibers and the collagenous fibers. The PAS-positive rim of connective tissue beneath the epidermis is partly dis-

TABLE 26–4   HISTOLOGIC COMPARISON OF LICHEN SCLEROSUS ET ATROPHICUS AND
CIRCUMSCRIBED SCLERODERMA*

	Lichen Sclerosus et Atrophicus	Circumscribed Scleroderma
Epidermis	atrophic, disturbed keratinization, in early stages acanthotic	less atrophic, rather stretched
Basement membrane	divided into fibers and PAS-positive material, curled, split, partially absent in final stages	usually normal
Corium		
1. Upper portion	characteristic	later affected, same changes as in other layers of the corium or less
Hale-pos. and Azan blue material	only slightly stained, rather increased	early lesions increased, late lesions decreased
PAS-pos. material	diminished in pseudosclerosis	increased in collagen bundles
Reticular fibers	degenerating, no isolated fibers in pseudosclerosis	increased number
Collagen fibers	as reticular fibers	thicker than normal, sclerotic
Elastic fibers	(1) pushed aside in edema; (2) destroyed in pseudosclerosis	mostly normal
X-ray absorption	decreased	increased or not significant
2. Middle portion	pronounced shell-like infiltrate around pseudosclerosis	same involvement as other layers of corium, earliest changes
3. Deeper portion	occasionally involved when affected like upper corium	always pronounced changes present
Blood vessels	normal	pathologic changes present
Infiltrate	absent	present
Appendages		
1. Hair follicles	present; follicular hyperkeratosis and plugging	atrophic, vanished
2. Eccrine sweat glands	preserved	surrounded by sclerotic collagen often atrophic

From Steigleder and Raab: Arch. Dermatol., 84:219, 1961. Copyright 1961, American Medical Association.

solved at the beginning and sometimes destroyed in later stages of the disease. In early stages the epidermis is acanthotic and hyperkeratotic with follicular plugging; in later stages the epidermis is atrophic with dissolution of the basal cells (Klug and Sönnichsen, 1972).

In early LSA the thickening of the epi-

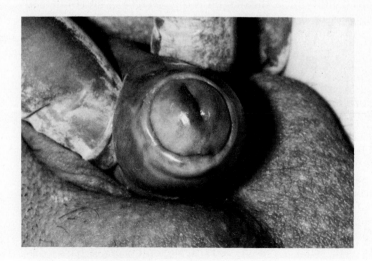

Figure 26–4 LSA of the penis. There is red edema around the external urethral orifice, white patches on the glans, and narrowing of the preputium.

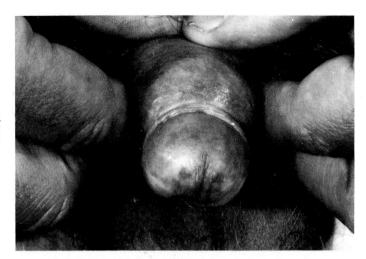

Figure 26-5 LSA of the penis. Preputial sack retracted, glans of the preputium involved (so-called balanitis xerotica obliterans).

dermis and the hyperkeratosis may result in a misdiagnosis of leukoplakia, especially if the dermis is not carefully examined or is not present in the specimen. The infiltrate itself has a lymphadenoid structure and is mostly called a round cell type infiltrate. Apparently in the area of infiltration, new connective tissue fibers are formed (Steigleder and Raab, 1961), as can also be seen with the electron microscope (Forssmann et al., 1964). In the genital area the typical findings are sometimes masked by more pronounced infiltrates, especially by plasma cells (Steigleder et al., 1965). At the beginning the nerve corpuscles are found to be unchanged, but the nerve fibers actually increase, though later they degenerate and disappear (Zeitz and Rösler, 1962). This finding is confirmed by measuring the chronaxia, which is pro-

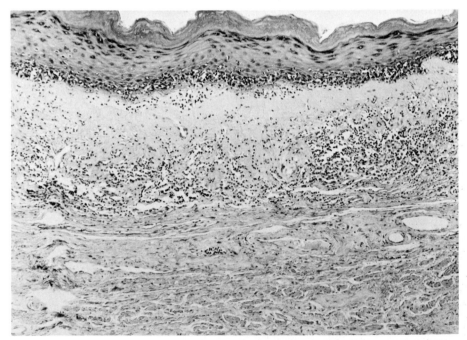

Figure 26-6 Histology of LSA. The epidermis is hyperkeratotic with a pronounced granular layer, liquefaction of the basal cells, and atrophy of germinal layers. Beneath the epidermis, a pseudosclerotic zone with dilated blood vessels appears separated from the deeper dermis by a perivascular infiltrate made up predominantly of round cells. ×125.

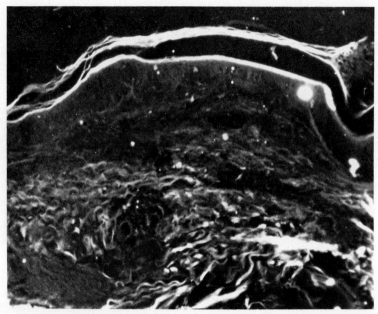

Figure 26–7 A microradiograph of an LSA lesion, in which good permeability to rays appears black and bad permeability white. The horny layer and the collagenous bundles in the deeper dermis are white, and the pseudosclerotic zone reveals good permeability in contrast to the picture seen in true sclerosis. The permeability of the epidermis is increased. × *100*.

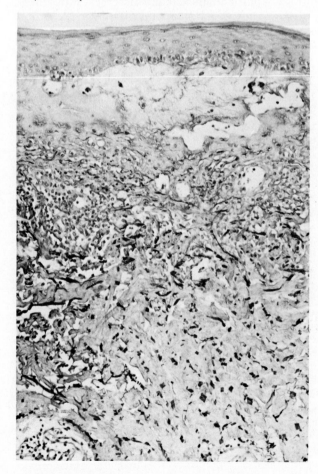

Figure 26–8 Elastic fibers in LSA. In the pseudosclerotic zone the fibers have disappeared. A very small blister is found beneath the atrophic epidermis. *Resorcin, fuchsin, and van Gieson,* × *about 100.*

longed but only in the LSA lesion, whereas in circumscribed and systemic sclerosis, the chronaxia is found to be impaired over the entire skin (Haustein and Sönnichsen, 1968. Meffert et al., 1968). Studies of ^{32}P uptake in LSA of the vulva have revealed inconsistent results (Clarke et al., 1960; Kaufman et al., 1967).

COURSE IN THE GENITAL AREA

Data concerning the course of LSA are contradictory. Of 1528 patients, LSA was reported to have disappeared from only 32. At least in the early stages the lesions may heal without atrophy. The duration of LSA was reported to be a few months or several decades, according to the completely accidental time of examination. Spontaneous resolution is possible but rare.

PROGNOSIS

The prognosis of LSA is good as far as longevity is concerned, but very bad in regard to healing. LSA of mucous membranes and especially of the female genitalia has to be carefully watched, since malignant degeneration is possible in that area. Recently we observed a squamous cell carcinoma of the tongue on LSA in a female.

Malignant Degeneration in the Genital Area

Leukoplakia was found in 93 patients out of 1528; there were four cases of malignant degeneration in the male genital area, and 94 in the female genital area. In Cologne we observed one carcinoma on vulval LSA in 44 patients (Fig. 26–1); in Frankfurt we noted four carcinomas in 30 women with LSA. According to Wallace and Whimster (1951), leukoplakia coexisted with vulval LSA in about 25 percent of the patients; two out of 20 patients revealed a carcinoma. Janowski and Ames found two patients with LSA out of 83 with squamous cell carcinoma of the vulva. Suurmond (1964), in a study of all patients at the dermatologic and gynecologic de-

partments of the municipal hospital in The Hague from 1950 to 1960, reported that of 55 patients with LSA eight had vulval carcinoma, and only 11 patients had carcinoma of the vulva without evidence of LSA. Tritsch (1968) even described an adenoid squamous cell carcinoma on the mucosa of the fossa navicularis in association with LSA.

INCIDENCE IN FAMILIES

Incidence of LSA is reported in only two families (Barker and Gross, 1962). Once a mother and daughter and once two sisters were involved. One of my own patients with LSA of the genital area brought her daughter for examination with possible primary symptoms of LSA in the vulval area. Wüstner and Gartmann (1974) observed LSA of the palms and soles and of the genitals in female monozygotic twins.

COEXISTENCE WITH OTHER DISEASES

In 15 patients the differential diagnosis between LSA and localized scleroderma could not be made. No mention of the coexistence of systemic scleroderma and LSA is to be found in the literature. Unfortunately the differential diagnosis can be made only by exact analysis of the behavior of the fibers in the dermis (see Table 26–1). The statistical correlation of LSA and circumscribed scleroderma has been claimed (Wallace, 1971), but in our opinion it was not proved, even in well-documented patients (Hauser, 1956).

Lichen planus, induratio penis plastica, and alopecia areata were found coexisting with LSA. Eczema was often found in patients with LSA, as mentioned above. Involvement of the internal organs was not mentioned; other internal diseases, however, were seen, such as diabetes (in 15 patients) and gastrointestinal complaints. Apparently these were no more frequent with LSA, however, than is to be expected in a normal population. Wallace (1971) found a probably significant correlation between vitiligo and LSA.

Disturbances of the urogenital system

are mentioned—such as 20 patients with urethritis and seven with cystitis. These might be considered as complications of LSA; in six cases, however, a gonorrheal urethritis also coexisted with LSA (Catterall and Oates, 1962). Malformations of the urogenital tract were found four times (Clark and Muller, 1967). There is mention of LSA beginning in puberty, with menopause, and after menopause. A relation between LSA and hormonal disorders has been mentioned but not proved (Novak and Woodruff, 1974).

Curth (1973) has seen LSA associated with internal malignant tumors. The parallelism of the conditions in two cases went so far that there was improvement of LSA when the tumor was removed and reappearance of the cutaneous lesions when the tumor reappeared.

THERAPY

Several therapeutic measures have been recommended, of which the best seems to be local injection of a suspension of fluorinated steroids (Grimmer, 1970; Steigleder et al., 1965). Lesions may be treated locally by alcoholic solutions combined with subsequent applications of creams containing fluorinated steroids. In addition, symptomatic treatment of the pruritus is recommended, using antihistamines, sedative procedures, and intradermal injection of local anesthetics and of alcohol.

Special Treatment in the Male Genital Area

Circumcision of the sclerotic and narrowed preputium is recommended; if necessary, the preputial sac should be enlarged by plastic surgery. Extension of the external orifice of the urethra by mechanical means is sometimes necessary (Catterall and Oates, 1962), or even incision down to the fossa navicularis (meatomy). In addition, some authors recommend surgical undermining of the skin of the vulva and penis, and some even the resection of the pudendal nerve in special cases.

Special Treatment in the Female Genital Area

Vulvectomy is in most cases contraindicated, since LSA is a generalized disease. Only in cases of precancerous or carcinomatous changes is it recommended. Injections of steroid suspensions are extremely valuable, together with the local treatment recommended above. Of course, secondary infection should also be treated, especially infection by *Candida* and infection of the vagina. In addition, antigens such as anesthetics, which cause an allergic contact eczema of the vulva, should be avoided.

REFERENCES

Barclay, D. L., Macay, H. B., and Reed, R. J.: Lichen sclerosus et atrophicus of the vulva in children. Obstet. Gynecol., 27:637, 1966.

Barker, L. P., and Gross, P.: Lichen sclerosus et atrophicus of the female genitalia Arch. Dermatol., 85:362, 1962.

Borda, J. M.: Formas clinicas del liquen escleroso y atrófico. Z. Haut. Geschlechtskr., 109:121, 1961.

Catterall, R. D., and Oates, J. K.: Treatment of balanitis xerotica obliterans with hydrocortisone injections. Br. J. Vener. Dis., 38:75, 1962.

Chernosky, M. E., Derbes, V. J., and Burks, J. W.: Lichen sclerosus et atrophicus in children. Arch. Dermatol., 75:647, 1957.

Clark, J. A., and Muller, S. A.: Lichen sclerosus et atrophicus in children. Arch. Dermatol., 95:476, 1967.

Clark, D. G. C., Zumoff, B., Brunschwig, A., and Hellman, L.: Preferential uptake of phosphate by premalignant and malignant lesions of the vulva. Cancer, 13:775, 1960.

Curth, H. O.: Discussion of Abrahams, I.: LSA. Arch. Dermatol., 108:433, 1973.

Feldman, F. F., and Lerner, A. G.: Bullous lichen sclerosus et atrophicus. Arch. Dermatol., 83:705, 1961.

Findley, G. H.: Lichen sclerosus et atrophicus. Med. Proc., 15:195, 1969.

Forssmann, W. G., Holzmann, H., and Cabré J.: Elektronenmikroskopische Untersuchungen der Haut beim Lichen sclerosus et atrophicans. Arch. Klin. Exp. Dermatol., 220:584, 1964.

Grimmer, H.: Lichen sclerosus et atrophicus (Kraurosis) vulvae (mit besonderer Berücksichtigung der subfokalen Corticoidtherapie). Z. Haut. Geschlechtskr., 45:535, 1970.

Harkness, A. H., and Haber, H.: Constricting meatopathy of the male urethra. Proc. 11th Internatl. Congr. Dermatol., 1957. Acta Derm. Venereol. (Stockh.), 3:1002, 1960.

Hauser, W.: Zur nosologischen Stellung des Lichen sclerosus et atrophicus. Arch. Klin. Exp. Dermatol., 208:44, 1956.

Haustein, U. F.: Sklerosierende Genitalatrophien als Ursache von Phimosen: Kraurosis penis — BXO — Lichen sclerosus et atrophicus. D. Gesundheitsw., 23:2081, 1968.

Haustein, U. F., and Sönnichsen, Klinische und pathophysiologische Befunde bei Lichen sclerosus et atrophicus. Arch. Klin. Exp. Dermatol., 231:187, 1968.

Höfs, W.: Lichen sclerosus et atrophicus, Kraurosis vulvae und Balanitis xerotica obliterans. Dermatol. Wochenschr., 149:217, 1964.

Janovski, N. A., and Ames, S.: Lichen sclerosus et atrophicus of the vulva: A poorly understood disease entity. Obstet. Gynecol., 22:697, 1963.

Kaufman, R. H., Gardner, H. L., and Johnson, P. C.: ^{32}P uptake in lichen sclerosus et atrophicus of the vulva. Am. J. Obstet. Gynecol., 98:312, 1967.

Klug, H., and Sönnichsen, N.: Elektronenoptische Untersuchungen bei Lichen sclerosus et atrophicus. Dermatol. Monatsschr., 158:641, 1972.

Layman, C. W., and Freeman, C.: Relationship of balanitis xerotica obliterans to lichen sclerosus et atrophicus. Arch. Dermatol., 49:57, 1944.

Meffert, H., Sönnichsen, and Rietschel, L.: Vergleichende Messungen der sensitiven Chronaxie bei verschiedenen Sklerodermie-Formen sowie Lichen sclerosus et atrophicus. Dermatol. Wochenschr., 2:25, 1968.

Miller, R. F.: Lichen sclerosus et atrophicus with oral involvement: Histopathologic study and dermabrasive treatment. Arch. Dermatol., 76:43, 1957.

Montgomery, H.: Dermatopathology. New York, Harper & Row, Publishers, Inc., 1967.

Montgomery, H., and Hill, W. R.: Lichen sclerosus et atrophicus. Arch. Dermatol. Syph. (Berl.), 42:755, 1940.

Nicolau, S. G., and Balus, L.: Sur la localisation vulvaire du lichen scléro-atrophique. Dermatologica, 132:27, 1966.

Novak, E. R., and Woodruff, J. D.: Gynecologic and Obstetric Pathology. Ed. 7. Philadelphia, W. B. Saunders Company, 1974.

Oberfield, R. A.: Lichen sclerosus et atrophicus and kraurosis vulvae. Arch. Dermatol., 83:806, 1961.

Perry, H. O., and Homme, D. V.: Personal communication mentioned by Hunt, A. B., in discussion with J. D. Woodruff. Am. J. Obstet. Gynecol., 91:816, 1965.

Purres, J., and Krull, E. A.: LSA involving the palms. Arch. Dermatol., 104:68, 1971.

Steigleder, G. K., and Raab, W. P.: Lichen sclerosus et atrophicus. Arch. Dermatol., 84:219, 1961.

Steigleder, G. K., Scheicher-Gottron, E., and Kloss, D.: Die Lichenatrophie, ein häufig verkanntes Krankheitsbild. Med. Welt, 10:469, 1965.

Steppert, A., Wruhs, O., and Zandanell, E.: Lichen sclerosus et atrophicus penis. Münch. Med. Wochenschr., 112:1349, 1970.

Streitmann, B.: Lichen sclerosus und Vulvaatrophie. Arch. Dermatol. Syph. (Berl.), 198:199, 1954.

Suurmond, D.: Lichen sclerosus et atrophicus of the vulva. Arch. Dermatol., 90:143, 1964.

Tritsch, H.: Adenoid squamous cell carcinoma in lichen sclerosus et atrophicus. Arch. Klin. Exp. Dermatol., 232:187, 1968.

Wallace, H. J.: Lichen sclerosus et atrophicus. Trans. St. John's Hosp. Dermatol. Soc., N. S., 57:9, 1971.

Wallace, H. J., and Whimster, I. W.: Vulval atrophy and leukoplakia. Br. J. Dermatol., 63:241, 1951.

Wilkinson, D. S., and Sanderson, K. V.: Diseases of the perianal and genital regions. *In* Rook, A., Wilkinson, D. S., and Ebling, F. J. G. (Ed.): Textbook of Dermatology. Vol. II. Oxford, Blackwell Scientific Publications, 1968, pp. 1522-1563.

Wüstner, H., and Gartmann, H.: Palmoplantarer und genitoanaler LSA bei einigen Zwillingen. Z. Haut. Geschlechtskr., 1974 (in press).

Zeitz, H., and Rösler, Morphologische Veränderungen der Nervenstrukturen bei kraurosis vulvae. Arch. Gynaekol., 197:157, 1962.

Complete References

Kloss, D.: Der Lichen Sclerosus et atrophicus als Krankheit des Bindegewebes. Inaugural-Dissertation, D 6 Frankfurt, 1964.

Schlüter, M.: Der Lichen sclerosus et atrophicus. Inaugural-Dissertation, D 5 Köln, 1971.

27

Bowen's Disease and Erythroplasia

John M. Knox, M.D., and L. M. Joseph, M.D.

BOWEN'S DISEASE

Definition

Bowen's disease represents an intraepidermal squamous cell carcinoma involving the skin or mucous membranes. The mucous membrane lesions may involve the mouth, anus, or genitalia. Clinically the lesion usually appears as a solitary, sharply marginated dull red plaque, often with areas of crusting and oozing. The cutaneous lesions are sometimes associated with internal malignancy.

History

Bowen (1912) described two cases of chronic atypical epithelial proliferation of the skin which he termed a precancerous dermatosis. Clinically the nodules were so puzzling that their appearance suggested a late manifestation of syphilis, while histologically they shared many characteristics of the lesions of Paget's disease and arsenical keratosis. The lesions appeared as soli-

tary, well circumscribed, dull erythematous papulonodules with scattered superficial crusting. Darier (1914) gave the name "dermatose precancereuse de Bowen" to the dermatosis and reported three additional cases with a description of two clinical types: (1) lenticular or discoid papules, as described by Bowen, and (2) multiple, nonelevated, scaly or crusted plaques. Histologically the latter lesions were indistinguishable from those reported originally by Bowen. Bowen (1915), in reporting the sixth case, noted that the patient developed a carcinoma of the pylorus two years after apparent cure of the cutaneous tumor. At that time the internal cancer was considered unrelated to the primary skin tumors. When Mount (1921) compiled a complete survey of the literature, only 11 cases had been reported. By that time the concept was well established that Bowen's disease was a precancerous dermatosis, frequently, but not always, resulting in invasive cancer.

Bowen's disease of the oral mucosa was first reported by Lacronique and Dechaume (1932). By 1965 only 24 cases involving the oral mucosa had been re-

646

ported. It is doubtful that the condition is this rare, since some cases are probably mistaken for leukoplakia, white folded nevus, lichen planus, or oral florid papillomatosis. In addition, some patients are probably examined or diagnosed late when invasive carcinoma has already occurred.

Although Bowen's disease was first described as early as 1912, it was not until almost a decade later that the first case involving the vulva was reported (Jessner, 1921). Recognition of the relative infrequency of the disease in this location was documented by the finding of only 40 cases in a recent review (Lewis, 1964).

Etiology

Arsenic. There is a striking similarity in the natural histories of patients with Bowen's disease and those who have had prolonged contact or treatment with inorganic arsenicals. The average latent period of six to eight years from onset of the Bowen's lesions until skin and internal carcinomas appear is characteristic of the long latent period of the carcinogenic action of arsenic. However, in 95 percent of patients with Bowen's disease, there is no history of ingestion of or external exposure to arsenic; yet arsenic exposure may unknowingly occur from medicinal and occupational exposure.

Since arsenic is a known chemical carcinogen widely found in nature, Graham et al. (1961) looked for its presence in the lesions of 50 patients with Bowen's disease as compared with other types of lesions from control patients. The author found increased levels of arsenic in 82 percent of Bowen's lesions as compared to only 30 percent in controls.

Domonkos (1959) analyzed lesions of Bowen's disease from five patients with histories of arsenic exposure and lesions from two patients without such a history and found normal tissue levels of arsenic in all patients. Ferguson et al. (1960) similarly reported no increase in arsenic content in the lesions of six patients with Bowen's disease. The absence of elevated arsenic levels in Bowen's disease noted by

Domonkos and Ferguson could be explained by the relatively small number of lesions analyzed by them.

Since arsenic may be a cause of Bowen's disease, the internal and cutaneous cancers present in these patients may also represent the activity of this potent chemical carcinogen.

Sunlight Exposure. Bowen's disease occurs equally on exposed and covered areas. If clinically typical actinic keratoses that have a bowenoid histology are included in this group, then sunlight would be considered an important cause.

Viruses. Mierowsky et al. (1954) implanted filtered and unfiltered specimens from two cases of Bowen's disease on the allantois and yolk sac of chick embryos. The resulting histologic changes were essentially those of Bowen's disease. Similar histologic changes occurred with the injection of serum. Since the changes could be produced in passages with filtered material, a viral etiology was suggested. However, serologic evidence for an association of an infectious agent and disease in the patient remains to be found.

Electron microscopy has revealed the presence of viruslike particles within the cytoplasm of epithelial cells of Bowen's disease (Olson et al., 1968; Nordquist et al., 1970). In six of seven lesions of Bowen's disease, cytoplasmic particles measuring 800 to 1100 Å in diameter were demonstrated in the basal and malpighian layers of the epidermis. These viruslike particles appear to arise by budding from the plasma membrane or from tubular structures adjacent to the plasma membrane. No similar particles were found in normal skin or other epidermal diseases studied as controls.

Trauma. Stauffer and Lutz (1957) reported a case of histologically proven Bowen's disease at the site of a tick bite. Histologic studies approximately 1½ years after the bite revealed an unusual vacuolation of the epidermal cells. Subsequent biopsies revealed typical Bowen's disease. Early vacuolization in Bowen's disease has been noted previously.

Papa and Kennedy (1968) reported a case of Bowen's disease which occurred on the hip of an 83 year old white man 50 years after he was kicked while playing soccer. A scaling plaque developed at the site shortly after the injury.

Graham and Helwig (1961) obtained information from 111 patients with Bowen's disease regarding possible etiologic factors prior to the onset of the condition, and 37 (33 percent) indicated some variety of trauma to the involved site. Even though they were unable to obtain a large enough series to prove that injury was a statistically significant cause of Bowen's disease, it was their opinion that trauma could act as a triggering or promoting factor in the initiation of Bowen's disease in a predisposed individual. Trauma, however, is such a common occurrence that its role is difficult to evaluate.

Heredity. There is a definite predilection for Bowen's disease to occur in the fair-complexioned individual of Anglo-Saxon ancestry.

Prognosis

Eighty percent of all patients who have Bowen's lesions excised can expect to live for 15 years or longer without having a recurrence. In those patients who have a recurrence of the lesion, 50 percent of recurrences can be expected to appear within 10 months after excision. The five-year mortality from cancer in patients with Bowen's disease and concomitant systemic cancer is 50 percent. In one series, patients who de-

veloped an internal cancer in addition to their Bowen's disease exhibited a median survival time of only 4.6 years (Graham and Helwig, 1961).

Bowen's disease of the skin is not an aggressive carcinoma until it involves the dermis. In Graham and Helwig's series of 155 patients, the dermis was invaded in 8 (5.2 percent) of the patients. In 3 there was deep invasion and metastases to internal organs. Dermal invasion occurred in only 1 of the 38 patients reported by Hugo and Conway (1967). In this case metastases from lesions on both lower extremities to the inguinal areas resulted in the death of the patient.

Clinical Features

Age of Onset. Bowen's disease may occur at almost any age. The average age at onset is 48 years. In 60 percent of patients the onset is between ages 30 to 60. It is uncommon for the disease to begin prior to age 20; only 2 percent of patients were below age 20 at the time of onset (Graham and Helwig, 1961). The age distribution for vulvar lesions is generally between the third and sixth decades of life (Abell and Gosling, 1961); however, one case was reported in an 81 year old woman (Jeffcoate et al., 1944). Therefore, it may be concluded that each age group—reproductive, menopausal, and postmenopausal—is represented. The tendency, however, ap-

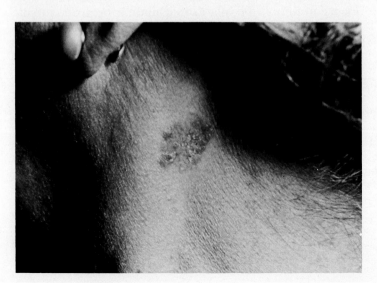

Figure 27–1 Bowen's disease of the neck. The lesion was originally mistaken for a perfume contact dermatitis.

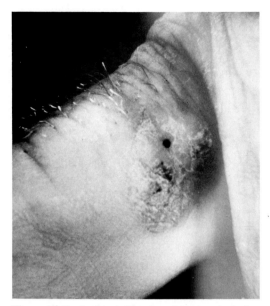

Figure 27–2 Scaling infiltrative plaque on the index finger.

with perhaps a slight predominance in men. There appears to be a striking predominance among Caucasians. Of 155 patients reported by Graham and Helwig (1961), only 7 (5 percent) were non-Caucasians.

Sites of Predilection. Bowen's disease may occur anywhre on the skin surface or on mucosal surfaces. Sites of predilection include the face, ears, neck (Fig. 27–1), lower abdomen, lower back, buttocks, extensor aspect of the thighs and legs, and extensor aspect of the hand and fingers (Fig. 27–2). One-third of all lesions occur on the head and neck. Occurrence is equal on exposed and nonexposed areas. Mucous membrane lesions occur in the mouth, vulva, and anus. Involvement of the glans penis should be considered separately as erythroplasia of Queyrat.

pears to be toward the latter two groups. Bowen's disease associated with pregnancy or diagnosed immediately after pregnancy has not been reported.

Sex and Racial Incidence. Although two large series (Graham and Helwig, 1959; Graham and Helwig, 1961) show a marked male preponderance, the data are probably biased since the major sources of patients were the armed forces. Other studies (Peterka et al., 1961; Hugo and Conway, 1967) have reported approximately equal distribution of the sexes

Clinical Description

Bowen's Disease of the Skin Surfaces. Initially, lesions appear as small erythematous scaling plaques which gradually enlarge in an irregular manner (Fig. 27–3). Graham and Helwig (1959) found a range of 0.7 to 13 cm., with a median diameter of 1.9 cm., among 24 patients. The scale, which appears white or yellow, may be removed without much difficulty to yield an erythematous, moist, granular surface with little or no bleeding. The plaques may be fissured, crusted, eroded, or ul-

Figure 27–3 Slightly scaling, crusted plaque of Bowen's disease on the forehead.

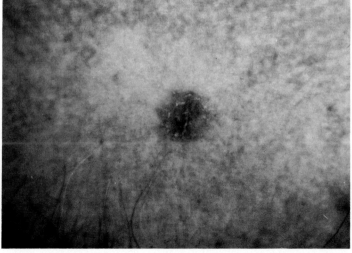

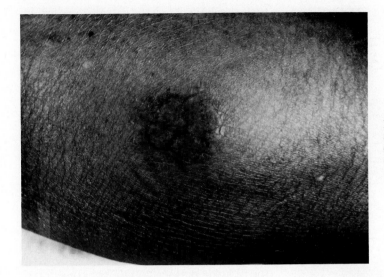

Figure 27–4 Sharply marginated lesions with thick overlying crust on the thigh of an elderly male.

cerated and on palpation feel firm, rough, and granular. The margin is sharp with the surface slightly raised and flat, but it may become irregularly elevated and nodular (Fig. 27–4). Ulceration is usually a sign of invasive growth (Fig. 27–5). Invasion, however, may be delayed for many years after the initial appearance of the condition. The clinical appearance depends somewhat upon location and other extrinsic factors, such as exposure, irritation, trauma, and treatment. Multiple types can occur either widely spaced or in close proximity and may become confluent (Fig. 27–6).

Bowen's Disease of the Oral Mucosa. Bowen's disease of the oral mucosa has a more variable clinical presentation than when it occurs on the skin surface. The appearance of lesions ranges from delicate, opaque, epithelial thickening to pronounced polypoid vegetations. Punctate, streaked, confluent, or chalk-white irregular mucosal opacities also occur. Erosive plaques are considerably less frequent, and their presence suggests transformation into invasive carcinoma.

Bowen's Disease of the Vulva. Bowen's disease, whether it appears on the mucocutaneous or skin surface of the vulva, manifests itself as a rough-surfaced, thick white or reddish brown plaque that slowly enlarges. It is often intensely pruritic. Occasionally the lesions may show ero-

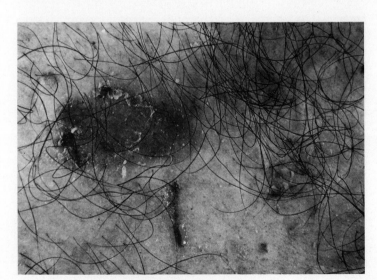

Figure 27–5 Slight scaling and multiple sites of ulceration at the margin of a lesion of the thigh.

sions and ulcerations prior to dermal invasion.

Haber's Syndrome. A variant of Bowen's disease, this syndrome is a rare and persistent familial, rosacea-like eruption involving the face with a tendency to develop intraepidermal epitheliomata on covered areas (Sanderson and Wilson, 1965). Onset is in early life and is characterized by redness of the forehead, cheeks, chin, and nose, which becomes worse after sunlight exposure. In addition to diffuse facial erythema, patchy scales, follicular papules, depressed scars, and telangiectasia are found. In one of the reported cases the trunk was the site of scaly or warty lesions which had the histologic features of atypical Bowen's disease with nests of clear cells.

Symptoms

The lesions are usually asymptomatic but occasionally pruritic or painful. Infrequently, episodes of minor bleeding occur, particularly following trauma. The relative absence of symptoms is supported by the fact that 23 of 35 patients reported by Graham and Helwig (1959) had an interval of 5 to 30 years from onset to removal of the lesions.

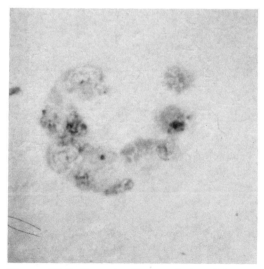

Figure 27–6 Bowen's disease of the abdomen. Multiple sharply marginated, scaling lesions have coalesced to form an annular plaque.

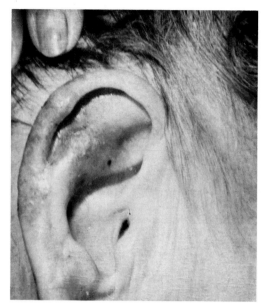

Figure 27–7 Widespread involvement of the helix and antihelix of the right ear.

Differential Diagnosis

Superficial basal cell epithelioma may appear as scaly, crusted, and eroded plaques that mimic Bowen's disease. Usually, however, the overlying epidermis is atrophic in the center, and the tumor is bounded peripherally by a slightly raised threadlike margin. In addition, pigmentary changes may be a prominent feature.

Actinic keratosis often resembles Bowen's disease; however, the former occurs only on exposed areas and usually has a more irregular, poorly defined border and a more erythematous base. Bowen's disease may occur on exposed or covered areas of the body.

Psoriasis occasionally is mistaken for Bowen's disease. Bowen's disease, with its characteristic white or yellow scale, will sometimes look like psoriasis. The scale in Bowen's disease, however, detaches without much difficulty to give a moist, erythematous surface without bleeding. Psoriatic scales when removed yield characterisitic minute bleeding points (Auspitz sign).

Eczema may clinically resemble Bowen's disease when it appears moist and crusted or scaly. Eczema, however, lacks the sharp and slightly elevated margin of Bowen's disease. If the diagnosis is uncertain on initial examination, the lack of improvement after a reasonable course of topical steroid therapy is suggestive of Bowen's disease.

Paget's disease usually first appears as a crusted, intermittently moist lesion on the nipple or genital or perianal region which gradually spreads to produce an eczematous appearance. Later the involved area is erythematous and crusted. If the crusts are removed, a red, glazed, moist or vegetating surface is apparent. Despite the clinical similarities between Paget's disease and Bowen's disease, the latter rarely, if ever, involves the nipple or areola.

Leukoplakia on the vulva usually presents as one or more well demarcated, thickened, greyish white plaques. Its appearance has been likened to white paint that has hardened and cracked. Bowen's disease, when on the vulva, characteristically appears as a raised velvety red or indurated lesion.

Lichen sclerosus et atrophicus involving the vulva presents initially as ivory-colored papules with follicular plugging and hyperkeratosis. Lesions are present in other areas of the body in one-third of the patients. Late lesions appear as plaques of ivory-white atrophic skin with characteristic cigarette paper surface atrophy. Bowen's disease lacks both the ivory color and cigarette paper atrophy.

Oral epithelial nevus, also known as white sponge nevus, may be present at birth or appear in childhood. Extensive areas of the oral mucosa are usually involved and manifest a deeply folded, corrugated, soft white surface. Bowen's disease of the oral mucosa appears much later in life and usually involves only a small localized area.

Oral florid papillomatosis, also a premalignant condition, presents as multiple whitish, friable, papillomatous plaques over extensive areas of the oral mucosa. The surface is much more papillomatous in appearance than a lesion of Bowen's disease.

Relationship to Internal Malignancy

Graham and Helwig (1959) studied 35 patients with Bowen's disease of the skin who either came to autopsy or were known to have died after surgical specimens were examined. Twenty-eight (80 percent) of the 35 patients developed one or more primary internal malignancies or a primary malignancy of the skin with metastasis at an average of 8.5 years after onset of Bowen's disease. Biologically the internal cancers were highly aggressive, since over 90 percent of the patients with primary internal cancers had metastatic lesions or generalized spread. Furthermore, 15 (43 percent) of the group developed a total of 49 premalignant and malignant cancers of the skin that appeared on an average of 6.2 years later than their Bowen's disease. Cancer proneness in this series is even more striking when one considers that 31 (89 percent) of the patients had primary cancer in one or more locations. All three germ layers were affected, with involvement of the respiratory, gastrointestinal, and genitourinary systems occurring in decreasing order of frequency.

Statistical analysis reveals that the difference between Bowen's disease and senile keratosis in relation to the incidence of primary internal malignancy is not significant (Graham and Helwig, 1959). Patients with Bowen's disease, however, are more likely to have primary internal cancer than those with squamous cell carcinoma of the skin.

Bowen's disease appears before the detection of cutaneous premalignant and malignant lesions in approximately 75 percent of patients. Senile keratosis, basal cell epithelioma, and squamous cell carcinoma appear approximately six years after the onset of Bowen's disease, internal cancer and skin cancers with metastasis an average of 8.5 years. Therefore, the time relationship between Bowen's disease and other malignant lesions points to the possibility of a common mechanism for development and perhaps individual predisposition toward cancer.

Hugo and Conway (1967) studied a series of 38 patients with Bowen's disease and found 6 (15.8 percent) to have systemic cancer. There was, however, no relationship between the time of appearance of the Bowen's disease and the diagnosis of the systemic cancer. The incidence of cancer in this group, with an average age of 62 years, was nine times the expected incidence of cancer of all sites and types. Graham and Helwig (1961), in a more comprehensive review of 155 patients with Bowen's disease, detected primary internal cancer in 37 (24 percent).

Peterka et al. (1961) found a significant difference in the incidence of internal cancer, depending upon whether the lesions of Bowen's disease were on unexposed (trunk, arms, legs) or exposed areas (face, neck, hand). When the lesions occurred on exposed areas, there was often difficulty in the histologic differentiation between Bowen's disease and actinic keratosis with bowenoid dyskeratosis. In the group with lesions on unexposed areas, 11 of 33 (33. 3 percent) had an associated internal malignancy. Consequently, convincing evidence exists that the patient with Bowen's disease is disposed to develop internal cancer.

Histopathology

Light Microscopy. Bowen's disease is an intraepidermal squamous cell carci- noma designated also as squamous cell carcinoma in situ. The epidermis is acanthotic with varying degrees of hyperkeratosis and parakeratosis. The malpighian layer shows a disorderly arrangement, and various stages of individual cell keratinization are observed. Many of these keratinized cells are large and round and have a pyknotic nucleus surrounded by an eosinophilic cytoplasm. Such individual cell keratinization is often referred to as malignant dyskeratosis, for it is characteristically found in senile keratosis and squamous cell carcinoma. Other prickle cells have large hyperchromatic nuclei. Giant epithelial cells with prominent mitotic figures are often present and lie adjacent to relatively normal-appearing epidermal cells. Abnormal cells appear to be randomly distributed throughout the full thickness of the epidermis (Fig. 27–8). The rete ridges are elongated and thickened, often reducing the dermal papillae to thin strands. In true Bowen's disease the basal layer remains intact, but in a small proportion of cases the basement membrane is broken through

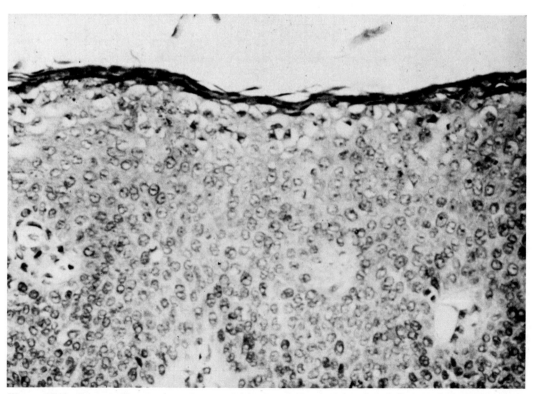

Figure 27–8 Bowen's disease. Note the completely disorderly arrangement of cells in the malpighian layer.

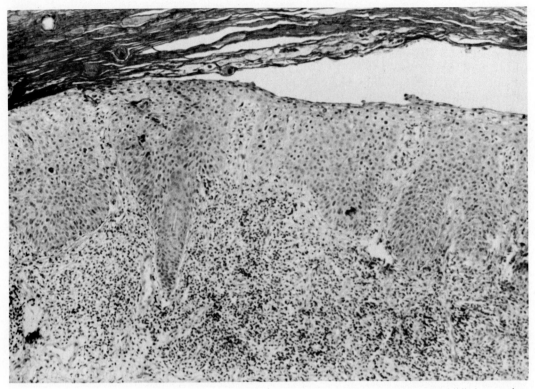

Figure 27-9 Bowen's disease. The epidermis is thickened, and the cells of the stratum malpighii lie in complete disorder. Several multinucleated cells and mitotic figures are present in the malpighian layer. The basal layer is intact. A moderately dense upper dermal infiltrate composed primarily of lymphocytes is present.

and invasive squamous cell carcinoma results.

The upper dermis usually shows a moderate amount of inflammatory infiltrate, primarily lymphocytic in nature but containing some plasma cells (Fig. 27–9). As long as Bowen's disease remains intraepidermal, metastases do not occur; however, when invasion occurs, the likelihood of lymph node metastasis is rather great. Widespread metastasis has been reported in exceptional cases. Invasion may occur initially in only one area or in several areas. For this reason it is almost mandatory, in advanced lesions, that serial sections through the tissue block be examined in order not to overlook such areas.

Electron Microscopy. Electron microscopic observation of Bowen's disease lesions reveals the basal and suprabasal squamous cells to be almost normal. The tonofilaments in these cells are, however, slightly aggregated in a fascicular form. Desmosomes located within squamous cells at the lower part of the epidermis are fewer than normal and poorly developed. These cells represent the dyskeratotic squamous cells seen on light microscopy. In dyskeratotic squamous cells undergoing mitosis, the cell surfaces appear very irregular. Large spaces occur between the mitotic cells and adjacent squamous cells. The most striking feature of these mitotic cells is the characteristic distribution of many fasiculated tonofilaments surrounding condensed chromosomes. Since these displaced fasicles of tonofilaments are entangled with the mitotic apparatus, they may interfere with the normal process of cell division. In some apparently normal cells, large keratinous masses consisting of loosely aggregated tonofilament and dense nuclear substances are present. Such cells probably correspond to the individual cell keratinization observed on light microscopy.

Since keratohyalin granules and membrane coating granules are not present in these abnormal dyskeratotic cells, the dyskeratotic process in Bowen's disease (Seiji and Mizuno, 1969) appears significantly different from that of benign dyskeratosis as observed in Darier's disease (Cauldfield and Wilgram, 1963).

Histopathologic Differential Diagnosis.

In the differential diagnosis, the bowenoid type of actinic keratosis, arsenical keratosis, leukoplakia, and Paget's disease should be considered. The bowenoid type of actinic keratosis differs from Bowen's disease by the presence of atypical cells in the basal layer. Characteristically within the epidermis a carcinoma in situ is found with disorderly, atypical malpighian cells, just as in Bowen's disease.

Arsenical keratoses also show atypical cells in the basal layer but in addition reveal marked vacuolization of malpighian cells. These vacuolated cells have darkly staining nuclei. Although vacuolated epidermal cells occur occasionally in Bowen's disease, they are usually less conspicuous.

In Paget's disease large pale-staining cells are present too, but there is no dyskeratosis, and the cells of the basal layer may appear to be compressed by the large Paget cells. Paget's cells, in contrast to the vacuolated cells in Bowen's disease, contain PAS-positive, diastase-resistant material. Furthermore, Bowen's disease, but not Paget's disease, may show clumping of nuclei within multinucleated epidermal cells and individual cell keratinization.

Therapy

Surgical Therapy. In one large series 36 of 48 Bowen's disease lesions were treated via surgical excision (Graham and Helwig, 1959). Six of these recurred. Two were treated by electrodesiccation, curettage, or both, and each recurred. Graham and Helwig (1961) reviewed therapeutic results of 83 patients who had a five-year follow-up or recurrences or both. Excision of the lesion alone resulted in a cure rate of 80 percent. Desiccation and curettage yielded a success rate of only 27.3 percent. Possibly the results of curettage in Graham and Helwig's series are not truly represent-

ative, because the clinical dermatology staff of Baylor College of Medicine routinely treats cutaneous Bowen's disease by curettage and electrodesiccation, obtaining a cure rate over 90 percent.

The consensus in the obstetric and gynecologic literature regarding vulvar lesions is that vulvectomy is the treatment of choice (Woodruff and Novak, 1962; Collins and Barclay, 1963). The necessity for adequate removal is indicated by the fact that these lesions may become invasive squamous cell carcinomas and subsequently metastasize. Radiation therapy of the vulva is contraindicated.

Good results have been achieved by the use of dermabrasion (Ridley, 1966). In contrast to radiotherapy, which produces scars on the trunk which tend to be thick, scaly, telangiectatic, and unsightly, dermabrasion produces scars which are usually inconspicuous, smooth, soft, and supple.

Topical Therapy. Topical 5-fluorouracil in propylene glycol appears to be effective therapy for Bowen's disease when the size of the lesion, the number of lesions, or the patient's refusal to accept surgery precludes the surgical approach. Jansen et al. (1967) reported that lesions in 9 of 13 patients responded promptly after one month of treatment with complete clearing. In three cases, however, small recurrent areas required reapplication of the medication. Topical 5-fluorouracil in propylene glycol under occlusion has been successfully used to resolve a large, protuberant 8 × 10 cm. lesion of Bowen's disease on the thigh of an elderly patient (Fulton et al., 1968). Occlusion enhances the effect of topical 5-fluorouracil.

Lever has successfully used topical cantharidin, 0.7 percent, in equal parts of acetone and collodion under occlusion for the treatment of lesions involving the fingers (Sweeney and Mescon, 1965). Several separate areas were treated every two weeks. Although the treatment required several months, there was complete healing with no recurrence.

Radiation (Grenz Ray and X-Ray). Bowen's disease responds poorly to x-ray. In a series of five patients treated with cancericidal doses of x-ray, one lesion recurred and four were completely unaltered, as proved by follow-up biopsies

(Graham and Helwig, 1959). A larger series with five-year follow-up reviewed by the same authors revealed a cure rate of only 12.5 percent (Graham and Helwig, 1961).

The successful treatment of Bowen's disease involving the palm utilizing Grenz ray has been reported after a total dose of 6400 R. in eight evenly divided doses over a three-week period (Schonberg and Litt, 1961). A recurrence, however, was noted after treatment of a penile lesion with 6500 R. in 13 equally divided doses of Grenz ray (Brauer and Fried, 1960).

ERYTHROPLASIA OF QUEYRAT

Definition

Erythroplasia of Queyrat is the term used to designate Bowen's disease when it is found on the glans penis. Most American and English authors use the term Bowen's disease for similar lesions occurring on the vulval, oral, and anal mucosa. The disease usually appears as well-defined, red, smooth, velvety plaques with little or no induration. Histologically, the lesions are identical to those of Bowen's disease; however, a higher propensity for dermal invasion with subsequent metastasis exists. Unlike Bowen's disease, there is no known increased incidence of internal malignancy and no established association with arsenic ingestion.

History

Fournier and Darier (1893) were the first to report a case under the title of "Epithelioma benign syphiloide de la verge" (benign syphiloid epithelioma of the penile shaft). The syphilitic implication incorporated into the original title was soon realized to be a chance, unrelated finding.

Queyrat (1911) coined the term "erythroplasia" and applied the name to distinctive, shiny, erythematous lesions of the glans penis on four patients. He considered the condition to be precancerous.

However, a biopsy was performed on the lesion in only one of the four cases, and it showed no definite characteristic of malignancy. Therefore, these early reports did not illustrate a precise relationship between erythroplasia and malignancy (Blau and Hyman, 1955).

Subsequently Hudelo and Cailleau (1933) and Jessner (1921) described cases of mucosal and mucocutaneous lesions with the clinical features of erythroplasia and the histologic features of Bowen's disease. Pautrier (1928) emphasized that erythroplasia and Bowen's disease of the glans penis were one and the same disease and that the condition was a cancer from the onset and not merely precancerous.

The first report in the American literature of erythroplasia was by Sulzberger and Satenstein (1933). The case, however, presented neither clinical nor histologic features of malignancy. In retrospect many of the early reports of "erythroplasia" in the American literature appear to have been benign conditions simulating erythroplasia of Queyrat clinically. For example, Sachs and Sachs (1948) described 10 cases of so-called erythroplasia of Queyrat occurring on both glans penis and glabrous skin of the scrotum. In none of these cases was there histologic evidence of malignancy or premalignancy. Clinical cure was attained with topical arsenical therapy.

Clinical Features

The glans penis represents by far the most common site of occurrence. Of extrapenile locations the vulvar mucosa is prominent, particularly in the foreign literature (Barbier, 1927; Barbier, 1928; Cartraud, et al., 1950); it however, is rarely reported in the American literature (MacDonald, 1941). Other rare sites of occurrence include the anal (Lutz, 1941) and oral mucosa (Darier et al., 1924; Sezary, 1932; Touraine and Solente, 1936).

The classical lesion appears as a solitary, smooth, red, velvety plaque (Fig. 27–10). The plaques are usually flat or slightly raised with a typically moist, glistening, lacquered appearance (Fig. 27–11). One case report describes a patient with nine individual tumors which eventually fused into one (Sezary, 1932).

Erythroplasia always begins on a mucosal surface but may subsequently spread to glabrous skin. The plaque is usually sharply marginated from the surrounding normal skin and may be round, oval, or irregular in shape. Early, normal mucosa may be seen within the plaques. Invasive change is indicated by ulceration, induration, or verrucous appearance.

Age at the time of diagnosis varies from the third to the eighth decades of life with the median age being 52 years. Duration of a lesion at the time of diagnosis may vary from several months to 25 years with a median duration of 2 years. Most cases reported in the foreign literature occurred after the age of 45 (Touraine and Solente, 1936; Jorno, 1938). In the American literature one-half occurred under 50 years of age; however, many of these causes did not represent true erythroplasia. No authentic case of the disease has been reported in men circumcised in infancy. Ninety-five percent of the cases occur in men who have not been circumcised prior to onset of the lesion (Graham and Helwig, 1963). There is no evidence for an increased incidence of skin lesions of Bowen's disease in patients with erythroplasia.

Occasionally the patients complain of mild pruritus, but pain and tenderness are absent. The relative absence of symptoms

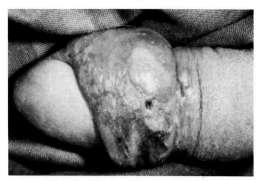

Figure 27–11 Slightly scaling infiltrated plaque of erythroplasia of Queyrat on the prepuce.

often allows the disease to be overlooked or unattended.

Clinical Differential Diagnosis

Nonspecific balanitis presents as a bright red, moist dermatitis involving the glans penis and often the adjacent foreskin, and is associated with a creamy secretion and offensive odor. The condition responds to cleansing and cool compresses.

Zoon's balanitis (Zoon, 1952) appears as a persistent inflammation on the inner surface of the prepuce and the glans. The lesion is erythematous, moist, and shiny in contrast to the velvety appearance of erythroplasia of Queyrat. Biopsy readily distinguishes the two diseases. Zoon's balanitis is best considered a benign yet persistent, usually plaquelike, chronic type of balanitis.

Squamous cell carcinoma of the glans penis may be preceded by leukoplakia, erythroplasia, a chronic ulcer, or a warty excrescence. Invasive change in erythroplasia is evidenced by ulceration, induration, or nodularity.

Lichen planus involving the glans usually appears as chronic violaceous papules. Typical plaques present elsewhere readily differentiate this condition from erythroplasia of Queyrat.

Psoriasis may appear on the glans as a solitary nonhealing plaque. The color of the lesion and its sharp border are usually distinctive, and plaques in other areas confirm the diagnosis.

Circinate balanitis of Reiter's syndrome first appears as a small, opaque vesicle which

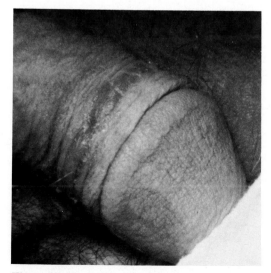

Figure 27–10 An early superficial plaque of erythroplasia involving the prepuce.

rapidly ruptures to form a painless, superficial erosion with only slight surrounding erythema. Coalescence of multiple lesions results in a circinate pattern involving the coronal margin of the prepuce and glans penis (Montgomery et al., 1959). The disease often resolves spontaneously in one to two weeks but may become chronic.

Granuloma inguinale is a venereal disease caused by *Donovania granulomatis.* The lesions appear as sharply marginated areas of granulation tissue having a livid hue. The tissue is friable and bleeds easily. Smears stained with Giemsa reveal the characteristic Donovan bodies. This disease responds to tetracycline.

Exudative discoid and lichenoid chronic dermatosis of Sulzberger and Garbe represents a variant of nummular eczema occuring in middle-aged Jewish males. Sharply demarcated, erythematous, scaling plaques, occasionally crusted, occur on the penis, scrotum, extensor aspect of extremities, and upper chest. Pruritus is severe and paroxysmal. The condition responds to topical or systemic steroids.

Histopathology

The surface may be denuded of stratum corneum and stratum granulosum, or it may be covered by a parakeratotic scale or a crust. The epidermis appears irregularly acanthotic with bulbar downward proliferation, often quite deep in the dermis. The acanthosis is similar to that of Bowen's disease, characterized by variation in cell and nuclear size, increased numbers of mitotic figures, multinucleated cells, and dyskeratotic cells (Fig. 27–12). These features therefore represent Bowen's disease of the mucosal surface. If erythroplasia of Queyrat persists, invasion of the dermis may occur along with the histologic features of squamous cell carcinoma. Occasionally even invasive lesions retain these bowenoid characteristics. When metastasis

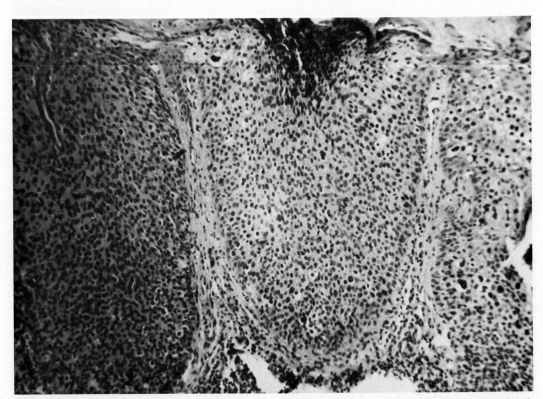

Figure 27–12 Erythroplasia of Queyrat. Note the prominent acanthosis. The rete ridges are elongated and thickened to such an extent that the dermal papillae are reduced to thick strands. The cells of the malpighian layer lie in complete disorder.

to regional lymph nodes occurs, the metastatic lesions show the histology of squamous cell carcinoma.

Histologic Differential Diagnosis

Balanitis circumscripta has a flat epidermis which may appear spongiotic. The upper dermal infiltrate is composed primarily of plasma cells. Inflammatory reactions occurring on the glans penis show a prominent plasma cell infiltrate (Korting and Theisen, 1963).

Zoon's balanitis usually manifests a more irregular acanthosis of the epidermis and lacks the disorderly arrangement of the malpighian layer as well as multinucleated cells and individual cell keratinization. A prominent plasma cell infiltrate in the dermis is also characteristic.

Lichen planus shows hyperkeratosis, sawtoothing of the rete ridges, destruction of the basal layer, and a bandlike upper dermal infiltrate. A granular layer, usually absent on the glans penis, may be present. In erythroplasia of Queyrat the basal layer is intact, the cells of the malpighian layer lie in complete disorder, and the rete ridges appear bulbar rather than saw-toothed.

Psoriasis presents a regular elongation of the rete ridges with overlying parakeratosis. Munro microabscesses may be found within this parakeratotic horny layer. The malipighian layer lacks the disorderly appearance, multinucleated cells, frequent mitotic figures, and dyskeratosis of erythroplasia.

Circinate balanitis of Reiter's syndrome shows the characteristic spongiform pustule of Kogoj in the upper epidermis.

Exudative discoid and lichenoid chronic dermatosis of Sulzberger and Garbe (1959) shows a more prominent and somewhat irregular acanthosis, characterized by migration of many inflammatory cells through the epidermis. None of the other epidermal changes so characteristic of erythroplasia is seen.

Prognosis

If erythroplasia of Queyrat persists long enough, frankly invasive squamous cell carcinoma will occur. Erythroplasia invades the dermis as squamous cell carcinoma (14 percent) more often than do the lesions of Bowen's disease (5.2 percent) (Graham and Helwig, 1963). Once invasion has occurred, there is a higher propensity for metastasis than in Bowen's disease.

Therapy

Surgical Therapy. If the process is confined to the mucous membrane, excision of a superficial part of the glans penis extending down to the corpus cavernosum is adequate. If deeper structures are involved, penile amputation is indicated (Andersson et al., 1967). Urologists almost routinely amputate the penis. Amputation probably is not necessary because only rarely is lymphatic extension present. Invasive erythroplasia of Queyrat can also be treated with chemosurgery as a means of salvaging the penis (Mohs, 1956). If the tumor does extend far back along the penis, it can be pursued selectively with the chemosurgical technique.

Regional node dissection is performed if lymph nodes are enlarged and there is likelihood of lymph node metastasis. The determination of whether enlarged, regional nodes are due to metastasis or inflammation is often difficult. However, the likelihood of positive nodes varies directly with the grade of the primary tumor and also with its size (Taylor and Nathanson, 1942). Usually the physician can be quite certain that metastases are present in the inguinal region on the basis of enlarged nodes, grade of malignancy of the tumor, and absence of infection. When doubt exists because of infection, it is preferable to amputate the penis and observe the nodes. If they do not regress in several weeks, bilateral lymph node dissection is done (Buddington et al., 1963).

Topical Therapy. Because of the successful use of topical 5-fluorouracil for Bowen's disease of the skin, this treatment has been advocated for erythroplasia involving the glans penis. Jansen et al. (1967) were the first to suggest the topical application of 5-fluorouracil in the treatment of erythroplasia of Queyrat. In each of two cases treated with 5 percent 5-FU ointment twice daily for four weeks, clearing of the lesion was observed. In both cases reapplication of 5-FU to small areas of residual or recurrent disease was necessary six to nine months later. Hueser and Pugh (1969) reported a case in which 2 percent 5-FU ointment was applied once daily for five days and then increased to twice daily for a total of 12 days of therapy. Two months after cessation of treatment, a repeat biopsy revealed no carcinoma. However, until the long-term efficacy of topical chemotherapy is known, particularly in terms of recurrence rates, this form of therapy can only be recommended with reservations. Particular attention must be given to the treated site, and frequent follow-up examinations must be made.

X-Ray Therapy. X-ray therapy preceded by circumcision can be recommended as a second choice if partial amputation is refused. Circumcision is necessary because of the possibility of phimosis developing after radiation.

Shapiro et al. (1962) reported a case of invasive erythroplasia successfully treated with a total dose of 4950 R. of x-ray fractionated into 40 daily treatments. Possible sequelae of this mode of therapy include stricture of the urethral meatus, impaired sensation in the glans penis, and failure to achieve successful erection.

REFERENCES

Bowen's Disease

Abell, M. R., and Gosling, J. R. G.: Intraepithelial and infiltrative carcinoma of vulva; Bowen's type. Cancer, 14:318, 1961.

Bowen, J. T.: Precancerous dermatoses: A study of 2 cases of chronic atypical epithelial proliferation. J. Cutan. Dis., 30:241, 1912.

Bowen, J. T.: Precancerous dermatoses: A sixth case of a type recently described. J. Cutan. Dis., 33:787, 1915.

Brauer, E. W., and Fried, S.: Bowen's disease of the penis: Response to Grenz ray therapy. In Society Transactions. Arch. Dermatol., 82:288, 1960.

Cauldfield, J. B., and Wilgram, G. F.: An electron-microscopic study of dyskeratosis and acantholysis in Darier's disease. J. Invest. Dermatol., 41:57, 1963.

Collins, C. G., and Barclay, D. L.: Cancer of the vulva, and cancer of the vagina in pregnancy. Clin. Obstet. Gynecol., 6:927, 1963.

Darier, J.: La dermatose precancereuse de Bowen, dyskeratose lenticulaire et en disques. Ann. Dermatol. Syphiligr. (Paris), 5:449, 1914.

Domonkos, A. N.: Neutron activation analysis of arsenic in normal skin, keratoses and epitheliomas. Arch. Dermatol., 80:672, 1959.

Ferguson, A. G., Dewar, W. A., and Smith, H.: Arsenic values in various skin diseases: Estimated by activation analysis. Arch. Dermatol., 81:931, 1960.

Fulton, J. E., Carter, D. M., and Hurley, H. J.: Treatment of Bowen's disease with topical 5-FU under occlusion. Arch. Dermatol., 97:178, 1968.

Graham, J. H., and Helwig, E. B.: Bowen's disease and its relationship to systemic cancer. Arch. Dermatol., 80:133, 1959.

Graham, J. H., and Helwig, E. B.: Bowen's disease and its relationship to systemic cancer (review). Arch. Dermatol., 83:738, 1961.

Graham, J. H., Mezzanti, G., and Helwig, E. B.: Chemistry of Bowen's Disease: Relationship to arsenic. J. Invest. Dermatol., 37:317, 1961.

Hugo, E., and Conway, H.: Bowen's disease: Its malignant potential and relationship to systemic cancer. Plast. Reconstr. Surg., 39:190, 1967.

Jansen, G. T., Dillaha, F. T., and Honeycutt, W. M.: Bowenoid conditions of the skin: Treatment with topical 5-FU. South. Med. J., 60:185, 1967.

Jeffcoate, T. N. A., Davie, T. B., and Harrison, C. V.: Intra-epidermal carcinoma (Bowen's disease) of the vulva. J. Obstet. Gynaecol. Br. Emp., 51:377, 1944.

Jessner, J.: Die Bowensche Krankheit. Arch. Dermatol. Syph. (Berl.), 134:361, 1921.

Lacronique, G., and Dechaume, M.: Maladie de Bowen de la muqueuse buccale. Rev. Stomatol. Chir. Maxillofac., 34:95, 1932.

Lewis, T. L. T.: Carcinoma of the vulva. In Progress in Clinical Obstetrics and Gynecology. Ed. 2. Boston, Little, Brown and Company, 1964.

Mierowsky, E., Freeman, L. W., and Woodard, J. S.: The response of embryonic chick membrane to Bowen's intraepithelial cancer. J. Invest. Dermatol., 22:417, 1954.

Mount, L. B.: The Bowen type of epithelioma. Arch. Dermatol. Syph., (Berl.), 4:769, 1921.

Nordquist, R. E., Olson, R. L., Everett, M. A., and Condit, P. T.: Virus-like particles in Bowen's disease. Cancer Res., 30:288, 1970.

Olson, R. L., Nordquist, R. E., and Everett, M. A.: An ultrastructural study of Bowen's disease. Cancer Res., 28:2078, 1968.

Papa, C. M., and Kennedy, R.: Bowen's disease case presentation. In Society Transactions. Arch. Dermatol., 97:84, 1968.

Peterka, E. S., Lynch, F. W., and Goltz, R. W.: An association between Bowen's disease and internal cancer. Arch. Dermatol., 84:623, 1961.

Ridley, B. M.: The treatment of epitheliomata by dermabrasion. Br. J. Dermatol., 78:149, 1966.

Sanderson, K. V., and Wilson, H. T. H.: Haber's syndrome. Familial rosacea-like eruption with intraepidermal epithelioma. Br. J. Dermatol., 77:1, 1965.

Schonberg, I. L., and Litt, J. Z.: Bowen's disease of the palm treated with Grenz rays. In Society Transactions. Arch. Dermatol., 84:144, 1961.

Seiji, M., and Mizuno, F.: Electron microscopic study of Bowen's disease. Arch. Dermatol., 99:3, 1969.

Stauffer, H., and Lutz, W.: Bowen's disease after tick bite. Dermatologica, 115:656, 1957.

Sweeney, T., and Mescon, H.: Actinic keratoses, some

with bowenoid features. *In* Society Transactions. Arch. Dermatol., 91:79, 1965.

Woodruff, J. D., and Novak, E. R.: Premalignant lesions of the vulva. Clin. Obstet. Gynecol., 5:1102, 1962.

Erythroplasia of Queyrat

Andersson, L., Jonsson, G., and Brehmer-Andersson, E.: Erythroplasia of Queyrat—Carcinoma *in situ*. Scand. J. Urol. Nephrol., 3:303, 1967.

Barbier, M. G.: Erythroplasie vulvaire. Presse Med., 35:360, 1927.

Barbier, M. G.: Erythroplasie vulvaire. Marseille Med., 3:184, 1928.

Blau, S., and Hyman, A. B.: Erythroplasia of Queyrat (review). Acta Derm. Venereol. (Stockh.), 35:341, 1955.

Buddington, W. T., Klickham, C. J., and Smith, W. E.: An assessment of malignant disease of the penis. J. Urol., 89:442, 1963.

Carteaud, A., Meyer, J. J., and Lebrun, F.: Erythroplasie vulvaire. Bull. Soc. Fr. Dermatol. Syphiligr., 57:321, 1950.

Darier, J., Lemaitre, F., and Monier, L.: Les modes de debut des cancer de la bouche et des machoires. Bull. Assoc. Fr. L' etude Cancer, 13:256, 1924.

Fournier, A., and Darier, J.: Epithelioma benign syphiloide de la verge. Bull. Soc. Fr. Dermatol. Syphiligr., 4:324, 1893.

Graham, J., and Helwig, E. B.: National Cancer Institute Monograph No. 10. Washington, D. C., United States Public Health Service, 1963, p. 323.

Hudelo, L., and Cailleau, P.: Maladie de Bowen des muqueuses. Ann. Dermatol. Syph., 4:813, 1933.

Hueser, J. N., and Pugh, P. R.: Erythroplasia of Queyrat treated with topical 5-fluorouracil. J. Urol., 102:595, 1969.

Jansen, G. T., Dillaha, C. T., and Honeycutt, W. M.: Bowenoid conditions of the skin: Treatment with topical 5-fluorouracil. South Med. J., 60:185, 1967.

Jessner, M.: Die Bowensche Krankheit. Arch. Dermatol. Syph., 134:161, 1921.

Jorno, J. F.: Contribution a l' etude de l'erythroplasie de Queyrat. Acta Derm. Venereol. (Stockh.), 19: 123, 1938.

Korting, G. W., and Theisen, H.: Circumscripta plasmacellulare Balanoposthitis and conjunctivitis bei derselben Person. Arch. Klin. Exp. Dermatol., 217:495, 1963.

Lutz, W.: Bowen's disease of vulva and anus. Schweiz. Med. Wochenschr., 71:1298, 1941.

MacDonald, W. I.: Erythroplasia of Queyrat. Arch. Dermatol. Syph. (Berl.), 43:919, 1941.

Mohs, F. E.: Chemosurgery. *In* Cancer, Gangrene and Infection. Springfield, Ill., Charles C Thomas, Publisher, 1956.

Montgomery, M. M., Poske, R. M., Barton, E. M., Foxworthy, D. T., and Baker, L. A.: The mucocutaneous lesions of Reiter's syndrome. Ann. Intern. Med., 51:99, 1959.

Pautrier, L. M.: Cancer epitheliale. Brux. Med., 9:51, 1928.

Queyrat, L.: Erythroplasia du gland. Bull. Soc. Fr. Dermatol. Syphiligr., 22:378, 1911.

Sachs, W., and Sachs, P. M.: Erythroplasia of Queyrat: Report of 10 cases. Arch. Dermatol., 58:184, 1948.

Sezary, M. A.: Erythroplasie develope sur l'emplacement d'un chancre syphilitique. Bull. Soc. Fr. Dermatol. Syphiligr., 39:605, 1932.

Sezary, M. A., Horowitz, A., and Levy-Coblentz, G.: Erythroplasie avec epithelioma ganglionaire du penis. Bull. Soc. Fr. Dermatol. Syphiligr., 39:514, 1932.

Shapiro, L., Boyarsky, S., and Roberts, T. W.: Carcinoma developing in Queyrat's erythroplasia. N.Y. State J. Med., 62:2999, 1962.

Sulzberger, M. A., Mareh, C., and Gay, C.: Distinctive exudative discoid and lichenoid chronic dermatoses. Z. Haut. Geschlechtskr., 27:223, 1959.

Sulzberger, M. B., and Statenstein, D. L.: Erythroplasia of Queyrat. Arch. Dermatol. Syph. (Berl.), 28:798, 1934.

Taylor, G. W., and Nathanson, I. T.: Incidence and Surgical Treatment in Neoplastic Disease, Lymph Node Metastases. New York, Oxford University Press, 1942.

Touraine, A., Solente, G.: L'erythroplasie. Presse Med., 44:1830, 1936.

Touraine, A., Solente, G., and Renault, P.: Deux cas d'erythroplasie de type hyperplasique chez des syphilitiques. Bull. Soc. Fr. Dermatol. Syphiligr., 42:339, 1935.

Zoon, J. J.: Balanoposthite chronique circonserite benigne a plasmocytes. Dermatologica, 105:1, 1952.

28

Extramammary Paget's Disease

Georg Klingmüller, M.D., and Yasumasa Ishibashi, M.D.

Based on the clinical and histologic criteria for mammary Paget's disease, extramammary Paget's disease can be seen as a similar, perhaps identical, disease. Its most important characteristics are appearance in older age groups, extended course, similar macroscopic structure of the efflorescence, and similar histologic and, in our opinion, submicroscopic features. Extramammary Paget lesions are, however, mostly verrucous and thicker, and the accompanying inflammatory reaction is more clearly defined. In a manner similar to mammary Paget, the extramammary form can also be observed as having underlying, previous, simultaneous, or later-occurring malignant tumors, especially adenocarcinomas. The pathogenesis of the disease is not clear. While some believe it is an epidermal "parasitic" spreading of a ductal carcinoma, others hold it to be a localized, epidermal dedifferentiation, which then affects the epidermis and gland ducts or the glands themselves in these particular regions.

Until recently, no spontaneous recovery has been seen. After a positive diagnosis, the disease has always taken a progressive course, if no restraints were placed through early treatment. The malignancy of this disease is thereby sufficiently emphasized.

The most noticeable clinical symptom is the localization, which applies to both forms, mammary as well as extramammary Paget's. In the first, the characteristic site is the mammary areola, associated with the apocrine glands (of Montgomery). The preferred localization of the extramammary form is wherever apocrine odorous and sweat glands are found. The embryonic relationship between the apocrine and mammary glands was recognized early as a factor in this localization.

Mammary Paget is a rare disease. Adamsons and Reisfield (1964) reported the incidence as 70 cases in 1909 dermatologic patients, and of patients examined in the Bonn dermatology clinic from 1946 to 1973, 29 were seen with Paget's disease. Only four had an extramammary localization: 77, 75, and 55 year old men and a 72 year old woman. Burdick and Warner (1964) observed over 100 patients up to 1963. Gunn and Fox (1971) counted 52 perianal occurrences up to 1971. Lüders compiled a list of 84 cases of extramammary Paget's disease in 1968. Since then a number of important observations have been made. Today, a certain

662

diagnosis is more frequently achieved owing to the increased tendency to carry out rapid biopsies. In this manner at least 50 further patients could be reported, while at the same time the diagnosis of more than 150 patients in the literature could be refuted. An individual presentation of all cases is no longer possible, particularly since no further features of significance can be expected.

HISTORY

According to Treves (1954), alterations of the mamillae were first noted in the 14th century by Johannes von Arderne, then by Velpeau in 1840, later by Lorain and Robin in 1854, and by Porter in 1872. The groundwork, however, was laid by Paget's paper in 1874 reporting on 15 patients. After a recommendation by Erichsen in 1879 at a meeting of the Royal Society of Medicine and Surgery, the disease was designated "Paget's disease of the nipple." This became generally known with Munro's publication (1880). The initial histologic description was made by Butlin (1876) and by Thin (1881). Soon thereafter similar processes were observed in male patients (11 cases listed by Treves in 1949) and then also in extramammary locations. Crocker in 1889 and Wickham in 1890 described Paget's disease on the scrotum. Further reports were published by Pick (1891), Tommasoli (1893), Neisser (1892), Darier (1925), Kren (1914), Graske (1912), Poland (1914), and others. The first description of vulvar Paget's disease was made by Dubreuilh in 1901. Paget himself had already observed similar clinical alterations on the penis: "I have seen a persistent 'rawness' of the glans penis, like a long-enduring balanitis, followed after more than a year's duration by cancer of the substance of the glans." However, at the time, the case was not accompanied by a histologic description. This was done by Crocker to render a definite classification possible. In more recent years, special mention could be given to the work of Satani (1920), Weiner (1937), Prose and Hyman (1959), Huriez et al. (1971), Murrell et al. (1962), Helwig and Graham (1963), and finally Lüders (1968)

(with detailed literature). For a long period of time no unity of opinion in recognition of extramammary Paget's disease could be achieved, as seen from the critical observations of Weiner (1937), Pinkus and Gould (1939), Pinkus and Mehregan (1963), Parsons and Lohlein (1943), and Allen and Spitz (1954).

CLINICAL OBSERVATIONS

Lüders (1968), then Jacobsen and Haavelsrud (1969), stated that sex ratios often given as 2 to 1 in favor of women are deceptive. According to Gunn and Fox (1971), perianal Paget's disease has the inverse relationship: the incidence is twice as great in men. It is universally reported that the disease primarily appears after 60 years of age. Helwig and Graham (1963) state the mean age as being over 62 years, and Gunn and Fox (1971) for perianal localization, as 63.9 years. These results were summarized by Lüders in a chart from which no new diagnostic criteria were recognizable. The earliest recorded cases are in a 34 year old woman and a 48 year old man; at the other extreme are the oldest patients, an 84 year old woman and an 86 year old man.

From these observations it could correctly be assumed that we are dealing with a more or less pronounced disease of old age, which also holds true for mammary Paget, in which the median patient age, after Stankovic (1963) reported on 177 patients, could be calculated as 57.1 years.

Macroscopic Appearance

The disease begins insidiously with itching and burning sensations similar to those of mammary Paget's disease. Erythema is seen and can be bright red or beefy red. Flaking, more or less intensive oozing, and macerations with subsequent verrucous and frequently vegetating alterations are also observed. Commonly there is a single initial lesion which spreads in area and becomes polycyclic with mostly sharp borders. With an increasing infectious reaction and broad, loose acanthosis accompanied by papillomatosis, the originally soft plaques become denser and harder.

Erosions, excoriation, and ulcerations are also present, caused by the itching and consequent scratching. The occasionally distended ulcerous margins flatten out and form a scar, or the ulcerations become confluent. A bright red color is maintained, and the lesion can also be covered with whitish macerations or barklike flakes. Secondary alterations include eczema, impetigo, and minimal tissue destruction, which nevertheless does not belong to the original epidermal degeneration. Depending on the location, symptomatic variations can be observed (Figs. 28–1 and 28–2).

This stage of extramammary Paget's disease can be brief or may endure for a number of years, in one patient for 31 years, according to Helwig and Graham (1963) or Jakobsen and Haavelsrud (1969), gradually increasing in area up to 20 × 30 cm.

Preclinical symptoms of Paget's disease have received considerable attention, and occasionally in such early stages, an already widespread mammary adenocarcinoma has been found (Dockerty and Pratt,

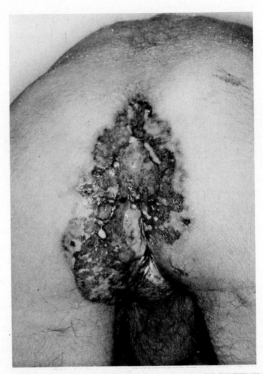

Figure 28–2 Extramammary Paget's disease in a 55 year old male treated for five years for anal eczema and hemorrhoids. Death was due to tumor metastases.
(See also Color Plate I-C.)

1952). As opposed to this, epidermal changes can occur without any participation by the adjacent glands. This also holds true for extramammary Paget's disease.

Localization

Apocrine Glands. The conspicuous degree of localization of mammary and extramammary Paget's disease has always attracted much attention. The embryonic similarity between the apocrine sweat or odorous glands and the mammary glands has already been mentioned in this connection. The holocrine sebaceous glands and apocrine sweat glands develop in the third month of gestation as epithelial thickenings from lateral offshoots of the hair buds (Bargmann, 1951). As these glands open to the hair follicle or out to the epidermal surface, where apocrine cells or their predecessors already lie normally, they can be affected by specific dedifferentiation (Jacobsen and Haavelsrud,

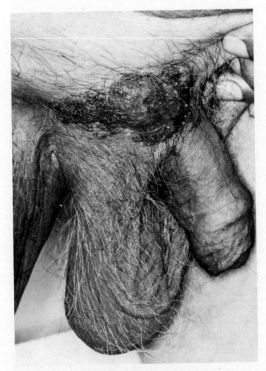

Figure 28–1 Extramammary Paget's disease in a 77 year old male. Onset was in right lower pubic region. Probable initiation was three years previously. (See also Color Plate I-B.)

1969), just like their epidermal equivalents.

Mammary Ridge. It is to be expected that Paget's disease can also occur on accessory nipples. Crosti (1932) expressed the view that the extramammary disease was localized along the mammary ridge. Perhaps the localization of extramammary Paget's disease in the vicinity of the navel could be so classified, but no further observations have been made to support this assumption.

Helwig and Graham (1963) discussed the possibility that, in the anal and perineal regions as well as the genitalia, portions of entoderm persist into adult life. Such transitional epithelia, as ontogenetically similar cells, may then be affected by an unknown carcinogenic stimulus.

Apocrine glands are hormonally influenced, their functions beginning during puberty and ceasing with old age. The appearance of extramammary Paget's disease seems to depend on reduced sex hormone functions. Clear-cut experimental observations supporting these clinical impressions are not available.

The most frequent site is the vulvar region (Falkinburg and Hoey, 1958; Duperrat and Mascaró, 1965; Lüders, 1968; and others). In men, the anogenital area is most often affected, then the axillae, the penis and less frequently the navel or the eyelid (Whorton and Patterson, 1955; Knauer and Whorton, 1963). The malignant processes are most frequently found in the area of anal transitional epithelium.

Exceptional Cases

Most frequently, extramammary Paget's disease is found in only one site. Duperrat and Mascaró reported a patient with genital Paget's disease who later developed a second lesion with a deep-seated apocrine epithelioma in the right axilla. Extramammary Paget's disease was seen by Kawatsu and Miki (1971) in the genital region and both axillae of a 77 year old Japanese farmer. Localization to the eyelids was attributed by Knauer and Whorton (1963) to the presence of Moll's glands. Of particular interest is the appearance of lesions in the larynx and esophagus, as described by Yates and Koss (1968). Other sites are unknown, and if a lesion of this type is found elsewhere, it is most likely a melanoma (Stout, 1938; Zieler, 1904; Adamsons and Reisfield, 1964; Allen and Spitz, 1954). The same holds true for the case of the 9 year old girl described by Komori (1938), who probably had a juvenile melanoma.

In the initial stages the lymph nodes may be involved by secondary infectious processes and then become enlarged. Untreated, the primary focus changes in the classic process of malignant tumorous proliferation, with solid, deep-seated nodes in the vicinity and regional lymph node infiltration. Distant metastases appear, and there is a decline in overall condition. Deterioration and death invariably occur (Lüders, 1968), and spontaneous recovery is unknown.

In 50 percent of 73 cases of mammary Paget's disease seen by Lattes and Haagensen (1958), regional lymph node metastases were established. This important finding can be attributed to the thoroughness of the operation, with removal of the accompanying lymph nodes. Such a procedure is not always carried out in cases of extramammary Paget's disease, but it should be a basic principle.

According to Dockerty and Harrington (1951), Dockerty and Pratt (1952), Bennett (1943), Culberson and Horn (1956), and Wessel, underlying carcinoma is frequently discovered in cases of mammary Paget's disease, but not in extramammary Paget's disease (Taki and Janovski, 1961). Willis (1960) conjectured that extramammary Paget's disease is merely a structural variant of an intraepithelial carcinoma such as Bowen's disease. Burdick and Warner (1964) saw a patient with Bowen's and Paget's lesions. Falkinburg and Hoey (1958) listed additional cases of extramammary Paget's disease. Nevertheless the sweat glands participate up to 25 percent in the dedifferentiation, as demonstrated by Cawley (1957) in the axillary region.

During the formation of metastases an epidermal carcinoma "en cuirasse" is seen to underlie formation of additional characteristic Paget cells (Miescher and Ceelen, 1952). By invasive growth, the customary lymphocellular and plasmacellular infiltrate seen in malignant processes is found as well in Paget's disease, which is significant in view of its primarily epidermal localization.

The mean survival time of patients with anogenital Paget's disease was given as 7 years after initial biopsy by Helwig and Graham. The prognosis is much poorer for patients with underlying carcinoma. Recently, Paget's disease extending over 20 to 30 years has been described.

HISTOLOGIC FINDINGS

After the initial histologic description by Butlin (1876) and Thin (1881), Darier (1925) and Wickham (1890) were particularly interested in the histology, and Unna (1894) also reported extensively. Like Thin, Duhring, and Wile (1884), and then Karg (1892), Unna observed the most important change to be a characteristic degeneration of the squamous cells. Karg had observed that these large cells were squeezed together at the basal

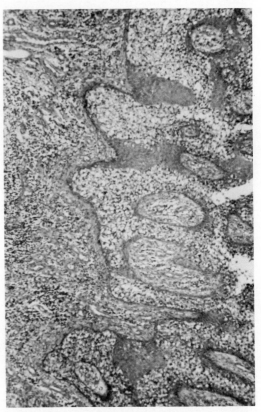

Figure 28-4 Biopsy from patient shown in Figure 28-1. Acanthotic proliferation of the epidermis with large, mostly similar, light Paget cell complexes. *H & E.* (See also Color Plate I-D.)

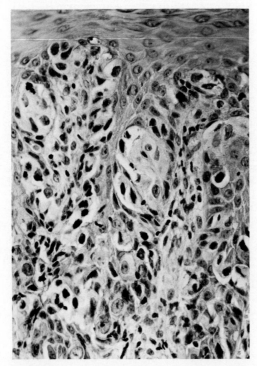

Figure 28-3 Anal extramammary Paget. Acanthotic papillary epidermis. In the basal cell region are clusters of or various single Paget cells. These seem to replace the normal-appearing epidermal cells rather than to displace them.

regions and on the outer borders of the epidermal ridges, which appear very light. Unna also reported that, where a cell swells, its filamental system disappears. The cells undergo metaplasia.

Histologically, the only epidermal change is an acanthotic widening or thickening (Figs. 28-3 and 28-4). The specific signs lie in the basal cell layer (Karg, 1892; Montgomery, 1967; and others), occasionally directly above the basal membrane (Ishibashi et al.), but mostly somewhat higher (Figs. 28-5 and 28-6). These relatively large, round or polyhedral, light cells, which stain poorly with hematoxylin and eosin, are the so-called Paget cells (Fig. 28-7). They lie isolated or in small groups, mostly extending in bands on the surface. Often they are found in trabeculae or clusters, massive, mixed, or budding (Mori, 1965). The nuclei are large, pale, and clearly more lightly stained. They are frequently pressed to the edge (Ceelen, 1952). Mitoses are

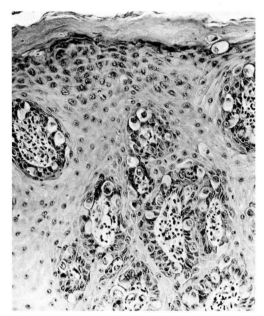

Figure 28–5 Anal extramammary Paget. In an oblique tangential section, large Paget cells can be found, primarily in the basal cell region.

more frequently observed, in part, of an atypical form which is responsible for the numerical increase. Of note is that the Paget cell is adjacent to a normal-appearing keratinocyte (Gans and Steigleder, 1957; Montgomery, 1967; and others) (Fig. 28–8). Only rarely are intercellular connections suggested. According to Pinkus, Paget cells nevertheless are of an adnexal nature and have intercellular bridges (Fig. 28–9).

The number of cells decreases toward the surface of the skin, but they are readily seen throughout the well-defined granular layer. They hardly appear keratinized—that is, they remain seemingly dedifferentiated. Generally, the dermal border is intact, though often papillomatous, warped, and wavy.

In addition to these, other types of cells (Huber et al., 1951; Prose and Hyman, 1959; Satani, 1920; Strauss, 1957; and others) or several different cell forms (Helwig and Graham, 1963; Mori, 1965; Weiner, 1937) can be specifically designated as Paget cells. It remains unclear whether these cells should be seen as "altered" or merely "other" Paget cells (Mori, 1965). Strauss (1957) histochemically differentiates two cell forms. His A cells are supposedly typical Paget cells with larger chromatin-poor nuclei and foamy, light cytoplasm; the B cells are "anaplastic" and

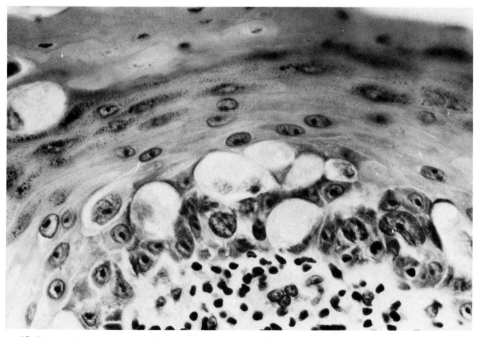

Figure 28–6 Anal extramammary Paget. Several Paget cells seem to lie directly on the corium (on the basal membrane). Single cells migrate, dedifferentiated, through the granular cell layer into the stratum corneum. In the corium, limited round cell infiltrate.

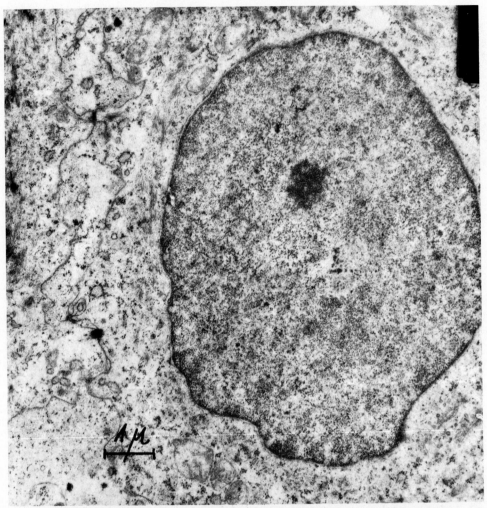

Figure 28–7 Electron microscopic view of a Paget cell in extramammary Paget's disease. This big, light cell (Paget cell) has a large nucleus, loosened tonofilaments, and rudimentary desmosomes.

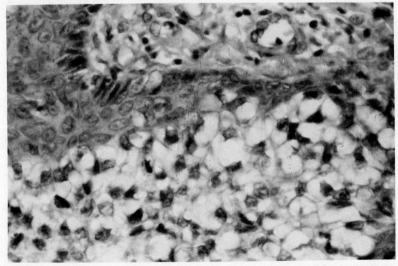

Figure 28–8 Portion of Figure 28–4. Vacuolar cytoplasm of the Paget cell complex. The Paget cells border on the corium and lie directly adjacent to normal-appearing keratinocytes. (See also Color Plate I-E.)

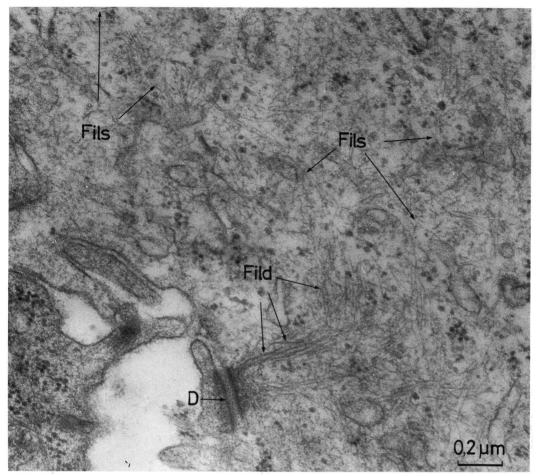

Figure 28–9 Portion of a Paget cell in extramammary Paget's disease. In the Paget cell, irregular filaments of varying thickness are seen (*Fils:* approximately 60 to 70 Å; *Fild:* approximately 70 to 100 Å thick). Nearby, normally structured desmosomes (D).

have a small hyperchromatic nucleus with shrunken cytoplasm. Around these cells there is an optically empty region. Mori (1965) listed six morphologically different cell forms with transitional states. He also described connections between the Paget cells and their neighboring epidermal cells, a feature which has been disputed (Lüders, 1968).

In extramammary Paget's disease, infiltrative tumor cell growth into the corium is seldom seen, and neither is lymphatic spread, as in carcinoma erysipeloid.

Histochemical Findings

The Paget cells in mammary as well as in extramammary Paget's disease contain mucin, perhaps with certain quantitative variations (Hertig and Gore, 1960; Lund, 1957; Lübschitz, 1944; Neubecker and Bradshaw, 1961: Montgomery, 1967; Cawley, 1957; Fisher and Beyer, 1959; Helwig and Graham, 1963; Lennox and Pearse, 1954; Mori, 1965; Strauss, 1957; and others). Paget cells possibly also contain protein, mucoprotein, glycoprotein, acid and neutral mucopolysaccharides, and sulfated acid mucopolysaccharides (Helwig and Graham, 1963; Andrade, 1964). Staining methods that have been used are the mucicarmine method according to Mayer, alcian blue, Gomori's aldehyde-fuchsin reaction, and PAS before and after diastase treatment (Jakobsen and Haavelsrud, 1969; Pievard et al., 1958; Taki, 1961; Weiner, 1937).

Paget cells do not exhibit a positive reaction to dihydroxyphenylalanine (DOPA) (Woodruff and Pauerstein, 1966), which can be seen as an important differential diagnostic criterion in intraepithelial melanoma (Burdick and Warner, 1964). Melanin is found in Paget cells (Adamsons and Reisfield, 1964; Helwig and Graham, 1963; Madsen, 1965; Komori, 1938; Gargiulo, 1956; Strauss, 1957; Bontke, 1958; Ishibashi et al.; Montgomery, 1967; Kawamura, 1962), which is not surprising if one assumes formation and proliferation of Paget cells in the epidermal basal cell layer (Fig. 28–10).

In the vacuolized cytoplasm, further profuse glycogen deposits can be found, perhaps even lying somewhat higher in the germinative cell layer (Arnd, 1926; Braun-Falco and Rathjens, 1955; and others) (Figs. 28–8, 28–11, and 28–12).

It cannot be decided with certainty whether it is possible, based only on histologic and histochemical methods, to distinguish between an immature Paget cell and a more clear-cut Paget cell (Adamsons and Reisfield, 1964), or between two different cell types, as assumed by Strauss (1957). Overall, it can be said that histochemical methods cannot determine an absolutely certain diagnosis. Borderline situations will always be present on examination of histologic sections alone. Histochemical reactions are naturally based on the spectrum of cell components, which initially form a seemingly uniform Paget cell. This is more clearly recognized in ultrastructural examination.

Electron Microscopic Pathology

Extramammary Paget's disease, as an entity, can be clinically and histologically comprehended, yet it must be conceded that neither the clinical nor the histologic findings clarify the pathogenesis and nature of the disease or give clues to the significance of the characteristic Paget cell. Extramammary Paget's disease was first examined electron microscopically in 1963 by Sagami and then in conjunction with mammary Paget's disease by Califano and Caputo (1968), Ebner (1969), Ishibashi et al. (1969, 1970a, 1970b, and 1972); Ofuji and Takeda (1969), again by Sagami et al. (1967), Toker (1961), Ikeda et al. (1970), Koss et al. (1968), Mishima and Matsumaka (1969), Medenica and Sahihi (1972), Uyeda et al. (1972), Hollmann et al. (1969), Gros and Girardie (1971), Sagebiel (1969), Gunn and Fox (1971), and Huriez et al. (1971).

The Paget Cell. In the lower malphigian cell layer and eventually on the basal membrane, abnormal epidermal cells with intact or slightly regressive desmosomes can be found. Their tonofilaments are reduced, loose, or bristle in an electron-

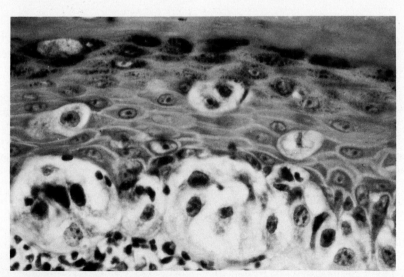

Figure 28–10   Malignant melanoma with pagetoid structure (superficial spreading type) in a 36 year old male. The patient died.
(See also Color Plate I-F.)

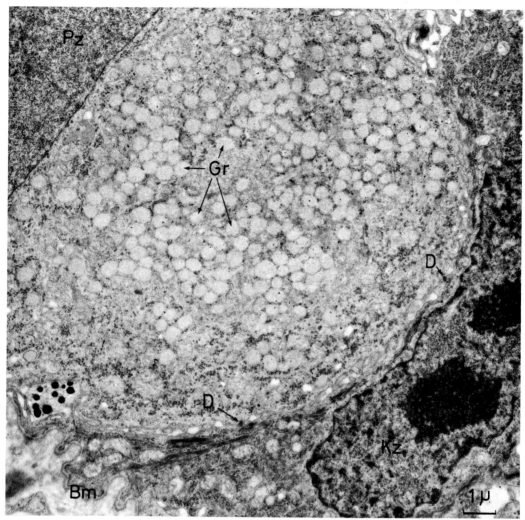

Figure 28-11   Vacuolar granula *(Gr)* in a Paget cell. These lie directly on the basal membrane *(Bm)*. Adjacent, minimally altered keratinocyte *(Kz)*. Desmosomes *(D)*.

thin cytoplasm. Glycogen granula, approximately 200 to 300 Å in size, are recognizable aggregated around the nucleus, as well as in the Paget cell cytoplasm. Similar observations can be made of the neighboring, seemingly normal, epidermal cells. The dilated intercellular spaces contain a granular substance with smaller granula-like ribosomes. Their significance is unclear. A number of cells have increased keratinosomes and isolated bodies like lysosomes as well as vacuolar endoplasmic reticulum without granula. Other large ballooned cells do not possess keratinosomes. The number of desmosomes is greatly reduced. They are frequently rudimentary, but are clearly recognizable be-

tween the Paget cells and between Paget cells and keratinocytes. Intracellular tonofilament-desmosome complexes are occasionally observed in keratinocytes neighboring Paget cells. Similar findings have been reported in squamous cell carcinoma (Klingmüller et al., 1970), Bowen's disease (Seiji and Misune, 1969), and keratoacanthoma (von Bülow and Klingmüller, 1971; Takasi et al., 1971), as well as in varicella. Most likely, their presence signifies altered characteristics of the cellular surface. That is, these findings are not specific for Paget cells.

Furthermore, in the cytoplasm, fine fibrillar elements can be found. This supports the assumption that in Paget cells

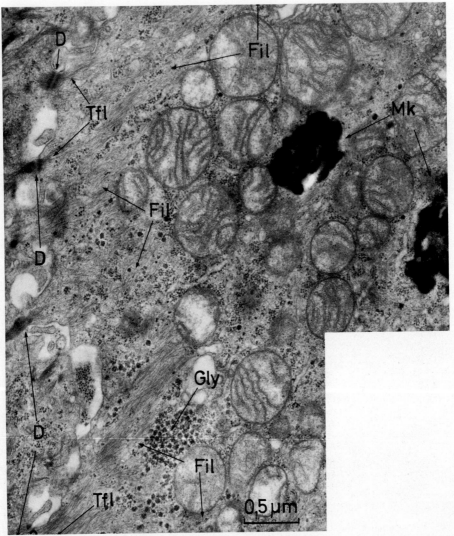

Figure 28–12 Portion of a Paget cell in extramammary Paget's disease. In the cytoplasm, continuous interconnections between tonofilaments (*Tfl*) and between desmosomes (*D*) with intracytoplasmic filaments (*Fil*). Melanosome complexes (*Mk*) and glycogen granula (*Gly*) in the cell.

some disrupted tonofilament formation stages are present. Frequently, increased ribosomes and endoplasmic reticula are seen, as well as a clearly defined Golgi apparatus. These are of note only in a quantitative sense.

Mitochondria can be giant, ballooned, or deformed (Caputo and Califano, 1970; Medenica and Sahihi, 1972) and contain tubular or paracrystalline deposits. In many Paget cells inter- as well as intracellular canaliculi with well-developed longer microvilli are recognizable. Clearly dif-

ferent from the normal keratinocyte, these cells correspond to those previously described by Sagami (1963), Ofuji and Takeda (1965), and Ebner (1969). Between these ballooned Paget cells and the epidermal cells lying above them, transitional regions are occasionally seen, which vary from case to case. Hori et al. (1970) and Ishibashi et al. (1969, 1970a, 1970b, and 1972) have also described Paget cells with a darker cytoplasm than that of keratinocytes.

The mechanism of the submicroscopic

precipitation of the mucin substance is still in question. While Koss and Brockunier (1969) differentiate between secretory and nonsecretory Paget cells, "secretory granula" have been described by Toker (1961 and 1967) and Ofuji and Takeda (1965). Such granula are surrounded by a double membrane and show an internal fine fibrillary structure. They are thought to represent the histochemically demonstrable mucin in Paget cells, and these results make it clear that Paget cells can exhibit a certain stage of differentiation toward glandular cells, particularly apocrine sweat glands.

Summarizing the manifold results, one can state that Paget cells display extremely variable structures in various patients or disease forms. This is particularly true for extramammary Paget's disease. These cells are not necessarily similar in their structure or composition. They are, however, always distinguishable from normal keratinocytes in all epidermal layers, as they show a seemingly characteristic alteration of the cell organelles and various cellular products. It has not been possible to determine whether Paget cells always must display cellular differentiation toward glandular cells or whether they merely are defectively differentiated epidermal cells which can retain their structure (Figs. 28–7, 28–9, 28–11, and 28–12).

Interpretation of Electron Microscopic Findings

Ishibashi's observations suggest the following assumptions:

1. In extramammary Paget's disease, we are dealing with a cellular differentiation process. The characteristic Paget cells wander from the lower malpighian layer upward, finally into cells of the horny layer. Perhaps that is why such cells are no longer readily observable in the granular and horny layers in extramammary Paget's disease. Clusters of cells and "cast off" phenomena (Mori, 1965) of the Paget cells can be seen as residues of this differentiation process.

2. Paget cells do not spread from one area to another, but instead appear in various regions independently through a similar stimulus.

3. The epidermal alterations must be seen as a morphologic as well as cytochemical differentiation of the epidermis which varies from the norm.

4. In mammary Paget's disease, Paget cells display pleomorphism. This indicates a differentiation in the direction not of keratinization, but more likely of secretion.

5. Melanosomes and melanosome complexes in Paget cells show that these cells have phagocytic capacity.

6. Paget cells exhibit a quantitative, defective, and eventually intracytoplasmic desmosome formation. The capacity for normal desmosome formation is not totally lost. This allows conjecture on cell membrane alterations.

7. In several cases of extramammary Paget's disease, not only are typical Paget cells observed, but a certain degeneration of all epidermal cells in this region can also be seen. It is possible that, when this observation is made, one is in fact dealing with an unspecific concomitant symptom.

CAN EXTRAMAMMARY PAGET'S DISEASE BE SEEN AS PRECANCEROUS?

If one observes only the epidermal alterations in extramammary Paget's disease and the appearance of malignant Paget cells, it is entirely correct to designate it as a precancerous condition like Bowen's disease or senile keratoma. Precancerous is dermatologically defined as involving an exceedingly long, progressive, malignant process within the epidermis. Here, however, the invasive growth is not present. Following Broder's (1932) logic, extramammary Paget's disease must certainly be seen as a carcinoma in situ. Montgomery (1967) regarded Paget's disease as merely a precancerous dermatosis. Bennett (1943) relates that, in mammary Paget's disease, an underlying adenocarcinoma could invariably be found. In his opinion, the classical definition of a precancerous condition was exceeded with this observation.

The increased mitotic rate, the irregular ultrastructure, the nuclear alterations, and the multinuclear (Bowen-like) giant cell formation led Ishibashi et al. (1969, 1970a, 1970b, and 1972) to consider extramammary Paget's disease as carcinomatous.

DIAGNOSIS AND DIFFERENTIAL DIAGNOSIS

The diagnosis of extramammary Paget's disease is chiefly based on uncharacteristic clinical findings in typical locations. A longer case history, deficient changes in response to external therapy, and particularly further invasive growth require biopsy. The diagnosis is then secured histologically (Dockerty and Pratt, 1952; Berggren and Bogg, 1962; Miescher, 1957). Butlin (1876) first attracted attention to the typical cell picture, which has also held true for extramammary Paget's disease, though a certain caution is advisable. A false diagnosis of Paget's disease is possible in cases of junctional nevi and superficial spreading melanoma when their cells differentiate intraepidermally. This eventually led Allen and Spitz (1954) to diagnose extramammary Paget's disease only with the greatest care and reticence. The presence of large clear cells in the vulvar epithelium histologically offers two diagnostic possibilities: intraepidermal nevus or malignant melanoma of the superficial spreading type, and extramammary Paget's disease or the closely related Bowen's disease. The differentiation between Bowen's disease and erythroplasia of Queyrat is exceedingly difficult (Jacobsen and Haavelsrud, 1969). Dockerty and Pratt (1952) examined sections of a so-called transitional cell carcinoma of the bladder which grew into the abdominal wall and produced Paget cells in the suprapubic skin. Occasionally, uniformly large clear cells can be seen in the upper walls of eccrine sweat glands or the apocrine glands.

In contrast to the situation in Bowen's disease or senile keratoma, in extramammary Paget's disease, more noticeable cell types, nuclear clumping, dyskeratotic cells, or individual cellular keratinization is not present. Montgomery (1967), however, occasionally observed benign dyskeratotic cells outside the Paget cells and also found round bodies or grains.

The following theories on the pathogenesis and nature of the Paget cells have been proposed:

We are dealing with a metastatic migration of epidermal cells from an already present underlying adenocarcinoma, as described earlier by Thin (1881) and Crocker (1888), later by Ribbert (1905), Masson (1925), Pautrier (1928), Jacobäus (1904), Muir (1935), and Adamsons and Reisfield (1964). Dockerty and co-workers, in particular, lean toward this notion. Among 100 cases of mammary Paget's disease, not one was free of a so-called deep-seated carcinoma of the glandular ducts or acinar system. The search for such a deep-seated carcinoma must be carried out with great care (Casper, 1948). If one assumes migration, then active ameboid movement of the Paget cells must be imagined (see Dockerty, 1951 and 1952). This special cancer cell type must, according to Pinkus and Gould (1939), have particular affinity to the epidermis. These authors assume that Paget cells and epidermal cells exist in a system of imperfect symbiosis, leading to eczema, itching, or irritation of the skin. Grimes (1959) has also observed such migration in a prostate carcinoma.

Adamsons has cast doubt on the idea of migration of the Paget cells within the epidermal borders. An extreme opinion is that it involves cells completely heterogeneous to the epidermis (Bowman and Hartman, 1954)—that is to say, cells which by themselves cannot develop independently from epidermal cells. Pinkus and Mehregan (1963) designated Paget's disease an "epidermotropic adnexal carcinoma" and extramammary Paget's disease as an "epidermotropic apocrine adenocarcinoma." They presume that cell migration can also begin in the poral portion of the glands.

Lüders (1968) summarized these opinions as follows:

1. Paget's disease originates in the epithelium of apocrine secretory glands of similar ontogenetic origin. In extramammary Paget's disease the Paget cells migrate from the secretory ducts of these glands via the hair follicles centrifugally into the epidermis, the cells of which they force out. Finally they exhibit a noticeable epidermal tropism, without possessing characteristics of epidermal origin. As a summarized definition, Lüders proposed, after Pinkus, the designation "adenocarcinoma apocrinocellulare epidermotropicum." However, based on the electron micro-

scopic findings, this name no longer has any significance.

2. The Paget cells dedifferentiate by themselves in the epidermis. Such local transformations were held by Arzt and Kren (1925) to be possible only in rare instances. Then Helwig and Graham (1963), Madsen (1965), and Jacobäus (1904) described extramammary Paget's disease exclusively in the epidermis. They were of the opinion that Paget cells were altered keratinocytes and that their presence caused a further transformation of epidermal basal cells into Paget cells.

Paget cells could develop from pluripotential undifferentiated elements of the primary developmental layer (Kaufman et al., 1960) or from an intermediary cell (Taki and Janovski, 1961). Careful light microscopic (Mori, 1965) as well as electron microscopic examinations (Sagami, 1963) have shown that Paget cells have desmosomes as well as tonofilaments. This would be an important argument for the theory of an independent epidermal formation of Paget cells.

3. Epidermis and underlying appendages are altered together or sequentially. An unknown carcinogenic stimulus induces cancerous transformation of epidermal cells and glands (Butlin, 1876; Montgomery, 1967; Helwig and Graham, 1963). Under closer scrutiny, however, this hypothesis is found to be implicit in the "local transformation" theory already mentioned.

Another theory is that Paget cells are actually epidermal nonkeratinocytes, which are similar to Langerhans cells, and which proliferate under certain conditions (Hollmann et al., 1969). However, further investigations have not been able to support this opinion (Ishibashi et al., 1969, 1970a, 1970b, and 1972).

THERAPY

Therapy of extramammary Paget's disease can be briefly summarized. It includes measures normally utilized in treating all other cancerous alterations over larger or smaller areas, depending on the extent of the process. Surgical treatment should be considered first (Helwig and Graham, 1963; Muri, 1960), and has been developed

in particular by Adamsons and Reisfield (1964). The regional lymph nodes should be included as far as possible, although this is frequently difficult in the affected locations. One must remember that in mammary Paget's disease there is metastasis to regional nodes in 50 percent of cases (Lattes and Haagensen, 1958). Corresponding findings could also be expected in extramammary Paget's disease. Most patients usually come for treatment at a late stage of their disease. Duperrat and Mascaró (1965) are of the opinion that extirpation does not always lead to positive results, perhaps owing to the multicentric character of extramammary Paget's disease. Therefore, regional radiation therapy with deep irradiation of the corresponding lymph nodes should be used as well.

REFERENCES

Adamsons, K., Jr., and Reisfield, D.: Observations on intradermal migration of Paget cells. Am. J. Obstet. Gynecol., 90:1274, 1964.

Allen, A. C., and Spitz, S.: Histogenesis and clinopathologic correlation of nevi and malignant melanomas. Arch. Dermatol, 69:150, 1954.

Andrade, R.: Die präcanceröse und canceröse Wucherung von Epidermis und Anhangsgebilden. *In* Jadassohn's Handbuch der Haut- und Geschlechtskrankheiten. Ergänzungswerk I/2. Berlin Springer-Verlag, 1964.

Arnd, W.: Über die Pagetsche Erkrankung der Brustwarze. Virchows Arch., 261:700, 1926.

Arzt, L., and Kren, O.: Die Paget disease mit besonderer Berücksichtigung ihrer Pathogenese. Arch. Dermatol. Syph. (Berl.), 148:284, 1925.

Bargmann, W.: Histologie und mikroskopische Anatomie des Menschen. Stuttgart, Thieme, 1951.

Bennett, W. A.: Pathologic study of Paget's disease of the nipple. Master's Thesis, University of Minnesota, 1943.

Berggren, O.G.A., and Bogg, A.: Extramammary localisation of Paget's disease. Acta Derm. Venerol. (Stockh.), 42:72, 1962.

Bontke, E.: Vergleichende Betrachtungen über die Paget-Erkrankungen der Mamma und Vulva. Geburtsh. Frauenkrkh., 18:185, 1958.

Bowman, H. E., and Hartman, F. W.: Extramammary Paget's disease of the vulva. Arch. Pathol., 58:304, 1954.

Braun-Falco, O., and Rathjens, B.: Histochem. Untersuchungen über Lokalisation und Grösse der Bernsteinsäuredehydrogenase-Aktivität bei M. Paget, Basaliom und spinocellulärem Carcinom. Arch. Dermatol. Syph. (Berl.), 199:152, 1955.

Broders, A. C.: Carcinoma in situ contrasted with benign penetrating epithelium. J.A.M.A., 99:1670, 1932.

Bülow, M. von, and Klingmüller, G.: Elektronenmikroskopische Untersuchungen des Keratoakanthoms. Vorkommen intracytoplasmatischer Desmosomen. Arch. Dermatol. Forsch., 241:292, 1971.

Burdick, C. O., and Warner, P.O.: Simultaneous vulvar Bowen's disease and Paget's disease. J. Obstet. Gynecol., 23:396, 1964.

Butlin, H. T.: Proc. R. Med. Clin. Soc. (Lond.), 8:37, 1876.

Califano, A., and Caputo, R.: La Microscopia Electronica nello studio delle precancerosi epiteliali cutanee. Minerva Dermatol., 43:568, 1968.

Caputo, R., and Califano, A.: Ultrastructural features of extramammary Paget's disease. Arch. Klin. Exp. Dermatol., 236:121, 1970.

Casper, W. A.: Paget's disease of the vulva. Arch. Dermatol., 57:668, 1948.

Cawley, L. P.: Extramammary Paget's disease. Am. J. Clin. Pathol., 27:559, 1957.

Ceelen, W.: Über den Paget-Krebs. Dermatol. Wochenschr., 126:820, 1952.

Crocker, R.: Disease of the Skin. London, H. K. Lewis, 1888.

Crosti, A.: Il morbo di Paget cutaneo interpretato quale epitelioma epidermotropo dell'apparato ghiandolare sudorale (Ghiandola mammaria, ghiandole sudorifere). G. Ital. Dermatol. Sif., 73:1021, 1932.

Culberson, J. D., and Horn, R. C.: Paget's disease of the nipple; review of twenty-five cases with special reference to melanin pigmentation of Paget's cells. A.M.A. Arch. Surg., 72:224, 1956.

Darier, J.: Note sur la dyskératose en particulier dans la maladie de Paget. Bull. Soc. Fr. Dermatol., 32:R.S.1, 1925.

Dockerty, M. B., and Harrington, S. W.: Preclinical Paget's disease of the nipple. Surg. Gynecol. Obstet., 93:317, 1951.

Dockerty, M. B., and Pratt, J. H.: Extramammary Paget's disease. A report of four cases in which certain features of histogenesis were exhibited. Cancer, 5:1161, 1952.

Dubreuilh, W.: Paget's disease of the vulva. Br. J. Dermatol., 13:407, 1901.

Duhring, L. A., and Wile, H.: On the pathology of Paget's disease of the nipple. Am. J. Med. Soc., July, 1884.

Duperrat, B., and Mascaró, J. M.: Maladie de Paget extra-mammaire. Presse Med., 73:1019, 1965.

Ebner, H.: Zur Ultrastruktur des Morbus Paget mamillae. Z. Haut. Geschlechtskr., 44:297, 1969.

Falkinburg, L. W., and Hoey, W. O.: Paget's disease of the vulva. Report of a case and review. Am. J. Obstet. Gynecol., 75:189, 1958.

Fisher, E. R., and Beyer, F.: Extramammary Paget's disease. Am. J. Surg., 94:493, 1957.

Fisher, E. R., and Beyer, F.: Differentiation of neoplastic lesions characterized by large vacuolated intraepidermal (pagetoid) cells. A.M.A. Arch. Pathol., 67:140, 1959.

Gans, O., and Steigleder, G. K.: Histologie der Hautkrankheiten. Die Pagetsche Krankheit. Berlin, Springer-Verlag, 1957.

Gargiulo, F.: Morbo di Paget vulvare. Clin. Obstet. Gynecol., 59:333, 1956.

Graske, E.: Über Pagetsche Krankheit usw. Dissertation, Königsberg, 1912.

Grimes, O. F.: Extramammary Paget's disease. Surgery, 45:569, 1959.

Gros, M. C., and Girardie, J.: Données ultrastructurales concernant l'origine des cellules de Paget du mamelon. Ann. Dermatol. Syphiligr. (Paris), 98:57, 1971.

Gunn, A., and Fox, H.: Perianal Paget's disease. Br. J. Dermatol., 85:476, 1971.

Helwig, E. B., and Graham, J. H.: Anogenital (extramammary) Paget's disease. Cancer, 16:387, 1963.

Hertig, A. T., and Gore, H.: Tumors of the female sex organs. Armed Forces Institute of Pathology, Sect. 9, Fas. 33, Part 2, 15, 1960.

Hollmann, K. H., Verley, J. M., and Civatte, J.: La maladie de Paget du mamelon. Étude de deux cas au microscope électronique. Ann. Dermatol. Syphiligr. (Paris), 96:37, 1969.

Hopsu-Havu, V. K., and Sonck, C. E.: The problem of extramammary Paget's disease; report of four cases with "pagetoid" cells. Z. Haut. Geschlechtskr. 46:41, 1971.

Hori, Y., Ishibashi, Y., Ikeda, S., Niki, F., and Miyasato, H.: Anal Paget's disease. Tokyo Dermatol. Soc., 479th Meeting, 1970.

Huber, C. P., Gardiner, S. H., and Michael, A.: Paget's disease of the vulva. Am. J. Obstet. Gynecol., 62:778, 1951.

Huriez, C., Mazzuca, M., Nenoit, M., Bombart, M., and Thomas, P.: Maladie de Paget mammaire et extramammaire. Encyclopédie Medico-Chirugicale (Paris), 12:755, Alo -lo, 1971.

Ikeda, S., Tajima, K., Ishibashi, Y., Mizutani, H., Miyasato, H., Niimura, M., Imai, S., Nishiwaki, M., and Torii, Y.: Extramammary Paget's disease. Jap. J. Clin. Dermatol., 24:15, 1970.

Ishibashi, Y., Jäger, G., and Klingmüller, G.: Elektronenmikroskopische Untersuchung eines extramammären Morbus Paget. Arch. Klin. Exp. Dermatol., 234:293, 1969.

Ishibashi, Y., Miyasato, H., Ikeda, S., Niki, F., and Klingmüller, G.: Elektronenmikroskopische Untersuchungen eines mammären Morbus Paget. Arch. Klin. Exp. Dermatol., 238:258, 1970a.

Ishibashi, Y., Ikeda, S., and Klingmüller, G.: Weitere Untersuchung eines extramammären Morbus Paget mit besonderer Berücksichtigung elektronenmikroskopisch erkennbarer granulärer Substanzen in Pagetzellen. Arch. Klin. Exp. Dermatol., 238:366, 1970b.

Ishibashi, Y., Niimura, M., and Klingmüller, G.: Elektronenmikroskopischer Beitrag zur Morphologie von Paget-Zellen. Arch. Dermatol. Forsch., 245:402, 1972.

Jacobäus, H. C.: Paget's disease und ihr Verhältnis zum Milchdrüsen-Karzinom. Virchows Arch., 178:124, 1904.

Jacobsen, K. B., and Haavelsrud, O. J.: Extramammary Paget's disease, a case report. Acta Derm. Venerol. (Stockh.), 49:87, 1969.

Karg, C.: Über das Carcinom. Dtsch. Z. Chirurgie, 34:133, 1892.

Kaufman, R. H., Boice, E. H., and Knight, W. R.: Paget's disease of the vulva. Am. J. Obstet. Gynecol., 79:451, 1960.

Kawamura, T.: On certain aspects of the pathogenesis of the ectodermal skin growths. Jap. J. Dermatol., 72:513, 1962.

Kawatsu, T., and Miki, Y.: Triple extramammary Paget's disease. Arch. Dermatol., 104:316, 1971.

Klingmüller, G., Klehr, H. U., and Ishibashi, Y.: Desmosomen im Cytoplasma entdifferenzierter Keratinocyten des Plattenepithelcarcinoms. Arch. Klin. Exp. Dermatol., 238:356, 1970.

Knauer, W. J., and Whorton, C. M.: Extramammary Paget's disease originating in Moll's glands of the lids. Trans. Am. Acad. Ophthalmol. Otolaryngol., 67:829, 1963.

Komori, S.: On extramammary Paget's disease. Mitt. Med. Akad. Kioto, 24:42;267, 1938.

Koss, L. G., and Brockunier, A.: Ultrastructural aspects of Paget's disease of the vulva. Arch. Pathol., 87:592, 1969.

Koss, L. G., Ladinsky, S., and Brockunier, A.: Paget's disease of the vulva; report of 10 cases. Am. J. Obstet. Gynecol., 31:513, 1968.

Kren, O.: Pagetsche Erkrankung am Anus und Genitale. Wien. Klin. Rdsch., No. 5, 1914.

Lattes, R., and Haagensen, C. D.: International Symposium on Mammary Cancer. Perugia:189, 1958.; cit. Adamsons et al.

Lennox, B., and Pearse, A. G. E.: Histochemical characterization of specific cells in Paget's disease of vulva. J. Obstet. Gynaecol. Br. Emp., 61:758, 1954.

Lübschitz, K.: Paget's disease with special consideration of clinical course and therapy. Acta Radiol. (Stockh.), 25:127, 1944.

Lüders, G.:Zur Pathologie und Genese des extramammären Morbus Paget. Arch. Klin. Exp. Dermatol., 232:16, 1968.

Lund, H. Z.: Tumors of the Skin. Armed Forces Institute of Pathology; Washington, D. C., 1957.

Madsen, A.: Paget's disease of the vulva. Acta Derm. Venerol. (Stockh.), 45:84, 1965.

Masson, P.: Consideration sur la maladie de Paget. Bull. Soc. Fr. Dermatol., 32:R.S.6, 1925.

Medenica, M., and Sahihi, T.: Ultrastructural study of a case of extramammary Paget's disease of the vulva. Arch. Dermatol., 105:236, 1972.

Miescher, G.: Zwei Fälle von vegetierendem Morbus Paget der Genitalregion. Dermatologica, 108:309, 1954.

Miescher, G.: Morbus Paget der Genitalregion mit Beteiligung von Haut und Schweissdrüsen mit Pigmentierungen vom Aussehen der melanotischen Präkanzerose. Dermatologica, 114:193, 1957.

Mishima, Y., and Matsunaka, N.: Paget's disease. Hifuka no Rinsho., 11:792, 1969.

Montgomery, H.: Dermatopathology. Vol. II. New York, Harper and Row, 1967, p. 1007.

Mori, S.: Studies of the extramammary Paget's disease. Part I. Review of literature and difference between primary Paget's disease and secondary Paget's disease. Jap. J. Dermatol., Ser. B, 75:44, 1965. Part II. Pathogenesis of primary Paget's disease. Jap. J. Dermatol., Ser. B., 75:56, 1965.

Muir, R.: Pathogenesis of Paget's disease of the nipple and associated lesions. Br. J. Surg., 22:728, 1935.

Muir, R.: Further observations on Paget's disease of the nipple. J. Pathol. Bacteriol., 49:299, 1939.

Munro, R.: Paget's disease of the nipple. Glasgow Med. J., 16:342, 1880.

Muri, O., Jr.: Paget's disease of the vulva. Acta. Pathol. Microbiol. Scand., 49:401, 1960.

Murrell, T. W., and Mcmullan, F. H.: Extramammary Paget's disease: a report of two cases. Arch. Dermatol., 85:600, 1962.

Neisser, A.: Verh. Dtsch. Ges., Dermatol. 80, 1892.

Neubecker, R. D., and Bradshaw, R. P.: Mucin, melanin and glycogen in Paget's disease of the breast. Am. J. Clin. Pathol., 36:40, 1961.

Ofuji, S., and Takeda, T.: An electronmicroscopic observation on genital Paget's disease. Acta Dermatol. (Kyoto), 60:209, 1965.

Paget, J.: On disease of the mammary areola preceding cancer of the mammary gland. St. Barth. Hosp. Rep., 10:87, 1874.

Parsons, L., and Lohlein, H. E.: Paget's disease. Arch. Pathol., 36:424, 1943.

Pautrier, L. M.: Paget's disease of the nipple: a true cancer tending to invade the epidermis and necessitating total and early amputation of the breast. Arch Dermatol., 17:767, 1928.

Pick, F. J.: Der Befund von Psoropsermien in einem Falle von Paget-Krankheit an der Glans penis. Prag. Med. Wochenschr., 282, 1891.

Pierard, J., Thiery, M., Boddaert, J., and Smet, H.: Maladie de Paget de la vulve avec métastases viscérales. Arch. Belg. Dermatol., 14:87, 1958.

Pinkus, H.: Genital Paget's disease. Arch. Dermatol., 82:863, 1960.

Pinkus, H., and Gould, S. E.: Extramammary Paget's disease and intraepidermal carcinoma. Arch. Dermatol., 39:479, 1939.

Pinkus, H., and Mehregan, A. H.: Epidermotropic eccrine carcinoma: A case combining features of eccrine poroma and Paget's dermatosis. Arch. Dermatol., 88:597, 1963.

Polland, R.: Paget's disease an der Wange. Dermatol., 21:983, 1914.

Prose, P. H., and Hyman, A. B.: Extramammary Paget's disease. Arch. Dermatol. Syph. (Chic.), 80: 398, 1959.

Ribbert, H.: Über den Paget-Krebs. Dtsch. Med. Wochenschr., 31:1218, 1905.

Rosenberg, J.: Zur Pagetschen Krankheit Mh. Prakt. Dermatol., 49:235, 1909.

Sagami, S.: Electron microscopic studies in Paget's disease. Med. J. Osaka Univ., 14:173, 1963.

Sagami, S., Horiki, M., and Tabata, M.: Cellular pathology of Paget's disease. Jap. J. Clin. Dermatol. (Suppl.), 21:377, 1967.

Sagebiel, R. W.: Ultrastructural observations on epidermal cells in Paget's disease of the breast. Am. J. Pathol., 57:49, 1969.

Satani, J.: Extramammary Paget's disease of the axilla. Br. J. Dermatol., 32:117, 1920.

Seiji, M., and Misune, F.: Electron microscopic study of Bowen's disease. Arch. Dermatol., 99:3, 1969.

Stankovic, P.: Über die Pagetsche Krankheit. Dissertation, Göttingen, 1963.

Stout, A. P.: The relationship of malignant amelanotic melanoma (nevocarcinoma) to extramammary Paget's disease. Am. J. Cancer, 33:196, 1938.

Strauss, G.: Histochemische Untersuchungen bei Pagetscher Erkrankung der Vulva. Z. Krebsforsch., 61:632, 1957.

Strauss, R.: Extramammary Paget's disease of the anus. Am. J. Proctol., 15:36, 1964.

Takaki, Y., Masutani, M., and Kawada, A.: Electron microscopic study of keratoacanthoma. Acta Derm. Venereol. (Stockh.), 51:21, 1971.

Taki, I., and Janovski, N. A.: Paget's disease of the vulva: presentation and histochemical study of four cases. Obstet. Gynecol., 18:385, 1961.

Thin, G.: On the connection between disease of the nipple and areola and tumors of the breast. Trans. Pathol. Soc., London, 32:218, 1881.

Toker, C.: Some observations on Paget's disease of the nipple. Cancer, 14:653, 1961.

Toker, C.: Further observations on Paget's disease of the nipple. J. Nat. Cancer Inst., 38:79, 1967.

Tommasoli, P.: Malattia di Paget della verge. G. Ital. Mal. Ven., Vol. 28, 1893.

Treves, N.: Paget's disease of the male mamma: A report of two cases. Cancer, 7:325, 1954.

Unna, P. G.: Paget's Carcinom der Brustwarze. *In* Die Histopathologie der Hautkrankheiten. Berlin, Hirschwald, 1894, p. 737.

Uyeda, K., Nakayasu, K., and Hasegawa, M.: Genital Paget's disease associated with Candida infection—Case report with electron microscopic observation. Klin. Dermatol. (Tokyo), 26:417, 1972.

Weiner, H. A.: Paget's disease of the skin and its relation to carcinoma of apocrine sweat glands. Am. J. Cancer, 21:373, 1937.

Wessel, W.: Personal communication.

Whorton, C. M., and Patterson, J. B.: Carcinoma of Moll's gland with extramammary Paget's disease of the eyelid. Cancer, 8:1009, 1955.

Wickham, cit. Unna: Pathologische Anatomie der Paget' schen Krankheit. Internatl. Kongr. Dermatol., Paris, 1889. Med. Exp., 1, 1890.

Wile, U.: Bowen's disease and Paget's disease of the nipple. Arch. Dermatol., 18:826, 1928.

Willis, R. A.: Pathology of Tumors. Washington, D. C., Butterworth, 1960.

Woodruff, J. D.: Paget's disease of vulva: Report of two cases. Obstet. Gynecol., 5:175, 1955.

Woodruff, J. D., and Pauerstein, C. J.: Differential metabolic activity in Paget's cell and associated epithelia of the vulva. Obstet. Gynecol., 28:663, 1966.

Woodruff, J. D., and Richardson, E. H., Jr.: Malignant vulvar Paget's disease. Obstet. Gynecol., 10:10, 1957.

Yates, D. R., and Koss, L. G.: Paget's disease of the esophageal epithelium. Arch. Pathol., 86:447, 1968.

Zieler, K.: Über die unter dem Namen "Paget's disease of the nipple" bekannte Hautkrankheit und ihre Beziehungen zum Karzinom. Virchows Arch. [Pathol. Anat.], 177:293, 1904.

29

Circumscribed Precancerous Melanosis (Dubreuilh)

Rafael Andrade, M.D.

This disease is known under several synonyms, such as senile freckle, melanotic freckle, infective melanotic freckle (Hutchinson's), lentigo malin des vieillards, mélanose circonscrite précancéreuse (Dubreuilh), lentigo maligna, melanosis premaligna (Gans and Steigleder), melanosis circumscripta preblastomatosa (Schuermann), precancerous non-nevoid melanocytoma (Mishima).

DEFINITION

Circumscribed precancerous melanosis is a long-standing, slowly progressing, pigmented, very sharply outlined lesion with a play of colors from pale tan to brown. Periods of growth may alternate with periods of quiescence and even with periods of spontaneous regression in some areas of the lesion. The lesions are often located on the face and may undergo transformation into malignant melanoma. Apparently the prognosis, at least for facial lesions, is not so poor, even if regional metastases—which are rare—are present.

HISTORY

Hutchinson (1892a and 1892b) described this entity as a senile freckle or infective (spreading) melanotic freckle. Dubreuilh, in 1894, presented four cases under the name of "lentigo malin des vieillards." In 1912, this author presented a masterly analysis of 35 cases (30 of them from other authors) and coined the descriptive and most appropriate term of "mélanose circonscrite précancéreuse." Since then several authors, most of them dermatologists, have studied this condition.

EPIDEMIOLOGY AND INCIDENCE

Circumscribed precancerous melanosis occurs approximately equally in males and females, and more frequently after middle age. It has been described in younger patients, however. Duration may be as long as 35, 50, and 60 years. Approximately 60 to 70 percent of the cases involve the face. Practically all cases have

679

been described in Caucasians or people with a light complexion. To date, about 800 cases, including those complicated with malignant melanomas, have been reported.

Clark and Mihm (1969) presented a table with a list of cases previously reported, including their own cases. The total was 202 cases of precancerous melanosis and 396 cases with melanoma (lentigo maligna melanoma). They included lesions of the conjunctiva (Reese and Morgan, 1967). To this should be added 14 cases with melanoma and 17 cases of precancerous melanosis (Schuermann, 1963); 21 cases of precancerous melanosis published by Jardak (1969); 17 cases from the study of Jung and Koelzsch (1968); two cases involving the fingertip published by Lupulescu et al. (1973); 69 cases of precancerous melanosis and 19 cases with malignant melanoma published by Arma-Szlachcic et al. (1970); and Maillard's 30 cases with malignant melanoma (1971). Grinspan et al. (1969) mentioned eight cases of precancerous melanosis with malignant melanoma of the oral mucosa, and McGovern (1970) listed 20 further cases of malignant melanoma on precancerous melanosis. The approximate total of published cases would thus be 328 precancerous melanoses and 487 cases of precancerous melanosis accompanied by melanoma. To this should be added the 26 cases of precancerous melanosis and 10 cases with malignant melanoma which we have seen at the Skin and Cancer Unit of New York University Medical Center. In the precancerous stage the incidence is certainly higher, however, since many cases remain unpublished. Many patients afflicted with the disease will probably never ask for medical advice, and of those who do, many probably have died for reasons unrelated to precancerous melanosis. The large number of cases with malignant melanoma can probably be attributed to the tendency to report these complicated cases more readily than others.

ETIOLOGY AND PATHOGENESIS

The etiology is unknown. The predominance of lesions on the face suggests a relationship to sun exposure, a point on which many authors are agreed. Because of this relationship, it would be advisable to group the lesions occurring on the face separately from those in other locations until we have more cases of and experience with this last group. It has been maintained that there is a relationship between circumscribed precancerous melanosis and nevus cell nevus. Gartmann (1962) considered a circumscribed precancerous melanosis and an active junctional nevus to be histologically similar. Mishima (1960), Pinkus and Mishima (1963), and Pinkus (1967) considered this condition to be derived from abnormal dendritic melanocytes, which are different from nevus cells, and referred to it as a precancerous, non-nevoid, melanocytic tumor. According to Mishima, all other malignant melanomas derive from nevus cells, a fact which he feels explains their different biologic behavior. Clark, From, Bernardino, and Mihm (1969) considered all malignant melanomas to be derived from epidermal melanocytes and not from nevus cells. By studying the melanocytes in the basal layer of the lesion and in the basal layer of the adjacent surrounding epidermis in melanocytic and nonmelanocytic tumors, Cochran (1971) has found consistent differences: in circumscribed precancerous melanosis he found an increase in the number of melanocytes, which can be normal or pleomorphic, scattered or in clusters, but there was no junctional activity.

McGovern (1970) studied the incidence of associated intradermal nevi and found intradermal nevi in 5 percent of the cases of circumscribed precancerous melanosis with melanoma, in 34 percent of the cases of superficial malignant melanoma, and in 24 percent of the cases of nodular melanoma. Wayte and Helwig (1968) found a benign intradermal nevus underneath the area of the lesion in eight cases of their 85 circumscribed precancerous melanoses and considered them as separate entities. In a few of our cases, we have occasionally found typical nests of nevus cells at the junction area (see Fig. 29–10). We cannot exclude the possibility that the nests of nevus cells found in an area of precancerous melanosis are there by coincidence. Their growth might also be stimulated by

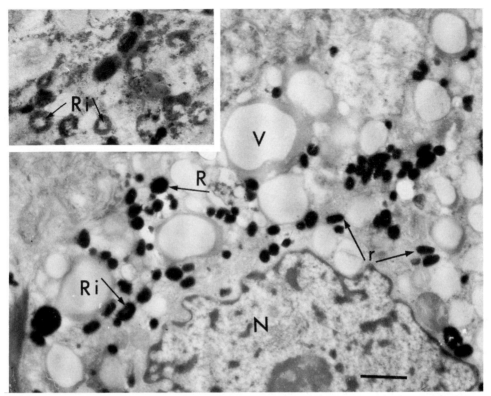

Figure 29–1   Melanocyte of an advanced stage of Dubreuilh's precancerous melanosis, revealing melanosomes which appear rod-shaped (*r*) when sectioned along their short axis and round (*R*) when cut parallel to their long axis. They exhibit a ringlike appearance (*Ri*) when partially melanized. The melanocytes from earlier stages of circumscribed precancerous melanosis also contain elongated granules similar to those of normal melanocytes. Large vacuole-like structures (*V*) are seen. *N*, nucleus; fixed with OsO$_4$. *Phosphotungstic acid and uranyl acetate,* ×*12,000 (inset* ×*21,700). (From* Mishima: Arch. Dermatol., 91:519, 1965.)

the neighboring melanocytic prolifer-ation. Our findings do not contradict ei-ther Mishima's or Clark's hypothesis.

The cells are DOPA-positive and often show a positive tyrosinase reaction (Mi-shima, 1960 and 1967). Mishima (1965 and 1970), using the electron microscope, found that melanosomes synthesized by these cells were distinctly different from those synthesized by junctional nevus cells (Fig. 29–1). This supports Mishima's con-clusion that precancerous melanosis is not a variety of junctional nevus cell nevus. According to Mishima (1970) there ap-pear to be two different types of melano-somes in the melanocytes of Dubreuilh's melanosis, depending on the age of the lesion. Moreover, there are ultrastructural differences between the anaplastic dendri-tic melanocytes invading the upper epi-dermis and the normal melanocytes lo-cated in the junction area.

Oberste-Lehn has recently studied the epidermal-dermal interface in this condi-tion (see Chapter 9, pp. 207, 208) (Fig. 29–2). Clark and Bretton (1971) have shown ultrastructural differences between the intraepidermal melanocytes in lentigo maligna melanoma (circumscribed pre-cancerous melanosis with melanoma), a relatively benign melanoma, and super-ficial spreading melanoma (premalig-nant melanosis or pagetoid melanoma [McGovern, 1970]), which is potentially aggressive. In the former, melanosome formation is essentially normal, with or-derly progression through the various melanosomal stages. In contrast, the latter shows a strikingly disordered melanoso-mal structure. Pinkus (1967) pointed out that in circumscribed precancerous mel-anosis the regular relationship which exists within the epidermal biologic unit formed by basal cells and melanocytes

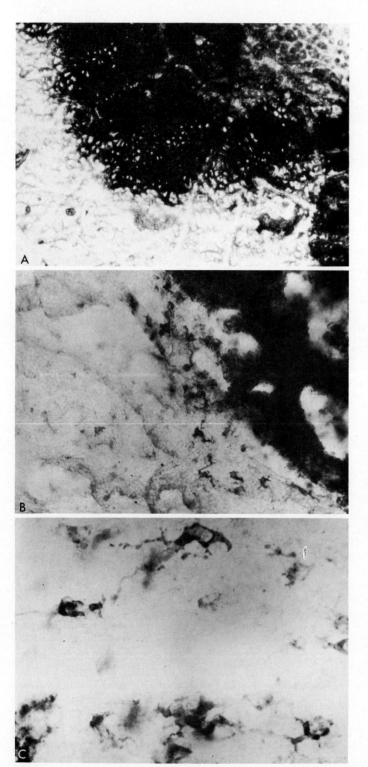

Figure 29–2 Dermal-epidermal separation in a case of precancerous melanosis with malignant melanoma in another area of the lesion. Cheek of 77 year old white woman.

A, This preparation is from the border area of the precancerous melanosis, showing the general configuration of normal skin and of the pigmented skin corresponding to the lesion. *DOPA, ×12.5.*

B, Higher power view of the border between normal skin and the pigmented lesion with numerous large, isolated, dendritic melanocytes in that area. *DOPA, ×100.*

C, High-power view of several of the melanocytes. *DOPA, ×450.* (Histologic preparations by Dr. J. Jelinek, Skin and Cancer Clinic, New York University Medical Center, for a study of dermal-epidermal separation in pigmented lesions.)

(Fitzpatrick and Breathnach, 1963) is probably lost. Since the melanocytes become more numerous and larger, they no longer respect the territory of the neighboring cells, and this might be the first indication of an escape from regulatory influences. For Pinkus (1967), circumscribed precancerous melanosis commonly lacks the third (rapid growth) and the fourth (metastasis) of Warren's four criteria, and "definitely occupies the border zone between cancer and noncancer, gradually making its way from benign hyperplasia to malignant invasion, but rarely and only late does it progress to dissemination and death."

CLINICAL DESCRIPTION

Precancerous melanosis is essentially a *clinicopathologic entity* (Fig. 29–10). In the 80 years since Hutchinson and Dubreuilh described and clearly defined it, it has found but poor acceptance outside of dermatologic circles. It was not until recently (Ollstein et al., 1966; Clark, 1966; Wayte and Helwig, 1968; Clark and Mihm,

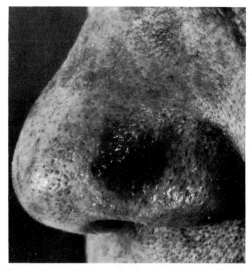

Figure 29–3 Circumscribed precancerous melanosis on left side of nose in an 80 year old man. Asymptomatic, mottled, pigmented macule, 1 × 1 cm., of several years' duration. Biopsy confirmed clinical diagnosis. (Private patient of Dr. Leonard C. Harber, New York.)

1969; McGovern, 1970) that surgical pathologists and surgeons began to accept this condition as a separate entity and gave dermatology credit for having sepa-

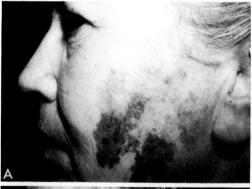
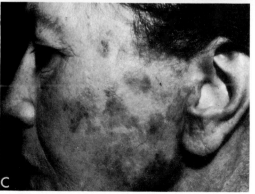
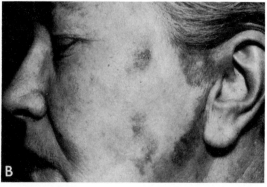

Figure 29–4 A 73 year old white woman. Patient stated that the lesion started at age 14 as a small brown area that progressively grew to present size and appearance. First seen at the Skin and Cancer Clinic, New York University Medical Center, in 1956 at age 59 (*A*) with an 84-mm. asymptomatic lesion. Two biopsies confirmed the diagnosis of circumscribed precancerous melanosis. Patient had never been treated before. Treated at the Skin and Cancer Clinic three times with electrodesiccation and curettage. Each time there were recurrences in different areas and the lesion extended at the periphery (*B* and *C*). In 1966 and 1967, the pigmented area was treated with Miescher's technique (grenz ray) with good results. No recurrence in 1970. (See Figure 3 in Petratos et al.: Treatment of melanotic freckle with X-rays. Arch. Dermatol., *106*:189, 1972; fourteen years of follow-up.)

rated it from superficial malignant melanoma. We wonder how many previously published cases of so-called malignant melanoma of the face and neck were really cases of precancerous melanosis.

An established circumscribed precancerous melanosis has a very peculiar, distinctive clinical picture, which makes it relatively easy to differentiate from superficial malignant melanoma. In the early stage, there is a small, round or oval, tan, sepia, or brown, sharply outlined macule of about 8 to 10 mm. in diameter (Fig. 29–3), which progressively extends at the periphery in a very irregular fashion. It may also be the result of a fusion of several pigmented areas. Many years may pass before the patient seeks medical treatment. As the years go by, the color range becomes wider—tan, dark brown, grayish, bluish, and black—and the lesion may show some scaly and erythematous areas, which give it a mottled appearance (Figs. 29–4, 29–5, 29–10, 29–16, 29–17, and 29–18). In general, the lesion enlarges progressively, but it may also become stationary. Periods of progression may alternate with periods of quiescence and periods of regression, since pigmented areas may spontaneously regress, leaving a very superficial atrophy (Fig. 29–4). The spontaneous regression of an entire lesion has been reported on rare occasions. This changeability is character-

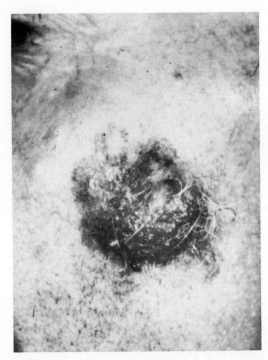

Figure 29–6 Melanoma arising in circumscribed precancerous melanosis of many years' duration. Note the nodular lesion surrounded by an irregularly pigmented area. (*From* Andrade: Lentigo maligna— Hutchinson's freckle. *In* Demis, Crounse, Dobson, and McGuire (Eds.): Dermatology, Vol. 2, Unit 11-54. New York, Harper & Row, 1972, pp. 1–6.)

istic of the condition. The lesion sometimes involves a wide area, such as an entire cheek (Fig. 29–4).

Some of the dark brown and mainly the arciform, black areas may become infiltrated, show surface irregularities, and form frank tumoral nodules. There may be areas of hypopigmentation, and the surface may be verrucous, eroded, or crusted, bleeding easily. In these cases, the transformation into a malignant melanoma is a distinct possibility (Figs. 29–6 and 29–7).

Although circumscribed precancerous melanosis is more frequent in the face, it may also be present on the trunk and extremities, mostly on the dorsa of the hands (Figs. 29–8 and 29–9) and feet. The incidence of precancerous melanosis in the conjunctiva varies according to the authors (Reese, 1943 and 1966; Greer, 1956; Reese and Morgan, 1967; see Henkind and Friedman, Chapter 57). It is exceptional in the mucous membranes of the mouth and vulva (Duperrat, 1959)

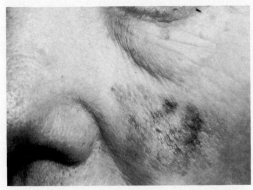

Figure 29–5 A 70 year old white woman presented with a macular, slowly growing, 25-mm. lesion in two years' duration. Biopsy confirmed the diagnosis of circumscribed precancerous melanosis. Treated with electrodesiccation and curettage, with recurrence in the pigmented areas one year later. Refused treatment. Follow-up for two years, then lost to follow-up. (Case from the Oncology Section, Skin and Cancer Clinic. New York University Medical Center.)

and the penis (Relias and Sakellarion, 1963). In the oral mucosa it is probably more frequent (Grinspan et al., 1969). More observation of these extracutaneous locations is needed for a better appreciation of the incidence and prognosis of the disease.

Even if malignant melanoma develops, years may pass before regional metastases appear. If they do appear, the prognosis is apparently more favorable than in other cases of malignant melanoma, at least in cases involving the face. Many cases of so-called superficial malignant melanoma of the face are probably really circumscribed precancerous melanosis. Statistics on malignant melanoma do not always clearly distinguish between this

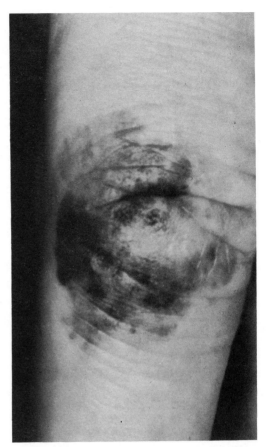

Figure 29–8 Lesion on knuckle of right fourth finger of a 75 year old woman. Duration about three years. Area of pigmentation had slowly increased in size. Microscopically, the rete ridges were elongated, and the basal layer contained an increased number of pleomorphic melanocytes. (*From* Andrade: Lentigo maligna—Hutchinson's freckle. *In* Demis, Crounse, Dobson, and McGuire (Eds.): Dermatology, Vol. 2, Unit 11-54. New York, Harper & Row, 1972, pp. 1–6.)

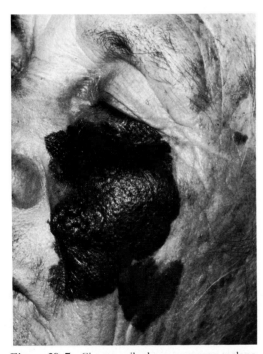

Figure 29–7 Circumscribed precancerous melanosis with malignant melanoma in a 74 year old woman. Left cheek. Hyperpigmented lesion, 8 cm. × 6 cm., with a nodular, crusted neoformation of 2.2 cm. in diameter and 0.3 cm. thick between ala nasi and corner of the mouth. Patient complained of pruritus in this area. The nodular lesion appeared three years ago and grew slowly to present size. The flat, pigmented lesion began many years back as a 1 cm. × 1 cm. tan plaque which grew slowly. No adenopathy. Surgically excised with plastic repair. Pathology confirmed the clinical diagnosis of circumscribed precancerous melanosis with malignant melanoma. Patient was lost to follow-up. (Case of Dr. Jorge Peniche, Oncology Section, Department of Dermatology, Hospital General de México, S.S.A.)

condition and malignant melanoma, so that errors may creep into the statistical evaluations. (Figure 29–10 illustrates the life history of a case of circumscribed precancerous melanosis.)

The transformation into malignant melanoma, according to Miescher, occurs in approximately one-third of the cases. The statistics oscillate, however, below and above this estimate. The duration of the lesion at the time of biopsy obviously affects the histopathologic findings, so that the assessment of a precancerous or cancerous stage in any series would become very difficult to evaluate (Wayte and Helwig, 1968). In the study by Wayte and Helwig, the average duration of the lesion

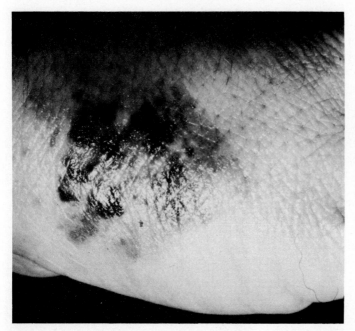

Figure 29–9 Lesion of eight years' duration on dorsum of hand of a 58 year old white woman seen at the Oncology Section, Skin and Cancer Clinic, New York University Medical Center. Patient claims that since onset there has been little change in size, shape, and surface characteristics. Some of the hyperpigmented brown-black areas are barely elevated on palpation. Asymptomatic. Two biopsies were taken at different levels. Consistent with circumscribed precancerous melanosis with areas of transformation into early superficial malignant melanoma. No adenopathy. Treatment consisted of surgical excision with plastic repair. Some of the sweat ducts showed nests of nevus cells in the junction area. (Case presentation at Dermatological Society of Greater New York, March 18, 1965, by A. W. Kopf, R. Andrade, and N. Pensley.)

was 14 years. In cases showing a malignant melanoma, it was 18 years. Lesions greater than 4 cm. in diameter were more likely to contain melanoma than smaller lesions. According to the authors, these two findings suggest that the older and larger the lesion, the greater the incidence of malignant melanoma. This is an interesting suggestion, which might also be applicable to other precancerous conditions.

The malignant transformation may occur a few or many years after onset, up to 34, 50, and 60 years later (Dubreuilh, 1894 and 1912; Miescher, 1954; Klauder and Beerman, 1955; Duperrat, 1962; Clark and Mihm, 1969; Mihm et al., 1971; McGovern, 1970; Andrade, 1964 and 1972; Sulzberger et al., 1959; Mishima, 1970). The average is 10 to 14 years after onset. In Dubreuilh's series, 23 out of 35 cases (including five of his own, 10 of Hutchinson's, and the rest from other sources) showed malignant melanoma. Justitz (1935) reported seven malignant melanomas in a series of 10 cases of precancerous melanosis; Klauder and Beerman (1955) had four malignant melanomas in five cases of precancerous melanosis; Schuermann (1955) reported nine malignant melanomas out of 25 cases

of precancerous melanosis, his material having enlarged by 1963 to include 56 cases with a 41 percent incidence of malignant melanoma; Grinspan and Abulafia (1956) had 10 cases with malignant melanoma; Costello, Fisher, and DeFeo (1959) had four out of 10 cases; Jackson, Williamson, and Beattie (1966) had 21 cases with melanoma; and Friederich and Schneider (1966) had 29 cases out of 61. In the series of 85 cases of the Armed Forces Institute of Pathology (Wayte and Helwig, 1968), malignant melanoma was present in 45. Arma-Szlachcic, Ott, and Storck (1970) published 88 cases of precancerous melanosis from the Clinic in Zurich, including the cases previously studied by Miescher; 69 of these cases were in the precancerous stage and 19 occurred with malignant melanoma. Seventy-four of these patients were observed for five years or more.

Clark and Mihm (1969) published a study of 13 patients with circumscribed precancerous melanosis and 35 patients with circumscribed precancerous melanosis plus malignant melanoma. For this last condition they coined the new name of lentigo maligna melanoma and felt that it deserved special consideration within the group of malignant melanomas.

Text continued on page 692

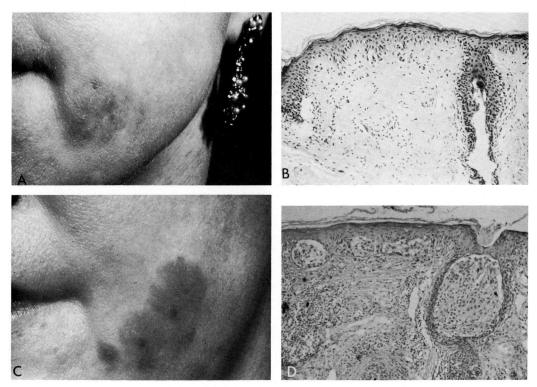

Figure 29–10 This case illustrates the life history of circumscribed precancerous melanosis as a clinicopathologic entity. This patient was seen in 1956 at age 49 at the Oncology Section of the Skin and Cancer Clinic, New York University Medical Center, five years after onset of the lesion. At that time the patient rejected all treatment. The patient was followed for six years, and periodic biopsies were obtained until she accepted local destruction of the lesion. Six punch biopsies were taken just before electrocauterization. These simultaneous biopsies representing different areas of the lesion 11 years after onset illustrate all stages from a benign junctional proliferation to a frank superficial malignant melanoma. The exclusively local treatment documents the peculiar, benign behavior of this lesion, since even in the presence of one spot of superficial malignant melanoma, a superficial destructive method such as electrocauterization could *cure* it, without recurrence of pigmentation or cellular proliferation nine years after treatment. This case illustrates very well the peculiar place precancerous melanosis of the *face* in adults and elderly people should occupy, compared with an active junction nevus and a superficial malignant melanoma of covered areas of the body.

A, This was the appearance of the lesion at the time of consultation at the Skin and Cancer Clinic, at age 49, five years after onset. The plaque measured 2 × 3 cm. and showed erythema, some slightly pigmented areas, and some slightly scaly ones.

B, Histologically there was a junction nevus with a few nests of nevus cells and isolated melanocytes involving the junction area of the epidermis and of a hair follicle infundibulum. There was very little pigment and a very mild, diffuse, lymphocytic infiltrate. *H & E, ×125.*

C, This clinical photograph shows the lesion three years later (1959). The lesion had enlarged; there were more areas with varying shades of pigmentation.

D, The biopsy showed more clearly than the previous one a typical junction nevus involving the hair follicle infundibula. There was a moderate inflammatory infiltrate formed by lymphocytes and histiocytes. Some dilated capillaries were present, which explains the erythematous aspect of the lesion. *H & E, ×125.*

Illustration continued on following page.

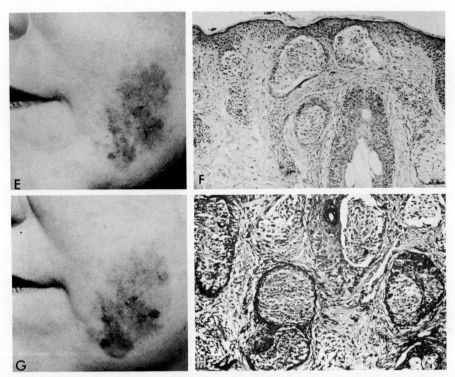

Figure 29–10 *Continued*   One year later, in 1960 (*E* and *F*), and two years later, in 1961 (*G* and *H*), the lesion had enlarged; it showed still more marked color changes, and its erythematous background had persisted. In 1961, in the central area, one could feel on palpation a slightly elevated area a few mm. in size. Histologically, both biopsies, in 1960 and 1961, showed a frank junction nevus. They showed junctional nests, partly pigmented, and isolated large melanocytes. The hair follicle infundibula were involved. There was a patchy, round-cell, inflammatory infiltrate in the dermis. *H & E, ×125; H & E, ×250.*

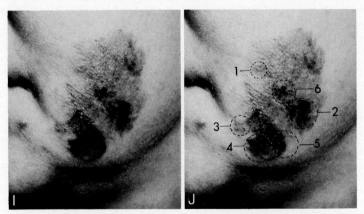

Figure 29–10 *Continued*   In 1962, at age 55, 11 years after the first lesion appeared, there was a change again in the size and appearance of the lesion (*I*). Immediately before treatment, six punch biopsies of 3 mm. in diameter were taken from the pigmented areas, the erythematous area, and the small infiltrated area (*J*).

Illustration continued on opposite page.

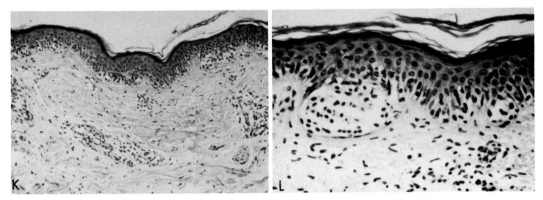

Figure 29–10 *Continued*   This biopsy corresponds to the tan area (site of biopsy No. 1) and shows poorly pigmented nests of nevus cells and large isolated melanocytes in the junction area. The inflammatory infiltrate is mild, *K, H & E, ×125; L, H & E, ×250.*

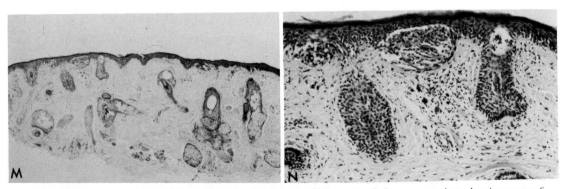

Figure 29–10 *Continued*   *M, N,* Dark pigmented area, site of biopsy No. 2. Low-power view, showing nests of cells in the junction area. *M, H & E, ×25.* High-power photograph, showing the lack of cohesion of the cells, the nuclear hyperchromatism, involvement of the hair follicle infundibulum, and the degree of the inflammatory infiltrate containing melanophages. *N, H & E, ×125.*

Illustration continued on following page.

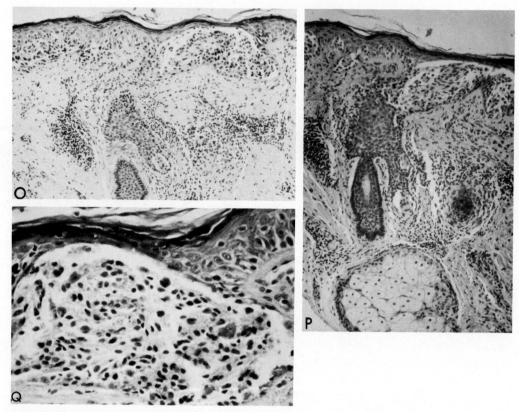

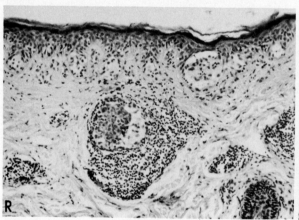

Figure 29–10 *Continued   O, P, Q,* Tan pigmented area, site of biopsy No. 3. Low-power view, showing poorly pigmented nests of cells (*O* and *P*). Note the abundant perifollicular inflammatory infiltrate. The hair follicle infundibula show junctional proliferation of cells. *H & E, ×125.* High-power view (*Q*). Note the separation from the epidermis, the pale abundant cytoplasm of the cells, and the slight nuclear pleomorphism. *H & E, ×500.*

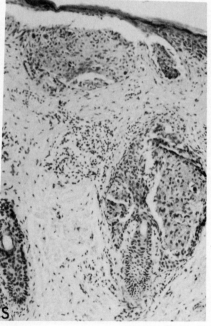

Figure 29–10 *Continued   R,* Encircled pigmented area, site of biopsy No. 4. Figure showing junctional proliferation with a dense, patchy, perifollicular, inflammatory infiltrate. There are isolated melanophages, poorly limited cell nests with peripheral cleavage, nuclear pleomorphism, and abundant, dustlike, pigmented cytoplasms. *H & E, ×250.*

S, Pigmented, harmless looking area, site of biopsy No. 5. Figure showing active junctional proliferation with hair follicle involvement and a patchy, round-cell, inflammatory infiltrate. There is peripheral cleavage around the cell nests and nuclear pleomorphism. The cells show a poorly limited, dustlike cytoplasm. *H & E, ×125.*

Illustration continued on opposite page.

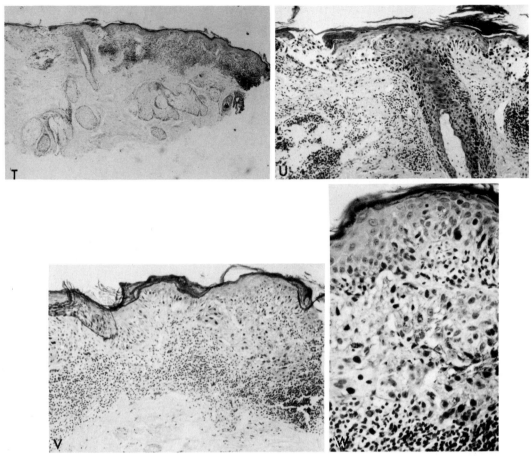

Figure 29–10 *Continued   T through W,* Moderately pigmented area, corresponding to the small, infiltrated area noticeable on palpation only, site of biopsy No. 6. Low-power view (*T*) showing an area of dermal invasion, junctional proliferation, and epidermal compression. *H & E, ×25.* Microphotograph (*U*) showing junctional proliferation, epidermal compression, and disruption. Note the poorly outlined nests of cells and the nuclear pleomorphism. The dermis shows at this level a bandlike, round-cell, inflammatory infiltrate. *H & E, ×250.* Microphotographs showing the area of dermal invasion, with nuclear pleomorphism; hyperchromatism; pale, abundant, dustlike cytoplasms; and occasionally an isolated mitotic figure. A dense, bandlike, inflammatory infiltrate outlines this area of invasion, which was diagnosed as superficial malignant melanoma. *V, H & E, ×250; W, H & E, ×500.*

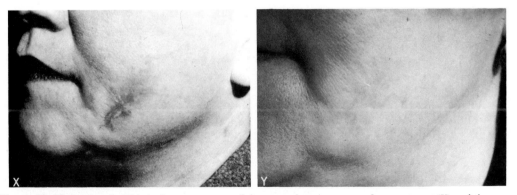

Figure 29–10 *Continued*   This is the appearance of the treated area *one year* after treatment (*X*) and *three years* after treatment (*Y*). Since then, nine years (1971) after treatment, there has been no recurrence, and the area seems to have healed.

In the series of cases we saw at the Skin and Cancer Clinic in New York between 1955 and 1968, there were seven cases of malignant melanoma out of 23 cases of circumscribed precancerous melanosis. In this series, 17 cases concerned patients in the fifth and sixth decades. The youngest was 27 years old and the oldest 70, at the moment of diagnosis. There were seven men and 16 women. In 18 cases the lesions were located on the face, and in 14 of these on the cheeks. The average size was 2 to 3 cm. in 14 cases. The smallest was 0.8 cm. and the largest 8.4 cm. The growth was slow in all cases. The duration of the lesions was from six months to 25 years. In 13 cases the lesions had been present for more than five years. The follow-up was more than five years in seven cases, and between one and five years in 13. In the seven cases with malignant melanoma, the lesion was surgically excised; one of the seven was located on the trunk, the other six on the face. From 1968 to 1971, we had collected 13 additional cases of precancerous melanosis, three of which showed evidence of early invasive malignant melanoma.

In the Department of Dermatology of the Mexico City General Hospital S.S.A., there have been 12 cases, two of them with malignant melanoma, during a 15-year period (Peniche).

In 1969, Grinspan, Abulafia, Diaz, and Berdichesky published one case of melanoma in Hutchinson's melanotic freckle of the oral mucosa, and mentioned seven more which they had found in their literature review (Fig. 29–11).

PATHOLOGY

As mentioned above, circumscribed precancerous melanosis is essentially a *clinicopathologic entity* (Fig. 29–10). Dubreuilh's report in 1912 contains a classic description of the microscopic features. The histologic features are those of widespread junctional proliferation and can be interpreted only on the basis of the clinical findings. The degree of junctional proliferation varies according to the age of the lesion and the clinical appearance of the biopsy area (pale, erythematous, tan, brown, black, flat, or infiltrated). The darker areas are related not only to a

greater cellular proliferation in the junction area but also to the amount of pigment in the junction area itself, in the basal layer, upper epidermal layers, and/or in the dermis, where it may be very abundant. In the early stage, and in the tan areas of old lesions, the junction area shows an increased number of isolated, normal (Miescher, Haeberlin, and Guggenheim, 1936), and abnormal large melanocytes containing little or no melanin and a nucleus, which may be larger than that of the average melanocyte (Figs. 29–10 and 29–17). The nucleus may show hyperchromatism and a distinct nucleolus. The atypical melanocytes can be arranged in a palisade-like distribution with a honeycomb appearance (Mishima, 1970). A few of the abnormal cells are sometimes multinucleated. The dendrites of normal and abnormal melanocytes may be prominent in tan, brown, or black areas (Mishima, 1970; Clark and Mihm, 1969). Clark and Mihm found that the most distinctive feature is the pleomorphism of the melanocytes and the presence of bizarre, large, and strikingly atypical melanocytes side by side with normal ones. This is valid for circumscribed precancerous melanosis and for the noninvasive areas of circumscribed precancerous melanosis with melanoma. Korting and Hassenpflug (1966) have described typical hematoxylin bodies in a lesion of circumscribed precancerous melanosis. They felt, however, that the question whether these hematoxylin bodies play a role in an immunologic mechanism has to be left open.

The cells can also be grouped in small nests (Wayte and Helwig, 1968; Graham et al., 1972) (Fig. 29–10; see discussion under Etiology and Pathogenesis). The junction area of the sweat ducts and hair follicles can be involved. This would explain recurrences following superficial destruction of the lesion. The upper dermis shows some dilated capillaries, sometimes numerous melanophages, depending on the degree of clinical pigmentation, and a mild, perivascular, inflammatory infiltrate consisting of lymphocytes, histiocytes, and plasma cells (Fig. 29–10). Usually there are no mitotic figures. In general, the darker the area, the more marked the cellular proliferation and the cellular abnormalities, but they are still located

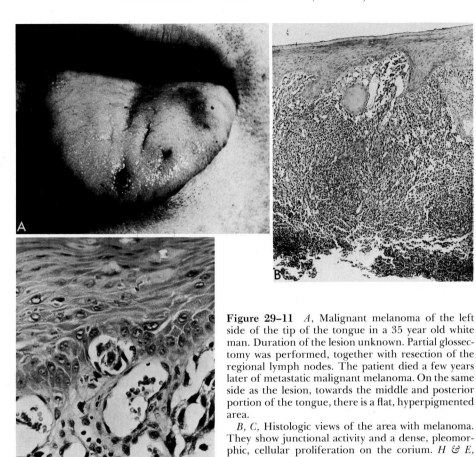

Figure 29–11 *A,* Malignant melanoma of the left side of the tip of the tongue in a 35 year old white man. Duration of the lesion unknown. Partial glossectomy was performed, together with resection of the regional lymph nodes. The patient died a few years later of metastatic malignant melanoma. On the same side as the lesion, towards the middle and posterior portion of the tongue, there is a flat, hyperpigmented area.

B, C, Histologic views of the area with melanoma. They show junctional activity and a dense, pleomorphic, cellular proliferation on the corium. *H & E, ×125 and ×600.*

Figure 29–11 *Continued   D, E,* Histologic views of the flat, pigmented area. The number of melanocytes in the basal layer is increased, and there is a tendency to form nests. These findings suggest that this malignant melanoma of the tongue either developed close to a circumscribed precancerous melanosis or started from a small spot of circumscribed precancerous melanosis on the tip of the tongue. *H & E, ×250 and ×600.* (Case from the Oncology Section, Skin and Cancer Clinic, New York University Medical Center.)

above the basement membrane (Clark and Mihm, 1969). The proliferating, abnormal, melanin-synthesizing, dendritic melanocytes can also be found in the upper layers of the epidermis (Mishima, 1970). The areas where the pigmentation regresses spontaneously are characterized by the disappearance of proliferating melanocytes and by less atypical individual melanocytes; DOPA-positive melanocytes are again limited to the junction layer and are separated by an interval of five to seven basal cells; residual melanophages are seen in the dermis (Mishima, 1970).

The following may be considered as early signs of malignant transformation: poorly outlined junction nests invading the superficial dermis, increase in the degree of cellular pleomorphism, presence of mitotic figures, invasion of the upper layers of the epidermis, and presence of an intense inflammatory reaction in the dermis (Fig. 29–10). The epidermis may show some acanthosis with areas of pseudoepitheliomatous hyperplasia and areas of compression and atrophy. The epitheliomatous hyperplasia may become so intense that there have been isolated reports of association with a squamous cell carcinoma (Vilanova and Cardenal, 1958; Grinspan and Abulafia, 1956; Duperrat, 1962). Duperrat (1959) has reported cases of association with trichoepithelioma. Elastic tissue degeneration is present, depending on the site of the lesion and the patient's age. It is especially marked in cases located in the face. A few authors (Clark and Mihm, 1969; Conley et al., 1971) have mentioned that a melanoma arising in precancerous melanosis often shows a spindle cell type.

DIAGNOSIS

The diagnosis is based on the duration and size of the lesion, its sharp, irregular outline, its color range, and its characteristic changeability, manifested by periods of progression, quiescence, and even regression. The early small lesion is probably often diagnosed clinically as an early junction nevus (see Table 29–1), senile lentigo, ephelis, seborrheic keratosis, ac-

TABLE 29–1   DISTINCT DIFFERENTIATING FEATURES OF DUBREUILH'S MELANOSIS AND JUNCTION NEVUS*

	Dubreuilh's Precancerous Melanosis	Junction Nevus
1. Usual development	old age	childhood
2. Solar exposure	etiologic	nonetiologic
3. Radiosensitivity	sensitive	nonsensitive
4. Malignant transformation	frequent	not frequent

*From Mishima, Y.: Changes in the current concept of malignant melanoma. *In* Current Problems in Dermatology, Vol. 3. Basel, S. Karger, 1970, p. 51.

tinic keratosis, and pigmented superficial basal cell epithelioma.

Special attention should be called to the differential diagnosis from the so-called flat type of seborrheic keratosis (Figs. 29–12 to 29–15), which probably represents, at least in a few cases, a large senile lentigo (Fig. 29–13). It is not frequent and usually occurs in the face (mainly on the cheeks and forehead). It is more regular in color, tan to brown, fixed, well outlined (Figs. 29–13 and 29–14), and has a rough surface, which can be appreciated upon palpation. There may be local areas of growth, which clinically look like isolated seborrheic keratosis (Fig. 29–13*A*). I have seen seven cases of this type of large flat

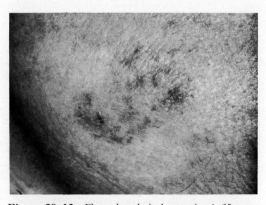

Figure 29–12   Flat seborrheic keratosis. A 65 year old woman with a mottled, brown to sepia-colored, hyperpigmented macule on the right cheek, 3 × 2.2 × 2 cm., of five years' duration. Clinical impression: Hutchinson's freckle or seborrheic keratosis. The biopsy confirmed the diagnosis of seborrheic keratosis. (Case from Oncology Section, Skin and Cancer Clinic, New York University Medical Center.)

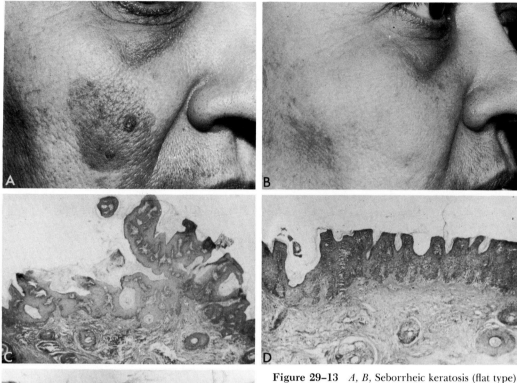

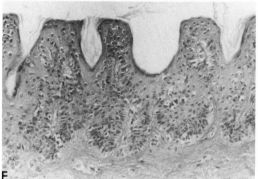

Figure 29–13 *A, B,* Seborrheic keratosis (flat type). A 58 year old woman showed a 2.5 × 2 cm. hyperpigmented, flat, sharply outlined plaque on the right cheek. Slow growth, 15 years' duration. A few years ago, there appeared within the plaque three verrucous, hyperpigmented lesions of about 0.3 to 0.4 cm. in diameter, which clinically and histologically were seborrheic keratoses (*A*). The histologic appearance of the surrounding flat pigmented area suggested a senile lentigo. Light desiccation and curettage produced excellent results. No atrophy, no residual pigmentation one year later (*B*).

C, Low-power histologic view of verrucous area in the center of the lesion. *H & E,* ×25.

D, E, Low- and high-power histologic views of surrounding, flat, pigmented area. The regular acanthosis, the elongated thin rete ridges, the hyperpigmentation, and the increased number of melanocytes in the basal layer suggest a senile lentigo. *H & E,* ×75 and ×200. (Case of Dr. Jorge Peniche, Oncology Section, Department of Dermatology, Hospital General de México, S.S.A.)

seborrheic keratosis. Miescher et al. pointed out the possibility of this differential diagnosis in 1936, but it has not generally been given attention in studies of circumscribed precancerous melanosis.

When the precancerous lesion has attained its distinct characteristics, the clinical diagnosis is evident. A superficial malignant melanoma (superficial spreading melanoma: Clark and Mihm, 1969; premalignant melanosis or pagetoid melanoma: McGovern, 1970) has a shorter duration, is usually smaller, does not show the wide color range and changeability, is uniformly darker, brown or black, is sharply and more regularly outlined, may show some leakage of pigment at the periphery, and often is mildly elevated and therefore palpable.

Several authors have discussed the clinical and pathologic differential diagnosis with extramammary Paget's disease (Allen, 1949 and 1954; Allen and Spitz, 1954; Stout, 1938; Miescher, 1957; Pinkus and Gould, 1939; Steigleder, 1958; Strauss, 1957; Taki and Janovsky, 1961;

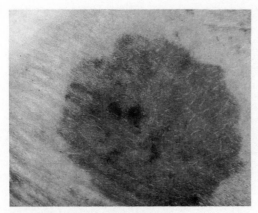

Figure 29–14   Flat seborrheic keratosis. A regularly pigmented, well limited, brown to sepia-colored patch, 3.5 cm. in diameter, with two keratotic papules, each measuring 2 mm. in diameter, in the center. Several years' duration. Right cheek of a 69 year old woman. Clinical impression was Hutchinson's freckle or seborrheic keratosis. (Private patient of Dr. Morris Leider, Skin and Cancer Clinic, New York University Medical Center.)

anosis or pagetoid melanoma: McGovern, 1970) should be treated as separate entities, because they are different in prognosis, age incidence, regional distribution, and probably also in etiologic mechanisms. Clark (1966), Clark and Mihm (1969), and Mihm, Clark, and From (1971) have stressed the pathologic differential diagnosis between these two entities, beyond the ultrastructural characteristics mentioned above. "The neoplastic cells of any kind of malignant melanoma invasive to levels III, IV or V may be similar, regardless of whether the entire lesion was classified as superficial spreading melanoma, nodular melanoma or lentigo maligna melanoma. However, lesions of lentigo maligna, a considerable portion of the primary lesions of lentigo maligna melanoma and superficial spreading melanoma are located intraepidermally. Multiple sections through these intraepidermal portions are required to distinguish the processes from each other" (Clark and Mihm, 1969).

Table 29–2 summarizes the clinical and pathologic differential diagnosis between the three types of malignant melanoma.

Wayte and Helwig, 1968). Now, with the help of highly developed histochemical methods (Steigleder, 1958; Wayte and Helwig, 1968) and ultrastructural studies, these diagnostic problems can be avoided (see Chapter 28). Mishima (1960 and 1970), Pinkus and Mishima (1963), Clark (1966), Clark and Mihm (1969), McGovern (1970), Lupulescu et al. (1973), and the author feel that circumscribed precancerous melanosis with melanoma (lentigo maligna melanoma: Clark and Mihm, 1969) and superficial malignant melanoma (superficial spreading melanoma: Clark and Mihm, 1969; premalignant mel-

TREATMENT

Because of the slow, chronic course of circumscribed precancerous melanosis, superficial destruction (electrodesiccation and curettage, electrocautery) has been advocated (Costello et al., 1959; Klauder and Beerman, 1955). Pigment may reap-

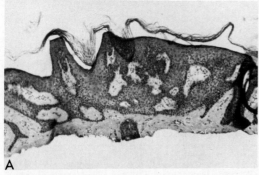
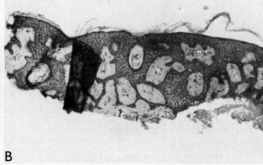

A   B

Figure 29–15   Two histologic views of a flat seborrheic keratosis of the face; left temporal area in a 65 year old white woman; five years' duration, slow growth; tan to sepia-colored, well outlined, 1.5 × 1.7 cm. in size. In the center there was a flat, verrucous area (site of biopsy). The figures show the reticulated pattern, consisting of small basal cell–like cells, the hyperkeratosis with pseudo–horn cyst formation, and papillomatosis. There are also areas of hyperpigmentation of the epidermal cells. *H & E*, ×75.

TABLE 29–2 DIFFERENTIAL CLINICAL AND HISTOLOGIC FEATURES*

Type of Melanoma	Location	Median Age (yr.)	Sex Predilection	Duration†	Margin of Lesion	Color	Histologic Characteristics of noninvasive Areas
Lentigo maligna	usually on exposed surfaces—head and neck (less commonly, hands and legs)	70	none	usually 5–15 yr.	flat	various shades of brown and black; frequent hypopigmentation (regression)	cellular pleomorphism; normal and bizarre melanocytes side by side, principally in basal regions
Superficial spreading	all body surfaces	56	lesions of lower legs predominate in women	1–5 yr.	distinctly palpable	various shades of brown and black; gray and pinkish rose common; occasional depigmented, irregular halo	diffuse intraepidermal distribution of relatively monomorphous, large, malignant melanocytes in noninvasive areas
Nodular	all body surfaces	49	none	months–2 yr.	palpable	uniform bluish black; occasional depigmented, irregular halo	no noninvasive areas in epidermis; invasion of dermis coexistent with intraepidermal neoplasm

*From Mihm, Clark, and From: Reprinted, by permission. From the New England Journal of Medicine, 284:1078, 1971.
†Figures represent common duration of various types; we have encountered neoplasms of each type with much shorter and much longer durations.

pear in some areas of the treated lesion or at the immediate periphery, and these areas can be retreated with the same methods. It is advisable to treat also a safe margin of normal surrounding skin. In very old patients with a wide, flat lesion, some authors recommend watching the lesion and would consider treatment only if signs of malignant degeneration appear (Klauder and Beerman, 1955; Degos, 1953). Miescher (1954 and 1960) recommended grenz ray in high doses (2.000 R., 12 kv., HVL 0.050 AL, 1.0 mm. cellon filter, ma. 15; four- to five-day intervals, five doses, total 10.000 R.) and reported

good results. After the radiation reaction, the pigmentation disappears progressively. Follow-up of 88 cases from the Zurich Skin Clinic (Arma-Szlachcic et al., 1970), which were all treated with this method, established it as the treatment of choice. Arma-Szlachcic et al. (1970) reported 69 cases; 68 of them were treated with varying doses (two with 6.000 R., nine with 8.000 R., 44 with 10.000 R., 11 with 12.000 R., and two with 14.000 R.). Of these, 65 had never had any previous treatment; three had been previously and unsuccessfully treated by other methods. One of the 69 cases was treated with an-

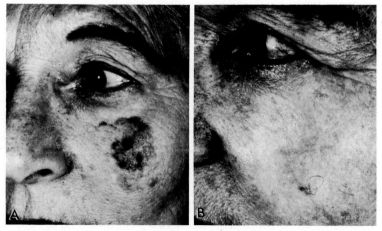

Figure 29–16 Case of precancerous melanosis before treatment (*A*) and two years after treatment (*B*) with grenz ray therapy (Miescher's technique). (Case from the Oncology Section, Skin and Cancer Clinic, New York University Medical Center.)

other method. Fifty-nine patients were observed for five years or more and are alive and cured; eight died of other diseases during the five years of follow-up, without recurrences of the lesion. Two patients had recurrences one year and five years after treatment, respectively, and the recurrences were successfully eradicated by other methods. The good results obtained with this therapy have been confirmed by other authors (Schuermann, 1955 and 1963). Since 1966, eight cases have been treated at the Skin and Cancer Unit in New York with the Miescher method (Petratos et al., 1972). In six of these the response was excellent, and the pigment took two to three weeks to disappear. One patient who had previously had numerous electrodesiccation procedures did not respond. One had a recurrence three years after an excellent response (Figs. 29–16, 29–17 and 29–18).

Miescher (1960) reported late radiation sequelae in 54 patients who were treated by his method and observed for five years or more: hyperpigmentation in one patient, hypopigmentation in 11 patients, leukomelanoderma in five, telangiectasia in five, and atrophy in three patients. Petratos et al. (1972), in four years of observation, reported no radiation sequelae aside from hypopigmentation and a few telangiectasias. These authors observed in several patients that hair continued to grow after use of the Miescher technique.

According to Gladstein (1971) and Petratos et al. (1972), similar radiation results can be obtained by adding a 0.6-mm. cellulose acetate filter to a standard grenz ray machine. Petratos et al. (1972) mentioned several possible reasons for the effectiveness of this method of x-ray radiation. It has been suggested that this method be used in cases of intraoral pre-

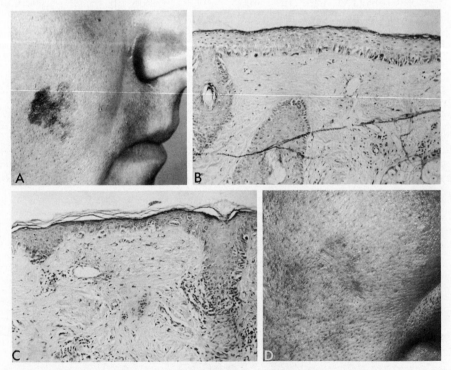

Figure 29–17   A 27 year old white man, seen in 1966 at the Oncology Section, Skin and Cancer Clinic, New York University Medical Center, had a 20-mm. slowly growing lesion of three years' duration on the right cheek (*A*). Biopsy confirmed the diagnosis of circumscribed precancerous melanosis with atypical, large, isolated melanocytes in the basal layer of the pigmented area (*B*) and a few isolated nests of nevus cells (*C*). Treated with grenz ray (Miescher's technique) with good results. Excellent result one year later (*D*). Note the normal beard growth in treated area. In March, 1971, there appeared in this area an ill-defined tan macule 1.5 cm. in diameter. Biopsy confirmed the diagnosis of circumscribed precancerous melanosis. (See Figure 5 in Petratos et al.: Treatment of melanotic freckle with X-ray. Arch. Dermatol., 106:189, 1972.)

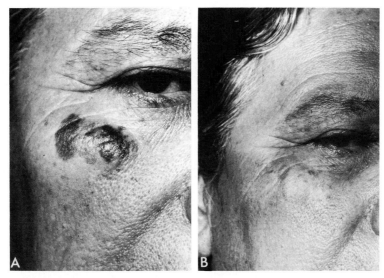

Figure 29–18 Circumscribed precancerous melanosis. A 65 year old woman showed a typical pigmented lesion, 2.5 × 1.5 cm., of several years' duration and very slow progressive growth in the right malar area. Biopsy in two different areas confirmed the clinical diagnosis (*A*). Two years after superficial x-ray therapy, she presented only a few tan residual areas (*B*). (Case of Dr. Jorge Peniche, Oncology Section, Department of Dermatology, Hospital General de México, S.S.A.)

cancerous melanosis (Malkinson and Pearson, 1973).

In our series of 23 cases (1955 to 1968, Skin and Cancer Unit, New York University Medical Center), nine were treated with different locally destructive methods (desiccation and curettage, cryotherapy, electrocautery, trichloroacetic acid), 10 were surgically excised and two of these had a graft, two had grenz ray treatment after a recurrence, and one had first desiccation and curettage, then grenz ray treatment, and finally, after a recurrence, surgical excision. In this series, all cases with malignant melanoma were surgically excised.

Some authors have used surgical excision as the only treatment in the precancerous stage, with or without plastic repair, depending on the size of the lesion. When signs of malignant transformation are present, treatment is the same as for malignant melanoma. Regional lymph nodes are not excised, unless there are signs of invasion.

PROGNOSIS

When the lesion is diagnosed and treated in time, the prognosis is good. If a malignant melanoma develops, the prog-

nosis is apparently better than that for a malignant melanoma developed in normal skin or in a junction nevus, even in the rare cases in which regional lymph node metastases are present. This impression concerns mainly lesions located on the face. We have less valid data on other sites.

Clark and Mihm (1969) reported survival data on 35 patients with malignant melanoma: three died of metastatic malignant melanoma; three developed lymph node metastases, and one of these died of causes unrelated to malignant melanoma; the other two were alive and well after two and four years, respectively, with no evidence of malignant melanoma. Nine patients died of causes unrelated to malignant melanoma, and five were lost to follow-up. The remaining 15 patients were alive and well. The average follow-up period was 5.2 years.

In a series of 85 cases of circumscribed precancerous melanosis published by Wayte and Helwig (1968), malignant melanoma was present in 45. Of these 45 patients, 14 were followed for longer than five years, and 26 were followed for longer than two years. In four patients of the group of 45, there were metastases. The survival rate was 73 percent for those followed five years or longer, and 88 percent for those followed two years or longer. These survival rates, significantly higher than those for malignant melanoma in general, would be in favor of classifying the malignant melanoma that arises in lentigo maligna separately from other melanomas.

In 74 of the 88 cases of circumscribed precancerous melanosis published by Arma-Szlachcic, Ott, and Storck in 1970, the follow-up had been five years or more. In 69 of these cases, the lesions were in the precancerous stage. Sixty-one patients were alive and cured; eight had died during the five years of observation of other diseases, but without recurrences of their lesions. Nineteen of the 88 patients had malignant melanoma; of these, 13 (78 percent) were free of melanoma after five years or more. Of the remaining six, one died shortly after treatment of myocardial infarction, and five had metastases shortly after treatment. Of these, four died the same year, and one died after six years.

McGovern (1970) studied 20 cases of malignant melanoma in precancerous melanosis, 12 women and eight men. Eighteen of the lesions occurred on the head and neck, and two on the dorsa of the wrists. The five-year survival rate was higher in women: 100 percent as compared with 50 percent for the men. The combined percentage was 80 percent (four men and 12 women). This five-year survival rate was significantly higher than that in the superficial spreading melanoma (69 percent) and nodular melanoma (53 percent). Maillard (1971) computed a 66 percent five-year survival rate in 30 cases of circumscribed precancerous melanosis with melanoma. Survival curves (McGovern, 1970) have shown that the observations of Clark and Mihm (1969) are valid, depending on the depth of the invasion of the melanoma. According to these authors, the stages of invasion should be divided as follows: (1) melanoma cells confined to the epidermis of premalignant melanosis (superficial spreading melanoma or pagetoid melanoma); (2) invasion of the papillary zone of the dermis; (3) invasion up to the level of the subpapillary plexus of vessels; (4) invasion of the reticular layer; and (5) invasion of the subcutaneous fat. According

to this classification, the five-year survival rates are 69 percent for stage one (superficial spreading melanoma) and 53 percent for nodular melanoma, which has a higher proportion of tumors in stage five.

McGovern and Lane Brown (1969) have worked out a histologic grading table for malignant melanoma: grade 1, melanoma cells which resemble intradermal nevus cells; grade 3, highly anaplastic cells; and grade 2, tumors with cells that resemble neither grade 1 nor grade 3. Their contention is that there is an overall increase in mortality with higher degrees of cell anaplasia. Nodular melanoma has a higher proportion of grade 3 tumors than melanoma developing from premalignant melanosis (superficial spreading melanoma), while none of the melanomas arising from circumscribed precancerous melanosis was grade 3 (McGovern, 1970).

In our own above-mentioned series of 23 cases, there were three deaths. The patients had only had lesions in the precancerous stage, two of them for five years and one for four years, and died of causes unrelated to malignant melanoma. Of these 23, seven patients had malignant melanomas, which were surgically excised. One of these died of unknown causes one year after treatment; the other six were alive (in 1968) after a follow-up of 12, four, four, three, and two years, and six months in one case. One of the patients followed for four years had had a positive lymph node verified by pathology at the time of surgical excision.

We can conclude with Schuermann (1955) and Arma-Szlachcic, Ott, and Storck (1970) that the diagnosis and rather simple treatment of circumscribed precancerous melanosis play a positive, contributive role in the prophylaxis of malignant melanoma.

REFERENCES

Allen, A. C.: A reorientation on the histogenesis and chemical significance of cutaneous nevi and melanomas. Cancer, 2:28, 1949.

Allen, A. C.: The Skin. St. Louis, Mo., C. V. Mosby Company, 1954.

Allen, A. C., and Spitz, S.: Histogenesis and clinico-pathological correlation of nevi and malignant melanoma. Arch. Dermatol. Syph., 69:150, 1954.

Andrade, R.: Präcanceröse und canceröse Veränderungen von Epidermis und Anhangsgebilden.

In Handbuch der Haut- und Geschlechtskrankheiten. I, 2: 344, Berlin, Springer-Verlag, 1964.

Andrade, R.: Lentigo maligna (Hutchinson's freckle). *In* Demis, J. D., Crounse, R. G., Dobson, R. L., and McGuire, J. (Eds.): Clinical Dermatology, Vol. 2, Unit 11–54. New York, Harper & Row, 1972.

Arma-Szlachcic, M., Ott, F., and Storck, H.: Zur Strahlentherapie der melanotischen Präcancerosen (Studie anhand von 88 nachkontrollierten Fällen). Hautarzt, 21:505, 1970.

Clark, W. H., Jr.; A classification of malignant melanoma in man correlated with histogenesis and biological behavior. *In* Montgomery, W., and Hu, Funan (Eds.): Advances in Biology of the Skin, Vol. 8: The Pigmentary System. New York, Pergamon Press, 1966, pp. 621–647.

Clark, W. H., Jr., and Bretton, R.: A comparative fine structural study of melanogenesis in normal human epidermal melanocytes and in certain human malignant melanoma cells. *In* Helwig, E. B., and Mostofi, F. K. (Eds.): The Skin. Baltimore, The Williams & Wilkins Company, 1971, pp. 197–214.

Clark, W. H., Jr., and Mihm, M. C., Jr.: Lentigo maligna and lentigo maligna melanoma. Am. J. Pathol., 55:39, 1969.

Clark, W. H., Jr., From, L., Bernardino, E., and Mihm, M. C., Jr.: The histogenesis and biologic behavior of primary human malignant melanomas of the skin. Cancer Res., 29:705, 1969.

Cochran, A. J.: Studies of the melanocytes of the epidermis adjacent to tumors. J. Invest. Dermatol., 57:38, 1971.

Conley, J., Lattes, R., and Orr, W.: Desmoplastic malignant melanoma. Cancer, 28:914, 1971.

Costello, M. J., Fisher, S. B., and DeFeo, C. P.: Melanotic freckle (lentigo maligna). Arch. Dermatol., 80:753, 1959.

Degos, R.: La mélanose circonscrite précancéreuse de Dubreuilh. *In* Dermatologie. Paris, Ed. Med. Flammarion. 1953.

Dubreuilh, M. W.: Lentigo malin des vieillards. Bull. Soc. Fr. Dermatol. Syphiligr., August 4, 1894, pp. 460–467.

Dubreuilh, M. W.: De la mélanose circonscrite précancéreuse. Ann. Dermatol. Syphiligr. (Paris), 3:129, 1912.

Duperrat, B.: La mélanose de Dubreuilh. *In* Dermatologie. Paris, Masson & Cie. 1959, pp. 810–812.

Duperrat, B.: Mélanose circonscrite précancéreuse de Dubreuilh – Etude histologique. Ann. Dermatol. Syphiligr. (Paris), 89:319, 1962.

Fitzpatrick, T. B., and Breathnach, A. S.: Das epidermale Melanin-Einheiten-System. Dermatol. Wochenschr., 147:481, 1963.

Friederich, H. C., and Schneider, H. J., Jr.: Ergebnisse der operativen Behandlung der Melanosis circumscripta preblastomatosa Dubreuilh. Vorläufige Mitteilung. Med. Welt., 46:2495, 1966.

Gartmann, H.: Besteht ein histologischer Unterschied zwischen der präblastomatösen Melanose und dem "activated junctional nevus" (Allen)? Hautarzt, 13:507, 1962.

Gladstein, A. H.: Discussion of a case of Hutchinson's freckle treated by the Miescher technique utilizing a Grenz-Ray machine adapted for the purpose. Arch. Dermatol., 103:456, 1971.

Graham, J. H., Johnson, W. C., and Helwig, E. B.: Melanotic freckle of Hutchinson. *In* Dermal Pathology. New York, Harper & Row, 1972, p. 490.

Greer, C. H.: Precancerous melanosis of the conjunctiva. Aust. N. Z. J. Surg., 25:258, 1956.

Grinspan, D., and Abulafia, J.: Lentigo maligna de Hutchinson (melanosis circunscrita precancerosa de Dubreuilh) – Clínica, Histología, Diagnóstico diferencial. Arch. Argent. Dermatol., 6:351, 1956.

Grinspan, D., Abulafia, J., Diaz, J., and Berdichesky, R.: Melanoma of the oral mucosa. A case of infiltrating melanoma originating in a precancerous melanosis. Oral Surg., 28:1, 1969.

Hutchinson, J.: Senile freckle on tissue dotage. Arch. Surg., 3:315, 1892a.

Hutchinson, J.: On senile moles and senile freckles and on their relationship to cancerous processes. Arch. Surg., 2:218, 1892b.

Jackson, R., Williamson, G. S., and Beattie, W. G.: Lentigo maligna and malignant melanoma. Can. Med. Assoc. J., 95:846, 1966.

Jardak, H.: Über das Schicksal der Patienten mit melanotischer Präkanzerose und Melanom, welche in den letzten 20 Jahren an der Städt. Poliklinik für Hautkrankheiten Zürich behandelt wurden. Dermatologica, 139:92, 1969.

Jay, B.: Naevi and melanomata of the conjunctiva. Br. J. Ophthalmol., 49:169, 1965.

Jung, H. D., and Koelzsch, J.: Zur Epidemiologie von Präcancerosen und bösartigen Tumoren der Haut V. Melanosis circumscripta praecancerosa und malignes Melanom. Hautarzt, 19:350, 1968.

Justitz, H.: Melanotische Präcancerose. Dissertation, Zurich, 1935 (quoted by Wayte and Helwig).

Klauder, J. V., and Beerman, H.: Melanotic freckle (Hutchinson), mélanose circonscrite précancéreuse (Dubreuilh). Arch. Dermatol., 71:2, 1955.

Korting, G. W., and Hassenpflug, K. H.: Über das Vorkommen von "Haematoxylin-Körpern" bei einem Naevuszellennaevus und einer Melanosis Dubreuilh Arch. Klin. Exp. Dermatol., 224:81, 1966.

Lupulescu, A., Pinkus, H., Birmingham, D. J., Usndek, H. E., and Posch, J. L.: Lentigo maligna of the fingertip – Clinical histologic and ultrastructural studies of two cases. Arch. Dermatol., 107:717, 1973.

Maillard, G. F.: Etude statistique de 623 mélanomes malins cutanés. Ann. Dermatol. Syphiligr. (Paris), 98:5, 1971.

Malkinson, I. D., and Pearson, R. W.: Editor's note. Year Book of Dermatology. Chicago, Year Book Medical Publishers, 1973, p. 58.

McGovern, V. J.: The classification of melanoma and its relationship with prognosis. Pathology, 2:85, 1970.

McGovern, V. J., and Lane Brown, M. M.: The Nature of Melanoma, Springfield, Ill., Charles C Thomas, Publisher, 1969, Chapter 7. pp. 100–106.

Miescher, G.: Die präcanceröse Stufe des malignen Melanoms: präcanceröse Melanose. *In* Jadassohn, J. (Ed.): Handbuch der Haut- und Geschlechtskrankheiten. XII, 3:1085, Berlin, Springer-Verlag, 1933.

Miescher, G.: Über fleckförmige Alterspigmentierungen. Ihre Beziehungen zur melanotischen Präcancerose und zur senilen Keratose. Arch. Dermatol. Syph. (Berl.), 174:105, 1936.

Miescher, G.: Über melanotische Präcancerose. On-cologia, 7:92, 1954.

Miescher, G.: Morbus Paget der Genitalregion mit Beteiligung von Haut und Schweissdrüsen mit Pigmentierung vom Aussehen der melanotischen Präcancerose. Dermatologica, 114:193, 1957.

Miescher, G.: Die Behandlung der malignen Mela-nome der Haut mit Einschluss der melanotischen Präkanzerose. Strahlentherapie, 46:25, 1960.

Miescher, G., Haeberlin, L., and Guggenheim, L.: Über fleckförmige Alterspigmentierungen. Ihre Beziehungen zur melanotischen Präcancerose und zur senilen Warze. Arch. Dermatol. Syph. (Berl.), 174:105, 1936.

Mihm, M. C., Jr., Clark, W. H., Jr. and From, L.: The clinical diagnosis, classification, and histogen-etic concepts of the early stages of cutaneous malignant melanoma. New Engl. J. Med., 284:1078, 1971.

Mishima, Y.: Melanosis circumscripta praecancerosa (Dubreuilh). A nonnevoid premelanoma distinct from junction nevus. J. Invest. Dermatol., 34:361, 1960.

Mishima, Y.: Macromolecular changes in pigmented disorders. Arch. Dermatol., 91:519, 1965.

Mishima, Y.: Melanotic tumors. In Zelickson, A. S. (Ed.): Ultrastructure of Normal and Abnormal Skin. Philadelphia, Lea & Febiger, 1967, pp. 388–424.

Mishima, Y.: Changes in the current concept of malignant melanoma. In Current Problems in Der-matology, Vol. 3. Basel, S. Karger, 1970, pp. 51–81.

Ollstein, R. N., Kaplan, H. S., Crikelair, G. F., and Lattes, R.: Is there a malignant freckle? Cancer, 19:767, 1966.

Peniche, J.: Personal communication.

Petratos, M. A., Kopf, A. W., Bart, R. S., Grisewood, E. N., and Gladstein, A. H.: Treatment of melano-tic freckle with X-rays. Arch. Dermatol., 106:189, 1972.

Pinkus, H.: The borderline between cancer and non-cancer. In Kopf, A. W., and Andrade, R. (Eds.): Year Book of Dermatology, 1966–67. Chicago, Year Book Medical Publishers, 1967, pp. 5–34.

Pinkus, H., and Gould, S. E.: Extramammary Paget's disease and intraepidermal carcinoma. Arch. Der-matol. 39:479, 1939.

Pinkus, H., and Mishima, Y.: Benign and precan-cerous nonnevoid melanocytic tumors. Ann. N.Y. Acad. Sci., 100:256, 1963.

Reese, A. B.: Precancerous melanosis and the result-ing malignant melanoma (cancerous melanosis) of conjunctiva and skin of lids. Arch. Ophthalmol., 29:737, 1943.

Reese, A. B.: Precancerous and cancerous melanosis of the conjunctiva. Am. J. Ophthalmol., 61:1272, 1966.

Reese, A. B., and Morgan, W. E.: Precancerous and cancerous melanoses of skin and mucous mem-branes. In Cobley, J. (Ed.): Proceedings of the In-ternational Workshop on Cancer of the Head and Neck. Washington, D.C., Butterworth, 1967, pp. 253–256.

Relias, A., and Sakellarion, G.: Mélanoses circon-scrites précancéreuses de Dubreuilh balaniques et préputiales. Ann. Dermatol. Syphiligr. (Paris), 90:45, 1963.

Schuermann, H.: Melanosis circumscripta praecan-cerosa. Arztl. Wochenschr., 10:49, 1955.

Schuermann, H.: Zur Nosologie der melanosis cir-cumscripta praeblastomatosa. Hautarzt, 14:56, 1963.

Steigleder, G. K.: Pseudo-Paget des Scrotums. Me-lanotische Präcancerose unter dem klinischen Bild eines superfiziellen Carcinoms, die histologisch einen Morbus Paget nachahmt. Dermatologica, 117:165, 1958.

Stout, A. P.: The relationship of malignant amelanot-ic melanoma (naevocarcinoma) to extramammary Paget's disease. Am. J. Cancer, 33:196, 1938.

Strauss, G.: Histochemische Untersuchungen bei Pagetscher Erkrankung der Vulva. Z. Krebs-forsch., 61:632, 1957.

Sulzberger, M., Kopf, A. W., and Witten, V. H.: Pig-mented nevi, benign juvenile melanoma and cir-cumscribed precancerous melanosis. Postgrad. Med., 26:617, 1959.

Taki, I., and Janovsky, N. A.: Paget's disease of the vulva: Presentation and histochemical study of four cases. Obstet. Gynecol., 18:385, 1961.

Vilanova, X., and Cardenal, G.: Über einen stachel-zelligen Krebs, der sich auf einer präcancerösen Dubreuilhschen Melanose entwickelte. Arch. Der-matol. Syph. (Berl.), 200:416, 1958.

Wayte, D. M., and Helwig, E. B.: Melanotic freckle of Hutchinson. Cancer, 21:893, 1968.

30

Intraepidermal Epithelioma

Amir H. Mehregan, M.D.

Intraepidermal epithelioma, also called intraepidermal basal cell epithelioma and Borst-Jadassohn epithelioma (Risold, 1961), is a superficial cutaneous neoplasia in which nests of morphobiologic, deviating, epithelial cells are found in the form of well-defined islands within the epidermis.

Borst (1904) described an interesting histologic phenomenon occurring at the border of an ulcerated carcinoma of the lip. Sharply defined nests of anaplastic tumor cells were found within the hyperplastic normal epidermis surrounding the carcinomatous ulcer. Borst used this demonstration as an argument for propagation of carcinoma through multiplication of its own cells and against the widely held opinion that cancer grows by continuous conversion of normal cells into malignant ones. Jadassohn (1926), in a general discussion of superficial basal cell epithelioma 22 years later, called attention to a case in which nests of basaloid tumor cells were present exclusively within the epidermis and were completely surrounded by epidermal cells. Jadassohn called this phenomenon "intraepidermal basal cell epithelioma" and interpreted it as supporting the concept of multicentric origin of these tumors.

Formation of nests of epithelial cells within the epidermis may either occur through invasion of the epidermis from without by a malignant neoplasm or originate within the epidermis of a benign or premalignant tumor. The presence of intraepidermal nests is not an uncommon finding in dermal pathology. Mehregan and Pinkus (1964) found 85 specimens with histopathologic features corresponding to intraepidermal epithelioma in a review of 45,000 skin specimens. They suggested that intraepidermal nests may take their origin from two major sources:

1. From cells of the epidermis or its normal symbionts (see Chapter 4), such as intraepidermal sweat duct unit (acrosyringium), follicular infundibulum (acrotrichium), or melanocytes.

2. From completely foreign strains of cells, usually of malignant nature, that invade the epidermis from below. In Table 30–1 various epithelial tumors which may form intraepidermal nests are listed and classified under three categories: benign primary, malignant primary, and malignant secondary.

703

TABLE 30–1 TUMORS OF THE SKIN WITH INTRAEPIDERMAL NESTS

Benign Primary	Malignant Primary	Malignant Secondary
Seborrheic verruca	Bowen's disease	Epidermotropic carcinomas
Verrucous epidermal nevus	Actinic keratosis	Paget's disease
Hidroacanthoma simplex	Squamous cell carcinoma	Extramammary Paget's disease
Junction nevus	Basal cell epithelioma	
	Malignant melanoma	

In the remainder of this chapter clinical features and histopathologic findings of tumors which may exhibit the phenomenon of intraepidermal nest formation are discussed.

PRIMARY BENIGN EPITHELIAL TUMORS WITH INTRAEPIDERMAL NESTS

Seborrheic Verruca (Seborrheic Keratosis)

The formation of intraepidermal nests in seborrheic verruca can be satisfactorily explained if one considers these superficial neoplasms as a papillomatous epidermal growth exhibiting retarded maturation of epidermal cells. In a typical lesion, the papillomatous epidermis consists mainly of immature cells resembling epidermal basal cells (basal cell papilloma of Lever, 1949). Transition to large and pale-staining prickle cells and to granular cells occurs only in areas near the surface or around the intraepidermal horn cysts. Intraepidermal nests are formed in seborrheic verruca under two circumstances: in association with inflammation and without inflammation.

The histopathology of seborrheic verruca may change when the lesion is irritated following an infection, by accidental injury, or by experimental trauma. The number of basaloid cells is markedly diminished, and prickle cells become more numerous (acanthoma of Williams, 1956). Occasionally, maturation of basaloid cells begins in numerous small foci characterized by formation of squamous eddies, and such lesions may resemble Helwig's (1955) inverted follicular keratosis (Mehregan, 1964). On the other hand, maturation of basaloid cells may take place unevenly, and

while the bulk of tumor consists of large and light-staining prickle cells, isolated islands of basaloid cells persist in various areas. There is usually a gradual transition between the small basaloid cells at the periphery of the intraepidermal nests and the surrounding larger and light-staining prickle cells. Signs of inflammation, such as dilated capillaries and perivascular inflammatory cell infiltrate, are usually present in the underlying dermis.

In the second type of disease, intraepidermal nests occur in flat lesions of seborrheic verruca which occur most commonly over the upper and lower extremities in the form of yellowish brown, well-defined, keratotic growths. In this form of seborrheic verruca, islands and nests of basaloid cells are separated from each other by deepened papillae and by the normal-appearing epithelium of infundibulum and intraepidermal sweat duct units (Fig. 30–1). These nests are more or less sharply defined from the surrounding epidermal cells and are best demonstrated when the tumor cells show melanin pigmentation; they are also associated with proliferation of dendritic melanocytes (Fig. 30–2). It has been demonstrated that activation of these lesions experimentally or following infection will lead to maturation of the basaloid cells and complete disappearance of the tumor islands (Mehregan and Pinkus, 1964; Morales and Hu, 1965).

Hidroacanthoma Simplex

Under this term Smith and Coburn (1956 and 1957) suggested that some of the intraepidermal epitheliomas may be of sweat gland origin. Since the upper part of the eccrine sweat duct actually lives in a symbiotic fashion within the epidermis, one may expect neoplasia of this portion of

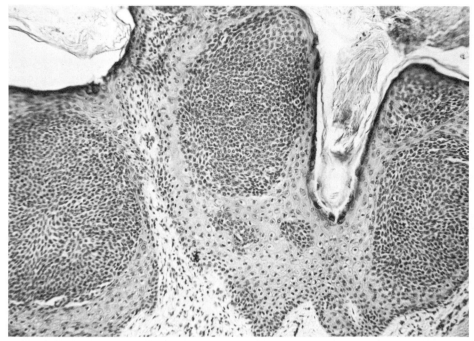

Figure 30-1 Seborrheic verruca with intraepidermal nests. The tumor nests consist of small basaloid cells and are well-differentiated from the surrounding epidermis. *H & E, ×180.*

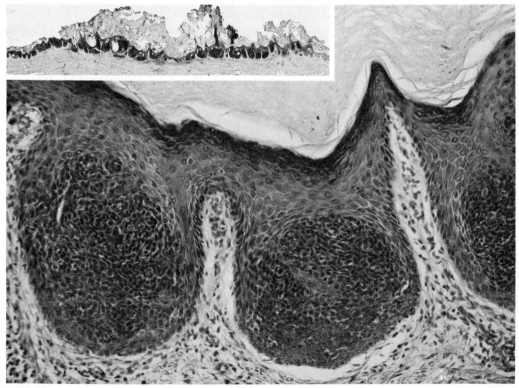

Figure 30-2 Flat type of seborrheic verruca with intraepidermal nests. The tumor nests consist of heavily pigmented basaloid cells and also show proliferation of dendritic melanocytes. *H&E, ×180.*

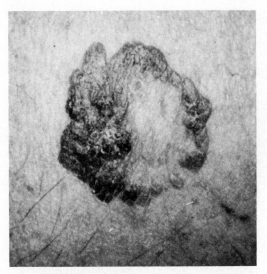

Figure 30–3 Hidroacanthoma simplex. A ring-like keratotic lesion of the thigh. (*From* Mehregan and Levson: Arch. Dermatol., 100:303, 1969.)

sweat duct to form a superficial tumor partially or completely in the confines of the epidermis.

Hidroacanthoma simplex appears in the form of a flat and irregularly keratotic patch, usually singular and located over the extremities (Fig. 30–3). Histologically it is characterized by formation of numerous well-defined islands of tumor cells within an unevenly acanthotic and hyperkeratotic

epidermis (Mehregan and Levson, 1969). The tumor islands consist of small and evenly sized cells and are sharply demarcated from the surrounding epidermis (Fig. 30–4). In areas where tumor islands are exposed to the surface, the tumor cells shrink to form parakeratotic bodies. The PAS reaction shows large amounts of PAS-positive and diastase-digestible material (glycogen) within the tumor islands. In addition to morphologic resemblance of the tumor cells and the presence of glycogen, Holubar (1969) and Holubar and Wolff (1969) have demonstrated similarity of enzyme pattern between hidroacanthoma simplex and eccrine poroma and have considered this neoplasia as an intraepidermal form of eccrine poroma.

Verrucous Epidermal Nevus

On rare occasions nests of immature basaloid cells may be present within the hyperplastic epidermis in verrucous epidermal nevi. A case of this type, reported by Sachs (1952), occurred on the scalp of a 16 year old girl. Similar observation was made by Winer and Levine (1961) in an adult with an organoid nevus (nevus sebaceus) of the scalp in which a basal cell epithelioma was also found in the corium.

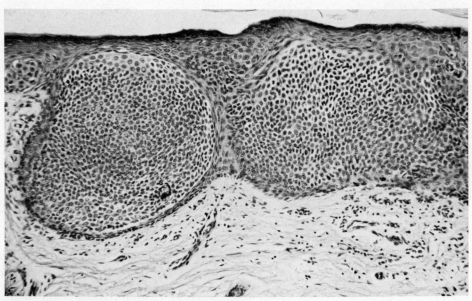

Figure 30–4 Hidroacanthoma simplex. The intraepidermal tumor islands uniformly consist of small cells and are sharply defined from the surrounding epidermis. *H&E, ×135.*

Junction Nevus

Well-defined nests of nevus cells in these nevi are usually located at the dermoepidermal junction and only on rare occasion are found within the epidermis. Pigment formation and other cellular characteristics of nevus cells facilitate differential diagnosis from other neoplasms.

PRIMARY MALIGNANT EPITHELIAL TUMORS WITH INTRAEPIDERMAL NESTS

Bowen's Disease

The anaplastic epithelium in Bowen's precancerous dermatosis is characterized by the presence of cells with irregularly large and hyperchromatic nuclei, atypical mitotic figures, and dyskeratotic cells. The anaplastic epithelium replaces the entire thickness of the epidermis and is usually sharply defined from the normal epidermis at the periphery of the lesion and also from the intraepidermal portion of sweat ducts. The infundibulum of hair follicles, however, may become completely replaced by the anaplastic epithelium (Graham et al., 1961).

Intraepidermal nest formation is not very rare in Bowen's disease and occurs in areas where the epidermis is hyperplastic. In these areas, multiple nests of cells with large and hyperchromatic nuclei are found sharply defined from the surrounding epidermal cells (Fig. 30–5). In rare cases intraepidermal nests of anaplastic epithelium of Bowen's disease consist of large cells with abundant and pale-staining cytoplasm resembling Paget's disease (Fig. 30–6). These lesions can be differentiated from Paget's disease by the presence of intercellular connections between the anaplastic tumor cells and their surrounding epidermal cells and also by negative histochemical findings.

Keratosis Senilis

In rare cases, the light-staining anaplastic epithelium of actinic keratosis forms nests surrounded by the normal epithelium of the follicular infundibulum and the intraepidermal sweat duct units.

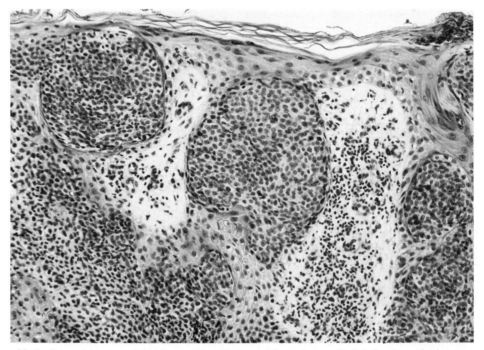

Figure 30–5 Bowen's precancerous dermatosis with intraepidermal nests. Well-defined anaplastic tumor nests consist of cells with irregular and hyperchromatic nuclei. *H & E, ×180.*

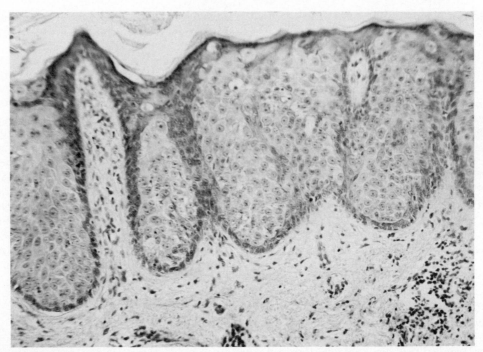

Figure 30–6   Bowen's precancerous dermatosis with nests of large and light-staining cells resembling Paget's disease. *H & E, ×180.*

Squamous Cell Carcinoma

Intraepidermal spread of anaplastic cells at the periphery of an area of ulceration in squamous cell carcinoma is best designated as Borst phenomenon. Individual cells or nests of cells with large and hyperchromatic nuclei are found within the irregularly acanthotic epidermis (Fig. 30–7). The anaplastic tumor cells appear to have intercellular connections between each other and also with the normal-appearing surrounding epidermal cells.

Basal Cell Epithelioma

Jadassohn's epithelioma has been considered a variant of superficial basal cell epithelioma in which proliferation of basalioma cells occurs in the form of well-defined nests within an acanthotic epidermis. Histologic studies of early lesions and of the superficial form of basal cell epithelioma by Zackheim (1963) and by Madsen (1955) suggest that, from the beginning, basal cell epithelioma is a fi-broepithelial growth and is characterized by proliferation of small basalioma cells surrounded by the specific mesodermal stroma. While partial replacement of the infundibular portion of hair follicles or the overlying epidermis by nests of tumor cells may occur, development of completely intraepidermal tumor nests is unlikely. It is most likely that cases described as Jadassohn's intraepidermal epithelioma are examples of either seborrheic verruca with nest formation, Bowen's disease, or hidroacanthoma simplex.

Malignant Melanoma

The type of malignant melanoma which deserves discussion in connection with the other forms of tumors described in this chapter is the so-called superficially spreading variety (Clark and Mihm, 1969). These lesions occur most commonly over the covered portion of the body and appear as flat and irregularly pigmented growths. They are characterized histologically by the occurrence of nests of anaplastic melanoma cells at the dermoepidermal

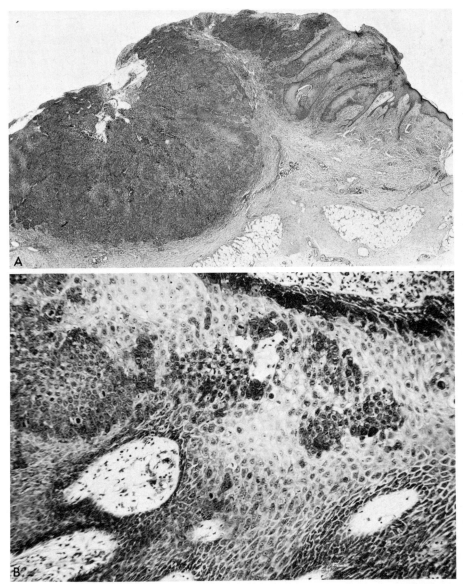

Figure 30–7 *A,* Invasive squamous cell carcinoma with a central area of ulceration surrounded by irregularly acanthotic epidermis. *H&E,* ×*20. B,* Nests of anaplastic tumor cells spreading within the hyperplastic epidermis at the periphery of the ulcer (Borst phenomenon). *H&E,* ×*180.*

junction and also intraepidermally. The tumor nests consist of cells with hyperchromatic nuclei and abundant and light-staining cytoplasm with dustlike pigment granules (Fig. 30–8). Scattered mitotic figures are present, and other signs of activity and malignancy include upward transmigration of tumor cells within the epidermis and the presence of inflammatory reaction in the underlying dermis.

SECONDARY MALIGNANT EPITHELIAL TUMORS WITH INTRAEPIDERMAL NESTS

Epidermotropic Carcinomas

The term "epidermotropic" has been used to specify the propensity of certain strains of tumor cells to invade and to set

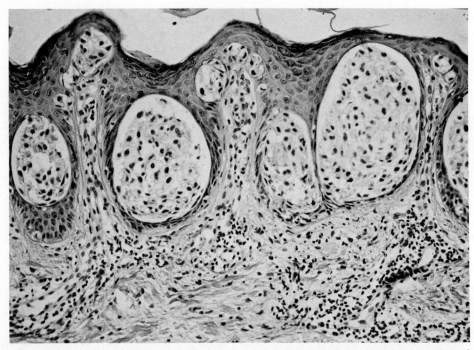

Figure 30–8 Superficially spreading form of malignant melanoma with junctional and intraepidermal nests of melanoma cells. *H & E, ×180.*

up housekeeping within the epidermis (Mehregan, 1970). An outstanding example of this phenomenon was observed in metastatic spread of an eccrine carcinoma of the foot (Pinkus and Mehregan, 1963) (Fig. 30–9). Invasion of the epidermis by nemerous nests of anaplastic tumor cells occurred through involvement of superficial dermal lymphatics, producing a histologic picture resembling Paget's disease of the breast (Paget phenomenon, Pinkus,

1968) (Fig. 30–10). Similar observation was made in a cutaneous metastatic lesion of carcinoma of the bladder (Eversole, 1952). In this case, in addition to the involvement of the corium by solid and cystic tumor masses, numerous nests of anaplastic tumor cells were also found within the overlying epidermis (Fig. 30–11). Involvement of the epidermis is also a feature not uncommonly observed in metastatic carcinoma of breast.

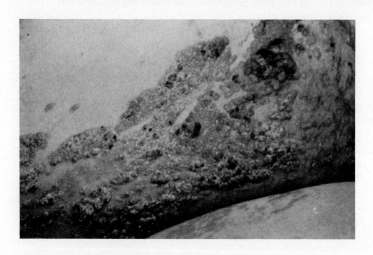

Figure 30–9 Cutaneous metastases of an epidermotropic eccrine carcinoma, forming closely aggregated keratotic nodules on the upper thigh.

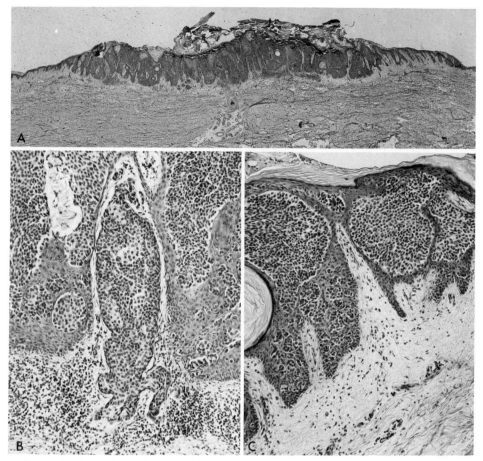

Figure 30–10 *A*, Metastatic epidermotropic eccrine carcinoma, entire nodular lesion. *B*, Extension of the anaplastic tumor nests from the superficial dermal lymphatics into the overlying epidermis. *H&E*, ×90. *C*, Periphery of the lesion shows tumor nests in confine of the hyperplastic epidermis (Paget phenomenon). *H & E*, × 90. (*From* Pinkus and Mehregan: A Guide to Dermatohistopathology, 1969. Courtesy of Appleton-Century-Crofts, Publishing Division of Prentice-Hall, Inc., Englewood Cliffs, N. J.)

Paget's Disease of the Breast

In mammary Paget's disease, the epidermal rete ridges are transformed into bags containing masses of light-staining anaplastic Paget cells (Fig. 30–12). The origin of the Paget cell is still not clear. Whether these cells invade the epidermis from an underlying tumor or develop primarily within the epidermis is debatable.

Extramammary Paget's Disease

Extrammary Paget's disease occurs most commonly over the anogenital area or in skin areas containing apocrine glands. Similar to the situation with mammary lesions, involvement of the epidermis occurs through the presence of numerous nests of light-staining anaplastic cells (Murrell and McMullan, 1962) (Fig. 30–13). The underlying tumor in these cases may be an apocrine carcinoma or carcinoma of the rectum. The tumor cells in extramammary Paget's disease contain varying amounts of acid mucopolysaccharide, which is PAS-positive, diastase-resistant (Helwig and Graham, 1963), and alcian blue and aldehyde fuchsin–reactive, and has the histochemical properties of sialomucin.

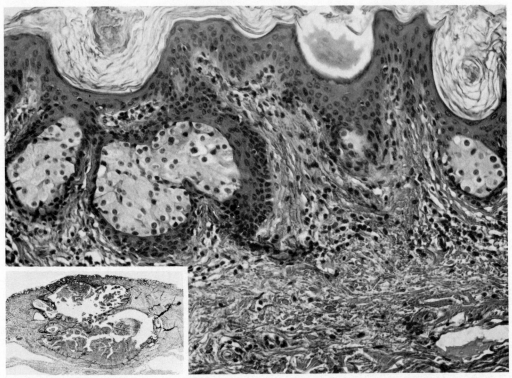

Figure 30–11 Carcinoma of urinary bladder which has metastasized to the skin. In addition to invasion of the corium by solid and cystic tumor masses, nests of anaplastic tumor cells are also present within the overlying epidermis. *H&E, ×180.*

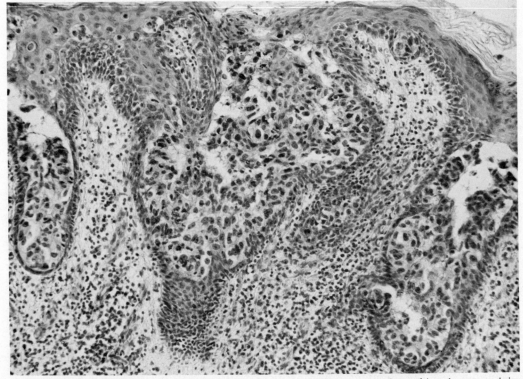

Figure 30–12 Paget's disease of the nipple. The epidermal rete ridges are transformed into bags containing light-staining Paget cells. *H&E, ×180.*

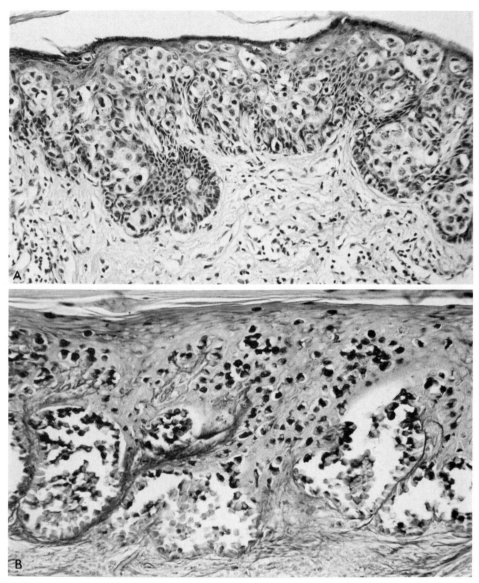

Figure 30–13 Extramammary Paget's disease. *A*, The epidermis is diffusely invaded by small nests and individual tumor cells. *H&E, ×180. B*, The tumor cells contain PAS-positive and alcian blue–reactive material. *Alcian blue–PAS, ×180.*

SUMMARY

It has been suggested that the so-called Borst-Jadassohn epithelioma cannot be considered a distinctive entity. Borst described invasion of the epidermis by tumor cells at the periphery of a carcinomatous ulcer, a feature which may also occur in Bowen's precancerous dermatosis and deserves the designation of Borst phenomenon. Jadassohn assumed multicentric origin of basal cell epithelioma within the epidermis, and neoplasms resembling those he described include seborrheic verruca with nests and hidroacanthoma simplex. Other tumors which form intraepidermal nests include junction nevi, malignant melanoma, epidermotropic carcinomas, and mammary and extramammary forms of Paget's disease.

REFERENCES

Borst, M.: Ueber die Möglichkeit einer ausgedehnten intraepidermalen Verbreitung des Hautkrebses. Verh. Dtsch. Pathol. Ges., 7:118, 1904.

Clark, W. H., Jr., and Mihm, M. C., Jr.: Lentigo maligna and lentigo maligna melanoma. Am. J. Pathol., 55:39, 1969.

Eversole, J. W.: Extra-mammary Paget's disease: Discussion of pathogenesis. South. Med. J., 45:28, 1952.

Graham, J. H., Mazzanti, G. R., and Helwig, E. B.: Chemistry of Bowen's disease: Relationship to arsenic. J. Invest. Dermatol., 37:317, 1961.

Helwig, E. B.: Inverted follicular keratosis. *In* Helwig, E. B.: Seminar on Skin Neoplasms and Dermatoses. Proceedings of the Twentieth Seminar of the American Society of Clinical Pathologists, Sept. 11, 1954. American Society of Clinical Pathologists, 1955, p. 38.

Helwig, E. B., and Graham, J. H.: Anogenital (extramammary) Paget's disease; clinicopathological study. Cancer, 16:387, 1963.

Holubar, K.: Das intraepidermale epitheliom (sog. Borst-Jadassohn): Verkörpert dieser begriff eine entität im histopathologischen sinne oder nich? Z. Haut. Geschlechtskr., 44:391, 1969.

Holubar, K., and Wolff, K.: Intraepidermal eccrine poroma, a histochemical and enzyme-histochemical study. Cancer, 23:626, 1969.

Jadassohn, J.: Demonstration von selteneren Hautepitheliomen. Beitr. Klin. Chir., 136:345, 1926.

Lever, W. F.: Histopathology of the Skin. Ed. 1, Philadelphia, J. B. Lippincott Co., 1949.

Madsen, A.: Histogenesis of superficial basal-cell epitheliomas; unicentric or multicentric origin. A.M.A. Arch. Dermatol., 72:29, 1955.

Mehregan, A. H.: Inverted follicular keratosis. Arch. Dermatol., 89:229, 1964.

Mehregan, A. H.: Transepidermal elimination. *In* Current Problems in Dermatology. Basel, S. Karger, 1970.

Mehregan, A. H., and Levson, D. N.: Hidroacanthoma simplex. A report of two cases. Arch. Dermatol., 100:303, 1969.

Mehregan, A. H., and Pinkus, H.: Intraepidermal epithelioma: A critical study. Cancer, 17:609, 1964.

Morales, A., and Hu, F.: Seborrheic verruca and intraepidermal basal cell epithelioma of Jadassohn. Arch. Dermatol., 91:342, 1965.

Murrell, T. W., Jr., and McMullan, F. H.: Extramammary Paget's disease. A report of two cases. Arch. Dermatol., 85:82, 1962.

Pinkus, H.: Epidermotropism in sweat apparatus tumors. Jap. J. Dermatol., Series B, 78:244, 1968.

Pinkus, H., and Mehregan, A. H.: Epidermotropic eccrine carcinoma; case combining features of eccrine poroma and Paget's dermatosis. Arch. Dermatol., 88:597, 1963.

Risold, J. C.: L'Épithélioma intra-épidermique de "Borst-Jadassohn;" est-il un cancer? M.D. thesis, Faculté de Médecine, Strasbourg, France, 1961. Unpublished. Abstr. in Z. Haut. Geschlechtskr., 110:264, 1961.

Sachs, W.: Intraepidermic nevus. A.M.A. Arch. Dermatol., 65:110, 1952.

Smith, J. L. S., and Coburn, J. G.: Hidroacanthoma simplex; assessment of selected group of intraepidermal basal cell epitheliomata and of their malignant homologues. Br. J. Dermatol., 68:400, 1956.

Smith, J. L. S., and Coburn, J. G.: Hidradenoid vestibuloacanthoma; benign neoplasia of extraapocrine sites. Br. J. Dermatol., 69:197, 1957.

Williams. M. G.: Acanthomata appearing after eczema. Br. J. Dermatol., 68:268, 1956.

Winer, L. H., and Levin, G. H.: Pigmented basal-cell carcinoma in verrucous nevi; report of 2 cases. Arch. Dermatol., 83:960, 1961.

Zackheim, H. S.: Origin of human basal cell epithelioma. J. Invest. Dermatol., 40:283, 1963.

31

Benign Juvenile Melanoma

Clinical Aspects

Alfred W. Kopf, M.D.

Since we have already presented a thorough review of this subject as the leading article of the 1965–66 Series of the Year Book of Dermatology (Kopf and Andrade, 1966), extensive quotations have been used in this chapter. In addition, the literature has been brought up to date to include the newer findings which have been published since this review, and the subject of malignant melanoma in children has been included to contrast with benign juvenile melanoma.

SYNONYMS

Benign juvenile melanoma (Kopf and Andrade, 1966; McWhorter and Woolner, 1954; Steigleder and Wellmer, 1956) has also been called juvenile melanoma (Spitz, 1948); spindle cell and epithelioid cell nevus (Helwig, 1955); spindle cell, epithelioid cell, and round cell juvenile melanoma (Gartmann, 1962); pseudomelanoma (Grupper and Tubiana, 1955); naevus prominens et pigmentosus (Du Bois, 1938); naevus cellulaire prepubertaire (Degos, 1958); and nevus with large cells (Duverne and Pruniéras, 1956b).

DEFINITION

Benign juvenile melanoma is a type of nevus cell nevus (melanocytic nevus, pigmented nevus, mole) which occurs mostly in children. It typically presents as a pink raised nodule on the face but may have a broad spectrum of clinical features and occur on any cutaneous site. The most significant feature of this lesion is its frequent histologic resemblance to malignant melanoma. Despite this similarity microscopically, the lesion, with rare exceptions, is biologically benign in that metastases do not occur. Benign juvenile melanoma, therefore, is one of the so-called "pseudocancers" of the skin which has been resurrected from the malignant melanomas by careful clinicopathologic correlation (Andrade, 1970).

HISTORICAL ASPECTS

Prior to 1948, when Spitz clearly delineated the concept of benign juvenile melanoma, observers had commented on the puzzling features and behavior of tumors considered on histologic grounds to be

715

malignant melanomas in children. The comments and quotations which follow are not meant to be an exhaustive review but rather to represent certain highlights which set the foundation for the final resolution of benign juvenile melanoma as a clinicopathologic entity.

Darier and Civatte (1910) described an 8 month old child who, for two months, had had a red, elevated, rapidly growing lesion situated on the nose. Histologically, it was considered to be a malignant melanoma, and yet the authors stated: ". . . but we must ask if [it will be clinically] benign or malignant." Unfortunately, lack of details in description and of photographic documentation of the histologic features leaves us in doubt as to whether this lesion really was a benign juvenile melanoma.

Miescher (1933) described, under the title "Faszikularer Typus des Pigmentzellennaevus," three lesions which had as their outstanding feature large, sometimes gigantic, spindle cells with large round and oblong nuclei. While these lesions had a strong resemblance to the fascicular type of malignant melanoma, he recognized their benign nature. Unfortunately, little clinical data are presented (although one lesion had angiomatous features), and the drawings of the microscopic morphology do not permit acceptance of these lesions as indubitable benign juvenile melanoma.

Du Bois (1938) presented a clinical photograph under the title of "naevus prominens et pigmentosus." The accompanying photomicrographs strongly suggested that this lesion was a benign juvenile melanoma.

In 1939, Pack and Anglem reviewed 483 lesions histologically diagnosed as malignant melanomas and found that only 12 (2.7 percent) had occurred in patients under 16 years of age. They stated: "Although malignant melanomas are found in infancy and childhood they are of low-grade malignancy and seldom metastasize. Under the microscope these tumors may be indistinguishable from other melanomas occurring in adult life which exhibit a high degree of malignancy."

Woringer (1939) described an 8 year old girl who had on her hand a slightly elevated, pea-sized, rose-colored growth of a few months' duration. Histologic examination of this tumor revealed a nevus cell nevus with certain unusual features, including a few large theques, numerous dilated capillaries, a lymphocytic infiltrate, and a peculiar morphology of the nevus cells. The latter, which included cells of both round and fusiform types, were larger than usual nevus cells, and some showed certain nuclear monstrosities. Because of the relatively few mitoses, the author suspected that the lesion was benign. He suggested that it could represent a nevus cell nevus being formed in a burst of growth which gave it an unusual picture resembling malignant melanoma.

In 1944, Webster and coworkers remarked: "There are certain lesions, usually of a pinkish-fawn color, noted in children, giving the histologic appearance of malignant melanomas which, in our experience, rarely metastasize."

Pack et al. (1947) reported on 862 patients in whom the histologic diagnosis of malignant melanoma had been made. Of these, 15 were prepubertal, and of them they wrote:

Although the microscopic appearance of these pigmented tumors is so identical with their cogeners of adult life that pathologists cannot distinguish between them, their behavior is not in keeping with their anatomic structure. None of these melanomas metastasized and all the patients have survived indefinitely. Inasmuch as the behavior of this tumor is so benign and the prognosis is so good, it would be well to classify it separately as prepubertal melanoma.

Again, in 1948, Pack stated:

There is one important type of pigmented nevus which bears such close resemblance to malignant melanoma that it is not possible, clinically, to distinguish the two. This nevus is found in children from the ages of 1 to the time of puberty. When this tumor is excised. . . and submitted to pathologists for diagnosis, they are frequently unable to state whether the neoplasm is benign or malignant, inasmuch as the histologic criteria—are practically identical with the malignant variety of melanomas as encountered in adults. Our experience . . . has been that none of these melanotic tumors of infancy and childhood has metastasized to regional lymph nodes, although many of them have been labeled as malignant melanoma by extremely competent pathologists. We might adopt such a term as prepubertal melanoma to indicate the group of tumors which resemble malignant melanoma histologically but do not behave as such.

Ackerman (1948), considering lesions of the type in point, remarked: "malignant changes may appear to develop in a prepubertal child but these changes, in this age group, are usually not clinically significant."

According to Gartmann (1962), other case reports were also probably benign juvenile melanomas rather than malignant melanomas (Bieberstein, 1925; Carol, 1931; Milian et al., 1932).

The largest series of benign juvenile melanomas published to date include the following: 308 cases, Allen (1963); 91 cases (26 adults), Echevarria and Ackerman (1967); 67 cases, Gartmann (1962); 50 cases, Jakubowicz (1965); 48 cases, Andrade (1968); 40 cases, Duperrat and Dufourmentel (1959); 40 cases, Kopf and Andrade (1966).

EPIDEMIOLOGY

Benign juvenile melanomas have been reported from all over the world and in many races. Epidemiologic factors do not seem to play a role in the development of such lesions.

ETIOLOGIC FACTORS

As with other nevus cell nevi, there are no known etiologic factors. It is generally accepted that such lesions belong to the broad group of *nevoid* tumors (i.e., con-

genitally determined, circumscribed, benign neoplasms of the skin). Hereditary factors do not play a significant role in such lesions, although a few familial cases have been published (Kopf and Andrade, 1966).

At times benign juvenile melanomas arise in giant nevus cell nevi (so-called bathing trunk nevi). In this clinical setting, the differential diagnosis between malignant melanoma and benign juvenile melanoma can pose a difficult problem, since the former occurs relatively frequently (see Clinical Differential Diagnosis) and requires an aggressive surgical approach, whereas the latter is treated conservatively. As with all nevus cell nevi, the problem of trauma in relation to malignant transformation must be considered. Currently, the weight of evidence seems to indicate that trauma is probably not a major factor in such transformation (Kopf, 1962).

INCIDENCE

The prevalence of benign juvenile melanoma in the general population is unknown. Stegmaier and Montgomery (1953) examined histologically 100 selected pigmented nevi excised from children 1 to 10 years of age. In only one instance were there features of benign juvenile melanoma. Clearly this type of study would have to be considerably expanded to assess the true prevalence of this type of lesion. More information is available concerning the prevalence of benign juvenile melanoma among surgical specimens. It should be pointed out, however, that lesions are removed in children usually for

TABLE 31–1 INCIDENCE OF BENIGN JUVENILE MELANOMAS IN SEVERAL SERIES OF SURGICALLY REMOVED AND HISTOLOGICALLY EXAMINED LESIONS CLINICALLY DIAGNOSED AS NEVUS CELL NEVI IN CHILDREN

Authors	Number of Nevi Examined	Benign Juvenile Melanoma	
		Number	*Per Cent*
Stegmaier and Montgomery (1953)	100	1	1
Schumachers-Brendler (1963)	1600	24	1.5
Kernen and Ackerman (1960)	2600	27	1
McWhorter and Woolner (1954)	156	11	7
Spitz (1948)	100	8	8
Total:	4556	71	1.6

such specific reasons as unusual growth, bleeding, peculiar clinical features, mistaken diagnosis, or cosmetic purposes. Thus this type of material is obviously select. Table 31–1 presents a summary of some of the published series of this sort and indicates that 1 to 8 percent of all nevus cell nevi in this age group, removed surgically and subjected to histologic examination, are benign juvenile melanomas.

It is evident that in children benign juvenile melanoma occurs much more frequently than does malignant melanoma. For example, Allen (1963) has seen 308 benign juvenile melanomas in all age groups (19 percent in adolescents and adults) compared with 29 malignant melanomas in children. Kernan and Ackerman (1960) saw 27 benign juvenile melanomas but not a single prepubertal malignant melanoma in their series. Only one of the 13 cases reviewed by Spitz (1948) was considered a malignant melanoma. Woringer (1956) reviewed seven lesions previously diagnosed as malignant melanoma in children and found that six were benign juvenile melanomas. McWhorter and Woolner (1954) reviewed the world's literature to 1954 and found only 18 cases acceptable by their criteria as malignant melanoma in children. This emphasizes the extreme rarity of this tumor in this age group. In contrast, they were able to find 11 cases of benign juvenile melanoma in their own material alone.

The conclusion is that benign juvenile melanoma is an uncommon lesion compared with other types of nevus cell nevi, which occur with tremendous frequency. However, in comparison with malignant melanoma in childhood, benign juvenile melanoma is encountered much more frequently. The precise incidence will not be known, however, until more careful studies are conducted.

CLINICAL DESCRIPTION

Most nevus cell nevi have as a component of their clinical character various shades of tan, brown, blue, or black. Be-

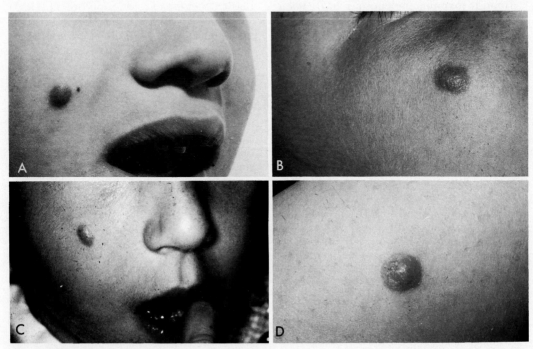

Figure 31–1 Examples of typical benign juvenile melanomas in children. Clinically all lesions were pink raised nodules.(*A* and *B from* Benign Juvenile Melanoma by Kopf, Alfred W., and Andrade, Rafael, *In* 1965–66 Year Book of Dermatology by Kopf, A. W., and Andrade, R. (Eds.). Copyright © 1966 by Year Book Medical Publishers, Inc., Chicago. Used by permission.)

nign juvenile melanoma is often an exception to this rule, since such shades of color are usually but not always absent. Instead, the most common clinical appearance which the benign juvenile melanoma presents is that of a smooth-surfaced or slightly scaly, raised, round or oval, moderately firm to rubbery hard, nonhairy, pink or purplish red asymptomatic nodule (Fig. 31–1). A clinical feature, insufficiently stressed in the literature, is overlying telangiectasia together with a certain grayish or pearly translucency on diascopy, at times even suggestive of basal cell epithelioma. In general, the lesion tends to be somewhat larger and more elevated than ordinary nevus cell nevi in children. Such are the gross features that permit the clinical diagnosis of benign juvenile melanoma. Because of the lack of discernible pigment, cursory inspection usually suggests such diagnoses as keloid, juvenile xanthogranuloma, a solitary nodule of urticaria pigmentosa, or a granuloma. However, once aware of the features of benign juvenile melanoma, this diagnosis can be entertained in many typical cases. Indeed, it was considered in 15 of our 43 lesions (Kopf and Andrade, 1966).

Although the tumors are generally asymptomatic, they may be attended by such symptoms as bleeding, pruritus, and tenderness.

Although the pink nodule noted above is the most common clinical form, many other clinical types have been described. Thus macular, polypoid, and verrucoid surfaces, tan to dark brown or black colors, multiple lesions, and hairiness are characteristics of some benign juvenile melanomas. If we add artifacts of traumatic erosion or ulceration leading to crusting and secondary infection, further diagnostic pitfalls are compounded. Table 31–2 summarizes the clinical features of the 43 lesions reported in our series.

Duperrat and Dufourmentel (1959) delineated four clinical types of benign juvenile melanoma:

1. The *light-colored and elastic form* is a pink or chamois-colored, elastic, sometimes soft, smooth elevation which flattens almost completely under the pressure of a diascope (Fig. 31–1).

2. The *light-colored and hard form* resembles a small cutaneous nodule (histiocytoma) or keloid (Fig. 31–2). The presence of a halo of fine telangiectatic vessels is not uncommon. Probably in this group

TABLE 31–2 CLINICAL FEATURES OF 43 BENIGN JUVENILE MELANOMAS*

Shape:			Consistency:	
Dome-shaped	13		Firm	20
Sessile	4		Soft	5
Polypoid	3			
Pedunculated	2		Hair:	
			Absent	15
Surface:			Present	1
Smooth	16			
Scaly	8			
Verrucous	4		Other Features:	
Crusted	2		Telangiectases	9
Eroded	1		Translucent	4
Mamillated	1			
			Symptoms:	
Color:			Asymptomatic	11
Red	14		Pruritus	6
Pink	14		Bleeding	5
Mottled brown	12		Tenderness	3
Brown	7			
Black	3			

*Data were obtained from reviewing the patients' records and are incomplete since not all had complete descriptions. Often multiple features were described, e.g., "pink color with superimposed mottled brown spots." (*From* Benign Juvenile Melanoma by Kopf, Alfred W., and Andrade, Rafael, *In* 1965–66 Year Book of Dermatology by Kopf, A. W., and Andrade, R. (Eds.). Copyright © 1966 by Year Book Medical Publishers, Inc., Chicago. Used by permission.)

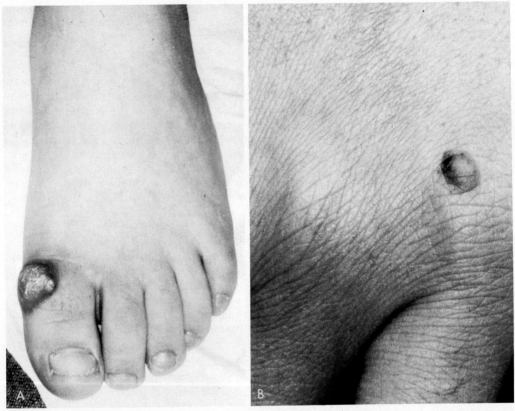

Figure 31-2   Benign juvenile melanomas resembling cutaneous nodules ("light colored and hard" form of Duperrat and Dufourmentel). (*B from* Benign Juvenile Melanoma by Kopf, Alfred W., and Andrade, Rafael, *In* 1965–66 Year Book of Dematology by Kopf, A. W., and Andrade, R. (Eds.). Copyright © 1966 by Year Book Medical Publishers, Inc., Chicago. Used by permission.)

belongs the type which was called "compact" juvenile melanoma by Schumackers-Brendler (1963).

3. The *dark form* is more variable. Many benign juvenile melanomas are not even as dark as a café au lait spot. Others are deeply pigmented and present a transition in clinical morphology to nevus cell nevi. Their surfaces are hairless, smooth, sometimes scaly, and, exceptionally, crusted. Pigmented lesions have been reported by Spitz (1948), Kernen and Ackerman (1960), Gartmann (1962), and others. Three of our 43 lesions were of this type. One of these presented as a raised brown nodule encircled by a pigmented halo (Fig. 31–3*A*).

4. The *multiple and agminated form* is a very special type. Its evolution is as follows: the patient is born with what appears to be a café au lait spot. During the early years of life, multiple, red-brown nodules appear on the surface of the tan

patch. These nodules have the histologic features of benign juvenile melanoma. We have seen two such cases (Fig. 31–4*A*). Others have been reported by Traub (1949) and Grupper and Tubiana (1955). Possibly the lesions of patients described by Cahalane and Meenan (1969), Doepfmer (1960), Jakubowicz (1965), and Winkelmann (1961, Case 2) also should be included here. We have seen several examples of *multinodular* benign juvenile melanomas not associated with café au lait spots (Fig. 31–4*B*).

Because of their experience with the multiple and agminated form of benign juvenile melanoma, Duperrat and Dufourmentel (1959) queried the parents of their other patients with benign juvenile melanomas and found that mothers often recalled that a small freckle or lentigo preceded the onset of the nodular lesion of benign juvenile melanoma. Oddoze (1959) reported another patient in whom

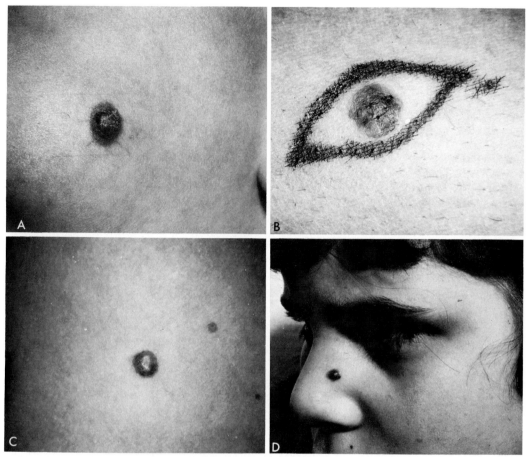

Figure 31–3 Pigmented benign juvenile melanomas. *A,* Central raised nodule surrounded by pigmented halo. *B,* Mottled tan to dark brown. *C,* Dark brown. *D,* Black. (*A from* Benign Juvenile Melanoma by Kopf, Alfred W., and Andrade, Rafael, *In* 1965–66 Year Book of Dermatology by Kopf, A. W., and Andrade, R. (Eds.). Copyright © 1966 by Year Book Medical Publishers, Inc., Chicago. Used by permission.)

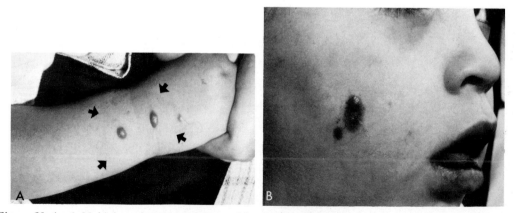

Figure 31–4 *A,* Multiple and agminated form of benign juvenile melanoma. Lesion began as a congenital macular café au lait spot upon which multiple pink nodules arose. Arrows indicate outline of light tan macule. *B,* Multinodular benign juvenile melanoma. No café au lait spot noted. (From Benign Juvenile Melanoma by Kopf, Alfred W., and Andrade, Rafael, *In* 1965–66 Year Book of Dermatology by Kopf, A. W., and Andrade, R. (Eds.). Copyright © 1966 by Year Book Medical Publishers, Inc., Chicago. Used by permission.)

a lentigo was associated with a benign juvenile melanoma.

A unique benign juvenile melanoma presenting 25 tumor nodules superimposed on an area of depigmentation has been described under the name "melanoma juvenile leucodermicum multiplex" (Korting et al., 1968).

Finally, there are still other unusual clinical types of benign juvenile melanoma. One variety closely resembles an angioma or granuloma telangiectaticum (Fig. 31–5). Some have occurred as part of bathing trunk nevi (Kernen and Ackerman, 1960; Greeley et al., 1965; McWhorter and Woolner, 1954; Pack and Davis, 1961; Reed et al., 1965). In one of the four cases of benign juvenile melanoma reported by Kawamura et al. (1962), the lesion was surrounded by a halo of hypopigmentation, resulting in the picture of leukoderma acquisitum centrifugum. Kopf et al. (1965) found some histologic features suggestive of benign juvenile melanoma in one of the cases of halo nevus in their series. Rarely have patients with multiple benign juvenile melanomas been reported. This has occurred in the multiple and agminated form and in the bathing trunk type of nevus cell nevus. Even less common are instances of multiple lesions arising on seemingly normal skin (Groothuis, 1959; Jakubowicz, 1965). We have seen multiple benign juvenile melanomas in dispersed locations on the skin in identical twins (Fig. 31–6).

It is evident from our own experience and from a review of the literature that in the past most benign juvenile melanomas have not been correctly diagnosed by clinicians. However, since the typical features of the more common types have become well known, the diagnosis of this tumor is being made correctly more often.

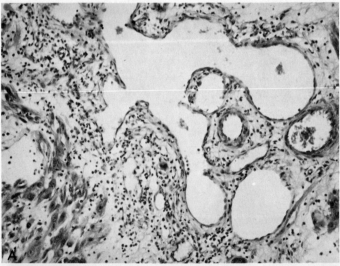

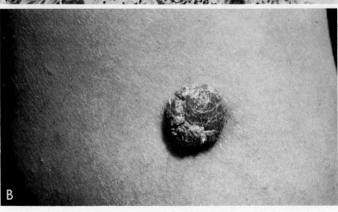

Figure 31–5 Granuloma telangiectaticum type of benign juvenile melanoma. *A,* Marked vascular ectasia associated with typical fusiform tumor cells in lower left portion of photomicrograph. *B,* Clinically this lesion was a bright red, spongy, vascular tumor. (From Benign Juvenile Melanoma by Kopf, Alfred W., and Andrade, Rafael, *In* 1965–66 Year Book of Dermatology by Kopf, A. W., and Andrade, R. (Eds.). Copyright © 1966 by Year Book Medical Publishers, Inc., Chicago. Used by permission.)

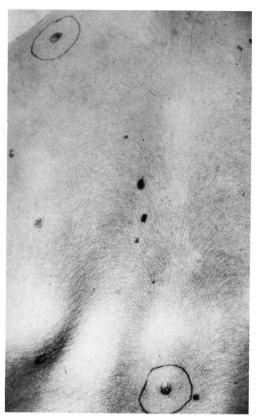

Figure 31–6 Multiple benign juvenile melanomas in 10 year old twin boy. Histologically the two encircled lesions were benign juvenile melanomas. His twin brother also had multiple benign juvenile melanoma. (From Benign Juvenile Melanoma by Kopf, Alfred W., and Andrade, Rafael, *In* 1965–66 Year Book of Dermatology by Kopf, A. W., and Andrade, R. (Eds.). Copyright © 1966 by Year Book Medical Publishers, Inc., Chicago. Used by permission.)

This is especially true for the usual form, *the raised, smooth-surfaced, pink facial nodule in a child.* To add to our clinical diagnostic problems, one of our patients had a classic pink, smooth-surfaced, nodular benign juvenile melanoma on the cheek. Four months later the clinical appearance had changed entirely to a mottled, tan to dark brown mass double the original size. The clinical features now were those of a typical pigmented nevus cell nevus of the ordinary type. Yet, the histologic appearance was that of benign juvenile melanoma.

In 1968 Andrade summarized our experience with benign juvenile melanomas. Briefly these are the findings: 51 lesions in 48 patients; average age at consulta-

tion, 10.3 years (range: 1 to 45 years); females, 27—males, 21; all Caucasians; average largest diameter, 7.3 mm. (range: 2 to 19 mm.); duration: ranged from two months to 22 years—37 in range two months to four years (average 11.1 months)—four present since birth—seven unknown duration; distribution: 19 face, 2 neck, 10 upper and 10 lower extremities, 9 back, 1 buttock; follow-up range, three months to 11 years (average three years). There were no serious sequelae or metastases in any of these patients.

Special mention should be made of benign juvenile melanomas in adults (Fig. 31–7). Echevarria and Ackerman (1967) reviewed the literature and added 26 cases of their own. In their experience almost 29 percent (26 of 91 benign juvenile melanomas) occurred in persons over 20 years of age. About half of these were in the third decade of life. The oldest patient was age 65. Clinically, the lesions tended to be dome-shaped and slowly enlarging, located on the face or extremities (Fig. 31–8), smaller than 1.5 cm., and more pigmented than those seen in the first two decades of life. Benign juvenile melanomas in adulthood arose de novo or were present since childhood and then enlarged and showed increased pigmentation. None spontaneously ulcerated. Local recurrences following inadequate excision were seen, but this did not imply malignancy. No lesions metastasized.

A few cases have been published of benign juvenile melanomas on noncutaneous sites: conjunctival (Gartmann and Thurm, 1960; Gartmann, 1962), uveal (Ellsworth, 1960), iridal (Samuels, 1963), and lingual (Jernstrom and Aponte, 1956). However, Allen (1963) stated that "none of the personally reviewed lesions has been on mucous membranes." Thus careful review of such lesions and further experience will be necessary before noncutaneous benign juvenile melanomas are accepted.

CLINICAL DIFFERENTIAL DIAGNOSIS

The principal points in the clinical differential diagnosis are presented in Table

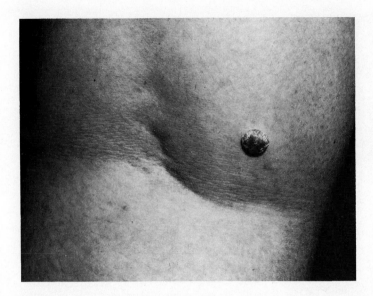

Figure 31–7   Benign juvenile melanoma of the popliteal area in a 45 year old woman.

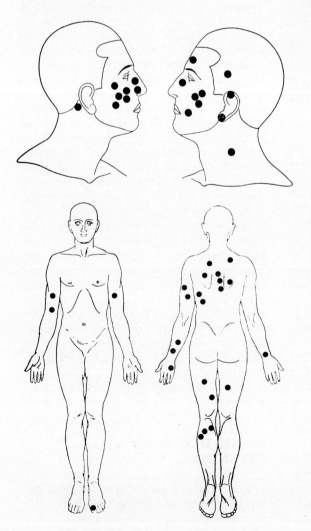

Figure 31–8   Anatomic sites of the 43 benign juvenile melanomas included in this report. (From Benign Juvenile Melanoma by Kopf, Alfred W., and Andrade, Rafael, *In* 1965–66 Year Book of Dermatology by Kopf, A. W., and Andrade, R. (Eds.). Copyright © 1966 by Year Book Medical Publishers, Inc., Chicago. Used by permission.)

TABLE 31–3 CLINICAL DIFFERENTIAL DIAGNOSIS OF BENIGN JUVENILE MELANOMA

	Nevus Cell Nevus	Benign Juvenile Melanoma	Malignant Melanoma
Age at Onset	first two decades of life	usually before puberty	after puberty
Location			
Head	44 to 64%*	40%**	28 to 31%*
Trunk	24 to 34%	20%	25 to 31%
Upper extremity	7 to 12%	20%	10 to 18%
Lower extremity	9 to 12%	20%	25 to 33%
Clinical Features			
Color	tan to black; some skin color	more than half are pink; rest tan to black	black, brown, tan (rarely amelanotic)
Surface	intact; variable smooth, verrucous, mamillated, etc.	intact; usually smooth, but can be verrucoid or polypoid	eroded or ulcerated; crusted, irregular, oozing
Inflammation	none	none	present
Pigment spread at periphery	none	none	present
Excess hair	may be present	rarely present	rarely present
Symptoms	usually none	usually none	pruritus, burning, stinging, bleeding, pain
Growth rate	relatively slow	usually slow, but may be fast	usually fast
Size	very variable; usually few mm. to few cm.; rarely giant	average about 1 cm.; may be few mm. to several cm.	usually over 0.5 cm.
Variants	very numerous sizes and shapes:† flat, slightly elevated, domed, verrucoid, polypoid, sessile, pedunculated	four forms: light-colored and elastic, light-colored and hard, dark, multiple and agminated	three principal forms:‡ lentigo maligna, superficial spreading, nodular
Changeability	slowly change over years	usually slowly change, but may show rapid change	usually shows rapid change
Satellitosis	no	no	yes
Multiplicity	numerous, fewer in early and late life§	usually single	usually single primary but may give rise to multiple nodules
Malignant Transformation	rare, but malignant melanoma is preceded by a "mole" in 25 to 50%	rare, but has been reported; very debatable subject; apparently none in a typical lesion before puberty (see p. 728)	
Metastasis	none	none	occurs frequently

*Szabó (1959)
**Andrade (1968)
†Shaffer (1957)
‡Clark et al. (1969)
§Stegmaier (1959)

31–3. The typical benign juvenile melanoma presents as an elevated pink nodule on the cheek of a child. Because of its usual lack of pigment (melanin), the possibility of a nevus cell nevus often does not occur to the inexperienced examiner. Instead, the diagnoses which might come to mind are keloid, angiofibroma, juvenile xanthogranuloma, cutaneous nodule, lymphocytoma cutis, adnexal tumors, or urticaria pigmentosa (especially the solitary nodular type). Often the correct diagnosis of benign juvenile melanoma is missed, as indicated by the correct clinical diagnosis reported in several large series: Kernen and Ackerman (1960), none of 27 lesions; Gartmann (1962), 18 of 67 lesions; Schumachers-Brendler (1963), 8 of 24 lesions; Jakubowicz (1965), 21 of 50 lesions; Kopf and Andrade (1966), 15 of 43 lesions. In addition to the above mentioned clinical diagnoses, others to be considered in the differential diagnosis are nevus cell nevus (especially if the benign juvenile melanoma is pigmented), cholin-esterase nevus (Winkelmann, 1960), gran-ulomas (e.g., insect bite), granuloma pyogenicum, hemangioma, fibroma, neurofibroma, facial granuloma, xanth-oma, eosinophilic granuloma, granular cell myoblastoma, and malignant melan-oma.

The clinicopathologic diagnosis of ma-lignant melanoma in children is of great importance because the outlook is poor. In addition to the spectrum of clinical fea-tures of adult malignant melanoma (see Chapter 42), several special clinical situa-tions exist in prepubertal malignant mel-anoma. The first is the neurocutaneous syndrome in which are combined central nervous system melanosis and large nevus cell nevi of the skin (Battin et al., 1968; Fox et al., 1964; Dailly et al., 1965). This syndrome has been included among the phakomatoses, i.e., those congenitally de-termined benign neoplasms which involve the central nervous system, skin, and/or eyes (Touraine, 1949; Van der Hoeve, 1923). In this clinical setting, malignant transformation of melanocytes can occur in the central nervous system. This is manifested by progressive enlargement of foci of tumor cells, leading to hydroce-phalus, convulsions, paralysis, and eventu-ally death of the child (Battin et al., 1968; Hoffman and Freeman, 1967; Reed et al., 1965; Touraine, 1949).

The second special clinical variant of malignant melanoma of childhood is its occurrence in *bathing trunk nevi*, i.e., giant nevus cell nevi (Bandiera, 1967; Fuste and Morales, 1944; Fish et al., 1966; Gross and Carter, 1967; Lerman et al., 1970; Lorétan and Delacrétaz, 1967; Schultz, 1961; Shaw, 1962). The prevalence of malignant transformation in these large pigmented nevi is reported to vary from 2 to 31 percent [10 percent of 56 patients, Greely and Curtin, 1966; 1.8 percent of 110 patients, Pers, 1963; 10 percent of 40 patients, Conway, 1939; 31 percent of 55 personal cases, Reed et al., 1965; 13 per-cent of 53 patients, Russell and Reyes, 1959; 17.5 percent of 57 patients, Pack and Davis, 1961; 19.5 percent of 200 cases, Reed et al., 1965 (review)]. Those reports which suggest higher rates of ma-lignant transformation are based on liter-ature reviews which probably are biased samples, since there is much greater ten-dency to report those patients who have unusual courses. What is needed is a Cen-tral Registry of all cases of giant nevus cell nevi and good follow-up of such patients over many years to collect sufficient data for analysis. Until such time, there is a dis-tinct impression that the chance of malig-nant melanoma occurring in bathing trunk nevi is significantly greater in child-hood than in the general population.

A third clinical setting in which malig-nant melanoma can supervene in child-hood is *xeroderma pigmentosum* (McGovern and Goulston, 1963). In this recessively inherited condition, skin cancers of sev-eral types including malignant melanomas arise following sun exposure. A major breakthrough in understanding the patho-mechanism of this disease is the discov-ery by Cleaver (1968) that such patients have a defective DNA repair mechanism following ultraviolet light exposure.

A final unique type of malignant melan-oma in children is *transplacental metastases*. These primary malignant melanomas oc-curred in the pregnant mother and gave rise to metastases via the placenta to the child (Brodsky et al., 1965; Cavell, 1963; Dargeon et al., 1950; Freedman and Mc-Mahon, 1960; Holland, 1949; Weber et al., 1930). In a review of the world's litera-ture on this subject, Potter and Schoene-man (1970) reported 24 cases of metas-tasis of maternal cancer to the placenta; in 11 of these 24, the tumor was malignant melanoma. Of the eight cases in which transplacental metastasis to the fetus oc-curred, seven involved malignant melan-oma.

TREATMENT

It should once again be stressed that be-nign juvenile melanomas, like other nevus cell nevi, are localized growths which only rarely give rise to malignant melanoma. Certainly there is no justification for the radical surgical and radiation therapy which has been used for some benign ju-venile melanomas in the past (Allen, 1963; Duperrat, 1955; Echevarria and

Ackerman, 1967; Grupper and Tubiana, 1955; Kernen and Ackerman, 1960; Mc-Whorter et al., 1954; Saksela and Rintala, 1968). On the other hand, since the natural history and spontaneous course of benign juvenile melanoma is unknown, complete surgical excision conservatively performed is the treatment of choice. The surgical specimen should always be submitted for histologic examination by an experienced pathologist. In general, this method is preferred over the usual scalpel-shave technique so frequently used in the dermatologic treatment of nevus cell nevi.

Andrade (1968) summarized the treatment used for our 48 cases (51 lesions): conservative excision, 36 lesions, two of which recurred and were re-excised; shave biopsy and electrodesiccation, eight lesions, two of which recurred and were re-excised; no treatment after partial removal for biopsy, two lesions. No metastases occurred in these patients.

PROGNOSIS

The long-term spontaneous course of benign juvenile melanomas is unknown (Fig. 31–9). There are no reports of long-term follow-up of untreated lesions following incisional biopsy for verification of the diagnosis. However, one possible course is suggested by Woringer (1963), who reported on a 10 year old girl with a pea-sized rosy lesion on the left side of her face. The tumor was clinically diagnosed as benign juvenile melanoma, and avoidance of therapy was advised. After three years, during which time the lesion remained stationary, it flattened, leaving only a red spot. We had a similar case in which a clinically typical benign juvenile melanoma on the malar area of a 12 year old boy disappeared spontaneously in a four-month period. Of added interest is that this patient had a histologically proved benign juvenile melanoma removed from his left deltoid area.

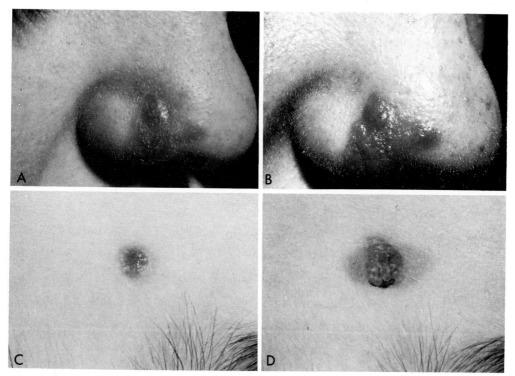

Figure 31–9   Course of untreated benign juvenile melanoma. *A,* Lesion on the ala nasi of a 16 year old girl. *B,* Five months later lesion shows considerable enlargement. *C,* Granuloma telangiectaticum type of benign juvenile melanoma in a 6 year old boy. *D,* Eight months later lesion is a markedly vascular, pedunculated mass. (*A* and *B from* Benign Juvenile Melanoma by Kopf, Alfred W., and Andrade, Rafael, *In* 1965–66 Year Book of Dermatology by Kopf, A. W., and Andrade, R. (Eds.). Copyright © 1966 by Year Book Medical Publishers, Inc., Chicago. Used by permission.)

Since benign juvenile melanomas are found predominantly in the first two decades of life, one wonders what happens to them thereafter. Several possible courses have been suggested. First, they may remain unchanged into adulthood. This might account for the reports of benign juvenile melanoma in later decades of life. About 15 percent to 30 percent occur in adolescents and adults (Allen, 1963; Echevarria and Ackerman, 1967). Secondly, they may undergo involution (Stegmaier, 1959) just as do other nevus cell nevi by processes of fibrosis, pedunculation, lipidization (e.g., balloon cell nevus, Hornstein, 1966), vacuolization (Andrade, 1968), and depigmentation followed by disappearance, as in the phenomenon of leukoderma acquisitum centrifugum (Kopf et al., 1965). Thirdly, the benign juvenile melanoma may transform into an ordinary intradermal nevus. This latter probability is supported by the observations of several authors, in which combinations of nevus cells of the benign juvenile melanoma type and ordinary nevus cells were demonstrated histologically (McWhorter and Woolner, 1954; Herzberg, 1956). These findings could be interpreted to indicate evidence for "maturation" on the histologic level. However, Kernen and Ackerman (1960) reasoned that, if benign juvenile melanomas tend to transform into ordinary nevus cell nevi in adults, then the adult lesions should show evidence of "maturation" more frequently than do the lesions in children. Since they did not find this to be the case, they felt that they could produce no evidence to support the hypothesis that such transformation occurs with age. Finally, these lesions may in rare instances give rise to malignant melanomas, as suggested by the histologic finding of remnants of benign juvenile melanoma features at the peripheral portions of some malignant melanomas (Allen and Spitz, 1953).

Much consideration has been given to the nature of benign juvenile melanoma. Several authors have raised the possibility that these lesions are in fact malignant melanomas and that these children are endowed with some unusual capacity to control the neoplasm and prevent it from metastasizing (Allen and Spitz, 1954; Attie and Khafif, 1964). Several possible mechanisms (e.g., hormonal, immunologic) for this type of "resistance" have been suggested. Considerable doubt has been cast on this concept by the increasing number of reports of benign juvenile melanomas in adults, indicating that this lesion is not limited to an age group peculiarly endowed with some mysterious capacity to confine true cancer.

Recurrences of benign juvenile melanomas following incomplete surgical removal have been reported (Becker, 1954; Dabska, 1956; Duperrat and Mascaro, 1961; Echevarria and Ackerman, 1967; Jones and Dukes, 1963; Kernen and Ackerman, 1960; McWhorter and Woolner, 1954; Schumachers-Brendler, 1963; Walther, 1959). In the series of 50 cases reported on by Jakubowicz (1965), eight recurred. Furthermore, two of these eight acted in a clinically aggressive manner. All eight recurrences occurred in lesions which had the following combination of features: (1) preponderance of spindle cells, (2) significant fibrosis of the connective tissue with a low cell count, and (3) insignificant junctional activity.

Four of the 51 benign juvenile melanomas included in our series recurred following therapy. Two reappeared after shave biopsy followed by electrodesiccation of the lesion base, and two recurred after an excision and graft had been performed. One of the latter lesions was of the multiple and agminated form. This child actually had two recurrences following surgery. Histologic examination of the surgical specimens revealed that the tumor had been cut through in depth, which probably was the reason for the recurrences.

Despite these occasional reports of post-treatment recurrences, Allen (1963) stated he was not aware of a single instance in which metastasis has occurred from a lesion fulfilling the histologic criteria of benign juvenile melanoma. None occurred in our 51 lesions

MALIGNANT TRANSFORMATION

Since most of the lesions now recognized as benign juvenile melanomas were at one time diagnosed as malignant melanomas, it is particularly difficult to interpret the cases reported prior to 1948, at which time Spitz firmly established the histologic criteria which separate the two. Ever since her important concept was proposed, difference of opinion has existed about malignant transformation of juvenile melanomas.

On the one hand, there are some who hold that juvenile melanoma has a distinct tendency to malignant change. Attie and Khafif (1964), for example, stated that "juvenile melanomas constitute a special kind of benign compound nevus with a high propensity of malignant change after puberty." This conclusion was presumably based on the fact that Allen and Spitz (1953) noted residual evidence of preexisting juvenile melanoma in 5.9 percent (21 of 362 cases) of malignant melanomas. However, before such a conclusion is reached, several critical considerations must be made with respect to these data. Kernen and Ackerman (1960) made a similar review of 430 malignant melanomas and failed to find a single case in which they were able to find remnants of juvenile melanoma in a malignant melanoma. Nevertheless, Allen (1963) stated that "a juvenile melanoma has essentially the same potentiality for undergoing cancerous change as any other compound nevus; no greater, no less. This incidence of malignant transformation of compound nevi is extremely low." The implication is that juvenile melanomas should be regarded as "benign" in the same way other compound nevi in general are considered benign lesions. This does not preclude the fact that rarely such lesions can give rise to malignant melanoma. In order to clarify this important point, we need to know the prevalence of benign juvenile melanomas in the population and compare it with the prevalence of remnants of such lesions in malignant melanomas. Even this type of study would be based on the possibly inaccurate assumption that the landmarks of the preexisting compound nevus or benign juvenile melanoma would be preserved in the same proportion of instances. Obviously, there are serious discrepancies in the interpretations by these various authors, and no

firm position can be taken at this time on this extremely important point. Nonetheless, one can conclude that most juvenile melanomas indeed act as benign lesions.

Kernen and Ackerman (1960) in their review concluded that in the few lesions reported since 1948 that were called juvenile melanoma and metastasized (Brunck, 1953; Yagawa and Nakamura, 1954), the diagnoses were in error. This leaves several reports in which it has been suggested that the lesions were combinations of benign juvenile melanoma and metastatic malignant melanomas (Delacrétaz, 1969; Duverne and Pruniéras, 1956a; Montgomery, 1958).

In correspondence with Allen in 1965, we asked the following question: "Have you encountered in your material or in the literature bona fide examples of malignant transformation of juvenile melanomas?" He replied:

It is my belief that juvenile melanomas are no more prone to undergo malignant transformation than any other compound nevus or junctional nevus. This likelihood is obviously extremely small in any of these instances. The statement that juvenile melanomas may become malignant should be viewed in the frame of reference of the likelihood just mentioned. When such malignant transformation does occur on occasion, it is for the reason that a junctional component is part of the juvenile melanoma; the cancer does not occur because the juvenile melanoma is more especially vulnerable than any other junctional component. I believe it is a disservice to endow the juvenile melanoma with a special cancerous potential. It is evident, however, from published statements and photomicrographs that some instances of so-called malignant transformation of juvenile melanomas were, in fact, malignant melanomas at the time of the first histologic examination.

Allen was further asked: "Please comment on your statement (Cancer, 6:1–46, 1953) to the effect that in 5.9 percent of 362 malignant melanomas 'there is noted residual evidence of preexisting juvenile melanoma.' Does this imply that juvenile melanomas have given rise to malignant lesions?" His reply was:

The incidence you mention of antedating juvenile melanomas is based, as we indicated, on the finding of a few landmarks suggestive of juvenile melanoma at the periphery of malignant melanomas. As I say, the juvenile melanomas are often difficult enough to diagnose when the entire, unaltered lesion is available for review, so that perhaps the figure of 5.9 percent is high from the point of view you mention. Again, the basic point, which this particular kind of partial evaluation should not be used to negate out of text, is that the juvenile melanoma is no more grave a lesion than the junctional nevus or compound nevus.

From all of the above we conclude that the consensus of most authors is that juvenile melanomas act as benign lesions in nearly all instances. The rare exceptions reported need critical review to determine if they indeed are indubitable examples of malignant transformation.

The importance of correct diagnosis of benign juvenile melanoma versus malignant melanoma is emphasized. The former is essentially a benign condition, whereas malignant melanoma in children carries with it a poor prognosis. Some earlier reports would suggest that the prognosis for prepubertal malignant melanoma was relatively good (Ackerman, 1948; Coffey and Berkeley, 1951; Pack, 1948; Pack and Scharnagel, 1951; Sylven, 1949). However, these reports undoubtedly were significantly weighted with patients who had benign juvenile melanomas. Reviews of histologic material from children originally diagnosed as having malignant melanoma have indicated significant error (Saksela and Rintala, 1968). The greatest factor in this error was the confusion between benign juvenile melanoma and malignant melanoma in children. When incorrect diagnoses are eliminated, it turns out that the prognosis of malignant melanoma in children is as poor as, or perhaps worse than, that in adults (Allen, 1960; Dobson, 1955; Fish et al., 1966; Lerman et al., 1970; Lorétan and Delacrétaz, 1967; McGovern and Goulston, 1963; McWhorter and Woolner, 1954; Montgomery, 1958). Several literature reviews would indicate that the total number of prepubertal children accepted to have malignant melanoma varies, depending on the criteria used by the author and the year of publication (55 cases, Fish et al., 1966; 11 cases, Hendrix, 1954; 45 cases, Skov Jensen et al., 1966; 62 cases, Lerman et al., 1970; 49 cases, Lorétan and Delacrétaz, 1967; 18 cases, McWhorter and Woolner, 1954). To these reviews can be added other more recently reported cases (Bandiera, 1967; Furuya et al., 1967; Lerman et al., 1970; Lyall, 1967; Oldhoff and Koudstaal, 1968; Saksela and Rintala, 1968; Van der Heul et al., 1966). Thus the total number of accepted cases of malignant melanoma reported to date is relatively small. However, there is the impression that the clinical course (i.e., presence or absence of metastases) may have influenced the inclusion or exclusion of cases in the categories of prepubertal malignant melanoma versus benign juvenile melanoma (Woringer and Alt, 1956). Lerman et al. (1970) summarized the problem in their discussion:

The only cases of malignant melanoma of childhood which are unequivocally acceptable are those that have documented metastatic disease. This situation exists because of 2 factors: the variety of malignant melanoma in childhood and the admitted difficulty in separating some cases from juvenile melanoma. Thus if one compares the survival of malignant melanoma of adulthood without specifying the stage of disease, a spurious conclusion may be reached that melanoma of childhood is a more malignant disease than melanoma of adulthood. In one of the largest series reported, Efskind and Nitter (1963) found a 5-year survival of 20 percent in 543 adults with malignant melanoma with regional metastases comparable to 19 percent in our own hospital (McNeer and Das Gupta, 1964). The 5-year survival of metastatic melanoma in children collected from a review of the literature in 1966 by Skov-Jensen et al. was 17 percent.

Thus the prognosis, at least of metastatic malignant melanoma of children, seems to closely parallel that of adults.

What is lacking is a specific and infallible method of differentiating these conditions. Until that time, there will continue to be borderline examples in which the present methods simply do not permit strict categorization. This in no way detracts from the major contribution made by Spitz (1948) and subsequent investigators, since in most instances we are now able to clearly distinguish the benign from the malignant melanocytic tumors in children based on current clinicopathologic criteria alone.

Pathology of Benign Juvenile Melanoma

Rafael Andrade, M.D.

The histologic features of benign juvenile melanoma are in most cases typical enough to make a microscopic diagnosis with reasonable certainty. There are 10 histologic characteristics, first published by Spitz in 1948, to which an eleventh characteristic was added by Allen in 1960: (1) nevus cells are present at the dermal-epidermal interface and in the cutis; (2) the process is superficial; (3) edema and telangiectases are present; (4) there is no cohesion between the nevus cells; (5) large nevus cells with an acidophilic cytoplasm (myoblastoid cells or "tadpole" cells) are present; (6) there are superficially located giant multinucleated nevus cells; (7) there is abrupt cleavage between the epidermis and the nevus cell nests in the junction area; (8) there is sparse pigment; (9) there is a chronic inflammatory infiltrate; (10) mitoses are present; and (11) there are changes in the epidermis, such as irregular acanthosis, pseudoepitheliomatous hyperplasia, and thinning (Table 31–4). Moreover, attention should be called to the fibrotic appearance of the stroma in the so-called "compact" benign juvenile melanoma (Schumachers-Brendler, 1963), which clinically resembles a cutaneous nodule (dermatofibroma) (see Clinical Aspects).

It is now generally accepted that benign juvenile melanoma is a sessile, pediculated, or dome-shaped compound nevus, i.e., a nevus involving the dermal-epidermal junction area and the dermis. It often reaches the lower levels of the dermis (Spitz, 1948) and may even penetrate the subcutis Helwig, 1955; McWhorter and Woolner, 1954; Gartmann, 1962) (Figs. 31–10 and 31–11). In 14 of our cases (2 adults, 12 children), the lesion involved the entire thickness of the dermis and reached the dermis-subcutis border.

One of our patients showed a lesion with a macular brown halo around its base and with nevus cell theques present at the junction in the halo area. Another patient presented only junctional nevus cell theques (Fig. 31–18). The nevus cells forming benign juvenile melanomas are either fusiform ("spindle-shaped") or polygonal ("epithelioid") (Figs. 31–12 and 31–13). These cells are the single most important histologic feature of the tumor. In most cases both types of cells are present, although the spindle-shaped cells seem to be more common (Helwig, 1955; McWhorter and Woolner, 1954; Kernen and Ackerman, 1960; Gartmann, 1962 and 1973; Coskey and Mehregan, 1973). Spitz (1948) and Allen (1960 and 1963) found this type of nevus cell in only 25 percent of their cases, however. In some rare cases, the nevus cells are exclusively epithelioid, and in other cases, the cells may be morphologically intermediate between the two principal types (Helwig, 1955; Gartmann, 1962). When interpreting such intermediate cells one has to bear in mind, however, that a spindle-shaped cell appears round when cut across its short axis. The nevus cells of the benign juvenile melanoma are found in nests sharply demarcated from the surrounding, usually scanty, stroma (Helwig, 1955). The spindle cells may occur in bundles of parallel cells in an irregular arrangement but still more or less perpendicular to the surface of the epidermis (Helwig, 1955; Kernen and Ackerman, 1960; Gartmann, 1962) (Fig. 31–12*A*). Toward the deepest part of the lesion the cells often become smaller and more similar to ordinary nevus cells (McWhorter and Woolner, 1954; Duperrat, 1955; Kernen and Ackerman, 1960; Gartmann, 1962). Some authors have interpreted this feature as a sign of cellular maturation. Gartmann (1962) described a third cell type in benign juvenile melanoma, the "round cell," which resembles an ordinary nevus cell very closely, has very little cytoplasm, and shows a well-differentiated nucleus. In this type of tumor, cells with giant nuclei and multinucleated giant cells can occasionally be found in the papillary bodies. Four out of Gartmann's 67 lesions were predominantly of the "round cell" type. In four cases this was combined with the spindle cell type and in five cases with the epithelioid type. Three of the lesions in

Text continues on page 736

TABLE 31-4 ANALYSIS OF THE INCIDENCE OF THE 11 HISTOLOGIC CHARACTERISTICS IN FOUR DIFFERENT PUBLICATIONS

11 Histologic Characteristics	67 Cases Gartmann, 1962	24 Cases Schumachers-Brendler, 1963	50 Cases Jakubowicz, 1965	43 Cases Kopf and Andrade, 1966
1. Compound nevus Spindle cells Epithelioid cells	+*	24	47	43
2. Superficial location	+	24	50	43
3. Edema and telangiectasia	35 (edema) 44 (telangiectasia)	20	38	36
4. Loss of cellular cohesion	+	18	25	43
5. Large nevus cells with acidophilic cytoplasm (myoblastoid-tadpole)	+	20	+	40 (numerous, 5;
6. Superficial multinucleated giant cells	+	17	25	39 (numerous, 19 few rate, 20)
7. Abrupt areas of cleavage (epidermis-junction nests)	+	21	46	38
8. Sparse pigment	sparse	15	in general	33 sparse 7 absent 3 abundant
9. Chronic inflammatory infiltrate	very variable	14	40	40 (4 mild, & 4 abundant)
10. Mitoses	31 after careful study of slides	5	20	33 (in 7 of them 1 mitosis in 6 sections)
11. Epidermal changes			variable	
pseudoepitheliomatous hyperplasia	35	8	3	4
acanthosis	8			23
compression	14			2
atrophy		8		13
tumoral	1			1
normal	9	8		

*Plus sign (+) indicates that histologic characteristics were mentioned, but no numbers were given.

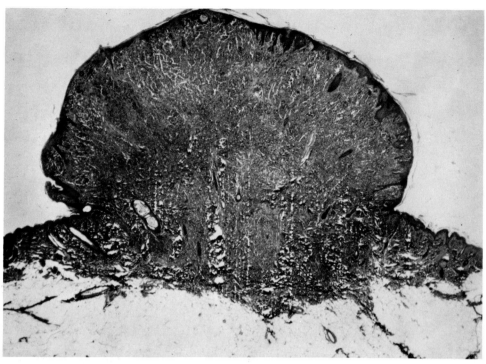

Figure 31–10 General view of a benign juvenile melanoma. Round, papular lesion rising above the surface of the epidermis and reaching the borderline with the subcutaneous tissue. *H & E, × 10.*

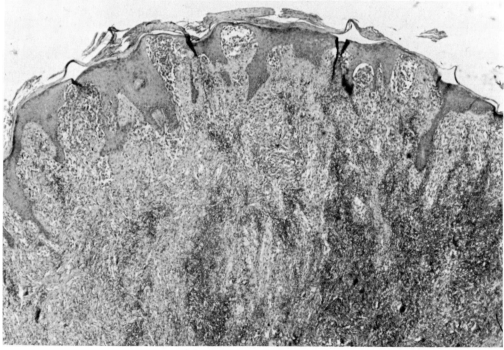

Figure 31–11 Low-power view, showing a compound nevus with marked acanthosis. The darker areas in the dermis correspond to the inflammatory cellular infiltrate. *H & E, × 25.*

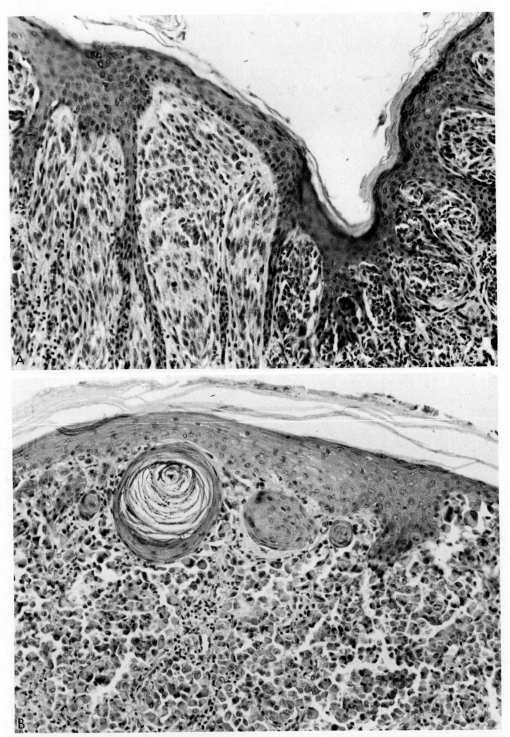

Figure 31–12   Two types of cells: spindle-shaped (*A*) and epithelioid (*B*). The latter shows the characteristics of these cells—abundant, well-outlined, eosinophilic cytoplasm and cellular segregation. *H & E, ×125*. (*From* Kopf and Andrade: Benign juvenile melanoma. *In* Year Book of Dermatology, 1965–1966. Chicago, Year Book Medical Publishers, 1966.)

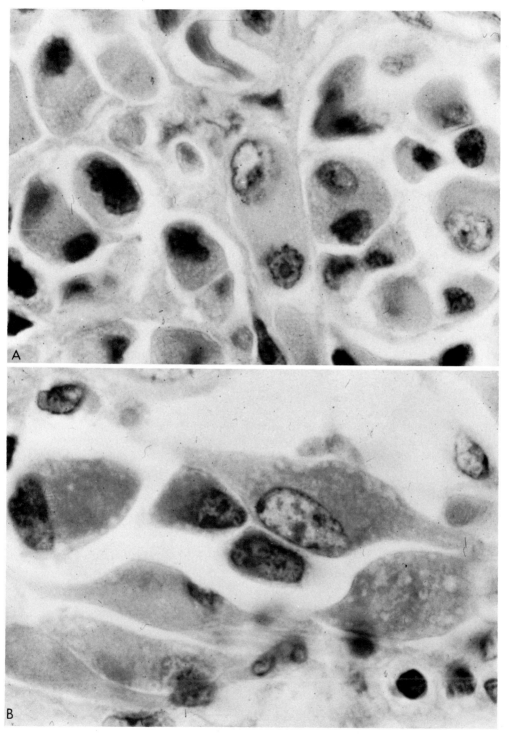

Figure 31–13 High-power views of the epithelioid (*A*) and spindle-shaped (*B*) cells. Note the cellular segregation and the nuclear pleomorphism. *H & E, × 1000.*

our series had such round cells. Schumachers-Brendler (1963) remained unconvinced of this third cellular type. Those cases may represent transitional forms between ordinary nevus cells and juvenile melanoma cells, since benign juvenile melanomas have occurred as part of a bathing trunk nevus (Kernen and Ackerman, 1960; Greeley et al., 1965; McWhorter and Woolner, 1954; Pack and Davis, 1961; Reed et al., 1965) and have been found to develop from dermal nevus cell nevus (Korting et al., 1968). In the deeper portion of the dermis, the nevus cells of a benign juvenile melanoma may be so narrow and fusiform that they are sometimes difficult to distinguish from fibroblasts (Miescher, 1933; Duperrat, 1955; Gertler, 1956; Delacrétaz and Jaeger, 1957).

In some benign juvenile melanomas, the *epidermis* is thinned or acanthotic and compressed, and very sparse isolated cells or cell nests are found in the junctional area. These cases have been considered examples of intradermal juvenile melanomas (Spitz, 1948; McWhorter and Woolner, 1954). Our series showed 14 lesions of this type. The *nuclei* of benign juvenile melanoma cells are large and often regular in size, contain fine chromatin and large acidophilic nucleoli, and may be vesicular and hyperchromatic (Spitz, 1948; Helwig, 1955; Kernen and Ackerman, 1960; Gartmann, 1962) (Figs. 31–12 and 31–13). Most authors find *mitotic figures* usually rare (Spitz, 1948; Woringer, 1956; Delacrétaz and Jaeger, 1957; Allen, 1963; Gartmann, 1962; Schumachers-Brendler, 1963; Jakubowicz, 1965). Helwig (1954), however, found mitoses almost always present and sometimes even numerous. Mitotic figures are mostly found in the upper portion of the lesion and are not confined to the junctional area. According to McWhorter and Woolner (1954), the number of mitoses in their material varied from 4 to 6 per section through the entire lesion to 1 to 2 per entire lesion. Atypical mitoses are extremely rare (Kernen and Ackerman, 1960; Jakubowicz, 1965). Even though there may be a few mitoses in benign juvenile melanoma lesions in adults, this is not to be interpreted as a sign of malignancy (Allen, 1963). There are some publications specifying the number of mitoses more precisely: Gartmann (1962) found rare mitotic figures in 31 out of 67 specimens; Schumachers-Brendler (1963) found mitoses in 5 out of 24 lesions (one of them with numerous mitoses); and Jakubowicz (1965) described numerous mitotic figures in 20 out of 50 lesions. In 33 of our own 43 lesions studied, mitotic figures were few or rare; in 7 of the 33 there was only one mitotic figure in the 4 to 6 sections of each specimen studied.

In general, the benign juvenile melanoma cells have an abundant, eosinophilic *cytoplasm* (Figs. 31–12 and 31–13). The epithelioid cells and the cells losing their cohesion have a more distinct cellular outline. In one of the lesions, we found in the upper dermis and in the papillary bodies several groups of nevus cells which showed large, empty, vacuolated spaces occupying almost the entire cytoplasm and compressing the nucleus. This picture resembles the round spaces in the cytoplasm of some ordinary nevus cells. These vacuolizations have been thought to indicate a fatty degeneration. Allen (1963) found an infrequent vacuolization of the nevus cells in the benign juvenile melanoma lesions of adults, of the kind described in association with hormonal changes during pregnancy and menarche, and occasionally in adolescent males. These changes are not the same as those that occur in the so-called foamy cell nevus (Miescher, 1933; Brunck, 1953 and 1957; Schrader and Helwig, 1967). Gartman (1962) found vacuolated cells in three of the lesions of his series.

An important clue to the diagnosis of benign juvenile melanomas, as already reported by Spitz in 1948, is the presence in the junction area and in the superficial dermis of variable numbers of two types of *giant nevus cells* (Figs. 31–14 and 31–15):(a) the *mononucleated* giant nevus cell with a large vesicular, often hyperchromatic, nucleus and an abundant, dense, eosinophilic cytoplasm, resembling a large neoplastic cell of fat or muscle origin (Allen, 1963); and (b) the *multinucleated* giant nevus cell, the cytoplasm of which is abundant, well-outlined, dense, eosinophilic, and sometimes granular. Schumachers-Brendler (1963) compared the shape of the mono-

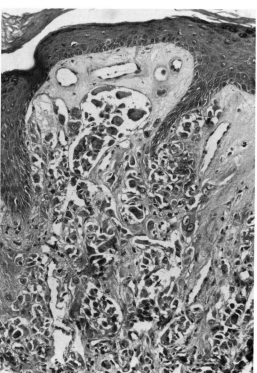

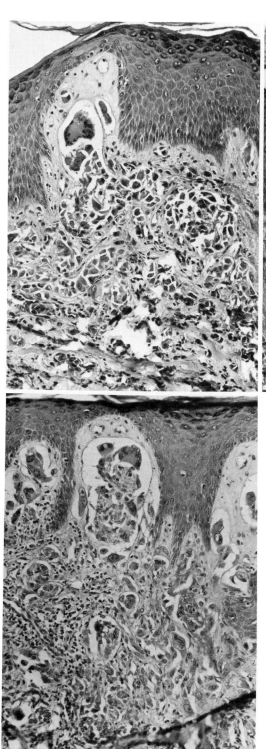

Figure 31–14 These pictures show moderate acanthosis, abundant papillary edema, epithelioid cells, giant cells of different sizes and shapes, cellular segregation, dehiscence of the stroma simulating lymphatic spaces, a few dilated capillaries, and foci of a round cell inflammatory infiltrate. *H & E, ×500.*

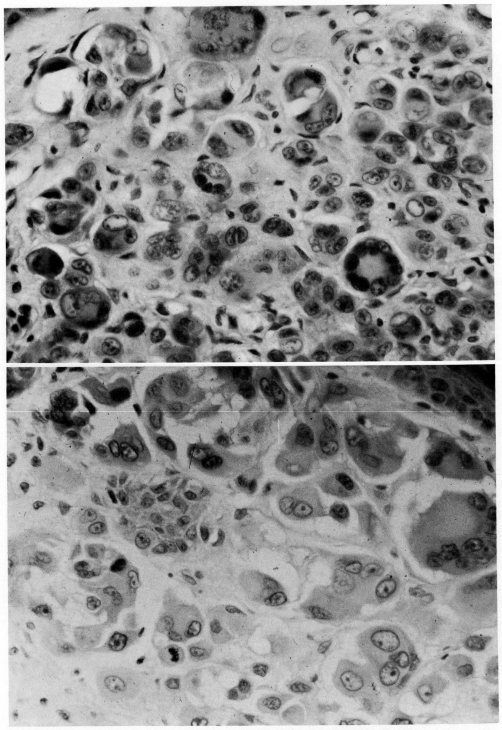

Figure 31–15 High-power view of several other types of giant multinucleated cells present in benign juvenile melanoma. *H & E, × 500.*

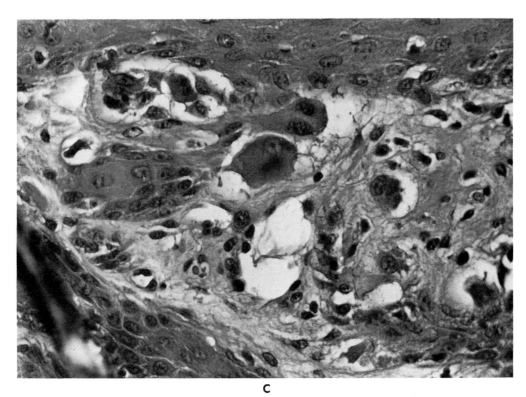

C

Figure 31-15 *Continued.*

nucleated giant nevus cell to a tadpole and reported such cells in 20 out of 24 benign juvenile melanomas. These cells were present in 40 out of 43 lesions in our series, rare or few in 20, and abundant in 5. Usually, the multinucleated giant nevus cell has 4 to 6 nuclei (Spitz, 1948) in peripheral arrangement, but there may be as many as 20 (Jakubowicz, 1965). Occasionally, the nuclei are clumped together in the center of the cell. These cells have been compared to Langhans' giant cells, to the giant cells found in measles, and even to Touton giant cells (Allen, 1963) (Figs. 31–14 and 31–15). Moreover, these cells may have large and eosinophilic nucleoli. The multinucleated giant nevus cells are irregularly round or oval but often show stellate cytoplasmic processes, especially when they are in contact with the epidermis (Spitz, 1948) (Fig. 31–15C). Their cytoplasm rarely contains pigment but is commonly vacuolated, suggesting the presence of lipid. Although giant cells may be a prominent feature in the epithelioid type of benign juvenile melanoma, they are not always present, and some authors feel that they have been overempha-

sized (McWhorter and Woolner, 1954; Duperrat, 1955). According to Schumachers-Brendler (1963), they are completely absent in the pure spindle cell type. Schumachers-Brendler found them present in 17 out of 24 lesions, and Jakubowicz (1965) in 25 out of 50 lesions. McWhorter and Woolner reported their presence in 9 out of 11 lesions, but prominent only in 2. We found them in 39 out of 43 lesions; in 20 of these they were rare or few in number. Allen (1963) stated: "In instances in which the resemblance of the giant cells of benign juvenile melanoma and malignant melanoma is close, the use of other histological criteria is required to establish the differential diagnosis."

The *epidermis* often shows reactive hyperplasia of such intensity that the diagnosis of squamous cell carcinoma is possible (Gartmann, 1962; Allen, 1963) (Figs. 31–11, 31–12, 31–16, and 31–17). There may also be areas of epidermal flattening and atrophy through compression. The compressed epidermis may become disrupted and ulcerated (McWhorter and Woolner, 1954; Woringer, 1956; Gartmann, 1962; Allen, 1963). Gartmann

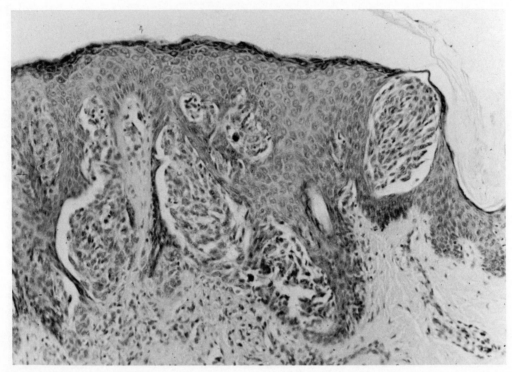

Figure 31–16   Irregular acanthosis with several nests of cells located at different levels inside the epidermis. Note the cleavage between the nests and the epidermis at the junction area. *H & E, × 125.*

(1962) found pseudoepitheliomatous hyperplasia in 35 lesions, thinning of the epidermis in 14, acanthosis alternating with areas of atrophy in 8, no changes in 9, and ulceration in one lesion. In the series of Schumachers-Brendler (1963), there were 8 cases with epidermal hyperplasia, 8 with atrophy, and 8 with normal epidermis. Pseudoepitheliomatous hyperplasia was present in 3 of 50 lesions described by Jakubowicz (1965), and there were various other epidermal changes. In our series, 27 lesions had different degrees of acanthosis, and of these, 4 showed pseudoepitheliomatous hyperplasia. A misdiagnosis of squamous cell carcinoma would have seemed possible in only one case, however. In 13 cases we found very mild acanthosis with other areas of epidermal thinning. Two specimens showed a compressed epidermis. In some rare cases there is a migration of tumor cells into the upper layer of the epidermis (Becker, 1954; Schumachers-Brendler, 1963). One of our cases showed such a migration. Another striking feature is the abrupt transition from junctional nevus cell nests to epidermal cells

(Allen, 1963), with formation of a crescent-like space between them (Figs. 31–11, 31–15*C*, 31–16, 31–18*D* and *E*). This feature was present in 21 of the 24 lesions of Schumachers-Brendler (1963), and in 46 out of 50 lesions of Jakubowicz (1965). We found it in 38 of our own 43 lesions. When studying the melanocytes in the basal layer of the overlying epidermis and of the normal surrounding epidermis, Cochran (1971) found consistent differences in melanocytic and in nonmelanocytic tumors. In benign juvenile melanomas as in compound nevi, he found an increased number of melanocytes in the overlying epidermis but very rarely in the normal surrounding epidermis. In the upper dermis, there is often *loss of cohesion* (Figs. 31–12 to 31–15) between the nevus cells after shrinkage or dissolution of some cells and flattening of others. These flattened cells can closely resemble endothelial cells lining vascular spaces, a feature conducive to the misdiagnosis of malignant melanoma with lymphatic invasion (Allen, 1963) (Figs. 31–14). In fact, however, these flattened cells are surrounded by a compressed dermal stroma and not by

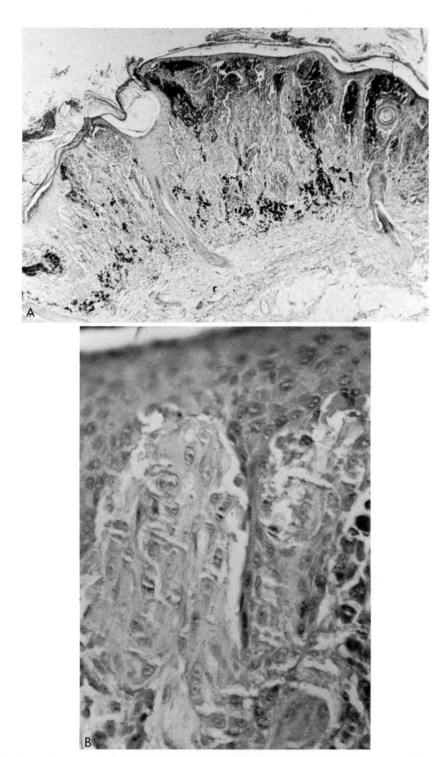

Figure 31–17 *A*, Low-power view of pigmented benign juvenile melanoma. *H & E*, × *25*. *B*, High-power view of a papilla following bleaching of the melanin. We see the characteristic eosinophilic, pale-staining, spindle-shaped cells with a pale nucleus. *H & E*, × *500*.

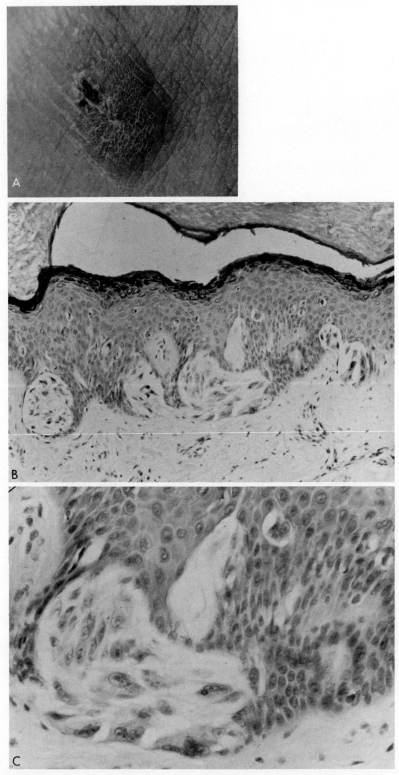

Figure 31–18 Peculiar benign juvenile melanoma of a pure junctional type. Clinically (*A*) it was considered a histiocytofibroma. Duration one year, located on the dorsum of the left foot of a 23 year old woman. The lesion was flat, 1 cm. in diameter, and brownish pink in color. Serial sections showed only junctional activity in an acanthotic epidermis (*B*). *H & E, ×125. C,* Characteristics of the cells. *H & E, ×500.*

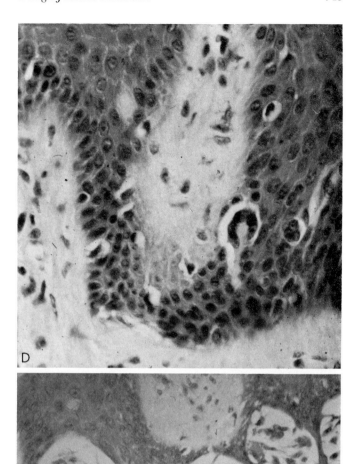

Figure 31–18 *Continued. D,* A giant multinucleated cell with an area of cleavage separating it from the epidermis. *H & E, × 500. E,* A giant multinucleated cell within a junctional nest.

vascular walls, as can be demonstrated with silver and elastic tissue stains (Allen, 1963). Loss of cellular cohesion was reported by Schumachers-Brendler (1963) in 18 out of 24 lesions, and by Jakubowicz (1965) in 25 out of 50 lesions. We found it present in all our lesions.

In the upper dermis we often see *dilated capillaries* and areas of *edema.* Vascular ectasias of subepidermal lymphatics and arterioles may be quite prominent, even cavernous (Allen, 1960 and 1963). A positive alkaline phosphatase reaction in the capillary walls emphasizes the increased vascularity of the lesion (Wells and Farthing, 1966). The edema is generally mild, but it can also be of such intensity that the tumor cells seem to be floating (Figs. 31–14 and 31–19). The pinkish, yellowish, or tan appearance that is so characteristic of the clinical lesion can be explained on the basis of these vascular alterations plus the absence or scarcity of melanin. These vascular features and the edema are not, however, specific for benign juvenile melanomas (McWhorter and Woolner, 1954). Gartmann (1962) found edema in 35 and telangiectasia in 44 of 67 lesions, Schumachers-Brendler (1963) in 20 out of 24 lesions, and Jakubowicz

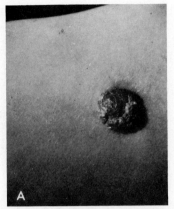

Figure 31-19 Pediculated benign juvenile melanoma in a 7 year old boy on exterior aspect of right arm. Duration six months. The lesion bled occasionally and was classified clinically (*A*) and pathologically (*B*) as granuloma telangiectaticum. Note the intense edema, numerous dilated capillaries, and numerous sweat ducts with branched and dilated structures. *H & E*, ×*10.*

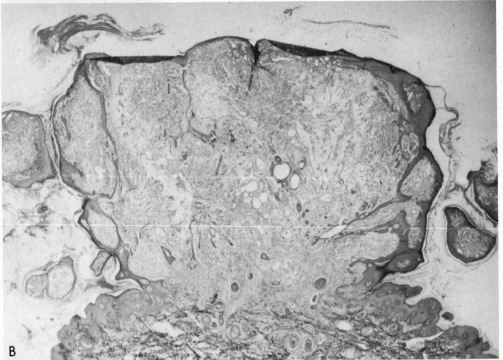

(1965) in 38 out of 50 lesions, and we found both features in 36 of our 43 cases. In one of these, the edema was very intense, and in another, edema and telangiectasia were clinically and histologically so striking that the lesion was called a granuloma pyogenicum (Fig. 31–19). In 10 other lesions of our series, telangiectasias were also prominent.

Frequently, there is an *inflammatory reaction* of variable intensity, usually consisting of lymphocytes, histiocytes, and a few plasma cells (Spitz, 1948; Allen, 1960; Gartmann, 1962) (Figs. 31–11 and 31–14). Schumachers-Brendler (1963) re-ported inflammatory infiltrates in 14 out of 24 lesions, and Jakubowicz (1965) in 40 out of 50 lesions. We found it present in 40 of our 43 lesions: very mild to moderate in 4 of these and abundant in 4. Whenever there is ulceration, varying numbers of polymorphonuclear neutrophils and eosinophils may be present.

Melanin is usually scanty (Spitz, 1948; Allen, 1960; McWhorter and Woolner, 1954; Gartmann, 1962; Schumachers-Brendler, 1963; Jakubowicz, 1965). Schumachers-Brendler (1963) found melanin in only 15 out of 24 lesions. In our own series, it was poor or scanty in 33, abun-

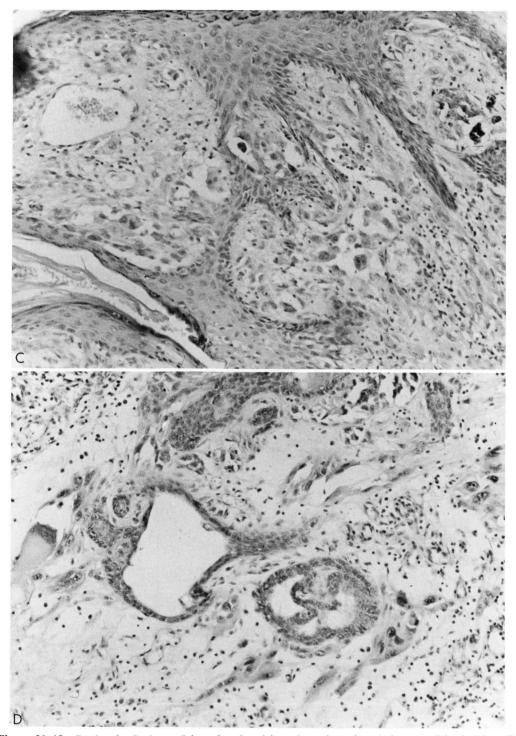

Figure 31–19 *Continued. C,* A careful study of serial sections showed typical nests of benign juvenile melanoma cells in the junction area. *H & E,* × *250. D,* In the center of the section there is a very edematous stroma. The figure shows a few isolated benign juvenile melanoma cells surrounding several tortuous, folded, dilated, excretory sweat duct structures. This case probably represents an association of benign juvenile melanoma with a sweat duct hamartoma. *H & E,* × *500.*

dant in 3, and absent in 7 cases. Lightly pigmented melanin granules in a few cells, especially those in the junction area and in the superficial dermis, can be made visible with the Masson-Fontana method. In some lesions, there is abundant melanin in the nevus cells, the epidermal cells, and the dermal melanophages (Spitz, 1948). There are cases in which the pigment is so dense that the cellular morphology cannot be studied unless the sections are bleached (Helwig, 1955). We had to bleach two of the heavily pigmented specimens in our series (Fig. 31–17).

No detailed study has yet been made of the presence of *neural fibrils*. Myelinated and nonmyelinated nerve fibers between, but not within, nevus cell groups have been reported by several authors, however (Steigleder and Wellmer, 1956; Gartmann, 1962). Neurinomatous and neural body–like structures, such as those seen in certain intradermal nevi, may be present (Gartmann, 1962). One of our lesions showed some structure with neuroid features in the mid dermis. Trichrome stains and reticulum stains show the same sharply outlined cellular nests we are used to seeing in nevus cell nevi. In several of our lesions, the *elastic tissue* was decreased in some areas and reduced to a few fine threads or completely absent in others.

The *cutaneous appendages* often remain intact in this tumor (Spitz, 1948). Sometimes there is some junctional activity along the hair follicles, but this is not as intense as at the dermal-epidermal junction. The sebaceous glands and sweat glands show no alterations except for some probably pressure-induced distortion.

The *regressive stage* is rarely seen. It is principally marked by involutional fibrosis of the stroma surrounding isolated small nests or cords of nevus cells or giant nevus cells. Four of the lesions included in our series were in this stage. Two of these occurred in children. One was a very firm lesion clinically diagnosed as a cutaneous nodule. A 22 year old woman had had a similar lesion on the dorsum of her hand for many years. A 34 year old man had such a lesion of one year's duration. It is difficult to affirm whether fibrosis represents a regressive stage or a clinical form of benign juvenile melanoma (com-

pact type, Schumachers-Brendler, 1963; hard type, Duperrat and Dufourmentel, 1959) (Fig. 31–20). Some authors (Allen and Spitz, 1953; Woringer, 1956; Allen, 1960; Gartmann, 1963) interpret the loss of junctional activity and transformation into an intradermal nevus as aspects of the regressive stage also. According to Allen (1963), benign juvenile melanoma lesions in adults can show some additional histologic characteristics. He found that these lesions tend to show involutional fibrosis and that the deeper isolated cells tend to have a more hyperchromatic nucleus and more prominent nucleoli and to extend deeper into the dermis than the usual benign juvenile melanoma in children. It is possible that other lesions disappear without traces at the approach of puberty or undergo pediculation, lipidization, vacuolization and edema, and depigmentation and finally vanish, as in the phenomenon of leukoderma acquisitum centrifugum (Kopf et al., 1965; Korting et al., 1968).

The so-called "balloon-celled nevus" (*Blasenzellennaevus*) is a rare entity (Hornstein, 1966; Schrader and Helwig, 1967). It is especially found in children and young adults. In a few cases, it may represent a regressive stage of a nevus or a benign juvenile melanoma (Hornstein, 1966; Andrade, 1968).

HISTOCHEMISTRY

Not many studies of the histochemistry of benign juvenile melanoma have been undertaken, and the results and interpretations they offer contain certain discrepancies. Wells et al. (1966), using histochemical and manometric methods, did not find any nonspecific cholinesterase activity. Winkelmann (1961), on the contrary, found nonspecific cholinesterase but no tyrosinase activity in two cases of benign juvenile melanoma. These findings led him to the conclusion that the cellular component of benign juvenile melanoma was more closely related to neural elements or intradermal nevus cells than to melanin-producing cells. He further suggested that the lack of tyrosinase activity in benign juvenile melanoma may be

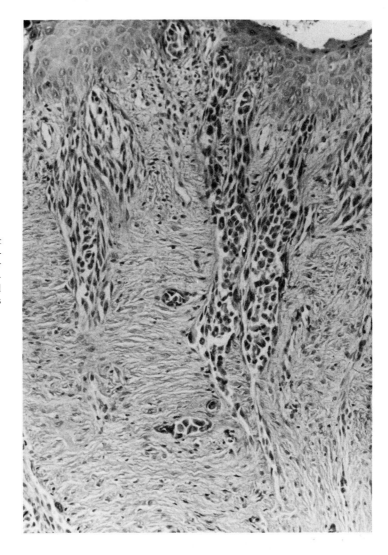

Figure 31–20 Hard, fibrotic type of benign juvenile melanoma. With a fibrotic cellular stroma, there are nests of epithelioid and spindle-shaped cells. There is slight acanthosis and junctional activity.

useful for differentiating this tumor from malignant melanoma. Woringer (1956) similarly found that the reaction of the benign juvenile melanoma cells to DOPA was negative. According to Wells and Farthing (1966), there is also a negative DOPA reaction or else a just barely discernible oxidase reaction in the cells immediately beneath the epidermis. Delacrétaz and Jaeger (1957) found no increase in the uptake of radioactive tyrosine in benign juvenile melanoma as compared with normal tissue. Other authors (Steigleder and Wellmer, 1956; Kawamura et al., 1962; Becker and Becker, 1965; Mishima, 1967) and we ourselves have demonstrated tyrosinase activity in benign juvenile melanoma, which casts some doubt

on the value of these stains in differentiating cell lineage.

Alkaline phosphatase and stains for polysaccharides and lipids (Winkelmann, 1961; Wells and Farthing, 1966) and for mucopolysaccharides and metachromatic material (Steigleder and Wellmer, 1956) have been negative. Steigleder and Wellmer (1956) have demonstrated fine, Sudan III–positive droplets in isolated cells. Wells and Farthing (1966) found faint cytoplasmic reactions for lipids and for nonspecific cholinesterases and a fairly strong reaction for acid phosphatases in some of the giant cells. Periodic acid–Schiff reactions sometimes showed an intact basement membrane outlining nests of nevus cells in the junction area

(Steigleder and Wellmer, 1956). Degos (1958) quoted a finding of Duverne and Pruniéras that in the nuclei of benign juvenile melanoma cells RNA is increased and DNA is decreased, as compared with an increase in both these nucleic acids in malignant melanoma. In contrast, nevus cells in ordinary nevus cell nevi have very little RNA but often a large amount of DNA.

The stroma of two of our lesions showed a moderate amount of Alcian blue–positive material, which was almost completely digested with hyaluronidase. Toluidine blue showed no metachromasia.

SPECIAL STUDIES

In a study of malignant melanoma with an *electrometer*, Melczer and Kiss (1958) found a decreased electrical resistance and consequently increased electrical conductivity in 14 cases. No similarly increased conductivity was demonstrable in 23 benign juvenile melanomas and 465 nevus cell nevi, however. Another benign juvenile melanoma, mentioned by the authors in the same publication but evidently not included in the above series, did show a small decrease of electrical conductivity.

The limitation of this highly interesting electrometric method is that it can be used only in lesions where the surface epidermis is intact, because erosion or ulceration of the skin reduces electrical resistance markedly. If this method can be shown to be accurate enough, it would be very valuable for differentiating at least between intact lesions of benign juvenile melanoma and malignant melanoma (see Chapter 12).

The *electron microscopic* features of a benign juvenile melanoma are illustrated in Figure 31–21, which Dr. Yutaka Mishima permitted us to reproduce. According to Mishima (1967), "the cytoplasm of juvenile melanoma cells can exhibit active melanosome synthesis by the presence of various developmental stages from small vesicles to mature melanosomes in the vicinity of the Golgi apparatus." Mishima's studies indicate that the subcellular organization of the juvenile melanoma cells,

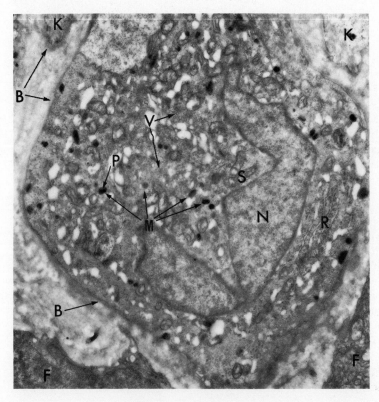

Figure 31–21 Electron micrograph of benign juvenile melanoma cell at the epidermal-dermal junction, which is in the process of "dropping off." Its active melanin biosynthesis is evidenced by the presence of melanosomes (M) in various developmental stages in close relationship to the Golgi vesicles (V). The melanosomes exhibit a distinct internal structure on which variously electron-dense melanin particles (P) are deposited: R, ergastoplasm; S, mitochondria; N, nucleus; B, basement membrane; K, basal cell; F, fibroblast. Fixed with OsO_4 and stained with phosphotungstic acid and lead citrate. Reduced from 10,100. (Courtesy of Y. Mishima, *from* Kopf and Andrade: Benign Juvenile melanoma. *In* Year Book of Dermatology, 1965–1966. Chicago, Year Book Medical Publishers, 1966.)

such as Golgi apparatus, mitochondria, endoplasmic reticulum, ribosomes, and general configuration, appears to be similar to, if not identical with, that of the intradermal nevus cells, although the latter show more melanized premelanosomes. Mishima concluded that benign juvenile melanoma seems to be a variant of nevus cell nevi and like these nevi has junctional, compound, and intradermal forms. According to Mishima's (1967) hypothesis, melanotic tumors like benign juvenile melanoma and nevus cell nevi would derive from the nevoblast rather than from the melanoblast.

HISTOLOGIC DIFFERENTIAL DIAGNOSIS

The diagnosis of a typical lesion of benign juvenile melanoma presents no problem for the experienced pathologist. There are, however, rare cases in which the degree of cellular pleomorphism and the absence of some of the important features discussed above make the differential diagnosis between benign juvenile melanoma and malignant melanoma quite difficult. These cases should be evaluated individually and considered as a separate group. They do not put the benignity of benign juvenile melanoma in question, especially not that of benign juvenile melanoma in children before puberty. In such difficult or ambiguous cases, the anamnesis and the clinical features acquire a particular importance. The value of the clinicopathologic correlation and the follow-up cannot be stressed enough.

One unusual benign juvenile melanoma in our series illustrates the problems that can be encountered. There was a well-limited area of cellular proliferation in the superficial dermis, compressing but not invading the epidermis. Junctional nevus cell theques were rare. The cellular pleomorphism seemed "frightening" to us and to Allen (personal communication). Clinically this lesion was a typical benign juvenile melanoma of several year's duration, excised from the back of an 11 year old boy (Fig. 31–22) who had had another benign juvenile melanoma removed from his shoulder. Both lesions were removed eight years ago, and neither has recurred

or given rise to metastases. This patient has two other clinically typical, pea-sized, benign juvenile melanomas on his back, which have not yet been excised. His twin brother has also had two clinically and histologically typical benign juvenile melanomas.

The principal features in the differential diagnosis of malignant melanomas have been evaluated in a number of classic publications (Unna, 1894; Darier, 1913; Miescher, 1933; Spitz, 1948; Allen and Spitz, 1953; Couperus and Rucker, 1954; McWhorter and Woolner, 1954; Duperrat, 1955; Woringer, 1956; Gans and Steigleder, 1957; Lane et al., 1958; Kernen and Ackerman, 1960; Gartmann, 1962; Lund and Kraus, 1962; Allen, 1963; Schumachers-Brendler, 1963; Lorétan and Delacrétaz, 1967; Saksela and Rintala, 1968). According to these authors, malignant melanomas possess the following characteristics: marked cellular pleomorphism, bizarre nuclei, prominent nucleoli, giant cells, frequency and atypia of mitotic figures, epidermal disintegration by migration of the tumor cells, leading to ulceration, inflammatory reaction, and depth of invasion.

As discussed above, one of the principal types of benign juvenile melanoma is the so-called spindle cell nevus type, in which most or all of the cells are fusiform. The unwary pathologist can easily confuse this with the uncommon spindle cell form of malignant melanoma. Couperus and Rucker (1954) reported that in their series of malignant melanomas only 3 percent of the primary lesions and 11 percent of the metastases were of the pure spindle cell type. Consequently, the pathologist will not come across this type of tumor often, and he may then misdiagnose it as benign juvenile melanoma.

Malignant melanomas with a few features of juvenile melanoma (Allen and Spitz, 1953) represent a separate problem, which is somewhat similar to the problem of malignant melanomas with "junction nevus" proliferation at the periphery or with nests of "nevus cells" in the dermis. It has not been resolved whether these associations represent malignant tumors arising from benign tumor cells, whether the malignant and benign cells arise inde-

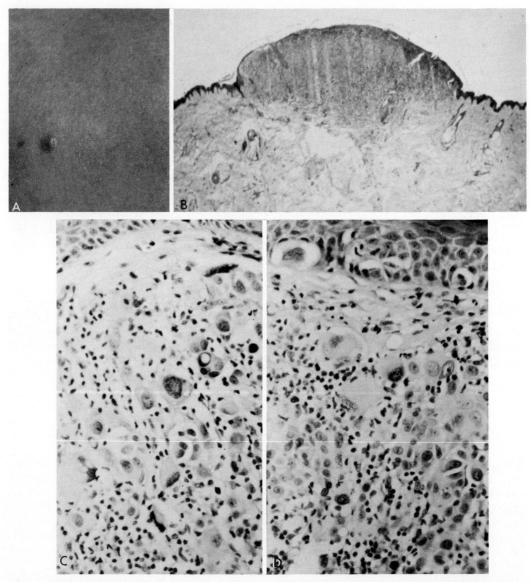

Figure 31–22 *A,* Benign juvenile melanoma of 0.5 × 0.5 × 0.2 cm. on left scapular area in an 11 year old boy. Several years' duration. *B,* General view of the section. The cellular proliferation invades the superficial dermis. *C, D, E, F, G,* High-power views of different areas of the sections, showing mono- and multinucleated cells with an abundant homogeneous, well-outlined, eosinophilic cytoplasm and nuclear pleomorphism. There are foci of lymphocytes. *H & E,* ×*320 and* ×*500.*

pendently, or whether such histologic interpretations are erroneous.

True malignant melanomas in children are exceptionally rare, and when they do occur, they show a histology very similar to that of the adult type and have the same prognosis (McWhorter and Woolner, 1954; Montgomery, 1958; Allen, 1963; McGovern and Goulston, 1963; Fish et al., 1966; Lorétan and De-

lacrétaz, 1967; Lerman et al., 1970). Allen (1963) has had the unique opportunity of studying 29 malignant melanomas in children. Fifteen of these were known to have been fatal; 8 were known to have developed metastases, and he had no follow-up on the remaining cases. Allen added: "None of these has shown any of the several morphologic landmarks of the juvenile melanoma.... This absence of fea-

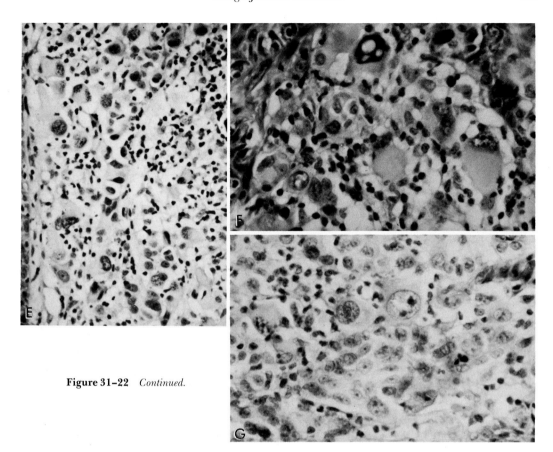

Figure 31–22   *Continued.*

tures of the juvenile melanoma in the melanocarcinomas of children completely comprises the core of the basis for the diagnosis of the tumors" (see Malignant Transformation, under Clinical Aspects).

Intermediate stages between benign juvenile melanomas and ordinary nevus cell nevi can be found, a fact that suggests their common origin. Thus the differential diagnosis between benign juvenile melanoma and nevus cell nevi presents less of a problem. Occasionally the following lesions have been considered in the histologic differential diagnosis of benign juvenile melanoma: pseudoepitheliomatous hyperplasia, squamous cell carcinoma, cellular blue nevus, cutaneous nodule, xanthoma, leiomyoma, angioma, granuloma telangiectaticum, juvenile xanthogranuloma, granular cell myoblastoma, reticulohistiocytoma, and histiocytosis X.

REFERENCES

Ackerman, L. V.: Malignant melanoma of the skin. Am. J. Clin. Pathol., 18:602, 1948.

Allen, A. C.: Juvenile melanomas of children and adults and melanocarcinomas of chidren. Arch. Dermatol., 82:325, 1960.

Allen, A. C.: Juvenile melanomas. Ann. N. Y. Acad. Sci. 100:29, 1963.

Allen, A. C., and Spitz, S.: Malignant melanoma. A clinicopathological analysis of the criteria for diagnosis and prognosis. Cancer, 6:1, 1953.

Allen, A. C., and Spitz, S.: Histogenesis and clinico-pathologic correlation of nevi and malignant melanomas. Arch. Dermatol., 69:150, 1954.

Andrade, R.: Benign juvenile melanoma: Several selected aspects from a study of 51 lesions. *In* XII Congressus Internat. Dermatol., München, 1967. Berlin, Springer-Verlag, 1968.

Andrade, R.: El Concepto de Seudomalignidad. Proc. VI Ibero-Latino Am. Congr. Derm. Barcelona, Editorial Cientifico-Médica, 1970, p. 333–348.

Attie, J. N., and Khafif, R. A.: Melanotic Tumors. Springfield, Ill., Charles C Thomas, Publisher, 1964.

Bandiera, D. C.: Névo giante pigmentado com transformacao maligna. Rev. Brasil. Cirurg., 54:120, 1967.

Battin, J., Vital, C., Alberty, J., Guyonnet-Duperat, J. P., Leger, H., and Fontan, A.: La melanose neuro-cutanee. Arch. Fr. Pediatr., 25:277, 1968.

Becker, S. W.: Pitfalls in diagnosis and treatment of melanomas. Arch. Dermatol., 69:11, 1954.

Becker, S. W., and Becker, S. W., Jr.: Personal communication to W. B. Reed. Giant pigmented nevi, melanoma and leptomeningeal melanocytosis. Arch.Dermatol., 91:100, 1965.

Bieberstein, H.: Naevotumor. Z. Haut. Geschlechtskr., 17:274, 1925.

Brodsky, L., Baren, M., Kahn, S., Lewis, G., Jr., and Tellum, M.: Metastatic malignant melanoma from mother to fetus. Cancer, 18:1048, 1965.

Brunck, J.: Über ein Metastasierenden, Aber Klinisch Gutartig Verlaufenden Naevus Mit Blasig Entarteten Naevuszellen und Über Deren Genese. Arch. Dermatol. Syph. (Berl.), 196:170, 1953.

Cahalane, S. F., and Meenan, F. O. C.: Benign juvenile melanoma: A clinical and pathological survey. Irish J. Med. Sci., 2:489, 1969.

Carol, W. L. L.: Amelanosarkom. Z. Haut. Geschlechtskr., 35:792, 1931.

Cavell, B.: Transplacental metastasis of malignant melanoma. Acta Paediatr. (Suppl.), 146:37, 1963.

Clark, W. H., Jr., From, L., Bernardino, E. A., and Mihm, M. C.: The histogenesis and biologic behavior of primary human malignant melanomas of the skin. Cancer Res., 29:705, 1969.

Cleaver, J. E.: Defective repair replication of DNA in xeroderma pigmentosum. Nature (Lond.), 218:652, 1968.

Cochran, A. J.: Studies of the melanocytes of the epidermis adjacent to tumors. J. Invest. Dermatol., 57:38, 1971.

Coffey, R. J., and Berkeley, W. T.: Prepubertal malignant melanoma: Report of a case. J.A.M.A., 147:846, 1951.

Conway, H.: Bathing trunk nevus. Surgery, 6:585, 1939.

Coskey, R. J., and Mehregan, A.: Spindle cell nevi in adults and children. Arch. Dermatol., 108:535, 1973.

Couperus, M., and Rucker, R. C.: Histopathological diagnosis of malignant melanoma. Arch. Dermatol., 70:199, 1954.

Dabska, M.: Melanoma juvenile. Nowotwory, 6:103, 1956.

Dailly, R., Forthhomme, J., Samson, M., Tayot, J., Clement, J. C., and Morin, C.: Melanose neuro-cutanée a l'évolution tumorale. Presse Med., 73:2867, 1965.

Dargeon, H. W., Eversole, J. W., and Del Duca, V.: Malignant melanoma in an infant. Cancer, 3:299, 1950.

Darier, J.: Des Naevocarcinomes. Bull. Assoc. Fr. Etude Cancer, 6:145, 1913.

Darier, J., and Civatte, A.: Naevus ou naevo-carcinome chez un nourisson. Bull. Soc. Fr. Dermatol. Syphiligr., 21:61, 1910.

Degos, R.: Naevus cellulaire prépubertaire. *In* Dermatologie. Paris, Flammarion, 1958, pp. 760a and 760b.

Delacrétaz, J.: Mélanome juvénile (mélanome de Spitz) à l'évolution maligne. Dermatologica, 139:79, 1969.

Delacrétaz, J., and Jaeger, H.: Sur deux cas de mélanomes juvéniles (de Spitz). Oncologia, 10:80, 1957.

Dickson, R. J.: Malignant melanoma. Am. J. Roentgenol., 79:1063,1958.

Dobson, L.: Prepubertal malignant melanomas. Am. J. Surg., 80:1128, 1955.

Doepfmer, R.: Sogenannte juvenile melanome. Hautarzt, 11:39, 1960.

Du Bois: Corpus iconum morborum cutaneorum. *In* Nekam, L. (Ed.): München, Johann Ambrosius Barth, 1938.

Duperrat, B.: Le mélanome juvénile. Bull. Soc. Fr. Dermatol. Syphiligr., 62:500, 1955.

Duperrat, B., and Mascaro, J. M.: Étude anatomo-clinique de quatre cas de "tumeur de Spitz" de l'adulte. Bull. Soc. Fr. Dermatol. Syphiligr., 68:472, 1961.

Duperrat, B., and Dufourmentel, C.: Étude du mélanome juvénile d'après 40 cas personnels. Minerva Dermatol., 34:190, 1959.

Duverne, J., and Pruniéras, M.: Trois cas de mélanome juvénile. Bull. Soc. Fr. Dermatol. Syphiligr., 63:259, 1956a.

Duverne, J., and Pruniéras, M.: Trois cas de mélanome juvénile. Lyon Med., 88:442, 1956b.

Echevarria, R., and Ackerman, L. V.: Spindle and epithelioid cell nevi in the adult—Clinicopathologic report of 26 cases. Cancer, 20:175, 1967.

Efskind, J., and Nitter, L.: A follow-up examination of 543 patients with malignant melanoma. Acta Un. Int. Cancr., 19:1542, 1963.

Ellsworth, R. M.: Juvenile melanoma of the uvea. Trans. Am. Acad. Ophthalmol., 64:148, 1960.

Fish, J., Smith, E. B., and Canby, J. P.: Malignant melanoma in childhood. Surgery, 59:309, 1966.

Fox, H., Emery, J. L., Goodbody, R. A., and Yates, P. O.: Neuro-cutaneous melanosis. Arch. Dis. Child., 39:508, 1964.

Freedman, W. L., and McMahon, F. J.: Placental metastasis. Obstet. Gynecol., 16:550, 1960.

Furuya, T., Kawada, A., Sekido, N., and Nobuko, S.: A case of malignant melanoma developing in giant nevus. Jap. J. Dermatol. (Series B), 77:94, 1967.

Fuste, R., and Morales, L. M.: Degeneración maligna de un nevi pigmentario giante de la espalda. Rev. Med. Cuba., 55:307, 1944.

Gans, O., and Steigleder, G. K.: Histologie der Hautkrankheiten. Berlin, Springer-Verlag, 1957.

Gartmann, H.: Das sog. Juvenile Melanom. Munch. Med. Wochenschr., 104:587, 1962.

Gartmann, H.: Benignes juveniles Melanom. *In* Braun-Falco, O., and Petzoldt, D. (Eds.): Fortschritte der praktischen Dermatologie und Venerologie. Vol. 7. Berlin, Springer-Verlag, 1973, pp. 66–72.

Gartmann, H., and Thurm, K: Juveniles Melanom der Augenbindehaut. Dermatol. Wochenschr., 142:805, 1960.

Gertler, W.: Faszikulaerer Spindelzellnaevus. Dermatol. Wochenschr., 133:110, 1956.

Greeley, P. W., and Curtin, J. W.: Giant pigmented nevi. GP, 34:132, 1966.

Greeley, P. W., Middleton, A. G., and Curtin, J. W.: Incidence of malignancy in giant pigmented nevi. Plast. Reconstr. Surg., 36:26, 1965.

Groothuis, F. B. G.: Melanomata juvenilia. Dermatologica (Basel), 119:61, 1959.

Gross, P. R., and Carter, D. M.: Malignant melanoma arising in a giant cerebriform nevus. Arch. Dermatol., 96:536, 1967.

Grupper, C., and Tubiana, R.: Mélanome juvénile

de Spitz ou pseudomélanome. Bull. Soc. Fr. Dermatol. Syphiligr., 62:300, 1955.

Helwig, E. B.: Seminar in skin neoplasms and dermatoses. *In* Proceedings of the Twentieth Seminar of The American Society of Clinical Pathologists, Washington, D.C., September 11, 1954, pp. 61–74. Washington, D.C., American Society of Clinical Pathologists, 1955.

Hendrix, R. C.: Juvenile melanomas, benign and malignant. Arch. Pathol., 58:636, 1954.

Herzberg, J. J.: Zur Diagnostik und Therapie der Melanocytoblastome. Arch. Klin. Exp. Dermatol., 203:142, 1956.

Hoffman, H. J., and Freeman, A.: Primary malignant leptomeningeal melanoma in association with giant hairy nevi. J. Neurosurg., 26:62, 1967.

Holland, E.: A case of transplacental metastasis of malignant melanoma from mother to foetus. J. Obstet. Gynaecol. Br. Emp., 56:529, 1949.

Hornstein, O.: "Blasenzell Naevus." Arch. Klin. Exp. Dermatol., 226:97, 1966.

Jakubowicz, K.: Uber Die Zugehorigkeit Des Sogenannten Juvenilen Melanomas Zur Gruppe de Aktiven Nevuszellnaevus. Hautarzt, 16:411, 1965.

Jernstrom, P., and Aponte, G. E.: Juvenile melanoma of the tongue. Am. J. Clin. Pathol., 26:1341, 1956.

Jones, S. T., and Dukes, T. E.: Juvenile melanoma of the eyelid. Am. J. Ophthalmol., 56:816, 1963.

Kawamura, T., Morioka, S., Kukita, A., Kawada, A., and Taniguchi, K.: So-called juvenile melanoma and its allied conditions. Jap. J. Dermatol., 72:67, 1962.

Kernen, J. A., and Ackerman, L. V.: Spindle cell nevi and epithelioid cell nevi (so-called juvenile melanomas) in children and adults. Cancer, 13:612, 1960.

Kopf, A. W.: Pigmented nevi and hemangiomas. *In* Traumatic Medicine and Surgery for the Attorney. London, Butterworth & Co., Ltd., 1962.

Kopf, A. W., and Andrade, R.: Benign juvenile melanoma. *In* Year Book of Dermatology, 1965–66. Chicago, Year Book Medical Publishers, 1966.

Kopf, A. W., Morrill, S. D., and Silberberg, I.: Broad spectrum of leukoderma acquisitum centrifugum. Arch. Dermatol., 92:14, 1965.

Korting, G. W., Brehm, G., and Nurnberger, F.: Zur Klinishen Variationsbreite Des Sog. Juvenilen Melanoms. Z. Haut. Geschlechtskr., 43:233, 1968.

Lane, N., Lattes, R., and Malm, J.: Clinicopathological correlations in a series of 117 malignant melanomas of the skin in adults. Cancer, 11:1025, 1958.

Lerman, R. I., Murray, D., O'Hara, J. M., Booner, K. J., and Foote, F. W., Jr.: Malignant melanoma of childhood. Cancer, 25:436, 1970.

Lorétan, R. M., and Delacrétaz, J.: Le prognostic du mélanome malin infantile. Ann. Dermatol. Syphiligr. (Paris), 94:465, 1967.

Lund, H. Z., and Kraus, J. M.: Melanotic tumors of the skin. Atlas of Tumor Pathology, Section 1, Fascicle 3. Washington, D.C., Armed Forces Institute of Pathology, 1962.

Lyall, D.: Malignant melanoma in infancy. J.A.M.A., 202:1153, 1967.

McGovern, V. J., and Goulston, E.: Malignant moles in childhood. Med. J. Aust., 1:181, 1963.

McNeer, G. P., and Das Gupta, T.: Prognosis in malignant melanoma. Surgery, 56:512, 1964.

McWhorter, H. E., and Woolner, L. B.: Pigmented nevi, juvenile melanomas, and malignant melanomas in children. Cancer, 7:564, 1954.

McWhorter, H. E., Figi, F. A., and Woolner, L. B.: Treatment of juvenile melanomas and malignant melanomas in children. J.A.M.A., 156:695, 1954.

Melczer, N., and Kiss, J.: Zur Frühzeitigen Erkennung von Melanoblastomen. Dermatologica, 117:242, 1958.

Miescher, G.: Melanom. *In* Jadassohn, J.: Handbuch der Hautund Geschlechtskrankheiten. XII, 3, Berlin, Springer-Verlag, 1933, p. 1005.

Milian, G., Perin, L., and Brunel: Naevo-carcinome de la région pariéto-temporale, chez un enfant de 12 ans. Bull. Soc. Fr. Dermatol. Syphiligr., 39:1327, 1932.

Mishima, Y.: Melanotic tumors, *In* Zelickson, A. S. (Ed.): Ultrastructure of Normal and Abnormal Skin. Philadelphia, Lea and Febiger, 1967.

Montgomery, H.: Die Histopathologische Unterscheidung der Pigmentnaevi, Juvenilen Melanome und Melanomalignome. Hautarzt, 9:52, 1958.

Montgomery, H.: In discussion of paper by Costello, M. J., Fisher, S. B., and De Feo, C. P.: Melanotic freckle. A. M. A. Arch. Dermatol., 80:768, 1959.

Oddoze, M. L.: À propos d'un cas de mélanome juvénile de Spitz. Bull. Soc. Fr. Dermatol. Syphiligr., 66:255, 1959.

Oldhoff, J., and Koudstaal, J.: Congenital papillomatous malignant melanoma of the skin. Cancer, 21:1193, 1968.

Pack, G. T.: Prepubertal melanoma of skin. Surg. Gynecol. Obstet., 86:374, 1948.

Pack, G. T., and Anglem, T. J.: Tumors of the soft tissues in infancy and childhood. J. Pediatr., 15:372, 1939.

Pack, G. T., and Davis, J.: Nevus giganticus pigmentosus with malignant transformation. Surgery, 49:347, 1961.

Pack, G. T., and Scharnagel, I. M.: Prognosis for malignant melanoma in the pregnant woman. Cancer, 4:324, 1951.

Pack, G. T., Perzik, S. L., and Scharnagel, I. M.: The treatment of malignant melanoma: Report of 862 cases. Calif. Med., 66:283, 1947.

Pers, M.: Naevus pigmentosus giganticus. Ugeskr. Laeger, 125:613, 1963.

Potter, J. F., and Schoeneman, M.: Metastasis of maternal cancer to the placenta and fetus. Cancer, 25:380, 1970.

Reed, W. B., Becker, J. W., Jr., Becker, S. W., Jr., Whiting, I., and Nickel, W. R.: Giant pigmented nevi melanoma, and leptomeningeal melanocytosis. Arch. Dermatol., 91:100, 1965.

Russell, J. L., and Reyes, R. G.: Giant pigmented nevi. J.A.M.A., 171:2083, 1959.

Saksela, E., and Rintala, A.: Misdiagnosis of prepubertal malignant melanoma. Cancer, 22:1308, 1968.

Samuels, S. L.: Juvenile melanoma of the iris. Trans. Am. Acad. Ophthalmol. Otolaryngol., 67:718, 1963.

Schrader, W. A., and Helwig, E. B.: Balloon cell nevi. Cancer, 20:1502, 1967.

Schultz, R. C.: Fatal malignant melanoma in children

with giant nevi. Plast. Reconstr. Surg., 27:551, 1961.

Schumachers-Brendler, R.: Beitrag zur Klinik und Histologie der Naevi Naevocellulares sowie des Juvenilen Melanoms. Arch. Klin. Exp. Dermatol., 217:600, 1963.

Shaffer, B.: The melanocytic (pigmented) nevus. J. Chronic Dis., 6:109, 1957.

Shaw, M. H.: Malignant melanoma arising from a giant hairy nevus. Br. J. Plast. Surg., 15:426, 1962.

Skov-Jensen, T., Hastrup, J., and Lambrethsen, E.: Malignant melanoma in children. Cancer, 19:620, 1966.

Spitz, S.: Melanomas of childhood. Am. J. Pathol., 24:591, 1948.

Stegmaier, O.: Natural regression of the melanocytic nevus. J. Invest. Dermatol., 32:413, 1959.

Stegmaier, O. C., and Montgomery, H.: Histopathologic studies of pigmented nevi in children. J. Invest. Dermatol., 20:51, 1953.

Steigleder, G. K., and Wellmer, K.: Zur Abtrennung Des Sogenannten Juvenile Melanom. Arch. Klin. Exper. Dermatol., 202:556, 1956.

Sylven, B.: Malignant melanoma of the skin. Acta Radiol. (Stockh.), 32:33, 1949.

Szabó, G.: Quantitative histological investigations on the melanocyte system of the human epidermis. *In* Gordon, M. (Ed.): Pigment Cell Biology. New York, Academic Press, 1959.

Touraine, A.: Les melanoses neurocutanées. Ann. Dermatol. Syphiligr. (Paris), 9:489, 1949.

Traub, E. F.: Melanoma. Arch. Dermatol., 59:349, 1949.

Unna, P. G.: Die Histopathologie der Hautkrankheiten. Berlin, A. Hirschwald, 1894.

Van der Heul, R. O., Blok, A. P. R., Zwaveling, A., and Westbroek, D. L.: Histologische Diagnostiek Van Maligne Melanoom BIJ Kinderen. Ned. Tijdschr. Geneeskd., 110:1376, 1966.

Van der Hoeve, T.: Eye diseases in tuberose sclerosis of the brain. Trans. Ophthalmol. Soc. U. K., 43:534, 1923.

Walther, D.: Juveniles Melanon (Randrezidiv un Narbe). Dermatol. Wochenschr., 140:801, 1959.

Weber, F. P. Schwarz, E., and Hellenschmied, R.: Spontaneous innoculation of melanomatic sarcoma from mother to foetus. Br. Med. J., 1:537, 1930.

Webster, J. P., Stevenson, T. W., and Stout, A. P.: The surgical treatment of malignant melanomas of the skin. Surg. Clin. North Am., 24:319, 1944.

Wells, G. C., and Farthing, G. J.: Juvenile melanoma, a histochemical study. Br. J. Dermatol., 78:380, 1966.

Wells, G. C., Magnus, I. A., and Farthing, G. J.: Cholinesterase in moles. Br. J. Dermatol., 78:376, 1966.

Winkelmann, R. K.: Cholinesterase nevus: Cholinestrases in pigmented tumors of the skin. Arch. Dermatol., 82:17, 1960.

Winkelmann, R. K.: Juvenile melanoma. Cancer, 14:1001, 1961.

Woringer, F.: À propos d'un naevus achromique de la joue chez une fillette de 8 ans. Bull. Soc. Fr. Dermatol. Syphiligr., 46:550, 1939.

Woringer, F.: Le mélanome juvénile de Spitz. Sem. Hôp. Paris, 32:1723, 1956.

Woringer, F.: L'évolution d'une tumeur de Spitz. Bull. Soc. Fr. Dermatol. Syphiligr., 70:246, 1963.

Woringer, F., and Alt, J.: À propos des mélanomes malins prépubertaires. Congres Derm. Syph. Lgue. Fr. Lausanne. IXe:152, 1956.

Yagawa, K., and Nakamura, K.: An autopsy case of the widely metastasized juvenile malignant melanoma arising from "naevus pigmentosus." Gann, 45:278, 1954.

32

Keratoacanthoma

Clinical Aspects

Alfred W. Kopf, M.D.

SYNONYMS

Keratoacanthomas have been described under a number of appellations, including crateriform ulcer of the face (Hutchinson, 1889); verrucome (Gougerot, 1929); kyste sébacé atypique (Dupont, 1930); multiple, primary squamous cell carcinomas of the skin with spontaneous healing (Smith, 1934); molluscum sebaceum (MacCormac and Scarff, 1936); tumorlike keratoses (Poth, 1939); idiopathic, cutaneous, pseudoepitheliomatous hyperplasia (Grinspan and Abulafia, 1955); keratoacanthosis (Helwig, 1955); molluscum pseudocarcinomatosum (Linell and Mansson, 1958); inverted wart (Brothers et al., 1960); and pseudocarcinoma (Peterkin et al., 1962).

DEFINITION

Keratoacanthoma is a benign neoplasm which, both clinically and histologically, closely resembles squamous cell carcinoma. Thus it is one of the lesions belonging to the group of pseudocancers or, in this case, pseudocarcinomas (Andrade,

1970). Its benign nature is indicated by the fact that spontaneous involution is the rule, and metastases do not occur.

HISTORY

St. Peregrine, the cancer saint, as a young priest suffered a cancer on his leg and was scheduled for operation. The night before he prayed fervently to be saved from amputation, and he dreamed he was cured. On awakening he discovered that it was more than a mere dream—he was completely cured. He lived to his 80th year, dying in 1345 without further evidence of cancer.

—Brown and Fryer, 1955

Probably the first descriptions of keratoacanthoma are to be found in the writings of Sir Jonathan Hutchinson (1888–1897). Originally, he reported cases (Fig. 32–1) under the names "peculiar form of skin cancer" and "acute epithelial cancer," but later settled on "crateriform ulcer." One wonders why these observations by this master clinician remained buried in the literature for so many decades

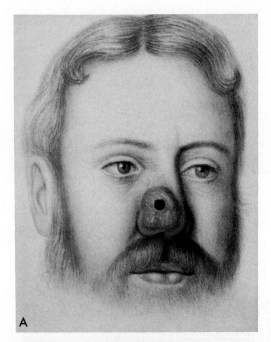

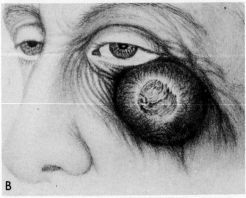

Figure 32–1 Hutchinson's illustrations of keratoacanthomas *(A,* 1888; *B,* 1889).

(Hjorth, 1960). Perhaps it was his use of the misleading word "ulcer" in the title he chose, since, as we shall see, keratoacanthomas rarely ulcerate. In 1893 Lassar described "cutaneous epitheliomas healed by arsenical," which Furtado (1962) believed were probable keratoacanthomas. Gougerot et al. (1929) mentioned under the title "verrucome" a number of patients who developed epitheliomatous structures that responded to the antisyphilitic therapy. Although these lesions were probably keratoacanthomas, it is disturbing to note that the patients pre-

sented with associated lymphadenopathy, a feature not encountered in patients with keratoacanthoma. Dupont (1930) described similar lesions as "atypical sebaceous cysts" (kyste sébacé atypique). Shortly thereafter, Dunn and Smith (1934) described a case under the title "self-healing primary squamous carcinoma of the skin," and MacCormac and Scarff (1936) called this tumor "molluscum sebaceum." The appellation "keratoacanthoma" was coined by Freudenthal in the late 1930's (for historical note see Baer and Kopf, 1963). Other terms include familial, primary, self-healing squamous epithelioma of the skin (Sommerville and Milne, 1950); diverticule epidermique à paroi végétante (Dupont, 1952); molluscum pseudocarcinomatosum (Editorial, Lancet, 1953); benign keratoacanthoma (Winer, 1955); idiopathic, cutaneous, pseudoepitheliomatous hyperplasia (Grinspan and Abulafia, 1955); and squamous cell pseudoepithelioma (Duany, 1958).

All the above terms refer to the "solitary" variety of keratoacanthoma. Historically, the "multiple" type was first described by Smith (1934) and the "eruptive" type by Grzybowski (1950). As the spectrum of clinical and histologic variants constantly broadens, the number of historical landmarks increases. Additional highlights and references are found under the section Unusual Variants of Keratoacanthomas in this chapter.

Probably the first American report on keratoacanthoma was that of Poth (1939), who described under the title "tumor-like keratoses" what appears to be a peculiar localized variant of multiple keratoacanthomas on the dorsa of the hands. Stenhouse and Becker (1942) reported the first American case of the Ferguson Smith type of keratoacanthoma. The greatest impetus to the flood of papers on this subject that appeared in the last 20 years was the paper of Levy et al. (1954).

Several reviews have recently appeared on the subject of keratoacanthoma which provide greater details on many aspects of this fascinating tumor (Baer and Kopf, 1963; Furtado, 1962; Lapière, 1965; Nazzaro and Tosti, 1968; Baptista, 1964; Rook and Champion, 1963).

EPIDEMIOLOGY

Apparently the same factors that predispose man to epithelial skin cancers play a role in solitary keratoacanthoma, since this tumor tends to afflict persons of light complexion on sun-exposed cutaneous sites (Whittle and Davis, 1957). Belisario (1959, 1965a and 1965b) noted that keratoacanthomas are more frequent in sunny Sydney than in less sunny Melbourne, Australia. Unfortunately, valid statistics concerning the worldwide prevalence of this tumor are not available, because the entity has been so confused with squamous cell carcinoma that meaningful statistics have not been accumulated and analyzed. Yet the distinct impression is that keratoacanthomas are far more common in Caucasians in sunny climates (Oettlé, 1963). The tumor has been reported in Japanese, Indian, Burmese, and Negro patients (Belisario, personal communication and 1965a and 1965b; Rajam et al., 1958). In a review of 592 solitary keratoacanthomas, only 20 were on non–sun-exposed cutaneous sites (Baer and Kopf, 1963). Rook and Champion (1963) found no keratoacanthomas in women on the ears or lips, which are relatively sun-protected areas in the sex. In contrast, of the keratoacanthomas in the men included their series, 11 percent were on the ear and 12 percent on the lips. This anatomic distribution reinforces the importance of exposure to the elements in the epidemiology of the solitary type of keratoacanthoma.

ETIOLOGIC FACTORS

Considerable evidence has accumulated to suggest that keratoacanthomas may be caused by a virus (Cipollaro, 1964; Ereaux et al., 1955; Forck et al., 1965; Sagebiel, 1966; Thivolet et al., 1966; Zelickson and Lynch, 1961; Zelickson, 1962). Clinically, an infectious agent is suggested by reports of juxtaposed ("kissing") lesions on the lips (Ereaux et al., 1955), by onset at sites of herpes simplex (Ereaux et al., 1955; Whittle and Davis, 1957), by the development of keratoacanthomas at sites of trauma (Clendenning and Auerbach,

1963; Elschner, 1956; Lloyd and Hall, 1969), by their appearance on donor or recipient graft sites, or both (Anderson, 1957; Brown and Fryer, 1955; Bruner, 1963; Diben and Fowler, 1955; Pillsbury and Beerman, 1958; Wilson, 1956), and by spontaneous involution.

Gay Prieto and coworkers (1964, 1969) reported electronmicroscopic findings of nuclear "viruslike" inclusion bodies in keratoacanthoma cells of five patients. In addition, dense, round, or oval elements were observed in the cytoplasm of such cells. They inoculated the tissues on HeLa or KB cell cultures, which resulted in severe cytopathogenic effect within four to five days. Inoculation of these cultures onto chick chorioallantoic membrane resulted in proliferation and acanthosis of the epithelium and appearance of histologically malignant epithelial tumors. These experimental tumors also had cellular inclusion bodies. When extracts from the chick eggs were reinoculated into the HeLa or KB cell cultures, cytopathogenic effects were again seen.

Despite these reports of the demonstration of virus or viruslike inclusions, repeated attempts to inoculate fragments of this tumor into normal skin in experimental animals (Gougerot, 1929; Grzybowski, 1950; Kopf and Silberberg, 1963; Marshall and Findlay, 1953; Poth, 1939) and in man (Beare, 1953; Binazzi & Finzi, 1960; Doepfmer, 1962; Ereaux et al., 1955; Ewing, 1956; Gay Prieto, 1964; Grzybowski, 1950; Kopf and Silberberg, 1963; Oliver, 1958; Poth, 1939) have failed to transmit this neoplasm. Some investigators have been unable to demonstrate virus or viruslike inclusion bodies in keratoacanthoma (Furtado, 1962; Jakubowicz et al., 1970), and others have found them in unrelated dermatoses, such as neurotic excoriations, psoriasis, and condyloma acuminatum (Nasemann, 1965). These reports cast doubt on the specificity of the virus-like inclusions reported in keratoacanthomas.

A number of other etiologic factors have been considered, including tar and oil products (Becker, 1955; Colomb et al., 1966; Ghadially, 1958 and 1959; Ghadially et al., 1963; de Moragas, 1966; Peterkin et al., 1962; Vickers and Ghadially,

1961), thermal burn or exposure (Baran, 1957; Ereaux et al., 1955; Pillsbury and Beerman, 1958), sunlight (Belisario, 1965b; de Moragas et al., 1958; Pillsbury and Beerman, 1958; Poth, 1939; Sommerville and Milne, 1950; Venkei and Sugár, 1958), trauma (Elschner, 1956; Friedman et al., 1965; Pillsbury and Beerman, 1958; Svejda and Schwartz, 1960), podophyllin (Nelson, 1959), smoking and air pollution (Ghadially et al., 1963), and carcinogens (Ghadially, 1958 and 1959; Prutkin and Gerstner, 1966; Rous and Kidd, 1941; Solomon and Beerman, 1964; Van Duuren et al., 1967; Whitely, 1957).

An immunologic response to extracts prepared from keratoacanthomas has been demonstrated (Nicolau et al., 1963), which raises hope for the development of a specific skin test in the future.

Hereditary (or familial) factors appear to play a role in the pathogenesis of multiple keratoacanthomas (Charteris, 1951; Machacek, 1957; Smith, 1948; Sommerville and Milne, 1950; Tarnowski, 1966). However, the precise mode of inheritance (or spread of an etiologic agent) has not been determined. Finally, a nevoid factor is suggested by those exceptional cases of unilateral distribution of keratoacanthomas (Marshall and Pepler, 1954).

INCIDENCE

There is a marked discrepancy in published figures on the relative incidence of keratoacanthoma versus squamous cell carcinoma. In our compilation of 17 publications on this subject, the authors reported 3866 squamous cell carcinomas versus 883 (18 percent) keratoacanthomas (for details see Baer and Kopf, 1963). In these reports the percentage of keratoacanthomas in the combined squamous cell carcinoma–keratoacanthoma figures varied from 2 percent to 62 percent. This wide range may reflect geographic, occupational, racial, or health-care differences, but undoubtedly it also involves an element of variability in interpretation, since the differential diagnosis of keratoacanthoma and squamous cell carcinoma clinically and histologically is difficult and open to personal interpretation.

In the Oncology Section of the Skin and Cancer Unit, of a total of 5719 lesions coded between 1955 and 1962, there were 219 (3.8 percent) squamous cell carcinomas and 55 (1 percent) keratoacanthomas. Thus, in our material, 20 percent of the combined squamous cell carcinoma–keratoacanthoma group were keratoacanthomas. It should be pointed out, however, that included in the squamous cell carcinomas above were a large number of lesions diagnosed as solar keratosis with "early squamous cell carcinoma," tumors which are rarely biologically aggressive in terms of metastases or lethal outcome. Huriez et al. (1961) reviewed 1002 tumors seen in the Lille Clinic in France during a six-year period and found 54.3 percent basal cell epitheliomas, 38.2 percent squamous cell carcinomas, 2.8 percent keratoacanthomas, 2.1 percent malignant melanomas, and 2.0 percent other cancers. On the other hand, Rook and Champion (1963) cited two large series in which the ratio of keratoacanthoma to squamous cell carcinoma was 1:3, and Rossman and coworkers (1964), in reviewing 1100 cases, found a ratio of 1:4.7.

Almost all the articles on keratoacanthoma have been written in the past two decades. This might imply that we are currently experiencing an "epidemic," which, if a viral etiology is correct, would be conceivable. However, Rook (1962), in reviewing old histologic material, concludes the incidence of keratoacanthoma has not increased, at least in Britain.

CLINICAL DESCRIPTION

There are three types of keratoacanthomas that have been described—*solitary, multiple,* and *eruptive* (Figs. 32–2 to 32–7). The solitary type is by far the most common, and thousands of cases have now been reported. In contrast, less than 100 cases of multiple keratoacanthoma and only seven cases of the eruptive variety are recorded. Table 32–1 summarizes the salient features of the two most common types.

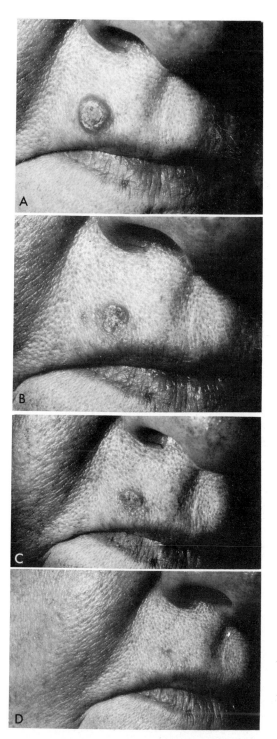

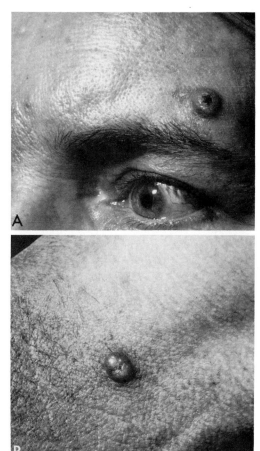

Figure 32–3 *A*, Typical keratoacanthoma with central keratotic core set into crater. *B*, Atypical keratoacanthoma with unusually small central opening.

Figure 32–2 Natural history of solitary keratoacanthoma. *A*, Typical lesion of two months' duration. Photograph taken 12/19/57. *B*, After incisional biopsy, removing only portion of tumor 1/9/58. *C*, Lesion disappearing 1/23/58. It was gone two weeks later. *D*, Follow-up. Complete spontaneous regression 6/5/58.

In the eruptive type of keratoacanthoma the patient develops thousands of lesions scattered over the integument (Grzybowski, 1950; Jolly and Carpenter, 1966; Rossman et al., 1954; Winkelmann and Brown, 1968; Witten and Zak, 1952). Unique features occurring in eruptive keratoacanthoma are: (1) generalized distribution, (2) innumerable lesions, (3) linear groups of lesions, (4) masked facies with ectropion, (5) mucosal lesions, and (6) severe pruritus. Of interest is the fact that at least four of the seven reported patients have died of various systemic ailments; none died of cutaneous cancer.

Whether solitary, multiple, or eruptive, the primary lesion of keratoacanthoma is identical. The tumor has its onset as a small red macule, which soon becomes a firm papule with scaling on its summit.

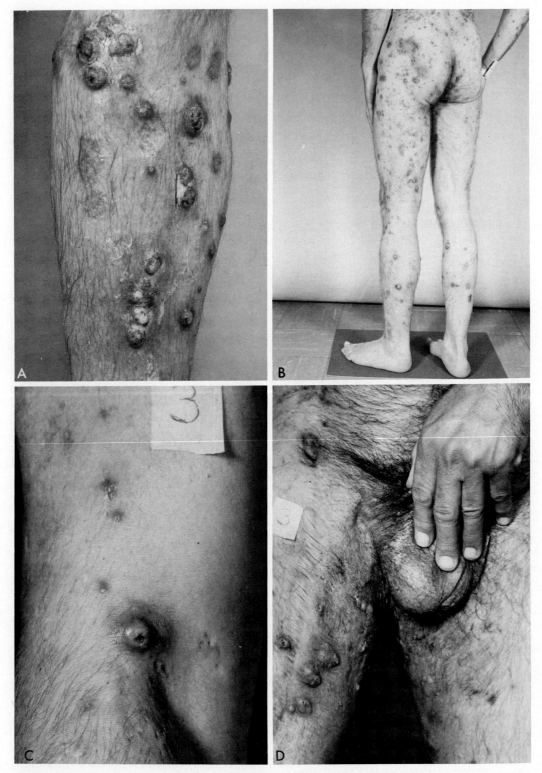

Figure 32–4   Multiple keratoacanthoma. *A* and *B*, Numerous nodules and scars from previous lesions that have regressed. *C* and *D*, Brother of patient depicted in *A* and *B*. (Courtesy of Dr. William Tarnowski. *A from* Tarnowski: Arch. Dermatol., 94:74, 1966.)

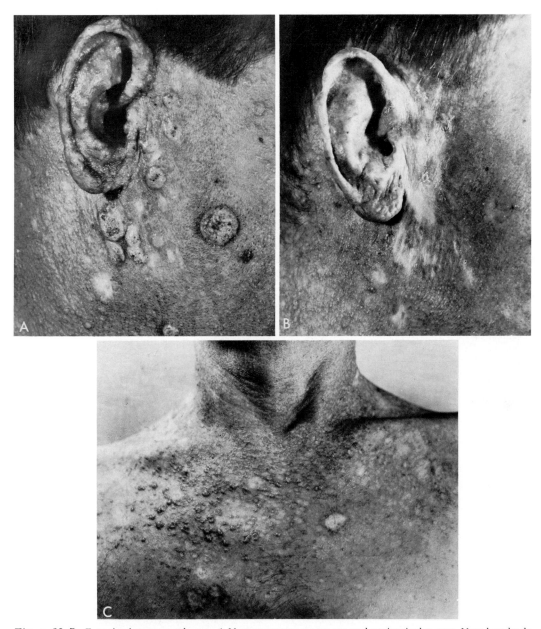

Figure 32–5 Eruptive keratoacanthoma. *A*, Numerous tumors on ear and periauricular area. Note hundreds of smaller papules in background. *B*, Scars at sites of previous larger nodules. *C*, Thousands of 1- to 4-mm. keratoacanthomas on neck and chest. (Courtesy of Dr. S. Jablonska. *From* Grzybowski: Br. J. Dermatol., 62:310, 1950, by permission of H. K. Lewis & Co., Ltd.)

This papule rapidly enlarges for approximately two to eight weeks and, already early in its course, presents as a round, firm, elevated, hemispheric, skin-colored to pink, asymptomatic (or slightly tender or pruritic) nodule with a central plug of keratin in its summit (Figs. 32–2 and 32–3). Thus the lesion can be likened to a giant molluscum contagiosum or to a volcano with a stopper of hardened lava in its central crater. The keratinous plug is usually firmly imbedded in its cup-shaped crater. The fully developed keratoacanthoma is 0.5 to 2.0 cm. in diameter and has gently sloping, smooth, shiny, nontranslucent borders which merge imperceptibly

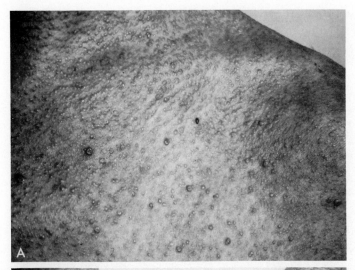

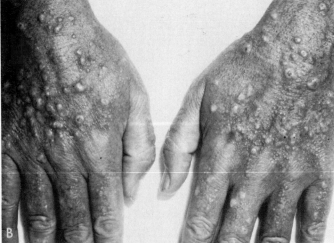

Figure 32–6 Eruptive keratoacanthoma. *A*, Myriad lesions on the chest. *B*, Numerous typical lesions on the dorsa of the hands. (*From* Witten and Zak: Cancer, 5:539, 1952.)

with the surrounding normal skin. At times the base of the lesion is surrounded by a zone of erythema. Fine telangiectases often run up over the surface of the tumor from its border. With rare exceptions, the tumor remains freely movable over the underlying structures. Following the period of maximal growth, the lesion remains stationary for a two- to eight-week period, after which it slowly undergoes spontaneous involution over another two- to eight-week period (Fig. 32–2). Thus the entire process from initiation to spontaneous disappearance can be divided into three phases: (1) growth phase, (2) stationary phase, and (3) phase of spontaneous involution. All this occurs in two to eight months and is often accomplished without bleeding at any stage.

However, it should be pointed out that some keratoacanthomas require much longer to involute (e.g., Venkei and Sugár, 1958, record a lesion requiring five years), and some to ulcerate. Involution takes place by expulsion of the corneous plug and resorption of the tumor mass. At the site a characteristic, somewhat depressed, often crenellated, hypopigmented, alopecic scar remains (Fig. 32–2). The borders are often slightly overhanging, which gives the scar such a characteristic appearance that the experienced observer will consider the diagnosis based on the healed scar alone.

The *age distribution* for solitary keratoacanthoma is wide, but most lesions occur in patients in the sixth and seventh decades of life. Almost all patients are over

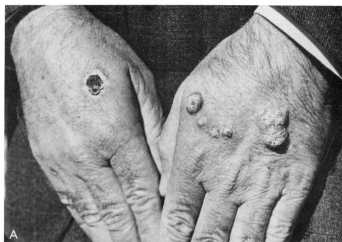

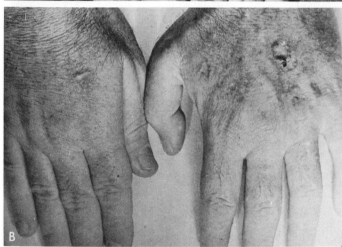

Figure 32–7 Tumorlike keratoses. (*From* Poth: Arch. Dermatol., 39:228, 1939.)

age 45. However, the tumor has been reported in children and even infants (Binazzi and Finzi, 1960; Binazzi and Miranda, 1965; Brown and Rentiers, 1969; Carteaud and Baptista, 1962b; Champion and Rook, 1963; Jackson and Williamson, 1961; Lapière, 1954 and 1955; Thompson, 1958).

The *anatomic distribution* of solitary keratoacanthomas involves primarily sun-exposed sites. In our review of 592 lesions (Baer and Kopf, 1963), the following distributions were reported: *face* (71 percent)—cheeks (27.2 percent), nose (16.9 percent), eyelids (5.6 percent), forehead (3.9 percent), lips (3.4 percent), chin (3.4 percent), temples (2.2 percent), eyebrows (0.3 percent), unspecified sites (8.1 percent); *sites other than the face*—hands (10.3 percent), wrists (4.4 percent), forearms (4.0 percent), neck (4.0 percent), ears (2.9

percent), trunk (1.4 percent), mastoid (0.7 percent), scalp (0.7 percent), lower extremity (0.3 percent), perianal area (0.3 percent).

UNUSUAL VARIANTS OF KERATOACANTHOMA

In addition to the three principal types of keratoacanthoma (solitary, multiple, eruptive), unusual variants have been described as our clinical acumen sharpens concerning this unusual tumor. These variants are claimed to be keratoacanthomas based on clinicopathologic correlations. However, not until the etiology and pathogenesis of these lesions are established will we be in the position to verify these impressions.

TABLE 32–1 DISTINGUISHING CLINICAL FEATURES OF SOLITARY AND
MULTIPLE FORMS OF KERATOACANTHOMA

Feature	Localized Keratoacanthoma	Multiple Keratoacanthoma
Incidence	common, perhaps 1/10 to 1/2 in incidence of squamous cell carcinoma	rare (less than 100 cases reported)
Age of onset	usually in 6th and 7th decades	begins in adolescence or early adult life
Sex distribution	equal or slightly greater incidence in males	greater incidence in males (70 per cent)
Number of lesions	usually single, rarely more than three	multiple and at times numerous (hundreds)
Distribution of lesions	exposed areas (face, neck, ears, forearms, dorsa of hands)	exposed and nonexposed areas (scalp, face, ears, neck, hands, forearms, arms, legs, trunk, external genitalia, mouth, anus)
Spontaneous healing	yes	yes, but tendency may decrease with duration of condition
Scar formation	yes (variable) but tend to be more superficial	yes (variable), but tend to be deeper and more destructive
Multiple scars from previous lesions	no	yes
Precipitating factors	sunburn, oil, arsenic, x-ray, tar, aging	none described, possible hereditary influence
Family history	not present	common
Duration of condition	limited—months to several years	many years—throughout most of patient's lifetime
Mucous membrane involvement	rarely reported	occurs, but uncommon

*After Epstein, Biskind, and Pollack: Arch. Dermatol., 75:210, 1957.

Giant Keratoacanthoma

In this category are lesions over 2 to 3 cm. in diameter. A number of examples have been reported (de Arruda Zamith and Brandi, 1960; Belisario, 1959; Brown and Rentiers, 1969; Bruner, 1963; Garrett et al., 1967; Gilbert, 1959; Harmel et al., 1967; Kallos, 1958; Lapière, 1960 and 1965; Obermayer, 1964; Peterkin et al., 1962; Pisanty, 1966; Rook et al., 1967; Stevanovic, 1960; Thivolet et al., 1966; Vickers and Ghadially, 1961; Webb and Ghadially, 1966). The record is a lesion 6 × 7 *inches* in its diameter (Duany, 1958). One wonders if the condition "epithelioma cuniculatum" described by Aird et al. (1954) is giant keratoacanthoma.

Multinodular Keratoacanthoma

In this variant there is continued acquisition of new keratoacanthoma nodules at the periphery, while partial or complete spontaneous central involution occurs (Figs. 32–8 and 32–9). This variety has been described under various names by several authors (aggregated keratoacanthoma-Spier and Thies, 1956; coral-reef keratoacanthoma—Belisario, 1959; nodulovegetating keratoacanthoma—Grinspan and Abulafia, 1955; keratoacanthoma centrifugum—Miedzínski and Kozakiewicz, 1962; keratoacanthoma centrifugum marginatum—Belisario, 1965a; kératoacanthomes centrifuges aigus—Lapière, 1965).

Keratoacanthomas Superimposed on Other Dermatoses

Keratoacanthomas can arise from or be engrafted on a number of skin disorders (Figs. 32–10 and 32–11). The list is constantly enlarging but currently includes the following: eczematous dermatitis (Allington, 1957; Becker, 1955; Hellier and Rowell, 1962; Lockwood, 1956; Peterkin et al., 1962; Williams, 1956), drug eruptions (Elerding, 1960), erythema multiforme (Eldering, 1960), psoriasis (Baer and Kopf, 1963; Vickers and Ghadially, 1961), pus-

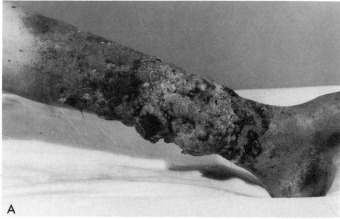

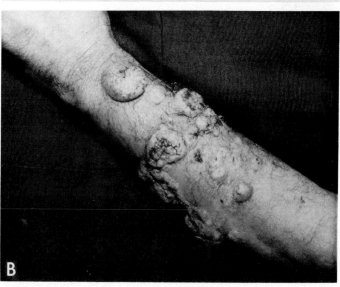

Figure 32–8 Multinodular keratoacanthoma. *A,* Case reported by Webb and Ghadially: J. Pathol. Bacteriol., 91:505, 1966. Reproduced by permission of E & S Livingstone. Leg finally required amputation. No metastases. *B,* Case reported by Hellier and Rowell: Arch. Dermatol., 85:485, 1962. Lesions on forearm. All lesions completely regressed (some spontaneously, others after being treated with 400 R: x-ray).

tular psoriasis (Clendenning and Auerbach, 1963), seborrheic dermatitis (Wilson, 1956), weather-beaten skin (this occurs often since keratoacanthomas frequently arise from exposed areas) (Poth, 1939), radiodermatitis (Baer and Kopf, 1963), xeroderma pigmentosum (Stevanovic, 1961), herpes simplex (Baer and Kopf, 1963; Ereaux et al., 1955), folliculitis (Stevanovic, 1962), acne conglobata (Ereaux et al., 1955), lichen simplex chronicus (Baer and Kopf, 1963), lichen planus (Peterkin et al., 1962), discoid lupus erythematous (Kopf and Andrade, 1968; Sklarz, 1955), sites of trauma (Lloyd and Hall, 1969; Thompson, 1958), miliaria (Witten and Zak, 1952), warty nevi (Peterkin et al., 1962), organoid nevi (Mehregan and Pinkus, 1965), and other miscellaneous conditions (Ghadially et al., 1963; Thompson, 1958).

Keratoacanthomas Arising on Mucous Membranes

There is a considerable amount of experimental and histologic evidence that keratoacanthomas arise from the infundibular portion of hair follicles (Calnan and Haber, 1955; Ghadially, 1958 and 1959; Grzybowski, 1950; Kalkoff and Macher, 1961; Oehlschlaegel, 1963; Baptista, 1964; Prutkin and Gerstner, 1966; Rigdon, 1960; Rossman et al., 1964; Witten and Zak, 1952). It is therefore of great interest to speculate on the histogenesis of the keratoacanthomas which have been re-

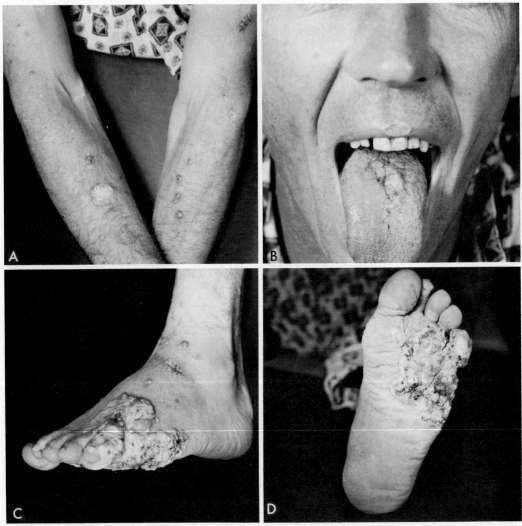

Figure 32–9   Multiple keratoacanthoma. *A,* Numerous crateriform nodules and scars at sites of previous tumors. *B,* Keratoacanthoma on tongue. *C* and *D,* Giant and destructive tumor of foot. This finally required amputation. (*From* Garrett et al.: Arch. Surg., 94:853, 1967. Copyright 1967, The American Medical Association.)

ported to arise on mucous and semimucous membranes (Fig. 32–12). They have been reported on the *conjunctiva* (Bellamy et al., 1963; Freeman et al., 1961; Friedman et al., 1965), *nasal mucosa* (Stevanovic, 1960), *lip* (Garrett et al., 1967; Silberg, Kopf, and Baer, 1962, Stevanovic, 1960; Vinton and Wilson, 1964), *perianal mucosa* (Elliott and Fisher, 1967), *anal mucosa* (Rook, 1956), *oral mucosa* (Winkelmann and Brown, 1968), *tongue* (Garrett et al., 1967), *palate* (Epstein et al., 1957), *gingiva* (Helsham and Buchanan, 1960), *palms and*

soles (Alessandrini, 1967; Dowling et al., 1954; Peterkin et al., 1962; Rossman et al., 1964), and *subungual region* (Lamp et al., 1965; Shapiro and Baraf, 1970). One possible explanation for finding such lesions on mucosal surfaces is the fact that ectopic sebaceous glands (i.e., portions of pilosebaceous units) have been reported on a number of mucous membranes (Guiducci and Hyman, 1962). Another explanation is that some of these lesions (e.g., lip, nasal mucosa, anal mucosa) actually arose in the skin and subsequently spread

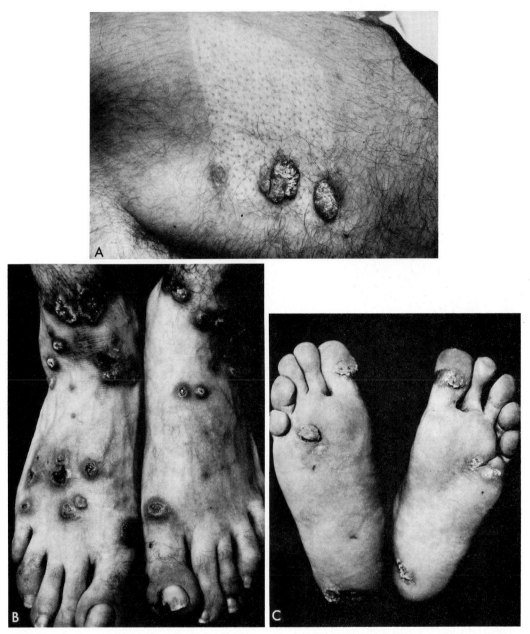

Figure 32–10   Multiple keratoacanthoma. Patient's sister has similar lesions. *A*, Keratoacanthomas on donor graft site. One tumor has already spontaneously disappeared, leaving typical scar with raised edges. *B*, Numerous keratoacanthomas of dorsa of feet. These lesions have virtually lost their propensity for spontaneous regression. *C*, Keratoacanthomas of soles.

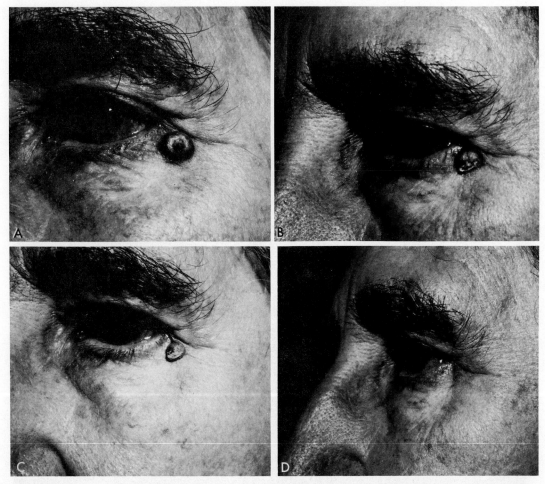

Figure 32–11 Keratoacanthoma arising at edge of area of radiodermatitis resulting from treatment two years previously of a basal cell epithelioma. *A,* Typical lesion with central keratotic plug. *B,* One week following partial removal of lower half of lesion for biopsy. *B,* Two weeks later. Partial involution noted. *C,* Seven weeks later. Complete involution.

onto the mucosal or semimucosal surfaces.

Keratoacanthoma Dyskeratoticum et Segregans

This type of keratoacanthoma was first reported by Stevanovic 1965a). It is recognized by its histologic features of acantholysis and dyskeratosis, thus simulating the adenoid type of squamous cell carcinoma (Muller et al., 1964). In some of the patients we have seen with this type of keratoacanthoma, the central plug in the crater was moistened by a serous exudate unlike the usual dry central kerato-

tic plug of the ordinary types of keratoacanthoma.

Subungual Keratocanthoma

This type of keratoacanthoma (Fig. 32–13) was first described by Fisher (1955) under the title of "distinctive destructive digital disease." These keratoacanthomas are often multiple (e.g., Fisher's patient eventually had at least six fingers involved by such lesions). Subungual keratoacanthomas can be very painful, as they slowly proceed to destroy the distal phalangeal bone by pressure necrosis. Keratoacanthomas in subungual locations can be

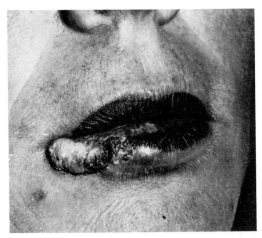

Figure 32–12 Multinodular keratoacanthoma on lip. (*From* Silberberg et al.: Arch. Dermatol., 86:44, 1962. Copyright 1962, The American Medical Association.)

seen independent of lesions elsewhere on the integument or in association with multiple keratoacanthomas. The differential diagnosis, especially in solitary lesions, between this type of digital keratoacanthoma and squamous cell carcinoma can be most difficult. Shapiro and Baraf (1970) recently reviewed the literature and their personal experience in relation to subungual keratoacanthomas (seven cases) subungual squamous cell carcinomas (44 cases). These authors found that *subungual squamous cell carcinoma* (1) is a very slow-growing tumor which masquerades for years as a chronic infection; (2) is less destructive locally; (3) occurs in older patients (average age 64); (4) destroys underlying bone in less than two-thirds of the cases; and (5) does not resolve spontaneously. In contrast, *subungual keratoacanthoma* (1)

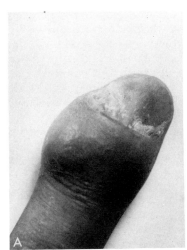

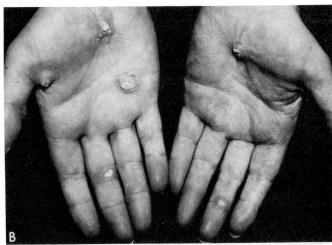

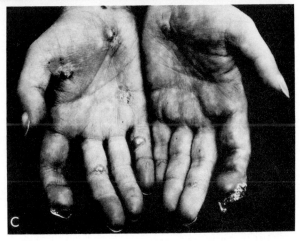

Figure 32–13 Distinctive destructive digital disease (subungual keratoacanthoma). *A*, Original lesion described by Fisher. (*From* Fisher: Arch. Dermatol., 71:73, 1955.) *B* and *C*, Progression of subungual keratoacanthomas, resulting in destruction of terminal phalanges over a two-year period.

grows rapidly; (2) is more destructive locally; (3) occurs in younger persons (average age 49); (4) destroys the underlying phalangeal bone in all reported cases; and (5) may resolve spontaneously. Interestingly, neither tumor metastasized in their review.

Verrucous Keratoacanthoma

The most typical lesion of keratoacanthoma is the hemispheric nodule with a central keratotic plug set into a crater in its summit. At times it presents as a verrucous papule or nodule. Histologically, such lesions have all the features of keratoacanthomas; however, the central cup-shaped invagination is missing. Instead the verrucoid surface gives rise to a keratotic mass resembling an early cutaneous horn with a benign hyperplastic epithelium at its base (Bart et al., 1968; Stevanovic, 1965b). These lesions are well known in multiple keratoacanthoma.

CLINICAL DIFFERENTIAL DIAGNOSIS

The most common and difficult problem in the clinical differential diagnosis of keratoacanthoma is squamous cell carcinoma. Since the latter is a potentially fatal malignancy and keratoacanthoma is benign, since the histologic features are at times closely similar or indistinguishable, and since these tumors can closely resemble one another, it is important for the clinician and pathologist to become familiar with the gross morphologic features of keratoacanthoma and squamous cell carcinoma. The salient features are enumerated in Table 32–2.

One important point in the distinction between keratoacanthoma and squamous cell carcinoma is that keratoacanthoma, with rare exception, is a *dry* lesion from its inception to its spontaneous involution. The central plug is a *keratotic plug* occupying a cul-de-sac. In contrast, squamous cell carcinoma characteristically is centrally ulcerated, resulting in a *moist* serosanguineous *crust*. It should also be stressed that the clinical features of these two neoplasms may overlap (Beare, 1955; Zoon et al., 1954). Except under unusual circumstances, their true natures should be substantiated by histologic examination. For the purposes of clinical investigation, we have developed the paracentral-fusiform-biopsy technique (Fig. 32–14), in which only the central portion of the lesions is excised and subjected to histologic examination (Popkin et al., 1966). Thus this technique provides the pathologist with a prime biopsy specimen through the heart of the tumor, and yet it allows the clinician to observe the subsequent course of spontaneous involution of the lesion (Fig. 32–14). An alternate method is excision of one-half of the lesion (Fig. 32–15). In our hands this biopsy technique has served us well in the clinical

TABLE 32–2 CLINICAL DIFFERENTIATION BETWEEN KERATOACANTHOMA AND SQUAMOUS CELL CARCINOMA*

Factor	Keratoacanthoma	Squamous Cell Carcinoma
Rate of growth	relatively faster (weeks)	relatively slower (months)
Relative size (for duration)	large	small
Average age of onset	55 years	70 years
Spontaneous involution	characteristically occurs	rarely, if ever, occurs
Shape	crateriform; exophytic	irregular; exophytic or endophytic
Central portion of tumor	keratotic plug	necrotic ulcer with crust
Borders	well circumscribed	often ill-defined
Resemblance to molluscum contagiosum	often	seldom
Surrounding skin	often normal	often shows "precancerous" changes
Lymph node involvement	absent	occurs
Progression	reaches maximum size, then does not progress further	tendency to progress indefinitely
Origin on mucosae	rare	common

*After Bowman and Pinkus: Arch. Pathol., 60:19, 1955.

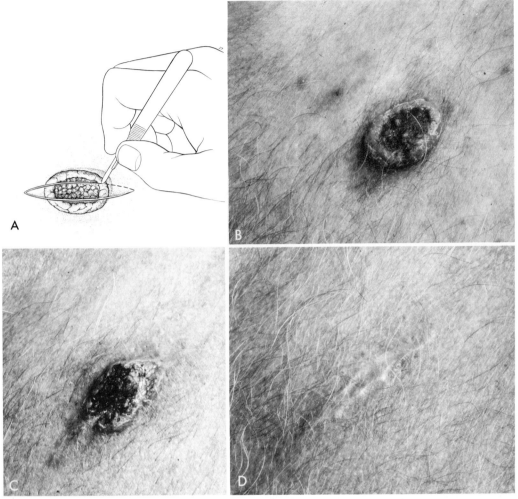

Figure 32–14 Paracentral, fusiform incisional biopsy technique. *A*, The central portion of the lesion is excised as shown. *B*, Prior to biopsy. *C*, One month after biopsy. *D*, Complete spontaneous regression three months after biopsy. (*From* Popkin et al.: Arch. Dermatol., 94:191, 1966.)

investigation of these tumors. However, it should be stressed that considerable expertise in clinical and histologic oncology is needed before this method of biopsy is used, since the lesion is only partially removed. Error in judgment could lead to a serious outcome if the lesion is a squamous cell carcinoma.

Other conditions which must be considered in the clinical differential diagnosis of keratoacanthoma include pseudoepitheliomatous hyperplasia, pseudoepithelioma of Azúa (Loewenthal, 1958), postradiation pseudorecidive (Herold and Nelson, 1957; Nelson, 1959), papillomatosis cutis carcinoides (Heite and Hintz, 1965; Nazzaro and Tosti, 1968), papillomatosis mucosae carcinoides (Tappeiner and Wolff, 1969), cutaneous horn (rarely keratoacanthoma can produce a central horny mass which projects from the summit of the lesion), iododerma and bromoderma, solar and seborrheic keratoses, inverted follicular keratosis (Helwig, 1955), arsenical keratosis, chondrodermatitis nodularis helicis chronicus (Peterkin et al., 1962), warty dyskeratoma (Szymanski, 1957), isolated dyskeratosis follicularis (Graham and Helwig, 1958), pityriasis rubra pilaris (Winkelmann and Brown, 1968), molluscum contagiosum (Peterkin et al., 1962; Tzanck et al., 1950), verruca vulgaris (Peterkin et al., 1962), orf (Peterkin et al., 1962), adnexal tumors (De-

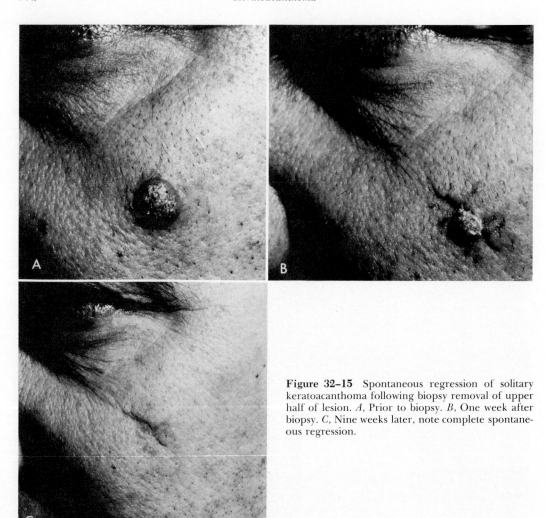

Figure 32–15 Spontaneous regression of solitary keratoacanthoma following biopsy removal of upper half of lesion. *A*, Prior to biopsy. *B*, One week after biopsy. *C*, Nine weeks later, note complete spontaneous regression.

lacrétaz and Leresche, 1965), trichoepithelioma, pilomatrixoma, sebaceous or epithelial cyst, basal cell epithelioma (Peterkin et al., 1962), insect bites, granulomas (Rocha and Fraga, 1962; Hewitt et al., 1960; Kanan, 1970), chancriform pyoderma (Frain-Bell, 1957), eosinophilic granuloma (Kresbach and Nürnberger, 1967), neurotic excoriations, prurigo nodularis, hypertrophic lichen planus, pyoderma vegetans, and cutaneous metastases (Jackson and Williamson, 1961; Winer and Wright, 1960).

MANAGEMENT

The proper management of keratoacanthomas requires background in clinical differential diagnosis and knowledge of the biologic behavior of the common and uncommon variants of this polymorphous tumor. With these prerequisites, *each lesion should be approached as an independent therapeutic problem.* The treatment of the various types of keratoacanthomas differs considerably.

Treatment of Solitary Keratoacanthoma

The current treatment of choice for most lesions is complete but conservative surgical excision. The specimen should be submitted for histologic examination. A number of other approaches have been advocated, including electrodesiccation and curettage (Rook et al., 1967), intralesional injection of corticosteroids (Belisario, 1965a and 1965b; Friedman et al., 1965; Gay Prieto et al., 1964; McNairy, 1964), topical application of chemotherapeutic agents (Belisario, 1959, 1965a, 1965b, and 1970; Grupper, 1968; Lloyd and Hall, 1969; Tarnowski, 1966), cryotherapy (Zacarian, 1969), chemosurgery, podophyllin resin (Cipollaro, 1964; Ereaux et al., 1955), and x-ray therapy (Alessandrini, 1967; Stevanovic, 1969; Thomson, 1958) and chemosurgery.

Since solitary keratoacanthomas spontaneously involute, one might question the logic of "watchful waiting." If total excision of the lesion would leave a marked cosmetic deformity and if the patient is apprised of the expected natural history of these lesions, the paracentral-fusiform-incisional biopsy technique can be used to permit histologic examination and observation of the subsequent clinical course of the lesion (Popkin et al., 1966). However, experience has taught that patients may refuse this "watchful waiting" approach once they are informed that (1) the lesion may take months to undergo spontaneous resolution, (2) the differential diagnosis between cancer and noncancer is not always possible by the pathologist, (3) the lesion can rarely grow to large size, and (4) the scar after spontaneous involution may be less acceptable cosmetically than that following treatment (Grant et al., 1962; Peterkin et al., 1962).

Treatment of Multiple Keratoacanthoma

The management of this type of keratoacanthoma is much more difficult, since the lesions are numerous, are very destructive in certain areas (particularly on acral sites, such as the nose, ears, digits), and eventually lose their initial capacity for complete spontaneous involution. These tumors often destroy underlying structures, including cartilage and bone, resulting in serious cosmetic deformity. New lesions continue to crop up over many years in relentless fashion (Ereaux and Schopflocher, 1965). Therapy includes the above approaches enumerated under the solitary type. In addition, in this clinical setting one is justified in observing lesions of multiple keratoacanthoma once the histologic diagnosis has been established. Some have advocated systemic chemotherapy with methotrexate alone (Rossman et al., 1964) or in combination with systemic antibiotics (Tarnowski, 1966). Ephraim and Kaufman (1958) reported success with intramuscular bismuth injections, but this report remains unconfirmed.

A particularly tragic type of lesion which can occur in multiple keratoacanthoma is "distinctive destructive digital disease" (Fisher, 1955), which may require amputation of several digits because of marked pain and deformity of the terminal phalanges.

Treatment of Eruptive Keratoacanthoma and of the Unusual Variants

The treatment of these lesions will depend on the clinical situation. For the eruptive type, systemic chemotherapy might be considered, since surgical or radiologic approaches for the myriad tumors is not possible except for the larger ones. Winkelmann and Brown (1968) reported some success with the local application of vitamin A. For the other less common variants of keratoacanthoma (giant, multinodular, mucosal), surgical excision with or without graft has been our general therapeutic approach.

PROGNOSIS

Although keratoacanthoma is a benign (pseudoepitheliomatous) tumor that does not metastasize or directly cause death, the prognosis concerning cosmetic disfigurement is less certain. Usually, in the *solitary* type, the cosmetic defect is minimal after spontaneous involution or after therapeutic intervention. In the unusual variants, the prognosis for a good cosmetic result is uncertain, since we are not dealing with a destructive process which involves large areas of skin (giant and multinodular keratoacanthomas) or important regions (periungual keratoacanthomas).

The prognosis for *multiple* keratoacanthoma is much more guarded, because these tumors often continuously form throughout the lifetime of the patient, causing considerable scarring and deformity, particularly of the acral parts (ears, nose, lips, digits). For example, in the patient of Marshall and Findlay (1953), both earlobes were penetrated. In the patient of Pillsbury and Beerman (1958), the keratoacanthoma invaded to the tendons of the wrists. In the patient of Stevanovic (1960), the ala nasi was perforated. In the patient of Smith (1948), the nose was destroyed. In the patient described by Garrett et al. (1967), the giant keratoacanthoma required amputation of the foot (Lloyd and Hall, 1969). And in the patients described by Obermayer (1964) and Boniuk and Zimmerman (1967), the eyelids involved with keratoacanthomas were destroyed.

Recurrences following attempted destruction of keratoacanthomas have been reported (Ayres, 1948; Beare, 1955; Brauer, 1962; Burman et al., 1956; Charteris, 1951; Civatte et al., 1951; Church, 1955; Degos et al., 1958; Diben and Fowler, 1955; Duperrat and Goetschel, 1966; Ephraim and Kaufman, 1958; Epstein et al., 1957; Ereaux et al., 1955; Feldman, 1956; Kuske and Baumgartner, 1962; Lapière, 1960, 1961, and 1965; Linell and Mansson, 1958; Peterkin et al., 1962; Silberberg et al., 1962; Simpson, 1955; Szymanski, 1962; Van der Meiren et al., 1956). In one review, recurrences occurred in 5 percent of 404 keratoacanthomas (Rook et al., 1967). These authors also pointed out that digital keratoacanthomas, although rare, represented

5.9 percent of the recurrences; lesions of the lips represented only 5.5 percent of the tumors but had a 28 percent recurrence rate; only 1 percent of keratoacanthomas of the cheek recurred. Most recurrent lesions were of average size, but giant keratoacanthomas seemed to recur more frequently. Recurrences often occurred at the borders of the lesions but had unusual clinical features, often slowly growing, firm nodules (Fig. 32–16). Yet histologically, the primary and recurrent lesions were similar, and all recurrence proved to be benign.

According to Stevanovic's (1969) review, 80 percent of recurrences occur in the first three months after treatment (curettage), and 98 percent in the first six months.

We have witnessed several lesions which underwent spontaneous involution follow-

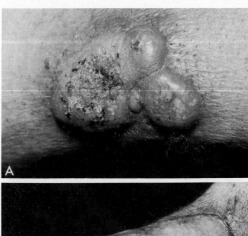

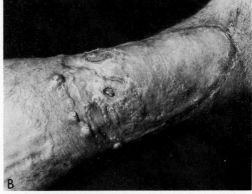

Figure 32–16 Recurrent multinodular keratoacanthoma. *A,* Lesion prior to surgical excision and graft. *B,* Multiple recurrent nodules at edge of graft. (*From* Pillsbury and Beerman: Am. J. Med. Sci., 236: 614, 1958.)

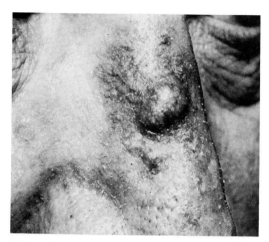

Figure 32–17 Recurrent keratoacanthoma following electrodesiccation and curettage of clinically and histologically typical lesion. The recurrent nodule spontaneously disappeared. (Courtesy of Dr. Earle Brauer.)

ing recurrence (Fig. 32–17). However, since the differential diagnosis between squamous cell carcinoma and keratoacanthoma is so difficult at times (Carteaud and Baptista, 1962a), recurrence should put one on guard that the lesion in question may be malignant, and it should be treated accordingly.

A few reports have appeared in which keratoacanthomas have been found in association with other malignant tumors (e.g., with basal cell epithelioma—Baptista, 1964; Burge and Winkelmann, 1969; Einaugler et al., 1968; Hadida and Sayag, 1964; Many et al., 1967; and with systemic cancers—Muir et al., 1967). Of special interest, however, are those publications which report clinical confusion between keratoacanthoma and squamous cell carcinoma or imply malignant transformation of keratoacanthomas to squamous cell carcinomas (Anderson, 1957; Baptista, 1964; Beare, 1953; Belisario, 1954, 1959, 1965a, and 1965b; Burge and Winkelmann, 1969; Charteris, 1951; Cramer and Weiss, 1965; Dupont, 1954 and 1960; Flegel, 1957; Huriez et al., 1954; Kopf and Andrade, 1968; Lapière, 1965; Lockwood and Baxter, 1959; Middleton and Curtin, 1966; Muller at al., 1964; Nicolau et al., 1963; Peterkin et al., 1962; Sklarz, 1955 and 1960; Vaccari and Tagliavini, 1955; Zimmerman, 1956; Zoon et al., 1954). In reviewing these

reports there are several possible explanations for these occasional observations: (a) malignant transformation to squamous cell carcinoma actually did take place; (b) the appearance of the two tumors in the same location was fortuitous, as occurs in mixed metatypical epithelioma (i.e., a basal cell epithelioma juxtaposed to a squamous cell carcinoma); and (c) the histologic interpretation is incorrect (i.e., the lesion never was a keratoacanthoma, or it really did not give rise to a squamous cell carcinoma). The latter explanation seems to be a major stumbling block in the diagnosis, since keratoacanthomas, especially in the early growth phase, can be indistinguishable from squamous cell carcinomas on histologic grounds using routine staining methods. Perhaps some newer approaches, such as the immunofluorescence technique now under investigation, may serve in the future to distinguish these closely similar tumors (de Moragas et al., 1970; Jordon et al., 1970).

Experimental evidence suggests the theoretic possibility of malignant transformation of keratoacanthoma to squamous cell carcinoma. Chemical carcinogens will produce keratoacanthomas (Ghadially et al., 1963) and, on continued application, will transform such lesions into frank squamous cell carcinomas (Ghadially, 1959; Rook and Champion, 1963). However, Champion and Rook (1963) reviewed the published cases up to 1962 and came to the conclusion that there was not a single case on record of a keratoacanthoma in which malignancy developed biologically (i.e., with distant metastases) as distinct from histologically. Similarly, careful review of cases published since 1962 leaves doubt that biologic malignancy has developed in a bona fide keratoacanthoma, although the data are suggestive in several instances. For example, Jackson (1969) described four cases initially diagnosed as keratoacanthoma but which "turned out to be squamous cell carcinoma." The first patient had a rapidly growing tumor of the right cheek, which was clinically and histologically a keratoacanthoma. Subsequently, metastatic squamous cell carcinoma was demonstrated in a lymph node removed from the neck. However, this patient later was shown to have primary bronchial carcinoma. The second patient had a keratoacanthoma (clinically) or low grade squamous cell carcinoma (histologically) which did not metastasize. The third patient developed lymph node and cerebral metastases from a neoplasm on the cheek. The primary lesion was never biopsied. The fourth patient had an *ulcerated* lesion on the ear which was clinically thought to be a keratoacanthoma but histologically was found to be an anaplastic squamous cell carcinoma. It metastasized and caused the patient's demise. No histology was depicted in this paper. Thus, in none of the four cases reported was there an unblemished record of a clinically documented (by photography), histologically verified keratoacanthoma which subsequently gave rise to metastases. This is not to say that such an occurrence cannot happen. However, if malignant transformation of keratoacanthoma to squamous cell carcinoma does occur, it must be exceedingly uncommon, since there now have been thousands of keratoacanthomas reported and only a few, usually poorly documented, cases of malignant transformation resulting in metastases or death.

REFERENCES

Aird, I., Johnson, H. D., Lennox, B., and Stanfeld, A. G.: Epithelioma cuniculatum: A variety of squamous carcinoma of the foot. Br. J. Surg., 42:245, 1954.

Alessandrini, A.: Contributo allo studio del cheratoacanthoma disseminato. Anthologica M. Santoriana, 82:80, 1967.

Allington, H. V., In discussion of paper by Epstein, N. N., Biskind, B. R., and Pollack, R. S.: Multiple primary self-healing squamous cell "epithelioma" of the skin. Arch. Dermatol., 75:210, 1957.

Anderson, N. P., In discussion of paper by Epstein, N. N., Biskind, B. R., and Pollack, R. S.: Multiple primary self-healing squamous cell "epithelioma" of the skin. Arch. Dermatol., 75:210, 1957.

Andrade, R.: Concepto de Pseudomalignidad. Proc. VI. Ibero-Latin Am. Congr. Dermatol. Barcelona, Edit. Cientifico. Medica, 1970, pp. 333–348.

de Arruda Zamith, V., and Brandi, A. J.: Ceratoacantoma gigante do nariz. Arq. Hosp. S. Casa S. Paulo, 6:45, 1960.

Ayres, S., Jr.: Squamous cell epithelioma (self-healing type). Arch. Dermatol. Syph., 58:584, 1948.

Baer, R. L., and Kopf, A. W.: Keratoacanthoma. *In* 1962–63 Year Book of Dermatology. Chicago,

Year Book Medical Publishers, Inc., 1963, pp. 7–41 (review).

Baptista, A. P.: Querato-acantoma. Coimbra, Portugal, Coimbra Editura Limitada, Ed., 1964.

Baran, M. L. R.: Kérato-acanthome. Rôle déclencant d'une brûlure. Bull. Soc. Fr. Dermatol. Syphiligr., 64:96, 1957.

Bart, R. S., Andrade, R., and Kopf, A. W.: Cutaneous horns: A clinical and histologic study. Acta Derm. Venereol. (Stockh.), 48:507, 1968.

Beare, J. M.: Molluscum sebaceum. Br. J. Surg., 41:167, 1953.

Beare, J. M.: Recurrent molluscum sebaceum. Lancet, 1:182, 1955.

Becker, S. W., In discussion of papers by Binkley and Johnson (1955) and Ereaux et al. (1955).

Belisario, J. C.: Discussion. Aust. J. Dermatol., 2:147, 1954.

Belisario, J. C.: Cancer of the Skin. London, Butterworth & Co., Ltd., 1959.

Belisario, J. C.: Brief review of keratoacanthomas and description of keratoacanthoma centrifugum marginatum, another variety of keratoacanthoma. Aust. J. Dermatol., 8:65, 1965a.

Belisario, J. C.: Keratoacanthoma and its incidence as affected by sunlight in the tropical and subtropical areas of Australia. Dermatologia Internationalis, 4:53, 1965b.

Belisario, J. C.: Ten year's experience with topical cytotoxic therapy for cutaneous cancer and precancer. Cutis, 6:293, 1970.

Bellamy, E. D., Allen, J. H., and Hart, N. L.: Keratoacanthoma of the bulbar conjunctiva. Arch. Ophthalmol., 70:512, 1963.

Binazzi, M., and Finzi, A. F.: Disseminated keratoacanthoma (apropos of an observation in an infant). Minerva Dermatol., 35:1, 1960.

Binazzi, M., and Miranda, R.: Cheratoacanthoma: Analisi e contributo casistico. Riv. Omnia Med. Therapeut., 43:355, 1965.

Binkley, G. W., and Johnson, H. H.: Keratoacanthoma (molluscum sebaceum). Arch. Dermatol., 71:66, 1955.

Boniuk, M., and Zimmerman, L. E.: Eyelid tumors with reference to lesions confused with squamous cell carcinoma. III. Keratoacanthoma. Arch. Ophthalmol., 77:29, 1967.

Bowman, H. E., and Pinkus, H.: Keratoacanthoma. Natl. Cancer Inst. Monogr., 10:257, 1963.

Brauer, E.: Keratoacanthoma vs. prickle-cell epithelioma. Arch. Dermatol., 86:144, 1962.

Brothers, W. S., New, W. A., and Nickel, W. R.: Keratoacanthoma. Arch. Dermatol., 81:369, 1960.

Brown, J. B., and Fryer, M. P.: Fallacy of the term "self-healing epidermoid carcinoma" and limitation of microscopy interpretations. Surg. Gynecol. Obstet., 100:179, 1955.

Brown, J., and Rentiers, P.: Solitary keratoacanthoma. Cutis, 5:1243, 1969.

Bruner, J. M.: Keratoacanthoma. Plast. Reconstr. Surg., 31:281, 1963.

Burge, K. M., and Winkelmann, R. K.: Keratoacanthoma: Association with basal and squamous cell carcinoma. Arch. Dermatol., 100:306, 1969.

Burman, S. O., Buckwalter, J. A., and Carter, J. R.: Molluscum pseudocarcinomatosum. Surg. Gynecol. Obstet., 102:574, 1956.

Calnan, C. D., and Haber, H.: Molluscum sebaceum. J. Pathol. Bacteriol., 69:61, 1955.

Carteaud, A., and Baptista, A. P.: Difficultés diagnostiques du kérato-acanthome. Press Méd., 70:2747, 1962a.

Carteaud, A., and Baptista, A. P.: Kérato-acanthome chez une enfant de 4 ans. Bull. Soc. Fr. Dermatol. Syphiligr., 69:254, 1962b.

Champion, R. H., and Rook, A.: Keratoacanthoma. *In* Pillsbury, D. M., and Livingood, C. S. (Eds.): Proc. XII Internatl. Congr. Dermatol. Amsterdam, Exerpta Medica Foundation, 1963.

Charteris, A. A.: Self-healing epithelioma of the skin. Am. J. Roentgenol., 65:459, 1951.

Church, R. E.: Molluscum pseudocarcinomatosum. Lancet, 1:460, 1955.

Cipollaro, A.: Keratoacanthoma recurring in a surgical scar. Arch. Dermatol., 90:438, 1964.

Civatte, A., Melki, G. R., and Goestschel, G. E.: Cas pour diagnostic (verrucome?). Bull. Soc. Fr. Dermatol. Syphiligr., 58:532, 1951.

Clendenning, W. E., and Auerbach, R.: Keratoacanthoma in generalized pustular psoriasis. Acta Derm. Venereol. (Stockh.), 43:68, 1963.

Colomb, D., Descos, L., and Gauthier, D.: Kératoacanthomes multiples et maladie du brai de houille. Rev. Lyon. de Méd., 15:449, 1966.

Cramer, H. J., and Weiss, H.: Zur Katamnese Und Klinik Der Keratoakanthomas. Dermatol. Wochenschr., 151:449, 1965.

Currie, A. R., and Smith, J. F.: Multiple primary spontaneous-healing squamous-cell carcinomata of the skin. J. Pathol. Bacteriol., 64:827, 1952.

Degos, R., Cottenot, F., and Civatte, J.: Kératoacanthome reformé asprès abrasion: Étapes successives suivies pendant 4 mois. Bull. Soc. Fr. Dermatol. Syphiligr., 65:122, 1958.

Delacrétaz, J., and Leresche, A.: Myoépithelioma atypique? Dermatologica, 130:274, 1965.

Dibden, F. A., and Fowler, M.: The multiple growth of molluscum sebaceum on donor and recipient sites of skin graft. Aust. N. Z. J. Surg., 25:157, 1955.

Doepfmer, R.: Experiences in transplantations of skin-exisates from person to person in erythema chronicum migrans, pityriasis rosea, lichen ruber planus, and keratoacanthoma. Proc. XII Internatl. Congr. Dermatol. Amsterdam, Exerpta Medica Foundation, 1962.

Dowling, G. B.: Personal communication, 1962.

Dowling, G., Galnan, C., and Tipping, D.: Self-healing squamous cell epithelioma of the ferguson smith type. Trans. St. John's Hosp. Dermatol. Soc., 33:60, 1954.

Duany, N. P.: Squamous cell pseudoepithelioma (keratoacanthoma). Arch. Dermatol., 78:703, 1958.

Dunn, J. S., and Smith, J. F.: Self-healing primary squamous carcinoma of the skin. Br. J. Dermatol., 46:519, 1934.

Duperrat, B., and Goetschel, G. E.: Forme récidivante de kérato-acanthome avec chondrite du tragus. Bull. Soc. Fr. Dermatol. Syphiligr., 73:242, 1966.

Dupont, A.: Kyste sébacé atypique. Bull. Soc. Belge Dermatol., 1930, p. 177.

Dupont, A.: Kystes sébacés végétants, kérato-acanthomes, verrucomes. Bull. Soc. Fr. Dermatol. Syphiligr., 59:340, 1952.

Dupont, A.: Le kérato-acanthome (kyste sébacé végétant; molluscum sebaceum). Ann. Dermatol. Syphiligr. (Paris), 81:621, 1954.

Dupont, A.: A propos du kérato-acanthome. Bull. Soc. Fr. Dermatol. Syphiligr., 67:297, 1960.

Editorial: Molluscum pseudocarcinomatosum. Lancet, 2:816, 1953.

Einaugler, R. B., Henkind, P., de Oliveira, L. F., and Bart, R. S.: Keratoacanthoma with basal cell carcinoma. Am. J. Ophthalmol., 65:922, 1968.

Elerding, C. E.: Multiple keratoacanthoma. Arch. Dermatol., 81:914, 1960.

Elliott, G. B., and Fisher, B. K.: Perianal keratoacanthoma. Arch. Dermatol., 95:81, 1967.

Elschner, H.: Molluscum pseudocarcinomatosum (Keratoacanthom) nach Trauma. Hautarzt, 7:368, 1956.

Ephraim, A. J., and Kaufman, J. J.: Multiple keratoacanthoma. Arch. Dermatol., 77:191, 1958.

Epstein, N. N., Biskind, B. R., and Pollack, R. S.: Multiple primary self-healing squamous-cell "epitheliomas" of skin. Arch. Dermatol., 75:210, 1957.

Ereaux, L. P., and Schopflocher, P.: Familial primary self-healing squamous epithelioma of skin. Arch. Dermatol., 91:589, 1965.

Ereaux, L. P., Schopflocher, P., and Fournier, C. J.: Keratoacanthomata. Arch. Dermatol., 71:73, 1955.

Ewing, M. R., In personal communication with Burman et al. (1956).

Feldman, F. F., In discussion of case of Wilson, J. W.: Multiple keratoacanthomata. Arch. Dermatol., 74:326, 1956.

Fisher, A. A.: A distinctive destructive digital disease. Arch. Dermatol., 71:73, 1955.

Fisher, A. A.: A distinctive destructive digital disease: Follow-up presentation. Arch. Dermatol., 86:800, 1962.

Flegel, H.: Molluscum pseudocarcinomatosum und Karzinom. Dermatol. Wochenschr., 135:153, 1957.

Forck, G., Fromme, H. G., and Jordan, P.: Zur Virusatiologie des Keratoakanthoms. Hautarzt, 16:153, 1965.

Frain-Bell, W.: Pyodermia chancriformis faciei. Br. J. Dermatol., 69:19, 1957.

Freeman, K., Cloud, T., and Knox, J.: Keratoacanthoma of the conjunctiva. Arch. Ophthalmol., 65:817, 1961.

Friedman, R. P., Morales, A., and Burnham, T. K.: Multiple cutaneous and conjunctival keratoacanthomata. Arch. Dermatol., 92:162, 1965.

Furtado, T. A.: Ceratoacanthoma e processos afins. Estudo clínico, histopathológico e experimental. Belo Horizonte, Brazil, Univ. Belo Horizonte, 1962.

Garrett, W. S., Ware, J. L., and Thorne, F. L.: Keratoacanthoma. Arch. Surg., 94:853, 1967.

Gay Prieto, J., Rodriguez Perez, P., Rubio Huertos, M., and Jaqueti, G.: On the virus etiology of keratoacanthoma. Acta Derm. Venereol. (Stockh.), 44:180, 1964.

Gay Prieto, J., González, G., and Garcia Gancedo, P.: Nuevas aportaciones al studio del queratoacanthoma. Med. Cután., 3:353, 1969.

Ghadially, F. N.: A comparative morphological study of the keratoacanthoma of man and similar experimentally produced lesions in the rabbit. J. Pathol. Bacteriol., 74:441, 1958.

Ghadially, F. N.: The experimental production of keratoacanthomas in the hamster and the mouse. J. Pathol. Bacteriol., 77:277, 1959.

Ghadially, F. N., Barton, B. W., and Kerridge, D. F.: The etiology of keratoacanthoma. Cancer, 16:603, 1963.

Gilbert, A. E.: Giant keratoacanthoma: The surgical significance of a benign lesion. Northwest Med., 58:373, 1959.

Gougerot, H. (in collaboration with Clara, Bournier, Paul Blum, Cousin, Eliascheff, Rist, and Joyeus): Verrucome avec adenite, à structure épithéliomatiforme curable par le 914. Arch. Derm.-Syph. (Paris), 1:374, 1929.

Gougerot, H., Blum, P., et Cousin: Un nouveau cas de verrucome avec adéite d'origine indéterminee á structure epithéliomatiforme curable par le 914. Bull. Soc. Fr. Dermatol. Syphiligr., 36:255, 1929.

Graham, J. H., and Helwig, E. B.: Isolated dyskeratosis follicularis. Arch. Dermatol., 77:377, 1958.

Graham, J. H., and Helwig, E. B.: Cutaneous precancerous conditions in man. *In* Urbach, F., and Stewart, H. L. (Eds.): Conference On Biology Of Cutaneous Cancer. Bethesda, Md., National Cancer Institute Monograph No. 10, 1963.

Grant, G. A., MacMillan, J. B., and Maclean, S.: Pseudo-carcinoma of skin: Follow-up of cases of keratoacanthoma seen in the 10 years 1951–1960. Scott. Med. J., 7:27, 1962.

Grinspan, D., and Abulafia, J.: Idiopathic cutaneous pseudoepitheliomatous hyperplasia. Cancer, 8:1047, 1955.

Grupper, C.: International conference on 5-fluorouracil ointment in dermatology, Rome, 1968.

Grzybowski, M.: A Case of peculiar generalized epithelial tumors of the skin. Br. J. Dermatol., 62:310, 1950.

Guiducci, A. A., and Hyman, A. B.: Ectopic sebaceous glands. Dermatologica, 124:44, 1962.

Harmel, L., Kalis, B., and Mallet, P.: Kératoacanthome géant. Essai de corticothérapie locale. Bull. Soc. Fr. Dermatol. Syphiligr., 74:48, 1967.

Heite, H. J., and Hintz, H.: Papillomatosis Cutis—Eine Analytische-Nosologische Studie. Arch. Klin. Exp. Dermatol., 222:254, 1965.

Hellier, F. F., and Rowell, N. R.: Giant keratoacanthoma complicating dermatitis. Arch. Dermatol., 85:485, 1962.

Helsham, R. W., and Buchanan, G.: Keratoacanthoma of the oral cavity. Oral. Surg., 13:844, 1960.

Helwig, E. B.: Inverted follicular keratosis. *In* Seminar On The Skin: Neoplasms and Dermatoses. Proceedings, 20th Seminar, Am. Soc. Clinical Pathologists, International Congress Clinical Pathology, Washington, D.C., 1954, Am. Soc. Clin. Pathol., 1955.

Herold, W. C., and Nelson, L. M.: Pseudoepitheliomatous reaction (pseudorecidive) following radiation therapy of epitheliomata. Acta Derm. Venereol. Proc. 11th Internatl. Congr. Dermatol. Vol. II, 1957, p. 426.

Hewitt, J., Kaufmann, P., and Le Grand, P.: Granulo-acanthomes multiples successies. Bull. Soc. Fr. Dermatol. Syphiligr., 67:502, 1960.

Hjorth, N.: Keratoacanthoma: A historical note. Br. J. Dermatol., 72:292, 1960.

Huriez, C., Driessens, J., Clay, A., and Desmons, F.: A propos d'une observation de kératoacanthoma. Bull. Soc. Fr. Dermatol. Syphiligr., 61:13, 1954.

Huriez, C., Desmons, F., and Benoit, M.: Lex faux cancers cutanés. Rev. Prat. (Paris), 7:1, 1957.

Huriez, C., Benoit, M., and Lebeurre, R.: Sur 1,002 cas de tumeurs cutanees malignes observees en 6 ans a la clinique dermatologique de Lille. Lille Med., 6:133, 1961.

Hutchinson, J.: A Smaller Atlas of Illustrations of Clinical Surgery: A Peculiar Form of Cancer of the Skin. Vol. 2, Plate 92. Philadelphia, Blakiston & Company, 1888.

Hutchinson, J.: The crateriform ulcer of the face: A form of epithelial cancer. Trans. Pathol. Soc. Lond., 40:275, 1889.

Hutchinson, J.: The crateriform ulcer (acute epithelial cancer), Plate 11. Arch. Surg. (Lond.), 1889–1890.

Hutchinson, J.: The crateriform ulcer, Plate XI. Arch. Surg. (Lond.), Vol. 1, 1890.

Hutchinson, J.: Syphilis No. XXIX. The crateriform ulcer simulated by syphilitic indurations. Arch. Surg. (Lond.), 3:245, 1891–1892.

Hutchinson, J.: The crateriform ulcer: Microscopic examination. Arch. Surg. (Lond.), 7:88, 1896a.

Hutchinson, J.: Crateriform ulcer of the forehead and epithelioma (rodent ulcer) on the cheek. Clin. J., 8:271, 1896b.

Hutchinson, J.: The crateriform ulcer (epithelial cancer), Plate CXXXI. Arch. Surg. (Lond.), Vol. 8, 1897.

Jackson, I. T.: Diagnostic problem of keratoacanthoma. Lancet, 1:490, 1969.

Jackson, R., and Williamson, G. S.: Keratoacanthoma: Incidence and problems in diagnosis and treatment. Can. Med. Assoc. J., 84:312, 1961.

Jakubowicz, K., Biczysko, W., and Dabrowski, J.: Studies on the ultrastructure of keratoacanthoma in man. Acta Derm. Venereol. (Stockh.), 50:89, 1970.

Jolly, H. W., and Carpenter, C. L.: Multiple keratoacanthoma. Arch. Dermatol., 93:348, 1966.

Jordon, R. E., Winkelmann, R. K., and de Moragas, J. M.: The study of skin tumors by indirect immunofluorescence using antibodies to basement-membrane and cell-surface antigens. J. Invest. Dermatol., 54:352, 1970.

Kalkoff, K. W., and Macher, E.: Zur Hitogenese der Keratoakanthoms. Hautarzt, 12:8, 1961.

Kallos, A.: Giant keratoacanthoma. Arch. Dermatol., 78:207, 1958.

Kanan, M. W.: Torulosis of the skin. Dermatologica, 141:15, 1970.

Kopf, A. W., and Andrade, R.: Editorial comment. *In* 1967–68 Series Year Book of Dermatology. Chicago, Year Book Medical Publishers, Inc., 1968, p. 160.

Kopf, A. W., and Silberberg, I.: Keratoacanthoma. *In* 1962–63 Series Year Book of Dermatology. Chicago, Year Book Medical Publishers, Inc., 1963, p. 25.

Kresbach, H., and Nürnberger, F.: Echthyma-Und

Keratoakanthom-Ähnliche Eosinophile Granuloma Der Haut. Arch. Klin. Exp. Dermatol., 230:286, 1967.

Kuske, H., and Baumgartner, P.: Multiple rezidivierende Kerato-acanthome. Dermatologica, 124:316, 1962.

Lapière, S.: Contribution à l'étude du kérato-acanthome. Arch. Belg. Dermatol. Syphiligr., 10:185, 1954.

Lapière, S.: Über Kerato-Acanthome. Hautarzt, 6:38, 1955.

Lapière, M. S.: Récidive sous forme géante mais benigne de trois kérato-acanthomes insuffisamment traites par clivage. Bull. Soc. Fr. Dermatol. Syphiligr., 67:302, 1960.

Lapière, S.: Kérato-acanthome à évolution clinique et histologique d'allure maligne se terminant par guerison spontaneé. Bull. Soc. Fr. Dermatol. Syphiligr., 68:783, 1961.

Lapière, S.: Quinze ans d'experience du kérato-acanthome. Bull. l'Acad. R. Med. Belg., VII Serie, Tome V, No. 6–7, 1965, p. 615.

Lassar, O.: Zur Therapie Der Hautkarzinome. Berl. Klin. Wochenschr., 30:587, 1893.

Levy, E. J., Kahn, M. M., Shaffer, B., and Beerman, H.: Keratoacanthoma. J.A.M.A., 155:562, 1954.

Linell, F., and Mansson, B.: Molluscum pseudocarcinomatosum. Nord. Med., 59:226, 1958.

Lloyd, K. M., and Hall, J. H.: Ferguson Smith syndrome of multiple keratoacanthoma. Cutis, 5:1093, 1969.

Lockwood, J. H., In discussion on Wilson, J. W.: Multiple keratoacanthomata. Arch. Dermatol., 74:326, 1956.

Lockwood, J. H., and Baxter, D. L.: Squamous cell carcinoma, formerly presented as keratoacanthoma. Arch. Dermatol., 80:637, 1959.

Loewenthal, L. J. A.: Pseudoepithelioma of Azúa. Acta Derm. Venereol. (Stockh.), 38:78, 1958.

Lund, H. Z.: Epidermal tumors: Some special considerations. *In* Helwig, E. B., and Mostofi, F. K. (Eds.): The Skin. Baltimore, The Williams & Wilkins Company, 1971, pp. 476–489.

MacCormac, H., and Scarff, R. W.: Molluscum sebaceum. Br. J. Dermatol., 48:624, 1936.

Machacek, G. F.: Familial multiple recurrent keratoacanthomatosis (so-called self-healing squamous-cell epithelioma), in Society Transactions. Arch. Dermatol., 75:446, 1957.

McNairy, D. J.: Intradermal triamcinolone therapy of keratoacanthomas. Arch. Dermatol., 89:136, 1964.

Marshall, J., and Findlay, G. H.: Multiple primary self-healing squamous epithelioma of the skin (Ferguson Smith) and its relationship to molluscum sebaceum. S. Afr. Med. J., 27:1000, 1953.

Marshall, J., and Pepler, W. J.: Mollusca pseudocarcinomatosa: Discussion of a case of the Ferguson Smith type of unilateral distribution. Br. J. Cancer, 8:251, 1954.

Mehregan, A. H., and Pinkus, H.: Life history of organoid nevi. Arch. Dermatol., 91:574, 1965.

Middleton, A. G., and Curtin, J. W.: Keratoacanthoma or squamous cell carcinoma? A surgeon's dilemma. Plast. Reconstr. Surg., 38:56, 1966.

Miedzínski, F., and Kozakiewicz, J.: Das Keratoa-kanthoma Centrifugum—Eine Besondere Varietät Des Keratoakanthoms. Hautarzt, 13:348, 1962.

de Moragas, J. M.: Multiple keratoacanthoms: Relation to Jamarson therapy of pemphigus foliaceus. Arch. Dermatol., 93:679, 1966.

de Moragas, J. M., Montgomery, H., and McDonald, J. R.: Keratoacanthoma versus squamous-cell carcinoma. Arch. Dermatol., 77:390, 1958.

de Moragas, J. M., Winkelmann, R. K., and Jordon, R. E.: Immunofluorescence of epithelial skin tumors. Cancer, 25:1399, 1970.

Muir, E. G., Bell, A. J. Y., and Barlow, K. A.: Multiple primary carcinomas of colon, duodenum and larynx associated with keratoacanthoma of the face. Br. J. Surg., 54:191, 1967.

Muller, S. A., Wilhelms, C. M., Harrison, C. M., and Winkelmann, R. K.: Adenoid squamous cell carcinoma (adenoacanthoma of Lever). Arch. Dermatol., 89:589, 1964.

Nasemann, T.: Electronenoptische Beobachctungen An Einen Acanthom Mit Sicherer Virusatiologie in Analogie Zu Befunden am Keratoakanthom. Hautarzt, 16:156, 1965.

Nazzaro, P., and Tosti, A.: Le pseudo-cancerosi cutanée. Minerva Dermatol., 52:617, 1968.

Nelson, L. M.: Self-healing pseudocancers of the skin. Calif. Med., 90:49, 1959.

Nicolau, S. G., Badanoiu, A., and Balus, L.: Untersuchungen Über Spezifische Anti-Tumorale Reactionem Bei an Keratoakanthom leidenden kranken mit einigen Betrachtungen bezüglich des Eingreifens von Immunitätsprozessen bei der spontanen Heilung dieser Geschwulste. Arch. Klin. Exp. Dermatol., 217:308, 1963.

Obermayer, M. E.: Das Keratoakanthom: Sein zur Gewebsdestruktion Fuhrende Wachstumskapazitat. Hautarzt, 15:628, 1964.

Oehlschlaegel, G.: Zur Histogenese und Nosologischen Stellung der Keratoakanthoms. Hautarzt, 14:156, 1963.

Oettlé, A. G.: Skin cancer in Africa. Bethesda, Md., National Cancer Institute Monograph No. 10, 1963, p. 197.

Oliver, J. O.: Personal communication to Thomson, S.: Ann. R. Coll. Surg. Engl., 22:382, 1958.

Peden, A. S.: Molluscum sebaceum (keratoacanthoma): Its etiology and relationship to early squamous carcinoma, whether self-healing or not. S. Afr. Med. J., 36:1091, 1962.

Peterkin, G. A. G., Macmillan, J. E., and Maclean, S.: Pseudocarcinoma of skin: Follow-up of keratoacanthoma seen in the 10 years (1951–1960). Scott. Med. J., 7:27, 1962.

Pillsbury, D. M., and Beerman, H.: Multiple keratoacanthoma. Am. J. Med. Sci., 236:614, 1958.

Pisanty, S.: Keratoacanthoma of the face. Oral Surg., 21:505, 1966.

Popkin, G. L., Brodie, S. J., Hyman, A. B., Andrade, R., and Kopf, A. W.: A technique of biopsy recommended for keratoacanthomas. Arch. Dermatol., 94:191, 1966.

Poth, D. O.: Tumor-like keratoses: Report of a case. Arch. Dermatol., 39:228, 1939.

Prutkin, L., and Gerstner, R.: A histochemical study of the keratoacanthoma, experimentally produced. Dermatologica, 132:16, 1966.

Rajam, R. V., Thambiah, A. S., and Anguli, V. C.: Keratoacanthoma on the skin of the face. Indian J. Dermatol. Venereol., 24:13, 1958.

Reed, R. J.: Actinic keratoacanthoma. Arch. Dermatol., 106:858, 1972.

Rigdon, R. H.: Histopathogenesis of "keratoacanthoma" induced with methylcholanthrene. Arch. Dermatol., 81:381, 1960.

Rocha, G., and Fraga, S.: Sea urchin granuloma of the skin. Arch. Dermatol., 85:406, 1962.

Rook, A.: Kérato-acanthome et états pseudo-carcinomateux voisins. IX Congrès Assoc. Dermatol. Syphiligr. Langue Francaise. Lausanne, Geneva, Editions Médecine et Hygiène, 1956, p. 221.

Rook, A.: Personal correspondence with the author, 1962.

Rook, A., and Champion, R. H.: Keratoacanthoma. *In* Conference on Biology of Cutaneous Cancer. Bethesda, Md., National Cancer Institute Monograph No. 10, 1963, p. 257.

Rook, A., and Whimster, I.: Le Kérato-acanthome. Arch. Belg. Dermatol. Syphiligr., 6:137, 1950.

Rook, A., Kerdel-Vegas, F., and Young, J. A.: Recurrences in keratoacanthoma. Med. Cutan., 11:17, 1967.

Rossman, R. E., Freeman, R. G., and Knox, J. M.: Multiple keratoacanthomas. Arch. Dermatol., 89:374, 1964.

Rous, P., and Kidd, J. G.: Conditional neoplasms and subthreshold neoplastic states. J. Exp. Med., 73:365, 1941.

Sagebiel, R. W.: Non-specific inclusions in epidermal cells of keratoacanthoma. J. Invest. Dermatol., 46:293, 1966.

Shapiro, L., and Baraf, C. S.: Subungual epidermoid carcinoma and keratoacanthoma. Cancer, 25:141, 1970.

Silberberg, I., Kopf, A. W., and Baer, R. L.: Recurrent keratoacanthoma of the lip. Arch. Dermatol., 86:44, 1962.

Simpson, J. R.: Molluscum pseudocarcinomatosum. Lancet, 1:569, 1955.

Sklarz, E.: Tumorbildung auf Lupus Erythematodes. Z. Haut. Geschlechtskr., 19:321, 1955.

Sklarz, E., In discussion of paper by Foelsche-Halle, O. A.: Histochemische Untersuchungen der Molluscum Pseudocarcinomatosum. Arch. Klin. Exp. Dermatol., 211:210, 1960.

Smith, J.: A case of multiple primary squamous-celled carcinomata of skin in a young man, with spontaneous healing. Br. J. Dermatol., 46:267, 1934.

Smith, J. F.: Multiple primary, self-healing squamous epithelioma of the skin. Br. J. Dermatol. Syph., 60:315, 1948.

Solomon, L. M., and Beerman, H.: Der einflus von Keratoakanthomen auf die Entwicklung von Shope-Papillomen beim Kaninchen. Hautarzt, 15:86, 1964.

Sommerville, J., and Milne, J. A.: Familial primary self-healing squamous epithelioma of the skin. Br. J. Dermatol. Syph., 62:485, 1950.

Spier, H. W., and Thies, W.: Aggregierte Keratoacanthome (Mollusca Pseudocarcinomatosa). Hautarzt, 7:206, 1956.

Stenhouse, E. E., and Becker, S. W.: A case for diagnosis (pseudoepitheliomatous hyperplasia? Benign squamous cell tumor? Multiple squamous cell epithelioma?). Arch. Dermatol., 45:999, 1942.

Stevanovic, D. V.: Keratoacanthoma: Mucous membranes at the site of its localization. Dermatologica, 121:278, 1960.

Stevanovic, D. V.: Keratoacanthoma in xeroderma pigmentosum. Arch. Dermatol., 84:53, 1961.

Stevanovic, D. V.: Keratoakanthome Nach Folliculitis Barbae. Hautarzt, 13:286, 1962.

Stevanovic, D. V.: Keratoacanthoma Dyskeratoticum and Segregans. Arch. Dermatol., 92:666, 1965a.

Stevanovic, D. V.: A comparative morphological and dynamic study of the pseudocarcinomatous process of man and hairless mouse. Dermatologica, 131:367, 1965b.

Stevanovic, D. V.: Récidives du kérato-acanthome: Reformation, exacerbation, recroissance, keratoacanthomata duplex. Ann. Dermatol. Syphiligr. (Paris), 96:415, 1969.

Svejda, J., and Schwartz, A.: Molluscum Pseudocarcinomatosum Labii. Czas. Stomatol., 13:263, 1960.

Szymanski, F. J.: Warty dyskeratoma. Arch. Dermatol., 75:567, 1957.

Szymanski, F. J., In discussion of Cases Presented in Society Transactions. Arch. Dermatol., 86:109, 1962.

Szymanski, F. J.: Keratoacanthoma and squamous cell carcinoma. South. Med. J., 56:609, 1963.

Tappeiner, J., and Wolff, K.: Papillomatosis mucosae carcinoides ("Oral florid papillomatosis"). Hautarzt, 20:102, 1969.

Tarnowski, W. M.: Multiple keratoacanthoma: Response to systemic chemotherapy. Arch. Dermatol., 94:74, 1966.

Teller, H.: Molluscum pseudocarcinomatosum with special reference to its microhistory. Z. Haut. Geschlechtskr., 20:217, 1956.

Thivolet, J., Leung, T. K., Moulin, G., Sepetdjan, M., and Lieux, J. M.: Kérato-acanthome géant, aspects en microscopie électronique. Ann. Dermatol. Syphiligr. (Paris), 93:137, 1966.

Thompson, S.: Molluscum sebaceum and its surgical significance. Ann. R. Coll. Surg. Engl., 22:282, 1958.

Tzanck, A., Sidi, E., and Melki, G.: Trois cas de molluscum contagiosum unique, avec réaction ganglionnaire importante. Ann. Dermatol. Syphiligr. (Paris), 10:263, 1950.

Vaccari, R., and Tagliavini, R.: Il keratoacanthoma. Arch. Ital. Dermatol. Sif., 27:239, 1955.

Van der Meiren, L., Mestdagh, G. H., and Achten, G.: Étude clinique et histologique du kérato-acanthome. Assoc. des Dermatologistes et Syphiligraphes de Langue Francaise. IX Congrès Lausanne, 1956, pp. 244–247.

Van Duuren, B. L., Langseth, J., Goldschmidt, B. M., and Orris, L.: Carcinogenicity of epoxides, lactomes and peroxy compounds. VI. Structure and carcinogenic activity. J. Natl. Cancer Inst., 39:1217, 1967.

Venkei, T., and Sugár, J.: Über Keratoakanthome von Präkarzinomatosem Charakter (Keratoakantom A und B). Dermatol. Wochenschr., 138:957, 1958.

Vickers, C. F. H., and Ghadially, F. N.: Keratoacanthomata associated with psoriasis. Br. J. Dermatol., 73:120, 1961.

Vinton, R. A., Jr., and Wilson, L. H.: Keratoacanthoma of the vermilion border. J. Florida Med. Assoc., 51:363, 1964.

Webb, A. J., and Ghadially, F. N.: Massive or giant keratoacanthoma. J. Pathol. Bacteriol., 91:505, 1966.

Whiteley, H. J.: The effect of the hair growth cycle in experimental skin carcinogenesis in the rabbit. Br. J. Cancer, 11:196, 1957.

Whittle, C. H., and Davis, R. A.: Kerato-acanthoma of lower-lip red margin. Lancet, 272:1019, 1957.

Williams, M. G.: Acanthomata appearing after eczema. Br. J. Dermatol., 68:268, 1956.

Wilson, J. W.: Multiple keratoacanthomata. Arch. Dermatol., 74:325, 1956.

Winer, L. H., In discussion of papers of Binkley, G. W., and Johnson, H. H., and Ereaux et al.: Arch. Dermatol., 71:66, 1955.

Winer, L. H., and Wright, E. T.: Uber Den Sekundären (Metastatischen) Hautkrebs. Hautarzt, 11:22, 1960.

Winkelmann, R. K., and Brown, J.: Generalized eruptive keratoacanthoma. Arch. Dermatol., 97:615, 1968.

Witten, V. H., and Zak, F. G.: Multiple primary self-healing prickle-cell epithelioma of the skin. Cancer, 5:539, 1952.

Zacarian, S. A.: Cryosurgery of Skin Cancer and Cryogenic Techniques in Dermatology. Springfield, Ill., Charles C Thomas, Publisher, 1969.

Zelickson, A. S.: Virus-like particles demonstrated in keratoacanthomas. Acta Derm. Venereol. (Stockh.), 42:23, 1962.

Zelickson, A. S., and Lynch, F. W.: Electron microscopy of virus-like particles in a keratoacanthoma. J. Invest. Dermatol., 37:79, 1961.

Zimmerman, M., In discussion of case presentation by Wilson, J. W.: Multiple keratoacanthomata. Arch. Dermatol., 74:326, 1956.

Zoon, J. J., Jansen, L. H., and Van Baak, J.: Le molluscum sebaceum (kérato-acanthome). Dermatologica, 108:81, 1954.

Histopathology of Keratoacanthoma

A. Bernard Ackerman, M.D.

Keratoacanthoma is a singular neoplasm. No other cutaneous new growth evolves so rapidly and yet resolves so predictably and completely. The histologic concomitants of this extraordinary crescendo and diminuendo are the subject of this account. The prototype for this discussion is the solitary keratoacanthoma. What is written about it also applies, in general, to the familial and eruptive types of keratoacanthomas.

The observations which follow are based on my own experience with partially biopsied, proved cases of keratoacanthoma, i.e., lesions that resembled keratoacanthoma grossly and microscopically and which subsequently underwent total regression.

The initial histologic changes of keratoacanthoma appear to be downward and outward extensions of epithelial cells that emanate from several contiguous pilar in-

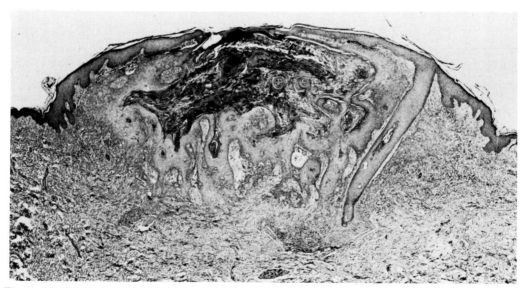

Figure 32–18 The initial histologic changes of keratoacanthoma appear to be downward and outward extensions of epithelial cells that emanate from several contiguous pilar infundibula ×6.

fundibula, the funnel-shaped upper segments of hair follicles. (Fig. 32–18). As the epithelial cells proliferate, they also differentiate and cornify. Increasing numbers of ortho- and parakeratotic cells are added to the progressively widened infundibula. These contiguous, horn-filled infundibula form a cornified mass within a concavity in the center of the tumor, which even at this beginning stage rises as a small dome above the skin surface (Fig. 32–19). These very early events establish the pattern for subsequent histologic developments during the evolutionary phase of keratoacanthoma. The tumor, almost from the outset, has an exo- and endophytic configuration, growing both above and below the skin surface. The exophytic epithelial component produces a dome-shaped nodule within which is a central cup containing cornified cells, whereas the endophytic epithelial component extends as a heart-shaped wedge pointing in the direction of the subcutaneous fat (Fig. 32–20). At the sides and base of this advancing wedge, strands, cords, and "tongues" of epithelial cells interpose themselves between collagen bundles (Fig. 32–21).

The width of the keratoacanthoma is probably determined by the number of adjacent hair follicles involved in the tumor's histogenesis (Figs. 32–22 and 32–23). Depending upon the number and kinds of pilar units involved, some keratoacanthomas are predominantly oriented in a hor-

izontal direction, others are mostly vertical, and still others have vertical and horizontal boundaries that are approximately equidistant. As the infundibular epithelial cells continue to proliferate, the keratoacanthoma expands in all directions—downward, sideward, and upward. The centrifugal spread stretches the epidermis that surrounds the several dilated, horn-plugged infundibula that are involved. This taut epidermis surrounding and overlying the keratoacanthoma is seen in histologic cross-sections as two thin lips which gently rise toward each other but fail to meet, being separated by a variously sized chasm that houses the central cornified mass (Fig. 32–24).

There is wide cytologic variation among keratoacanthomas and sometimes within the epithelium of the same tumor. The cells that constitute most keratoacanthomas are large and spinous, with such abundant pale-staining, glycogen-containing, eosinophilic cytoplasm that they resemble the cells of mucous membrane epithelium (Fig. 32–25). The nuclei of these cells are commonly well differentiated, similar to those of normal epidermal and infundibular epithelium. By contrast, evolving keratoacanthomas can be composed of cells that have less abundant and darker staining eosinophilic cytoplasm, strikingly large, pleomorphic, vesicular, atypical nuclei, and numerous differently sized nucleoli (Figs. 32–26 and

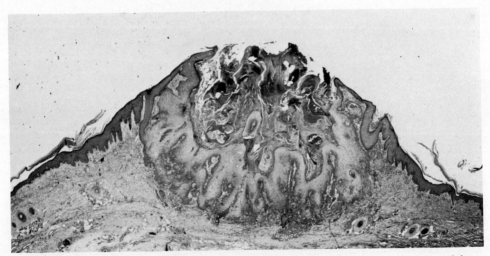

Figure 32–19   The contiguous, horn-filled infundibula form a cornified mass within a concavity of the tumor, which even at this early stage rises as a small dome above the skin surface ×3.

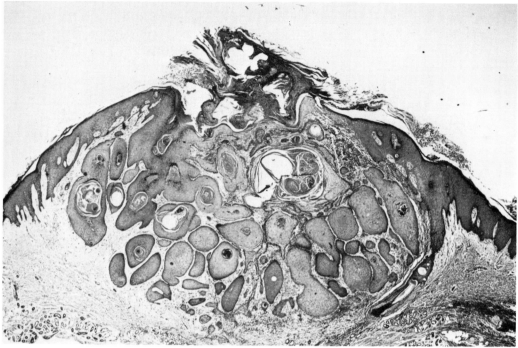

Figure 32–20 The exophytic component of a keratoacanthoma produces a dome-shaped nodule within which is a central cup containing cornified cells, whereas the endophytic component extends as a heart-shaped wedge pointing in the direction of the subcutaneous fat ×6.

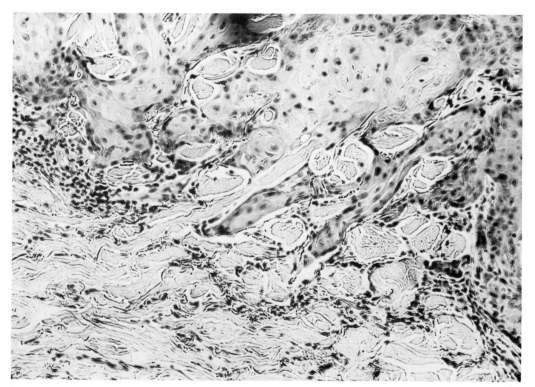

Figure 32–21 At the sides and base of the advancing wedge, strands, cords, and "tongues" of epithelial cells interpose themselves between collagen bundles ×20.

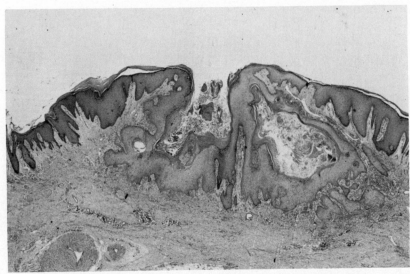

Figure 32–22   Only a few horn-filled, widened pilar infundibula are involved in this keratoacanthoma ×3.

32–27). Some cells contain several atypical nuclei. Numerous mitotic figures, often 10 or more per high power field, some highly atypical, may also be seen. Necrotic and dyskeratotic cells pepper the neoplastic epithelium. Acantholytic cells may appear within spaces that simulate glandular lumina. Occasionally, in a single specimen, a portion of the epithelium surrounding the cornified crater of an evolving keratocanthoma may consist of cells having abundant, pale-staining cytoplasm and relatively small, uniform nuclei, whereas the remaining portion may consist of cells that are startlingly atypical. At the junction between these portions, atypical keratinocytes merge and mingle with well-differentiated ones.

In addition to the epithelial changes of evolving keratoacanthomas, there are significant stromal alterations. The earliest inflammatory cells to appear are lymphocytes and some histiocytes. As the tumor grows, increasing numbers of plasma cells, eosinophils, and neutrophils arrive. Eventually, the neutrophils and eosinophils may predominate. Within well-developed and fully developed keratoacanthomas, these inflammatory cells can be found not only in the stroma but also within the spinous and cornified epithelium (Figs. 32–28 and 32–29). Neutrophils form intraepithelial abscesses, within which there often are nuclear dust, dyskeratotic and necrotic keratinocytes, and acantholytic cells (Figs. 32–30 and 32–31). In some in-

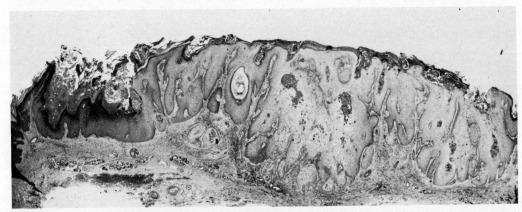

Figure 32–23   Many pilar infundibula are involved in this keratoacanthoma, which has a mostly horizontal orientation. The individual infundibula are in different stages of evolution and resolution ×2.5.

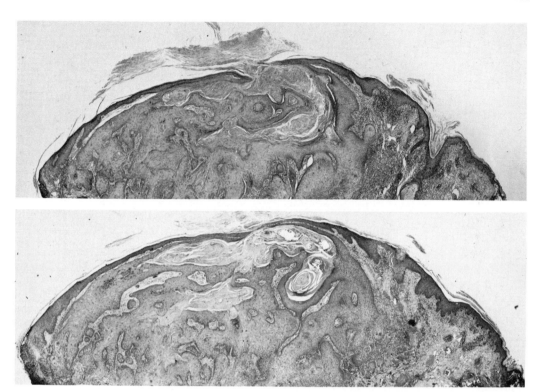

Figure 32–24 The epidermis that surrounds and overlies the keratoacanthoma is seen as two thin lips which gently rise toward each other but fail to meet, being separated by a variously sized chasm that houses the central cornified mass. Serial sections through the specimen show how closely the "lips" come to actually meeting ×7.2.

stances, these inflammatory and altered epithelial cells are also observed within widely dilated eccrine sweat ducts, into whose lumina project papillary epithelial buds. If a keratoacanthoma encroaches upon or enters the subcutis, inflammatory cells appear in the subcutaneous fat. The density of the inflammatory cell infiltrate

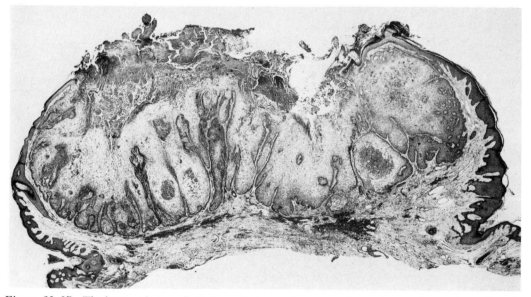

Figure 32–25 The large, spinous cells that constitute most keratoacanthomas have such abundant pale-staining, glycogen-containing cytoplasm that they resemble the cells of mucous membrane epithelium ×4.

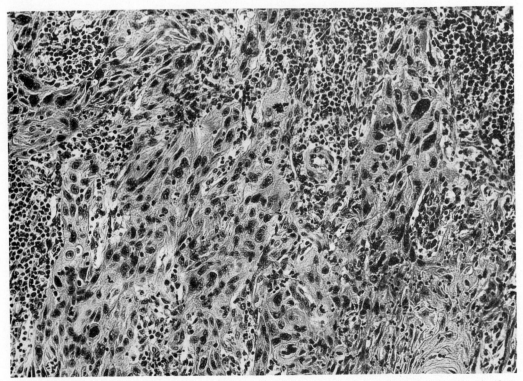

Figure 32–26　Some keratoacanthomas are composed of cells with large, pleomorphic nuclei, prominent nucleoli, and numerous atypical mitotic figures ×40.

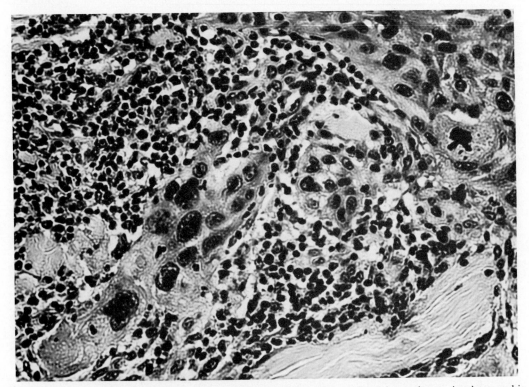

Figure 32–27　Epithelial aggregates in an evolving keratoacanthoma have large, hyperchromatic, pleomorphic nuclei and are surrounded by a dense predominantly lymphocytic infiltrate ×100.

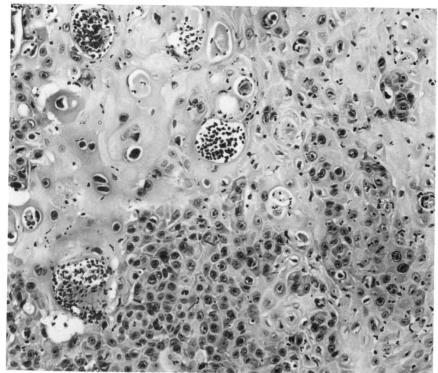

Figure 32–28 Abscesses containing neutrophils and eosinophils within the atypical epithelium of a well-developed keratoacanthoma. Necrotic and dyskeratotic cells pepper the neoplastic epithelium ×20.

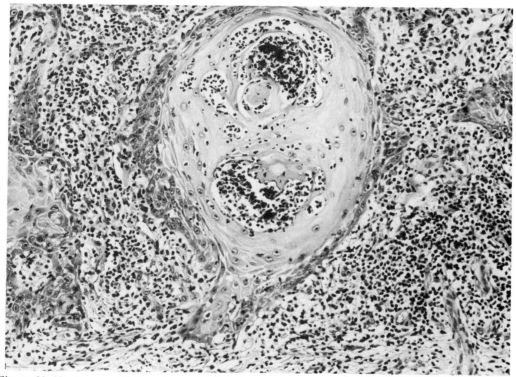

Figure 32–29 Neutrophils form intraepithelial abscesses in this fully developed keratoacanthoma. A dense, polymorphous, inflammatory cell infiltrate surrounds dilated blood vessels that are lined by plump endothelial cells ×9.

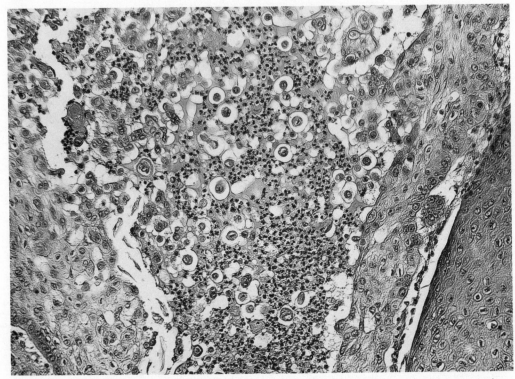

Figure 32–30   Intraepithelial abscess within which there are neutrophils, nuclear dust, and dyskeratotic and necrotic keratinocytes, as well as acantholytic cells ×20.

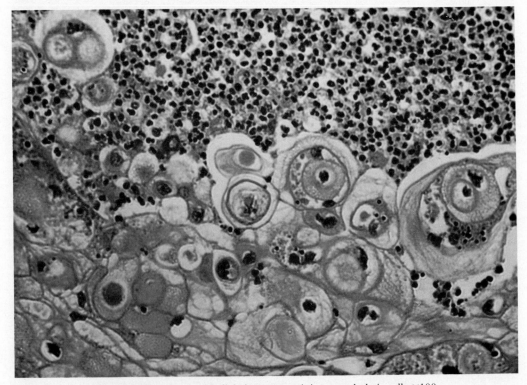

Figure 32–31   Intraepithelial abscess containing acantholytic cells ×100.

in keratoacanthoma may vary from sparse to massive.

Resolution of a keratoacanthoma is heralded by the presence of granulation tissue at the advancing edge of epithelial growth. The edematous dermis then contains an increased number of blood vessels lined by plump endothelial cells. A dense, polymorphous, inflammatory cell infiltrate of neutrophils, eosinophils, plasma cells, mast cells, lymphocytes, and histiocytes obscures the interface between the advancing epithelium and the adjacent dermis (Fig. 32–32). Numerous necrotic keratinocytes come to be intermingled with the inflammatory and endothelial cells (Fig. 32–33). The necrotic cells, as well as numerous cornified cells, become surrounded by histiocytes and multinucleated histiocytes (histiocytic giant cells), as a foreign body granulomatous reaction ensues (Fig. 32–34). To this mélange of cells are now added robust fibroblasts. Resolution of keratoacanthoma begins with granulation tissue, progresses to granulomatous inflammation, and ends in fibrosis (Fig. 32–35). New collagen fibers are formed from below, starting at the base of the tumor,

and are sequentially deposited at increasingly higher levels. The entire epithelial component of the keratoacanthoma retreats before the granulomatous and fibrosing onslaught. Some epithelial cells are destroyed by inflammatory cells, and the horn-containing crater is gradually pushed upward by the fibrosis forming beneath it. Ultimately the cornified contents of the crater extend above the skin surface, giving the lesions the clinical appearance of a cutaneous horn (Fig. 32–36). Finally the horn plug is extruded from its cup-shaped socket, and the entire dermis is replaced by scar (Fig. 32–37). Some sweat ducts may be found within the scarred dermis, but there are no remnants of pilar units.

The epidermis overlying a keratoacanthoma may be relatively normal or show varying keratinocytic and melanocytic abnormalities. Because a solitary keratoacanthoma occurs almost exclusively on sun-damaged skin, solar keratosis (Fig. 32–38), basal cell carcinoma, squamous cell carcinoma, lentigo, and lentigo maligna may be found in juxtaposition to a solitary keratoacanthoma. Aggregates of basal cell

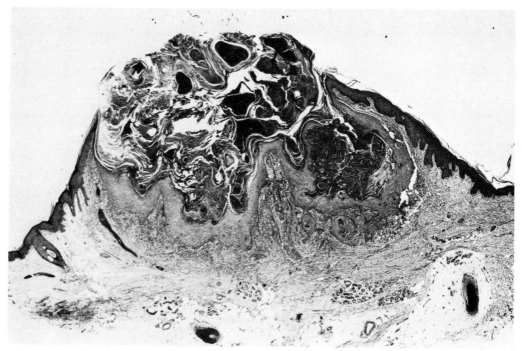

Figure 32–32   A dense, polymorphous, inflammatory cell infiltrate of neutrophils, eosinophils, plasma cells, mast cells, lymphocytes, and histiocytes obscures the interface between the epithelium and adjacent dermis of a resolving keratoacanthoma ×5.

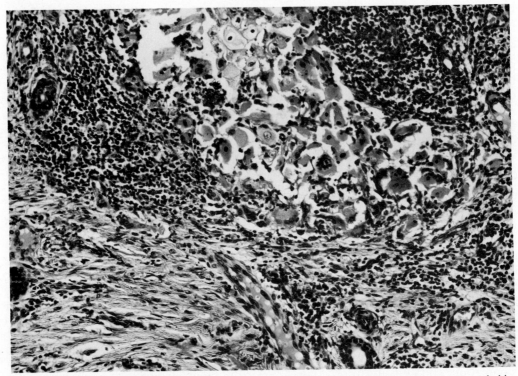

Figure 32–33 In this resolving keratoacanthoma, dyskeratotic and necrotic keratinocytes are surrounded by a dense, polymorphous, inflammatory cell infiltrate, beneath which is fibrosis ×20.

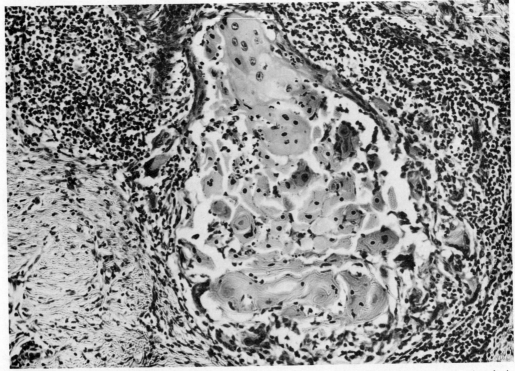

Figure 32–34 Foreign body granulomatous reaction to dyskeratotic cells and fibrosis are signs of an involuting keratoacanthoma ×20.

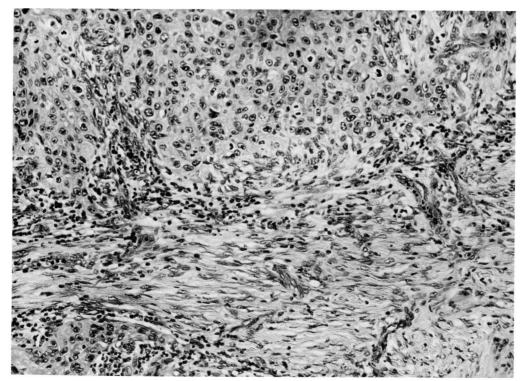

Figure 32–35 Fibrosis beneath a tumor of atypical keratinocytes is characteristic of resolving keratoacanthoma ×20.

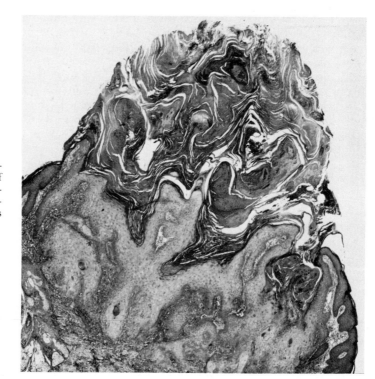

Figure 32–36 When the cornified contents are pushed out of the crater of a resolving keratoacanthoma, the tumor has the clinical appearance of a cutaneous horn ×5.

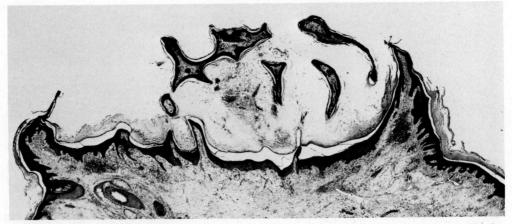

Figure 32–37   The entire dermis is replaced by fibrosis, but the epithelium retains its cup shape in this keratoacanthoma that has undergone almost total regression ×5.

carcinoma can also occur within the substance of keratoacanthoma. Dermal evidence of solar damage (elastotic material, solar elastosis) is consistently present in solitary keratoacanthoma.

The histologic diagnosis of keratoacanthoma can be made with certainty only if the overall configuration of the tumor can be studied. The histologic diagnosis of keratoacanthoma is made by pattern rather than cytology. It is essential that an adequate biopsy specimen be submitted if keratoacanthoma is to be distinguished from its cytologic look-alike, squamous cell carcinoma. A biopsy, ideal for this purpose, is taken with a scalpel and is done with an elliptical excision that stretches from normal skin to normal skin through the center of the lesion at its widest diameter and extends down to subcutaneous fat (Fig. 32–39). At the very least, an adequate

specimen is one that reaches from the center of the crater to the normal skin (Fig. 32–40). Such a biopsy will provide the critical information necessary to distinguish keratoacanthoma from squamous cell carcinoma by pattern. A punch biopsy may be worthless when attempting to differentiate keratoacanthoma from squamous cell carcinoma. If the specimen consists only of strikingly atypical keratinocytes, or even of well-differentiated ones, it is impossible to distinguish between keratoacanthoma and squamous cell carcinoma with certainty because the overall configuration of the tumor has not been presented to the pathologist for histologic examination.

Both keratoacanthoma and squamous cell carcinoma are characterized by varying degrees of atypical keratinocytic neoplasia, but their patterns in histologic cross-sections are very different. Evolving

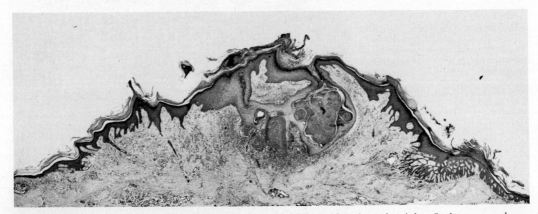

Figure 32–38   Hyperplastic solar keratosis emanating from the epidermis to the right of a keratoacanthoma ×2.5.

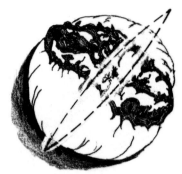

Figure 32–39 Ideal biopsy for histologic diagnosis of keratoacanthoma is taken with a scalpel in an elliptical excision that stretches from normal skin to normal skin through the center of the tumor at its widest diameter and extends down to subcutaneous fat.

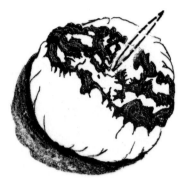

Figure 32–40 An adequate biopsy for histologic diagnosis of keratoacanthoma reaches from the center of the crater to the normal skin.

keratoacanthoma is distinguished by an epithelial tumor that extends as a dome above the skin surface and as a heart-shaped wedge into the dermis. The domed portion is a crateriform structure composed of multiple, widely dilated, horn-filled pilar infundibula. To either side of the crater and partly covering it is an epidermal "lip." This pattern is diagnostic of keratoacanthoma. Unfortunately, even in optimally obtained specimens, the characteristic central structure is not always seen. Sometimes the infundibula remain dis-

crete and do not coalesce to form a multiloculated, horn-filled crater (Fig. 32–41). If the biopsy is taken from the periphery rather than from the center of the keratoacanthoma, the characteristic architecture may not be visible at all (Figs. 32–42 and 32–43).

Often a keratoacanthoma has practically no nuclear atypia, but in some cases the degree of nuclear atypia is greater than in poorly differentiated squamous cell carcinoma. Nuclear features in themselves are irrelevant to distinguishing keratoacantho-

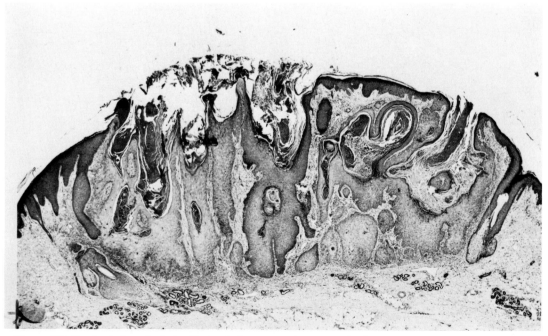

Figure 32–41 Sometimes the infundibula of a keratoacanthoma remain discrete and do not coalesce to form a central horn-filled crater ×4.

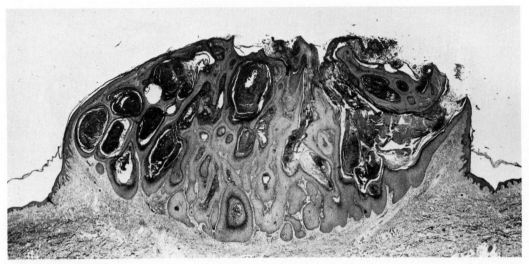

Figure 32–42 Biopsy specimen taken slightly peripheral to the central crater of a keratoacanthoma ×3.

ma from squamous cell carcinoma, but cytoplasm that is very abundant and pale-staining tends to favor the diagnosis of keratoacanthoma. Moreover, the presence of neutrophilic abscesses within epithelial aggregates favors the diagnosis of kerato-acanthoma rather than squamous cell carcinoma. Formation of pseudoglands con-

taining acantholytic cells, in the absence of an inflammatory cell infiltrate, is more indicative of squamous cell carcinoma. When acantholytic cells develop in keratoacanthoma, they are almost always within neutrophilic abscesses. Perineural location of tumor cells can be seen in both kerato-acanthoma (Fig. 32–44) and squamous cell

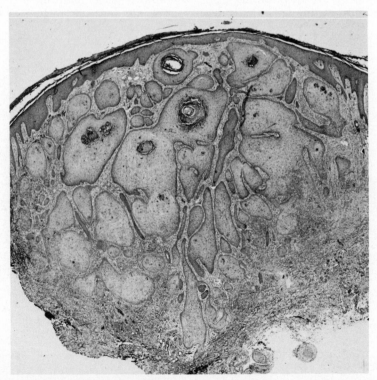

Figure 32–43 If the biopsy is taken from the periphery rather than from the center of a keratoacanthoma, the characteristic architecture may not be visible at all ×5.

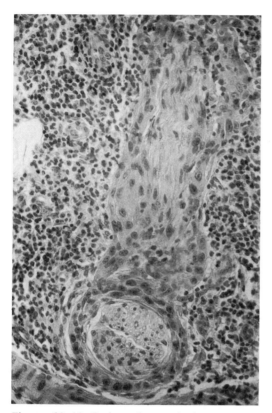

Figure 32–44 Perineural, neoplastic, squamous epithelial infiltration at the periphery of a keratoacanthoma. A dense, round cell, inflammatory infiltrate surrounds the structures. (*From* Baptista: Querato-Acanthoma. Coimbra, Portugal, Coimbra Editura Limitada, Ed., 1964, p. 385.)

carcinoma and therefore is not a helpful differential feature. Both keratoacanthoma and squamous cell carcinoma may extend into the subcutaneous fat and, exceptionally, into underlying skeletal muscle. Squamous cell carcinoma that develops on sun-damaged skin metastasizes with exceeding rarity, but keratoacanthoma, by definition, never metastasizes.

Resolution of a keratoacanthoma is recognized histologically by the fibrosis that forms immediately beneath the deepest epithelial component. The fibrosis develops in a band across the entire base of the tumor and, in time, consists of fibrillary collagen which is arranged parallel to the surface of the specimen and which bears dilated blood vessels orientated perpendicular to the skin surface. There may be a concurrent suppurative, granulomatous, and fibrosing reaction at the interface between epithelium and stroma in a

keratoacanthoma that is beginning to resolve. Stromal changes are an invariable accompaniment of all epithelial neoplasms, but the fibrosis of keratoacanthoma is distinctive. It begins at the base and sweeps upward. Fibrosis when associated with squamous cell carcinoma tends to surround irregularly shaped aggregates of atypical epithelium wherever they may be found in the dermis rather than in an orderly sequence beginning from below. The presence of fibrosis along the base of a tumor composed of atypical keratinocytes is a helpful diagnostic clue to involuting keratoacanthoma rather than squamous cell carcinoma.

In the ultimate analysis the clinicopathologic condition is essential, and the diagnosis of keratoacanthoma can only be made with absolute certainty by biologic behavior in the form of eventual involution. The diagnosis can be made histologically with near certainty on the basis of fulfillment of the criteria enunciated above, based upon careful study of partially biopsied specimens from lesions that have subsequently resolved. A biopsy specimen that does not have the typical histologic pattern of keratoacanthoma should not be certified indubitably as keratoacanthoma. Rather, the diagnosis should state no more than what the pathologist really knows, namely that the lesion probably is a keratoacanthoma but that a squamous cell carcinoma cannot be ruled out with certainty.

The principal neoplasm to be distinguished histologically from keratoacanthoma is squamous cell carcinoma. Rarely, verruca vulgaris and inverted follicular keratosis can pose problems in differential diagnosis from keratoacanthoma. Pattern again is the critical determining feature. Unlike keratoacanthoma, a verruca is predominantly exophytic and consists of digitate epidermal hyperplasia with peripheral rete ridges that point inward toward the center of the lesion. Inverted follicular keratosis is identified by prominent whorls of spinous cells ("squamous eddies") within a mostly endophytic and hyperplastic pilar epithelium. Giant molluscum contagiosum has a dome shape with a central horn-filled crater, but the epithelial cell cytoplasm houses characteristic molluscum bodies.

Several histologic findings support the hypothesis that keratoacanthoma is primarily a pilar neoplasm. The lesions almost always occur on hair-bearing skin. Well-defined hair follicles are usually seen to the sides of a keratoacanthoma, but identifiable hair follicles are rare or absent within the lesion itself, although hair erector muscles are commonly seen there. The crater of keratoacanthoma appears to consist of several contiguous, dilated pilar infundibula. The narrow orifice sometimes seen between the overriding "lips" above the crater of keratoacanthoma is similar to the narrow outlet in infundibular-type pilar cysts (epidermoid cysts). The apparent relationship of keratoacanthoma to hair follicle epithelium does not account for the rare reports of keratoacanthoma said to arise in non–hair-bearing sites, such as palms, soles, nail beds, and mucous membranes.

For additional reading see Baptista (1964), Bøwman and Pinkus (1963), Carteaud and Baptista (1962a), Jackson (1969), Lapière (1965), Lund (1971) Middleton and Curtin (1966), Peden (1962), Popkin et al. (1966), Read (1972), and Szymanski (1963).

33

Florid Oral Papillomatosis

Klaus Wolff, M.D., and Josef Tappeiner, M.D.

SYNONYMS

Florid oral papillomatosis has also been called papillomatosis mucosae carcinoides (Scheicher-Gottron, 1958) and oral florid verrucosis (Barnett and Hyman, 1968).

DEFINITION

Florid oral papillomatosis is a proliferative papillomatous hyperplasia of the oral cavity, characterized by a slow but relentless progression and a proclivity for recurrences; it may transform into carcinoma.

HISTORY

In 1960 Rock and Fisher described a 60 year old patient with papillomatous oral lesions which showed a tendency to recur but always exhibited a benign histology. The report contained two additional patients with laryngeal papillomas, and the disorder was designated as "florid papillomatosis of the oral cavity and larynx." A series of analogous cases have been reported since, and oral florid papillomatosis has become an accepted nosologic entity.

The disease is not "new" in the sense that similar patients were not seen prior to Rock's and Fisher's (1960) communication. Scheicher-Gottron (1958) had published an analogous case employing the designation "papillomatosis mucosae carcinoides," and several reports dealing with verrucous carcinoma of Ackerman contain cases that unequivocally fit the description of florid oral papillomatosis. In fact, and this will be elaborated in more detail later on in this chapter, it is very difficult, and at times impossible, to draw a distinct line between the two conditions.

Florid oral papillomatosis was originally considered a benign disorder (Rock and Fisher, 1960; Wechsler and Fisher, 1962), but today we know that it may transform into carcinoma (Samitz et al., 1967).

EPIDEMIOLOGY AND INCIDENCE

The number of cases reported so far is exceedingly small but, for various reasons, cannot be considered to reflect the true incidence of the disease. Photographs of florid oral papillomatosis are shown in the textbook of Schuermann, Greither and Hornstein (1966) and labeled as hyperplastic Bowen's disease of the oral mucosa (hyperplasie pure). Some patients with florid oral papillomatosis have been included in series of patients with verrucous carcinoma (Friedell and Rosenthal, 1941; Sorger and Myrden, 1960; Kraus and Perez-Mesa, 1966); others can be found in series of patients with papilloma or have been considered to have squamous cell carcinomas [possibly the patient reported by Schiller (1960)]. However, if it is taken into account that even verrucous carcinoma is infrequent in comparison to the more epidermoid carcinoma of the oral cavity,* the conclusion is justified that florid oral papillomatosis is indeed a rare disorder.

Table 33–1† summarizes 11 cases from the literature and 8 patients seen by us. Both sexes may be affected, although there appears to be a preponderance of males (12:7). The onset of the lesions falls into the higher age group, as all but two of the patients were older than 55 years when they developed the first symptoms. All patients were Caucasians, but this, of course, does not exclude the possibility that other races may be affected as well. Verrucous carcinoma occurs also in Negroes, and this is equally true for the giant papillomatous lesions of the genitals. There is no geographic prevalence.

ETIOLOGY AND PATHOGENESIS

Nature of the Disease

Since the original case was reported in conjunction with two patients exhibiting laryngeal papillomas (Rock and Fisher, 1960), oral florid papillomatosis has been considered an oral corollary of the laryngeal disease, and the two conditions have been regarded by some as manifestations of an identical pathologic process. This, however, may be more apparent

---

*In the series of Goethals et al. (1963), only 55 of 1217 cases of oral carcinoma fulfilled the clinical and histologic criteria of verrucous carcinoma.

†This list does not claim to be complete. The cases reported by Jaimovich et al. (1965), Knossew (1966), and Prokopcuk (1968) are not included, as sufficient data were not available to us. The patient of Roenigk and Lesowitz (1969) was omitted since, in our opinion, this patient probably had acanthosis nigricans of the oral mucosa.

than real. Multiple laryngeal papillomas are a fairly common disease in children; they are less common in adults, and in this age group they may evolve into carcinoma (Al-Saleem et al., 1968). The lesions are confluent, tend to recur (Stein and Volk, 1959; Rock and Fisher, 1960), and, very rarely, may be associated with multicentric papillary neoplasms of the trachea and bronchi (Buffmire et al., 1950; Moore and Lattes, 1959; Stein and Volk, 1959; Al-Saleem et al., 1968). None of the reported patients with florid oral papillomatosis had laryngeal lesions, and, conversely, oral changes are not mentioned in papers dealing with papillomas of the upper respiratory tract (Altmann et al., 1955; Al-Saleem et al., 1968). Florid oral papillomatosis occurs in old people, whereas the onset of multiple laryngeal papillomas is found in a much younger age group; thus, oral and laryngeal papillomatosis may have less in common than was believed originally.

Rock and Fisher (1960) followed their case for more than nine years without observing malignant changes and regarded the disorder as a wholly benign proliferative process. Several patients have since been seen in whom carcinoma eventually developed (Kaminsky et al., 1966; Samitz et al., 1967; Kanee, 1969; Tappeiner and Wolff, 1971), and, consequently, this view is not tenable any more. Today it is generally agreed that florid oral papillomatosis represents a precancerous condition, but it remains to be clarified whether it is benign initially, requiring a carcinogenic stimulus to transform into carcinoma, or whether it harbors malignant potentials ab initio.

We find it difficult to concur with Greither's and Hornstein's (1966) view that florid oral papillomatosis is a hyperplastic form of Bowen's disease of the oral mucosa. Bowen's disease is a carcinoma in situ, characterized by cell polymorphism, atypical mitoses, dyskeratotic changes, and disturbances of the intraepithelial architecture; all these features are characteristically absent from the lesions of florid oral papillomatosis. Andrade (1969) has included florid oral papillomatosis in the "giant mucocutaneous papillomatoses" which comprise verrucous papillomatous lesions of the mucous membranes and glabrous skin. They all exhibit florid growth patterns and have a tendency to recur; whereas some of them are benign, others may be malignant. It is evident from his classification (Table 33–2) that florid oral papillomatosis is thought to occupy a similar biologic position as the giant condylomata acuminata of Buschke and Löwenstein or papillomatosis cutis carcinoides of Gottron, i.e., similar growths occurring on the genital and glabrous skin, respectively. Indeed, Buschke-Löwenstein tumors may advance to frank carcinoma (Machacek and Weakley, 1960; Dawson et al., 1965), and the similarity of florid oral papillomatosis and papillomatosis cutis carcinoides has been underscored by the creation of the term "papillomatosis mucosae carcinoides" (Scheicher-Gottron, 1958). In our original publication we have favored this designation (Tappeiner and Wolff, 1969), but today we are less convinced of the merits of this term. Etymologically, "carcinoides" means cancerlike, whereas florid oral papillomatosis can progress into true carcinoma.

The possible interconversions of the disorders listed in the lower half of Table 33–2 into the carcinomas in the top row require clarification, and it may be that each condition has a different etiology (Andrade, 1969). It is our belief that the relationship of florid oral papillomatosis to Ackerman's (1948) verrucous carcinoma is a much closer one than has been appreciated so far, and Table 33–3 is shown to corroborate this view. Verrucous carcinoma is characterized by extensive, fungating, papillomatous growths of the oral mucosa. It is an extremely slow-growing tumor with a course extending over a number of years, and recurrences are common. There is only local invasion, and regional metastases are an exception. It is prevalent in elderly men and ofen found in an indigent population. Histologically, there is epithelial hyperplasia, hyperkeratosis, parakeratosis, and leukoedema, and the advancing border of the lesions is characterized by well-defined bulbus rete ridges, little cellular atypia, and only a moderate loss of polarity. All these features are also characteristic of florid oral

papillomatosis, and the differences may be more quantitative than qualitative in nature. Verrucous carcinoma is usually more aggressive, involving the surrounding soft tissues and the bone; this is usually not found in the more superficial lesions of florid oral papillomatosis, but in the cases of Wechsler and Fisher (1962) and Richter and coworkers (1972), erosions and even perforations of the mandible were observed. Verrucous carcinoma may contain foci of keratinization in the depth of the lesion; the polarity of basal cells is less well maintained than in florid oral papillomatosis, and although it does not grow destructively, it may infiltrate between preexisting structures. However, areas exhibiting just these features were present in the patients reported by Kaminsky et al. (1969) and by Kanee (1969), and in case no. 9 of Table 33–1. After X-ray irradiation, verrucous carcinoma may undergo anaplastic changes (Kraus and Perez-Mesa, 1966; Fonts et al., 1969), and in florid oral papillomatosis a similar switch to anaplasia was observed after aminopterin therapy (Samitz et al. 1967). Finally, a definite relationship exists between the pathogenesis of verrucous carcinoma and the exposure to tobacco (Friedell and Rosenthal, 1941; Kraus and Perez-Mesa, 1966; Fonts et al., 1969), and although such a relationship is not quite as evident in florid oral papillomatosis, the histories of most of these patients reveal long-term smoking habits.

Ackerman's (1948) verrucous carcinoma is quite distinct from the more common, "usual," epidermoid carcinoma of the oral cavity. This pertains both to the clinical and histologic manifestations and to the biologic behavior of this tumor. However, a careful review of the pertinent literature (Friedell and Rosenthal, 1941; Ackerman, 1948; Sorger and Myrden, 1960; Goethals et al., 1963; Kraus and Perez-Mesa, 1966; Cooke, 1969; Fonts et al., 1969) discloses that even this group is not quite homogeneous, and that the term verrucous carcinoma comprises a spectrum of biologically "almost benign", "not so benign," and low grade malignant tumors. In our opinion florid oral papillomatosis occupies the "benign" end of this spectrum.

TABLE 33–1

No.	Author	Age of Onset	Sex	Duration in Years	Tobacco	Dental Status	Localization	Treatment	Course	Histology	Final Outcome
1	Scheicher-Gottron, 1958	57	M	2	?	periodontitis ?	tongue, buccal mucosa, palate	X-ray, surgery declined	progressive	benign papillomatous	?
2	Rock and Fisher, 1960	60	M	9	cigarettes	?	mandibular recess, buccal mucosa, palate	X-ray, excision, electrocoagulation, maxillectomy	multiple recurrences	benign papillomatous	?
3	Wechsler and Fisher, 1962	81	F	4	?	edentulous, dentures	lower molar, buccal, sublingual mucosa, peripharyngeal fossa	podophyllin, electrocautery, curettage, X-ray, excision	multiple recurrences	benign papillomatous	?
4	Samitz and Weinberg, 1963; Samitz et al., 1967	55	M	10	pipe	edentulous, full dentures	buccal mucosa, lips	podophyllin, aminopterin, iridium 162	multiple recurrences	benign papillomatous; developed anaplastic squamous cell carcinoma	
5	Kaminsky et al., 1966	70	M	1	?	edentulous ?	buccal mucosa, lips	methotrexate	recurrences; involution after treatment	benign papillomatous; areas suggestive of low grade carcinoma	?
6	Barnett and Hyman, 1968	62	M	1	cigarettes	?	mandibular gingiva, lower gingival sulcus, lip vermilion border	methotrexate, electrodesication, curettage, excision	recurrences	benign papillomatous	
7	Tappeiner and Wolff, 1969	49	M	17	cigarettes	edentulous, full dentures	buccal mucosa, lips, vermilion border, oral commissure	electrocautery, excision	multiple recurrences	benign papillomatous	died of unrelated cause
8	Kanee, 1969	78	F	1	0	edentulous, full dentures	buccal mucosa, mandibular gingiva, floor of mouth, lip	excision, curettage, electrocautery, podophyllin, methotrexate	recurrences; improvement after methotrexate	benign papillomatous; areas suggestive of low grade carcinoma	died of unrelated cause

No.	Author, year	Age	Sex	Smoking	Years	Dentition	Location	Therapy	Course	Histology	Outcome
9	Tappeiner and Wolff, 1971	58	M	pipe	19	almost edentulous, remaining teeth decayed, broken	buccal mucosa, lips, tongue, oral commissurae	no therapy (declined), excision of nodular lesions, bleomycin	gradual progression	benign papillomatous; developed grade II carcinoma	alive; persistent lesions 1 year after excision of carcinoma; free of lesions after bleomycin (12 months)
10	Tappeiner and Wolff, 1971	37	M	pipe	20	almost edentulous, remaining teeth decayed, broken	buccal mucosa, lips	excision	gradual progression	benign papillomatous	alive; persistent lesions
11	Tappeiner and Wolff, 1971	89	F	0	4	edentulous, full dentures	tongue	no therapy	slowly but steadily progressive	benign papillomatous	alive; persistent lesions
12	Richter et al., 1972	71	F	?	2	edentulous	buccal mucosa, lips, tongue	electrocautery, excision, grafting, methotrexate	progression, recurrences; perforation of mandible	benign papillomatous	died, no autopsy
13	Eyre and Nally, 1971	58	M	?	26	edentulous	buccal mucosa	?	progression	benign papillomatous; squamous cell carcinoma	?
14	Kaulen-Becker, 1973	76	M	?	1	edentulous	buccal mucosa, alveolar process, palate	electrocautery	recurrences, progression	benign papillomatous	?
15	Kaullen-Becker, 1973	82	F	?	5	?	lips, palate	methotrexate, 5-FU, corticosteroids	recurrences, improvement after intralesional steroids	benign papillomatous	free of lesions (5 months)
16	Present authors	77	F	0	2	edentulous, plates	buccal mucosa, lips, alveolar process, palate	liquid nitrogen, podophyllin, excisions, resection of maxillary bone, grafting, bleomycin	recurrences, progression, recurrences within grafts, involution after bleomycin	benign papillomatous	free of lesions after bleomycin (18 months)
17	Present authors	63	M	pipe several years		edentulous	buccal mucosa	excision, grafting	free of lesions when last seen	benign papillomatous	?
18	Present authors	66	M	cigarettes several years		edentulous	maxillary gingiva, palate	no therapy (refused)	unchanged (6 months)	benign papillomatous	unchanged when last seen (6 months)
19	Present authors	57	M	1	—	edentulous	lower lip, vermilion border, buccal mucosa	liquid nitrogen	stable; then recurrences	benign papillomatous	recurrent lesions, presently stable

TABLE 33–2   CLASSIFICATION OF GIANT PAPILLOMATOSES OF SKIN
AND MUCOUS MEMBRANES*

Skin (General Expanse)	Mucous Membranes (Mainly Mouth)	Mucocutaneous Junctions (Lips, Lids, Urethra, Anus)
Verrucous (squamous cell) carcinoma	verrucous (squamous cell) carcinoma	verrucous (squamous cell) carcinoma
Pseudomalignant epitheliomatous hyperplasia†	florid verrucosis†	pseudomalignant epitheliomatous hyperplasia†
Papillomatous cutis carcinoides†	florid oral papillomatosis†	condyloma acuminatum, multiple, agminated†, and giant, of Buschke-Löwenstein†

*Modified from Andrade: Arch. Dermatol., 99:499, 1969. Copyright 1969, American Medical Association.
†Question of transition to malignancy.

Causative Factors

Really nothing is known about causative agents, and only assumptions can be made regarding the precipitating factors in this disease. A viral etiology has been implicated, as florid oral papillomatosis exhibits some similarities to verrucal lesions of viral origin and to canine oral papillomatosis, a condition induced by virus (Cheville and Olson, 1964). The alleged relationship of florid oral papillomatosis to laryngeal papillomas has also been taken to suggest a viral nature: viruslike structures have been observed with the electron microscope in laryngeal papillomas (Meesen and Schulz, 1957); papillomatous lesions were induced in human skin and in canine vagina by cell-free filtrates of laryngeal papillomas (Ullmann, 1923); and laryngeal papillomatosis has been noted to regress after treatment with a vaccine from bovine warts (Irvine et al., 1961). Structures probably belonging to the papovavirus group have also been observed in papillomas of the

TABLE 33–3   COMPARISON OF FLORID ORAL PAPILLOMATOSIS AND
VERRUCOUS CARCINOMA

	Florid Oral Papillomatosis	Verrucous Carcinoma
Age	old age	old age
Sex	M > F	M > F
Duration	years to decades	years
Tobacco	exposure common (cigarettes, pipe)	frequent and massive exposure (chewing, pipe, snuff)
Dental status	edentulous; plates	edentulous; plates
Preferential localization	buccal mucosa, gingiva, lips, floor of mouth	buccal mucosa, gingiva, lips, floor of mouth
Clinical appearance	papillomatous, vegetating, cauliflower-like; white, hyperkeratotic; leukoplakia	papillomatous, vegetating, cauliflower-like; white, hyperkeratotic; leukoplakia
Histology	papillomatosis; bulbous rete ridges, leukoedema, parakeratosis, hyperkeratosis; highly differentiated, little loss of polarity, well-defined margin to connective tissue, intact basement membrane; no keratinization in depth of epithelial masses; expansive but no infiltrative growth	papillomatous; bulbous rete ridges, leukoedema, parakeratosis, hyperkeratosis; highly differentiated, moderate loss of polarity, well-defined margin to connective tissue, basement membrane mostly intact, rare breaks occur; outline often irregular; keratinization may occur in depth of epithelial masses; some infiltrative growth
Course	gradual progression; recurrences	gradual progression; recurrences; may involve underlying soft tissue and erode bone
Anaplasia	extremely rare	rare
Metastases	not yet observed [probable in one case (Samitz et al., 1967)]	rare

human oral mucosa (Frithiof and Wersäll, 1967). These lesions bore no resemblance to florid oral papillomatosis, and papillomas caused by the wart virus are known to occur in the oral cavity. In contrast, there is neither histologic nor electron microscopic evidence for the presence of viral inclusions in florid oral papillomatosis, and attempts to recover a virus from the oral papillomas by tissue culture techniques were unsuccessful (Wechsler and Fisher, 1962). Moreover, therapeutic trials with autogenous papilloma tissue vaccine have failed (Wechsler and Fisher, 1962). The possibility still exists that a virus may have initially induced the tissue changes and subsequently became no longer extant (Wechsler and Fisher, 1962), but at present there is no cogent evidence for a viral etiology. Therefore, the term "oral florid verrucosis," as suggested by Barnett and Hyman (1968), does not appear advantageous, as it implies a viral cause.

The question has been raised whether trauma plays a role in the pathogenesis of this disease. Lacerations of the oral mucosa were experienced by two patients prior to the onset of their lesions (Barnett and Hyman, 1968; Tappeiner and Wolff, 1969), but these traumas cannot be held responsible for the papillomatous growths. The chronic, persistent irritations exerted by dentures may be more significant, and indeed most patients with florid oral papillomatosis have been edentulous or have worn dental plates for decades (Table 33–1). An analogous situation is encountered in patients with verrucous carcinoma: they are usually edentulous, have decayed or broken teeth, wear ill-fitting dentures, and exhibit poor oral hygiene (Fonts et al., 1969).

Tobacco may be another precipitating factor. Most patients with verrucous carcinoma are tobacco chewers or have been sucking snuff for many years (Friedell and Rosenthal, 1941; Ackerman, 1948; Kraus and Perez-Mesa, 1966; Fonts et al., 1969). Moreover, tobacco has been implicated as a cocarcinogenic agent in the pathogenesis of verrucous carcinomas in betelnut chewers (Sorger and Myrden, 1960; Cooke, 1969). A long-term exposure to tobacco is not quite as evident in florid oral papillomatosis, but 9 of 19 patients on

whom information is available have been cigarette or pipe smokers for many years. One of our patients, who had leukokeratosis nicotinica palati in addition to florid oral papillomatosis (Tappeiner, 1966), had been smoking 50 pipes (100 g. crude tobacco) per day for 58 years (case no. 9, Table 33–1), and another patient smoked 50 g. per day for 25 years (case no. 10, Table 33–1).

CLINICAL MANIFESTATIONS AND COURSE

Initially, the lesions may be solitary, but usually they arise in a multifocal pattern. The most common sites of involvement are the buccal mucosae (Figs. 33–1, 33–3, and 33–4), the upper and lower molar gingivae, and the floor of the mouth. The vegetating growths may spread to other areas of the oral cavity, extending to the palate, tongue (Fig. 33–5), peripharyngeal fossae, the lips, and the angles of the mouth (Figs. 33–1 and 33–2). The lesions appear as broad-based, papillary vegetations with a verrucous or polypoid surface and often evolve into fungating, cauliflower-like

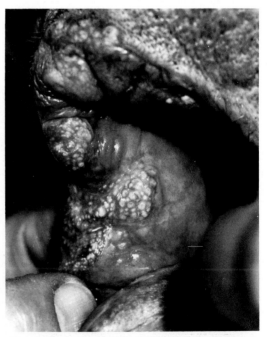

Figure 33–1　Florid oral papillomatosis of the buccal mucosa. Patient no. 7 (Table 33–1). (*From* Tappeiner and Wolff: Hautarzt, 20:102, 1969.)

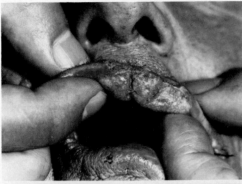

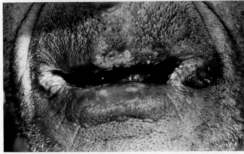

Figure 33–2 The same patient as in Figure 33–1. The upper lip is deeply infiltrated (*top*), and the oral commissurae exhibit nodular growths and hyperkeratotic fissures (*bottom*). (*From* Tappeiner and Wolff: Hautarzt, 20:102, 1969.)

masses which arise from a normal-appearing mucosa or from semiopaque and leukoplakic areas (Figs. 33–1 to 33–5). They may be red and beefy, assuming a raspberry-like appearance, but more fre-

quently they appear pearly white and hyperkeratotic. Hornlike lesions and nodular growths occur on the lips, and involvement of the oral commissurae results in deep fissures with hyperkeratotic margins (Fig. 33–2). Leukoplakia is common.

Initially the lesions are superficial, but as the process continues there is considerable infiltration of the tissue which, upon palpation, appears to be composed of hard, nodular, or platelike masses (Fig. 33–2).

The lesions are asymptomatic, but occasionally there may be soreness and a sensation of burning. Rarely, there is ulceration and, as bacterial infection supervenes, the lesions become painful, and there may be an inflammatory enlargement of the regional lymph nodes.

The course of these papillomatous proliferations is highly characteristic. They enlarge and spread very slowly but relentlessly, and, at least clinically, they seem to follow a locally aggressive growth pattern. In the patient reported by Wechsler and Fisher (1962), the papillomatous masses even extended into a fistula which had developed after surgical drainage of an inflammatory lymph node. Attempts to remove these vegetating masses by nonradical therapeutic measures are invariably followed by recurrences which, after variable periods of time, may arise either at the site of the original lesions, in

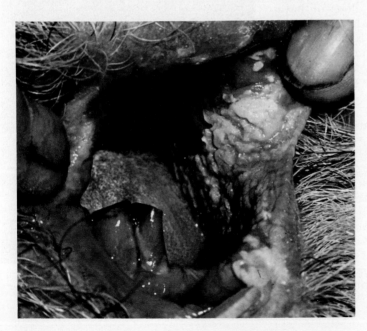

Figure 33–3 Vegetating, hyperkeratotic growths on the left buccal mucosa and lips (patient no. 9, Table 33–1).

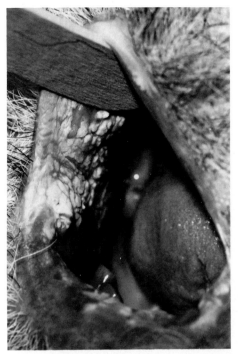

Figure 33–4 Right buccal mucosa of the patient shown in Figure 33–3 (case no. 9, Table 33–1). (*From* Tappeiner: Hautarzt, 17:152, 1966.)

their vicinity, or in a distant localization within the oral cavity.

Thus, the disease runs a protracted course which spans many years. In three patients followed by the present authors (cases no. 7, 9, and 10, Table 33–1), there

was a gradual progression for 17, 19, and 20 years, respectively.

Frank carcinoma does eventually supervene, but clinically it is difficult to assess the onset of the malignant change. Five cases have been reported so far in whom the diagnosis of carcinoma was finally established. The latency period varies within a wide range: in the two cases reported by Kaminsky et al. (1966) and Kanee (1969), a low grade carcinoma was diagnosed after a course of approximately one year; in the case originally observed by Samitz and Weinberg (1963), multiple biopsies had been taken during a span of 10 years and had revealed nothing but benign features. Eventually, an anaplastic carcinoma was demonstrated in a biopsy of an ulcerated lesion; in one case carcinoma developed after 26 years (Eyre and Nally, 1971); and in our case (case no. 9, Table 33–1; Figs. 33–3 and 33–4), a low grade squamous cell carcinoma was detected 19 years after the onset of the disease.

Metastases have not been described. Secondary malignancy may have been present in the regional lymph nodes of one patient (Samitz et al., 1967), but no biopsy was performed.

PATHOLOGY

The most striking and prominent histologic feature is the benign appearance of

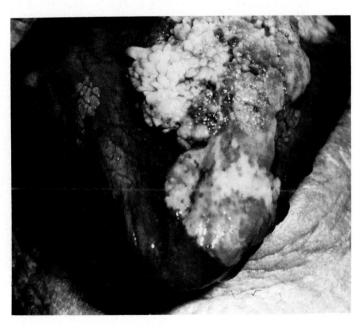

Figure 33–5 Florid oral papillomatosis of the tongue. The cauliflower-like surface is particularly evident in this tumor (patient no. 11, Table 33–1).

the lesions, which contrast with the impression gained by clinical inspection. Massive hyperplasia of the epidermis, bulbous rete ridges separated by slender strands of connective tissue, hyperkeratosis, and para-keratosis dominate the microscopic picture (Fig. 33–6).

The hyperplastic rete ridges are responsible for the papillary configuration of the lesions. They are aligned closely to each

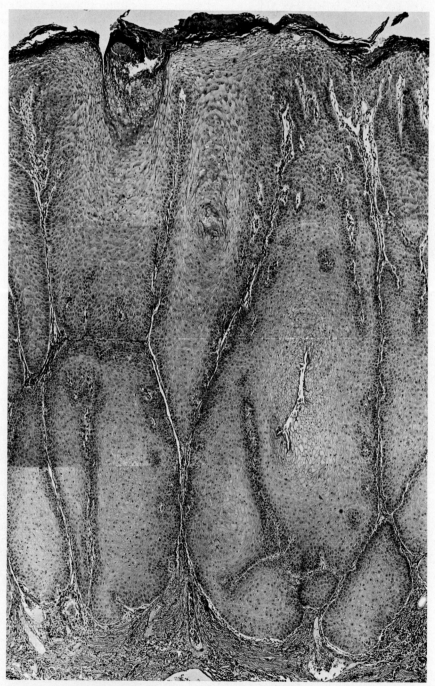

Figure 33–6 Low power photomicrograph of a typical lesion of florid oral papillomatosis (photomontage). There is a tremendous hyperplasia of the rete ridges, which are bulbous and swollen, but there are no signs of malignancy. ×50. (*From* Tappeiner and Wolff: Hautarzt, 20:102, 1969.)

other, advancing toward the underlying connective tissue in a broad front, and their rounded lower margins contrast with the uneven and jagged rete profiles usually present in the "ordinary" form of pseudoepitheliomatous hyperplasia (Fig. 33–6). Their margins are well defined, the basement membrane is intact, and the polarity of the basal zone is usually maintained (Figs. 33–7 and 33–8*A, C*). The basal cells are somewhat hyperchromatic; there is a moderate increase of mitotic figures, but abnormal mitoses are absent, and only occasionally are the basal cells poorly oriented. Suprabasally, there is no disorganization of the intraepithelial architecture and no disturbance of the epidermal stratification. There is neither cell polymorphism nor dyskeratosis (Figs. 33–6 to 33–8). The suprabasal cells exhibit normochromatic nuclei and ample eosinophilic cytoplasm which, in the upper strata, assumes an increasingly translucent and vacuolated appearance; in these layers the cells are swollen, the cell membranes are readily seen, and the nuclei become pyknotic (Figs. 33–8*B* 33–9) (leukoedema, Sandstead and Lowe, 1953). Keratohyalin is ab-

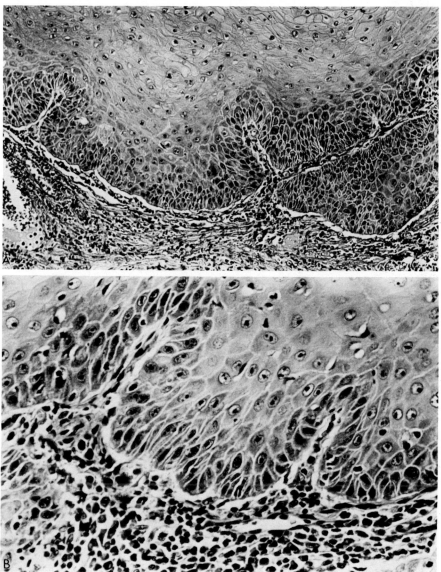

Figure 33–7 Border between proliferative epithelium and dermis. The basement membrane is intact, and the nuclei of basal cells are somewhat hyperchromatic, but there is neither a loss of polarity nor a disturbance of the epithelial stratification. *A, ×120. B, ×300. (B, From* Tappeiner and Wolff: Hautarzt, 20:102, 1969.)

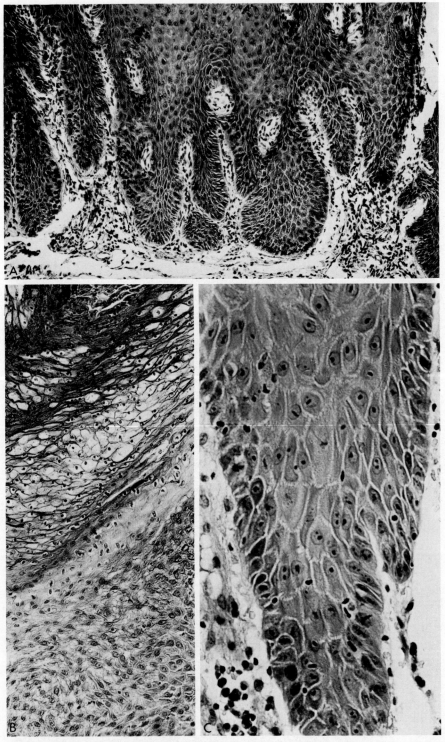

Figure 33–8 *A,* Lesion from the vermilion border of the lip. Note bulbous rete ridges, sharp margin to connective tissue, polarity of basal cells, and normal intraepithelial architecture. ×*120. B,* Superficial strata of mucosal lesion exhibiting a well-preserved stratification of the epithelium, leukoedema, and parakeratosis. ×*120. C,* High power view of margin between proliferative epithelium and dermis. There are no signs of malignancy. ×*300.*

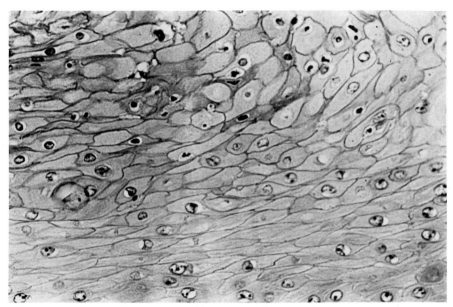

Figure 33–9 Superficial layer of mucosal lesion. Transition from leukoedema to parakeratosis. ×*300*. (*From* Tappeiner and Wolff: Hautarzt, 20:102, 1969.)

sent, and there is a gradual transformation of the viable epithelium into a thick, undulating, parakeratotic and hyperkeratotic, horny layer which may be infiltrated by polymorphonuclear leukocytes (Figs. 33–6 and 33–8*B*).

The dermal papillae represent extremely narrow and elongated strands of connective tissue, containing dilated blood vessels and extending between and separating the bulbous epithelial masses. An increased vascularity is also seen in the subjacent connective tissue, which contains a band of inflammatory infiltrate composed of lymphocytes, plasma cells, mast cells, and occasional polymorphs. The inflammatory infiltrate may extend into the epithelial masses.

It is obvious from this description that lesions of florid oral papillomatosis lack features of malignancy, and this may be true for years or even decades. In particular, the sharp margin of the epithelial-dermal interface is regularly maintained, and even repeated biopsies of different sites spaced over large periods of time fail to disclose a true neoplastic invasion. Sooner or later, however, such an invasion does occur, but the grade of anaplasia varies. Kaminsky et al. (1966) observed areas with cellular atypia, abnormal mitoses, and isolated nests of epithelial cells within the dermis, suggestive of low grade squamous

cell carcinoma, and similar changes were noted by Kanee (1969). The present authors observed a grade II squamous cell carcinoma within an area of otherwise typical florid oral papillomatosis (Table 33–1, case no. 9), and extreme anaplasia was present in the case reported by Samitz et al. (1967). A direct association of this carcinoma with previous lesions of florid oral papillomatosis was not unequivocally demonstrated in the sections but appears highly probable.

DIFFERENTIAL DIAGNOSIS

Squamous cell carcinoma of the oral cavity leads the list of conditions that have to be considered in the differential diagnosis. An exclusion of carcinoma is impossible on clinical grounds, but histologically the decision is easy. Cellular anaplasia, atypical mitoses, and infiltrative or aggressive growth patterns are not found in florid oral papillomatosis unless it has progressed to malignancy. On the other hand, it may be impossible to separate verrucous carcinoma of Ackerman and full-blown florid oral papillomatosis. The history and clinical manifestations of the two conditions are identical, and the course and histopathologic features are similar. Verrucous carcinoma should be considered if there is massive involvement of the underlying soft tissues or if erosions and destruction of the bony structures have occurred. The microscopic features favoring the diagnosis of verrucous carcinoma are: loss of polarity of the basal layer, foci of keratinization in the depth of the epithelial masses, disappearance of a regular and distinct demarcation between epithelial and connective tissues, and an infiltrating growth pattern.

Leukoplakia is easily excluded, as it represents a nonpapillary semiopaque or whitish plaque with a rough, brittle, and nonglistening surface. Histologically this clinical entity comprises rather superficial lesions, which lack the monstrous rete ridges of florid oral papillomatosis and exhibit cellular atypia, loss of polarity, and occasionally dyskeratosis (King, 1964). Leukokeratosis nicotinica palati is encountered in heavy smokers and may well occur concomitantly with florid oral papillomatosis (case no. 9, Table 33–1). It features multiple, confluent, whitish papules on the palate, each of which exhibits a small depression in the center. The depression corresponds to the orifices of mucous glands. Characteristically, these lesions involute spontaneously after the smoking habit is interrupted (Tappeiner, 1966).

Warts of the oral mucosa usually arise from a narrow base. They are few in number and not confluent; histologically, they exhibit a convergence of acanthotic rete ridges to a vascular base in the center. Although intranuclear inclusions are absent from many lesions, their presence excludes florid oral papillomatosis. Condylomata acuminata represent the prototype of papillary, digitate, cauliflower-like growths and thus resemble the lesions of florid oral papillomatosis. However, on the mucosal surfaces condylomata acuminata exhibit only a minimal degree of keratinization. Their color is usually pink or red, and they often feature a filiform surface. Histologically, the rete ridges are hyperplastic and bulbous, but often they anastomose, producing a retiform pattern. Nuclear inclusions may be rarely observed (Nasemann, 1961). In early lesions the general appearance is that of a richly vascularized stalk with a papillomatous growth, and there is little if any increase of the horny layer (Montgomery, 1967). However, in extensive and older lesions a histologic distinction from florid oral papillomatosis may be impossible.

The differential diagnosis also has to consider oral epithelial nevi [white sponge nevus; familial white folded dysplasia; white folded gingivostomatosis (Camon, 1935; Zegarelli et al., 1959; Cooke and Morgan, 1959)]. These are familial, their onset is in childhood, and there may be involvement of other mucous membranes (vagina, anus). The buccal mucosae or even the entire mucous membranes have a white folded or corrugated-like character, looking spongy and sodden in places or appearing as if they were covered by a milky film.

Focal epithelial hyperplasia (Tan et al., 1969) is also a nevoid lesion of the oral mucous membranes and consists of soft, sessile, plaquelike, and confluent lesions which exhibit the same color as the adjacent mucosa. The disorder is hereditary, occurring predominantly in individuals of Indian ancestry.

Acanthosis nigricans may produce considerable papillomatous lesions on the buccal mucosae, tongue, and lips. These are usually filiform or velvety; the characteristic lesions on the glabrous skin provide the correct diagnosis. Finally, secondary syphilis, lichen planus, and pemphigus vegetans will have to be excluded, but this will not present difficulties.

TREATMENT

Various therapeutic modalities have been tried, but the results are not too encouraging. The lesions may be removed by curettage, electrodesiccation, or electrocautery, but it is the experience of most physicians confronted with this problem that recurrences invariably ensue. Treatment with podophyllin or caustic measures, such as the application of trichloroacetic acid, are of no avail. Improvement has been noted by some after X-ray therapy (Rock and Fisher, 1960), while others have not seen beneficial results (Wechsler and Fisher, 1962). It should be emphasized that even doses which induce radiation damage cannot prevent recurrences. A note of caution appears appropriate in this context: there have been a number of instances in which irradiation of verrucous carcinoma of the oral cavity has been followed by highly anaplastic changes of the tumor as well as metastatic spread (Kraus and Perez-Mesa, 1966; Fonts et al., 1969), and there are reasons to believe that identical complications may ensue from X-ray therapy of florid oral papillomatosis.

The lesions can be removed by surgical excision, but this does not prevent the development of new growths in other areas of the mucous membrane. A partial maxillectomy was performed in Rock's and Fisher's (1960) patient, but the disease recurred in other sites. Nevertheless, wide surgical excision and grafting appear to be superior to all the other measures enumerated so far. Neck dissections are not necessary, since the probability of metastatic spread is low.

Chemotherapy appears to be the most promising approach for the future. Samitz and Weinberg (1963) introduced aminopterin into the therapy of florid oral papillomatosis and observed a complete involution of the lesions after repeated courses with this drug. Several recurrences were controlled in the same manner. Kaminsky et al. (1966) had excellent therapeutic results with methotrexate (three courses, 5 mg. b.i.d., for nine days each), and a similarly enthusiastic report is given by Kanee (1969): complete remissions were obtained after three courses of methotrexate given in weekly oral doses (10 mg. on two consecutive days a week), totaling 622. 5 mg. over a period of one year. However, it is still too early to reliably assess the long-term value of this type of treatment. Barnett and Hyman (1968) failed to obtain beneficial results, and the patients who apparently had shown a good response (Kaminsky et al., 1966; Kanee, 1969) have not been followed long enough. Of the five patients who have received methotrexate and who have been followed long enough, four have developed recurrences. Moreover, Samitz and Weinberg's (1963) patient, who initially responded so favorably, eventually developed a highly anaplastic squamous cell carcinoma (Samitz et al., 1967).

Though remote, the question arises whether aminopterin served as a trigger similar to X-ray in some cases of verrucous carcinoma.

Bleomycin has been reported to exert beneficial effects on squamous cell carcinomas of the oral cavity (Clinical Screening Co-operative Group, 1970). Our own experience with this drug is encouraging. Two patients have been treated so far (total dose, 4.5 mg. per kg.); they have responded surprisingly fast and have shown complete remissions. There have been no recurrences for 12 and 18 months, respectively. It remains to be seen whether this treatment will be equally successful in a large number of patients.

PROGNOSIS

Only scant information is available on the ultimate fate of the reported cases (Table 33–1). None of the patients on whom pertinent data are available died of their disease, and the deaths that have occurred are attributable to other causes. Of the eight patients observed by the present authors, one (no. 7, Table 33–1) died of an unrelated pulmonary condition, and seven (nos. 9, 10, and 11) are alive and well, but five have persistent lesions.

Extrapolating from what has been repeatedly stated in this article and considering the extremely long course of this disorder, it may be assumed that the prognosis of florid oral papillomatosis is probably much better than that of verrucous carcinoma in general.* However, many more cases will have to be observed before a definite stand can be taken in this matter.

---

*Goethals et al. (1963) reported on 55 patients with verrucous carcinoma of the oral cavity. Twenty-five out of 35 deaths were attributable to unrelated causes. Eleven patients were believed to have died of oral carcinoma, and in six of these the oral lesions were from distinctly separate (more undifferentiated) lesions that had metastasized. Other series (Kraus and Perez-Mesa, 1966; Cooke, 1969) give an even better prognosis.

REFERENCES

Ackerman, L. V.: Verrucous carcinoma of the oral cavity. Surgery, 23:670, 1948.

Andrade, R.: Giant mucocutaneous papillomatoses. Arch. Dermatol., 99:499, 1969.

Al-Saleem, T., Peale, A. R., and Norris, C. N.: Multiple papillomatosis of the lower respiratory tract. Clinical and pathologic study of eleven cases. Cancer, 22:1173, 1968.

Altmann, F., Basek, M., and Stout, A. P.: Papillomas of the larynx with intraepithelial anaplastic changes. A.M.A. Arch. Otolaryngol., 62:478, 1955.

Barnett, J. G., and Hyman, A. B.: Oral florid verrucosis. Arch. Dermatol., 97:479, 1968.

Buffmire, D. K., Clagett, O. T., and McDonald, J. R.: Papillomas of the larynx, trachea and bronchi: Report of a case. Proc. Mayo. Clin., 25:595, 1950.

Camon, A. B.: White sponge nevus of the mucosa (naevus spongiosus albus mucosae). Arch. Dermatol., 31:365, 1935.

Cheville, N. F., and Olson, C.: Cytology of the canine oral papilloma. Am. J. Pathol., 45:849, 1964.

Clinical Screening Co-operative Group of the European Organization for Research on the Treatment of Cancer: Study of the clinical efficiency of bleomycin in human cancer. Br. Med. J., II:643, 1970.

Cooke, B. E. D., and Morgan, J.: Oral epithelial naevi. Br. J. Dermatol., 71:134, 1959.

Cooke, R. A.: Verrucous carcinoma of the oral mucosa in Papua-New Guinea. Cancer, 24:397, 1969.

Davies, S. W.: Giant condyloma acuminatum: Incidence among cases diagnosed as carcinoma of the penis. J. Clin. Pathol., 18:142, 1965.

Dawson, D. F., Duckworth, J. K., Bernhardt, H., and Young, J. M.: Giant condyloma and verrucous carcinoma of the genital area. Arch. Pathol., 79:225, 1965.

Eyre, J., and Nally, F. F.: Oral candidosis and carcinoma. Br. J. Dermatol., 85:73, 1971.

Fonts, E. A., Greenlaw, R. H., Rush, B. F., and Rovin, S.: Verrucous squamous cell carcinoma of the oral cavity. Cancer, 23:152, 1969.

Friedell, H. L., and Rosenthal, L. M.: The etiologic role of chewing tobacco in cancer of the mouth. J. A.M.A., 116:2130, 1941.

Frithiof, L., and Wersäll, J.: Virus-like particles in papillomas of the human oral cavity. Arch. Virusforsch., 21:31, 1967.

Goethals, P. L., Harrison, E. G., and Devine, K. D.: Verrucous squamous carcinoma of the oral cavity. Am. J. Surg., 106:845, 1963.

Greither, A., and Hornstein, O.: *In* Schuermann, H., Greither, A., and Hornstein, O. (Eds.): Krankheiten der Mundschleimhaut und der Lippen. München-Berlin-Wien: Urban und Schwarzenberg, 1966, p. 437.

Irvine, E. W., Jr., Irvine, E. S., and Moffitt, O. P. Jr.: Treatment of laryngeal papillomas with bovine wart vaccine: A preliminary report of 4 cases. Cancer, 14:636, 1961.

Jaimovich, L., Abulafia, J., and Kaminsky, A.: Papillomatosis florida. Asoc. Argent. Dermatol., 24:4, 1965.

Kaminsky, de A. R., Kaminsky, C. A., Abulafia, J., and Kaminsky, A.: Papillomatosis florida oral: su tratamiento con methotrexate. G. Ital. Dermatol., 107:821, 1966.

Kanee, B.: Oral florid papillomatosis complicated by verrucous squamous carcinoma. Treatment with methotrexate. Arch. Dermatol., 99:196, 1969.

Kaulen-Becker, L.: Orale floride Papillomatose. Z. Haut. Geschlechtskr., 48:1, 1973.

King, O. H.: Intraoral leukoplakia. Cancer, 17:131, 1964.

Knossew, I. S.: Papillomatous granulomatosis (florid oral papillomatosis). Aust. J. Dermatol., 8:173, 1966.

Kraus, F. T., and Perez-Mesa, C.: Verrucous carcinoma. Clinical and pathologic study of 105 cases involving oral cavity, larynx and genitalia. Cancer, 19:26, 1966.

Machacek, G., and Weakley, D.: Giant condylomata acuminata of Buschke and Löwenstein. Arch. Dermatol., 82:41, 1960.

Meesen, H., and Schulz, H.: Elektronenmikroskopischer Nachweis des Virus im Kehlkopfpapillom des Menschen. Klin. Wochenschr., 35:771, 1957.

Montgomery, H.: Dermatopathology. Vol. I. New York, Hoeber Medical Division, Harper and Row, Publishers, 1967, p. 545.

Moore, R. L., and Lattes, R.: Papillomatosis of larynx and bronchi. Case report with 34-year follow-up. Cancer, 12:117, 1959.

Nasemann, T.: Die Viruskrankheiten der Haut und die Hautsymptome bei Richettsiosen und Bartonellosen. *In* Handbuch der Haut- und Geschlechtskrankheiten. Ergänzungswerk. Vol. 4/2, Berlin, Springer-Verlag, 1961, p. 413.

Prokopcuk, A. J.: Papillomatosis oralis florida. Derm. i. Vener. (Sofia), 7:193, 1968.

Richter, G., Engel, S., and Jacobi, H.: Zum Krankheitsbild der sogenannten oral florid papillomatosis. Dermatologica, 44:75, 1972.

Rock, J. A., and Fischer, E. R.: Florid papillomatosis of the oral cavity and larynx. Arch. Otolaryngol., 72:593, 1960.

Roenigk, H. H., and Lesowitz, S. A.: Acanthosis nigricans and oral florid papillomatosis. Arch. Dermatol., 99:119, 1969.

Samitz, M. H., and Weinberg, R. A.: Oral florid papillomatosis. Response to aminopterin. Arch. Dermatol., 87:478, 1963.

Samitz, M. H., Ackerman, A. B., and Lantis, L. R.: Squamous cell carcinoma arising at the site of oral florid papillomatosis. Arch. Dermatol., 96:286, 1967.

Sandstead, H. R., and Lowe, J. W.: Leukoedema and keratosis in relation to leukoplakia of buccal mucosa in man. J. Natl. Cancer Inst., 14:423, 1953.

Scheicher-Gottron, E.: Papillomatosis mucosae carcinoides der Mundschleimhaut bei gleichzeitigem Vorhandensein eines Lichen ruber der Haut. Z. Haut. Geschlechtskr., 24:99, 1958.

Schiller, F.: Zungencarcinom bei Epidermolysis bullosa dystrophica. Arch. Klin. Exp. Dermatol., 209,:643, 1960.

Shklar, G.: The precancerous oral lesion. Oral Surg., 20:58, 1965.

Sorger, K., and Myrden, J. A.: Verrucous carcinoma of the buccal mucosa in tobacco chewers. J. Can. Med. Assoc., 83:1413, 1960.

Stein, A. A., and Volk, B. M.: Papillomatosis of trachea and lung. Arch. Pathol., 68:468, 1959.

Tan, K. N., Medak, H., and Cohen, L.: Focal epithelial hyperplasia in a Mexican Indian. Arch. Dermatol., 100:474, 1969.

Tappeiner, J.: Zur Klinik und Pathogenese der Leu-kokeratosis nicotinica palati. Hautarzt, 17:152, 1966.

Tappeiner, J., and Wolff, K.: Papillomatosis mucosae carcinoides (oral florid papillomatosis). Hautarzt, 20:102, 1969.

Tappeiner, J., and Wolff, K.: Floride oral Papil-lomatose (oral florid papillomatosis). Wien Klin. Wochenschr., 83:795, 1971.

Ullmann, E. V.: On the aetiology of the laryngeal papilloma. Acta Otolaryngol., 5:317, 1923.

Wechsler, H. L., and Fisher, E. R.: Oral florid papillo-matosis. Arch. Dermatol., 86:480, 1962.

Zegarelli, E. V., Everett, F. G., Kutscher, A. H., Gor-man, J., and Kupferberg, N.: Familial white folded dysplasia of the mucous membranes. Arch. Derma-tol., 80:97, 1959.

34

Giant Condyloma of Buschke-Löwenstein

Alvin E. Friedman-Kien, M.D.

DEFINITION

Giant condyloma acuminatum (Buschke-Löwenstein tumor) is an unusual, exuberant, wartlike growth that penetrates the deeper tissues. It occurs mostly on the penis with only a few exceptions. Clinically, the tumor behaves like a malignancy, yet histologically it appears remarkably benign. Although it was initially reported by Buschke in 1896, the first detailed description of this lesion was presented in 1925 by Buschke and Löwenstein. Subsequent reports of similar tumors have been made with increasing frequency, so that at present there are over 70 cases reported in the medical literature. The Buschke-Löwenstein tumor has now gained acceptance as a distinct entity. It is known by different names, such as "carcinoma-like condyloma," giant condyloma of Buschke and Löwenstein, or "verrucose carcinoma."

ETIOLOGY

Giant condyloma acuminatum is thought to be an unusual variant of the ordinary human papillomavirus-induced warts, which are known as condylomata acuminata when they occur on the genitalia. These papillomata are sometimes called "venereal" warts, "fig" warts, or "moist" warts (Goldschmidt and Kligman, 1958; McCarron and Carlton, 1970; Powley, 1964). These simple, benign, noninvasive condylomata acuminata have a predilection for moist mucocutaneous or intertriginous surfaces, especially of the genital and anal regions of both males and females.

Human warts are caused by a DNA-containing virus, approximately 45 to 55 mμ in diameter, which is usually found in the nuclei of infected cells. It is classified under the papova virus group—a particular class of viruses, such as SV40 and polyoma, known to induce tumors in mammals. The viral etiology of human warts has been confirmed by electron microscopic evidence (Almeida, 1972) and by the successful transmission of warts to inoculated human volunteers using virus containing extracts of venereal and other types of warts (Serra, 1924; Goldschmidt and Kligman, 1958).

Different varieties of human warts are believed to be caused by the same species of human papillomavirus. The differences in wart morphology are thought to be due to a variation in the specific local tissue response to the infectious agent. Electron microscopic examination of tissue and extracts of various kinds of warts shows that condylomata acuminata are apparently much less abundant in virus particles than are most other verrucae, such as plantar warts. To date, there is no definite evidence for the viral etiology of the giant condyloma of Buschke-Löwenstein. However, it has been suggested that this "giant" wartlike tumor is a peculiar local variant of the simple condyloma acuminatum or that perhaps it is due to a particularly virulent strain of the human wart virus.

CLINICAL FEATURES

In the early stages giant condyloma acuminatum of Buschke-Löwenstein can be easily mistaken for the ordinary type of condyloma acuminatum. Common venereal warts are found as single, or more often multiple, discrete, superficial, verrucous growths which rarely attain a size greater than 1 cm. in diameter. These cauliflower-like lesions have a mucosal pink-red color and are rarely keratinized except when they occur on the glabrous skin of the genitalia or have been present on the mucosal surfaces for a prolonged period. Similarly, the giant condylomata of Buschke-Löwenstein may initially appear as a single or coalescent group of verrucous papules most often on the mucosal surface of the glans or preputial sac of the penis (Fig. 34–1).

Löwenstein stated that the essential difference between giant condyloma and simple condyloma acuminatum is that the former's growth is not confined to the surface but shows a marked tendency to penetrate into the deeper tissues. Due to the rapid proliferation, the giant condyloma of Buschke-Löwenstein forms a mushrooming, yellowish white, cornified mass which may reach the size of a golf ball or an even greater diameter, and which by extension may invade, distort, and eventually destroy the deeper tissues of the penile shaft. Ulceration and ureterocutaneous fistulae may occur, resulting in secondary infection which often produces a foulsmelling, purulent discharge. Simple condylomata do not behave in such an aggressive manner. Löwenstein explained that it was the invasive characteristics of the giant condyloma described above which led to the term "carcinoma-like con-

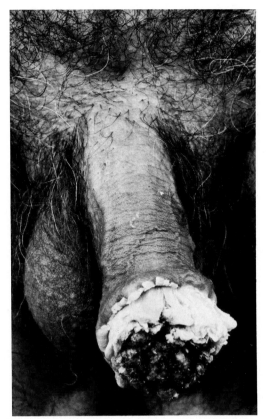

Figure 34–1 Giant condyloma of Buschke-Löwenstein involving the glans penis. [Photograph used by permission of New York University School of Medicine (Skin and Cancer Unit).]

dyloma." He pointed out that "the infiltration is not an active one; but one in which the lower condylomatous tissue has been displaced downward by the prolific growth of the condyloma above it. The ultimate effect of this process is to compress portions of the corpus cavernosum of the penile shaft. Nowhere are there abnormal tumor cells to be seen; neither in the tissue spaces, blood vessels, nor in the lymphatics." Most often the lesion appears under the prepuce of uncircumcised males, although a few cases occurring in circumcised individuals have been reported (Dreyfuss and Neville, 1955; Powley, 1964; Dawson et al., 1965).

Only five cases of giant condyloma of Buschke-Löwenstein involving the female vagina have appeared in the medical literature (Rosenthal and Wiese, 1923; Evans and Dische, 1969; Kraus and Perez-Mesa, 1966). A case of giant condyloma of Buschke-Löwenstein on the perianal skin was reported by Dawson et al. (1965), and two cases of giant condylomata actually involving the rectum were reported by Knoblich (1967) and DiCaro and Bernardini (1971). Greenberg and Wallace in 1963 reported a case of a giant wartlike growth, appearing on the skin of the shoulder and demonstrating a benign histopathologic picture, similar to that seen in association with giant condyloma of Buschke-Löwenstein on the penis.

RELATIONSHIP TO MALIGNANCY

The gross clinical appearance of the Buschke-Löwenstein tumor suggests a malignancy of the penis, most often thought to be a squamous cell carcinoma. Davies in 1965 studied 100 cases diagnosed as squamous cell carcinoma and found that 24 of these actually proved to be benign giant condylomata of Buschke and Löwenstein by histologic examination. One of these 24 cases showed early "malignant" changes, but for the most part almost all the reported cases paradoxically presented a remarkably orderly, benign, microscopic appearance very similar to, but not identical to, that of simple condyloma acuminatum. Machacek and Weakley in 1960, as well as others, have stressed the fact that a transition from the benign to the malignant state in either the simple or "giant" variety of condylomata is very unusual. One case has been reported in which the giant condyloma of Buschke-Löwenstein of the penis was associated with a metastatic carcinoma of an inguinal lymph node (Sims and Garb, 1962). Another case of typical penile giant condyloma acuminatum with metastatic lymph node invasion was reported by Dawson and associates in 1965, but in this case the question was raised whether this lesion was not actually a misdiagnosed carcinoma from its inception. A most unusual case of a giant condyloma of Buschke-Löwenstein arising in the inguinal fold, which developed distant metastases five years later, was described by Machacek and Weakley (1960). The authors of all of these reports believed the Buschke-Löwenstein tumor to be a relatively benign variant of squamous cell carcinoma.

Kraus and Perez-Mesa in 1966 reviewed 105 cases of what were called "verrucose carcinomas," closely resembling giant condylomata of Buschke-Löwenstein and involving the oral cavity, larynx, and genitalia. Progressive local invasion of bone cartilage and contiguous structures in patients with the oral lesions was found to be similar to the "compression invasion" seen with genital giant condylomata of Buschke and Löwenstein. Despite the aggressive behavior of these "verrucose carcinomas," they all presented a benign histologic picture very much like that seen with the simple condyloma acuminatum and giant condyloma of Buschke-Löwenstein. Ninety-five of Kraus's cases occurred in the oral cavity. Of the 10 reported on the genitalia, two of them appeared in the vagina of females, and the remaining eight occurred on the glans penis of males. In all these patients, lymph node metastases were extremely rare on initial examination regardless of tumor size. An especially surprising observation was made in that, following radiation treatment of "verrucose tumors" in four of these patients, a sudden alteration of the lesions was noticed, resulting in an anaplastic growth pattern with distant metastases. Excellent therapeutic results were obtained, however, when adequate surgical dissection and removal of these tumors were performed. Apparently regional lymph node dissection was not deemed necessary.

The unusual occurrence of malignant transformation within simple condylomata acuminata has been reported (Mariame, 1950; Friedberg and Serlin, 1963; Siegel, 1962), but this is apparently a very rare event. It may well be that a time lapse between the appearance of such a lesion and the actual obtaining of histologic evidence of malignancy does not permit an accurate initial diagnosis.

Although so few cases of the Buschke-Löwenstein tumor have been associated with malignancy, the "malignant potential" has been repeatedly emphasized in the literature (Gilbert, 1966). There is an unusual syndrome known as epidermodysplasia verruciformis described by Lewandowski and Lutz which is characterized by generalized and persistent verrucosis (see Chapter 24). This verrucosis is thought to be due to an unusual host response to the wart virus. In some exceptional cases of this syndrome, bowenoid changes and even squamous cell carcinoma have been observed to develop within what initially appear to be benign warts (Jablonskia and Milewski, 1957).

DIAGNOSIS

It is interesting to note that, although simple condylomata acuminata are exquisitely sensitive to, and rapidly destroyed by, the topical application of podophyllum and peltatins, the "active moieties" found in podophyllin resin, giant condylomata of Buschke and Löwenstein are not all affected by the cytotoxic effect of podophyllin. In the early stages when a small, wart-like Buschke-Löwenstein tumor may not be easily differentiated from an ordinary venereal wart, a positive response to podophyllin treatment will help to make the diagnosis in favor of a simple condyloma acuminatum.

It should be noted however that, not only does the giant condyloma of Buschke-Löwenstein resist podophyllin treatment, but also the application of this chemical resin, when applied to epithelium, induces the formation of "podophyllin cells," which can be easily confused with the atypical malignant cells seen in squamous cell carcinomas on microscopic examination (Sullivan, 1947; Saphir, 1958). The application of podophyllin should not be used if a biopsy and tissue examination are contemplated, since such treatment may affect the histologic picture and thereby obscure the true diagnosis.

Although "florid" growth and the clinically aggressive behavior of the Buschke-Löwenstein tumor resemble those of a low grade squamous cell carcinoma, the clinical appearance is not substantiated by the histologic criteria of malignancy. Since the histology of the giant condyloma acuminatum is similar to, but not exactly identical to, that of the benign simple condyloma acuminatum, it is extremely important to emphasize the importance of not only a skillful and thorough clinical examination, but also an extremely careful choice of exact biopsy site. Because there may be a transition from benign to malignant tissue beneath normal epithelium within a lesion which is actually a carcinoma, multiple biopsies from different sites are probably advisable to ascertain the correct tissue diagnosis. In the evaluation of such a peculiar lesion as the Buschke-Löwenstein tumor, the microscopic section should always be examined in context with the clinical picture. The pathologist receiving a histologic specimen taken from a patient with a giant condyloma of Buschke-Löwenstein without the benefit of either actually seeing the lesion or having an accurate description of the tumor will more likely than not make a histologic diagnosis of simple condyloma acuminatum (Gersh, 1963; Powley, 1964; Dreyfuss and Neville, 1955).

HISTOLOGY

Microscopically, the tumor of Buschke-Löwenstein appears as a fungating mass composed of increased papillomatosis with broadened papillary processes of hyperplastic squamous epithelium (Figs. 34–2 and 34–3). These exhibit marked hyperkeratosis and parakeratosis, resulting in elongated rete ridges that extend deep into the underlying tissue and produce a striking, convoluted mass with deep sulci. The histology is remarkably uniform, consisting of a regular arrangement of cells with an orderly pattern of maturation seen from the basal cell layer to a very thickened parakeratotic and hyperkeratotic statum corneum. The basal cells show little variation in size, staining quality, or arrangement. The epidermal cell intracellular bridges remain intact. Mitotic figures are infrequently seen in the basal layer and rarely in the prickle cell layers. Although quite distorted, the basement membrane of giant condyloma lesions is found to be intact; differentiation from low grade epidermoid carcinoma can be made on the basis of the intact basement membrane.

Essentially the histology is similar to, but exaggerates, that of simple condylomata acuminata. The most distinct difference in the histology of giant condyloma acuminatum of Buschke-Löwenstein is a marked vacuolization of the cells in the upper portion of the thickened epidermis. These cells are larger than those seen in the same location in simple condyloma and have a clear cytoplasm with hyperchromatic, pyknotic, centrally placed nuclei. In the sub-

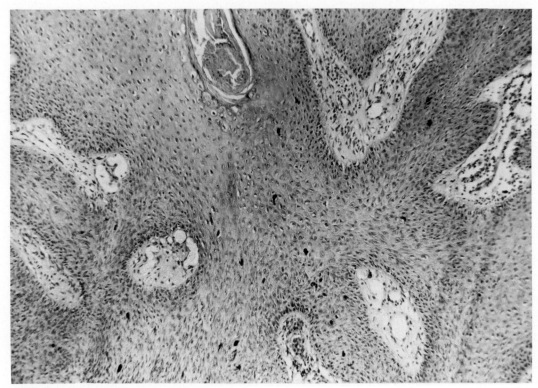

Figure 34–2   Microscopic section of giant condyloma of Buschke-Löwenstein. *Approximately ×15*. [Photograph used by permission of New York University School of Medicine (Skin and Cancer Unit).]

epidermis, dilated capillaries and chronic inflammatory cells, such as lymphocytes and occasional plasma cells, are frequently seen. The characteristic orderly arrangement and polarity of the cells, as well as the absence of invasion of the tumor into lymphatics, nerves, and blood vessels and of distant metastases to lymph nodes, support the relatively benign nature of the Buschke-Löwenstein giant condyloma.

TREATMENT

A review of the reported cases indicates that the only satisfactory treatment for giant condyloma of Buschke-Löwenstein is thorough but conservative surgical removal of the entire mass. This tumor does not respond to the topical application of chemical or caustic agents, such as podophyllin or trichloroacetic acid. Radiation therapy is not at all effective in arresting the growth of this tumor (Sampson and Watson, 1970). As indicated above, in a few cases reported by Kraus and Perez-Mesa in 1966, radiation was thought to be contraindicated because of an anaplastic transformation which was observed immediately following

the exposure of some of these tumors as well as related tumors to irradiation. In most cases thorough electrocautery and diligent, total surgical dissection of the tumor have been the most successful techniques used to treat these tumors. Partial penisectomy followed by skin grafting and, if necessary, plastic reconstruction, may be required. Total amputation of the penis is the only recourse when the tumor involves the bulk of the penile mass. In the few reported cases of giant condyloma of Buschke-Löwenstein located in the vaginal or rectal area, total surgical excision of the lesion has also been the treatment of choice. In very few of the surgically treated cases was lymph node dissection performed or found to be necessary. Caution must be taken that the true pathologic diagnosis be well established prior to treatment, that a low grade or "disguised" malignancy is not overlooked.

DIFFERENTIAL DIAGNOSIS

Although the giant condyloma acuminatum clinically behaves like a malignancy, it is important to recognize that the tumor

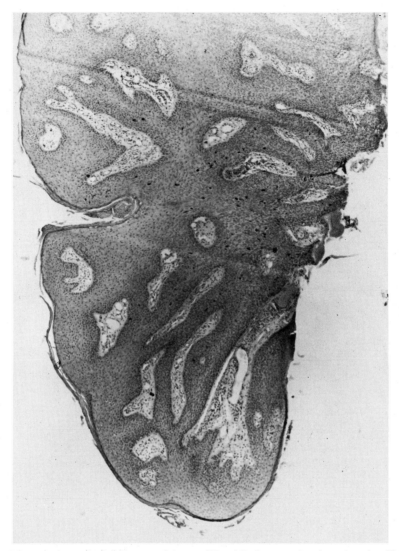

Figure 34–3 Microscopic section of giant condyloma of Buschke-Löwenstein. *Approximately* ×*50.* [Photograph used by permission of New York University School of Medicine (Skin and Cancer Unit).]

grows via local extension by compression and displacement, not by actual invasion. Differentiation from a malignant carcinoma can only be safely made by histologic examination of several biopsy specimens taken from different areas of the tumor.

Giant condyloma of Buschke-Löwenstein can be confused clinically with another rare, keratinizing, aggressive tumor, infrequently seen in the anogenital area, known as a keratoacanthoma. The keratoacanthoma and the giant condyloma are similar in gross appearance in that they are both large, fungating, cornified, friable masses. Microscopically their histologic patterns are quite different. The keratoacanthoma shows a microscopic pathologic

picture not unlike that seen in a squamous cell carcinoma. Despite a malignant histopathology, the keratoacanthoma clinically tends to resolve spontaneously even without treatment (see Chapter 32).

In evaluating the differential diagnosis of vaginal giant condyloma, one should consider the spectrum of benign and malignant tumors which occur in the vaginal area. These include various types of cancer, virus-induced condyloma acuminata, and the infectious secondary syphilitic lesion seen on the genitalia, known as a condyloma latum, which can also resemble, and is frequently mistaken for, the ordinary venereal wart.

Although only a few cases of giant condyloma of Buschke and Löwenstein have been seen in the rectal areas, one would have to entertain the diagnosis of syphilitic condyloma latum, as well as of a variety of both benign and malignant tumors that can occur in this region.

PROGNOSIS

The prognosis for giant condyloma of Buschke-Löwenstein is excellent, provided the tumor has been thoroughly removed. As more cases, reports, and follow-up evaluations become available, the nature of this peculiar tumor will be better understood.

REFERENCES

Almeida, J. D., Howatson, A. T., and Williams, M. G.: Electron microscopic study of human warts: Site of virus production and nature of the inclusion bodies. J. Invest. Dermatol., 38:337, 1972.

Becker, F. T., Walder, H. J., and Larson, D. M.: Giant condylomata acuminata. Arch. Dermatol., 100:184, 1969.

Bulkley, G., Wendel, R., and Grayhack, J.: Buschke-Löwenstein tumor of the penis. J. Urol., 97:731, 1967.

Buschke, A.: *In* Neisser, A. (Ed.): Stereoscopischer Medicinischer Atlas. Kassel, Fischer, 1896.

Buschke, A., and Löwenstein, L.: Uber Carcinomahnliche Condylomata Acuminata. Klin. Wochenschr., 4:1728, 1925.

Davies, S. W.: Giant condyloma acuminatum: Incidence among cases diagnosed as carcinoma of the penis. J. Clin. Pathol., 18:142, 1965.

Dawson, D. F., Duckworth, J. K., Bernhardt, H., and Young, J. M.: Giant condyloma and verrucous carcinoma of the genital area. Arch. Pathol., 79:225, 1965.

DiCaro, A., and Bernardini, R.: Buschke-Löwenstein condyloma. Minerva Chir., 26:1035, 1971.

Dreyfuss, W., and Neville, W. E.: Buschke-Löwenstein tumors (giant condylomata acuminata). Am. J. Surg., 90:41, 1955.

Evans, R. L., and Dische, F. E.: A large condyloma of the vagina. J. Obstet. Gynecol. Br. Commonw., 76:757, 1969.

Dunn, A. E. G., and Ogilvie, M. M.: Intranuclear virus particles in human genital wart tissue: Observations on the ultrastructure of the epidermal layer. J. Ultrastruct. Res., 22:282, 1967.

Friedberg, M. J., and Serlin, O.: Condyloma acuminatum: Its association with malignancy. Dis. Colon Rectum, 6:352, 1963.

Gersh, J.: Giant condyloma acuminatum (carcinoma-like condylomata or Buschke-Löwenstein tumors) of the penis. J. Urol., 69:164, 1963.

Gilbert, C. T.: Giant condyloma acuminatum (Buschke-Löwenstein tumor). Arch. Dermatol., 93:714, 1966.

Goldschmidt, H., and Kligman, A. M.: Experimental inoculation of humans with ectodermotropic viruses. J. Invest. Dermatol., 31:175, 1958.

Greenberg, S. D., and Wallace, S. A.: Giant cutaneous papilloma of the shoulder. Arch. Pathol., 76:446, 1963.

Jablonskia, S., and Milewski, B.: Generalized common and hypertrophic warts. Br. J. Dermatol., 69:273, 1957.

Knoblich, R., and Failing, J. F., Jr.: Buschke-Löwenstein tumor of the rectum. Am. J. Clin. Pathol., 40:427, 1963.

Knoblich, R., and Failing, J. F., Jr.: Giant condyloma acuminatum (Buschke-Löwenstein tumor) of the rectum. Am. J. Clin. Pathol., 48:389, 1967.

Kraus, F. T., and Perez-Mesa, C.: Verrucose carcinoma, clinical and pathologic study of 105 cases involving the oral cavity, larynx, and genitalia. Cancer, 19:26, 1966.

Lepow, H., and Leffler, N.: Giant condylomata acuminata (Buschke-Löwenstein tumor): Report of two cases. J. Urol., 83:853, 1960.

Litvak, A. S., Melnick, I., and Lieberman, P. R.: Giant condylomata acuminata associated with carcinoma. J. Med. Soc. N.J., 63:165, 1966.

Löwenstein, L.: Carcinoma-like condylomata acuminata of the penis. Med. Clin. North Am., 23:789, 1925.

McCarron, D. L., and Carlton, C. E.: Giant condylomata of the penis. J. Urol., 104:730, 1970.

Machacek, G. F., and Weakley, D. R.: Giant condylomata acuminata of Buschke and Löwenstein. Arch. Dermatol., 82:41, 1960.

Mariame, G.: Malignant transformation of venereal vegetations of the penis. Arch. Belg. Dermatol. Syph., 6:175, 1950.

Powley, J. M.: Buschke-Löwenstein tumor of the penis. Br. J. Surg., 51:76, 1964.

Rosenthal, F. (1923), and Wiese, B. (1926), cited by Freudenthal, W., and Spitzer, R.: Warzen und Kondylome. Handbuch der Haut- und Geschlechtskrankheiten, 12:33, 1933.

Saphir, O., Leventhal, M. L., and Kline, T. S.: Podophyllin induced dysplasia of the cervix uteri. Am. J. Clin. Pathol., 32:446, 1959.

Sampson, L. W., and Watson, E. C.: Buschke-Löwenstein tumor. Cutis, 6:1013, 1970.

Serra, A.: Studi sul virus della verruca, del papilloma, del condiloma accuminato. G. Ital. Mal. Vener., 65:1808, 1924.

Shabad, A. P.: On the nature of condyloma acuminatum of the penis. Vestn. Dermatol. Venerol., 37:53, 1963.

Siegel, A.: Malignant transformation of condyloma acuminatum. Am. J. Surg., 103:613, 1962.

Sims, C. F., and Garb, J.: Giant condyloma acuminatum of the penis associated with metastatic carcinoma of the right inguinal lymph node. Arch. Dermatol. Syph. (Berl.), 63:383, 1962.

Sullivan, M., and King, L. S.: Effects of resin of podophyllin on normal skin. Arch. Dermatol. Syph. (Berl.), 56:30, 1947.

CANCER *of the* SKIN

Index

Page numbers in italics indicate illustrations

Basal cell carcinoma (*Continued*)
  vs. squamous cell carcinomas, 411, 899, 903
  sunlight and, 416
  superficial, *485*
  tar warts and, *517*
  of upper lip, *470*
  in xeroderma pigmentosum, 580, 583, 589
  x-rays and, 420
Basal cell epitheliomas, 228, *249*, 394, 395,
    398–400, 474, 772, 821–842
  acid mucopolysaccharides in, 860
  acid phosphatase in, 862
  alkaline phosphatase in, 861–864
  atypical and nonconstant cells in, 250
  basal cell membrane and, 867
  basement membrane and, *868*
  biopsy in, 829
  blue cells in, *249*
  border of, 402
  carbohydrates in, 860
  cell necrosis in, *854*
  cells within clear nucleus in, 249
  cell types in, 845–846, *847*, 848
  cellular syncytia in, 249–250
  central cells in, 869, *870*
  chemosurgery in, 842, *1538*
  citric acid cycle in, 864
  clinical course of, 826–827
  complications of therapy and, 838
  concentrically arranged cell groups in, *851*
  crusted nodular, *825*
  cryosurgery for, *1585*
  cure rates for, 842
  curettage and electrodesiccation for, 832, *833*,
    836, 838, 839, 841, 1504, *1505, 1508, 1509*
  cutaneous horns in, 571
  cylindromatous degeneration in, 848, 852
  cytochromeoxidase in, 866
  cytodiagnosis in, 248–253
  dedifferentiated cell origin of, 875
  defined, 821
  degenerative alterations in, 877
  derivation of, 872–873
  desmosomes in, *871*
  differential diagnosis in, 827–829
  differentiating capacities of cells in, 849–851,
    869–870
  DNA and, 824, 861, 877
  electrodesiccation in. See *Basal cell epithelioma,
    curettage and electrodesiccation for.*
  electron microscopy in, 866–872
  energy-producing metabolism in, 864–866
  enzymes in, 861–866
  eosinophilic cells in, 250
  epidermal-dermal interface in, 209–211, *212*
  epidermis in, *867*
  esterases in, 862, *863*
  etiology of, 821–822
  evolution toward malpighian cell in, *871*
  excision of, *830, 831, 832*
  experimental production of, 874
  of eyelid, 1349–1355
  and fibroepithelioma of Pinkus, *827*, 858–859
  follicular atrophoderma and, 1305–1306
  glycogen and, 860, 876

Basal cell epitheliomas (*Continued*)
  glycolysis and, 864
  growth of, 828
  hair germ and, 873
  of hand, 1437–1438
  as hamartoma, 873–874
  hematoma in, 839, *840*
  histochemistry of, 860–866
  histogenesis of, 872–877
  histology of, 845–849, 1354
  hyaline degeneration in, 852
  hydrolytic enzymes in, 861–864
  hypertrophic scars and, 838, *839*
  incidence of, 822–824
  with intraepidermal nests, 708
  karyoplasm in, 870
  keloids and, 838
  keratinization in, 849, *850*
  laser surgery for, *1643, 1644*
  melanin in, 849, 872, 876
  melanocytes in, 250
  metastasizing of, 827
  metatypic epithelioma and, 841
  microscopic appearance and clinical aspect of,
    856–860
  morphea type of, 826, *827*, 828–829, 858, *859*
  NADPH-tetrazolium reductases and, 864
  naphthylamidases in, 864, *865*, 877
  nasal tumors and, 1406
  necrotic tumor cells in, *855*
  neutral polysaccharides in, 860
  nodular epithelioma in, 857, *858*
  nucleic acids and, 861
  pagetoid, 597
  pagetoid epithelioma and, 856
  palisade cells in, 867–869, *875*
  pathology of, 845–877
  peripheral and central cells of, *847*
  peritumoral lacunae in, *854–856*
  peritumoral stroma in, 848–849, 862
  pigmentation in, 849
  pilary formations in, 869, *872*
  planum cicatrisans of, 856
  polypoid, *1353*
  prekeratogenous zone in, 875
  primary hair buds in, *852*
  probe for, 1504
  pseudocysts in, 851, *853*, 857, 874
  radiation therapy in, 1512–1517
  radiodermatitis and, 837
  recurrences of, 841–842
  regression phenomena in, 870–872
  regressive changes in, 851–856
  response to radiation for, 1515–1516
  reticular or adenoid type, *846*
  RNA and, 861, 876
  on scalp, *822*
  sclerosing, *857*
  –SH and S-S groups in, 861
  shaving nicks and, 824
  skin pigmentation in, 823
  small cells in, 249
  smears in, 251
  solid or massive type, *846*
  spindle-shaped cells in, *850*

Circumscribed precancerous melanosis (Dubreuilh),
   237, *237*, 679–700, 683, *684, 685, 699*
  clinical description of, 683–692
  as clinicopathic entity, 692–694
  defined, 679
  dermal-epidermal separation in, 682
  diagnosis in, 694–696
  differential clinical and histogenic features of, 697
  epidemiology and incidence of, 679–680
  epidermal-dermal interface in, 207–208, *208*
  etiology and pathogenesis in, 680–683
  on hand, *686*
  history of, 679
  vs. junction nevus, 694
  on knuckle, *685*
  life history of, *687, 688, 689, 690, 691*
  melanocyte of, *681*, 692
  Miescher's technique in, *697, 698*
  pathology of, 692–694
  prognosis in, 699–700
  vs. seborrheic keratosis, 695
  spontaneous regression of, 684
  sunlight in, 680
  of tongue, 693
  treatment in, 696–699
Citric acid cycle, in basal cell epithelioma, 864
Clear cell malignant hidradenoma, 1054, *1061–1062*
Clear cell sarcoma, of tendons and aponeuroses,
  1147–1149
Cleavage lines. See *Langer lines.*
Clinitrochlorobenzene, in Kaposi's sarcoma, 1202
Cloacogenic carcinoma, 1395–1406
  transitional, 1400
Cloacogenic mucosa, *1396*
Club hair, 70, *71*
Coal products, in tar keratoses, 493
Coal tar
  carcinogenic factors in, 494
  exposure to, 413
  squamous cell carcinoma and, 920
Codominant, defined, 142
Coffee tar, as carcinogen, 494
Coilonychia, 36
Colchicine, in arsenical cancer, 489
Collagen, 61–62, 64, 105
  aging and, 163, 167–168
  amino acids and, 324
  atmospheric oxygen and, 324
  defined, 323
  in dermis, 323–324
  glycine content of, 324
  hydroxylysine in, 324
  hydroxyproline in, 324
  in neurofibromatosis, *368, 370*
  proline in, 324
  of skin, 322
  stability of, 324
  water in, 324
Collagenase activity, in tumor growth, 326–327
Collagen fibers
  in dermal connective tissue, 323
  in neurofibromatosis, *370*
  in perivascular space between capillaries, 358
Coloboma, in nevoid basal cell carcinoma syndrome,
  895

Colon carcinoembryonic antigen, 1649
Colon cancer, *1286, 1287,* 1649
Color top, in skin pigmentation studies, 29
Conductivity changes, in skin, 294
Condyloma, in squamous cell carcinoma, 923
Condylomata acuminata, 817
Congenital immune defect, 922
Conjunctiva
  carcinoma of, 1361–1365
  layers of, 1346–1347
  melanoma of, 1004, *1004,* 1005, *1005*
  nevi of, 1365–1366
  noncancerous lesions of, 1363–1365
  papillomas of, *1366*
  pigmented tumors of, 1365–1370
  precancerous melanosis of, *1369*
  squamous cell carcinoma of, *1363*
  in xeroderma pigmentosum, 583
Conjunctival lesions, 1361–1370
Conjunctivitis, 1351
Connective tissue reaction, in wound healing, 105
Connective tissue tumors
  cytodiagnosis of, 254–259
  dermatofibrosarcomas as, *256, 257*
  fibromas as, 254–255
  Kaposi's angiosarcoma as, 258
  melanoma cells of, 1026–1028
  pseudosarcomatous fascitis, as, 258
Contact dermatitis, of lips, 609
Contact inhibition, 154–155
Contraction, in wound healing, 104–105
Cornea, in xeroderma pigmentosum, 583
Corneal opacities, in nevoid basal cell
  carcinoma syndrome, 895
Corneocyte, 56
Cornified epithelioma, 916
Corticoids, in xeroderma pigmentosum, 591
Corticotropin defect, 577
Cortisone, 129, 131
  wound healing and, 108
Cosmetic surgery. See *Plastic surgery.*
Croton oil, 123, 128
  as promotion agent, 315
Cryoglobulinemia, in multiple myeloma, 1266
Cryosurgery, 1569–1587
  blister in, 1576
  bullous lesions in, 1585
  carbon dioxide snow in, 1570
  cold penetration measurement in, *1578*
  complications in, 1585–1586
  Cooper apparatus in, 1571
  cryobiological basis of, 1572–1574
  Cryoderm system in, *1572, 1573*
  current instrumentation in, 1571–1572
  diphosphopyridine nucleotide diaphorase in, 1575
  of eyelid, *1584*
  freezing of tissue in, 1573, *1576, 1577, 1578,*
    1579, 1581, 1582, 1583
  hemorrhage in, 1586
  history of, 1569–1571
  infection in, 1586
  injury in, *1578*
  lateral spread of freezing in, *1579*
  liquid nitrogen in, 1571
  for malignancies, 1580–1583

Leiomyosarcoma, 1103–1104, *1105*, 1106,
    1141–1142, *1142*, 1143, *1173*
  age and sex in, 1103
  clinical course in, 1106
  clinical features of, 1103–1104
  cytodiagnosis in, *262*
  pathology of, 1104–1106
  treatment in, 1106
Lenticular fibroma (histiocytoma), epidermal-dermal
    interface in, 216, *216*, 217
Lentigo maligna, 428, 1028, *1029, 1032*, 1033
  in melanotic tumors, 237
Lentigo senilis, 449, *451*
  squamous cell carcinoma and, *451*
Leprosy
  carcinoma in, 1304–1305
  Kaposi's sarcoma and, 1218
  squamous cell carcinoma and, 922
Letterer-Siwe disease, 1261–1263
Leukedema, leukoplakia and, 530
Leukemia, 1253–1261
  acute. See *Acute leukemia.*
  blast cell, 1253
  chronic lymphatic, 150
  granulocytic, 1257
  lymphocytic, 1254–1257
  monocytic, 1258
  nonspecific cutaneous lesions associated with,
    1258–1261
  pigmentation in, 1261
  plasma cell, 1263, 1267
  pyoderma in, 1261
  stem cell, 1253
  systemic chemotherapy in, 1602–1603
  trophic cutaneous changes in, 1261
Leukemia cutis
  BIKE program in, 1603
  POMP program in, 1603
  VAMP program in, 1603
Leukemia virus, 130
Leukemic reticuloendotheliosis, 1236–1237
Leukocyte culture test, 95
Leukokeratosis, 638
Leukokeratosis nicotinica, *527*
  smoking and, 810
Leukonychia, 36
Leukopenia, 1261
Leukoplakia, 524–553
  actinic, 531
  betel nut and, 531
  Bowen's disease and, 652
  carcinoma and, 532
  cell structure in, 529
  cheilitis and, 544
  clinical and epidemiological features in, 527–529
  cryosurgery for, 1580
  curettage and electrosurgery for, 1503
  cytologic examination of, 241
  defined, 524
  from dentures, 531
  differential diagnosis in, 529–531
  electrogalvanic, 531
  epidermolysis hereditaria bullosa dystrophicans
    and, 530
  etiology of, 531–532

Leukoplakia (*Continued*)
  of eyelid, 1363–1364, *1364*
  histopathologic features of, 531
  florid oral papillomatosis and, 810
  focal dysplasia in, 527
  idiopathic, 524, 528
  immunotherapy in, 1656–1657
  incidence of, 527
  irritative, *526*
  in lichen sclerosus et atrophicus, 638
  of lip, 309, *546*
  lip cancer and, *541*
  malignant, 532
  oral submucous fibrosis and, 530
  precancerous, 525, *527*, 528–529
  predisposition to, 530
  site of, 527
  speckled, 529, 533–534, *547*
  symptomatic, 524–525, *525*, 528
  symptoms of, 528
  therapy and prognosis in, 532
  tobacco and, 531
  of tongue, *525, 526*
  traumatic, 525, 528
Lexer's diverticulum, 1384
Lichen albus. See *Lichen sclerosus et atrophicus.*
Lichenatrophy, 636
Lichen nitidus, 1294
Lichen planopilaris, 1294
Lichen planus, 452, 810, 1293–1294
  carcinomas with, 1294
  erythroplasia of Queryat and, 657, 659
  hypertrophic, 772
  lichen sclerosus et atrophicus and, 643
  malignant degeneration in, 1293
  melanin deposit in, 227
  melanophages in, 228–229
  of oral mucosa, 1301
  of penis, *639*
  squamous cell carcinoma and, 922
Lichen planus-like granulosis, in tar warts, *508*
Lichen planus-like keratosis, 448–449, *449*
Lichen planus sclerosus. See *Lichen sclerosus et
    atrophicus.*
Lichen ruber planus, *197*, 198
Lichen sclerosus et atrophicus, 635–644, 1301
  Bowen's disease and, 652
  circumcision in, 644
  clinical features of, 636
  coexistence with other diseases, 643–644
  defined, 635–644
  differential diagnosis in, 638–639
  elastic fibers in, 642
  epidermal-dermal interface in, 213–214, *214*
  family incidence of, 643
  of female genitals, 637–639
  in genital area, 639, 643
  histology of, 639–640, *641*
  incidence of, 636
  lichen planus and, 643
  localization of, 637
  malignant degeneration in, 643
  meatomy in, 644
  of penis, 639, *640, 641*
  prognosis in, 643

Skin color, 29–30
Skin creases, in facial surgery, *911*
Skin cytology
    chondrocytes and, 232, *232*
    endothelial cells in, 230
    fibroblasts in, 229
    hair follicle cells in, 231
    hair sheath cells in, *231*
    mastocytes in, *232*
    melanocytes in, 227–228
    melanophages in, 228–229
    sebaceous cells in, 231
    smooth muscle cells in, 230
    sweat gland cells in, 230, *231*
Skin disease. See also *Skin cancer.*
    cancer and, 281–282
    decreased polarizability in, 298–299
    in diabetes, *283*
    giant melanocytes in, 228
Skin flaps
    contraindications for, 912
    in postchemosurgery repair, 1558–1561
Skin grafts
    bleeding in, 1494
    composite, 1490–1492, *1492*
    contracture of, 1494
    free, *1490*
    full-thickness, 1489–1490, *1491, 1492*
    in nevoid basal cell carcinoma syndrome, *889*
    in plastic surgery, 1489–1494
    in postchemosurgery repair, 1557
    split-thickness, 1490
    in squamous cell carcinoma, 911
    survival of, 1493
    whole-thickness, *1492*
Skin lesions. See also *Cutaneous lesions.*
    internal carcinoma and, 1308–1336
    malignant acanthosis nigricans and, 1309–1314
    precancerous, 393
Skin malignancies
    chronic radiodermatitis from treatment of, 465–467
    as manifestation of internal malignancies 289–291
Skin neoplasms. See also *Neoplasia; Neoplasms.*
    capillary hemangioma as, 356–360
    fibrous xanthoma as, 360
    keratoacanthoma as, 360–374
    leiomyoma cutis as, 351–356
    malignant, 375–384
    molluscum contagiosum as, 374–375
    neurofibromatosis as, 360
Skin pigmentation
    melanoma and, 427
    skin cancer and, 416
Skin polarizability
    calcium chloride solution and, 311
    diminution of in malignant growths, 306–312
    failure of in primary cancers and malignant melanomas, 307–308
    false-positive and false-negative results in, 310–312
    heat-induced diminution of, 299
    hyper- and hypopolarizability in, 312
    ionizing radiations in, 312
    in malignant melanoma, 310

Skin polarizability (*Continued*)
    ultraviolet and x-ray irriadiation in, 299–300
Skin polarization resistance. See also *Skin resistance.*
    potassium chloride in, 311
    sodium chloride in, 311
Skin potentials, measurement of, 293
Skin resistance
    diminution of, 311
    direct potentiometer measurement of, 301–303
    electrodermamometer in, 304
    electropermeagraph in, 304
    malignometer in, 306
    nonpolarizable electrodes in measurement of, 301–302
    oscillogram in, *305*
    Whelan apparatus in, 306
Skin reticulosis, cytodiagnosis of, 224–278. See also
    Histocytic medullary reticulosis.
Skin tension lines, in plastic surgery, *911*
Skin thickness measurement, 37–38, *39*
Skin tumors
    amelanotic melanoma as, 238
    biopsy and surgery for, 1496–1500
    cytodiagnosis of, 224–278
    cytology of, 233–240
    fibrosarcoma as, *257, 258*
    with intraepidermal nests, 704–707
    malignant. See *Malignant tumors.*
    in multiple myeloma, 1265
    pigmented melanomas as, 238
    tissue culture studies of, 1605–1606
Skull anomalies, in nevoid basal cell carcinoma syndrome, 893
Smoking. See also *Pipe smoking; Tongue cancer.*
    carcinoma and, 531
    in floral oral papillomatosis, 803
    leukokeratosis nicotinica palati and, 810
    leukoplakia and, 531
    palate cancer and, 552
    tongue cancer and, 549
Smooth muscle cells
    in leiomyomas, *355–356*
    in normal skin cytology, *230*
Snuff, in floral oral papillomatosis, 803
Sodium chloride, in skin polarization resistance tests, 311
Soft part sarcomas, 1126–1149. See also *Malignant soft tissue tumors.*
Solar keratoses, 405 n. See also *Keratosis(-es).*
    chemotherapeutic treatment of, 1589, *1589*, 1590, *1590*
    on covered skin, 443
    defined, 437
    development of, *440*
    of hand, 1436
    hyperplastic, *792*
    skin cancer and, 430
    squamous cell carcinoma and, 923, 925–926, 928, 933
    sun as etiologic agent in, 438
Solar radiation
    global distribution of, 410
    skin cancer and, 410–411
Somatic mutations, in carcenogenisis, 152–154, 335, 338–339, 391–392

Spastic paralysis, in xeroderma pigmentosum, 583

Specialized glands, 78

Spectrophotometer, 29

Spinalioma, 916

Spindle cell epidermoid carcinoma, 542

Spindle cell nevi, 1038–1039. See also *Benign juvenile melanoma.*

Spine anomalies, in nevoid basal cell carcinoma syndrome, 893

Spiradenoma, eccrine, 1045

Spiramycin, in chemotherapy, 1592

Split-thickness skin graft, in squamous cell carcinoma, 911

Squamous cell carcinoma, 245–246, *246, 247,* 247–248. See also *Keratoacanthoma.*

in acrodermatitis chronica atrophicans Herxheimer, *1300*

in actinic cheilitis, 615–616

actinic keratoses and, 454

adenoid, 925

in Africa, 417

age at onset of, 770

anal cancer and, 1400, *1401,* 1402, 1404

anaplastic, 923, 927, 936

anatomic distribution of, 412

arsenic and, 481–483, 488–489, 900

of auditory canal, 914–915

vs. basal cell carcinoma, 411, 899, 903

basal cell epithelioma and, 821, 926

benign juvenile melanoma and, 740

biopsy in, 905–906, 926, 928

of body and extremities, 916–930

bone and muscle involvement in, 929

and Bowen's disease, 646, 920, 922, 926, 933–934, 937, 1438

burn scars and, 902, 917, *920,* 921, 923

in cheilitis, 609, *616–620*

cheilitis glandularis and, *629, 630*

chemically induced, 120

chemotherapy in, 927–928

chromatin in, 233

chromoblastomycosis and, 922

chronic radiodermatitis from treatment of, 467

classification of, 916–917

clinical description of, 923–924

course of, 904–909

cryosurgery in, 927–928

cutaneous horns and, *557,* 558, 564–565, *565, 566, 567*

deaths from, 422, 929–930

delayed hypersensitivity to DNCB in, 923

dermatomyositis and, *1314*

desmosomes in, *377*

diagnosis of, 903–904

differential diagnosis in, 926–927, 937

differentiation in, 925

dyskeratosis and, 934

dystrophic epidermolysis bullosa and, 922

of ear, *309*

epidemiology of, 917–919

on epidermodysplasia verruciformis, 247, *248,* 599

epithelioma cuniculatum and, 923

epitheliomatous horn pearl and, *247*

Squamous cell carcinoma (*Continued*)

etiology and carcinogenesis of, 900–903, 919–923

exophytic, 924

of external ear canal, 1372, *1375,* 1376–1378

of eyelids, 912–913, 1355–1356, *1356, 1357,* 1363

on face, 928

Fanconi's anemia and, 919

fibroxanthomas and, 936

five-year survival rates in, 423

flaps for adjoining tissues in, 911–912, *913*

vs. florid oral papillomatosis, 809

of foot, 927

of forehead, 913–914

full-thickness skin graft in, 911

fungal infections and, 922

giant condylomata and, 923

granuloma inguinale and, 922

growth of, 899, 905, 925, 934

of hand, 1438

in head and neck, 418

hidradenitis suppurativa and, 923

histochemistry of, 937

histologic grading of tumor in, 905

histopathology of, 934–937

history of, 917

immunosuppressive drugs and, 922

immunotherapy in, 1656

impetiginization in, 443

inadequately excised, 906

incidence and distribution of, 900, 917–919

with incompletely keratinized cells, 247–248

induration in, 923

in situ, 904

internal cancer and, 900

intradermal lymphatic spread in, 907

invasive, 904

keratinization rate in, 233

keratinizing, 246–247

keratoacanthoma and, 758, 764, 770, 775, 792, 794–795, 904, 926–927

laser surgery for, 1641, 1643

on legs, 918–919, *921*

leg ulcers and, 929

in leprosy, 1305

lichen planus and, 922, 1294

in lichen sclerosus et atrophicus, *1302*

of lips, 607, *913*

local invasion by, 905–906

of lower eyelid, 910

lupus erythematosus and, 904, 922

lupus vulgaris and, 922

lymphatic metastases in, 906–909

in lymph nodes, 907, 924–925

of maxilla, 914

melanoma and, 1040

in men, 918–919

metastasis and, 421–422, 905–909, 924–925, 927

metastatic cancer nodes in, 908

microscopic types of, 936

Mohs' surgery for, 1537–1549

in moles, 933–934

mortality in, 904–905

multiple skin carcinomas and, 901

Subungual melanomas (*Continued*)
  onychomycosis nigricans and, 978
  paronychia and, 978
  pigmentation in eponychium of, 976
  pyogenic granuloma and, 978
  satellitoses in, 984, 986
  subungual glomus tumor and, 978
  surgical specimens in, *983, 986*
  symptoms in, 975
  of thumb, *977, 978, 979*
  of toes, *977, 979, 986*
  treatment in, 981–986
Subungual squamous cell carcinoma, 769
Sucquet-Hoyer canal, *53*, 54
Sulzberger and Garbe, dermatosis of, 658–659
Summer cheilitis, 610
Sunburn, keratoses or cancer from, 439
Sunlight. See also *Ultraviolet light.*
  age at exposure to, 418–419
  in basal cell epithelioma, 823
  in Bowen's disease, 647
  in cheilitis actinica, 610, 612, 615
  in circumscribed precancerous melanosis, 680
  excessive, 407
  keratoacanthomas and, 757
  melanomas and, 427, 950–951
  skin cancer and, 494–495
  in solar keratosis, 438
  in squamous cell carcinoma, 900–901, 933
  in tar keratosis, 496, 520–521
  in xeroderma pigmentosum, 589, 591
Supercilia, 49
Supernumerary digits, 54, *54*
Supernumerary nipples, 51
Surgery. See also *Chemosurgery; Cryosurgery;*
    Electrosurgery; Laser surgery.
  plastic. See *Plastic surgery.*
  for skin cancer, 1499–1500
  in squamous cell carcinoma, 910–912
  "tumor technique" in, 1499
Sutures
  in plastic surgery, 1480–1481
  wound healing and, 109
SV-40 virus, 139, 149, *149*
Sweat ducts, number of, 43
Sweat gland(s), 322
Sweat gland adenoacanthoma, 1045, 1060
  extramammary Paget's disease and, 1335
Sweat gland cancer, 903
Sweat gland carcinomas, 1053–1054, *1055, 1056,*
    1057, 1058
  adenoid basal cell epitheliomas and, 1060
  age and, 1054
  clinical study of, 1054–1055
  diagnosis in, 1060–1061
  epidermoid metaplasia and, 1058
  histologic study of, 1055–1060
  metastasizing in, 1059
  mimicking of, 1060
  tumor location in, 1059
Sweat gland cells, in normal skin cytology, 230, *231*
Sweating, in aging skin, 169
Synophrys, 49
Synovial sarcoma, 1132–1133, *1134*

Syphilis
  Bowen's disease and, 646
  penile cancer and, 1413
  squamous cell carcinoma and, 926
Syphilis tuberculosis, carcinomas in, 1304
Syringoma, epidermal-dermal interface in, 205, *205*
Systemic chemotherapy
  antimetabolites in, 1597–1598
  correlation results in, 1617
  cyclophosphamide in, 1596
  cytotoxic criteria in, 1616
  in Hodgkin's disease, 1600–1602
  hormones in, 1596–1597
  leukemia cutis in, 1602–1603
  in malignant melanoma, 1604–1605
  mycosis fungoides and, 1594–1600
  in squamous cell carcinoma, 1603–1604
  tissue culture and, 1594–1617
  triethylenemelamine in, 1596
Systemic endotheliomatosis, 1151–1152
Systemic reticulohistiocytosis, 1324
Systemizations, 44–45, *46, 47*

Taiwan, arsenic cancer in, 428–483, 489
Tar(s)
  carcinogenic, 494
  in keratoacanthomas, 757–758
Tar cancer. See also *Tar keratosis; Tar skin; Tar*
    warts.
  in chimney sweeps, 492
  coal and oil products in, 493
  development period in, 497
  in Europe, 493
  on face, 501
  scrotal cancer and, 592, 1430
  tar warts and, 500–501. See also *Tar warts.*
  ultraviolet rays and, 494, 501
Tar itch, 497
Tar keratosis, 492–522. See also *Tar skin.*
  age factor in, 495, 502, 522
  benzpyrene in, 496
  clinical features of, 497–502
  differential diagnosis in, 518–521
  epidemiology and incidence of, 493
  etiology of, 494–495
  exposure duration in, 522
  facial changes in, 497
  of hand, *516*
  histology in, 502–518
  itching in, 497
  pathogenesis in, 496–497
  photosensitizing chemicals in, 495
  pitch skin in, 500
  prognosis in, 522
  prophylaxis in, 521–522
  skin changes in, 498
  skin lipid content and, 496
  sunlight and, 496
  treatment in, 521
Tar noxae, 496
Tar painting, in animal experiments, 496
Tar products, photosensitivity effect in, 520–521

Umbilicus (*Continued*)
  lymphangiomas of, 1386
  malignant melanomas of, 1388–1389
  neoplasm origin in, 1391
  omphalomesenteric malformations in, 1384
  secondary tumors of, 1389–1392
  skin of, 51–52
  tumors of, 1383–1392
  ulcus rodens of, *1388*
  urachal cysts of, 1385
  vegetating exuberant metastasis of, *1390*
Undifferentiated reticular cell sarcoma, 271
United Kingdom, chemical carcinogenesis in, 404
Unna's cardlike scleroderma. See *Lichen sclerosus et atrophicus.*
Upper lip, squamous cell carcinoma of, 543. See also *Lip(s).*
Urachus, cysts of, 1385
Urinary bladder, carcinoma of, 712
Urine, melanoma and, 955
Urocanic acid, in epidermis, 328
Urogenital system, in lichen sclerosus et atrophicus, 644
Uronic acid, in scurvy, 326
Urticaria
  carcinoma and, 281
  in Hodgkin's disease, 1242
Uterine cancer
  dermatitis herpetiformis and, 1330
  herpes zoster and, 1327
UV. See *Ultraviolet radiation or light.*

Vaccination scars, basal cell epithelioma in, 825
Vagina. See also *Vulva.*
  anal cancer and, 1403
  Buschke-Löwenstein tumor of, 815
Vaginal giant condyloma, 815, 819
VAMP program, in systemic chemotherapy, 1603
Van de Graaff accelerator, 112, 115–116, *116*
Varicose ulcers, ulcus cruris and, 1302
Vascular alterations, in xeroderma pigmentosum, 584
Vascular dilatations, in xeroderma pigmentosum, 581
Vascular endothelium, diffuse malignant proliferation of, 1151–1170. See also *Angioendotheliomatosis proliferans systemisata.*
Vascular tissue tumors, 251–254
  angiomas as, *251,* 251–252
  glomus tumor as, 253–254
  granuloma pyogenicum in, 252–253
  hemangiopericytoma as, 254
  malignant hemangioendothelioma as, 253
Vater-Pacinian corpuscle, 80
Velban
  in Hodgkin's disease, 1602
  in mycosis fungoides, 1600
Vellus hair, 30, *66, 67*
Venereal papilloma, *245*
Venereal warts, 814
Vermilion, 50
Verruca plana, vs. tar warts, 520

Verruca seborrheica, cytodiagnosis of, 266
Verruca senilis, 438
Verruca vulgaris, 520, 596–597, 601
  in epidermodysplasia verruciformis, 599–601
Verrucae, skin polarizability in, 308
Verruciform lesions, in Bowen's disease, *599*
Verrucoma. See *Keratoacanthoma.*
Verrucous carcinoma, 552
  Buschke-Löwenstein tumor and, 816
  classification of, 802
  florid oral papillomatosis and, 799, 802
  growth of, 537
  hyperacanthosis in, 536
  hyperkeratosis in, *535, 537*
  misdiagnosis of, 537
  of oral cavity, 535–538
  of penis. See *Buschke-Löwenstein tumor.*
  of postcommissural mucosa, *535*
  treatment in, 538
Verrucous epidermal nevus, with interepidermal nests, 706
Verrucous keratomas, cryosurgery for, 1580
Verrucous lesions
  in epidermodysplasia verruciformis, *598*
  on hands, *597*
Verrucous papillomatosis, 798–799
Vertigo, in external ear canal cancer, 1375–1376
Vibrissae, of nose, 35, 49
Vinblastine, in Hodgkin's disease, 1602
Vinca alkaloids, in mycosis fungoides, 1600
Vincristine
  in POMP program, 1603
  in VAMP program, 1603
Viral carcinogenesis, 130–131
Virchow's cells, leprosy and, 1305
Viruses
  chromosome breaks and, 149, *149*
  classification of, 130
  interaction of with chemical carcinogens, 131
  in keratoacanthoma, 757
Visceral cancers, cutaneous metastases and, 1285–1287
Vitamin A
  in keratinization process, 328
  wound healing and, 108
Vitamin A deficiency
  follicular hyperkeratosis and, 326, 328
  in leukoplakia, 531
  in xeroderma pigmentosum, 586, 591
Vitamin B deficiency, leukoplakia and, 531
Vitamin C, wound healing and, 108
Vitamin C deficiency
  melanodermia and, 329
  in xeroderma pigmentosum, 519
Vitamin D, production of by skin, 322
Vitamin K, in chemotherapy, 1588
Vitamins
  in mucopolysaccharide metabolism, 326
  in tongue cancer, 549
Vitelline canal or duct, of umbilicus, 1383–1384
Vitiligo, vs. lichen sclerosus et atrophicus, 636
Voight lines, 45
Voltmeter-ammeter method, in skin resistance measurements, *301*